MedStud

Internal Medicine
2018 VIDEO BOARD REVIEW

COMPANION
SYLLABUS

© 2017 MedStudy®
ALL RIGHTS UNDER THE COPYRIGHT ARE RESERVED BY:
MedStudy® Corporation
1455 Quail Lake Loop, Colorado Springs, CO 80906
medstudy.com

1

Reinforce learning and solidify recall with our integrated review system

MedStudy's review system is designed with a variety of products that work together to help you understand and retain core knowledge. Our unique approach utilizes evidence-based learning techniques that ensure long-term durability and easy recall of what you learn.

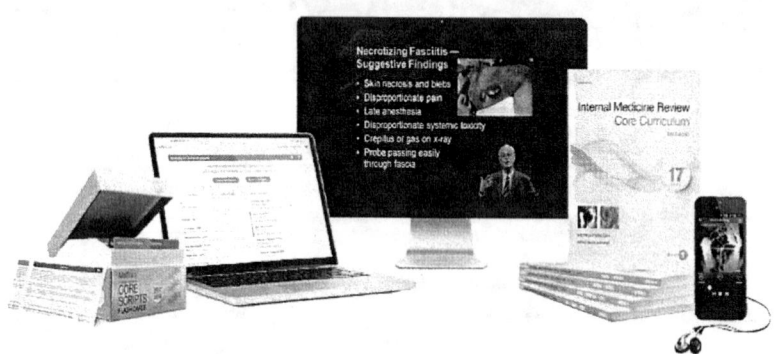

Other proven resources that reinforce Video Board Review knowledge:

Internal Medicine Review Core Curriculum — 17th Edition
Over 800 pages of clear, logically organized writing covering all internal medicine board exam topics, including 13 IM specialties/subspecialties. Includes memory-enhancing deep-learning tools and all-new hospitalist content.

Core Audio Pearls — Internal Medicine
Listen to 34 hours of high-yield, board-focused audio recordings by 12 internal medicine specialists, including every topic appearing on your ABIM or AOBIM exam.

2017–2018 Core Scripts® Flash Cards
Master 516 classic illness presentations likely to appear on your ABIM or AOBIM exam. Presentation or script appears on the front with the correct diagnosis and explanation on the reverse. Available in printed cards or online application.

Internal Medicine Board-Style Q&A Premium
This premium online application includes over 1,700 board-style questions and answers. Study on your PC, Mac, laptop, tablet, Kindle, or smartphone. Features include customizable practice tests, a running report card, and a realistic Board-Style Exam. Board-Style Q&As also available in books.

2018 Internal Medicine Accelerated Review Course
Attend a four-day crash course in IM review, featuring national experts who present high-yield, board-focused content. Perfect for exam prep or as a refresh for your practice. Available live or online.

2018 Internal Medicine Immersive Review Course
Take a deep dive into internal medicine at our nine-day live or online course. You'll gain a depth of understanding from national experts who provide board-relevant, comprehensive coverage of their specialty areas. Ideal for exam prep and physicians eager to ensure they are fully up to date on the latest practice guidelines.

ABIM MOC points available on most 17th Edition resources. Learn more at medstudy.com.

Additional copies of the Video Companion Syllabus are available for $230.

IMPORTANT: Available only to purchasers of the 2018 Internal Medicine Video Board Review video. Syllabus designed as an adjunct to the MedStudy *Internal Medicine Video Board Review* and is NOT an effective study tool when used separately.

To place your order or to learn more about any of these board-prep resources, visit **medstudy.com or call 1-800-841-0547.**

Good news! MedStudy products come with Free Shipping and Free CME (standard ground shipping to 48 states).

2

MedStudy

MedStudy

Internal Medicine Video Board Review

Table of Contents

Disclaimers

Content

The primary purpose of this activity is educational. Medicine and accepted standards of care are constantly changing. We at MedStudy do our best to review and include in this activity discussions of the standards of care, methods of diagnosis, and selection of treatments. However, the authors/presenters, editors, advisors, and publisher—and all other parties involved with the preparation of this work—disclaim any guarantee that the information contained in this activity and its associated materials is in every respect accurate or complete. MedStudy further disclaims any and all liability for damages and claims that may result from the use of information or viewpoints presented. MedStudy recommends you confirm the information contained in this activity and in any other educational material with current sources of medical knowledge whenever considering actual clinical presentations or treating patients.

Speakers

This program includes a diversity of presenters sharing their knowledge and expertise with viewers, listeners, and readers. The views and opinions expressed by these presenters are their own and not those of MedStudy.

ABIM

MedStudy has no affiliation with the American Board of Internal Medicine (ABIM) and no access to ABIM exam content. The material in this educational activity is developed as original work by MedStudy authors/editors, with additional input from expert contributors, based on their extensive backgrounds in professional medical education. This content is designed to cover subject matter typically included in certification and recertification exams as outlined in the ABIM's publicly available exam blueprints. It addresses the clinical knowledge reasonably expected to be tested on the Boards but makes no use of, and divulges no details of, ABIM's proprietary exam content.

Internal Medicine Video Board Review

Release Date: September 10, 2017   CME Expiration Date: September 10, 2020

CME Accreditation

MedStudy is accredited by the Accreditation Council for Continuing Medical Education (ACCME) to provide continuing medical education for physicians.

MedStudy designates this enduring material for a maximum of 62 *AMA PRA Category 1 Credits*™. Physicians should claim only the credit commensurate with the extent of their participation in the activity.

This credit may be submitted to the American Osteopathic Association (AOA) for category 2 credit. All other health care professionals completing this continuing education activity will be issued a certificate of participation.

ABIM MOC Points

Successful completion of this CME activity, which includes participation in the evaluation component, enables the participant to earn up to 62 Medical Knowledge MOC points in the American Board of Internal Medicine's (ABIM) Maintenance of Certification (MOC) program. Participants will earn MOC points equivalent to the amount of CME credits claimed for the activity. It is the CME activity provider's responsibility to submit participant completion information to ACCME for the purpose of granting ABIM MOC credit.

How to Apply for CME Credit and MOC Points

Please note: CME credit and MOC points are available only to the original purchaser of this product from MedStudy, and issuance of CME credit and submission of MOC points is subject to verification of product ownership. CME credits and MOC points will be available only after passing the required online posttest with a score of at least 70%. CME credits for the Internal Medicine Video Board Review will be available until September 10, 2020.

To claim your CME credits and/or MOC points:
1. Study the material as often as necessary in order to understand and master the content.
2. Go to www.medstudy.com and click on CME/MOC in the menu bar.
3. Follow the instructions for completing the CME credit and MOC point credit application, posttest, and product evaluation.

Note: For any questions, please email us at cme@medstudy.com or call 1-800-841-0547, ext. 3.

Learning Objectives

As a result of participation in this activity, learners will be able to:
- Integrate and demonstrate increased overall knowledge of Internal Medicine
- Identify and remedy areas of weakness (gaps) in knowledge and clinical competencies
- Describe the clinical manifestations and treatments of diseases encountered in Internal Medicine and effectively narrow the differential diagnosis list by utilizing the most appropriate medical studies
- Apply the competence and confidence gained through participation in this activity to both a successful Board exam-taking experience and daily practice

Target Audience

Participants in this educational activity are those physicians seeking to assess, expand, and/or reinforce their knowledge, decision-making strategies, and clinical competencies in Internal Medicine, focusing their learning on subjects that are directly relevant to clinical scenarios that will be encountered in the practice setting, as well as on the American Board of Internal Medicine (ABIM) Certification or Maintenance of Certification (MOC) Board exam.

Learner Participation

The content of this CME activity is intended to help learners assess their own key knowledge and clinical competencies with evidence-based standards of care, which are reflected on the Board exams and in clinical settings. View the presentations by specialty/subspecialty topic as often as needed to gain necessary competence and confidence in knowing the material. Since the ABIM typically cites in its exam blueprint that certain topic areas are emphasized more on the exam than others (e.g., Cardiology, Pulmonary Medicine, Infectious Disease, and Gastroenterology), MedStudy recommends that these topics in the Video Board Review be viewed at least twice. Use the accompanying eSyllabus as an outline guide for the presentations and as a place to document your personal study notes and/or highlight critical points of information as they are presented. Participants will be required to complete a posttest as part of the requirements for receiving CME credit for this product.

Course Director:

Robert A. Hannaman, MD
MedStudy
Colorado Springs, Colorado

Speakers:

Kathryn H. Dao, MD*
Associate Director of Clinical Rheumatology
Baylor Research Institute
Dallas, TX

Raj Dasgupta MD
Professor of Clinical Medicine
Keck School of Medicine of USC
Department of Medicine
Division of Pulmonary, Critical Care,
  and Sleep Medicine
Assistant Program Director of Internal
  Medicine Residency
Associate Program Director of the Sleep
  Medicine Fellowship
Los Angeles, CA

Jitesh Kar, MD, MPH
Clinical Assistant Professor,
  Department of Neurology
University of Alabama at Birmingham,
  Huntsville Regional Medical Campus
Huntsville, AL

Chris L. Knight, MD
Associate Professor of Medicine
University of Washington Medical Center
Seattle, WA

Nimisha K. Parekh, MD, MPH
Clinical Professor of Medicine
Program Director of Gastroenterology Fellowship
UC Irvine Health
Orange, CA

Course Co-Director/Speaker:

Aaron J. Calderon, MD*
Chairman, Department of Medicine
Program Director, Internal Medicine Residency,
  Saint Joseph Hospital
Clinical Professor of Medicine,
University of Colorado School of Medicine
Denver, CO

Doug Paauw, MD
Professor, Medicine
Director, Internal Medicine
  Medical Student Programs
University of Washington School of Medicine
Department of Medicine
Seattle, WA

Aric Parnes, MD
Instructor in Medicine — Harvard Medical School
Brigham & Women's Division of Hematology
Boston, MA

Rishi Sawhney, MD
Medical Director, Bayhealth Cancer Institute
Hematology/Medical Oncology
Dover, DE

Janet Schlechte, MD
Professor of Medicine
Department of Internal Medicine
University of Iowa Carver College of Medicine
Iowa City, IA

Matthew Sorrentino, MD
Professor of Medicine
Vice Chair for Clinical Operations
Department of Medicine, Section of Cardiology
University of Chicago Medicine
Chicago, IL

Manish Suneja, MD
Director, Internal Medicine Residency Program
Co-Strand Director, Clinical and Professional Skills
Professor of Internal Medicine
Dr. William and Sondra Myers Professor
University of Iowa Hospitals and Clinics
  & Carver College of Medicine
Iowa City, IA

Fred A. Zar, MD
Professor of Clinical Medicine
Program Director, Internal Medicine Residency
University of Illinois at Chicago
Chicago, IL

Note: Those speakers with an asterisk (*) after their names have disclosed relationships with entities producing, marketing, reselling, or distributing health care goods or services consumed by, or used on, patients. All others have documented they have **no** relationships with such entities.

MedStudy Disclosure Statement

MedStudy, including all of its employees, has **no** financial interest, arrangement, or affiliation with any commercial entity producing, marketing, reselling, or distributing health care goods or services consumed by, or used on, patients. Furthermore, MedStudy complies with the AMA Council on Ethical and Judicial Affairs (CEJA) opinions that address the ethical obligations that underpin physician participation in CME: 8.061, "Gifts to physicians from industry," 9.011, "Ethical issues in CME," and 9.0115, "Financial Relationships with Industry in CME."

MedStudy Disclosure Policy

It is the policy of MedStudy to ensure balance, independence, objectivity, and scientific rigor in all of its educational activities. In keeping with all policies of MedStudy and the ACCME, any contributor to a MedStudy CME activity is required to disclose all relevant relationships with any entity producing, marketing, reselling, or distributing health care goods or services consumed by, or used on, patients. Failure to do so precludes acceptance by MedStudy of any material by that individual. All contributors are also required to submit a signed Good Practices Agreement affirming that their contribution is based upon currently available, scientifically rigorous data; that it is free from commercial bias; and that any clinical practice and patient care recommendations offered are based on the best available evidence for these specialties and subspecialties. All content is carefully reviewed by MedStudy's CME Physicians Oversight Council, as well as on-staff copyeditors, and any perceived issues or conflicts are resolved prior to publication of an enduring product or the start of a live activity.

Speaker Disclosures: The following speakers have openly indicated affiliation with commercial entities.

Aaron J. Calderon, MD
Stockholder: Abbott, Merck, Medtronic, Pfizer

Kathryn H. Dao, MD
Grant/Research Support: AbbVie, AstraZeneca, Celgene, Janssen, Pfizer
Speakers' Bureau: ARTHROS

For Further Study

Print, Digital, and Audio Resources:
- *MedStudy Internal Medicine Review Core Curriculum*, 17th Ed. MedStudy, Colorado Springs, CO, 2016.
- *MedStudy 2017–2018 Core Audio Pearls – Internal Medicine.* MedStudy, Colorado Springs, CO, 2016.
- *MedStudy 2017–2018 Internal Medicine Board-Style Questions & Answers.* MedStudy, Colorado Springs, CO, 2016.
- *MedStudy Internal Medicine Core Scripts® Flash Cards*, 2017–2018 Ed. MedStudy, Colorado Springs, CO, 2016.

Online Resources:
- *MedStudy Internal Medicine Board-Style Q&A Premium*, MedStudy, Colorado Springs, CO.
- *MedStudy Heart Sounds™*, MedStudy, Colorado Springs, CO.
- *MedStudy Skin Signs™*, MedStudy, Colorado Springs, CO.

Web-Based Resources:
- National Guideline Clearinghouse: http://www.guideline.gov
- American College of Physicians Guidelines: http://www.acponline.org/clinical_information/guidelines
- American Board of Internal Medicine Internal Medicine Certification Examination Blueprint: http://www.abim.org/~/media/ABIM%20Public/Files/pdf/exam-blueprints/certification/internal-medicine.pdf
- American Board of Internal Medicine Maintenance of Certification (MOC) Examination Blueprint: http://www.abim.org/~/media/ABIM%20Public/Files/pdf/exam-blueprints/maintenance-of-certification/internal-medicine.pdf

Note: For any questions, please email us at cme@medstudy.com or call 1-800-841-0547, ext. 3.

MedStudy

Internal Medicine Video Board Review

Acid-Base Disorders

Presented by

Robert A. (Tony) Hannaman, MD
MedStudy
Colorado Springs, Colorado

Acid-Base Video Review

The 4-Step Method

Necessary labs to assess acid-base status:

ABGs: pH, PCO_2, HCO_3^- (not used)

Electrolytes:

$$\frac{Na^+ \quad | \quad Cl^-}{K^+ \quad | \quad HCO_3^-}$$

Note 1: Expected PCO_2 = $exPCO_2$ = HCO_3^- + 15

Note 2: Anion gap = $Na^+ - (HCO_3^- + Cl^-)$

The 4 Steps:

Steps 1–4: Write down pH, PCO_2, $exPCO_2$ (= 15 + HCO_3^-), HCO_3^-, and calculate AG (= $Na^+ - (HCO_3^- + Cl^-)$). Do this every time you have ABGs and electrolytes from your patient. And do it in the **same order** each time.

Then look at each filled-in term and consider the following:

Step 1. pH: 1° disorder is acidemia/alkalemia.

Step 2. PCO_2 is **higher**/lower/same than expected so patient has a **respiratory acidosis**/respiratory alkalosis/neither.

Step 3. HCO_3^- is **low**/high/normal, so patient has **metabolic acidosis**/metabolic alkalosis/neutral metabolic status.

Go on to step 4 only if you've determined that your patient has a metabolic acidosis.

Step 4a. AG1: If metabolic acidosis and AG is **high**/normal, patient has a **HAGMA**/NAGMA.

Step 4b. AG2: If there is a high anion gap, ensure that the drop in HCO_3^- is equal to the increase in AG (should be 1:1). If they are equally balanced, there is no additional metabolic disorder. If not, then there is an additional metabolic disorder, summarized as:

Drop in HCO_3^- is **more than**/ less than the increase in AG, so there is an additional **metabolic acidosis**/metabolic alkalosis. (Be sure this makes good sense to you before continuing!)

Each step of the 4-step method should be done in **all** acid-base cases. The following two options are done only as needed:

1. The osmolal gap (OG) if intoxicated or obtunded and source is not certain
2. The urine anion gap (UAG) if NAGMA to help determine the cause (GI bicarb loss [diarrhea] vs. RTA)

Option 1: Osmolal Gap (if intoxicated/obtunded)

OG = Measured P_{Osm} − Calculated P_{Osm}; Normal OG is < 10

Calculated P_{Osm} = 2[Na] + BUN/2.8 + Glucose/18

Or, using 3 and 20, for ease of calculating:

Calculated P_{Osm} = **2**[Na] + BUN/**3** + Glucose/**20**

Very high OG (> 25 mOsm/kg) plus a **HAGMA** is almost always due to **toxic alcohol poisoning**:
  − Methanol
  − Ethylene glycol
  − Propylene glycol

High OG plus a **HAGMA** can be caused by:
  − Chronic kidney disease
  − Lactic acidosis
  − Ketoacidosis (alcoholic ketoacidosis, DKA)

High OG with a **normal AG** status can be caused by toxic and nontoxic substances:
  − Toxic substances:
    • Isopropyl alcohol (can be > 25 mOsm/kg)
    • Ethanol
    • Acetone

  − Non-toxic substances:
    • Mannitol
    • Sorbitol
    • Glycerol

Option 2: Urine Anion Gap (if NAGMA)

The Urine Anion Gap (UAG) is used to evaluate the etiology of NAGMA to differentiate between gastrointestinal loss of HCO_3^- (diarrhea) and renal tubular acidosis. UAG is determined using the measured ions in the urine: Na^+, K^+, and Cl^-, expressed in mEq/L.

$$UAG = Na^+ + K^+ - Cl^-$$

UAG is an estimate of the unmeasured ions in the urine, the most important one being NH_4^+. In the setting of NAGMA due to extrarenal (e.g., GI) bicarbonate losses, renal H^+ excretion is increased, and this H^+ is excreted in the form of NH_4^+. We do not measure urine NH_4^+ directly; we estimate it indirectly using the UAG.

Since NH_4^+ is a cation:
- Normal value of UAG is close to 0.
- A normal/positive UAG value suggests low urinary NH_4^+ (e.g., **RTA**).
- A negative UAG value suggests high urinary NH_4^+ (seen in NAGMA due to HCO_3^- loss from diarrhea). Remember neGUTive UAG in cases of diarrhea.

In the setting of metabolic acidosis due to extra-renal bicarbonate losses, renal H^+ excretion should be high, and H^+ is excreted in the form of NH_4^+.

Putting It All Together

With hints:

pH PCO_2 exPCO_2 HCO_3^- AG   OG   UAG

Without hints:

pH PCO_2 exPCO_2 HCO_3^- AG   OG   UAG

Examples

Acid-Base 1

A 36-year-old man is brought to the ED following a shooting. He arrives with a BP of 60/P and an actively bleeding exit wound in the neck with a small-caliber bullet hole.

Hgb 12.0   Hct 38.2
Na 139   K 3.9   Cl 107 HCO_3 10
ABG: pH 7.22 PCO_2 25 HCO_3 12

What is the acid-base abnormality?
- A. NAGMA
- B. HAGMA
- C. HAGMA + respiratory acidosis
- D. HAGMA + respiratory alkalosis
- E. Metabolic alkalosis

pH PCO_2 exPCO_2 HCO_3^- AG   OG   UAG

Answer: _____

Acid-Base 2

A 43-year-old alcoholic is admitted to telemetry for chest pain. The morning after admission, the patient appears inebriated and is acting delirious. He has no tremor. His last drink was in the car before admission ~ 24 hours ago. He is receiving only aspirin, metoprolol, lovastatin, and nitro paste.

BP 110/85, HR 100, T 98° F (36.7° C), RR 10–12, pulse oximetry 92%; somnolent, laughing, and telling inappropriate jokes; uncoordinated attempts to interact with a nurse as she takes his vitals. Within a short period of time, he becomes obtunded. He is moved to the ICU for supportive care.

Na 139   Cl 107   K 3.7 HCO_3 23,
BUN 14   Creat 0.7   Glu 89
ABG: pH 7.33 PCO_2 45 PO_2 75
Blood alcohol level < 30 mg/dL
S_{Osm}: 305
CT head is normal.

Which of the following is the most likely diagnosis?
   A. Alcohol intoxication
   B. Carbon monoxide poisoning
   C. Isopropyl alcohol ingestion
   D. Delirium tremens
   E. Pneumonia and sepsis

1	2		3	4a	Opt1	Opt2
pH	PCO_2	$exPCO_2$	HCO_3^- 4b AG		OG	UAG

Answer: _____

Acid-Base 3

A 62-year-old acutely ill man is brought to the hospital by ambulance. He developed nausea, diarrhea, and a low-grade fever two days ago, and then developed progressive, severe abdominal pain.

PMH: No HTN or DM; glaucoma (acetazolamide); diverticulitis 1 year earlier

Gen: Extremely ill; BP 88/62; P 122; R 24

T 101.66° F (38.7° C)

Neck veins are not visible, even when he is supine; heart and lungs are clear; abdomen has absent bowel sounds with generalized rebound tenderness.

ABG: pH 7.12 PO_2 94 PCO_2 32
Hgb 13.1   Hct 39.6   WBC 22,300
Na 144   K 3.2   Cl 114 HCO_3 10
BUN 36   Cr 1.4
U/A: pH 5; SG 1.010, prot 1+, 2–4 hyaline casts

CXR nl   Upright Abd — air under diaphragm

What is the acid-base abnormality?
   A. HAGMA + NAGMA
   B. NAGMA + respiratory acidosis
   C. HAGMA + respiratory acidosis + NAGMA
   D. HAGMA + respiratory alkalosis + NAGMA
   E. HAGMA + respiratory acidosis

1	2		3	4a	Opt1	Opt2
pH	PCO_2	$exPCO_2$	HCO_3^- 4b AG		OG	UAG

Answer: _____

Acid-Base 4

A severely intellectually disabled 46-year-old male is brought to the ED by neighbors after he was found down in his garage. He is obtunded, and his clothing is very heavily soiled with liquid stool and urine. He is afebrile. Orthostatic vital signs show a change in blood pressure and pulse between lying and sitting. Kussmaul respirations are noted. Neurologic exam is nonfocal.
Na 130   K 3.0   Cl 109 HCO_3 10
BUN 52   Creat 3.4

U/A: pH 5.0   (normal 6, range 4.5–8)
Urine Na 6 mEq/L (normal > 20)
ABG: pH 7.26 PCO_2 23 HCO_3 10

What is the acid-base abnormality?
   A. HAGMA
   B. NAGMA
   C. HAGMA + respiratory acidosis
   D. HAGMA + respiratory alkalosis
   E. Metabolic alkalosis

1	2		3	4a	Opt1	Opt2
pH	PCO_2	$exPCO_2$	HCO_3^- 4b AG		OG	UAG

Answer: _____

Acid-Base 5

A 28-year-old man swallows a bottle of pills ("pain killers") in a fit of despondency after a break-up with his girlfriend.

ABG: pH 7.36 PCO_2 22
Na 138   Cl 107 HCO_3 12

What is the acid-base abnormality?
   A. HAGMA
   B. Respiratory alkalosis
   C. HAGMA + respiratory acidosis
   D. HAGMA + respiratory alkalosis
   E. Metabolic alkalosis

1	2		3	4a	Opt1	Opt2
pH	PCO_2	$exPCO_2$	HCO_3^- 4b AG		OG	UAG

Answer: _____

Acid-Base 6

A 45-year-old man with diabetes and hypertension stops taking all his medications for 1 week. He presents with extensive vomiting, thirst and polyuria. His blood glucose is 556!

ABG: pH 7.39 PCO_2 38

Na 145   Cl 100 HCO_3 22

What is the acid-base abnormality?
- A. HAGMA + metabolic alkalosis
- B. Metabolic alkalosis metabolic
- C. HAGMA + respiratory acidosis
- D. HAGMA + respiratory alkalosis
- E. Respiratory alkalosis

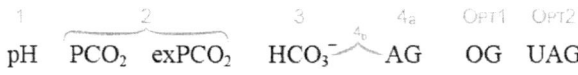

Answer: _____

Acid-Base 7

ABG: pH 7.49 PCO_2 20

Na 135   Cl 102 HCO_3 15

What is the acid-base abnormality?
- A. NAGMA
- B. HAGMA + respiratory alkalosis
- C. HAGMA + metabolic alkalosis
- D. Metabolic alkalosis
- E. Metabolic alkalosis + respiratory alkalosis + HAGMA

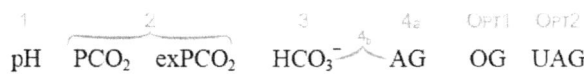

Answer: _____

Acid-Base 8

A 67-year-old man with chronic severe COPD and HF on diuretics presents with SOB, fever, and cough with purulent sputum.

Exam: T 102.3° F (39.06° C), BP 80/50, HR 135, RR 24, SPO_2 82% on RA

CXR: Severe multilobar pneumonia

ABG: pH 7.10 PCO_2 50

Na 145   Cl 100 HCO_3 15

What is the acid-base abnormality?
- A. HAGMA
- B. NAGMA
- C. HAGMA + NAGMA + respiratory acidosis
- D. HAGMA + metabolic alkalosis + respiratory acidosis
- E. Metabolic alkalosis

pH PCO_2 $exPCO_2$ HCO_3^- AG   OG   UAG

Answer: _____

Acid-Base 9

A 64-year-old obese lady with OHS and COPD has pulmonary hypertension and cor pulmonale treated with diuretics. She is having trouble breathing.

ABG: pH 7.39 PCO_2 60 PO_2 60

Na 135   K 3.1   Cl 91 HCO_3 35

What is the acid-base abnormality?
- A. NAGMA
- B. HAGMA + respiratory acidosis
- C. HAGMA + metabolic alkalosis
- D. Metabolic alkalosis
- E. Respiratory acidosis + metabolic alkalosis

pH PCO_2 $exPCO_2$ HCO_3^- AG   OG   UAG

Answer: _____

Acid-Base Answers

Acid-Base 1: B. HAGMA.

Acid-Base 2: C. Isopropyl alcohol ingestion (high OG + respiratory acidosis).

Acid-Base 3: E. HAGMA + respiratory acidosis.

Acid-Base 4: B. NAGMA.

Acid-Base 5: D. HAGMA + respiratory alkalosis.

Acid-Base 6: A. HAGMA + metabolic alkalosis.

Acid-Base 7: B. HAGMA + respiratory alkalosis. Classic salicylate OD presentation, which causes a HAGMA and also induces hyperventilation that more than compensates for the acidosis.

Acid-Base 8: D. HAGMA + metabolic alkalosis + respiratory acidosis.

Acid-Base 9: E. Respiratory acidosis + metabolic alkalosis.

MedStudy

Internal Medicine Video Board Review

Cardiology

Presented by

Matthew Sorrentino, MD
Professor of Medicine
Vice Chair for Clinical Operations
Department of Medicine, Section of Cardiology
University of Chicago Medicine
Chicago, Illinois

Table of Contents

Cardiology Abbreviations

ABI	Ankle-brachial index
ACEI	Angiotensin-converting enzyme inhibitor
ACHD	Adult congenital heart disease
ACS	Acute coronary syndrome
AF	Atrial fibrillation
ALT	Alanine aminotransferase
ANA	Antinuclear antibody
ANP	Atrial natriuretic peptide
APSAC	Anisoylated plasminogen-streptokinase activator complex
AR	Aortic regurgitation
ARB	Angiotensin receptor blocker
ARNI	Angiotensin receptor neprilysin inhibitor
AS	Aortic stenosis
ASCVD	Atherosclerotic cardiovascular disease
ASD	Atrial septal defect
ASO	Antistreptolysin O
AST	Aspartate aminotransferase
AV	Aortic valve
AVNRT	Atrioventricular nodal reentrant tachycardia
AVR	Aortic valve replacement
BMS	Bare metal stent
BNP	Brain natriuretic peptide
BUN	Blood urea nitrogen
CABG	Coronary artery bypass graft
CAC	Coronary artery calcification (score)
CAD	Coronary artery disease
CBC	Complete blood count
CHD	Coronary heart disease
CK	Creatine kinase
CKMB	Creatine kinase myocardial band
CKD	Chronic kidney disease
CO	Cardiac output
CRP	C-reactive protein
CRT	Cardiac resynchronization therapy
CTA	CT angiogram
CVA	Cerebrovascular accident
DES	Drug-eluting stent
DM	Diabetes mellitus
EBCT	Electron-beam computed tomography
ECG	Electrocardiogram
ETT	Exercise treadmill test
FDG	Fluorodeoxyglucose
FMC	First medical contact
GRACE	Global Registry of Acute Coronary Events
HACEK	*Haemophilus*, *Aggregatibacter* (*Actinobacillus*), *Cardiobacterium*, *Eikenella*, and *Kingella*
HCM	Hypertrophic cardiomyopathy
HDL	High-density lipoprotein
HF	Heart failure
HOCM	Hypertrophic obstructive cardiomyopathy
HTN	Hypertension
ICD	Implantable cardioverter defibrillator

ICT	Intrinsicoid deflection time
IE	Infective endocarditis
INR	International normalization ratio
IVC	Inferior vena cava
JVP	Jugular venous pressure
LA	Left atrium
LAD	Left anterior descending coronary artery
LBBB	Left bundle-branch block
LCX	Left circumflex (coronary artery)
LDH	Lactate dehydrogenase
LDL	Low-density lipoprotein
LICS	Left intercostal space
LLSB	Left lower sternal border
LV	Left ventricle
LVEDP	Left ventricular end diastolic pressure
LVEF	Left ventricular ejection fraction
LVH	Left ventricular hypertrophy
MAP	Mean arterial pressure
METs	Metabolic equivalents
MI	Myocardial infarction
MPI	Myocardial perfusion imaging
MR	Mitral regurgitation
MRA	Magnetic resonance angiogram
MS	Mitral stenosis
MTAP	Mitral, tricuspid, aortic, and pulmonic valves
MUGA	Radionuclide ventriculography
MVP	Mitral valve prolapse
NOACs	Novel oral anticoagulants
NSTE-ACS	Non–ST-elevation acute coronary syndrome
NSTEMI	Non–ST-elevation myocardial infarction
NTG	Nitroglycerin
$P2Y_{12}$	Inhibitors; antiplatelet agents (e.g., clopidogrel, prasugrel, ticagrelor)
PA	Pulmonary artery
PAD	Peripheral arterial disease
PCI	Percutaneous coronary intervention
PCWP	Pulmonary capillary wedge pressure
PDE	Phosphodiesterase
PET	Positron emission tomography
PFO	Patent foramen ovale
PMBC	Percutaneous mitral balloon commissurotomy
PR	Pulmonic regurgitation
PS	Pulmonic stenosis
PSVT	Paroxysmal supraventricular tachycardia
PTA	Percutaneous transluminal angioplasty
PURSUIT	Platelet glycoprotein IIb/IIIa in Unstable angina: Receptor Suppression Using Integrilin (eptifibatide) Therapy
PVCs	Premature ventricular contractions
QRS	Q, R, and S waves on ECG
RA	Right atrium
RBBB	Right bundle-branch block
RCA	Right coronary artery

RCT	Randomized clinical trial
RICS	Right intercostal space
RV	Right ventricle
RVH	Right ventricular hypertrophy
S_1	First heart sound
S_2	Second heart sound
S_3	Third heart sound
S_4	Fourth heart sound
SL	Sublingual
STEMI	ST-elevation myocardial infarction
SVC	Superior vena cava
SVT	Supraventricular tachycardia
TEE	Transesophageal echocardiogram
TIA	Transient ischemic attack
TIMI	Thrombolysis in myocardial infarction
tPA	Tissue plasminogen activator
TR	Tricuspid regurgitation
TS	Tricuspid stenosis
TSH	Thyroid stimulating hormone
UFH	Unfractionated heparin
USB	Upper sternal border
VF	Ventricular fibrillation
VSD	Ventricular septal defect
VT	Ventricular tachycardia
WPW	Wolff-Parkinson-White syndrome
XRT	External radiation therapy

Speaker Disclosure

Matthew Sorrentino, MD, has documented that he has no commercial relationships to disclose.

Cardiology

Cardiology Review Outline
- **Part 1:** Diagnostic Studies
- **Part 2:** Physical Examination
- **Part 3:** Coronary Artery Disease
- **Part 4:** Peripheral Arterial Disease
- **Part 5:** Valvular Heart Disease
- **Part 6:** Heart Failure, Miscellaneous
- **Part 7:** ECG, Arrhythmia Management

Suggested References
Go to www.acc.org, and you will be able to click on "Guidelines," the first header tab on the home page.

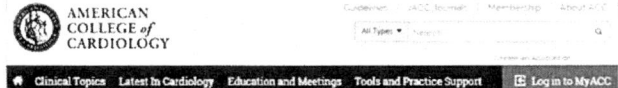

Suggested References

Guideline	Year	Format
ST-Elevation Myocardial Infarction	2012	Pocket Guide
Stable Ischemic Heart Disease	2013	Pocket Guide
Atrial Fibrillation	2014	Pocket Guide
Assessment of Cardiovascular Risk, Cholesterol	2013	Pocket Guide
Non–ST-Elevation Acute Coronary Syndrome	2014	Slide Set
Carotid and Vertebral Artery Disease	2011	Pocket Guide
Peripheral Arterial Disease	2011	Pocket Guide
Heart Failure	2013	Pocket Guide
Valvular Heart Disease	2014	Pocket Guide
Hypertrophic Cardiomyopathy	2011	Pocket Guide
Perioperative Cardiovascular Evaluation	2014	Pocket Guide

**Part 1:
Diagnostic Studies**

Chest X-ray

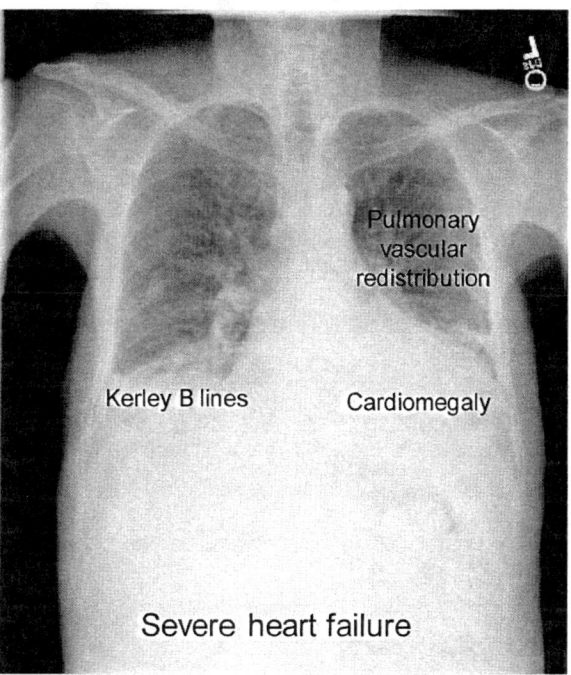

Severe heart failure

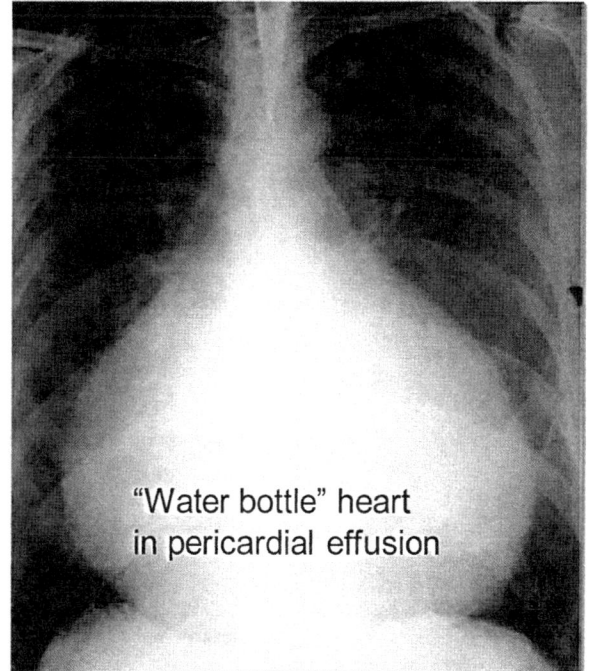

"Water bottle" heart in pericardial effusion

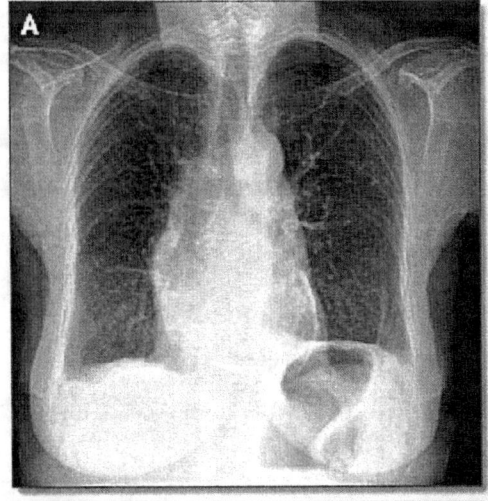

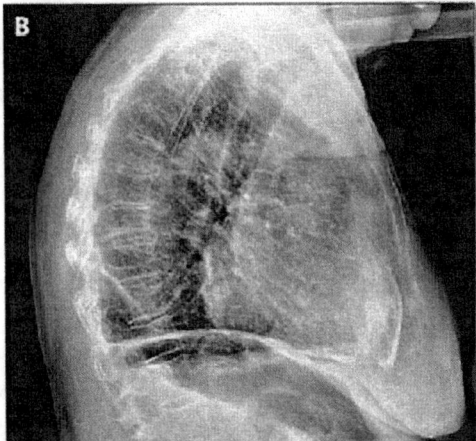

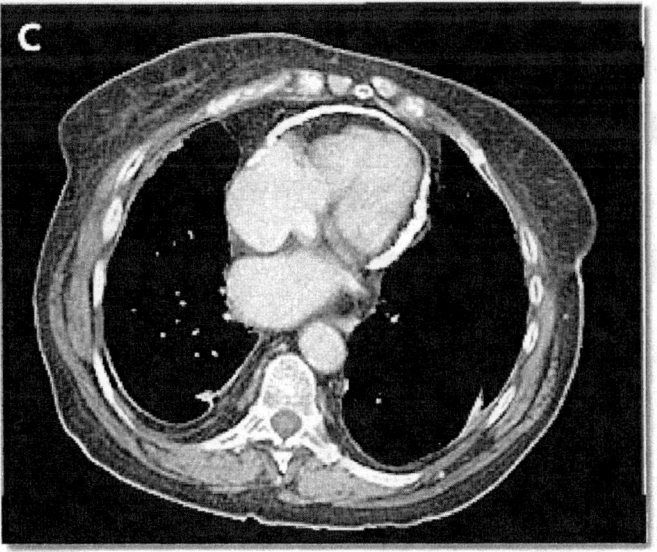

Pericardial calcification on x-ray and CT

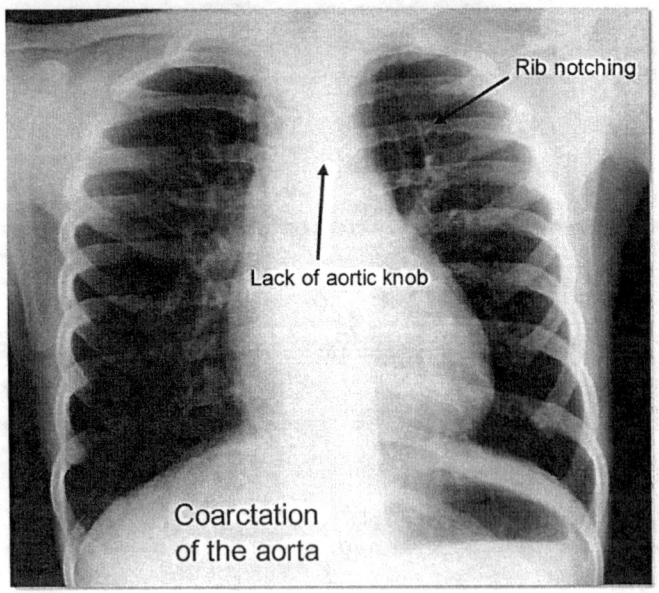

Rib notching

Lack of aortic knob

Coarctation of the aorta

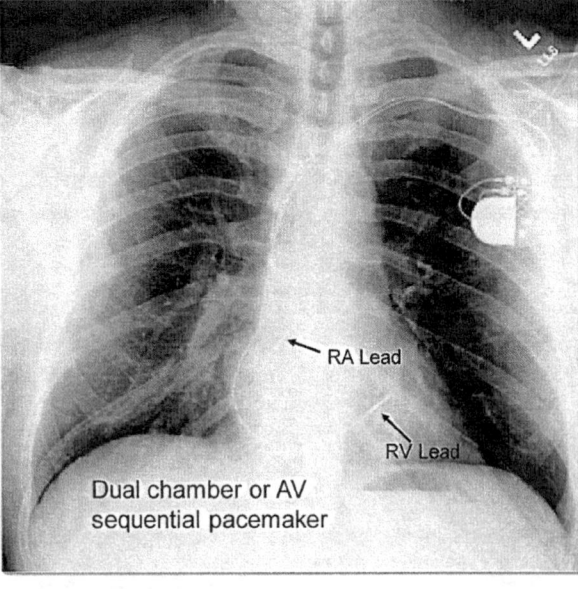

RA Lead

RV Lead

Dual chamber or AV sequential pacemaker

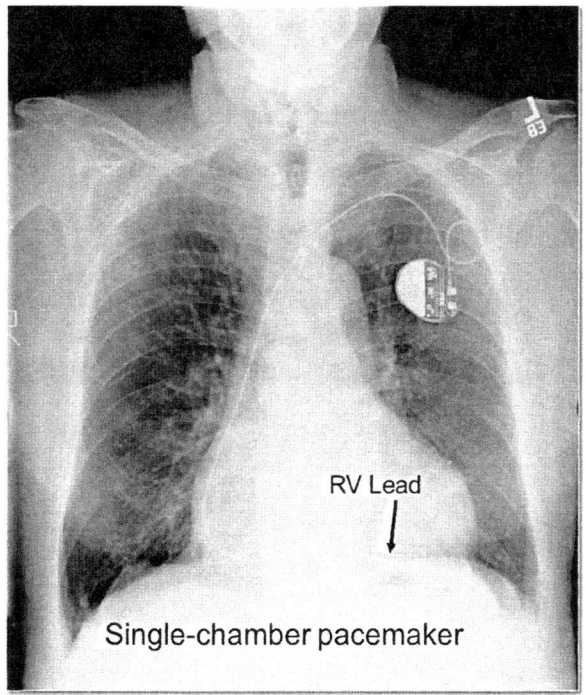

RV Lead

Single-chamber pacemaker

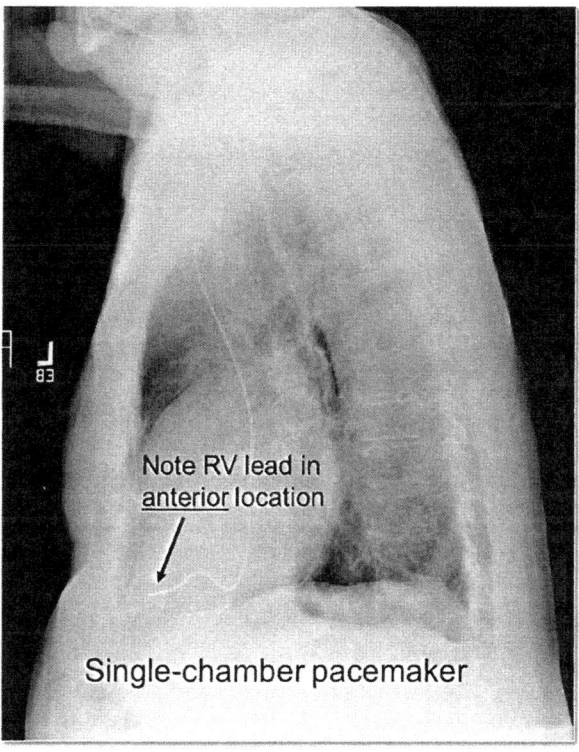

Note RV lead in anterior location

Single-chamber pacemaker

Echocardiography

There are no echo images on the exam, but several case studies **do** refer to echo findings.

Uses of Echo
- Cardiac function, chamber size, and wall thickness
- Valvular heart disease
- Congenital heart disease
- Aortic root disease
- Suspected pulmonary HTN
- Pericardial diseases
- Cardiac masses
- Descending aortic dissection (with TEE)
- HCM

Audience Response 1
A temporary transvenous pacemaker was placed in a patient in the CCU.
Minutes later, he developed hypotension and elevated neck veins, but lung fields remained clear.

What would an echocardiogram show?
A. Severe left ventricular dysfunction
B. Acute aortic regurgitation
C. Acute mitral regurgitation
D. Hypertrophic cardiomyopathy
E. A large pericardial effusion

Answer: _____

Pericardial Effusion

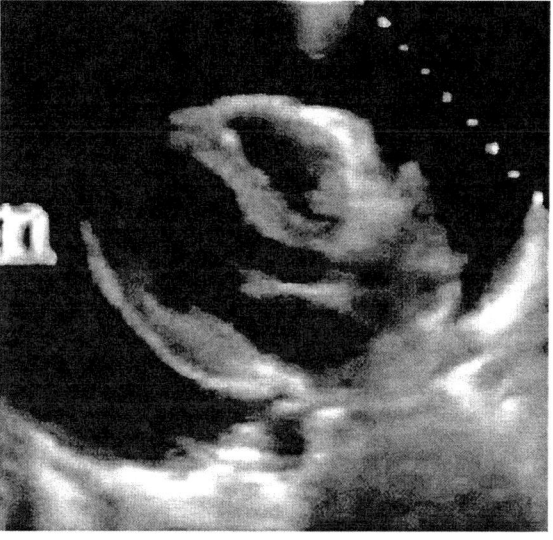

Other Common Echo Findings
- Hypertrophic cardiomyopathy (HCM)
- Aortic stenosis (AS)
- Aortic regurgitation (AR)
- Mitral regurgitation (MR)
- Mitral stenosis (MS)

Basic Findings — HCM
- Thickened septum
- Obstruction of left ventricular outflow tract
- Asymmetric LV hypertrophy

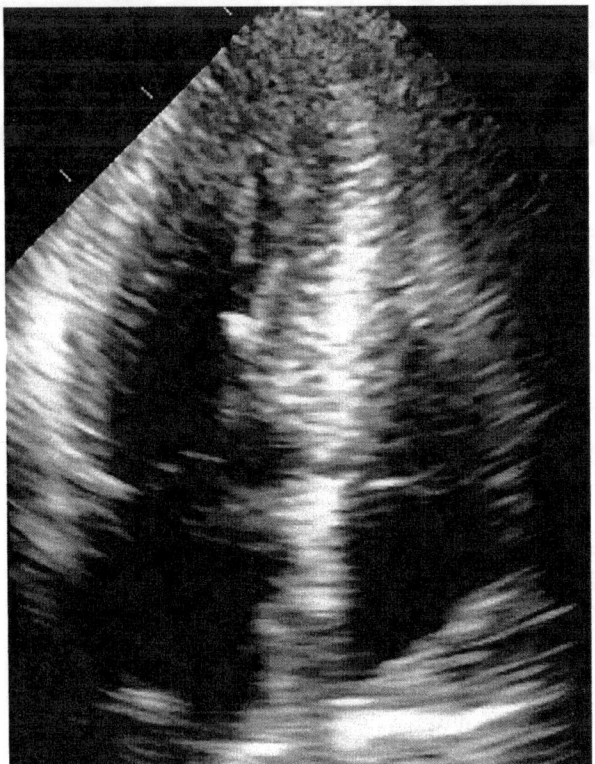

HCM

Basic Findings — AS
- Thickened, calcified aortic leaflets
- Bicuspid valve
- Reduced leaflet excursion
- Reduced leaflet mobility
- Severely reduced valve area

Aortic Stenosis

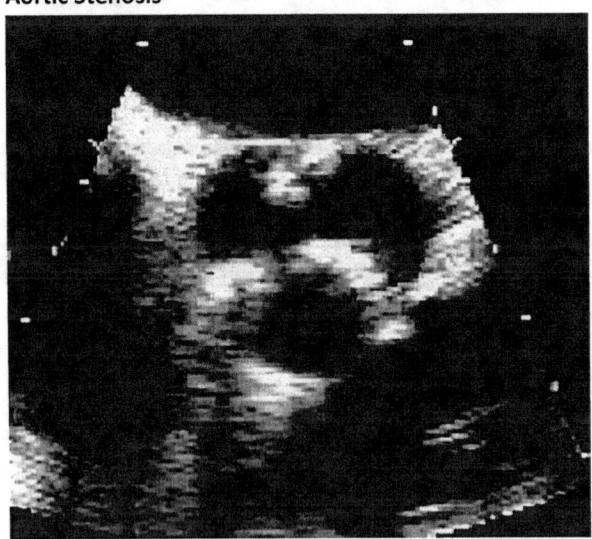

Basic Findings — MS
- Thickened leaflets
- Calcified leaflets
- Reduced leaflet excursion
- Severely reduced valve area

Mitral Stenosis

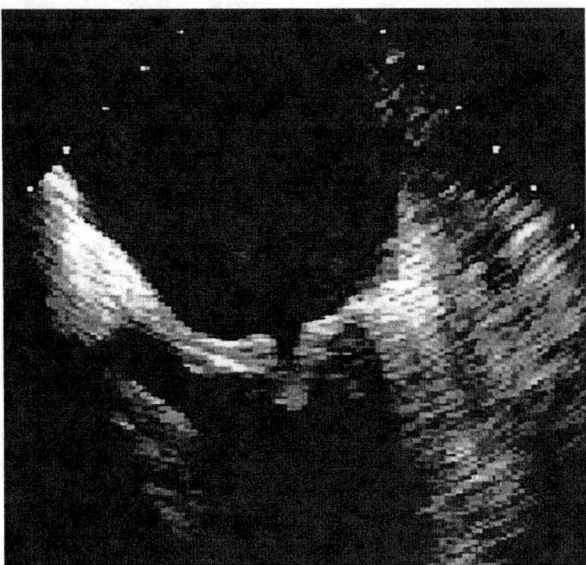

Basic Findings — AR
- Regurgitant jet
- Doppler shows regurgitant flow into the left ventricle
- Description of damaged valve or vegetation

Aortic Regurgitation

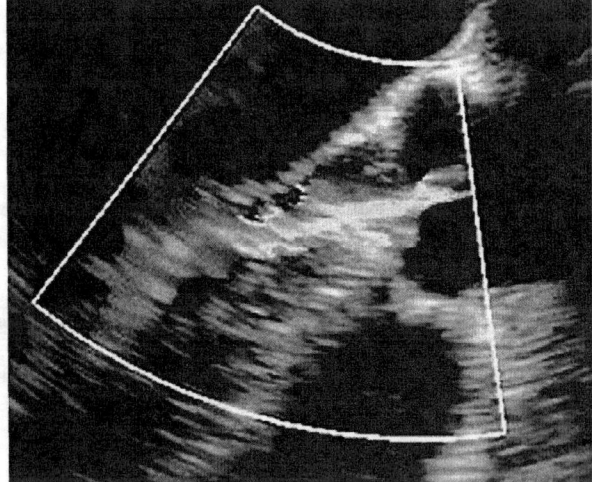

Basic Findings — MR
- Regurgitant jet(s)
- Doppler shows regurgitant flow into the left atrium
- Description of damaged valve or vegetation
- Tethered leaflet(s)
- Torn chordae
- Prior MI

Mitral Regurgitation

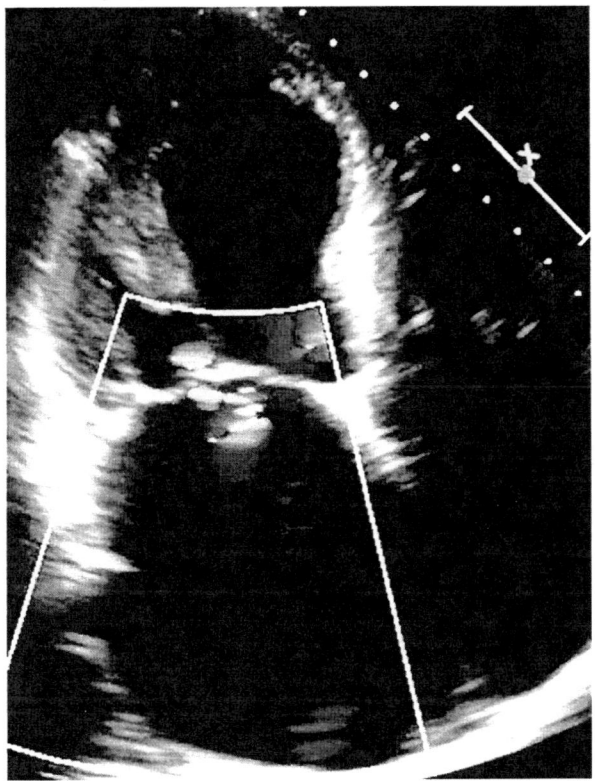

AR 2
A 55 yo woman with a history of bicuspid aortic valve presents with worsening dyspnea. A transthoracic echocardiogram shows calcification of the valve and reduced valve area.

Which of the following is most likely indicated?
A. Carotid endarterectomy.
B. Aortic valve surgery.
C. Mitral valve surgery.
D. Septal reduction therapy.
E. Observe and repeat echo in 6 months.

Answer: _____

AR 3
A 75 yo male with a h/o of prior MI presents with worsening dyspnea and fatigue. On exam, you detect a 2/6 holosystolic murmur best heard at the apex.

What should you order next?
A. An exercise treadmill test (ETT)
B. A transthoracic echocardiogram
C. A transesophageal echocardiogram
D. Ankle-brachial index (ABI)
E. A MUGA scan (radionuclide ventriculogram)

Answer: _____

Use of TEE
- Endocarditis
- Acute MR or AR
- Aortic dissection
- Prior to cardioversion for A-fib/flutter

AR 4
A 65 yo woman with DM and poorly controlled HTN presents with severe central chest pain.
Chest x-ray shows widening of the mediastinum. She states that the pain radiates down her back in a "ripping" or "stabbing" sensation.

What would you order next?
A. Anticoagulation with heparin
B. Emergency coronary angiography
C. Transesophageal echo
D. Barium swallow
E. Fibrinolytic therapy

Answer: _____

Stress Testing

Indications
- Suspected ischemic heart disease
- Risk stratification, particularly post-MI
- Assessment of the effectiveness of therapy (medical, PCI, surgery)
- Establishment of an exercise regimen

History

Classification of chest pain	Description	Precipitating and relieving factors
Typical angina	Yes	Yes
Atypical chest pain	Either Yes	Or Yes
Noncardiac chest pain	No	No

Pretest Probability of CAD

Age	Noncardiac Chest Pain		Atypical Chest Pain		Typical Angina	
	Women	Men	Women	Men	Women	Men
30–39	2	4	12	34	26	76
40–49	3	13	22	51	55	87
50–59	7	20	31	65	73	93
60–69	14	27	51	72	86	94

Bayes Theorem

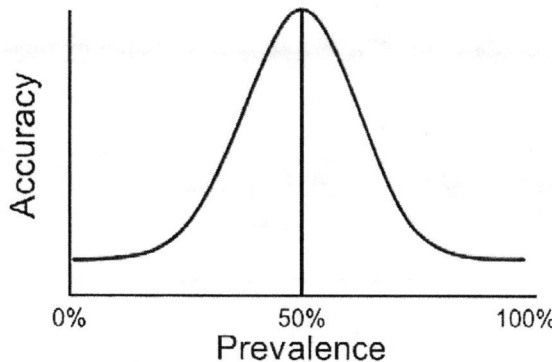

The accuracy of any test depends on the prevalence of the disease in the population studied.

Bayes Theorem and Stress Testing
- The greatest accuracy is obtained when the prevalence is 50%; e.g., in middle-aged men with atypical chest pain
- The false-positive rate is high (20%) in patients who are unlikely to have CAD
- The false-negative rate is high (25%) in patients who are very likely to have CAD

Why Use Exercise?
- Mimics normal patient activity
- Inexpensive
- **Gives additional important prognostic information**

ECG Changes During Exercise

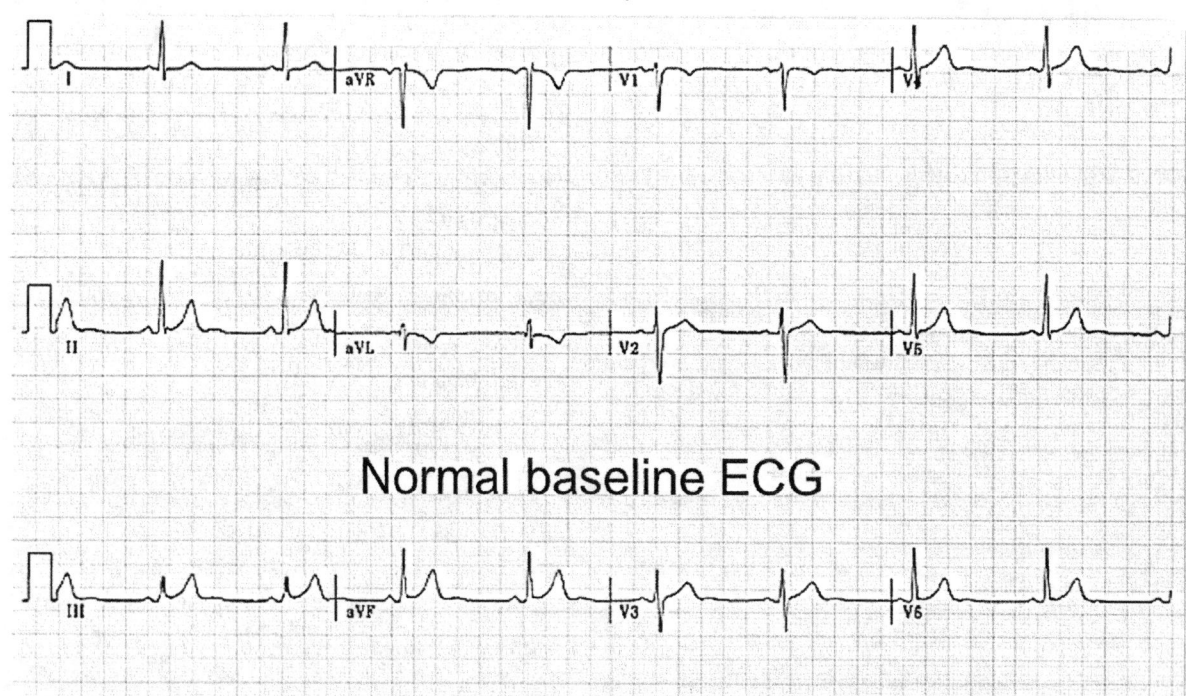

Normal baseline ECG

© 2017 MedStudy Internal Medicine Video Board Review – Cardiology • Matthew Sorrentino, MD

ECG Changes During Exercise (cont.)

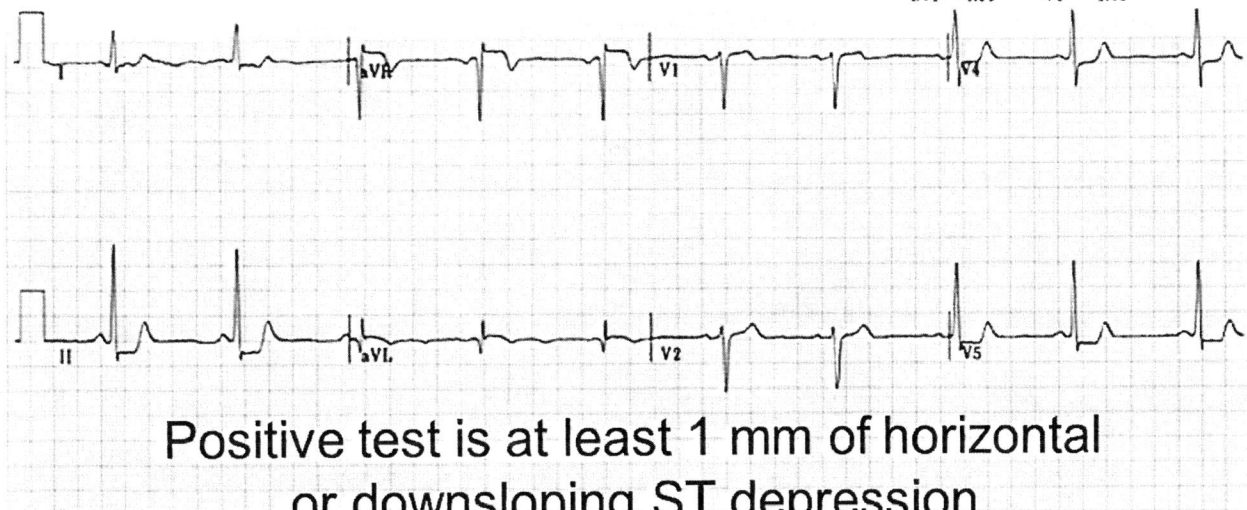

Positive test is at least 1 mm of horizontal or downsloping ST depression

Limitations of Exercise Stress Testing
- Many patients cannot exercise
- Specificity declines progressively as the baseline ECG is "uglier," roughly in this order:
  1) Nonspecific ST changes
  2) Digoxin therapy
  3) RBBB
  4) LVH
  5) WPW, LBBB, paced rhythm

Key Points
- If a patient can/is able to exercise, do everything you can to obtain the exercise portion of the test b/c of the invaluable prognostic information that it provides
- Let baseline ECG guide you as to whether to add imaging

Stress Testing Algorithm

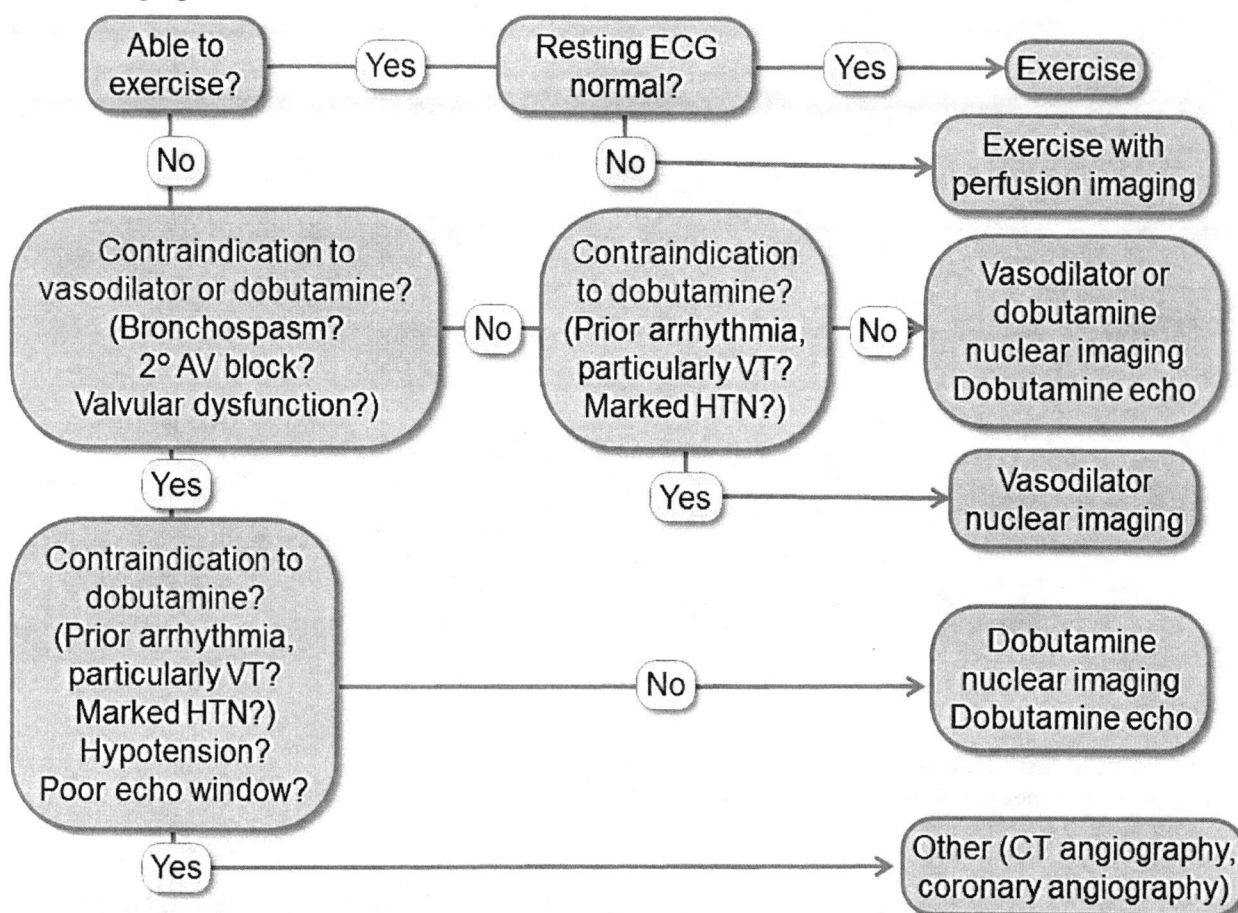

AR 5

A patient with risk factors for CAD presents with chest pain, and an MI has been ruled out. The baseline ECG shows LVH. Patient is able to exercise.

What stress test should be ordered?
A. A regular exercise treadmill test
B. An exercise stress test with nuclear perfusion imaging
C. A pharmacologic stress test with nuclear perfusion imaging
D. An ST-segment–sensitive Holter monitor
E. Cardiac catheterization

Answer: _____

AR 6

A patient has severe claudication and asthma. Baseline ECG shows LVH.

What stress test should you order?
A. A regular exercise stress test
B. An exercise test with nuclear perfusion imaging
C. An adenosine stress test with nuclear perfusion imaging
D. A dobutamine stress echo
E. Cardiac catheterization

Answer: _____

Pharmacologic Stress Testing
- Necessary if the patient cannot exercise
- Can be accomplished with vasodilators (adenosine, dipyridamole, regadenoson) or dobutamine
- Vasodilator stress imaging is particularly useful in patients with LBBB or paced rhythms

Myocardial Perfusion Imaging

- Stress is by exercise or chemical means (adenosine, dipyridamole, or dobutamine)
- ^{201}Thallium and ^{99m}technetium are distributed in the heart where there is adequate blood flow
- Uptake of the isotope is decreased during stress in ischemic zones
- In recovery, the ischemic myocardium recovers and takes up the isotope

- LV systolic function can be measured at rest and with stress
- Myocardial viability can be evaluated

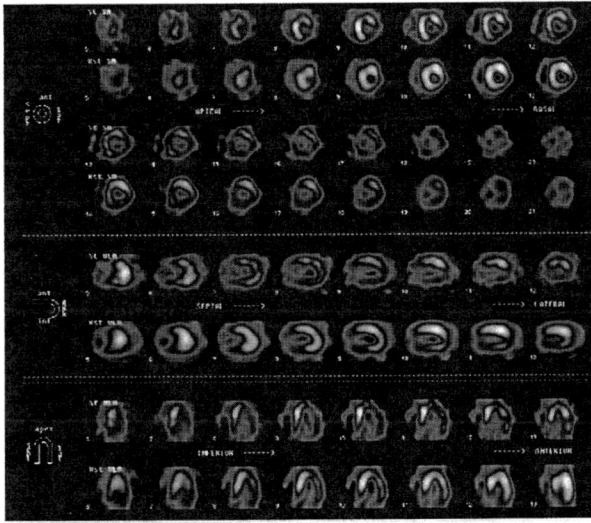

Stress Echocardiography

- Less expensive and more specific, but less sensitive, than nuclear imaging
- The choice of the 2 modalities usually depends on local expertise
- Not as useful in LBBB

Cardiac CT and MR

CT Modalities

Modality	Radiation Dose	Uses Contrast	Uses
Noncontrast CT (includes "EBCT")	Low	No	Detect coronary calcification
CT Angiography (CTA)	Moderate	Yes	Anatomy Function Evaluation of chest pain

Drawbacks of CTA

- Higher radiation dose
- Requires iodinated contrast
- Heart rate should be < 60 bpm
- Patient must be able to perform a 15-second breath hold

Noncontrast CT

- Mainly for detection of coronary calcification
- A high calcium score (> 100) indicates an increased risk of cardiac events
- Lack of coronary calcification is predictive of a very low risk of a cardiac event

Calcium Score and Risk of CAD

Calcium Score	Implication	Risk of Coronary Disease
0	No identifiable plaque	Very low; < 5%
1–10	Minimal plaque	Very unlikely; < 10%
11–100	Definite, at least mild atherosclerotic plaque	Minimal or mild coronary narrowings likely
101–400	Definite, at least moderate plaque	Mild CAD, significant narrowings possible
401 or higher	Extensive plaque	High likelihood of at least 1 significant coronary narrowing, odds ratio of ACS event > 10 to 1

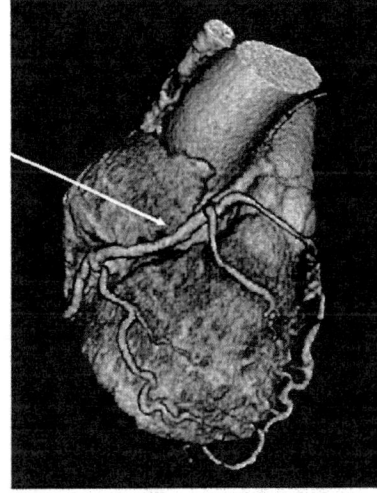

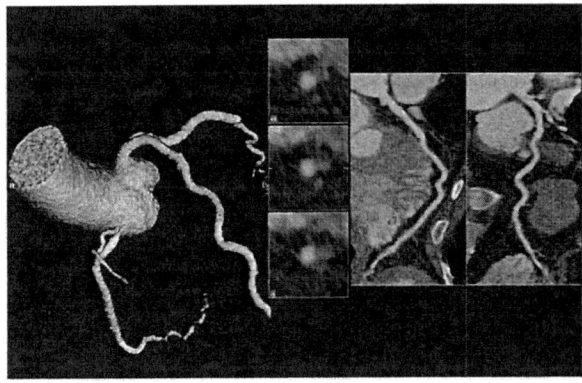

Coronary Calcification

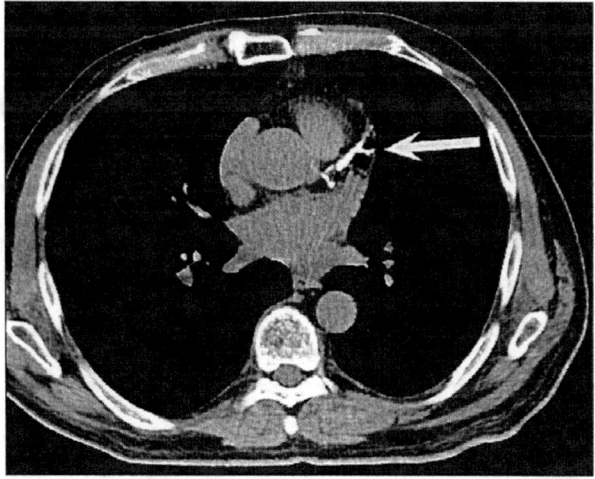

Uses of Cardiac MR
- LV function
- Valve function
- Tissue characterization (infiltrative cardiomyopathies; e.g., hemochromatosis)
- Myocardial masses
- Myocardial viability

Myocardial Viability

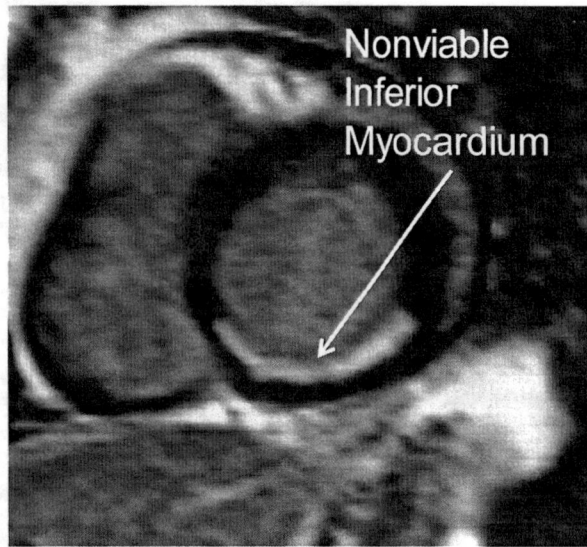

J Nucl Med. July 2007;48(7):1135–1146.

Myocardial Viability by PET

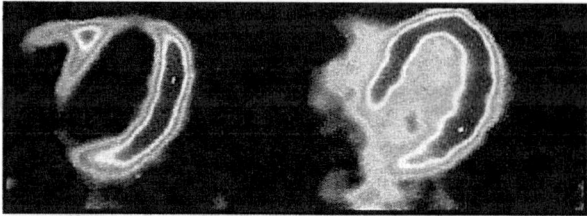

N^{13} Ammonia Scan   FDG Glucose Scan

J Nucl Med. July 2007;48(7):1135–1146.

AR 7

A 65 yo male with a history of MI in the past month and congestive heart failure, EF 30%, presents with a PET scan that shows viability in the anterior wall. He asks you if he should take his cardiologist's advice.

You tell him that, yes, he should follow his cardiologist's advice to:
A. Undergo coronary revascularization to the anterior wall.
B. Wear a 48-hour Holter monitor.
C. Get an ICD before doing anything else.
D. Get a pacemaker.
E. Have a TEE performed.

Answer: _____

Cardiac Catheterization

Left-Heart Catheterization
- All contraindications are relative
- Mortality is < 0.1%
- Ventriculography and aortography can also be performed in addition to coronary angiography

- Most common indication: CAD, coronary angiography
- Radial approach has less morbidity
- Possible complications:
  - Retroperitoneal hemorrhage
  - Coronary dissection
  - Cardiac tamponade
  - Cholesterol embolism/livedo reticularis

AR 8

A patient has coronary angiography from the femoral arterial approach. Immediately after the procedure, she develops sinus tachycardia and severe hypotension. A 12-lead ECG is otherwise normal. Stat CBC shows hemoglobin of 7 g/dL.

What is the most likely diagnosis?

A. Acute myocardial ischemia
B. Retroperitoneal hemorrhage
C. Cardiac tamponade
D. Pulmonary embolism
E. Tension pneumothorax

Answer: _____

AR 9

A 75 yo woman had a coronary angiogram 3 weeks ago. Over the past week, she noted discoloration and pain in the left foot.
Her laboratory data now shows a serum creatinine of 4.5 mg/dL.

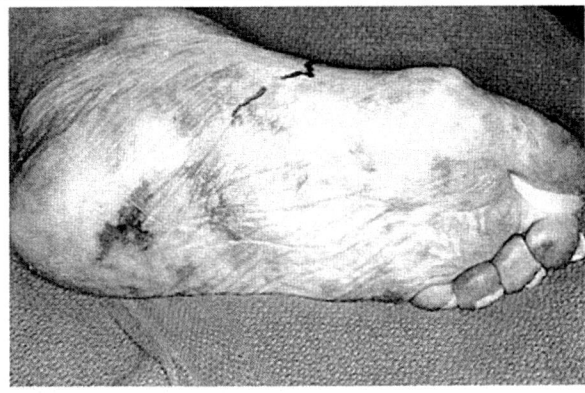

What is responsible for her renal failure?

A. Underlying interstitial kidney disease
B. Iodinated contrast nephropathy
C. Atherosclerosis of the renal arteries
D. An allergic reaction to iodinated contrast
E. Atherosclerotic embolization to the kidneys and systemically at the time of catheterization

Answer: _____

Right-Heart (PA) Catheterization

Pulmonary Capillary Wedge Pressure (PCWP)

- PCWP is a dampened form of LA pressure, which represents LVEDP
- Normal is < 12 mmHg
- Increases with:
  1) LVH
  2) LV failure
  3) Left-sided valvular disease
  4) Tamponade
  5) Constrictive pericarditis

PCWP

Acute increases in PCWP cause more symptoms at lower pressures than chronically elevated levels.

Pressure (mmHg)	Symptoms
> 12	Mild dyspnea on exertion
15–20	Dyspnea on exertion
25–35	Dyspnea at rest
> 35	Pulmonary edema

RA and RV Pressures

- Normal RA pressure is < 7 cm H_2O
- Jugular venous distention occurs at RA pressures > 7 cm H_2O (5 mmHg)
- Increased RA pressures are usually indicative of right-heart failure
- Normal RV systolic pressure is < 30 mmHg

**Examples of
Right-Heart Pressures**

Hemodynamic Examples

	RA Pressure	PA Pressure	PCWP	BP
1 (normal)	0–5	13–28/3–13	3–11	110/70
2	18	32/18	17	70/50
3	15	21/11	10	70/50
4	18	40/30	30	70/50
5	18	90/32	30	110/70
6	18	90/32	10	110/70

Example 2

	RA Pressure	PA Pressure	PCWP	BP
1 (normal)	0–5	13–28/3–13	3–11	110/70
2	18	32/18	17	70/50
3	15	21/11	10	70/50
4	18	40/30	30	70/50
5	18	90/32	30	110/70
6	18	90/32	10	110/70

Example 2 (cont.)

- RA, PA diastolic, and PCWP are equal
- The systemic blood pressure is low
- This combination is consistent with tamponade
- Tamponade and constrictive pericarditis produce equalization of diastolic pressures (see that section)

Example 3

	RA Pressure	PA Pressure	PCWP	BP
1 (normal)	0–5	13–28/3–13	3–11	110/70
2	18	32/18	17	70/50
3	15	21/11	10	70/50
4	18	40/30	30	70/50
5	18	90/32	30	110/70
6	18	90/32	10	110/70

Example 3 (cont.)
- RA much > PCWP
- Systemic blood pressure is low
- If this occurs in the setting of an inferior MI, these hemodynamics represent RV infarction

Example 4

	RA Pressure	PA Pressure	PCWP	BP
1 (normal)	0–5	13–28/3–13	3–11	110/70
2	18	32/18	17	70/50
3	15	21/11	10	70/50
4	18	40/30	30	70/50
5	18	90/32	30	110/70
6	18	90/32	10	110/70

Example 4 (cont.)
- The RA pressure is high, but the PCWP is extremely elevated
- The systemic blood pressure is low
- These hemodynamics represent cardiogenic shock, usually from an MI
- Expect cardiac output to be low

Example 5

	RA Pressure	PA Pressure	PCWP	BP
1 (normal)	0–5	13–28/3–13	3–11	110/70
2	18	32/18	17	70/50
3	15	21/11	10	70/50
4	18	40/30	30	70/50
5	18	90/32	30	110/70
6	18	90/32	10	110/70

Example 5 (cont.)
- The pulmonary systolic pressure and the PCWP are very high
- The systemic blood pressure is normal
- These hemodynamics are consistent with mitral stenosis

Example 6

	RA Pressure	PA Pressure	PCWP	BP
1 (normal)	0–5	13–28/3–13	3–11	110/70
2	18	32/18	17	70/50
3	15	21/11	10	70/50
4	18	40/30	30	70/50
5	18	90/32	30	110/70
6	18	90/32	10	110/70

Example 6 (cont.)
- The pulmonary artery systolic and diastolic pressures are very high, but the PCWP is normal
- These hemodynamics are consistent with pulmonary hypertension
- In all other conditions, the PA diastolic pressure and the PCWP are similar

Other — Endomyocardial Biopsy
- To evaluate etiology of cardiomyopathy or myocarditis
- Very useful in doxorubicin toxicity
- Evaluation of possible rejection in a transplanted heart
- A negative biopsy in sarcoidosis is not helpful
- Alcoholic cardiomyopathy is diagnosed from history

AR 10

A 35 yo woman presents with a history of a substernal pressure sensation, lasting from a few minutes to as long as 4 hours.
She does not get the pain with activity but occasionally has it when lying down.
Risk factors include HTN and obesity.

Which of the following is true?
A. She has a > 50% chance of having significant coronary disease.
B. An exercise stress test would have a high degree of accuracy in this patient.
C. Exercise duration would not be useful in predicting prognosis.
D. Nuclear perfusion imaging would improve the accuracy of the exercise study.

Answer: _____

AR 11

A 57 yo man with lung cancer presents with 24 hours of increasing dyspnea.
BP 85/40 mmHg
Neck veins are elevated.
Right-heart pressures follow.

Right-Heart Pressures

Location	Pressure (mmHg)
RA	21
PA	45/20
PCWP	21

What is the most likely diagnosis?
A. Pulmonary embolism
B. Acute myocardial infarction
C. SVC syndrome
D. Tamponade
E. Pneumonia

Answer: _____

Key Point
In cardiac tamponade, diastolic pressures are equalized in all 4 chambers.

AR 12
A 63 yo woman reports a history of effort-induced chest pain.
She is treated with low-dose aspirin, beta-blocker, and a statin.
On a treadmill, she exercises for 4 METs, peak HR of 110 bpm, and has her typical pain.
ECGs at rest and at peak exertion follow.

Resting ECG

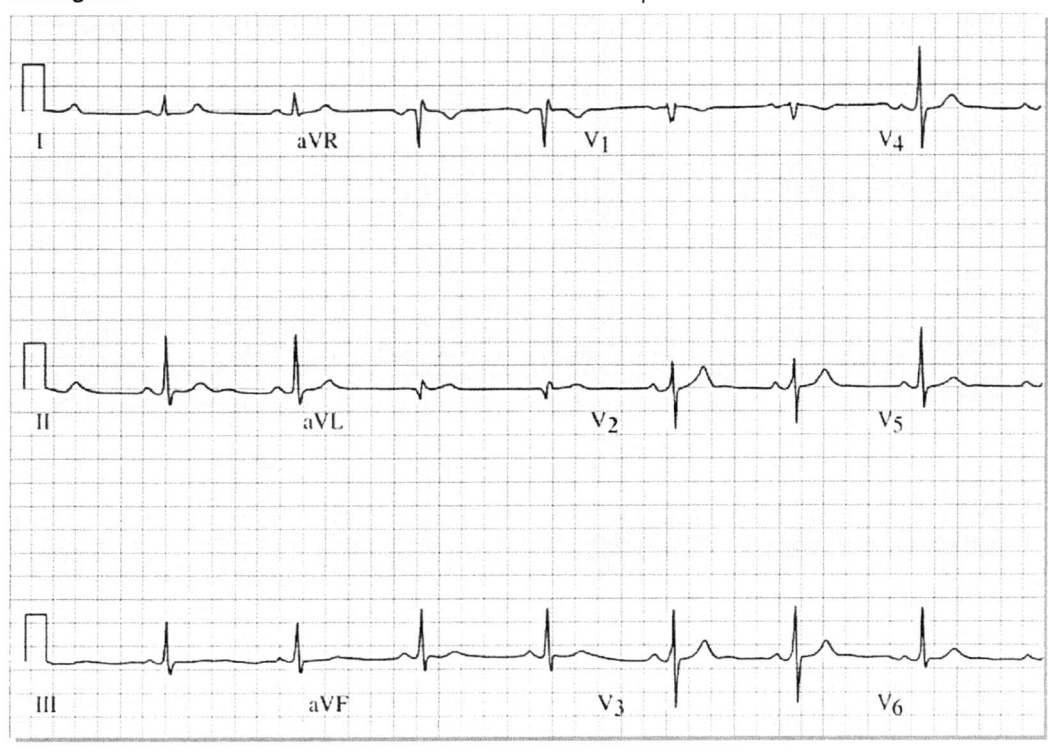

AR 12 (cont.)
Peak Exercise ECG

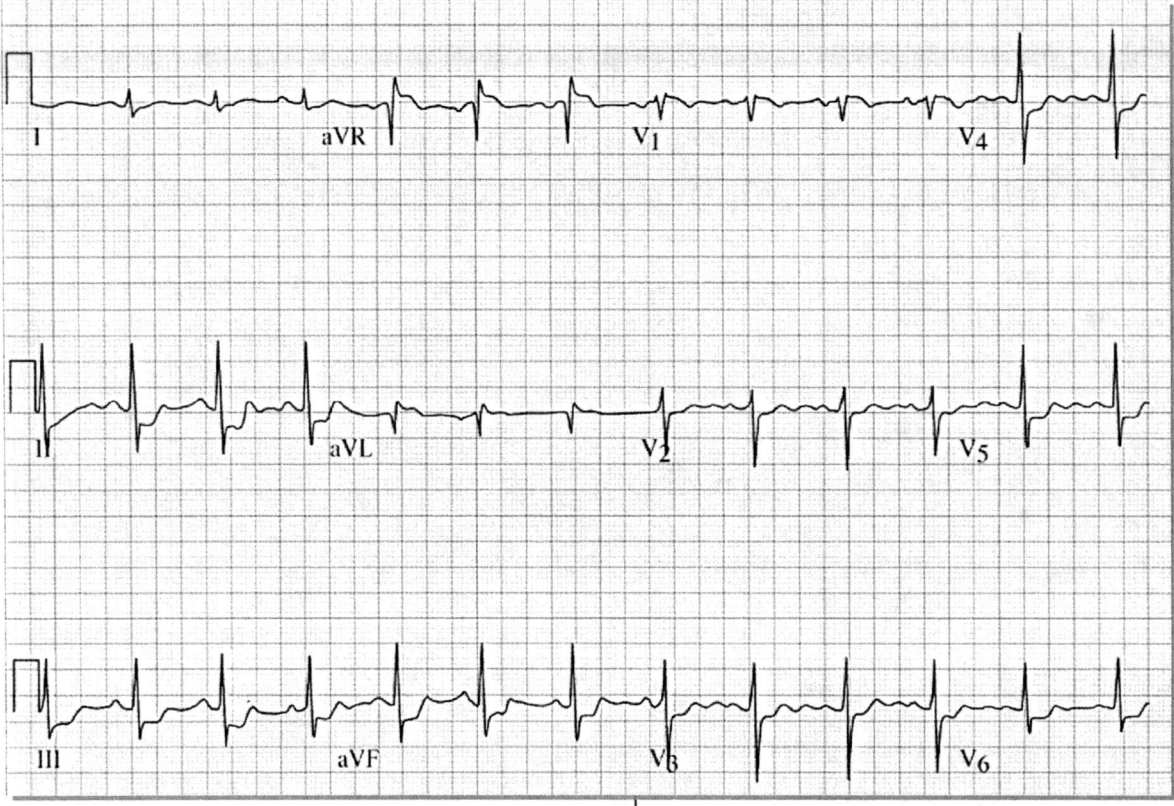

What do you recommend?
A. Reassure the patient, as this is a low-risk treadmill.
B. Repeat the test with nuclear perfusion imaging for greater accuracy.
C. Institute secondary prevention alone.
D. Refer her for urgent coronary angiography.
E. Refer her to a psychiatrist for treatment of an anxiety disorder.

Answer: _____

Part 2:
Physical Examination

Pulses

Pulsus Paradoxus
- Referred to on exam as an "inspiratory fall in systolic blood pressure"
  - Pericardial tamponade
  - Asthma
  - Tension pneumothorax

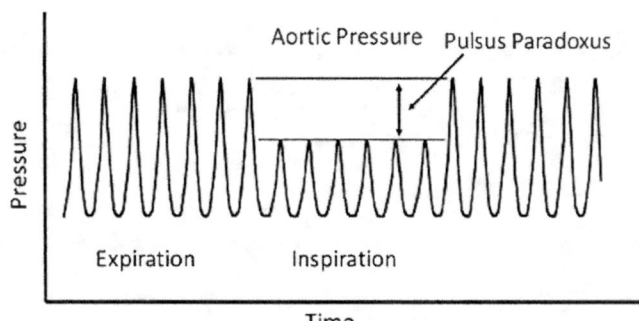

Bifid Arterial Pulse (Pulsus Bisferiens)
- Bifid pulse with 2 aortic peaks
  - Aortic regurgitation (AR)
  - Hypertrophic cardiomyopathy (HCM)

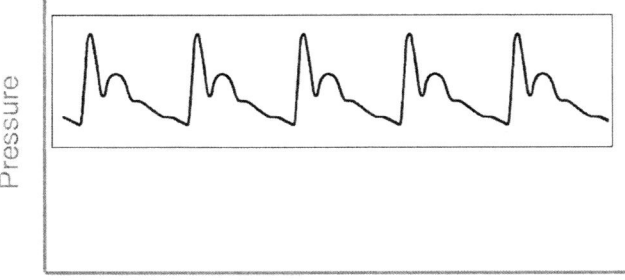

Alternating Arterial Pulse (Pulsus Alternans)
- Bigeminal premature ventricular contractions (PVCs)
  - Severe LV dysfunction
  - Severe AS

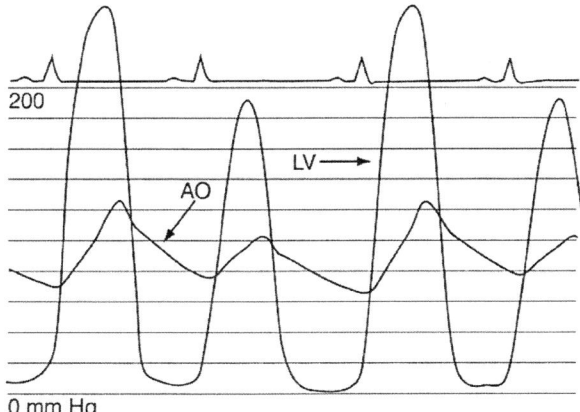

Decreased Rise Time and Volume of the Arterial Pulse
- Aortic stenosis (AS)
- May not be present in the elderly in spite of severe AS

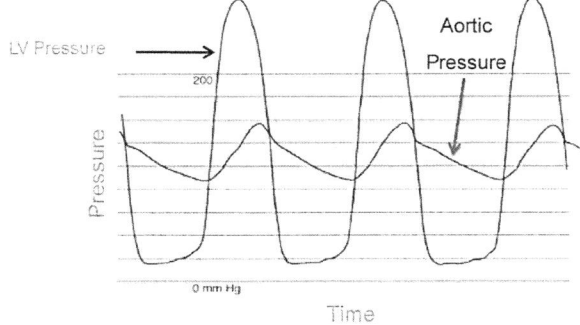

Other Pulse Abnormalities
- Aortic dissection causes asymmetrical pulses (normal in the upper extremities, absent in the lower)
- Peripheral arterial disease causes decreased or absent pulses in 1 or both legs

Jugular Venous Waveforms

Jugular Venous Pulse

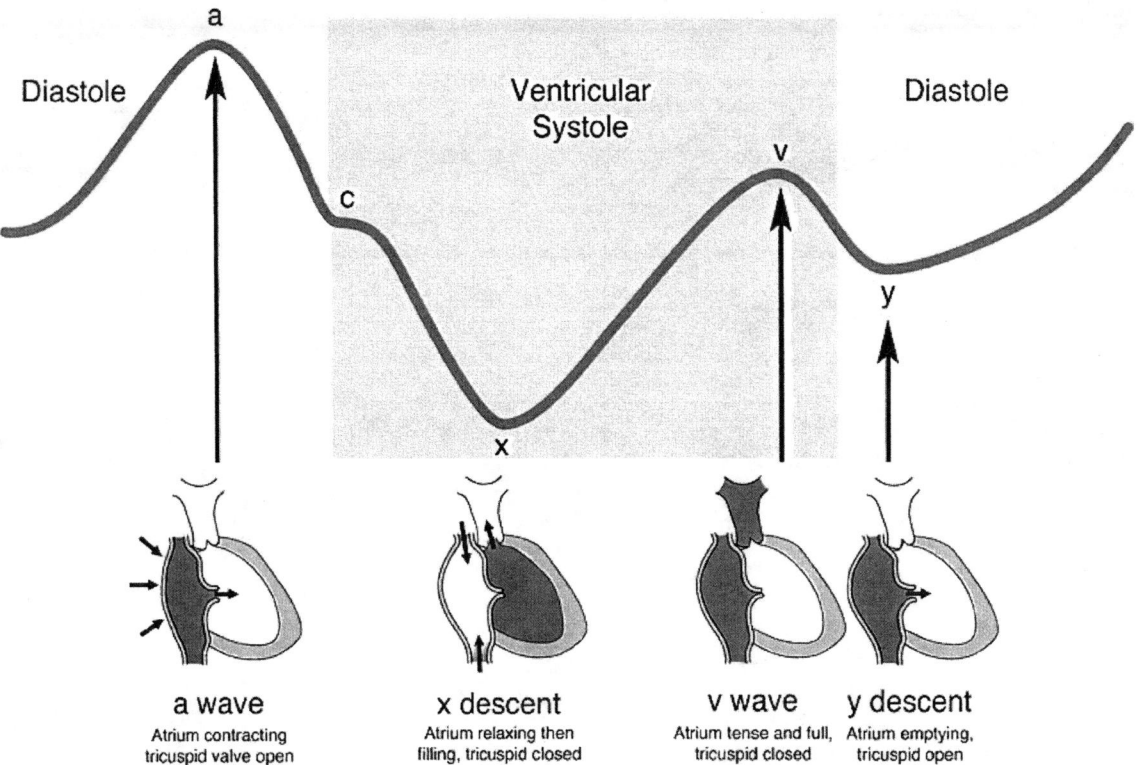

a wave
Atrium contracting
tricuspid valve open

x descent
Atrium relaxing then
filling, tricuspid closed

v wave
Atrium tense and full,
tricuspid closed

y descent
Atrium emptying,
tricuspid open

Large *a* Waves
- Tricuspid stenosis (TS)
- Severe pulmonic stenosis (PS)
- Severe, noncompliant RVH

Irregular Cannon *a* Waves
- Indicate A-V dissociation
- Occur in:
  - 70% of VT
  - 3rd degree AV block
  - Ventricular pacing in a patient with sinus rhythm and complete heart block

Irregular Cannon *a* Waves (cont.)

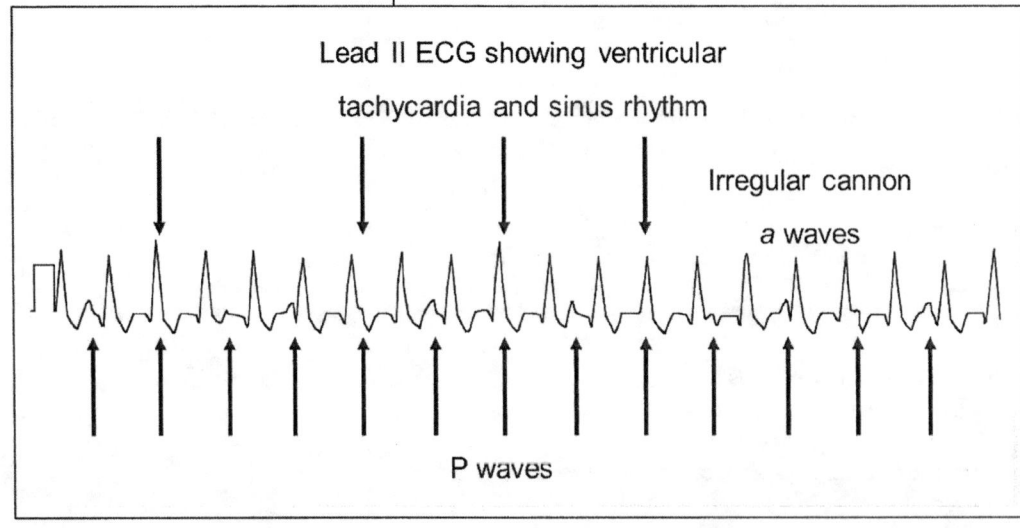

© 2017 MedStudy Internal Medicine Video Board Review – Cardiology • Matthew Sorrentino, MD

Irregular Cannon *a* Waves (cont.)

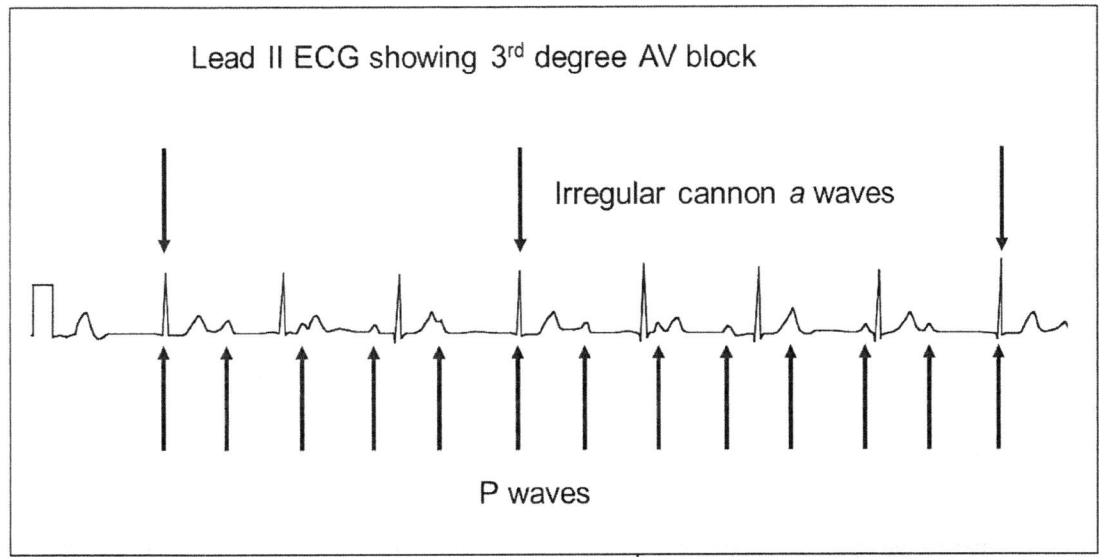

Lead II ECG showing 3rd degree AV block

Irregular cannon *a* waves

P waves

Rapid *x* and *y* Descents
- If both are present, think of constrictive pericarditis
- If only rapid *x* descent, think of tamponade (with loss of *y* descent)

Differential Diagnosis of Elevated Neck Veins

CONDITION	PHYSICAL EXAMINATION
RV infarction	Large *v* waves, Kussmaul sign
Tricuspid regurgitation	Large *v* waves
Tricuspid stenosis	Large *a* waves, slow *y* descent
Tamponade	Rapid *x* descent, pulsus paradoxus
Constrictive pericarditis	Rapid *x* and *y* descents, Kussmaul sign, may have a diastolic knock
Restrictive cardiomyopathy	Same as above, but no knock, and other systemic manifestations of primary illness
Superior vena cava syndrome	Large, possibly unilateral, nonpulsatile neck veins; May have facial edema and cyanosis
Tension pneumothorax	Large nonpulsatile neck veins, severe dyspnea and chest pain, unilateral lack of breath sounds
AV dissociation	Irregular cannon *a* waves

AR 13
A patient presents with complete heart block.

What pattern of neck vein elevation do you expect to see?
A. Absent *a* waves and a slow *y* descent
B. Large *a* waves and *v* waves
C. Rapid *x* and *y* descents
D. Cannon *a* waves
E. Distended neck veins with no pulsatile activity

Answer: _____

AR 14
A 45 yo male presents with several days of fever and tachypnea. History is positive for IV drug use. On exam, there are large *v* waves in the JVP. There is a 3/6 holosystolic murmur best heard at the LLSB that increases in intensity upon inspiration.

A transthoracic echo will most likely show which of the following?
A. Aortic stenosis
B. An anterior wall motion abnormality
C. Moderate-to-severe tricuspid regurgitation with a vegetation on the tricuspid valve
D. Cardiac tamponade physiology
E. Pulmonic stenosis

Answer: _____

Heart Sounds

Normal Mitral Valve Motion

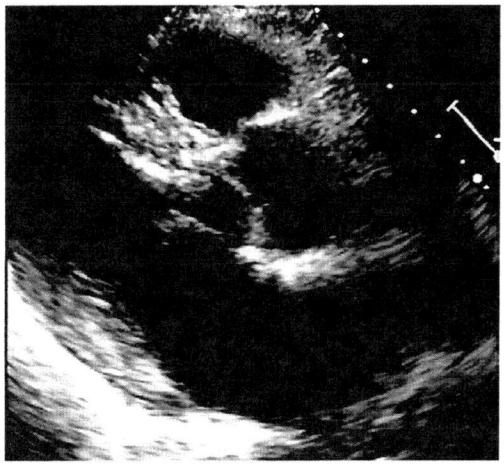

1st Heart Sound — S_1
- Occurs with closure of the mitral and tricuspid valves
- Changes in intensity of S_1 thus reflect processes that affect closure of these valves

Decrease in Intensity of S_1
- Prolonged PR interval
- Mitral regurgitation
- Acute aortic regurgitation
- Severely calcified mitral valve

Increase in Intensity of S_1
- Caused by closure of the mitral valve leaflets when they are stiffened (i.e., the mitral valve slams shut):
  - Short PR interval
  - Hyperdynamic LV function
  - Mitral stenosis (MS)

2nd Heart Sound — S_2
- Occurs with closure of the aortic (A_2) and pulmonic (P_2) valves
- To remember normal order of valve closure, think: **MTAP**

Physiologically Split S_2
- Normally, S_2 is single during expiration, and slightly split (A_2–P_2) during inspiration
- Increased venous return during inspiration causes:
  - Increased RV volume, which causes:
    - Delayed RV emptying and delayed P_2

Persistently Split S_2
- Splitting in expiration and inspiration (widens further during inspiration)
- Or "widened S_2" caused by delayed RV emptying:
  - Pulmonic stenosis (PS)
  - RBBB
- Early closure of the aortic valve (as in severe MR) may also cause a wide S_2

If associated with an ejection click that disappears with inspiration, think of **pulmonic stenosis.**

Paradoxically Split S_2
- Splitting occurs during expiration instead of inspiration
- Paradoxically split S_2, caused by delayed LV emptying and delay of aortic closure — P_2 occurs before A_2:
  - Severe AS
  - LBBB

Fixed Split S_2
- Present in inspiration and expiration; duration of splitting does not change throughout respiratory cycle
- Classically associated with an ASD

S_2 — Summary

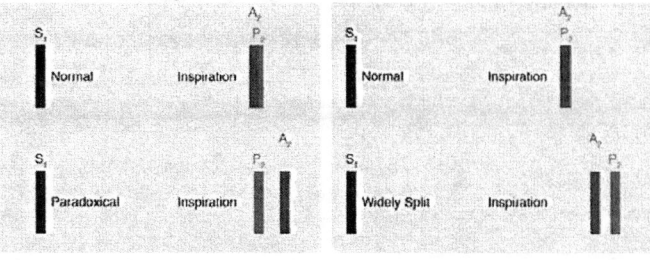

Pulmonic Ejection Sound
- Occurs with congenital pulmonic stenosis
- The only right-sided sound that becomes <u>softer</u> in inspiration; Hence, a favorite exam question

3rd Heart Sound — S_3
- Heard in early diastole with rapid passive filling of a stiff ventricle
- Normal in children and usually normal in pregnant women; abnormal over age 40
- Caused primarily by LV or RV dysfunction
- **A very bad prognostic sign in patients with known LV dysfunction or before surgery**

4th Heart Sound — S_4
- Heard in late diastole with rapid active filling of a stiff ventricle
- Associated with CAD, AS, MR, HCM, LVH
- When you would <u>not</u> hear an S_4:
  - Atrial fibrillation
  - Mitral stenosis

AR 15
A young patient presents with a 2nd heart sound that does not vary with respiration.
An ECG shows RVH and right-atrial enlargement.

What is the most likely diagnosis?
A. Mitral stenosis
B. Aortic stenosis
C. VSD
D. ASD
E. Pulmonic stenosis

Answer: _____

AR 16
A 22 yo woman presents with some mild dyspnea on exertion.
A 3/6 systolic ejection murmur is heard across the precordium, but best at the USB.
You notice that there is fixed splitting of S_2.

What diagnosis do you suspect?
A. Ventricular septal defect
B. Coarctation of the aorta
C. Atrial septal defect
D. Congenital pulmonic stenosis
E. Innocent, "benign" ejection murmur

Answer: _____

AR 17
On a preoperative evaluation, which of the following indicates the highest risk?
A. An S_3 on examination
B. An S_4 on examination
C. LBBB on an ECG
D. RBBB on an ECG
E. Left ventricular hypertrophy on an echo

Answer: _____

Murmurs
Will be Covered in Valvular Heart Disease

Part 3:
Coronary Artery Disease and Myocardial Ischemia

Overview

Angina
- Angina is caused by a mismatch of myocardial oxygen supply and demand
- Classified as:
  - Stable (usually due to concentric plaques)
  - Unstable (usually due to a ruptured plaque)
- Only about 20% of patients with ischemic ST changes have angina

Stable Plaque

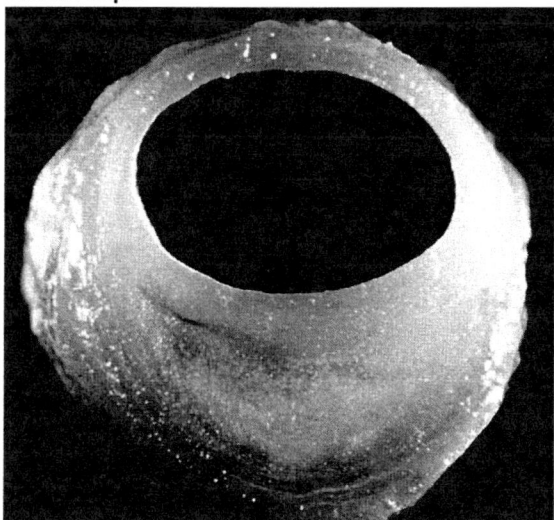

Ruptured Plaque

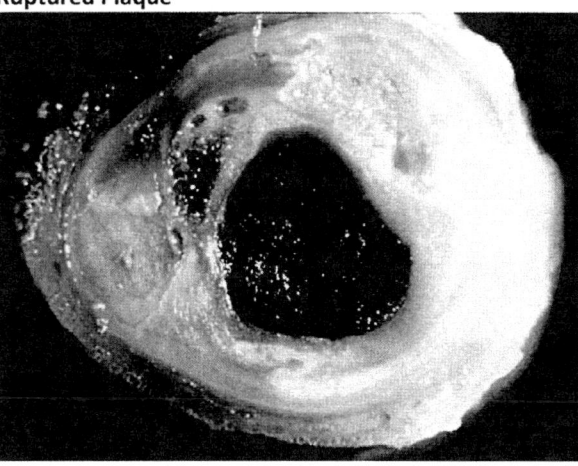

Prognosis in CAD
1) **LV function** — the most powerful risk stratification parameter in all of cardiology
2) **Exercise capacity** — (in METs) is highly predictive of prognosis
3) **Severity of angina**

Risk Assessment in Asymptomatic Patients

2013 Recommendations
- Risk scores should be calculated on **all asymptomatic adults** without a history of CHD
- Use one of the available scoring systems, such as the AHA/ACC ASCVD calculator based on the pooled cohort equations, or an older calculator such as Framingham or Reynolds

AHA / ACC Calculator

DOWNLOAD CV RISK CALCULATOR

Risk Factor	Units	Enter patient values in this column
		Value
Sex	M (for males) or F (for females)	M
Age	years	63
Race	AA (for African Americans) or WH (for whites or others)	AA
Total Cholesterol	mg/dL	275
HDL-Cholesterol	mg/dL	35
Systolic Blood Pressure	mm Hg	170
Treatment for High Blood Pressure	Y (for yes) or N (for no)	Y
Diabetes	Y (for yes) or N (for no)	Y
Smoker	Y (for yes) or N (for no)	Y

Calculated Risk

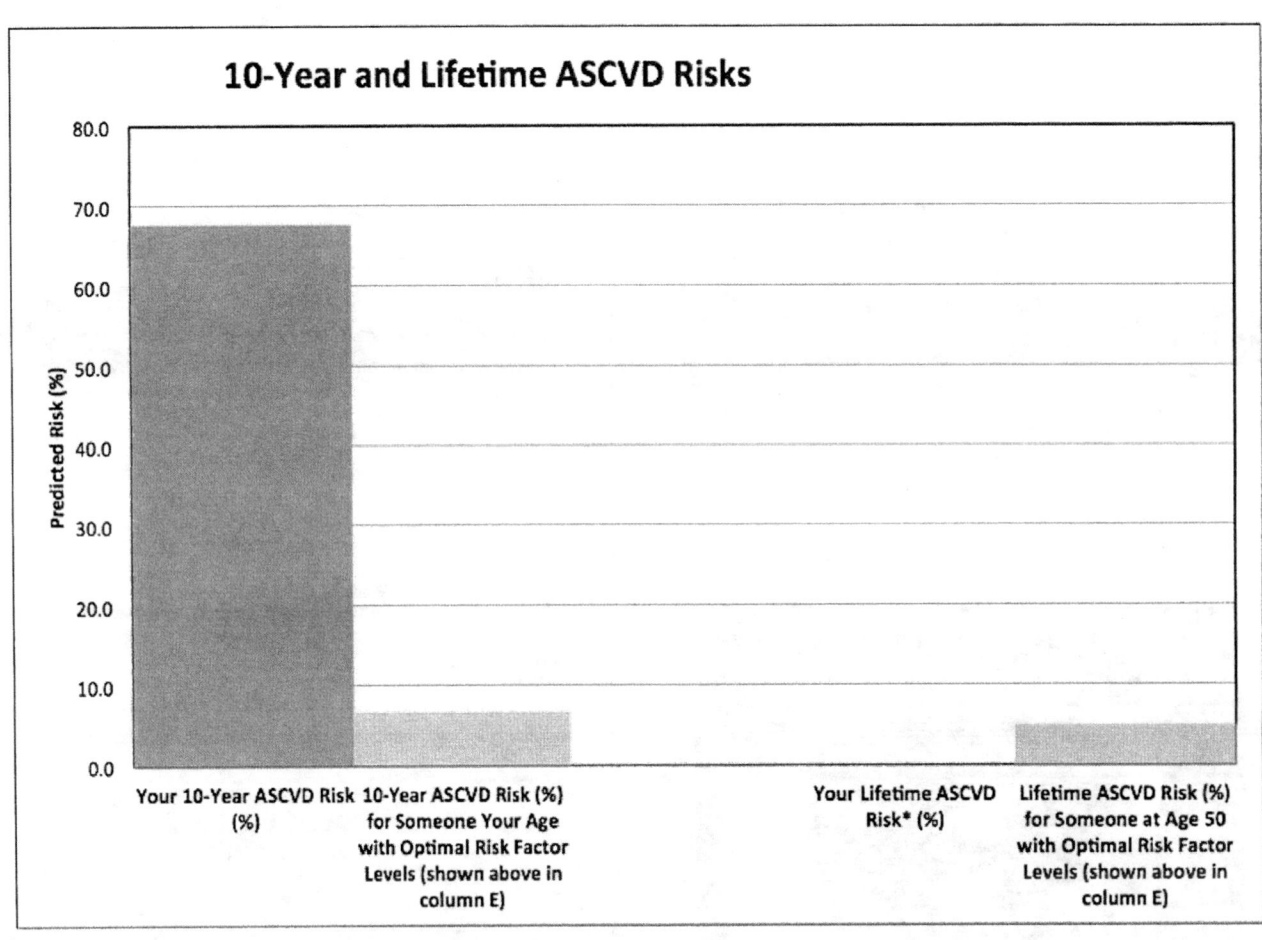

How to Use Risk Calculation
- For discussion regarding statin therapy — according to 2013 AHA/ACC Blood Cholesterol Guideline, statin therapy is recommended for anyone with a 10-year risk ≥ 7.5%
- For decisions regarding aggressiveness of treatment

Assignment of Risk
Risk of "Hard" CHD Event in 10 Years

Low Risk	< 10%
Intermediate Risk	10–20%
High Risk	> 20%

Recommended Assessments
- Family history of premature CVD
- Standard lipid profile
- Resting ECG in all patients with HTN or diabetes
- Measurement of ankle-brachial index is reasonable in patients at intermediate risk

- Measurement of coronary artery calcification (by CT) is reasonable for patients at intermediate risk
- In patients > age 40 with diabetes, measurement of coronary calcification is reasonable
- Remember that CAC score is different from CTA (!)

Not Recommended
- Measurement of advanced lipid parameters, including lipoproteins, apolipoproteins, particle size, and density
- CAD genotype testing
- Natriuretic peptide measurement
- C-reactive protein in high-risk patients
- CRP in younger low-risk patients

- Echo in patient without HTN
- Brachial/Peripheral arterial flow-mediated dilation studies
- Measures of arterial stiffness outside of research settings
- Stress echo in low- or intermediate-risk asymptomatic patients

- Stress MPI in low- or intermediate-risk asymptomatic patients
- Coronary calcification measurement in low-risk patients
- CT angio (CTA) in asymptomatic patients

Risk Modification and Prevention

Risk Factors for CAD
- Age
- Male sex
- Family history of premature CAD
- Dyslipidemia
- Smoking
- Chronic stress
- Sleep disorders

- HTN
- Diabetes
- Obesity
- Sedentary lifestyle
- Postmenopausal
- PAD
- Other known vascular Dz (e.g., CVA)
- CKD

AR 18
In a 55 yo man, which of the following risk factors is most predictive of the presence of coronary artery disease?
A. An LDL cholesterol of 120 mg/dL
B. A fasting blood glucose of 160 mg/dL
C. A 20-pack-year history of smoking, stopping 5 years previously
D. LVH on an ECG
E. Father died of an MI at age 68

Answer: _____

AR 19
A 30 yo woman with a BMI of 34.5 kg/m² and a family history of premature CAD presents for her annual visit. Her BP is 120/80 mmHg.
She has no complaints.

Which of the following should you recommend?
A. Coronary artery calcification (CAC) scoring
B. Exercise treadmill test
C. Right-heart catheterization to assess PA pressures
D. Weight loss counseling
E. Stress echo

Answer: _____

Statin Benefit Groups
1) Clinical ASCVD (e.g., CAD, CVA, PAD)
2) LDL ≥ 190 mg/dL
3) Ages 40–75 with DM and LDL 70–189 mg/dL
4) No known ASCVD or DM, but ages 40–75 with LDL 70–189 mg/dL and 10-yr risk of ≥ 7.5%

Statin Intensity
- High intensity: Lowers LDL cholesterol by at least 50% on average
  - Atorvastatin 40–80 mg
  - Rosuvastatin 20–40 mg
- Moderate intensity: Lowers LDL by 30% to < 50%

HDL Cholesterol
- Aerobic exercise and HDL cholesterol are inversely linked to CAD
- Increased by exercise, estrogens, and small amounts of alcohol
- Decreased by smoking and androgens
- Inverse relationship between triglycerides and HDL

Smoking Cessation
- Smoking cessation decreases mortality and decreases reinfarction rate by 50%
- Benefits of smoking cessation begin within 48 hours (!)

Blood Pressure Control
- Blood pressure control (according to JNC 7 guidelines) is recommended:
  - < 140/90 mmHg in all patients
  - < 130/80 mmHg in patients with diabetes or chronic kidney disease

Blood Pressure Control — SPRINT
- Landmark trial; results released in latter half of 2015
- Stopped early due to clear benefit
- Showed improved outcomes at BP < 120/80 mmHg
- Has been validated by a large Lancet meta-analysis, as well as smaller RCTs and registries

SPRINT
- Tested SBP target of < 140 vs. < 120
- Pts were ≥ 50 yo with increased risk for CVD
- < 120 mmHg resulted in:
  - 27% reduction in all-cause mortality
  - 38% reduction in heart failure

ASA for Primary Prevention
- According to most recent USPSTF recs, all adults at increased risk of CVD from age 50–69 who do not have increased risk of bleeding
- Insufficient evidence outside of that age range
- Dose is 81 mg daily

Diabetes Control
- HbA1c level of < 7%
- Diabetic patients should have aggressive management of other risk factors

Weight Management
- Normal BMI: 18.5–24.9 kg/m^2
- Waist circumference of < 40" in men and < 35" in women (Caucasian)

Waist Circumference
- Indicator of visceral obesity
- International Diabetes Federation:

Ethnicity	Men	Women
Europeans, East Mediterranean, Middle Eastern, and Sub-Saharan Africans	≥ 37 in (≥ 94 cm)	≥ 31.5 in (≥ 80 cm)
South Asians, Chinese, Japanese, First Nations, Ethnic South and Central Americans	≥ 35.5 in (≥ 90 cm)	≥ 31.5 in (≥ 80 cm)

http://www.idf.org/webdata/docs/MetSyndrome_FINAL.pdf — International Diabetes Federation

Depression
It is reasonable to refer/treat patients with depression.

Antioxidant Vitamin and Folic Acid
Antioxidant vitamin supplements (e.g., vitamins E, C, or beta-carotene) and folic acid (with or without B$_6$ and B$_{12}$) should not be used for secondary prevention.

AR 20
A 45 yo asymptomatic man presents for his annual visit. The ASCVD calculator indicates a 10-yr risk of 9% for a cardiovascular event.

Which of the following should you recommend?
A. An exercise treadmill test
B. Addition of a statin to his medication regimen
C. A coronary CTA
D. Cardiac catheterization
E. A transthoracic echo

Answer: _____

AR 21
A 55 yo woman with a history of diabetes presents at a routine visit with a BP of 150/88 mmHg. She is otherwise asymptomatic.
She is currently taking ASA 81 mg daily, metformin, and atorvastatin 40 mg.

Which of the following should you recommend next?
A. An exercise treadmill test
B. A carotid Doppler
C. Addition of lisinopril to her medication regimen
D. Addition of propranolol to her medication regimen
E. Addition of spironolactone

Answer: _____

AR 22
A 50 yo male who is asymptomatic presents for a routine annual visit. He asks you about preventing heart disease.

Based on current evidence, you can tell him:
A. Taking vitamin E daily has been shown to reduce cardiovascular events.
B. There is sufficient evidence to recommend that he begin taking ASA 81 mg daily for primary prevention.
C. There is no evidence that aggressively treating blood pressure to < 120/80 mmHg has any benefit for reducing CVD events.
D. A CTA is recommended for risk stratification.

Answer: _____

Acute Coronary Syndrome

Levels of Recommendations in ACC / AHA Guidelines

Class I	Class IIa	Class IIb	Class III No Benefit Or Class III Harm
Benefit >>> Risk	Benefit >> Risk	Benefit ≥ Risk	
Procedure/ treatment should be performed/ administered	It is reasonable to perform procedure/ administer treatment; additional studies needed	May be considered; additional studies needed	No benefit or harmful to patients

Levels of Evidence in ACC / AHA Guidelines

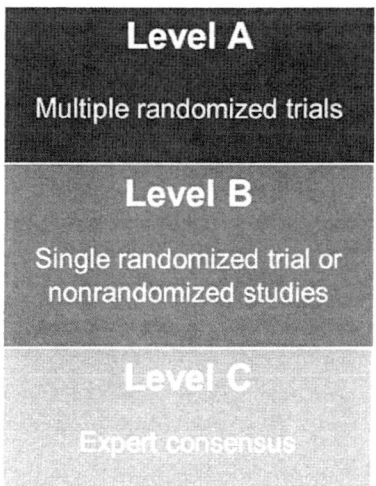

Level A — Multiple randomized trials

Level B — Single randomized trial or nonrandomized studies

Level C — Expert consensus

General Considerations

Infarction without Chest Pain
- Pain absent in > 15% of MIs
- More commonly absent in:
  - Elderly (2/3 of patients over 75)
  - Diabetics
  - Women
- Present with heart failure, atrial fib, etc.

Differential Diagnosis of Chest Pain
- Acute ischemia
- Aortic dissection
- Pericarditis
- Esophageal disorders
- Biliary disorders
- Pneumothorax
- Pulmonary embolism
- Pleurisy
- Chest wall pain
- Psychogenic

ACS — Classification

Spectrum of ACS

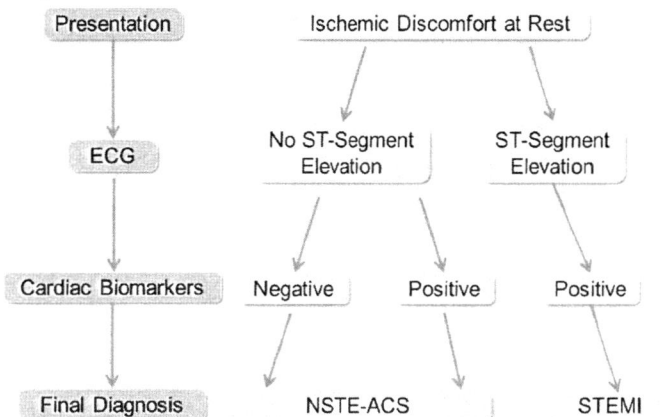

Non–ST-Segment Elevation Events
- Unstable angina or NSTEMI
- Patients usually have known CAD
- Involves less myocardium
- High risk of recurrent MI and death
- Even though initial prognosis is better, 1-year prognosis is the same as ST-elevation MI

Non–ST-Segment Elevation MI

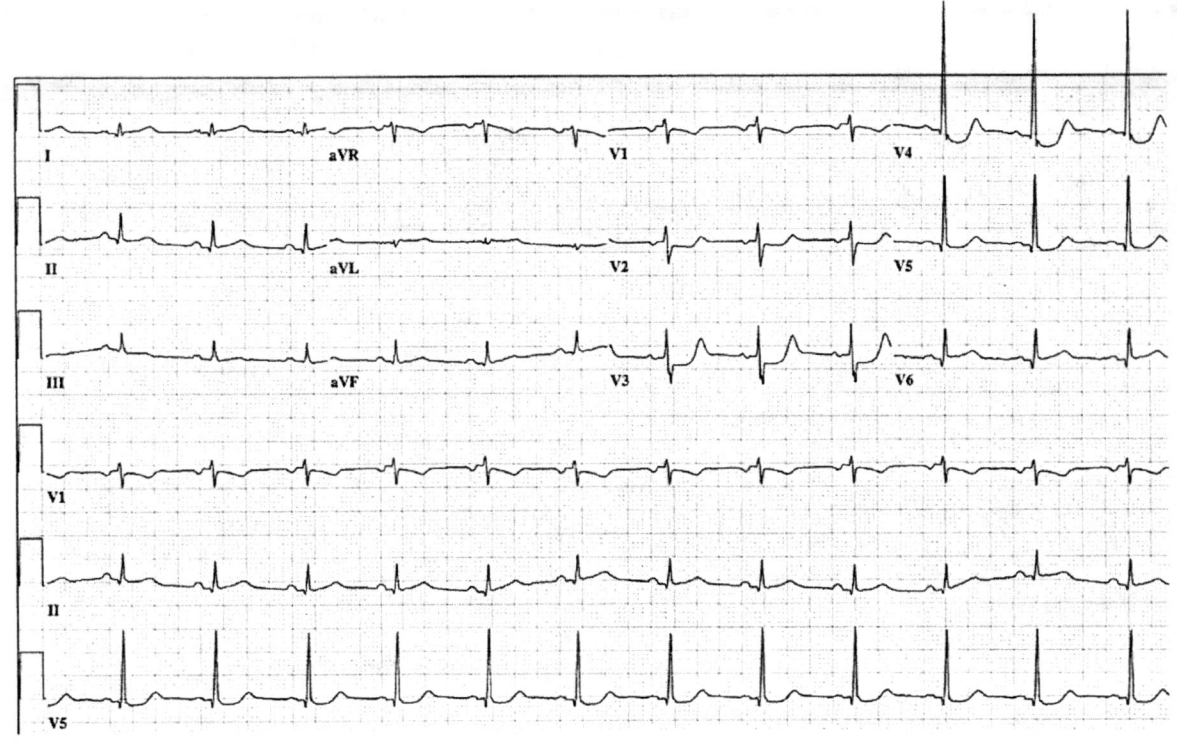

ST-Segment Elevation Events
- Hallmark is ST-segment elevation on ECG that localizes affected myocardium
- Usually develops a Q wave
- Infarct size is usually larger
- Initial prognosis is worse

Acute Anterolateral STEMI

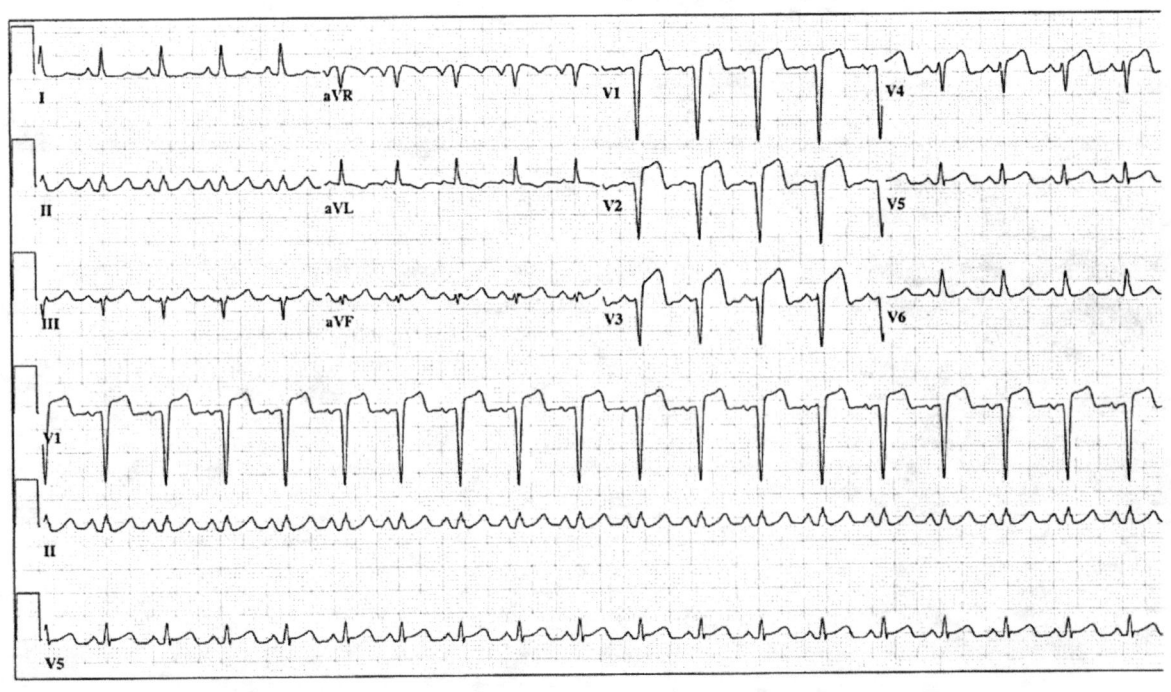

Distribution of MI Type

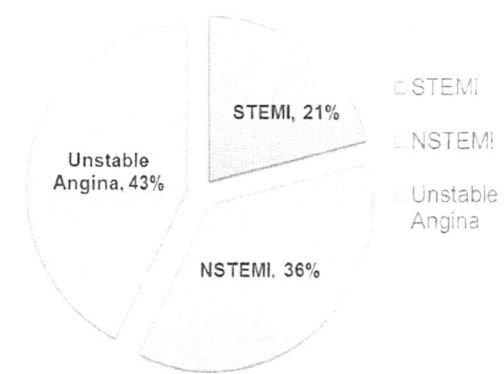

ACUTE CORONARY SYNDROME

STEMI, 21%
Unstable Angina, 43%
NSTEMI, 36%

- STEMI
- NSTEMI
- Unstable Angina

1.57 million Annual U.S. Hospital Admissions

Management of ACS

Prehospital NTG

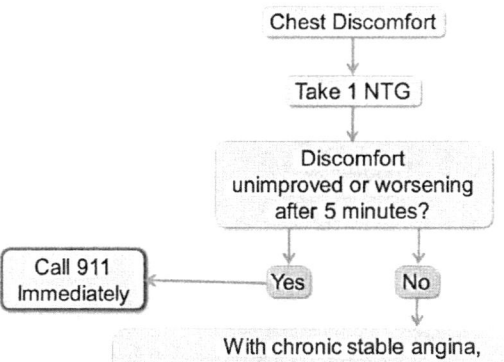

Chest Discomfort
↓
Take 1 NTG
↓
Discomfort unimproved or worsening after 5 minutes?
→ Yes → Call 911 Immediately
→ No
With chronic stable angina, if symptoms are improved after 1 NTG, repeat NTG every 5 minutes x 3; Call 911 if symptoms not completely resolved

Prehospital ECG
- EMS personnel should obtain a computerized 12-lead ECG
- If the ECG shows injury or ischemia, the receiving hospital should be notified

Out-of-Hospital Arrest
- In STEMI patients who have an out-of-hospital arrest because of VF or pulseless VT:
  - Comatose patients should have therapeutic hypothermia started as soon as possible
  - In resuscitated patients, immediate angiography and PCI should be performed

Critical Early Decisions
- Within 10 minutes after arrival in the ED with chest pain, patients must have:
  1) An ASA to chew
  2) An ECG interpreted
  3) A focused history and physical examination
  4) Cardiac markers drawn
  5) Evaluation of risk using TIMI, GRACE, or PURSUIT calculators

Symptoms and Signs Suggestive of ACS
- Nontraumatic chest or epigastric pain
  - Central/Substernal pressure, crushing, tightness, heaviness, cramping, burning, aching sensation
  - Unexplained indigestion, belching
  - Radiation to neck, jaw, shoulders, back, arms
- Associated with dyspnea, nausea/vomiting, diaphoresis

GRACE ACS Risk Calculator

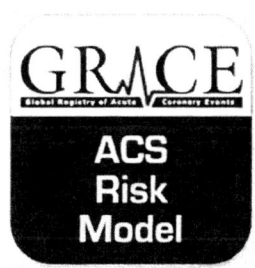

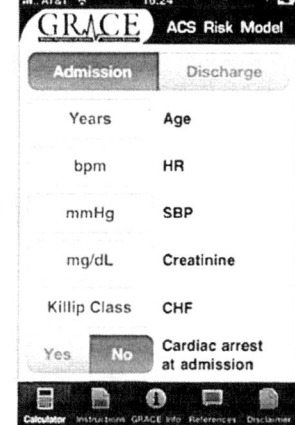

Available as an app for iPhone and Android

High-Risk Characteristics from TIMI, GRACE, PURSUIT
- Older age
- Heart failure
- Hypotension
- Angina
- ST-segment changes
- Positive markers

Biomarkers for Acute MI

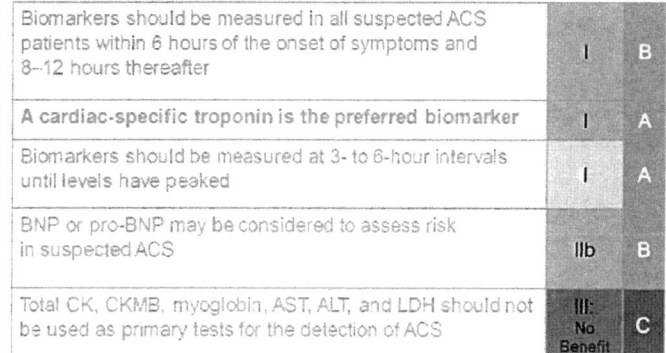

Biomarkers should be measured in all suspected ACS patients within 6 hours of the onset of symptoms and 8–12 hours thereafter	I	B
A cardiac-specific troponin is the preferred biomarker	I	A
Biomarkers should be measured at 3- to 6-hour intervals until levels have peaked	I	A
BNP or pro-BNP may be considered to assess risk in suspected ACS	IIb	B
Total CK, CKMB, myoglobin, AST, ALT, and LDH should not be used as primary tests for the detection of ACS	III: No Benefit	C

Timing of Cardiac Markers

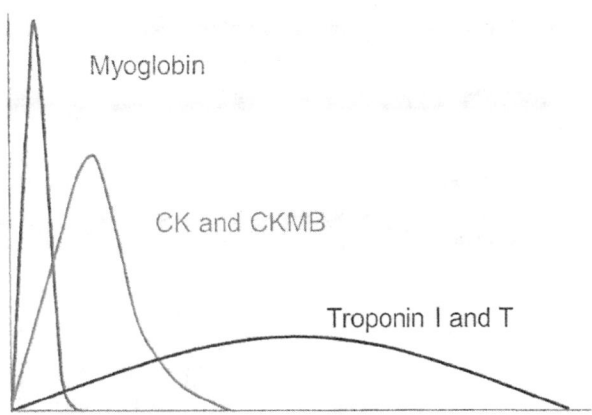

Myoglobin

CK and CKMB

Troponin I and T

Cardiac Markers
2014 AHA/ACC NSTE-ACS Guideline:
"With contemporary troponin assays, CKMB and myoglobin are not useful for diagnosis of ACS."

Symptoms Suggestive of ACS

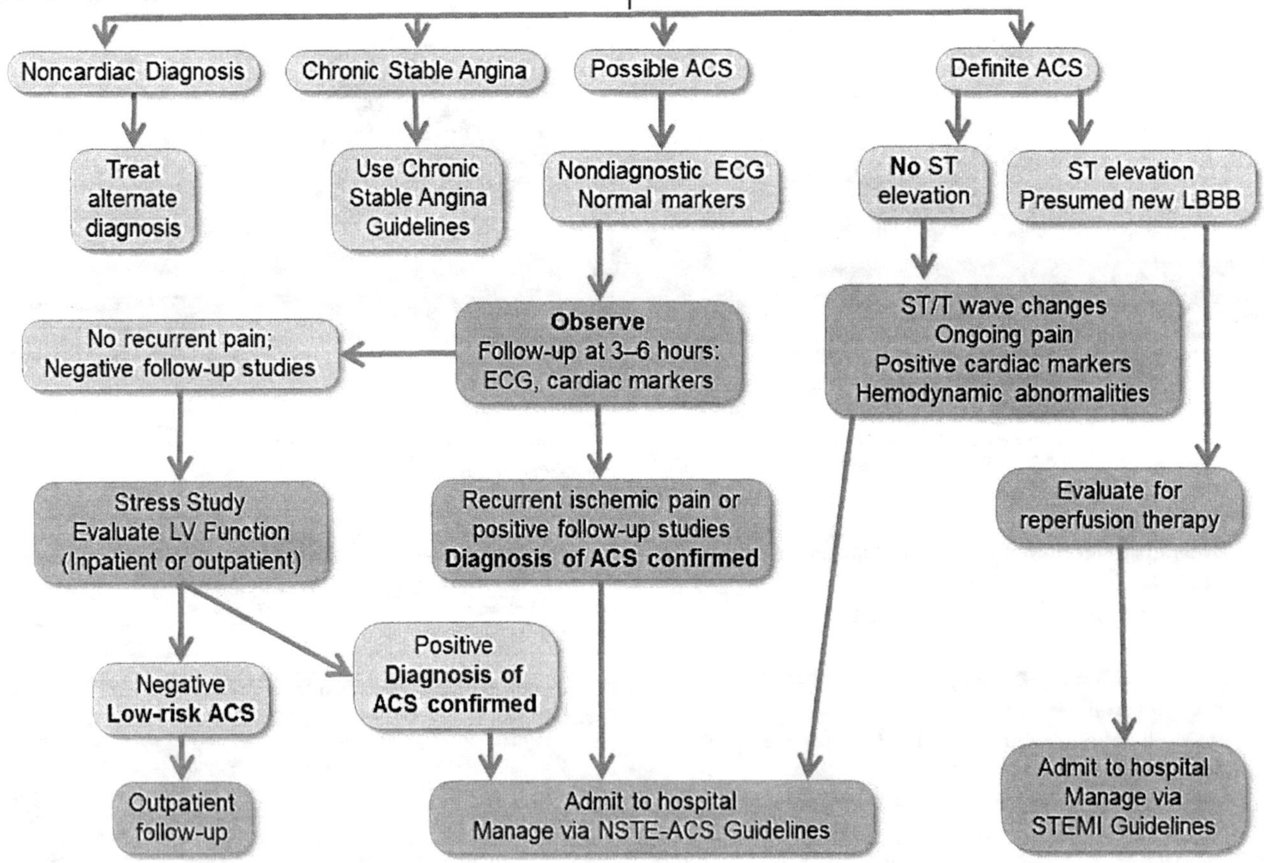

Noncardiac Diagnosis → Treat alternate diagnosis

Chronic Stable Angina → Use Chronic Stable Angina Guidelines

Possible ACS → Nondiagnostic ECG Normal markers → **Observe** Follow-up at 3–6 hours: ECG, cardiac markers

Definite ACS → **No ST** elevation / ST elevation Presumed new LBBB

Observe → No recurrent pain; Negative follow-up studies → Stress Study Evaluate LV Function (Inpatient or outpatient) → Negative **Low-risk ACS** → Outpatient follow-up

Stress Study / **Observe** → Positive **Diagnosis of ACS confirmed**

Observe → Recurrent ischemic pain or positive follow-up studies **Diagnosis of ACS confirmed** → Admit to hospital Manage via NSTE-ACS Guidelines

No ST elevation → ST/T wave changes Ongoing pain Positive cardiac markers Hemodynamic abnormalities → Admit to hospital Manage via NSTE-ACS Guidelines

ST elevation Presumed new LBBB → Evaluate for reperfusion therapy → Admit to hospital Manage via STEMI Guidelines

CT Angio in NSTE-ACS
- Acceptable alternative to a stress study **(IIa-B)**
- Ideal candidate is an intermediate-risk patient who is unable to exercise

AR 23
A 55 yo female with a history of cigarette smoking and a family h/o premature CAD presents to the ED with 2 hrs of crescendo angina.

Which of the following is an appropriate 1st line diagnostic test?
A. A 12-lead electrocardiogram
B. An exercise treadmill test
C. An EGD
D. A cardiac MRI
E. A pharmacologic nuclear stress test

Answer: _____

AR 24
A 55 yo male presents with typical angina and 2 mm of ST depression in the inferior leads (II, III, aVF) on ECG.

Which of the following should you order?
A. Total CK
B. CK-MB fraction
C. Cardiac troponin I
D. LDH
E. Amylase and lipase

Answer: _____

Early Hospital Care
- Supplemental O_2 only if $S_aO_2 < 90\%$, respiratory distress, or other high-risk features of hypoxemia
- NTG/nitrates contraindicated with recent use of PDE inhibitor

- Discontinue NSAIDs
- Initiate oral beta-blockers within first 24 hrs unless HF, low CO, risk for cardiogenic shock, or other contraindications to beta-blockade

- CCBs (diltiazem or verapamil) when beta-blockers unsuccessful or contraindicated
- Initiate high-intensity statin therapy

Antiplatelet / Anticoagulant Tx
- For patients with definite or likely NSTE-ACS and PCI:
  - Non–enteric-coated ASA 162–325 mg immediately after presentation
  - ASA 81 mg daily maintenance indefinitely
  - $P2Y_{12}$ inhibitor (clopidogrel, ticagrelor, prasugrel) loading dose and maintenance for up to 12 mo if no PCI; at least 12 mo if PCI

IV Anticoagulant Tx
- UFH vs. enoxaparin: Either can be used, but enoxaparin is preferred
- SC enoxaparin for duration of hospitalization or until PCI performed
- Bivalirudin until cardiac cath/PCI in patients with early invasive strategy

Fibrinolytics
***Do not use fibrinolytics in patients with NSTE-ACS (Class III: Harm)

AR 25
A 60 yo female with a history of DM presents to the ED with left jaw pain, mild dyspnea, and extreme fatigue. Her ECG shows a 2 mm of ST depression in the lateral leads (V5 and V6). Her 1st troponin is 4.1 ng/mL. Her S_aO_2 is 96% on room air.

Which of the following should you do?
A. Begin oxygen by nasal cannula.
B. Begin oxygen by face mask.
C. Give ASA 325 mg to chew.
D. Give fibrinolytic therapy (tPA).
E. Give amlodipine 10 mg.

Answer: _____

NSTE-ACS —
Invasive vs. Conservative Strategy

Select a Strategy

Preferred Strategy	Patient Characteristics
Invasive	• Recurrent angina or ischemia in spite of intensive medical therapy • Elevated biomarkers • New ST-segment depression • HF or worsening MR • High-risk noninvasive testing • Hemodynamic instability • Sustained VT • PCI within 6 Months • Prior CABG • High-risk score (TIMI, GRACE, PURSUIT) • Mild to moderate renal dysfunction • Diabetes • Decreased LV function (LVEF < 40%)
Conservative	• Low-risk score • Patient or physician preference

Specific STEMI Management

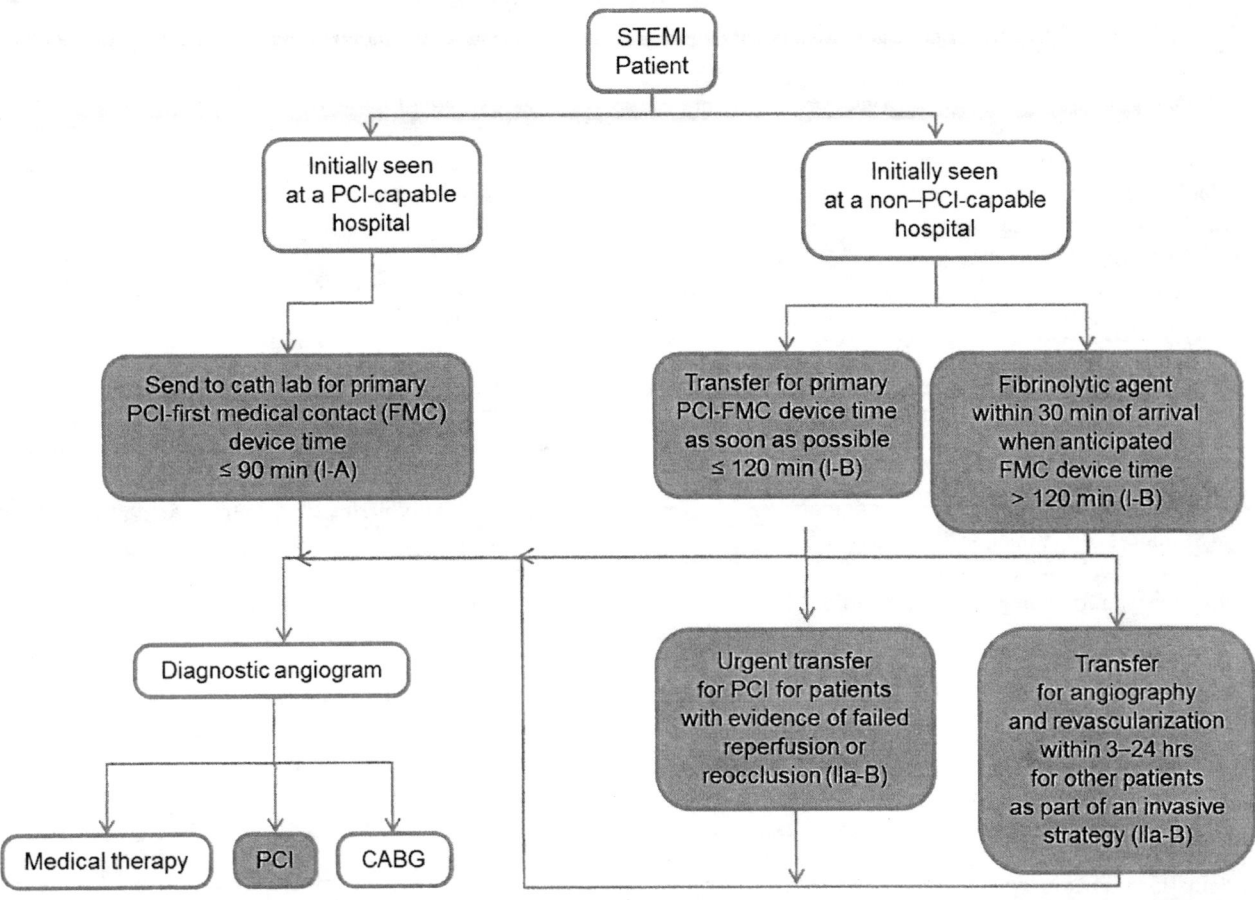

Statins in Secondary Prevention
All patients with CAD should receive a high-intensity statin, regardless of lipid levels.

Cardiac Rehab
All ACS patients should be referred for cardiac rehab!

AR 26
A 56 yo male presents with NSTE-ACS.
He was given ASA 325 mg in the field.
He is being prepped for cardiac catheterization.

Which of the following oral medications should be on his orders list?
A. Lisinopril 40 mg
B. Furosemide 20 mg
C. Atorvastatin 80 mg
D. Atorvastatin 10 mg
E. Lovastatin 20 mg

Answer: _____

AR 27
A 70 yo female presents with ST elevation in leads II, III, and aVF. She is at a PCI-capable facility.

Which of the following is recommended?
A. Due to age, she should not be referred for cardiac catheterization.
B. Due to gender, she should not be referred for cardiac catheterization.
C. She should be referred for immediate cardiac catheterization and primary PCI.
D. She should undergo a TTE.

Answer: _____

AR 28
A diabetic patient presents with unstable angina. The ECG shows new T wave inversion in the precordial leads.

What should be done next?
A. Immediate coronary angiography
B. Observation for 8–12 hours
C. A regular exercise stress test
D. A stress test with nuclear perfusion imaging
E. Dobutamine stress echo

Answer: _____

Antiplatelet and Anticoagulation Agents

Antiplatelet Agents
- ASA
- $P2Y_{12}$ inhibitors (clopidogrel, prasugrel, ticagrelor)
- IV GP IIb/IIIa receptor antagonists (abciximab, tirofiban, eptifibatide)

Anticoagulants
- Heparins (unfractionated heparin, and the low molecular weight heparins bivalirudin and fondaparinux)
- Warfarin
- NOACs

Mechanism of Action
- ASA — irreversibly inhibits cyclooxygenase, which is necessary for thromboxane synthesis; therefore, inhibits platelet aggregation
- $P2Y_{12}$ inhibitors — irreversibly binds to the $P2Y_{12}$ receptor on platelets, which inhibits cross-linkage

- Heparins
  - Unfractionated heparin binds to and activates antithrombin III, which inactivates thrombin and Factor Xa
  - Low-molecular–weight heparins bind directly to and inactivate Factor Xa

Warfarin — **inhibits the vitamin-K–dependent synthesis of the calcium-dependent clotting Factors II, VII, IX, and X**

Antiplatelet Therapy in Patients with PCI for Acute STEMI

Aspirin			165–325 mg load before procedure	I	B
			81–325 mg indefinite daily maintenance	I	A
			81 mg daily is the preferred maintenance dose	II a	B
$P2Y_{12}$ inhibitors	Loading doses		Clopidogrel 600 mg as soon as possible or at PCI	I	B
			Prasugrel 60 mg	I	B
			Ticagrelor 180 mg	I	B
	Maintenance dose and duration of therapy	DES placed; Continue therapy for 1 year	Clopidogrel 75 mg daily	I	B
			Prasugrel 10 mg daily	I	B
			Ticagrelor 90 mg bid	I	B
		BMS placed; Continue therapy for 1 year	Clopidogrel 75 mg daily	I	B
			Prasugrel 10 mg daily	I	B
			Ticagrelor 90 mg bid	I	B
		DES placed	Clopidogrel, prasugrel, ticagrelor beyond 1 year	II b	C
			Prasugrel in patients with prior stroke or TIA	III	B

Fibrinolytic Therapy

Reperfusion at a Non–PCI-Capable Hospital

Indications for fibrinolytic therapy when there is a > 120-minute delay from FMC to primary PCI		
Ischemic symptoms < 12 hours	I	A
Evidence of ongoing ischemia 12–24 hours after symptom onset and a large area of myocardium at risk or hemodynamic instability	IIa	C
ST depression, except when true posterior MI is suspected or when associated with ST elevation in lead aVR	III: Harm	B

Effectiveness of Reperfusion Therapy

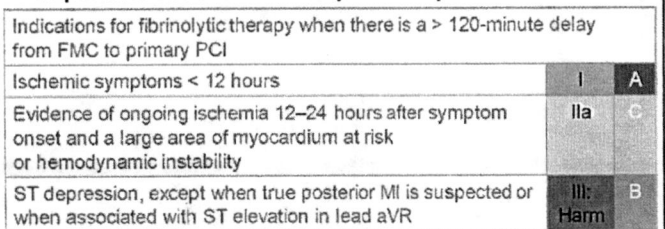

Fibrinolytic Agents
- Alteplase, reteplase, and tPA
- Anistreplase (anisoylated plasminogen-streptokinase activator complex [APSAC])
- Streptokinase and urokinase
- **tPA has the highest patency rates**

Effectiveness of Various Fibrinolytics
- Mortality is decreased the earlier fibrinolysis is given, particularly 1st hour
- In the GUSTO trial, the combination of **tPA and IV heparin** had a slight mortality advantage over other agents

Absolute Contraindications

Any prior intracranial hemorrhage
Known structural cerebral vascular lesion
Known malignant intracranial neoplasm
Ischemic stroke within 3 months
Suspected aortic dissections
Active bleeding or bleeding diathesis (except menses)
Significant closed head or facial trauma within 3 months
Intracranial or intraspinal surgery within 2 months
Severe uncontrolled hypertension (unresponsive to emergency therapy)
For streptokinase, prior treatment within the previous 6 months

Relative Contraindications

History of chronic, severe, poorly controlled HTN
Significant HTN on presentation (SBP > 180 mmHg or DBP > 110 mmHg)
History of prior ischemic stroke > 3 months
Dementia
Known intracranial pathology not covered in absolute contraindications
Traumatic or prolonged (> 10 min) CPR
Recent major surgery (< 3 weeks)
Recent (within 2–4 weeks) internal bleeding
Noncompressible vascular punctures
Pregnancy
Active peptic ulcer
Oral anticoagulant therapy

Indications for Transfer for Angiography Post Fibrinolysis

Immediate transfer for cardiogenic shock or severe acute HF irrespective of time delay from MI onset	I	B
Urgent transfer for failed reperfusion or reocclusion	IIa	B
As part of an invasive strategy in stable patients with PCI 3–24 hours after successful fibrinolysis	IIa	B

Indications for Angiography Post-Fibrinolysis or in Those Who Did Not Receive Reperfusion

Cardiogenic shock or acute severe HF that develops after initial presentation	I	B
Intermediate or high-risk findings on pre-discharge noninvasive ischemia testing	I	B
Spontaneous or easily provoked myocardial ischemia	I	C
Failed reperfusion or reocclusion after fibrinolytic therapy	IIa	B
Stable patients after successful fibrinolysis, before discharge, and ideally between 3 and 24 hours	IIa	B

Selected Routine Medical Therapies Post-STEMI

Indications	Dose	Avoid/Caution
Nitroglycerin		
• Ongoing chest pain • HTN and HF	• 0.4 mg SL every 5 min ≤ 3 doses as BP allows • IV dose to begin at 10 mcg/min; Titrate to desired BP effect	• Suspected RV infarction • BP < 90 mmHg or > 30 mmHg below baseline • Recent (24–48 hours) use of phosphodiesterase type 5 inhibitors
Oxygen		
• Clinically significant hypoxia (O_2 saturation < 90%) • HF • Dyspnea	• 2–4 L/min via nasal cannula • Increase rate or change to mask as needed	• Caution with COPD and CO_2 retention

Morphine in STEMI

- Morphine is indicated for relief of pain, anxiety, or pulmonary edema
- Dose
  - 4–8 mg IV initially, lower in elderly patients
  - 2–8 mg IV every 5–15 min if needed
- Avoid in lethargic, hypotensive, or bradycardic patients

Oral Beta-Blockers Post-STEMI

Oral beta-blockers should be started in the first 24 hours in patients without: • Signs of HF • Evidence of low cardiac output • Increased risk of cardiogenic shock • PR interval > 240 msec • 2nd or 3rd degree heart block • Active asthma or reactive airway disease	I	B
Beta-blockers should be continued after hospitalization	I	B
Patients with initial contraindications should be revaluated within 24 hours to assess subsequent eligibility	I	C
IV beta-blockers may be considered at presentation in patients with HTN or ongoing ischemia	IIb	B

Cardiogenic Shock Risk

- Patients with this combination are at increased risk of shock:
  - Age > 70
  - SBP < 120 mmHg
  - HR > 110 bpm
  - Long duration of time since onset of ACS

AR 29

A 65 yo female presented with anterior STEMI to a non-PCI facility and received tPA for reperfusion. 8 hours later, she continues to have a BP of 90/60 mmHg, and dopamine + dobutamine have been started.
HR is 120 bpm, sinus rhythm.

What should you do next?

A. Add vasopressin and epinephrine to her pressor regimen.
B. Give IV metoprolol.
C. Transfer her to a PCI-capable facility immediately.
D. Repeat the dose of tPA.
E. Begin CPR.

Answer: _____

AR 30

A 64 yo male presents to a PCI-capable hospital with STEMI, diagnosed by EMS in the field. Vital signs are currently stable.

Which of the following is recommended?

A. Administer streptokinase.
B. Administer tPA alone.
C. Administer tPA and IV heparin.
D. Refer for emergent PCI.
E. Obtain an urgent transthoracic echo.

Answer: _____

AR 31

An 80 yo male presents with inferior STEMI after 3 hours of nausea, vomiting, and dyspnea and is treated promptly with PCI to the RCA.

Which of the following is true?

A. Due to his gender, he is at higher risk of cardiogenic shock.
B. Due to his age, he is at higher risk of cardiogenic shock.
C. Due to not having received tPA, he is at higher risk of cardiogenic shock.
D. Because this was an inferior MI, he is not at any risk of cardiogenic shock.

Answer: _____

Renin-Angiotensin–Aldosterone System Inhibitors

An ACE inhibitor should be given to all patients who present with an anterior STEMI or an LVEF ≤ 40%	I	A
An ARB is an acceptable alternative for ACE-intolerant patients	I	B
An aldosterone antagonist is indicated in patients already receiving an ACE inhibitor and a beta-blocker with an LVEF ≤ 40% who have either symptomatic HF or diabetes	I	B
An ACE inhibitor is reasonable for all STEMI patients	IIa	A

Lipid Management Post-STEMI

High-intensity statin therapy should be started or continued in all STEMI patients	I	B
It is reasonable to obtain a fasting lipid profile, preferably within 24 hours	IIa	C

Risk Assessment after STEMI

Noninvasive testing for ischemia detection		
Prior to discharge in patients who have not had angiography and who do not have high-risk clinical features for which angiography would be indicated	I	B
To assess the significance of a noninfarct-related stenosis previously identified at angiography	IIb	C
To guide post-discharge exercise program	IIb	C
Assessment of LV function		
In all patients prior to discharge	I	C
Assessment of risk of sudden death		
Patients with an initially decreased LVEF who are possible candidates for ICD therapy should have reevaluation of LVEF 40 days after discharge	I	B

Cardiogenic Shock Post-STEMI

Emergency revascularization is recommended in patients in cardiogenic shock with either PCI or CABG irrespective of the time delay from MI onset	I	B

AR 32

A 66 yo female is admitted with an anterior STEMI.
She undergoes primary PCI to the LAD with 100% reflow (patency).
At the time of cath, her LVEF is noted to be 35%.

Which of the following is recommended based on current guidelines?

A. She should be referred for an ICD immediately.
B. She should receive beta-blockade to a target heart rate of 50 bpm.
C. She should be referred for CABG.
D. She should have lisinopril added to her medication list.
E. She should not be referred to cardiac rehab due to a good PCI result.

Answer: _____

Early Use of Pacing and ICDs

Temporary pacing is indicated in symptomatic bradycardia unresponsive to medical therapy	I	C
ICD implantation is indicated before discharge in patients who have had sustained VT/VF more than 48 hours after STEMI, provided the arrhythmia is not due to transient ischemia, reinfarction, or electrolyte abnormalities	I	B

ICDs Post-MI

- Patient must be at least 40 days post-MI
- LVEF ≤ 35% on optimal medical therapy
- Life expectancy of at least 1 year

Management of Pericarditis Post-STEMI

ASA is recommended	I	B
Acetaminophen, colchicine, or narcotics may be reasonable	IIb	C
Nonsteroidal antiinflammatory drugs or glucocorticoids are potentially harmful	III	B

Other Complications of Acute MI

Tachyarrhythmias
- Hemodynamically unstable tachyarrhythmias require immediate cardioversion (!)
- In stable patients, control ventricular response of atrial fibrillation with beta-blockers

RV Infarction
- Almost always:
  - Occurs with right coronary occlusion
  - Associated with an inferior-posterior MI
- Suspect RV infarction with the triad of:
  - Hypotension
  - Clear lung fields
  - Elevated JVP (Kussmaul sign)

- Transient ST elevation in right-sided chest leads (e.g., V4R)
- Treatment:
  - Fluids
  - Dobutamine, if hypotension persists
  - Avoid preload-reducing agents (e.g., nitrates)

AR 33

A patient is admitted to the CCU with chest pain and suddenly develops a narrow-complex–irregular tachycardia.
Systolic BP is 70 mmHg.

What is the next best step in management?
A. Administer intravenous adenosine.
B. Administer an intravenous beta-blocker.
C. Administer intravenous diltiazem.
D. Perform immediate synchronized electrical cardioversion.
E. Administer intravenous amiodarone.

Answer: _____

AR 34

A 74 yo female was admitted after 4 hours of substernal chest pain.
2 hours after admission, her blood pressure fell to 60/40 mmHg.
Neck veins are elevated.
ECG follows.

ECG

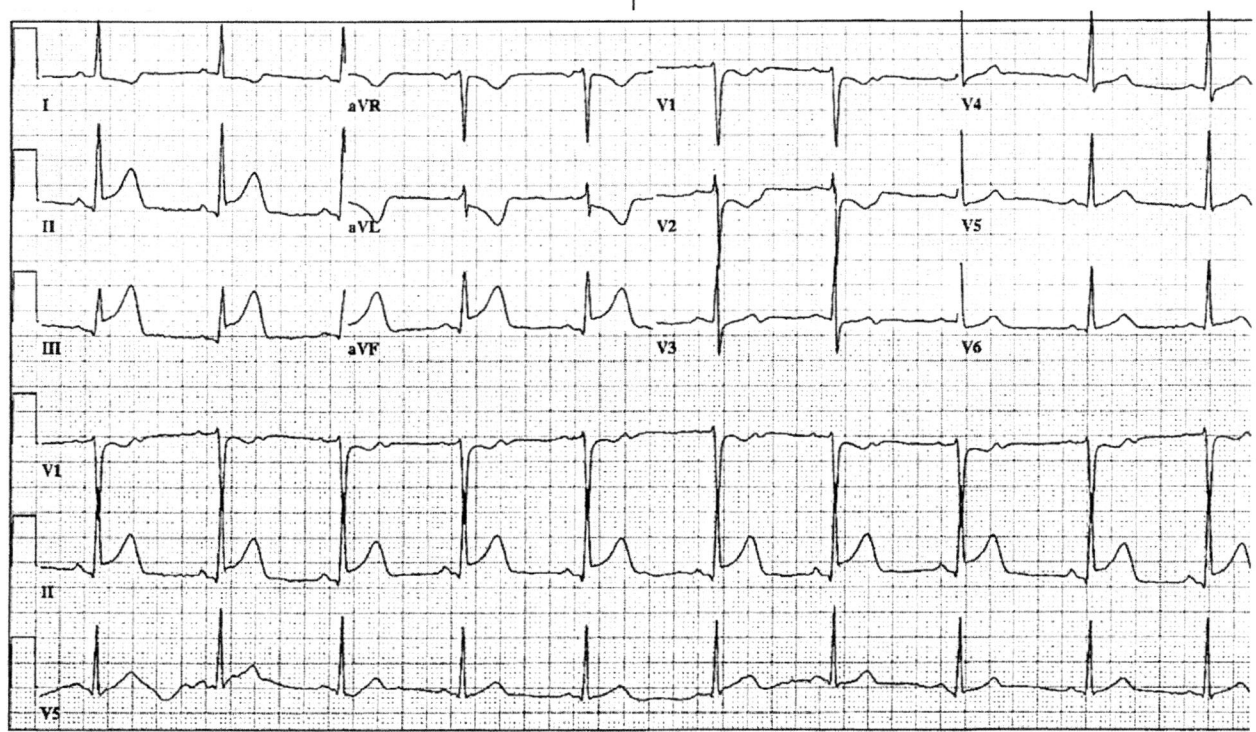

AR 34 (cont.)

A right-heart catheter is inserted, and the following pressures are obtained.

Position	RA	RV	PA	PCWP
Pressure (mmHg)	19	30/17	31/17	12

What is the diagnosis?
A. Tamponade
B. Cardiogenic shock
C. Papillary muscle dysfunction
D. RV infarction
E. VSD

Answer: _____

AR 35

A 56 yo man presents with an acute inferior MI by ECG and markers. Two hours after admission, he becomes profoundly hypotensive.

Which of the following features would not support the diagnosis of RV infarction?
A. A 3rd heart sound heard at the left sternal border
B. Neck vein distension on inspiration
C. Pulmonary congestion on auscultation
D. ST-segment elevation in right-sided chest leads
E. An echo showing RV dilation and hypokinesis

Answer: _____

VT / VF

Timing Post-MI	Implications
< 48 Hours	Does not affect prognosis
> 48 Hours	Associated with a poor prognosis (as it occurs with poor LV function)

Ventricular Tachyarrhythmias
- Cardiovert VF and unstable VT
- Stable VT can be treated with:
  - Amiodarone 150 mg infused over 10 minutes, repeated every 10–15 minutes
  - **Or**, 360 mg over 6 hrs (1 mg/min), then 540 mg over next 18 hrs (0.5 mg/min), not to exceed 2.2 g in 24 hrs

AR 36

A 72 yo woman is admitted with an acute inferior MI. 2 hours later, she develops a heart rate of 32 bpm, accompanied by lightheadedness and diaphoresis.

The most appropriate therapy would be:
A. Dopamine 4 µg/min/kg IV
B. Dobutamine 5 µg/min/kg IV
C. Esmolol 3 mg/kg/min IV
D. Atropine 0.5 mg IV
E. Digoxin 0.25 mg IV

Answer: _____

Pacing and MI
- Symptomatic bradycardia is always an indication for pacing
- 1° and 2° Type 1 block rarely requires pacing
- Higher grade AV block needs pacing only if the patient is **symptomatic**

Inferior vs. Anterior MI

	Infarct Size	Prognosis	AV Block	Prognosis With AV Block
Inferior MI	Smaller	Better	Fairly common	No effect
Anterior MI	Larger	Worse	Rare	Poor (associated with a very large MI)

© 2017 MedStudy Internal Medicine Video Board Review – Cardiology • Matthew Sorrentino, MD

The "Four Catastrophes"

	Free Wall Rupture	Papillary Muscle Dysfunction	VSD	Cardiogenic Shock
Setting	Anterior MI in old, hypertensive women	Inferior MI	Large anterior MI	Large anterior MI or MI with previous LV dysfunction
Presentation	Syncope, signs of tamponade	Shock	Shock	Shock
Physical Exam	Signs of tamponade	Systolic murmur, possibly with odd radiation	Loud systolic murmur heard widely	Signs of left heart failure
Diagnosis	Echo	Echo	Echo, O_2 saturation step up from RA to PA on right-heart cath	Echo
Management	A few heroic saves with urgent CT surgery	CT surgery	CT surgery	Supportive measures, primary PCI
Mortality	95%	50%	50%	85% (50% with primary PCI)

AR 37

A 73 yo man with typical angina for the past 12 hours is admitted to the ICU.
Initial physical exam is normal.
Troponin I peaked at 45.
He is treated with medical therapy.
ECG follows.

ECG

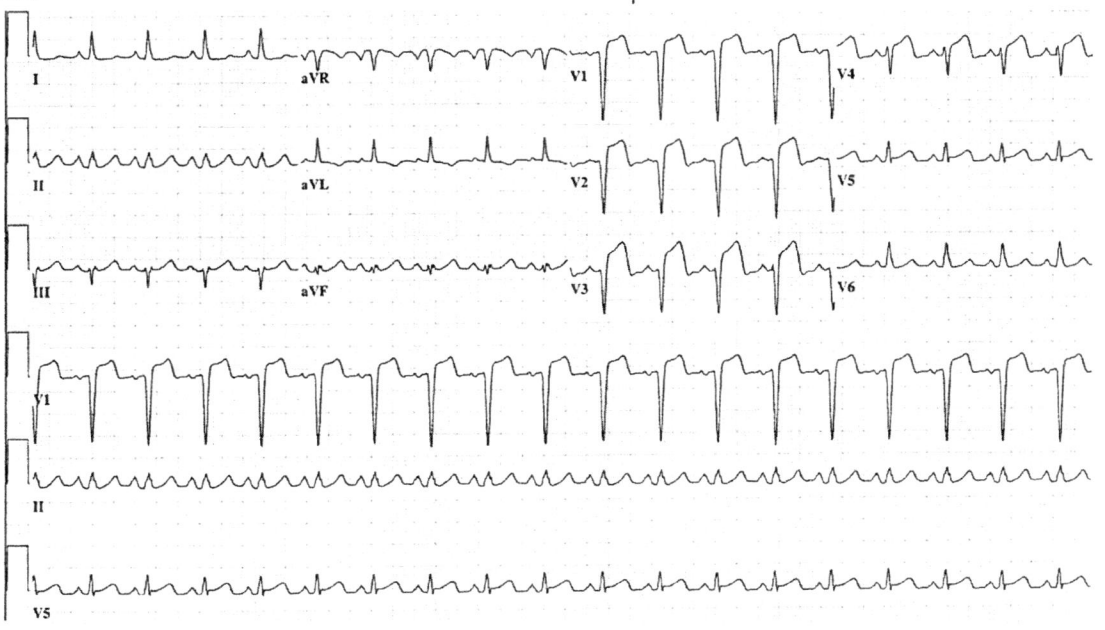

AR 37 (cont.)

Three days after admission, he suddenly develops severe hypotension and dyspnea.

Physical exam shows elevated neck veins, diffuse pulmonary crackles, a new 4/6 systolic murmur heard widely across the precordium and a left parasternal lift.

Chest x-ray is shown on the right.

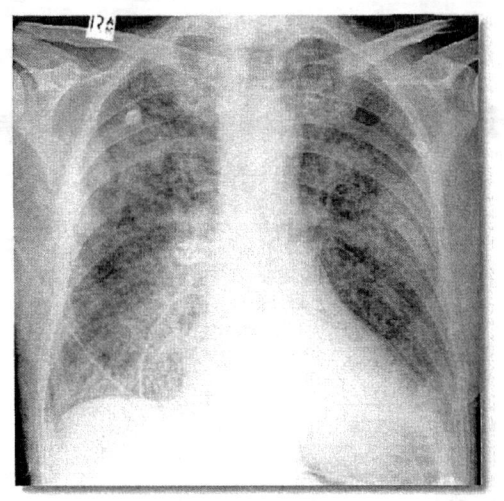

What is the most likely diagnosis?

A. Free wall myocardial rupture
B. Rupture of a papillary muscle
C. Acute VSD
D. Pulmonary embolism
E. RV infarction

Answer: _____

MEDICATION	NEGATIVE INO-TROPE	NEGATIVE CHRONO-TROPE	NEGATIVE DROMO-TROPE	VASO-DILATOR	ANTI-ANGINAL	PROLONG SURVIVAL POST-MI	PROLONG SURVIVAL IN HF	INDICATIONS
Digoxin	N	+	+	N	N	N	N	Systolic HF, arrhythmias
Beta-blockers	+++	+++	+++	N	Y	Y	Y	HTN, angina, HF, arrhythmias
Nifedipine	++	N	N	Y	Y	N	N	HTN, angina
Diltiazem	++	++	++	Y	Y	N	N	HTN, angina, arrhythmias
Verapamil	+++	+++	+++	Y	Y	N	N	HTN, arrhythmias
Nitrates				Y	Y	Y (with hydralazine)	Y (with hydralazine)	Angina, HF
ACEI				Y		Y	Y	HTN, HF
ARB				Y		Y	Y	HTN, HF
Hydralazine				Y		Y (with nitrates)	Y (with nitrates)	HTN, HF
Spironolactone Eplerenone						N	Y	HTN, HF
ASA						Y		CAD
Statins						Y		↑ Lipids

NSAIDs
- The issue of pain control for chronic musculoskeletal discomfort should be addressed prior to discharge
- NSAIDs should be avoided if possible
- If unavoidable, nonselective NSAIDs (e.g., naproxen) should be used

Older Patients
- Older patients with ACS should be evaluated in a manner similar to younger patients
- Decisions for management should consider general health, functional and cognitive status, comorbidities, life expectancy, and patient preferences

- Older ACS patients face increased early procedural risks with revascularization relative to younger patients
- However, overall benefits from invasive strategies are equal to or perhaps greater in older adults and are recommended

Drug-Induced MI: Cocaine
- Of the half million ED visits by cocaine users in 2005, 40% complained of chest pain
- Cocaine can cause ACS and aortic dissection, sometimes days after use
- NTG and calcium blockers are drugs of choice

Cocaine Users
- Coronary angiography is indicated if
  - Chest pain persists or
  - The ECG shows ST elevation or
  - Cardiac markers are elevated
- If none of these are present, the patient can be discharged after 9–12 hours
- The use of beta-blockers is controversial

Methamphetamine Users
It is reasonable to manage methamphetamine users in a manner similar to cocaine users.

AR 38

A 27 yo male presents with chest pain, agitation, confusion, tachycardia, and hypertension.
ECG follows.

ECG

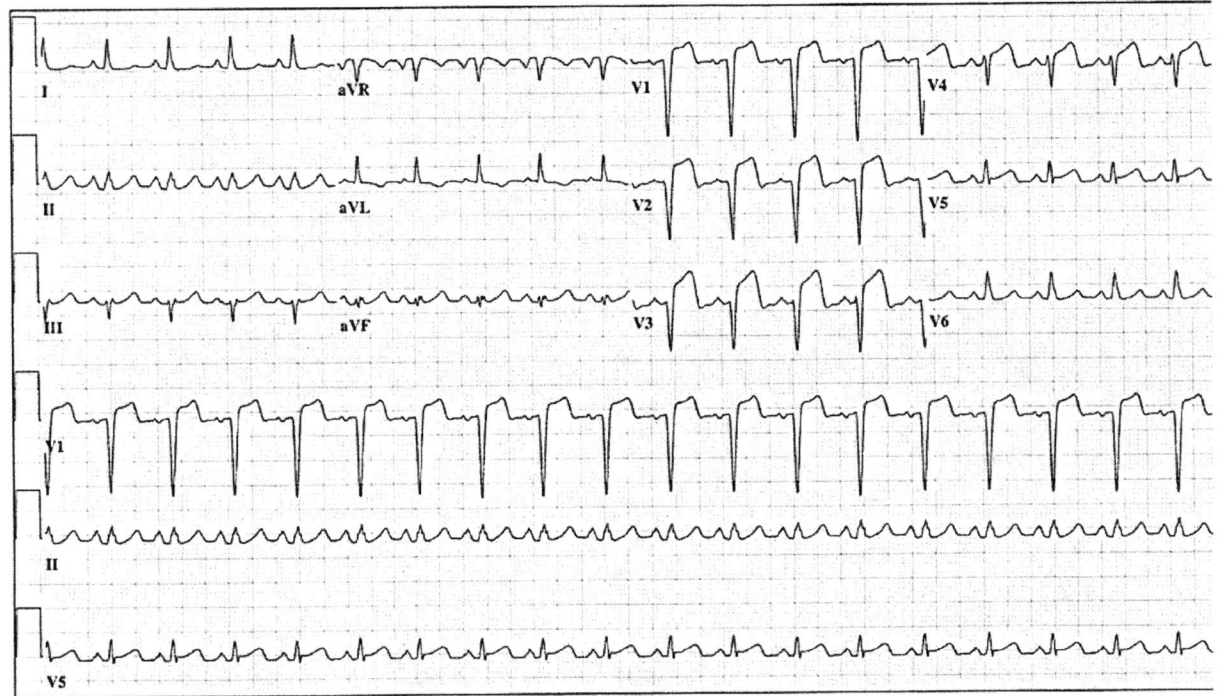

Which of the following should you order first?

A. Procainamide
B. Exercise stress test with nuclear imaging
C. NSAID
D. Urine drug screen
E. Cardiac MRI

Answer: _____

AR 39

Which of the following patients would be most appropriate for immediate reperfusion therapy?

A. A 47 yo man with a prior recent MI who presents with 1 mm of ST-segment elevation in leads I, II, III, aVF, and V1–V6
B. An 80 yo woman with a recent onset of right hemiparesis with 4 mm of ST-segment elevation from leads V1 to V6
C. A 65 yo man with 2 hours of chest pain and new left bundle-branch block
D. A 65 yo man with new T-wave inversion in leads V1 to V4
E. A 30 yo woman with a history of corrected tetralogy of Fallot and 2 hours of chest pain and palpitations

Answer: _____

AR 40

A 68 yo man comes to the ED with 12 hours of chest pain.

HR is 70 bpm and BP 90/50 mmHg.

There are irregular cannon *a* waves in the jugular venous pulse, and he has an apical 3rd heart sound.

His initial electrocardiogram follows.

ECG

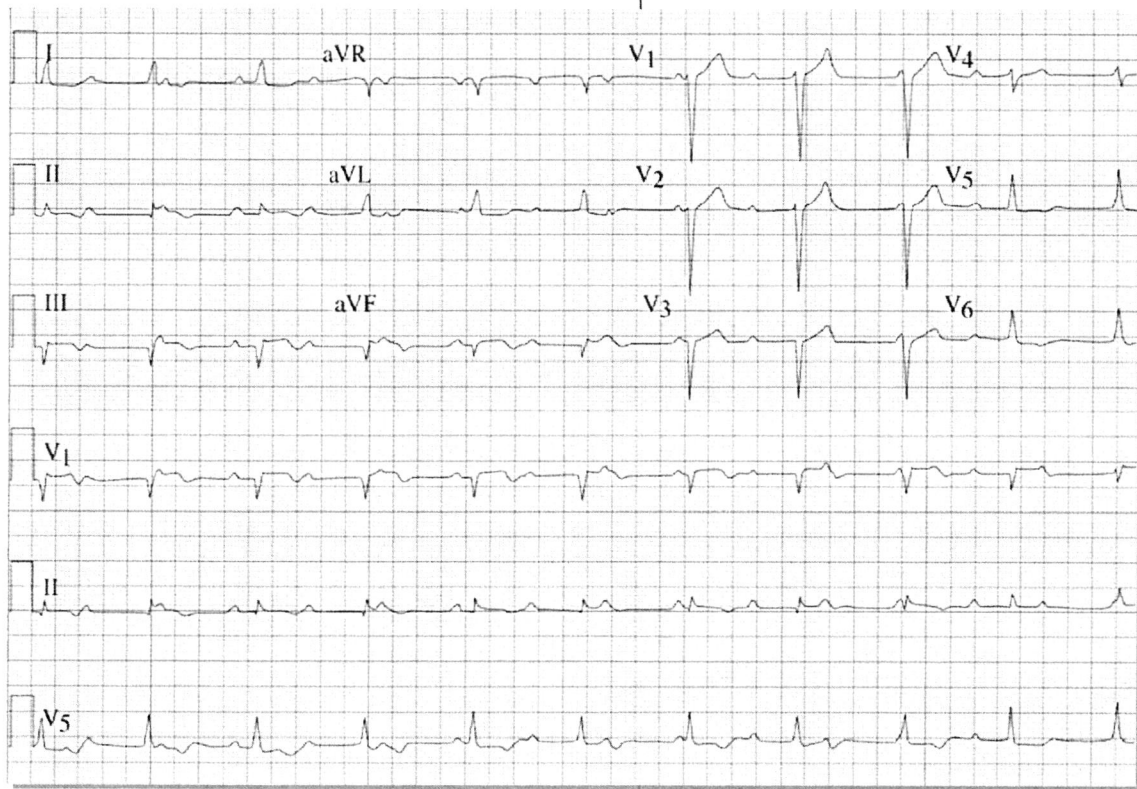

Which of the following statements is true?

A. Fibrinolytic therapy is likely to markedly decrease his 30-day mortality.

B. He is likely to require an ICD.

C. An exercise treadmill test would improve his rhythm.

D. An echo showing an LVEF of 30% would be an indication for coronary angiography.

E. This patient has an excellent prognosis.

Answer: _____

AR 41

A 56 yo man comes to the ED with 6 hours of constant, dull chest pain.

He has this pain at rest and with exercise, lasting 20 minutes to several hours.

His physical examination is normal.

Initial cardiac markers are negative, and his ECG is normal.

What should you do?

A. Discharge him with outpatient follow-up.

B. Start antianginal medications and arrange for outpatient follow-up.

C. Observe him for 8 hours, draw another set of markers, and obtain another ECG.

D. Admit him to the hospital and start on ASA, clopidogrel, and LMW heparin.

E. Immediate coronary angiography.

Answer: _____

AR 42

A 67 yo woman has had 3 hours of chest pain.
She has no contraindications to reperfusion therapy.
Her ECG follows.

ECG

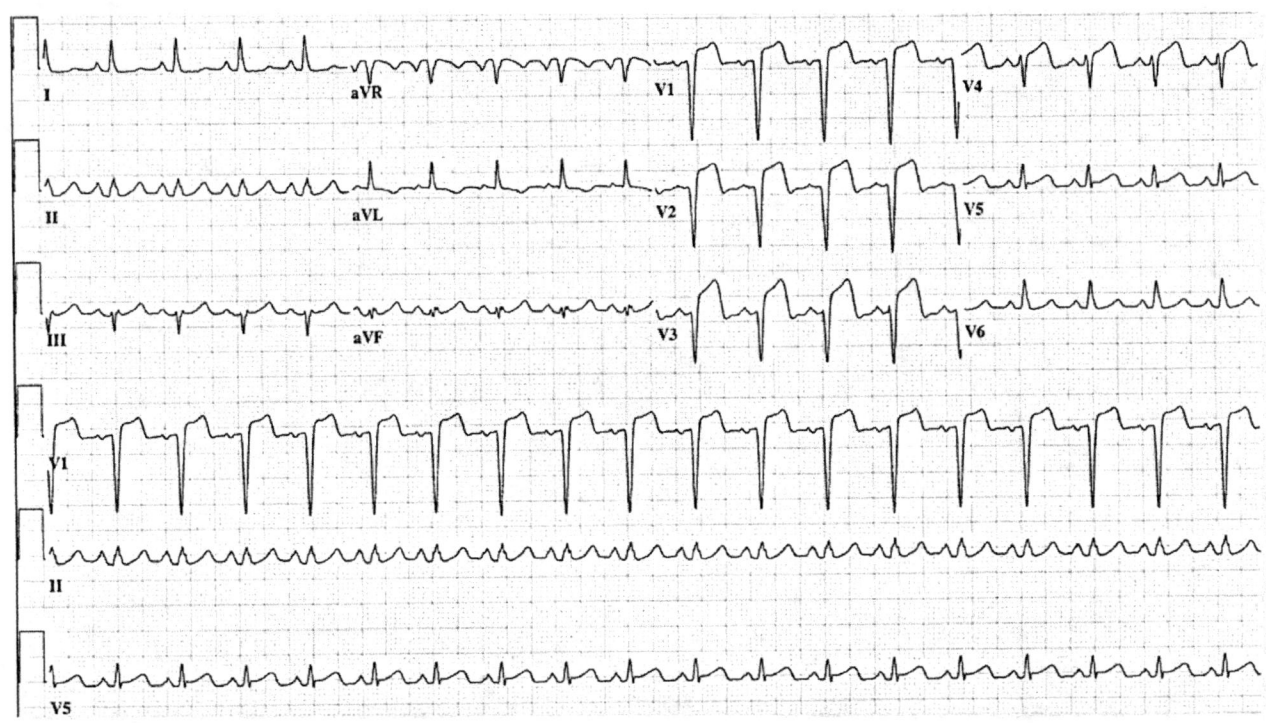

Which of the following agents has been shown to have the most favorable effect on prognosis?

A. Streptokinase alone
B. Streptokinase plus intravenous heparin
C. tPA alone
D. tPA plus subcutaneous heparin
E. tPA plus intravenous heparin

Answer: _____

AR 43

A 72 yo male with known CAD presents with 3 hours of chest pain.

HR is 85 bpm and BP 145/95 mmHg, and there is moderate elevation of the JVP.

His first troponin I level is 13.6 ng/mL.

His ECG follows.

ECG

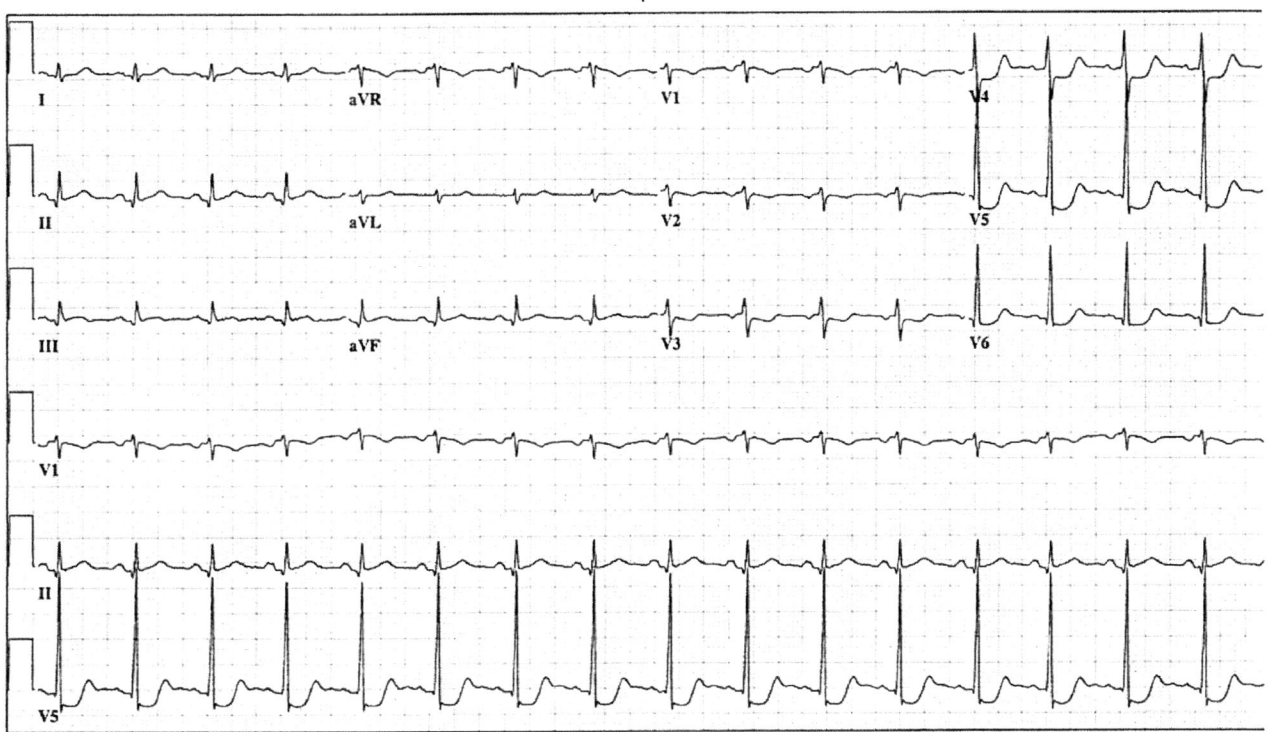

What would you do?

A. Reperfusion therapy with tPA and heparin.
B. Avoid beta-blockers because of his heart failure.
C. Perform a stress study to determine if coronary angiography is necessary.
D. Treat him with medical therapy alone.
E. Refer him for urgent coronary angiography.

Answer: _____

AR 44

A patient with a previous CABG has an LVEF of 25% by echo.

A 24-hour Holter monitor showed 4 episodes of nonsustained VT.

What treatment is appropriate?

A. Indefinite amiodarone therapy
B. A beta-blocker alone
C. An ACEI alone
D. ASA, beta-blocker, and ACEI
E. ASA, beta-blocker, ACEI, and referral for ICD placement

Answer: _____

AR 45

A 66 yo woman presents with 2 hours of substernal chest pain.
She has risk factors of diabetes, smoking, and dyslipidemia.
ECG follows.

ECG

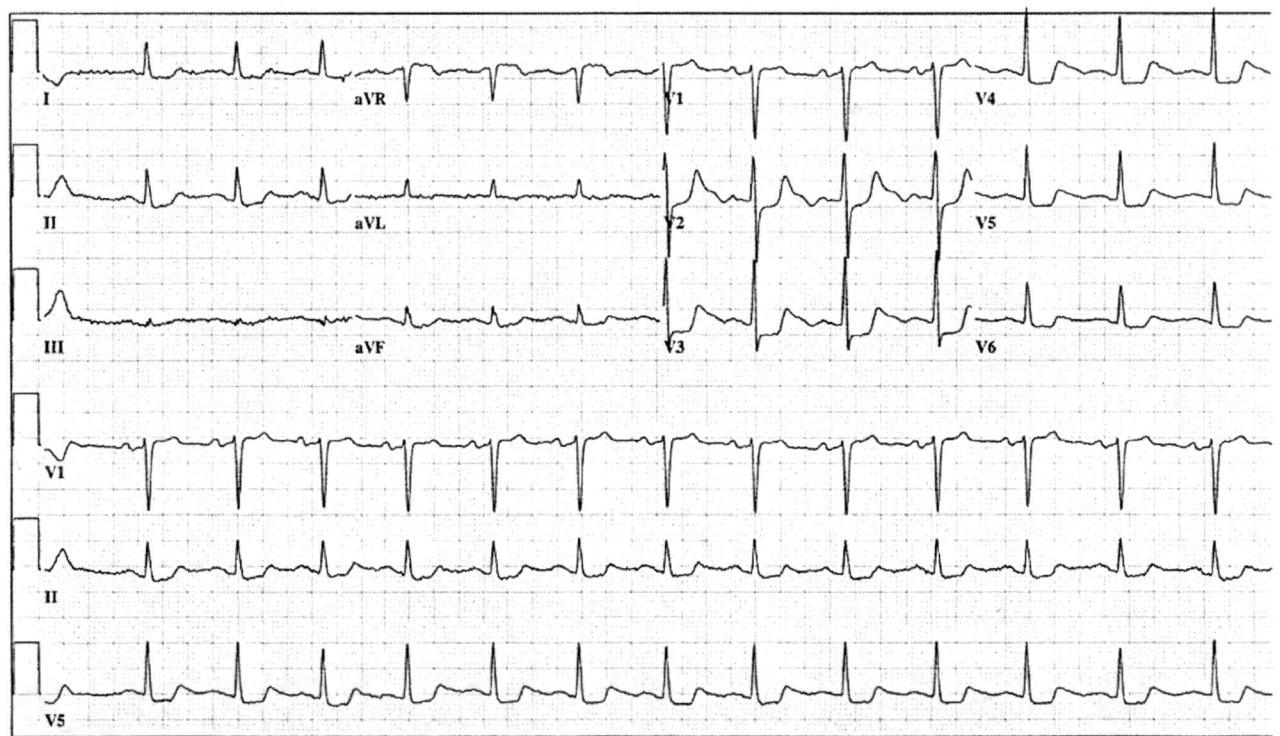

What should you do next?

A. Exercise stress test with nuclear perfusion imaging
B. CT angiography
C. Referral for catheter-based coronary angiography and possible PCI
D. Stress echocardiography
E. Radionuclide ventriculography (MUGA)

Answer: _____

AR 46

A 64 yo man had a STEMI and was treated with ASA, beta-blockers, an ACEI, and a statin.
He was standing at the nurses' station when telemetry showed the following:

What should you do?

A. Begin a dopamine infusion.
B. Refer for permanent pacemaker.
C. Electrophysiology study.
D. Decrease beta-blockers.
E. Coronary angiography.

Answer: _____

AR 47

A 74 yo woman comes to the ED with chest pain and dyspnea and is found to have an NSTEMI.
Physical exam and chest x-ray show pulmonary edema. She is given a beta-blocker, morphine, NTG, and 160 mg of furosemide.

She initially improves, but 1 hour later becomes hypotensive.
A right-heart catheter is inserted and the following pressures are obtained:

Location	RA	PA	PCWP
Pressure (mmHg)	2	20/10	6

What treatment is appropriate?

A. Intraaortic balloon pump
B. Emergency PCI
C. Fibrinolytic therapy
D. Slow infusion of normal saline
E. Blood cultures and empiric antibiotics

Answer: _____

Part 4:
Peripheral Arterial Disease

Clinical Presentation

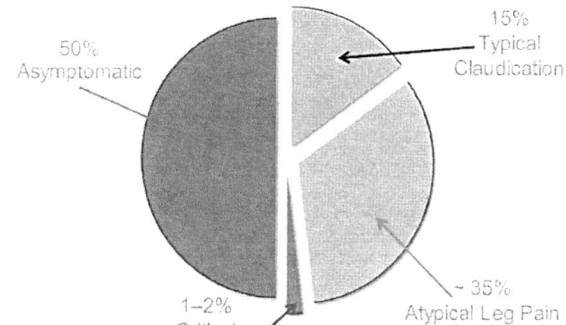

Diagnosis

- Claudication
- Brachial and ankle blood pressures before and after exercise are the best test of the degree of functional impairment
- Angiography is the best test for defining the location of the disease

Ankle-Brachial Index Interpretation

ABI	Interpretation
1.00–1.29	Normal
0.91–0.99	Borderline
0.41–0.90	Mild-to-moderate disease
≤ 0.40	Severe disease

Prevalence of PAD

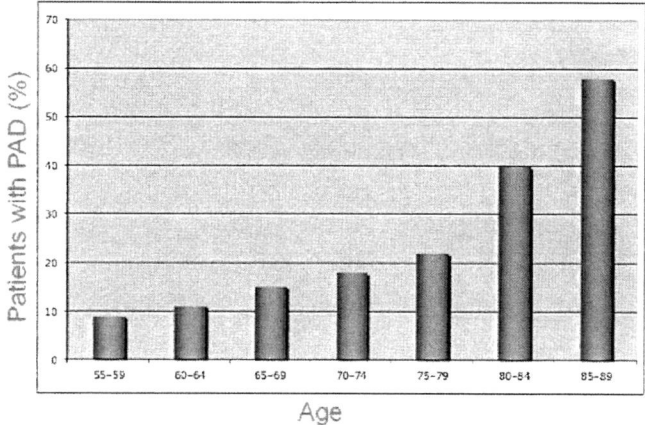

Gender Differences in PAD

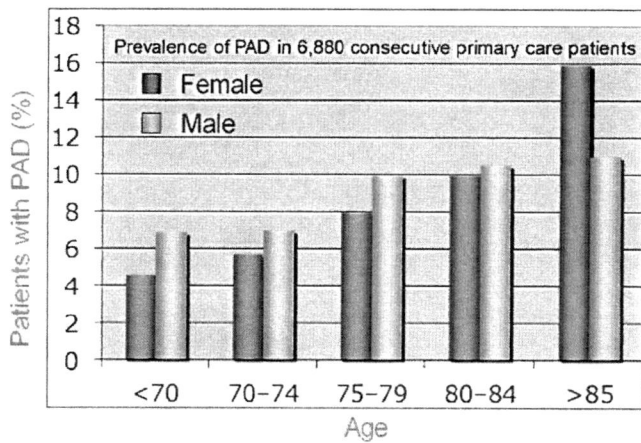

Ethnicity and PAD

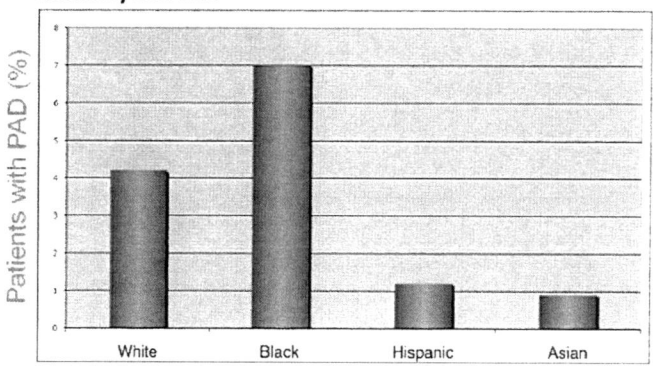

Risk Factors for PAD

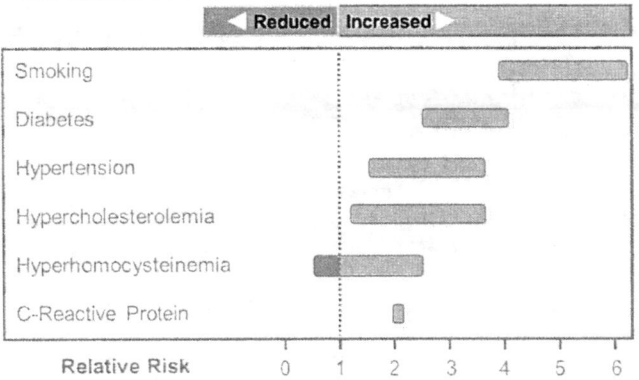

Relative Risk — Reduced ← → Increased

Smoking, Diabetes, Hypertension, Hypercholesterolemia, Hyperhomocysteinemia, C-Reactive Protein (Relative Risk scale 0 to 6)

At-Risk Population for PAD
- Age < 50 with DM and 1 additional risk factor
- Age 50–69 years and smoking or DM
- Age ≥ 70
- Claudication
- Abnormal lower extremity pulse exam
- Known atherosclerotic coronary, carotid, or renal artery disease

Long-term Survival with PAD

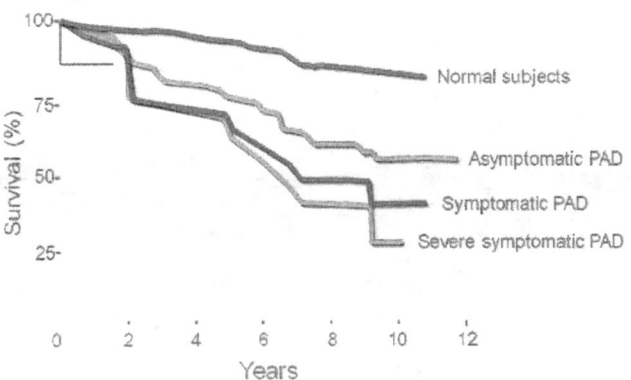

Survival (%) vs Years — Normal subjects, Asymptomatic PAD, Symptomatic PAD, Severe symptomatic PAD

MRA
- MRA has virtually replaced contrast arteriography for PAD diagnosis
- Excellent arterial picture
- No ionizing radiation

Source: ACC/AHA 2005 Guidelines for the Management of Patients with Peripheral Arterial Disease (Lower Extremity, Renal, Mesenteric, and Abdominal Aortic): A Collaborative Report From the AAVS/SVS, SCAI, SVMB, SIR, and the ACC/AHA Task Force on Practice Guidelines.

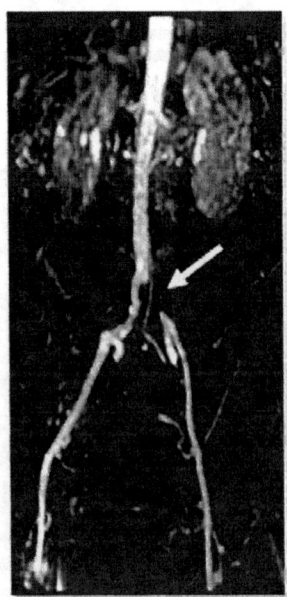

CT Angiography
- Requires iodinated contrast
- Requires ionizing radiation
- Produces an excellent arterial picture

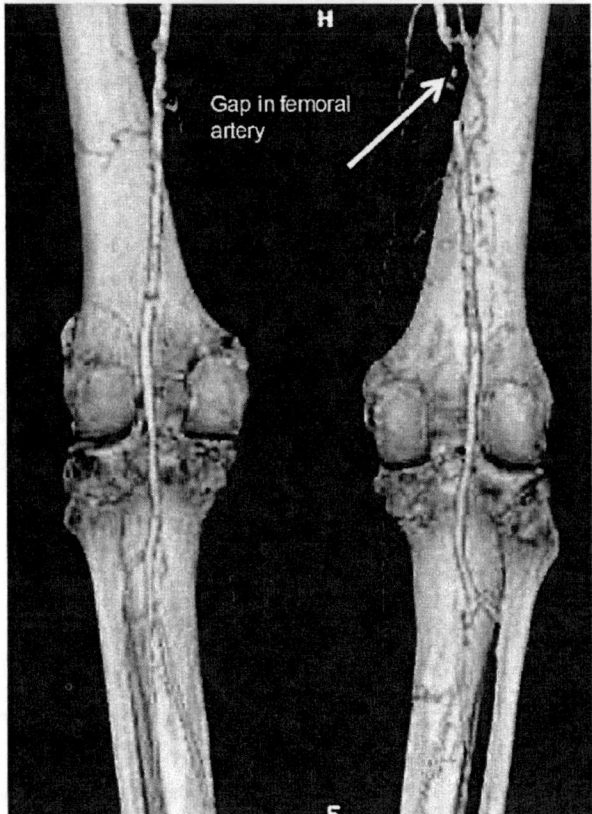

Gap in femoral artery

Source: ACC/AHA Guidelines

Treatment of PAD

Goals of Therapy

Limb Outcomes	Cardiovascular Outcomes
Improved ability to walk	Decrease in morbidity and mortality from stroke and MI
Improvement in quality of life	
Prevention of progression to critical limb ischemia and amputation	

Medical Therapy for PAD
- Smoking cessation
- Treatment of HTN
- Beta-blockers are not contraindicated
- High-intensity statin
- Treat diabetes aggressively

- ASA (75–325 mg/day) for all patients
- Clopidogrel (75 mg/day) is an effective alternative

- Cilostazol (100 mg bid) improves symptoms and increases walking distance (contraindicated in heart failure)
- Pentoxifylline (400 mg tid) is a 2nd line alternative with less effectiveness

Exercise Therapy for PAD
- Type of exercise: Walking to near-maximal claudication, 3–5 times per week for 35–50 minutes for 6 months
- Results: 100–150% improvement in walking distance and quality of life

AR 48
A 60 yo male with a history of smoking and diabetes presents with pain in his calves when walking farther than 2 blocks.
ABIs are 0.6 in the RLE and 0.7 in the LLE.

Which of the following is true based on current evidence?
A. Pentoxifylline 400 mg q a.m. is 1st line therapy for this condition.
B. He should be advised not to walk as fast or as far.
C. Cilostazol 100 mg bid can improve his symptoms and increase his walking distance.
D. Diabetes control to a HbA1c of 8.5% is in line with treatment goals.

Answer: _____

Indications for Revascularization in Patients with Claudication
- Lack of response to exercise therapy and claudication pharmacotherapies
- Presence of a severe disability
- Absence of other diseases that would limit exercise even if the claudication was improved
- Acceptable overall prognosis
- Favorable lesion morphology

Options in Limb Revascularization
- Endovascular reconstruction options
  - Percutaneous transluminal angioplasty (PTA)
  - Stents
- Surgical reconstruction options
  - Aortoiliac/Aortofemoral reconstruction
  - Femoropopliteal bypass (above knee and below knee)
  - Femorotibial bypass

Endovascular Management
- PTA is recommended for iliac, femoral, and popliteal lesions of < 3 cm in length
- Stenting is recommended for iliac lesions

Surgical Management
- Surgery is a reasonable alternative to PTA, particularly in patients with long or multiple lesions
- Surgical mortality ranges from 2–6%
- 5-year patency rates are about 80% for aortic, iliac, and femoral bypass, and about 60% for axillofemoral bypass

Acute Lower Limb Ischemia

Class	Prognosis	Symptoms	Sensory Loss	Muscle Weakness	Doppler Signals	
					Arterial	Venous
I. (Viable)	Not immediately threatened	Claudication	None	None	+	+
IIa. Marginal	Salvageable if promptly treated	Claudication	Toes or none	None	Often −	+
IIb. Immediate	Salvageable with immediate revascularization	Rest pain	More than toes	Mild to moderate	Usually −	+
III. Irreversible	Major tissue loss or nerve damage	None in the area	Anesthetic	Paralysis (rigor)	−	−

Source: Inter-society consensus for the management of peripheral arterial disease. *Int Angiol.* 2007 Jun;26(2):81–157.

Fate of Critical Limb Ischemia

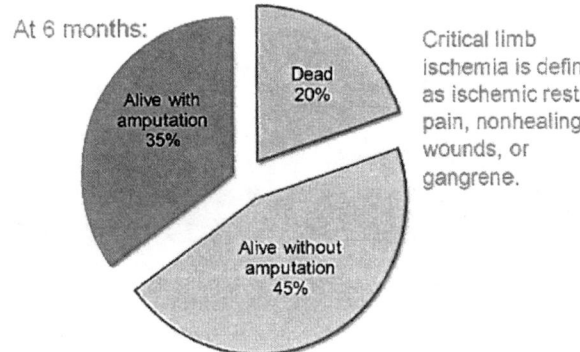

At 6 months:
- Dead 20%
- Alive with amputation 35%
- Alive without amputation 45%

Critical limb ischemia is defined as ischemic rest pain, nonhealing wounds, or gangrene.

Other Causes of PAD
- Arteritis (CT disease, giant cell, Takayasu)
- Trauma
- Buerger disease (usually male smokers < 30 years old)
- Entrapment

AR 49

A 28 yo male smoker presents with gangrene of the right foot and superficial thrombophlebitis.

What is the most likely diagnosis?
A. Buerger disease
B. Right iliofemoral atherosclerosis
C. Cardiac embolism to the right popliteal artery
D. Necrotizing fasciitis
E. Chronic pressure ulceration

Answer: _____

Buerger Disease
- Also called "thromboangiitis obliterans"
- Involves medium and small arteries
- Often affects the wrist (produces a positive Allen test) and hands

Buerger Disease

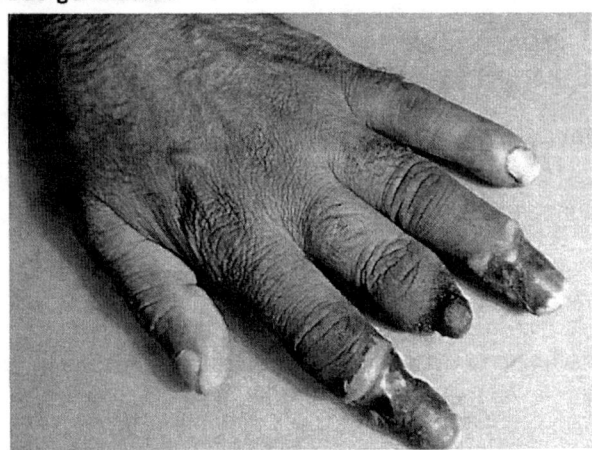

Entrapment
- Thoracic outlet syndrome
- Young men may have popliteal artery entrapment, which causes claudication of the arch of the foot with walking but not running (!)

Lumbar Stenosis vs. PAD
- Lumbar spinal stenosis produces pseudoclaudication
- Lumbar spinal stenosis is relieved by sitting down but not by standing still
- It is exacerbated by anything which compresses the spine, such as standing or walking (particularly downhill)

A young female patient presents with reduced left upper extremity pulsations and normal pulses in the right upper extremity and in the lower extremities.
The ESR is elevated.

What is the diagnosis?
A. Mitral stenosis with an embolism to the left subclavian artery
B. Atherosclerosis of the left subclavian
C. Coarctation of the aorta
D. Takayasu arteritis
E. Thoracic outlet obstruction

Answer: _____

Takayasu Arteritis

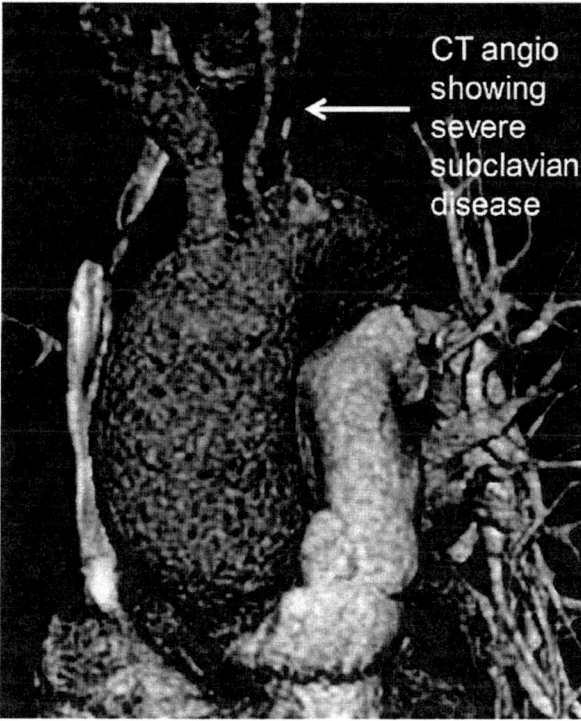

CT angio showing severe subclavian disease

Treatment
- Buerger's — stop smoking
- Arteritis — treat the disease

Venous Thrombosis
- Contrast venogram is still the gold standard
- Doppler ultrasound and impedance plethysmography are both good for above-the-knee thrombosis
- Color Doppler imaging can determine whether the thrombus is obstructive

Acute Arterial Occlusion
- Most arterial emboli to the legs come from the heart
- The aorta can be the source of atheromatous emboli
- Aneurysms of the limbs can produce emboli
- Heparin is useful in preventing new clot
- Embolectomy is the treatment of choice

Vasospastic Disease
- Primary Raynaud phenomenon (Raynaud disease)
  - Constriction of small arteries & arterioles when cold
  - Can lead to acrocyanosis
  - Involves digits of the hand
  - More common in women
  - Sometimes associated with livedo

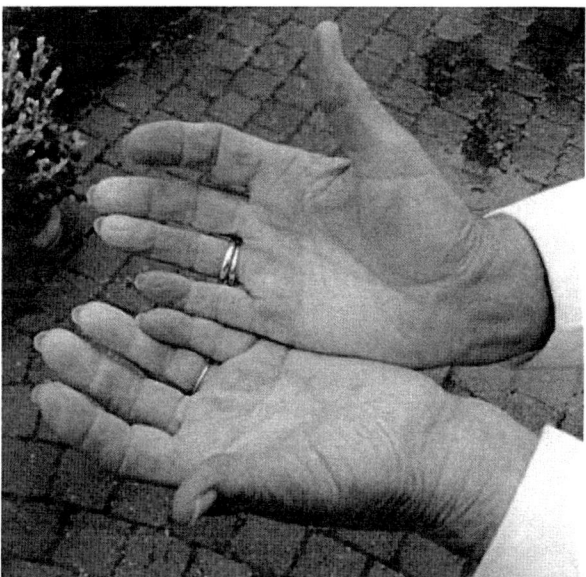

Coronary Vasospasm
- Prinzmetal angina
  - Transient dramatic ST elevation
  - Mainly at rest
  - Consider this in younger patient with transient ST elevation but normal cors

Vasospastic Disorders: Tx
- Calcium channel blockers
- Long-acting nitrates

AR 51

A 35 yo male presents with squeezing chest pressure at rest.
ECG follows.

ECG

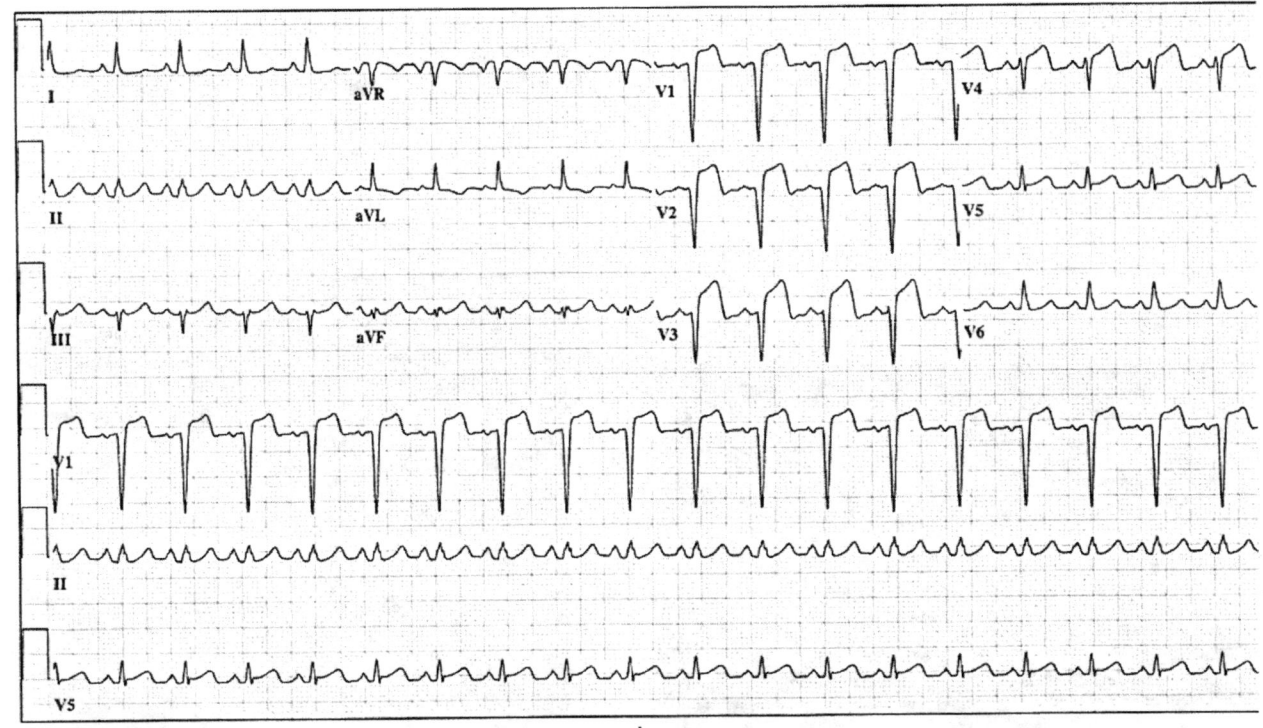

AR 51 (cont.)

He is sent to the cardiac cath lab ASAP, but the cardiologist calls you to report that his coronaries are completely normal. Left ventriculogram is also normal.

Which of the following is the most likely diagnosis?

A. Myocardial bridging
B. Prinzmetal angina
C. Buerger disease
D. Raynaud phenomenon
E. Takotsubo cardiomyopathy

Answer: _____

Carotid Artery Disease

Demographics of Stroke
- 3rd leading cause of death in the U.S.
- 1,000,000 stroke events/year:
  - 500,000 new strokes; 200,000 recurrent strokes; 240,000 TIAs
- Leading cause of serious long-term disability
- Atherosclerosis accounts for 1/3 of all strokes
- 55,000 more strokes in women per year than in men

Course of Carotid Disease
- In patients with a bruit, those who have a TIA are much more likely to have a stroke than those who are asymptomatic
- Patients with atherosclerotic carotid disease are more likely to have an MI than a TIA or stroke

Diagnosis
- Carotid ultrasound is probably indicated in patients with asymptomatic bruits and definitely with symptoms
- MRA and CT angio are acceptable alternatives
- Carotid angiography is definitive

Normal Carotid Ultrasound

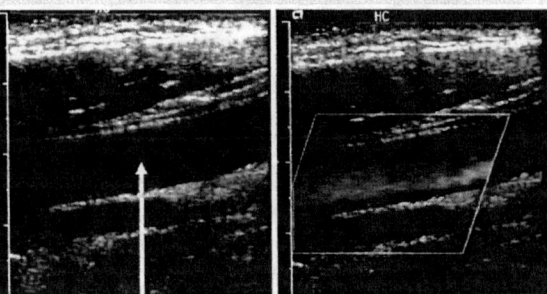

Right Common Carotid   Carotid Doppler

© 2017 MedStudy Internal Medicine Video Board Review – Cardiology • Matthew Sorrentino, MD

Abnormal Carotid Ultrasound

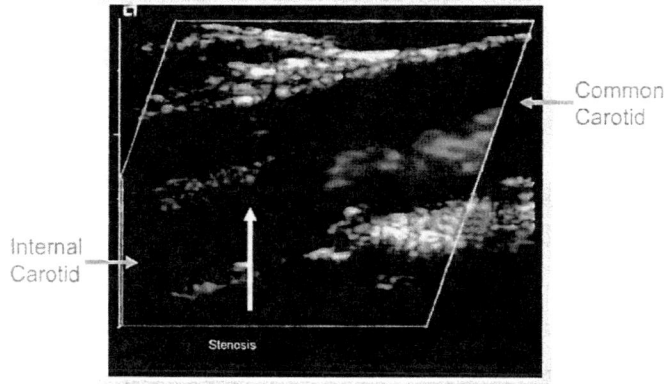

Carotid CT Angio

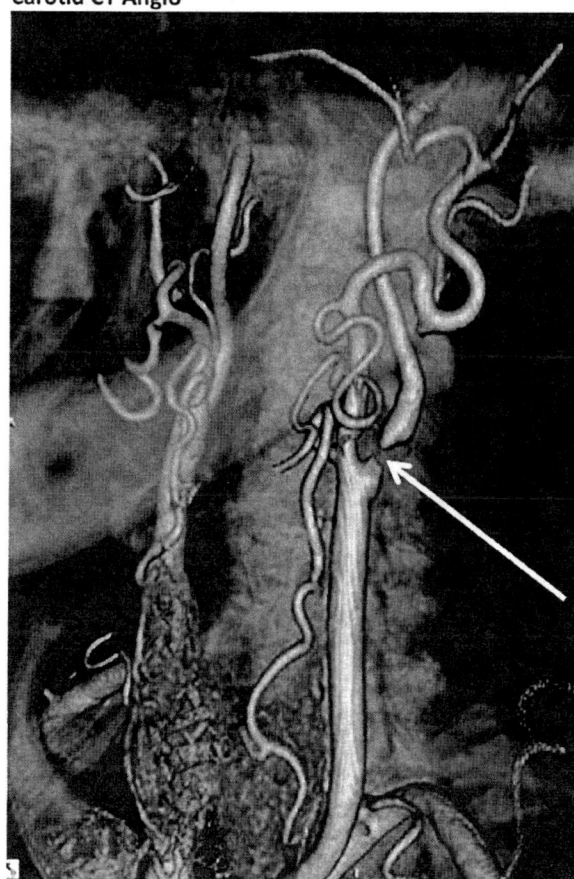

Carotid Angiography

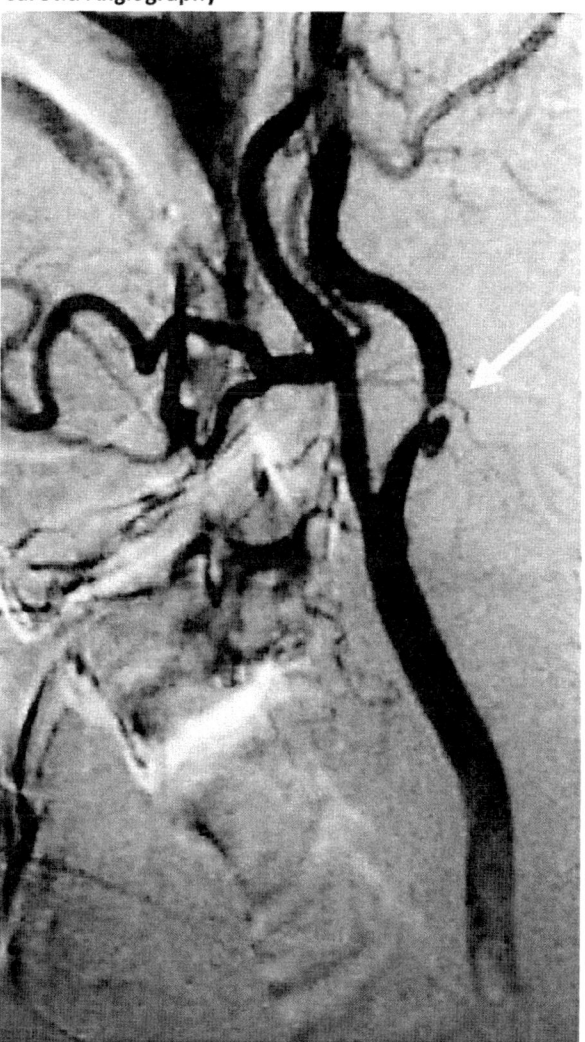

Indications for Carotid Endarterectomy
- Symptomatic patients with stenoses of 50–99%, as long as the risk of surgical mortality or stroke is < 6%
- Asymptomatic patients with stenoses of 60–99%, as long as the risk of surgical mortality or stroke is < 3%

Preventive Meds in PAD
- ASA 81 mg PO daily
- Clopidogrel if ASA cannot be taken
- High-intensity statin
- Aggressive HTN management
- Symptomatic Tx (i.e., cilostazol) for claudication

Aortic Dissection

Genetic Diseases Associated with Aortic Aneurysm and Dissection

Marfan's
- Features
  - Skeletal deformities
  - Dislocated lenses
- Aortic surgery is indicated if:
  - Aorta > 5.0 cm
  - Family history of dissection at < 5.0 cm
  - Rapidly expanding aneurysm
  - Significant AR

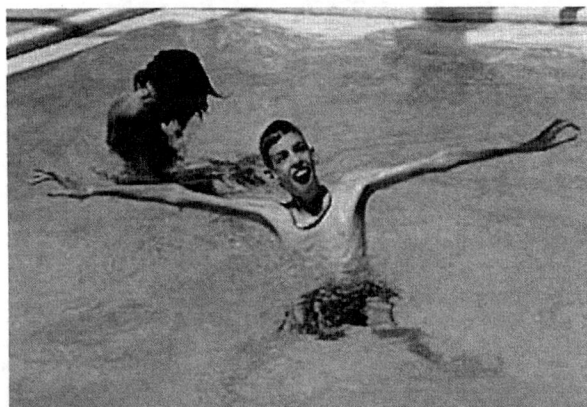

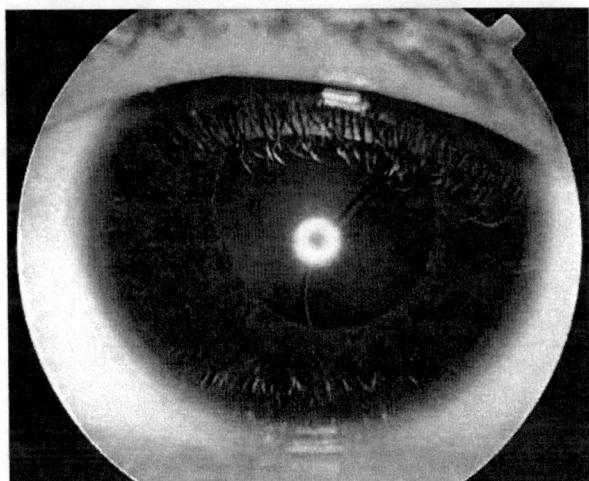

Dislocated lens

Loeys-Dietz
- Features — bifid uvula or cleft palate, arterial tortuosity, hypertelorism, skeletal features similar to Marfan's, aneurysms, and dissections of other arteries
- Aortic surgery is indicated if:
  - Aortic ≥ 4.2 cm by TEE
  - Aorta ≥ 4.4–4.6 cm by CT or MR

Loeys-Dietz

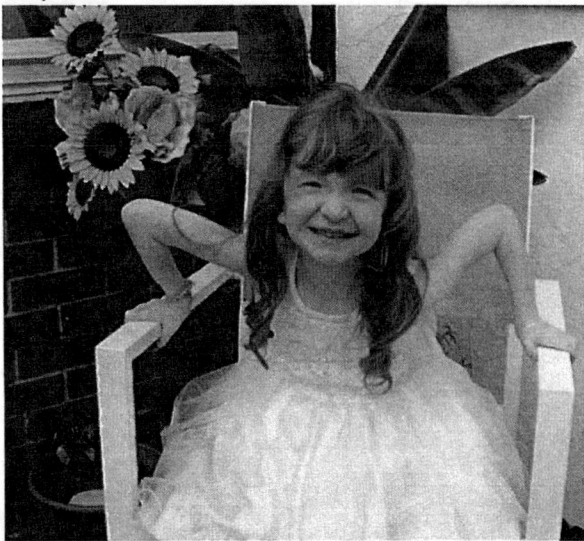

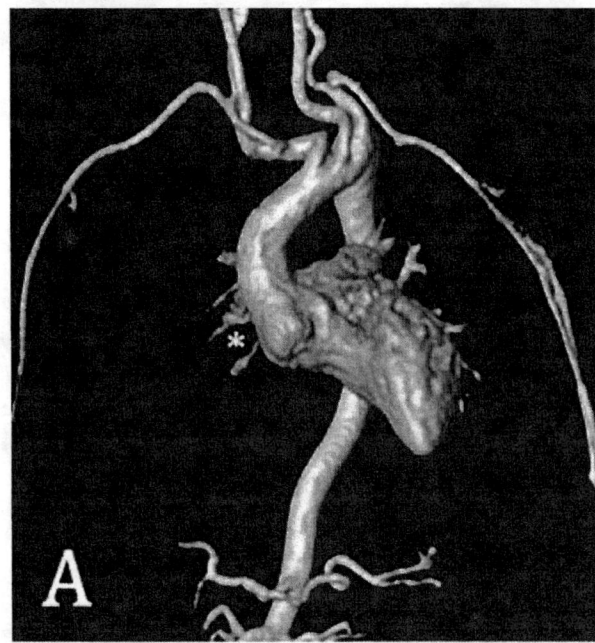

MR of tortuous great vessels in a child

Ehlers-Danlos
- Features — thin, translucent skin, GI rupture, rupture of the gravid uterus, rupture of medium-sized to large arteries
- Management
  - Surgical repair complicated by friable tissues
  - Noninvasive imaging recommended

Ehlers-Danlos (cont.)

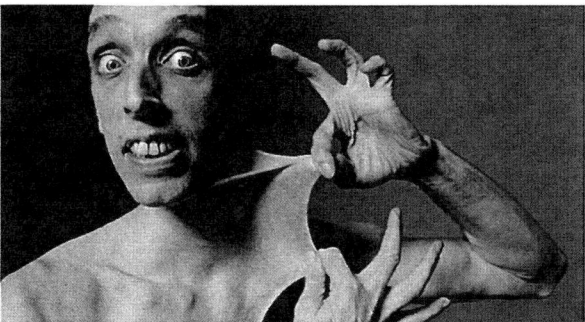

Turner's
- Features — short stature, primary amenorrhea, bicuspid aortic valve, coarctation, webbed neck, low-set ears, low hairline, broad chest
- Management — dissection risk increased with bicuspid aortic valve, aortic coarctation, HTN, or pregnancy

Features of Turner's

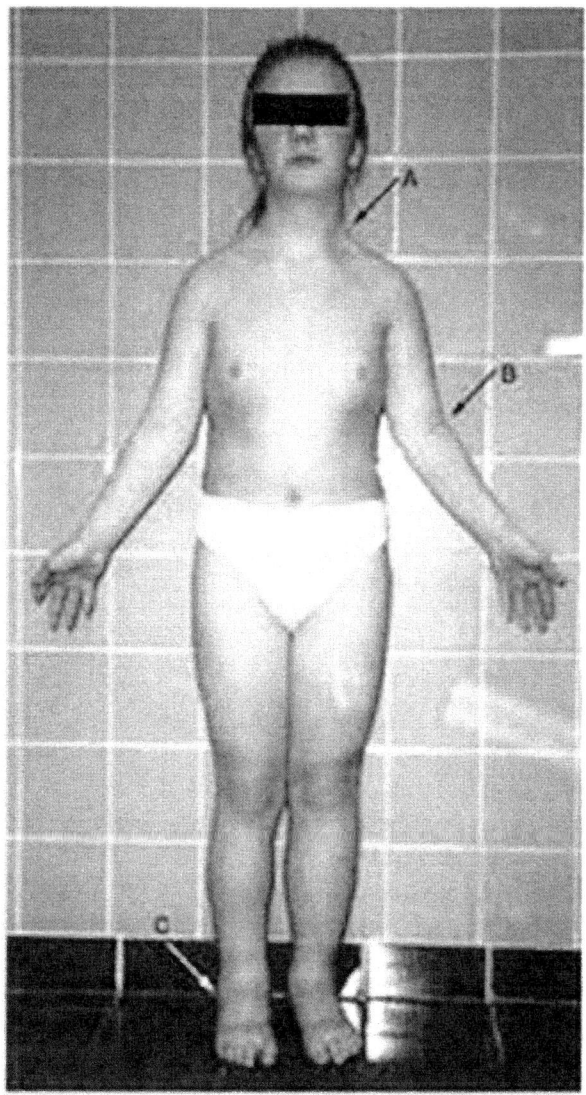

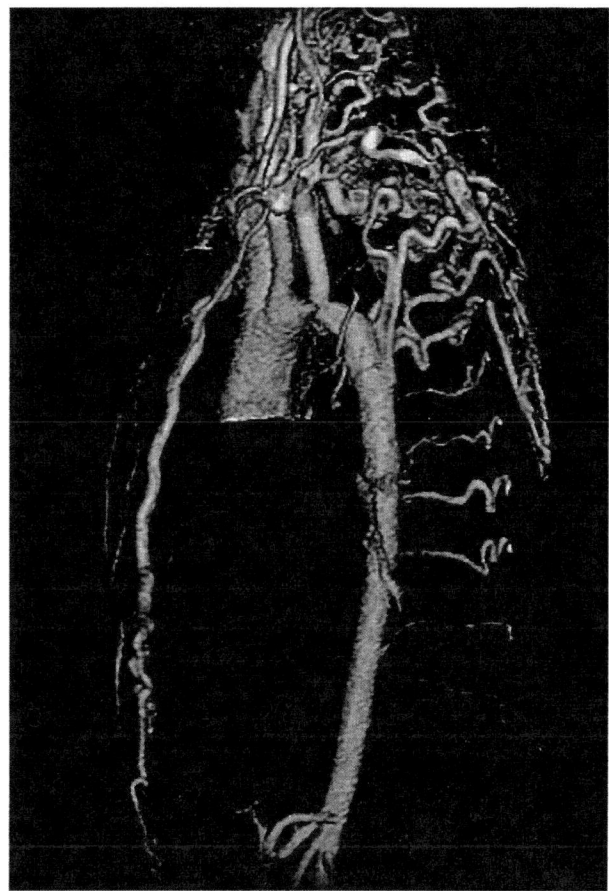

CT showing coarctation

AR 52

A tall, thin, 30 yo man complains of mid-back pain for 3 days, severe enough so that he has been unable to sleep. Physical exam shows a height of 6'8"; long, spindly fingers; and pectus excavatum.
Femoral pulses seem somewhat diminished.

Which of the following statements is true with respect to aortic dissection?
A. Dissection of the ascending aorta should be treated with medical therapy alone.
B. Appropriate medical therapy for dissection is intravenous nitroprusside alone.
C. Lowering the aortic systolic pressure is the most important aspect of medical therapy.
D. All descending thoracic aortic dissections require immediate surgery.
E. Dissection can occur in the 3rd trimester of pregnancy without any predisposing factors.

Answer: _____

**Aortic Dissection Pretest Risk Factors —
High-Risk Patient**
- Marfan's, Loeys-Dietz, Ehlers-Danlos, Turner syndrome, coarctation
- Family history of aortic disease
- Known aortic valve disease
- Recent aortic manipulation (surgery or catheter-based)
- Known thoracic aneurysm

Additional High-Risk Precipitating Factors
- Uncontrolled HTN
- Pheochromocytoma
- Cocaine or amphetamine use
- Weight lifting
- Chest trauma
- Takayasu or giant cell arteritis
- Pregnancy
- Polycystic kidney disease
- Chronic steroid or immunosuppressive therapy
- Bacteremia or extension of local infection

Pretest Risk Factors — High-Risk Pain Features
- Chest, back, or abdominal pain features described as pain that:
  - Is abrupt or instantaneous in onset
  - Is severe in intensity
  - Has a ripping, tearing, stabbing, or sharp quality

- Pulse deficit
- Systolic BP limb differential > 20 mmHg
- Focal neurologic deficit
- AR murmur (new or not known to be old and in conjunction with pain)

Diagnostic Evaluation

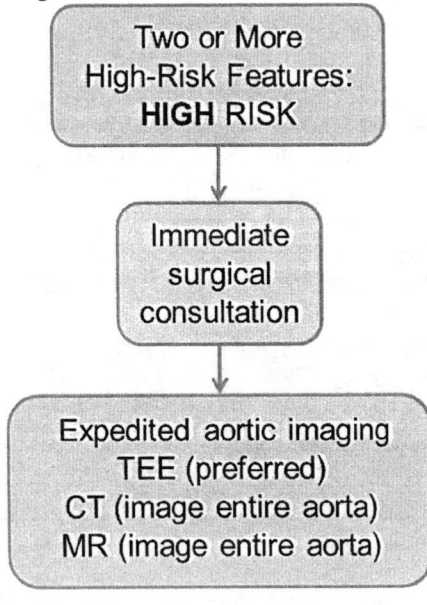

Initial Studies in Suspected Dissection
- ECG in all patients
- Chest x-ray in all intermediate- and high-risk patients
- TEE in all high-risk patients
- A second imaging study should be obtained in high-risk patients if the first is negative

Medical Management
- Beta-blockers to keep HR < 60 bpm
- Diltiazem or verapamil as an alternative if beta-blockers are contraindicated
- If systolic BP remains > 120 after adequate beta-blockade, begin ACE inhibitors and/or other vasodilators
- Goal is MAP of 70 mmHg

- Do not use beta-blockers in patients with acute AR
- Do not initiate therapy with vasodilators prior to beta-blockade

Indications for Surgery
- Ascending aortic dissections
- Coexistent coronary disease suitable for CABG
- Acute AR

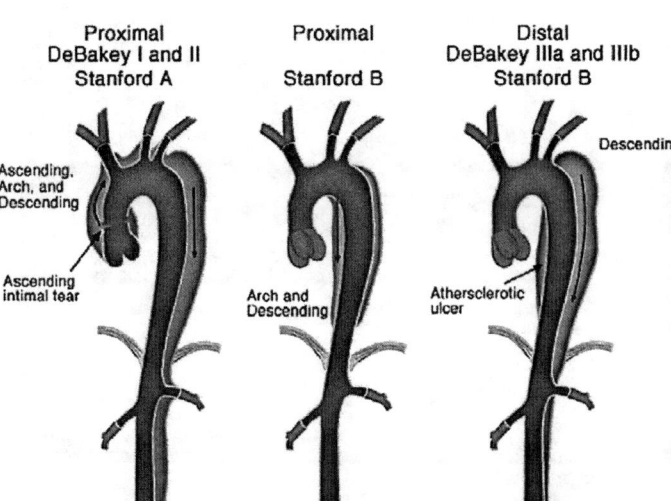

Classification
- DeBakey:
  - Type I — involvement of the ascending and descending aorta
  - Type II — ascending aorta alone
  - Type III — descending aorta alone
- Stanford:
  - Type A — any involvement of the ascending aorta
  - Type B — descending aorta alone

Management by Location
- Ascending dissections are at greater risk for rupture, and they are always an indication for surgery
- In general, descending dissections can be treated medically unless complications occur

Course
- Proximal dissection can cause AR, hemopericardium and tamponade, and severe anterior chest pain
- Descending dissection causes interscapular pain
- These pains are frequently migratory
- Dissections may reenter the aorta and obstruct an iliac artery

Aortic Coarctation
- A congenital condition that causes persistent HTN, even after surgery
- Associated with bicuspid aortic valve
- Blood pressure is higher in the arms than in the legs
- The ECG almost always shows LVH
- CXR shows rib notching

Takayasu and Giant Cell Arteritis
- These conditions should be treated initially with high-dose steroids
- Treatment should be monitored by sed rate or C-reactive protein
- Elective revascularization should be delayed until the acute inflammatory state is quiescent

Aortic Aneurysm

AAA Screening
- USPSTF:
  - Men ages 65 to 75 who have ever smoked cigarettes
  - One-time screening with abdominal ultrasound

Course
- Rupture is the biggest threat
- Another problem is atheroembolism; Signs include (in decreasing order):
  - Livedo reticularis
  - Blue toes
  - Ischemic ulceration
- Most emboli to the legs are from the heart
- HTN from renal failure may occur

Rupture
- May present with severe abdominal or back pain and syncope
- If the rupture is contained, local symptoms predominate subsequently
- Leukocytosis and anemia are common
- Diagnosis is by CT
- Treatment is urgent surgery

Indications for Surgery
- Any <u>thoracic</u> aneurysm > 6 cm, or:
  - An expanding aneurysm
  - If the aneurysm is putting pressure on other structures
  - If the aneurysm is traumatic in origin
- Any <u>abdominal</u> aneurysm > 5.0 cm, or any expanding aneurysm, regardless of size

AR 53
A 60 yo male with a history of Marfan syndrome presents to the ED with intense "stabbing, tearing" pain that radiates all the way down his back.

Which of the following diagnostic tests is indicated?
A. Plain x-rays of the lumbar spine
B. MRI of the spine
C. TEE
D. Pharmacologic nuclear stress test
E. Pulmonary angiography

Answer: _____

AR 54A
A 44 yo female with a history of bicuspid aortic valve and known ascending proximal aortic aneurysm presents with chest pain that radiates into her back. She describes the pain as "sharp, stabbing."
R arm BP is 160/80 mmHg;
L arm BP is 135/80 mmHg.
TEE shows a bicuspid aortic valve but is otherwise nondiagnostic.

Which of the following is indicated?
A. CT with imaging of the entire aorta
B. Reassurance that this is likely musculoskeletal in nature
C. LUE angiography
D. MRI of the entire spine
E. EGD

Answer: _____

AR 54B
Which of the following is recommended for the most likely diagnosis?
A. Careful observation
B. Medical therapy alone
C. Immediate cardiothoracic surgery
D. Immediate neurology consult

Answer: _____

AR 55

A 75 yo male with a history of smoking, diabetes, and CAD presents with severe abdominal pain that radiates to his lower back and an episode of syncope.
Labs show a Hgb of 11 g/dL, Cr 3.0 mg/dL, and leukocytosis.

Which of the following is recommended next?
A. Renal ultrasound
B. Coronary calcium scoring
C. CT with imaging of the entire aorta
D. Plain x-rays of the lumbar spine
E. Iliac angiography

Answer: _____

AR 56

Which of the following patients should be referred for urgent/emergent surgery?
A. 70 yo female with a history of stable AAA measuring 4.6 cm in diameter
B. 70 yo male with ascending aortic dissection identified on TEE
C. 40 yo female with bicuspid aortic valve and mild aortic regurgitation
D. 65 yo asymptomatic male with new 4.5-cm AAA identified on screening ultrasound

Answer: _____

Part 5:
Valvular Heart Disease

Infective Endocarditis

Classification
- Native valve
- IV drug abuse
- Prosthetic valve
- Culture-negative

Endocarditis Organisms

Group	Organism
All cases	*Streptococcus* and *Staphylococcus* — 80% of the total HACEK group *Streptococcus bovis* — GI malignancy *Enterococcus* — GI malignancy, GI, or GU procedure
Native valve	*Streptococcus viridans* — 50% *Staphylococcus aureus* — 20%
IV drug abuse	*Staphylococcus* — most common by far, 80% of tricuspid endocarditis Fungi (*Candida*)
Prosthetic valve	Early (< 2 months) *Staphylococcus epidermidis* Late (> 2 months) similar to native valve
Culture-negative	Previous antibiotic use — 60% of cases Fungi Fastidious, slow-growing organisms

Duke Endocarditis Criteria

Major Criteria	Minor Criteria
Positive blood cultures	Predisposing cardiac lesion
Evidence of endocardial involvement (echo, new regurgitant murmur)	Fever
	Vascular phenomena
	Immunological phenomena
	< 2 positive blood cultures
	Mild echo abnormalities

Diagnosis:	2 major criteria
	1 major plus 3 minor criteria
	5 minor criteria

Physical Exam of Endocarditis
- Fever
- Regurgitant murmur
- Osler nodes
- Petechiae
- Janeway lesions
- Roth spots
- Splenomegaly

Vascular Phenomena
- Major arterial emboli
- Septic pulmonary emboli
- Mycotic aneurysm
- Intracranial hemorrhage
- Janeway lesions

Janeway Lesions

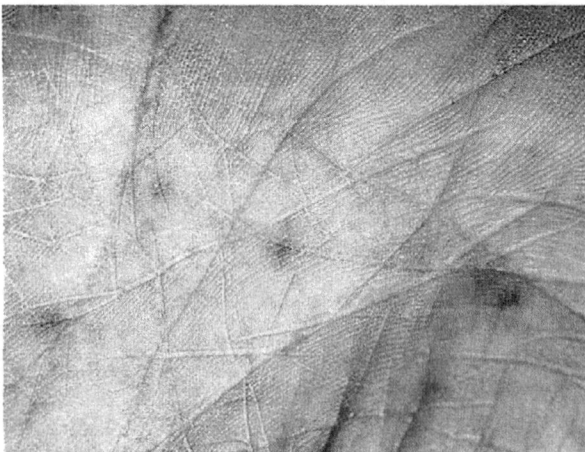

Flat, painless lesions on the palms and soles

Immunologic Phenomena
- Glomerulonephritis
- Osler nodes
- Roth spots
- Positive rheumatoid factor

© 2017 MedStudy Internal Medicine Video Board Review – Cardiology • Matthew Sorrentino, MD

Osler Nodes

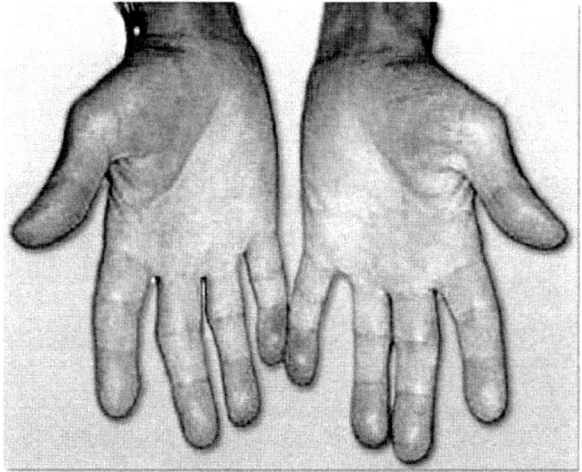

Painful raised lesions on the hands and feet

Roth Spots

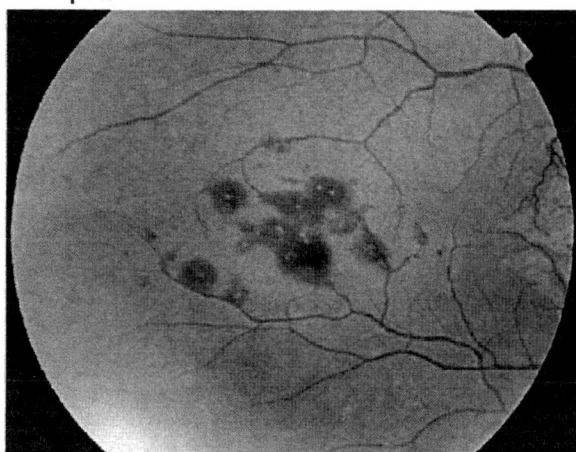

Retinal hemorrhages with white centers

Blood Cultures
- Blood cultures are positive in 95%
- Usually 2 cultures from different sites are sufficient to make a diagnosis

Indications for Surgery
- Heart failure
- Annular involvement or abscesses
- Fungal endocarditis
- Antibiotic resistant organisms
- Vegetation > 10 mm (?)
- Severe acute AR or MR
- Obstruction of prosthetic valve

Prosthetic Valve Endocarditis

Early (< 2 months)	Seeding of the valve at the time of surgery
	Usually skin contaminants; e.g., *S. epidermidis*
	Usually requires valve replacement
Late (> 2 months)	Involves typical endocarditis bacteria
	May respond to aggressive antibiotic therapy

Infective Endocarditis Prophylaxis

Current Guidelines
- Major changes in 2007 guidelines
- Changes based on the dubious benefit of traditional prophylaxis and the risk associated with antibiotic use
- Only highest-risk patients should now receive any form of IE prophylaxis

Highest-Risk Patients
- Prosthetic cardiac valve
- Previous infective endocarditis
- Congenital heart disease (CHD)
  - Unrepaired cyanotic CHD
  - Repaired CHD with prosthetic material or device that has residual leak
- Cardiac transplantation recipients who develop valvular disease

AR 57
A 32 yo woman presents with 3 weeks of weakness, fatigue, and arthralgias.
Roth spots on funduscopic exam are shown in a picture.

What test should be performed?
A. HIV titers
B. Toxoplasma serology
C. An ESR
D. Blood cultures
E. Treponemal-specific immunoassays

Answer: _____

AR 58
Patients with which of the following require antibiotic prophylaxis prior to a high-risk procedure?
A. Intracoronary stent
B. Mitral valve prolapse without MR
C. Prosthetic aortic valve
D. Permanent pacemaker
E. Uncomplicated repaired atrial septal defect

Answer: _____

AR 59

A young woman presents with a murmur during pregnancy.
Echo shows mild TR.

What antibiotic prophylaxis does she require prior to a dental extraction?

A. She does not require prophylaxis.
B. Amoxicillin 2.0 g orally.
C. Azithromycin 2.0 g orally if she is allergic to penicillin.
D. Intravenous ampicillin and gentamicin.
E. Intravenous vancomycin.

Answer: _____

Rheumatic Fever

Jones Criteria

Major	Minor
Carditis	Previous rheumatic fever
Polyarthritis	Arthralgias
Chorea	↑ sed rate, WBC, C-reactive protein
Erythema marginatum	Prolonged PR interval
Subcutaneous nodules	

Diagnosis	2 major criteria
	1 major and 2 minor criteria
	<u>And</u> positive Strep test or elevated ASO titers

Erythema Marginatum

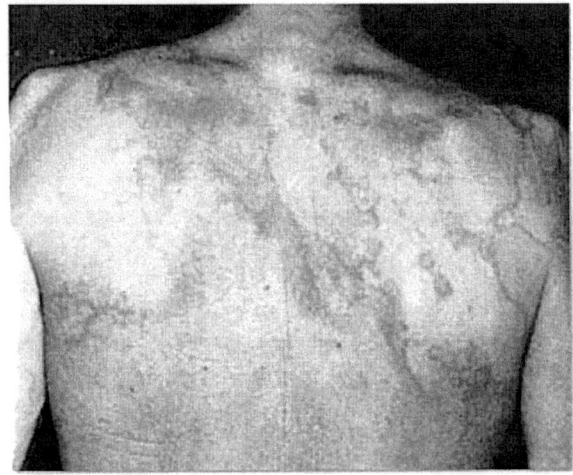

Course
- Rheumatic fever is reemerging
- Patients with pharyngitis should have a streptococcal screen
- Distinguished from rheumatoid arthritis by lack of joint deformities and a negative rheumatoid factor
- Most commonly affected valves: Mitral and aortic

Aortic Stenosis

Causes of Isolated AS

Age	Frequency of AS Patients	Status of Aortic Valve
< 50	7%	All either bicuspid or unicuspid
50–70	40%	67% bicuspid, 33% tricuspid
> 70	53%	40% bicuspid, 60% tricuspid

Bicuspid Aortic Valve
- Most common congenital cardiac anomaly (1 in 50 people)
- By age 45, half will have significant AS
- May be associated with ascending aortic aneurysm, so all patients with a bicuspid valve should have evaluation of the ascending aorta

Bicuspid Aortic Valve

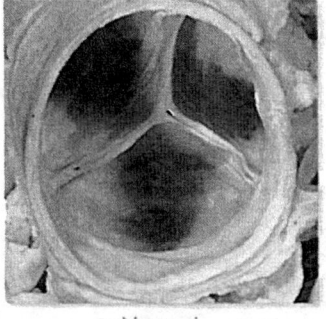

Normal

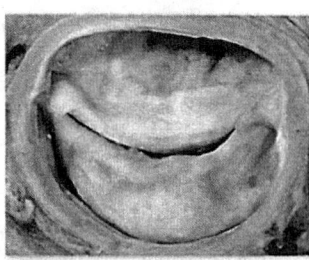

Bicuspid Valve with Severe AS

Bicuspid Aortic Valve

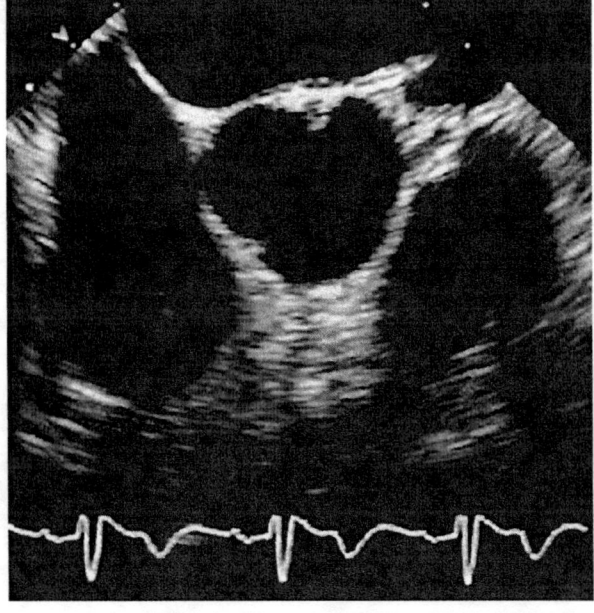

Senile Aortic Stenosis
- Trileaflet valves undergo degeneration in the 7th decade and later
- 80% men
- 25% of valvular heart disease

Course
- Long, asymptomatic latent period
- Symptoms often occur when the orifice size is reduced to 25% or less (orifice area < 0.7 cm^2; normal 2–4 cm^2)

Symptoms
- The average survival is:
  - 2 years with heart failure
  - 3 years with syncope
  - 5 years in patients with angina
- Sudden death occurs in 10% of patients, almost all of whom are symptomatic

Physical Examination
- Decreased rise time and volume in the carotid pulses (*pulsus parvus et tardus*)
- Systolic thrill or shudder in the carotids or the suprasternal notch
- 2nd heart sound paradoxically split or A_2 absent completely
- Murmur peaks after mid systole

Echo
- Most important test in valvular disease
- Echo can assess:
  - Chamber size
  - LV function
  - Valvular anatomy
  - Transvalvular gradients
  - Severity of regurgitant lesions
  - Pulmonary artery systolic pressure

Severe AS

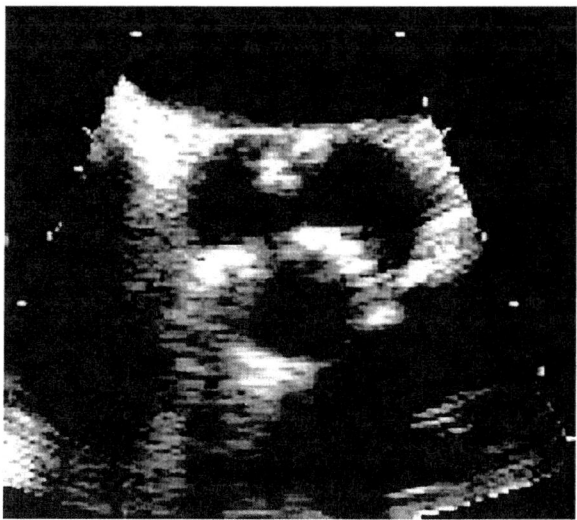

Cardiac Catheterization
- High prevalence of CAD mandates coronary angiography in patients with AS
- In severe AS, CAD is present in:
  - 33% of patients 40–59 years of age
  - 66% of patients > 60 years of age

Treatment
- Surgery is indicated in symptomatic patients with severe AS
- Most patients who have gradients of ≥ 50 mmHg are symptomatic
- Almost all sudden deaths occur in symptomatic patients
- AVR is often followed by dramatic improvement in LV function and symptoms

Transcatheter Therapy
- There are now prosthetic aortic valves that can be delivered by catheter-based systems
- These have been approved for patients with critical AS who are otherwise not candidates for surgery
- Survival is improved compared to medical therapy

AR 60
An 82 yo woman with a hip fracture is found to have severe AS on preoperative evaluation.
She reports progressive dyspnea over the past year, now occurring on activities of daily living.

What should be done next?
A. Refer to a skilled nursing facility, as it is too risky to perform hip surgery at any time.
B. Schedule cardiac catheterization in anticipation of aortic valve replacement.
C. Proceed with orthopedic surgery, but administer perioperative beta-blockers.
D. Proceed with surgery, but monitor the patient with a right-heart catheter.

Answer: _____

Chronic Aortic Regurgitation

Causes
- Congenital deformities
- Endocarditis
- Aortic root dilation (Marfan's, HTN)
- VSD
- Giant cell arteritis, relapsing polychondritis
- Syphilis
- Trauma

Course
- Long, asymptomatic latent period
- Exercise is well tolerated (as opposed to every other valvular disease) because of:
  - Peripheral vasodilation
  - Increased heart rate shortens diastole

Physical Examination
- Increased peripheral pulse pressure causes several examination findings
- High-pitched, blowing, decrescendo diastolic murmur at the lower left sternal border
- Murmur best heard when patient leans forward

Name	Physical Examination Finding
Watson's	"Water hammer" pulses
Corrigan's	Rapid rise and fall of pulses
De Musset's	Head bobbing
Quincke's	Pulsation of the nail beds
Traube's	Systolic and diastolic murmurs over the femoral arteries
Duroziez's	A double sound over the femorals when compresses distally
Lighthouse	Blanching and flushing of the forehead
Landolfi's	Constriction and dilation of the pupils
Becker's	Pulsation of the retinal arteries
Müller's	Undulation of the uvula
Mayen's	Drop in > 15 mmHg BP when arm is raised
Rosenbach's	Pulsatile liver
Gerhardt's	Enlarged spleen
Hill's	> 20 mmHg difference in popliteal and brachial pressures
Lincoln's	Pulsatile popliteal
Sherman's	Prominent dorsalis pedis pulse

Austin-Flint Murmur
- Low-pitched apical mid-diastolic rumble
- Caused by the AR jet hitting the anterior MV leaflet and forcing it into the posterior leaflet, causing functional mitral stenosis
- A systolic outflow murmur may occur, caused by the high velocity of blood through the aortic valve

Severe AR

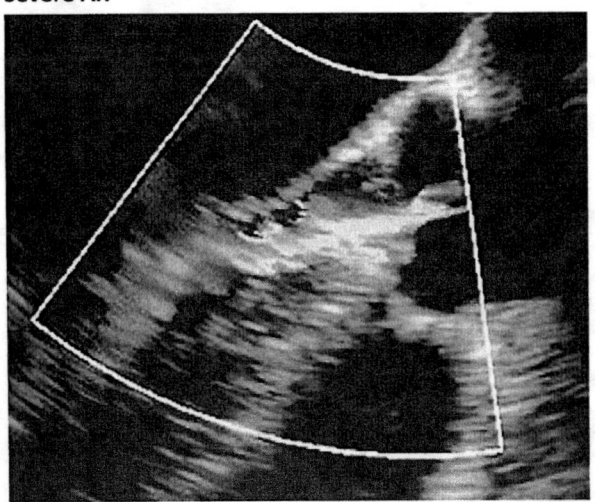

Indications for Surgery in Severe AR
- Symptomatic patients
- Asymptomatic patients
  - LVEF of < 50%
  - Other cardiac surgery already scheduled

AR 61
A 75 yo male with h/o hypercholesterolemia presents with intermittent chest pain that worsens with exertion and is accompanied by dyspnea and pre-syncope at times.

On physical exam, you detect a 2/6 crescendo systolic murmur best heard at the 2nd RICS but with radiation across the base.
Carotid pulses are low in amplitude and delayed.

Which of the following is true?
A. This patient has a benign "innocent" flow murmur.
B. This patient has classic signs of acute aortic regurgitation.
C. This patient will require cardiac catheterization.
D. This patient can undergo knee replacement surgery with no further workup.

Answer: _____

AR 62
A 50 yo female with h/o bicuspid aortic valve presents for annual exam and states she is asymptomatic.
On physical exam, you detect a 2/6 high-pitched, decrescendo diastolic murmur that is heard at the base and is heard even better when you ask her to lean forward.

You note that there is rapid rise and fall of her peripheral pulses. You also note a 2nd murmur on further auscultation, one which is best heard at the apex and resembles a low-pitched diastolic rumble.

Which diagnosis do you most suspect?
A. Mitral stenosis
B. Chronic aortic regurgitation
C. Chronic mitral regurgitation
D. Acute mitral regurgitation
E. Tricuspid stenosis

Answer: _____

Acute Aortic Regurgitation

Causes and Course
- Caused by:
  - Endocarditis
  - Trauma
  - Aortic dissection
- The sudden huge volume overload on the LV produces rapid decompensation, shock, and death

Acute AR — Endocarditis

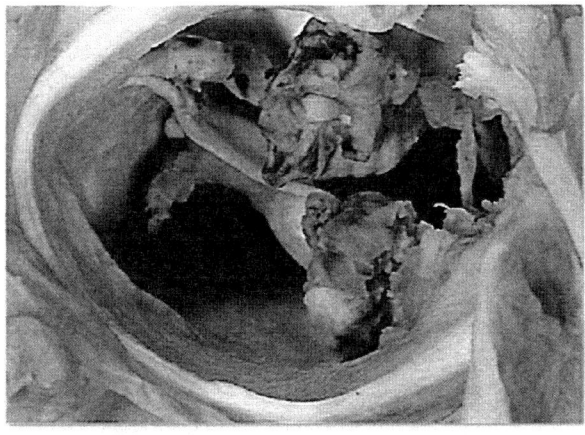

Physical Examination
- Tachycardia, hypotension, pulmonary edema, signs of vasoconstriction
- The murmur, if heard at all, is short, high-pitched, and decrescendo
- The bounding pulse pressure of chronic AR is not present

Diagnosis
- A high index of suspicion is needed in a patient who presents with shock and may possibly have 1 of the 3 causes
- Echocardiography, perhaps by TEE, is diagnostic

Treatment
- Urgent cardiothoracic surgical consult (!)
- Temporizing measures include positive inotropic therapy (dobutamine) and peripheral vasodilation (nitroprusside)

Mitral Stenosis

Cause
- Virtually always rheumatic in an adult
- Only 50% of patients remember an episode that could have been rheumatic fever

Course
- Two-thirds are female
- In temperate climates, there is a period of 10–20 years before symptoms appear
- The latent period is much shorter in tropical countries
- Often present with sudden onset of symptoms when atrial fibrillation occurs

Mitral Stenosis

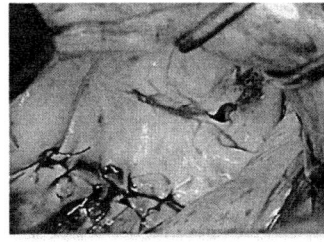
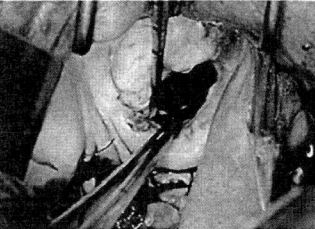

Post Commissurotomy

Course (cont.)
- Hemoptysis is fairly common in MS because of the very high pulmonary pressures
- Peripheral emboli, particularly stroke, occur in 20% of patients

Physical Examination
- An opening snap is heard at the apex
- S_1 may be loud
- A low-pitched diastolic rumble is heard at the apex with the bell
- Loud P_2 if pulmonary HTN

Diagnosis
- Diagnostic triad on chest x-ray:
  - Pulmonary artery revascularization
  - Large left atrium
  - Normal sized LV (!)
- Diagnosis and management are determined by echo, particularly TEE

Mitral Stenosis (cont.)

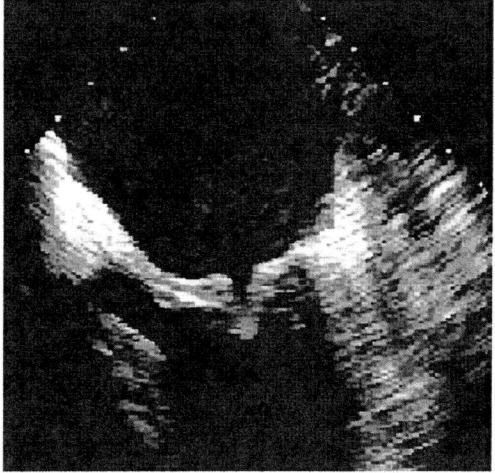

MS and Pregnancy
- May present with pulmonary edema at the onset of atrial fibrillation
- Cardioversion, procainamide, and verapamil are all safe during pregnancy

Treatment in Severe MS
Patients with any symptoms should have percutaneous mitral balloon commissurotomy (PMBC) or surgery (only if PMBC is not possible).

AR 63
A 33 yo woman presents with dyspnea and hemoptysis. Physical exam shows an irregularly irregular pulse, elevated JVP, loud P_2, and a diastolic murmur best at apex that has a low rumbling quality. Chest x-ray follows.

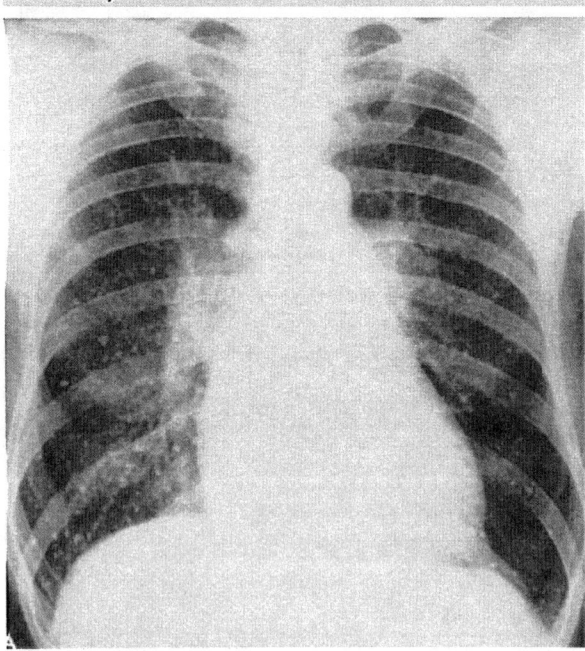

What is the diagnosis?
A. Acute AR
B. Chronic AR
C. Chronic MS
D. Bicuspid aortic valve with severe AS
E. Tricuspid stenosis

Answer: _____

AR 64
A 35 yo woman with known severe MS comes to the ED after the sudden onset of severe respiratory distress. Physical examination and chest x-ray show acute pulmonary edema.

What is the most likely cause of her sudden deterioration?
A. An acute viral pneumonia
B. Infective endocarditis of the mitral valve
C. Pulmonary hemorrhage
D. The onset of atrial fibrillation
E. Severe LV dysfunction

Answer: _____

Chronic Mitral Regurgitation

Causes
- Most common cause is LV dilation from CAD or HTN
- Other causes:
  - Rheumatic heart disease (more common in men)
  - Endocarditis
  - Various connective tissue and degenerative disorders, some represented by mitral valve prolapse
  - Ischemia of the papillary muscles

Severe MR

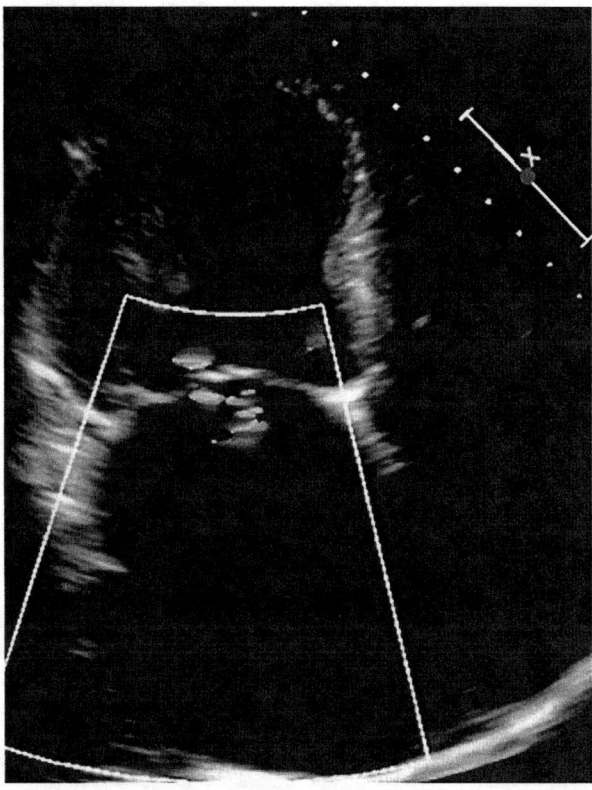

Physical Examination
- S_1 is soft
- The murmur is holosystolic and may be heard across precordium
- In severe MR, the aortic valve may close early, resulting in a widely split S_2
- S_3 is common in severe MR

AR 65
A 67 yo man presents with dyspnea.
Physical exam shows a soft S_1 and a holosystolic murmur that increases with handgrip.
The murmur does not change after an occasional premature beat.

What is the diagnosis?
A. Chronic MR
B. AS
C. Acute MR
D. Chronic AR
E. Hypertrophic obstructive cardiomyopathy

Answer: _____

AR 66
A 56 yo man presents with a holosystolic murmur.
Echo shows an LVEF of 50%, MVP, and severe MR.
He exercises for 4 minutes on a Bruce protocol, peak HR of 105 bpm, BP 130/80, stopping because of dyspnea.

What should be done next?
A. Dobutamine stress echo.
B. Observe for 6 more months.
C. Refer for mitral valve replacement.
D. Therapy with beta-blockers.

Answer: _____

Indications for Surgery in Severe Primary MR
- Symptomatic patients
  - LVEF > 30%

Surgery for Severe Secondary MR
- Persistent NYHA Class III–IV symptoms
- Otherwise, periodic monitoring and Tx of CAD, HF; Consider CRT

Mitral Valve Prolapse

AR 67
Mitral valve prolapse is identified on a routine echocardiogram.

What is the most common murmur associated with this condition?
A. Mid-diastolic rumble at the apex
B. Crescendo-decrescendo systolic murmur at the right sternal border
C. Blowing diastolic murmur at the lower left sternal border
D. Late systolic murmur at the apex

Answer: _____

Mild Form
- Very common: 10–20% of teenagers, mainly women, and 7% overall
- May or may not have clicks and murmurs
- There is no increase in conditions previously attributed to MVP, such as chest pain, dyspnea, panic attacks, etc.
- Tiny increase in stroke risk

Physical Examination
- There may be a midsystolic (not diastolic) click, which may be followed by a murmur
- The click becomes louder and moves earlier in systole with maneuvers that decrease LV volume, such as Valsalva or standing

Severe Form
- Congenital myxomatous degeneration of the chordae and mitral valve leaflets
- Some degree of chronic MR virtually certain
- Risk of acute MR from chordal rupture

Summary of MVP

Characteristic	Mild Form	Severe Form
Leaflets	May be slightly redundant	Thickened, redundant
Chordae	May be mildly elongated	Elongated, fragile
Population	Younger females	Men
Risk of chronic MR	Minimal	Virtually certain
Risk of acute MR	None	Moderate
Risk of endocarditis	Minimal	Small
Symptoms	None	Related to MR
Physical exam	May have click and murmur	MR murmur

Treatment
- The mild form does not require treatment
- MR, either chronic or acute, should be treated as in other causes of MR

Severe MVP

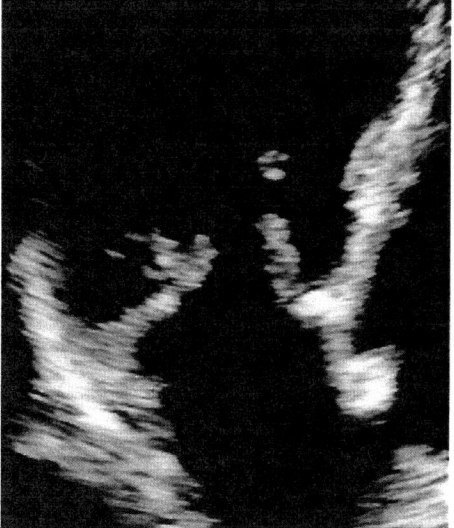

Cardiac Causes of Cerebral Embolic Events

Atrial fibrillation	45%
Acute MI	15%
LV aneurysm	10%
Mechanical valves	10%
Valvular heart disease, including endocarditis and MVP	10%
Other, including dilated cardiomyopathy and patent foramen ovale	10%

Acute Mitral Regurgitation

Causes and Course
- Causes:
  - Rupture of a myxomatous chordae
  - Endocarditis
  - Trauma
  - Acute ischemia of the papillary muscle
- Patients present with shock, like acute AR

Physical Examination
- Tachycardia, hypotension, pulmonary edema, signs of peripheral vasoconstriction
- The murmur, if heard at all, is short, early systolic, and a decrescendo

Treatment
- Urgent cardiothoracic surgical consult (!)
- Temporizing measures include positive inotropic therapy (dobutamine) and peripheral vasodilation (nitroprusside)

AR 68

A 72 yo female presents with an inferior STEMI. On her 3rd hospital day, you are called into her room because she suddenly sits upright in bed, gasping for air. You hear a new holosystolic murmur.

Which of the following should you do?
A. Call for an emergent cardiac cath.
B. Have the patient lie down and take deep breaths.
C. Obtain an emergent transthoracic echo and alert cardiac surgery.
D. Insert a transvenous pacemaker.

Answer: _____

Tricuspid Regurgitation

Causes
- Usually caused by whatever raises RV pressure and dilates the tricuspid annulus, including:
  - Left-heart failure
  - Chronic lung disease
  - Pulmonary emboli

- May be rheumatic, congenital, or from carcinoid
- IV drug abusers may develop tricuspid endocarditis, usually from *S. aureus*

Signs / Symptoms
- Severe TR can cause:
  - LE edema
  - Liver tenderness on palpation
  - Distended liver
  - Noticeable jugular venous pulsations
  - Abdominal distention
  - Fatigue

Physical Examination
- Large *v* waves in the neck
- Pulsatile liver
- Holosystolic murmur at the LLSB that increases with inspiration
- Other signs of pulmonary HTN are frequently present

Diagnosis
Echo defines the cause and the severity and can measure pulmonary systolic pressure.

Treatment
- Usually directed at the cause of pulmonary HTN
- Tricuspid valve removal may be necessary in endocarditis unresponsive to antibiotics
- Tricuspid annuloplasty using a metal ring may be appropriate with severe congestion

Severe TR

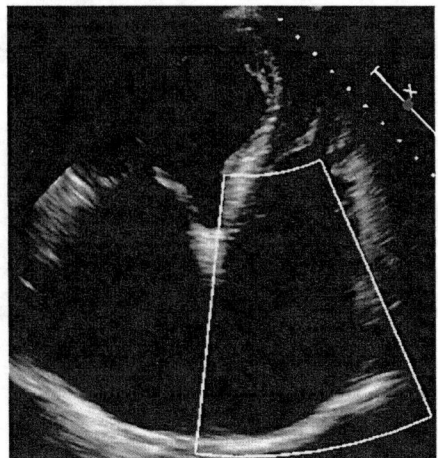

© 2017 MedStudy Internal Medicine Video Board Review – Cardiology • Matthew Sorrentino, MD

Pulmonic Stenosis

Causes
- Virtually always congenital
- Does not progress
- Usually not seen with other congenital defects, except Noonan syndrome
- May be seen in adults

PS — Symptoms & Signs
- Dyspnea
- Chest pain
- Syncope
- Cyanosis
- Abdominal distention
- Fatigue
- Sudden death

Physical Examination
- There may be a faint systolic murmur heard at the left sternal border/2nd LICS
- Usually there is a pulmonic ejection sound (remember, it gets softer on inspiration)
- Prominent a wave in the JVP

Diagnosis and Treatment
- Diagnosis is, of course, by echo
- Severe PS can be treated with balloon valvuloplasty

Ebstein Anomaly

Features
- Echo shows a redundant tricuspid leaflet arising lower in the ventricle than normal
- The RA, therefore, appears to be huge
- A TR murmur and a "sail" sound may be heard
- Frequently associated with PSVT or the WPW syndrome

AR 69
A 24 yo male presents with dyspnea.
He tells you he has "some" history of congenital heart disease but does not know what. On exam, you believe you detect a 1/6 systolic murmur at the 2nd LICS.

Which of the following would greatly increase your suspicion for pulmonic stenosis?
A. An accompanying holosystolic murmur at the apex
B. A flapping "sail" sound at the LLSB
C. The presence of WPW pattern on 12-lead ECG
D. An ejection sound at the 2nd LICS that gets softer upon inspiration

Answer: _____

Systolic Murmurs and Response to Maneuvers

	Post PVC	Valsalva	Handgrip	Standing	Squatting
AS	↑	↓	↓	↓	↑
MR	NC	↓	↑	↓	↑
HOCM	↑	↑	↓	↑	↓

AR 70
A 50 yo male presents with chest pain, dyspnea on exertion, and 1 recent episode of syncope. On physical exam, you detect a 2/6 systolic murmur best heard at the base, particularly the 2nd RICS. The murmur diminishes in intensity with Valsalva maneuver.

Which of the following should be in this patient's future?
A. Septal reduction surgery for HCM
B. Aortic valve replacement for bicuspid aortic valve
C. Mitral valve replacement for mitral stenosis.
D. EP study for WPW syndrome

Answer: _____

Valvular Surgery

General Principles
- Valve surgery, even though the mortality is high, is usually better than no surgery for patients who are symptomatic at rest
- Mitral valve repair for MR is preferable to replacement (decreased surgical mortality and better LV preservation)

Bioprosthetic and Mechanical Valves

	Bioprosthetic Valve	Mechanical Valve
Requires anticoagulation?	Usually not	Yes
Durability	10–15 years, less in dialysis patients and the young	Indefinite
Indications	• Chronic bleeding problem • Life expectancy < 5–10 years • Pregnancy • Pt preference re: anticoag	Everything else

Follow-up of Surgery
- Prognosis related to:
  - LVEF (of course)
  - Symptoms
  - Type of surgery (repair better than replacement)
- Echo is the best tool for following patients

AR 71

A 60 yo asymptomatic male presents with findings
of chronic MR on exam.
Echo shows severe MR and an LVEF of 50%.

What should you do next?

A. Prescribe an ACEI and see the patient in 6 months.
B. Refer for surgery now.
C. Perform an exercise stress test and refer for surgery
   if the LVEF falls.
D. Prescribe no medications and see the patient
   in 6 months.

Answer: _____

AR 72

A 26 yo IV drug user presents with dyspnea, fever,
and chills.
On exam, T is 102.3° F (39.1° C), and BP 110/60 mmHg.
He has large v waves in the JVP, a faint holosystolic
murmur at the LLSB that gets louder on inspiration,
and a few scattered rhonchi in his lung fields.

What is the diagnosis?

A. Endocarditis of the tricuspid valve
B. Endocarditis of the aortic valve
C. Endocarditis of the mitral valve
D. *Pneumocystis* pneumonia
E. *Cryptococcus* pneumonia

Answer: _____

AR 73

A 53 yo man presents with sudden onset of severe dyspnea.

In the ED, his BP is 70/30 mmHg, HR 156 bpm, T 97.0° F (36.1° C), and he is in severe respiratory distress.

JVP is elevated to the jaw in the sitting position; He has a faint apical systolic murmur and diffuse pulmonary crackles.

Troponin obtained at presentation is negative and other basic labs are normal.

His ECG and chest x-ray follow.

An echocardiogram is obtained.

ECG

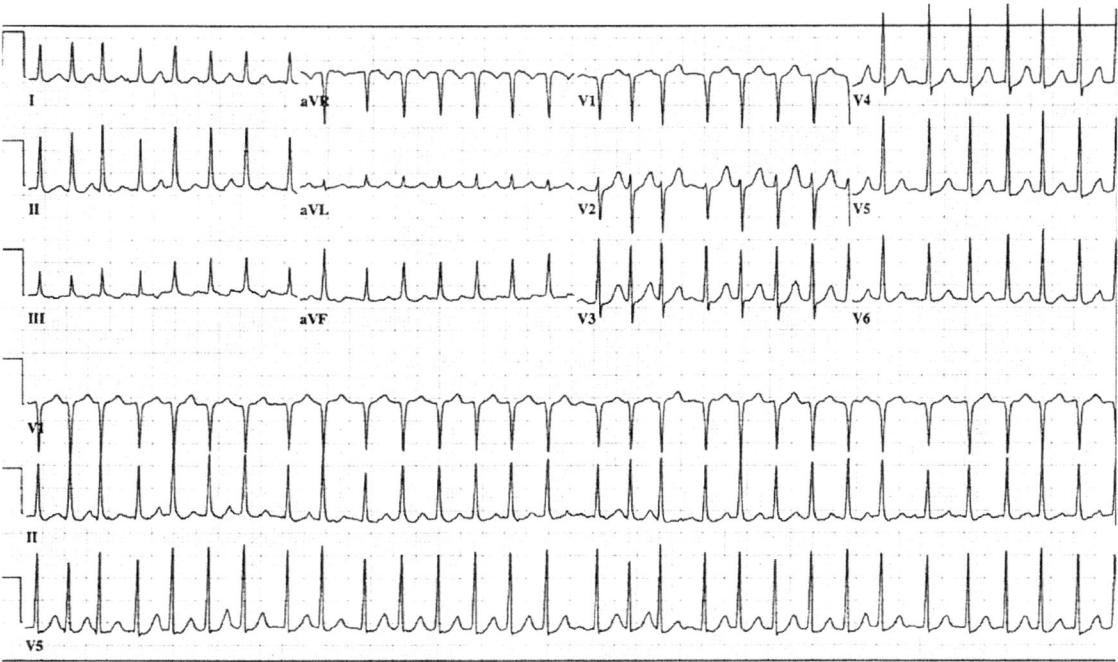

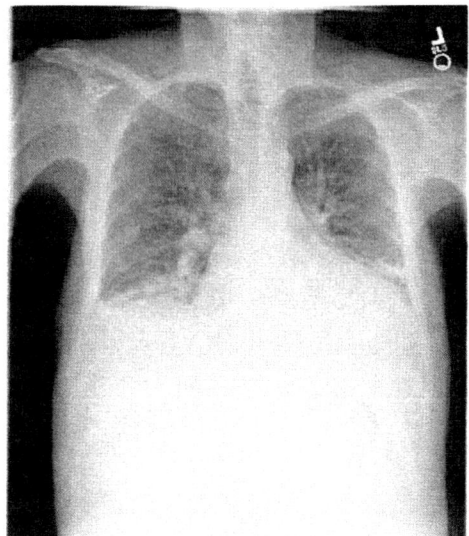

What is the diagnosis?

A. An acute anteroseptal STEMI
B. Acute tricuspid regurgitation
C. Acute MR due to chordal rupture
D. Acute aortic regurgitation
E. Pulmonary embolism

Answer: _____

AR 74

We have gone back in time to Paris in 1839 to the home of poet Alfred de Musset. M. de Musset is telling his companion, writer George Sand, that he could tell where the prostitutes were in Paris by listening to their earrings tinkle as their heads bobbed.

Which of the following physical examination findings would these ladies of the evening have?
A. Decreased rise time and volume in the carotid pulses
B. Low-pitched diastolic rumble at the apex
C. Late-peaking systolic ejection murmur in the 2nd right intercostal space
D. Slow y descent in the jugular pulse
E. Paradoxically split S_2

Answer: _____

AR 75

Which one of the following cardiac conditions tolerates exercise best?
A. AR
B. AS
C. MS
D. Hypertrophic cardiomyopathy
E. Eisenmenger syndrome

Answer: _____

AR 76

An 85 yo man reports several recent episodes
of exertional syncope and dyspnea.
Physical exam shows a normal carotid pulse, a single S_2,
and a long late-peaking systolic murmur at the right
2nd intercostal space.
His ECG follows.

ECG

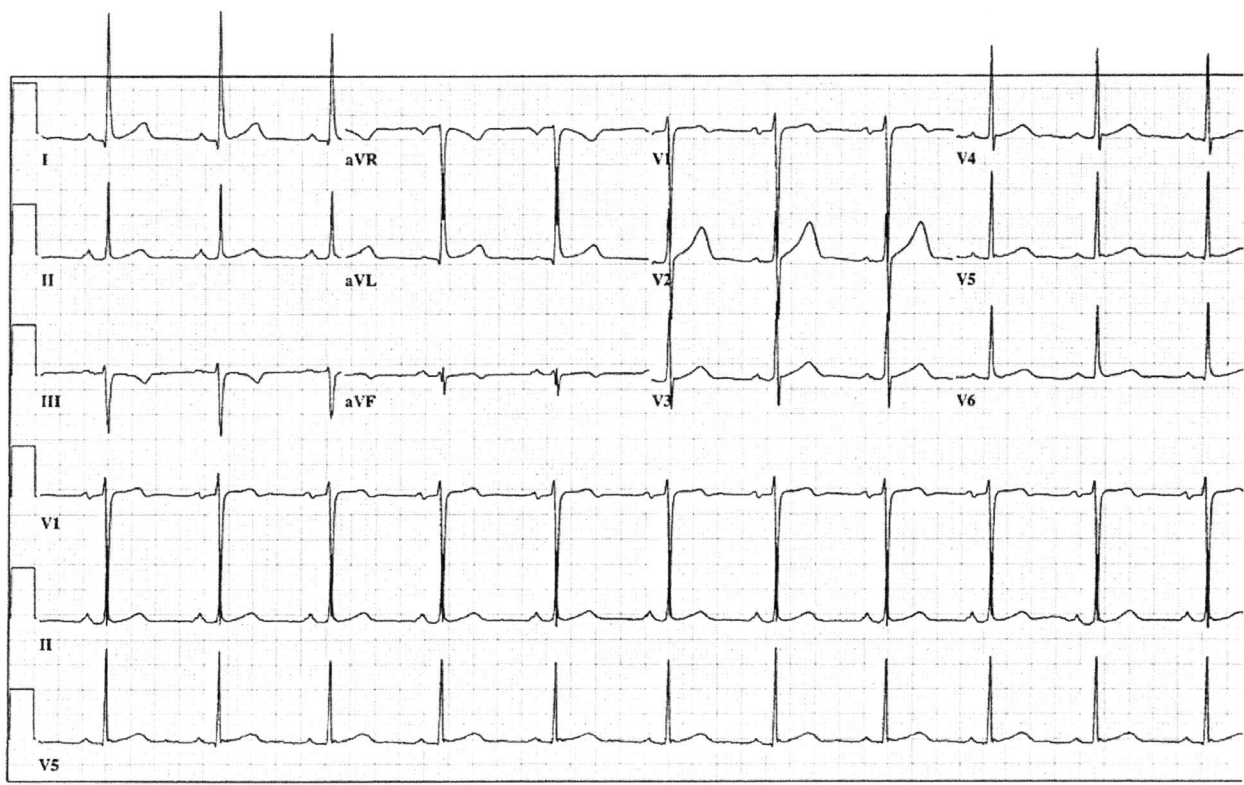

Which of the following statements is true?
A. Sudden death occurs in this condition.
B. The murmur would become louder
   with the Valsalva maneuver.
C. Treatment with an ACE inhibitor is indicated.
D. Conservative therapy is indicated for this very elderly
   patient.
E. If surgery were contemplated, echo alone would
   provide sufficient information.

Answer: _____

Part 6:
Heart Failure

**Classification of Heart Failure
by Hemodynamic Abnormality**

Diastolic Heart Failure
- About 30% of heart failure
- Characterized by impaired LV relaxation
  and an elevated LVEDP
- The elevated LVEDP causes increased left atrial
  and pulmonary capillary pressures

- Fluid leaks from the pulmonary capillaries, causing
  pulmonary edema and dyspnea
- Systolic performance is initially normal or
  hyperdynamic, but later falls
- Examples include hypertensive heart disease, HCM,
  and diabetic cardiomyopathy

High-Output Systolic Heart Failure
- Pure forms of systolic heart failure are uncommon and are characterized by:
  - Low LVEDP
  - Normal or hyperdynamic LV function
  - Tachycardia
  - Increased cardiac output

Causes of High-Output Failure

Peripheral shunting	Large AV fistulas Hepatic hemangiomas Paget disease
Decreased peripheral resistance	Gram-negative sepsis
Other causes of increased demand	Hyperthyroidism Beriberi Carcinoid Anemia

Systolic Heart Failure
- Systolic failure involves both decreased systolic function and an elevated LVEDP
- Decreased forward output causes weakness, fatigue, and fluid retention

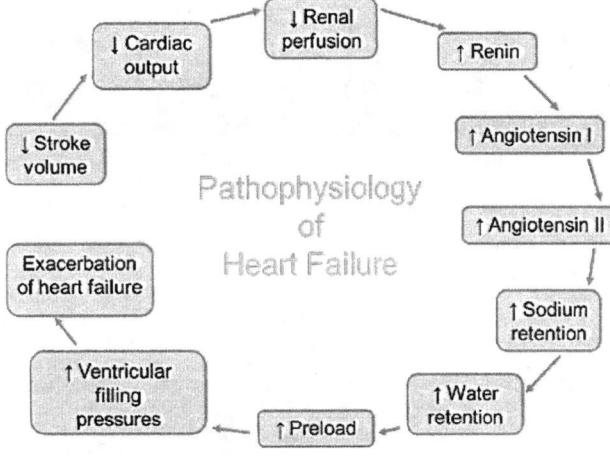

Pathophysiology of Heart Failure

Causes of Systolic Heart Failure

Coronary disease	40%
Dilated cardiomyopathy	30%
Valvular disease	15%
Hypertensive heart disease	10%
Restrictive cardiomyopathy	< 1%

Demographics
- Most expensive medical problem in the U.S.
- Most common diagnosis in hospitalized elderly patients

Mortality in HF
- 50% die with progressive heart failure
- 40% die of sudden death (VT/VF)
- **LVEF is the best predictor of prognosis (!)**
- Exercise tolerance does not predict outcome

Other Markers of Poor Outcome
- Low serum sodium
- High BUN
- Low potassium
- High or low magnesium
- High catecholamine levels

Summary

Type of HF	LVEDP	LVEF	Cardiac Output	Clinical Examples
Diastolic	High	Normal or increased	Normal	HTN HCM
"Pure" Systolic	Low	Normal or increased	Increased	AV fistula Anemia Hyperthyroidism Sepsis
Systolic	High	Decreased	Decreased	CAD Dilated cardiomyopathy Late HTN

Classification of Heart Failure by Myocardial Abnormality

Myocardial Abnormalities
- Ischemic
- Hypertensive
- Dilated
- Restrictive
- Hypertrophic

Ischemic Cardiomyopathy
- Caused by coronary disease
- Most common cause of systolic heart failure

© 2017 MedStudy Internal Medicine Video Board Review – Cardiology • Matthew Sorrentino, MD

Ischemic Cardiomyopathy

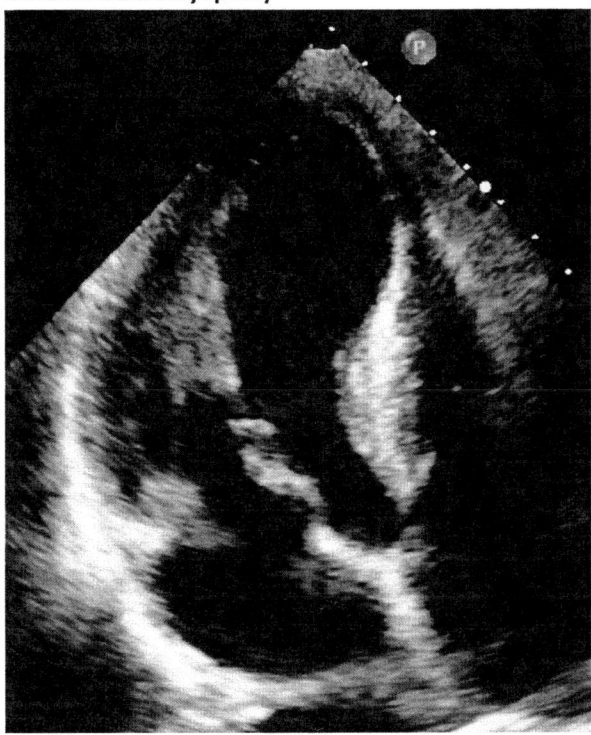

Hypertensive Cardiomyopathy
- Chronic HTN causes LVH, which increases LV stiffness and elevates LVEDP
- Systolic function may be normal, hyperdynamic, or, eventually, decreased
- Eventually leads to systolic failure and, at end-stage, a dilated cardiomyopathy

Severe LVH

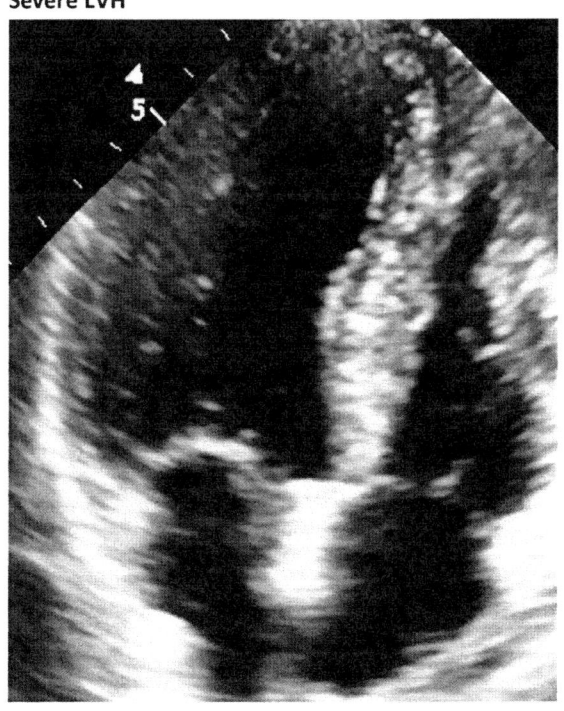

Dilated Cardiomyopathy
- 50% are idiopathic, presumably post viral
- Other causes include alcohol, cocaine, inhaled glue, chemotherapy, late hemochromatosis, and selenium and carnitine deficiencies

Dilated Cardiomyopathy

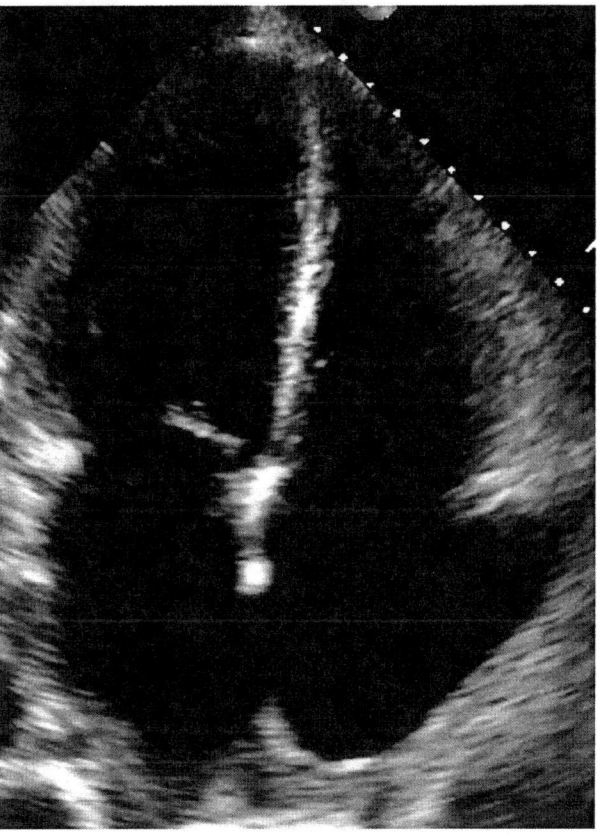

Peripartum Dilated Cardiomyopathy
- Occurs from the beginning of the 3rd trimester to 6 months postpartum
- Predilection for older women and African Americans
- About 2/3 resolve spontaneously
- Increased risk of recurrence with subsequent pregnancies

Takotsubo Cardiomyopathy
- Also known as "stress-induced cardiomyopathy" or "apical ballooning syndrome"
- Clinical presentation similar to MI, but clean cors
- Caused by extreme emotional or physical stress
- Often Sx of HF acutely
- More common in women; usually reversible

Takotsubo Cardiomyopathy (cont.)

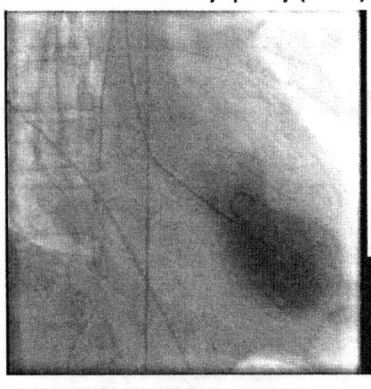
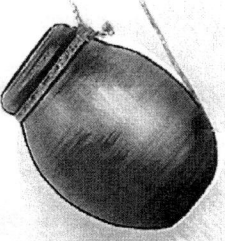

Restrictive Cardiomyopathy
- Caused by infiltrative diseases, such as amyloid and sarcoidosis
- Presents with signs of left- and right-heart failure, initially from diastolic dysfunction, but later from systolic failure

Echo Findings in Cardiomyopathies

Cardiomyopathy	Echo Appearance
Ischemic	Segmental wall motion abnormalities
Hypertensive	Concentric LVH
Dilated	4-chamber cardiac enlargement
Restrictive	Enlarged atria, normal ventricles

Diagnosis and Treatment of Restrictive Cardiomyopathy
- Must be differentiated from constrictive pericarditis (see that section)
- Treatment is standard heart failure care
- Once there is cardiac involvement, prognosis is very poor

Management of the Heart Failure Patient

Initial Lab Data
- CBC, U/A, electrolytes, BUN, creatinine, fasting glucose, HbA1c, lipid profile, liver function tests, TSH
- ECG
- Chest x-ray
- Transthoracic echo

ANP and BNP
- Atrial natriuretic peptide (ANP) and brain natriuretic peptide (BNP) are secreted in response to atrial stretch
- Increase excretion of salt and water, cause vasodilation, and inhibit the effects of aldosterone

BNP Levels
- BNP levels correlate roughly with the severity of heart failure and have moderate prognostic value
- BNP levels decrease in most patients with treatment of heart failure and can be useful in management

BNP
- Because BNP is excreted by the kidneys, the assay is not as helpful in patients with any degree of renal failure
- May be elevated in other causes of atrial stretch, such as lung disease
- BNP may not be elevated in patients with substantial obesity

Coronary Revascularization
"Coronary arteriography should be performed in patients presenting with HF who have angina or significant ischemia unless the patient is not eligible for revascularization of any kind."
Source: 2013 Focused Update: ACCF/AHA Guidelines for the Diagnosis and Management of Heart Failure in Adults

Stage A
- Patients at risk for heart failure but without structural heart disease, including:
  - HTN
  - Atherosclerotic disease
  - Diabetes
  - Metabolic syndrome
  - Using cardiotoxins
  - Family history of cardiomyopathy
  - Obesity

Therapy — Stage A
- Goals
  - Treat HTN
  - Smoking cessation
  - Treat lipid disorders
  - Encourage exercise, weight loss
  - Discourage alcohol/illicit drug use
  - Control metabolic syndrome
- Drugs
  - ACE inhibitors or ARBs

Stage B
- Patients with structural heart disease but without symptoms or signs of heart failure:
  - Previous MI
  - LV remodeling including LVH and low LVEF
  - Asymptomatic valvular heart disease

Therapy — Stage B
- Goals
  - All measures under Stage A
- Drugs
  - ACE inhibitors or ARBs
  - Beta-blockers
- Devices in selected patients
  - Implantable defibrillators

Stage C
- Patients with structural heart disease with prior or current symptoms of heart failure:
  - Known structural heart disease
  - Dyspnea, fatigue, and decreased exercise tolerance

Therapy — Stage C
- Goals
  - All measures under Stages A and B
  - Dietary salt restriction
- Drugs
  - Diuretics for fluid retention
  - ACE inhibitors
  - Beta-blockers
- Drugs in selected patients
  - Aldosterone antagonist
  - ARBs
  - Digitalis
  - Hydralazine/Nitrates
- Devices in selected patients
  - Resynchronization therapy
  - Implantable defibrillators

Stage D
- Patients with marked symptoms at rest in spite of maximal medical therapy:
  - Frequently hospitalized
  - Unable to be discharged without special interventions

Therapy — Stage D
- Goals
  - Appropriate measures under Stages A, B, and C
  - Decision regarding end-of-life issues
- Options
  - Compassionate end-of-life/hospice care
  - Extraordinary measures
    - Heart transplant
    - Chronic inotropes
    - Permanent mechanical support
    - Experimental drugs or surgery

Treatment of the Underlying Cause
- Ischemic — revascularize viable myocardium
- Hypertensive — treating HTN is effective
- Dilated — few are treatable; Stop EtOH
- Hypertrophic — septal ablation, transplant (when/if appropriate)
- Restrictive — usually no therapy works

Treatment of the Precipitating Cause
- Inappropriate reduction of therapy
- Dietary indiscretion
- Ischemia or infarction
- Arrhythmias (atrial fib)
- Systemic infection
- Pulmonary embolism
- Physical, environmental, or emotional stress
- High-output states (anemia)
- Poorly controlled HTN
- A new, unrelated illness
- Administration of a cardiac depressant drug
- Acquiring a 2nd form of heart disease
- Surgical procedure

NYHA Class
- Class I: Dyspnea only with extraordinary physical exertion; No limitation of physical activity
- Class II: Dyspnea with ordinary physical activity/exertion
- Class III: Dyspnea with less-than-ordinary exertion; Comfortable at rest
- Class IV: Dyspnea at rest

AR 77
A 35 yo male with a BMI of 40.0 kg/m^2 presents for annual visit.
BP is 130/80 mmHg; ECG is normal and he is asymptomatic.

Which of the following is true?
A. He has Stage A heart failure.
B. He has Stage B heart failure.
C. He has Stage C heart failure.
D. He has Stage D heart failure.
E. He does not have any stage of heart failure by current guidelines.

Answer: _____

AR 78
An 84 yo female with a history of systolic heart failure presents for routine follow-up. She states that she has symptoms of dyspnea and fatigue when getting up from her sofa and walking to the front door to let her dogs out. She is perfectly comfortable at rest, though.

What is her NYHA Class?
A. Class I
B. Class II
C. Class III
D. Class IV
E. She obviously doesn't have heart failure.

Answer: _____

AR 79

Which of the following combinations of medications has been shown to prolong survival in Class III–IV heart failure?

Medication	Choice 1	Choice 2	Choice 3	Choice 4
Digoxin	Yes	No	No	Yes
Spironolactone	No	Yes	Yes	No
Amlodipine	Yes	No	No	Yes
ACE inhibitors	No	Yes	Yes	Yes
Beta-blockers	Yes	Yes	No	Yes

A. Medication combination 1
B. Medication combination 2
C. Medication combination 3
D. Medication combination 4

Answer: _____

Medical Therapy of Heart Failure

Medications Known to Prolong Survival

Medication	Comments
ACE inhibitors	1st line vasodilator therapy for all patients
ARBs	Acceptable alternative in ACEI-intolerant patients
Hydralazine/ nitrates	Acceptable alternative vasodilator therapy; Should be added to ACEI therapy for patients of African descent
Beta-blockers	Bisoprolol, carvedilol, or sustained-release metoprolol for all patients except NYHA class IV
Spironolactone or eplerenone	For patients with increased preload and creatinine < 2.5 mg/dL and potassium < 5.0 mEq/L
ARNIs	Valsartan/sacubitril; For long-term treatment of chronic systolic heart failure; Trial showed benefit at EF ≤ 40%

Valsartan / Sacubitril
- First-in-class (ARNI)
- PARADIGM-HF trial
  - Over 8,000 patients with EF 40% or less
  - Reduction in mortality and HF hospitalizations as compared with enalapril
- Indicated for NYHA Class II–IV with reduced EF
- Do not use ACE or other ARB in combo

Medications for Symptom Control

Medication	Comments
Loop diuretics	For relief of dyspnea and peripheral edema, and for hypoxia due to pulmonary edema
Digoxin	May be useful for symptomatic patients with LVEF < 35%; Complex side-effect profile
Antiarrhythmic drugs	For control of symptomatic arrhythmias; May be proarrhythmic
Positive inotropes (dobutamine, dopamine, milrinone)	For selected refractory Stage D patients as palliation

Not Recommended
- Routine combined use of ACEI and ARB
- Routine use of calcium channel blockers
- Hormonal therapies
- Nutritional supplements

ICDs
- Indicated in nonischemic dilated cardiomyopathy <u>or</u> ischemic cardiomyopathy at least 40 days post-MI
- LVEF ≤ 35% on chronic medical therapy
- Life expectancy of at least 1 year

Resynchronization Therapy
- Indicated in patients with LVEF ≤ 35%
- Functional class II–III or ambulatory IV despite good medical therapy
- QRS duration ≥ 120 msec
- Usually in combination with an ICD

Other Therapies for Selected Patients
- Follow-up in a heart failure clinic
- Cardiac rehabilitation whenever possible
- Left ventricular assist devices
- Cardiac transplantation (survival 65% at 5 years and 55% at 10 years)

AR 80A

A 73 yo woman presents with increasing fatigue and peripheral edema.
Proteinuria was discovered on urinalysis.
Tongue photo follows.
ECG follows.

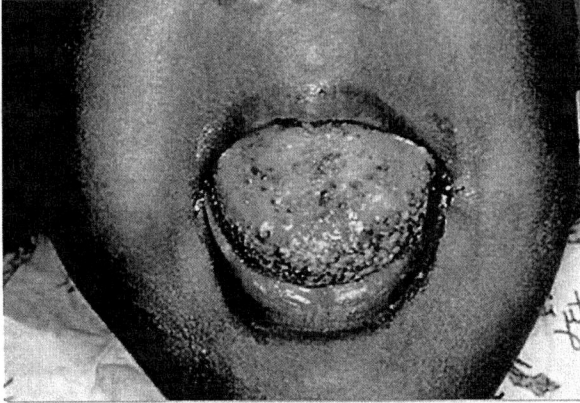

ECG

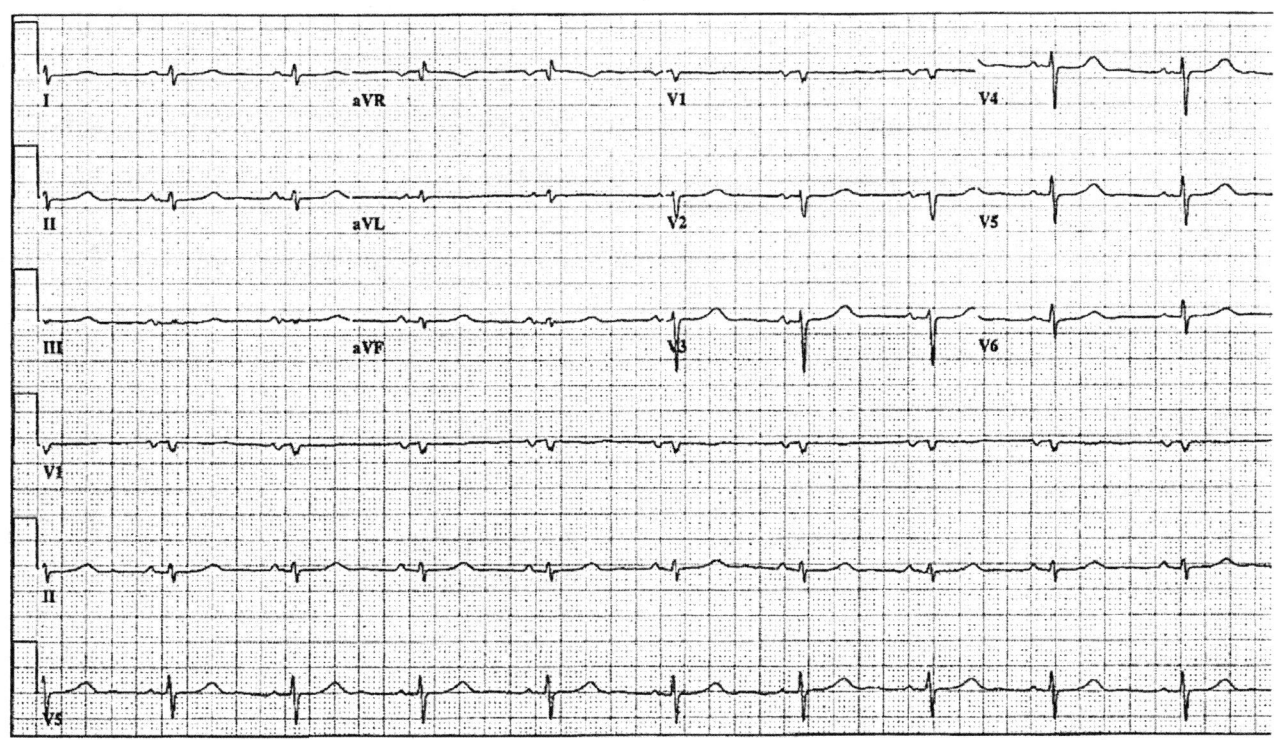

AR 80A (cont.)

What is the likely diagnosis?

A. Leprosy
B. Chagas disease
C. Severe COPD
D. Kawasaki disease
E. Amyloidosis

Answer: _____

AR 80B

What kind of cardiomyopathy does this disease cause?

A. Ischemic cardiomyopathy
B. Idiopathic dilated cardiomyopathy
C. Restrictive cardiomyopathy
D. Constrictive cardiomyopathy
E. Hypertensive cardiomyopathy

Answer: _____

Right-Heart Failure

- Usually from pulmonary HTN from left-heart failure or lung disease
- Multiple pulmonary emboli
- RV infarction
- If there are signs of right-heart failure and equalization of pressures in all 4 chambers, think of constriction or tamponade

The Hospitalized HF Patient

Initial Evaluation

- Determine if the event represents new or an exacerbation of chronic HF
- Rule out acute coronary syndrome
- Consider adequacy of systemic perfusion
- Determine volume status
- Consider precipitating factors of HF
- Chest x-ray, echo

Therapy

- Oxygen
- Loop diuretics to relieve symptoms and to reduce excess extracellular volume
- Daily intake and output and weights
- Daily electrolytes, BUN, and creatinine

Acute Pulmonary Edema

- 100% O_2, IV furosemide, morphine
- Stat echo; Direct treatment to the cause (!)
- Cardiovert tachyarrhythmias (atrial fib, atrial flutter, VT, VF)
- Intubate and ventilate if necessary

Hypertrophic Cardiomyopathy

Pathophysiology
- Disordered myocytes in the region of the hypertrophy, especially in the upper ventricular septum
- Other areas than the septum can be affected; Asians frequently have an apical form
- Occasionally presents as concentric LVH

Evaluation
- Symptoms include dyspnea, chest pain, or exercise-induced syncope
- Echocardiography is diagnostic
- The severity of the LV outflow gradient is not related to the risk of sudden death

Course
- Associated with sudden cardiac death (VT/VF), especially in exercising young people
- An ambulatory ECG that shows VT indicates a high risk for sudden death
- Atrial fibrillation is common because of high LVEDP

Physical Examination
- Harsh nonradiating midsystolic aortic murmur
- Murmur is louder with maneuvers that decrease LV volume (e.g., Valsalva)
- Carotid pulse has a rapid upstroke and is bifid in 2/3 of patients (as opposed to AS)
- Apical impulse may be double or triple

Maneuvers and Systolic Murmurs

	Post PVC	Valsalva	Handgrip	Standing	Squatting
AS	↑	↓	↓	↓	↑
MR	NC	↓	↑	↓	↑
HCM	↑	↑	↓	↑	↓

ECG
- If patients have septal hypertrophy, there may be inferolateral Q waves because of the thick septum
- The precordial lead voltage is usually high in the area of the hypertrophy

Echo

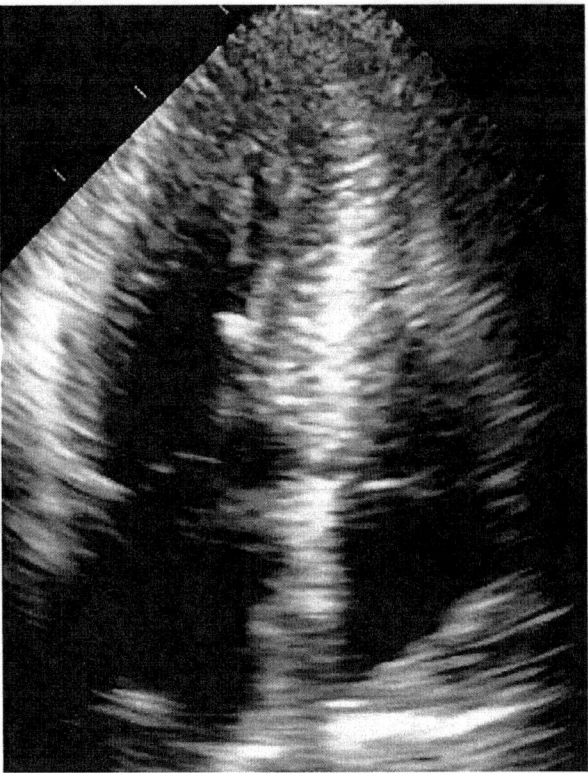

© 2017 MedStudy Internal Medicine Video Board Review – Cardiology • Matthew Sorrentino, MD

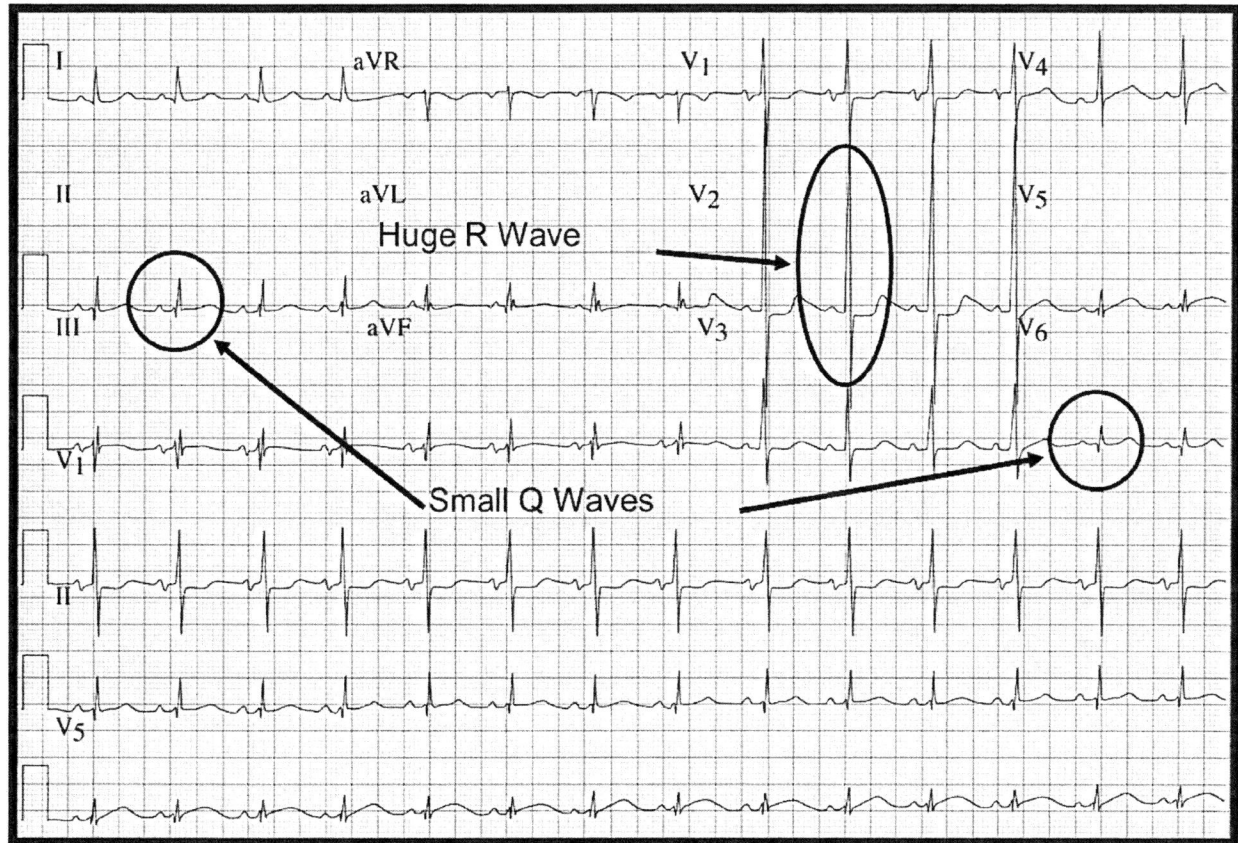

ECG labels: Huge R Wave, Small Q Waves

Therapy
- Beta-blockers, verapamil
- Resynchronization therapy
- Septal myomectomy
- Antiarrhythmic therapy (amiodarone) for symptomatic VT or atrial fibrillation
- No drug prolongs survival

- Decreasing ventricular volume (diuretics, nitrates, dehydration) is potentially dangerous
- Implantable defibrillators have been shown to reduce the incidence of sudden death
- No ultimate cure except heart transplant

Sudden Cardiac Death in Exercising Young People

HCM	36%
Coronary anomalies	19%
Cardiac hypertrophy	10%
Ruptured aorta	5%
Intramyocardial course of the LAD	5%
Aortic stenosis	4%
Others	17%

AR 81

A 43 yo man complains of intermittent palpitations and increasing dyspnea. He has a family history of premature sudden cardiac death.
He is found to have a systolic murmur that becomes softer on passive leg raising and deep inspiration and louder during the strain phase of the Valsalva maneuver.

What is 1st line symptomatic medical therapy for this condition?

A. Beta-blockers
B. ACE inhibitors
C. Neprilysin inhibitor
D. Pentoxifylline
E. Clopidogrel

Answer: _____

Pericardial Diseases

Nonconstrictive Pericarditis

Causes
- 90% idiopathic, presumably post viral, and often preceded by URI or gastroenteritis

- TB
- Connective tissue diseases
- Sepsis
- Uremia
- Cancer
- Post-MI (Dressler syndrome)
- Post cardiac surgery
- Procainamide
- Hydralazine

Dressler Syndrome and Post Cardiac Surgery
- These are caused by an autoimmune process and occur 1–2 weeks after the event
- Be sure to r/o new MI, pulmonary embolism, endocarditis, and postoperative infection

Acute Pericarditis
- Present with severe (usually pleuritic) chest pain, relieved by sitting forward
- Fever and tachycardia are common
- If present, a friction rub is diagnostic
- ECG usually shows diffuse ST elevation and PR segment depression, particularly in lead II

- CKMB/troponin may be slightly elevated if there is concomitant myocarditis
- Pericarditis should be differentiated from acute MI, as fibrinolytic therapy in the former could cause acute tamponade
- If in doubt, an echo would show a wall motion abnormality in acute MI

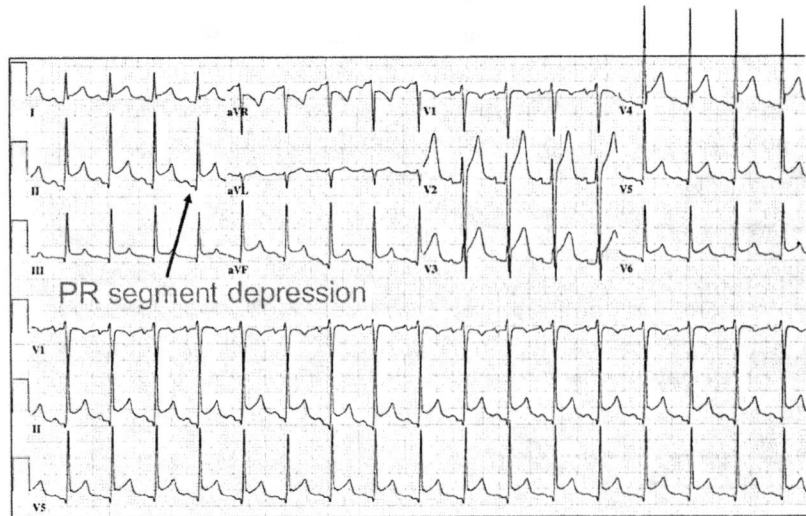

PR segment depression

Management
- Immediate therapy is high-dose ASA or NSAIDs
- Corticosteroids (used in the past) have been shown to increase the frequency of relapse
- Colchicine has emerged as the treatment of choice to prevent recurrent pericarditis

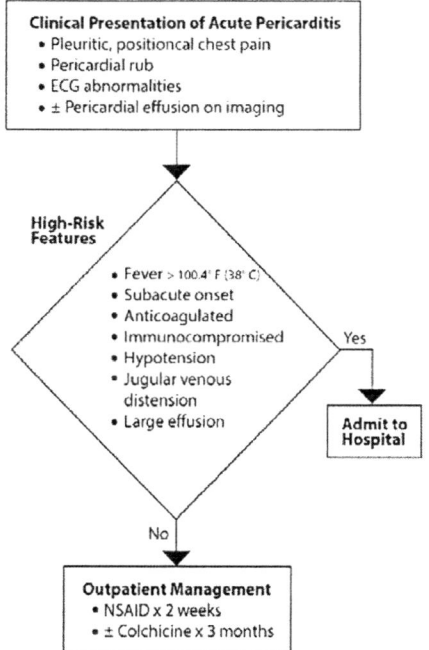

Source: AHA *Circulation*. 2013;127:1723–1726.

Constrictive Pericarditis

Causes
- 50% of cases in this country are idiopathic, presumably post viral
- In developing countries, TB is still the most common cause
- Other causes include cardiothoracic surgery, radiotherapy, and coccidiomycosis

Constrictive vs. Restrictive Cardiomyopathy
- Constriction and restrictive cardiomyopathy share many features
- It is imperative to differentiate these two, as the former is treatable with surgery (pericardial stripping)

Constrictive Pericarditis
- Kussmaul sign — an inspiratory rise in the jugular venous pulse
- Large, rapid x and y descents
- Pericardial knock in early diastole (just after S_2)

- Calcification of the pericardium on chest x-ray (particularly if TB is the cause)
- Thickened pericardium on CT or MR

Thickened Pericardium — MR

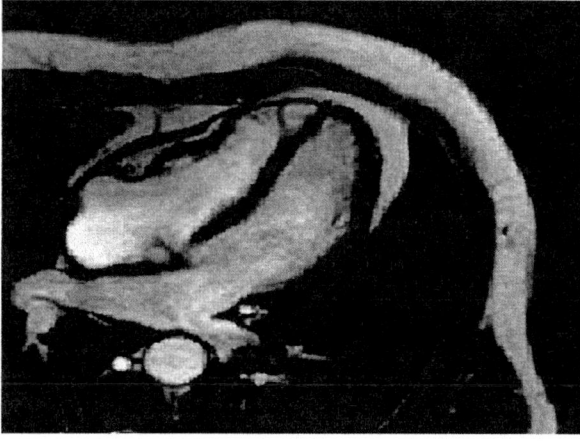

Thickened Pericardium — CT

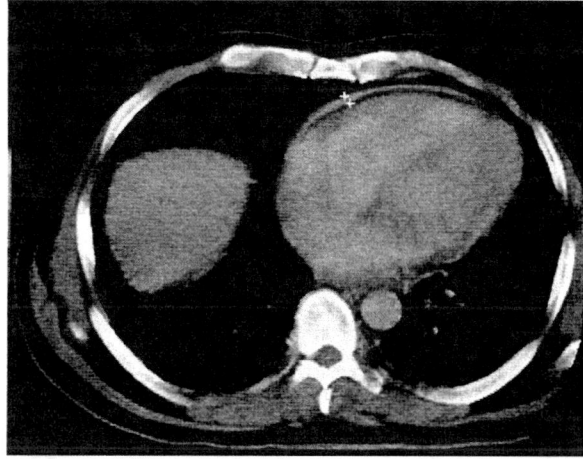

Pericardial Calcification — CT

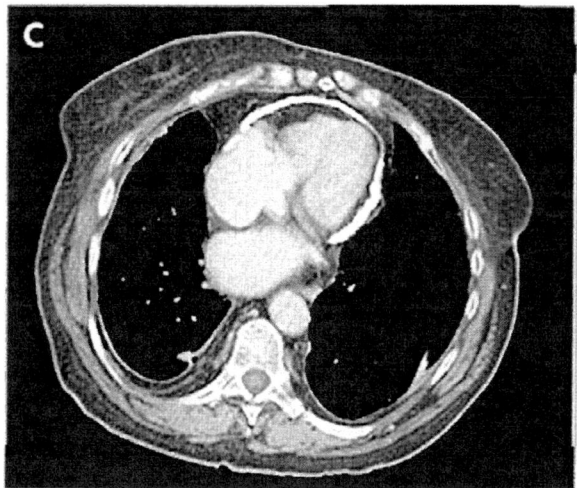

Calcification on Chest X-ray

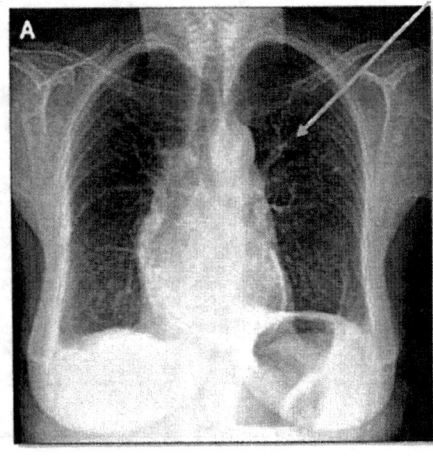
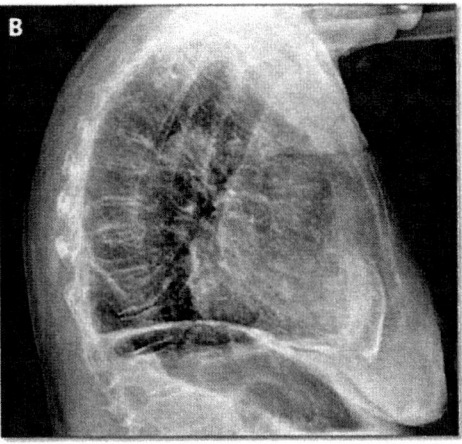

Right Atrial Pressure

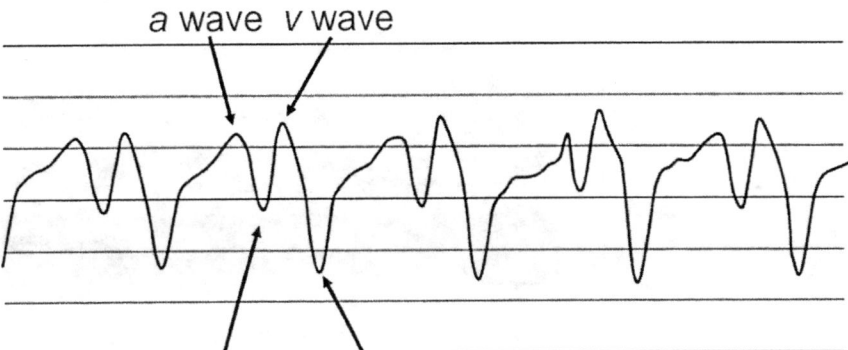

50

a wave v wave

x descent   y descent

0 mm Hg

Simultaneous Pressures

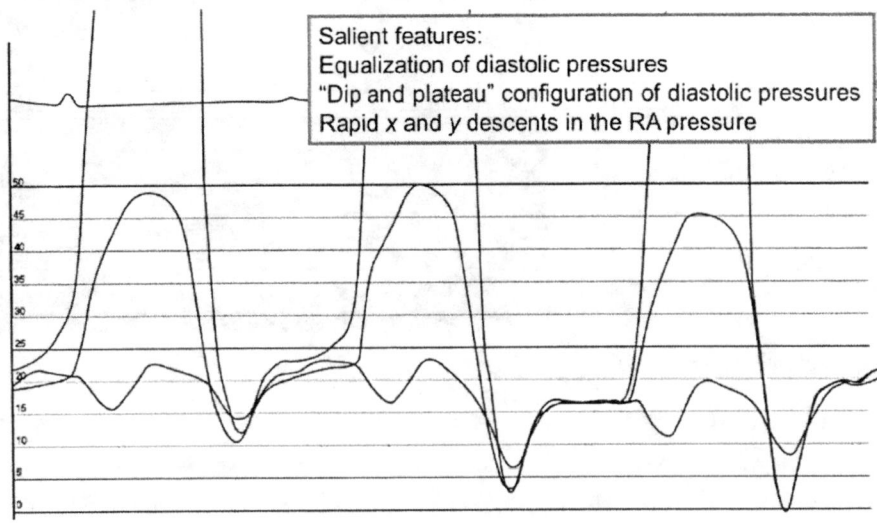

Salient features:
Equalization of diastolic pressures
"Dip and plateau" configuration of diastolic pressures
Rapid x and y descents in the RA pressure

Pericardial Effusion

AR 82

A 52 yo female with metastatic breast cancer is admitted with increasing dyspnea.
BP is 130/75 mmHg, falling to 110/65 mmHg on inspiration.
Neck veins are elevated.
Chest x-ray shows a large pleural effusion.
ECG follows.

ECG

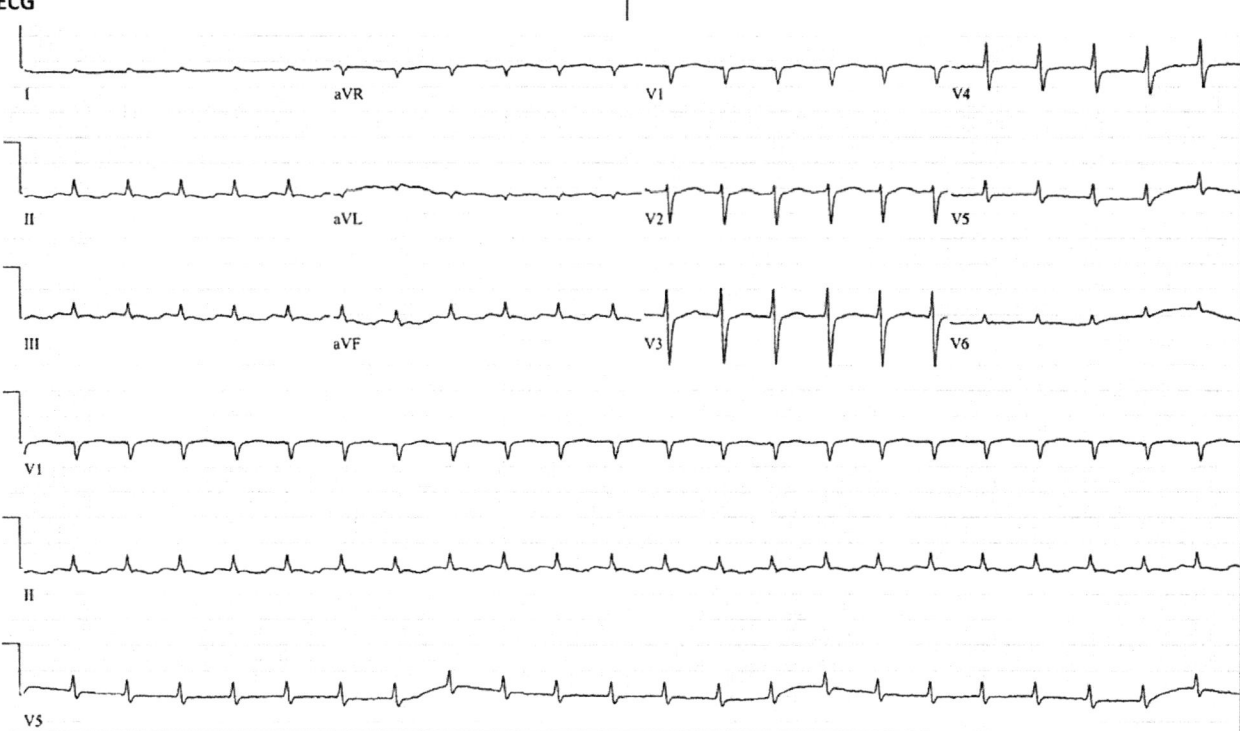

What test would confirm the diagnosis?

A. Pleural biopsy
B. Ventilation/Perfusion scan
C. Positron emission tomography (PET)
D. Echocardiogram
E. Sputum culture

Answer: _____

Pericardial Effusion — Causes

- Neoplasm, particularly from lung and breast
- Idiopathic
- Post viral
- Infectious (TB, other bacteria)
- Post-cardiothoracic surgery
- Penetrating chest trauma
- Uremia

Diagnosis

- Echo confirms the presence of fluid
- CT/MR may be better for localized pockets of effusion
- If the cause is not obvious (e.g., trauma), pericardiocentesis fluid yields a diagnosis < 10% of the time

Evaluation of a Persistent Effusion
- Serial echoes to assess size and possible progression to tamponade
- CBC, electrolytes, BUN, TSH, ANA
- TB skin tests
- Chest CT

Management of a Persistent Effusion
- If no cause can be found in an otherwise healthy person for an effusion that persists > 3 months, pericardiocentesis is indicated
- About 50% of patients with idiopathic effusions are cured

Tamponade

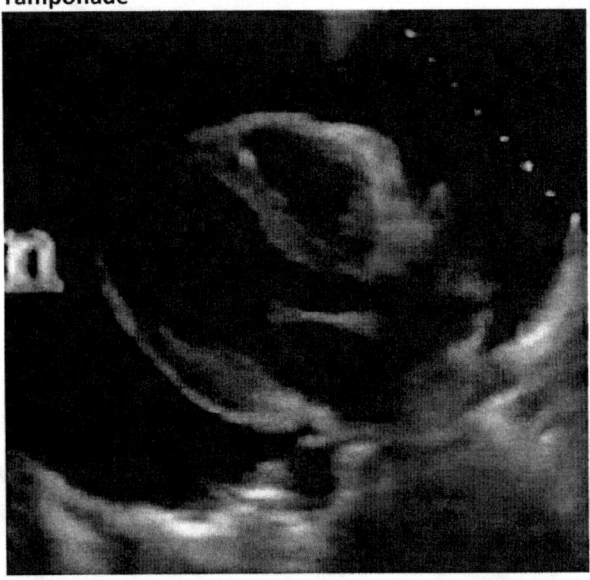

Tamponade (cont.)
- Tamponade can develop quickly if there is free wall rupture, a recent MI, or penetrating trauma
- Otherwise, pericardial fluid usually accumulates slowly

Diagnosis of Tamponade
- Echo shows pericardial effusion, diastolic collapse of the RA and perhaps the RV
- Physical exam shows pulsus paradoxus and jugular venous distention with a single rapid x descent
- Learn the difference between this and constrictive pericarditis (!)

Acute Tamponade
- 3 hallmarks:
  1) Hypotension and muffled heart sounds
  2) Pulsus paradoxus (systolic BP drops > 10 mmHg during inspiration)
  3) Jugular venous distention, no collapse in diastole

Jugular Venous Pulse

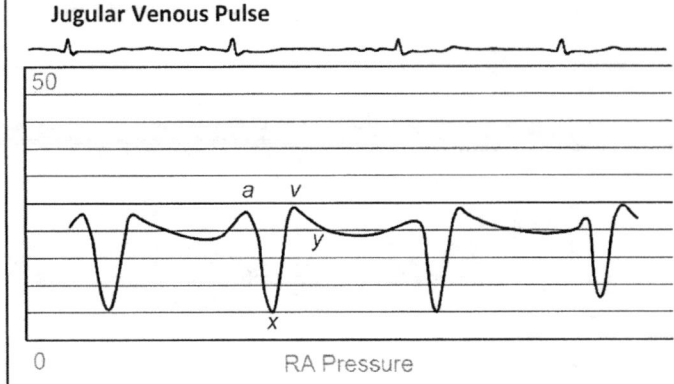

Tamponade vs. Constriction

Findings	Tamponade	Constrictive Pericarditis
Duration of symptoms	**Hours to days**	**Months to years**
Chest pain, friction rub	Often present	Absent
Pulsus paradoxus	**Present**	**Usually absent**
Kussmaul sign	**Absent**	**Usually present**
Diastolic knock	Absent	Often present
Pericardial calcification	Absent	Often present
Thickened pericardium on CT/MR	Absent	**Present**
Pericardial effusion	**Present**	Absent
Jugular venous waveforms	**Prominent x descent**	**Prominent x and y descents**
Diastolic pressures	**Equal**	**Equal**
Echo findings	**Pericardial effusion**, collapse of RV/RA	Marked respiratory variation in transmitral flow
Systemic disease	Cancer, uremia, recent CT surgery, chest trauma	TB, previous XRT, remote CT surgery

Jugular Venous Pulse

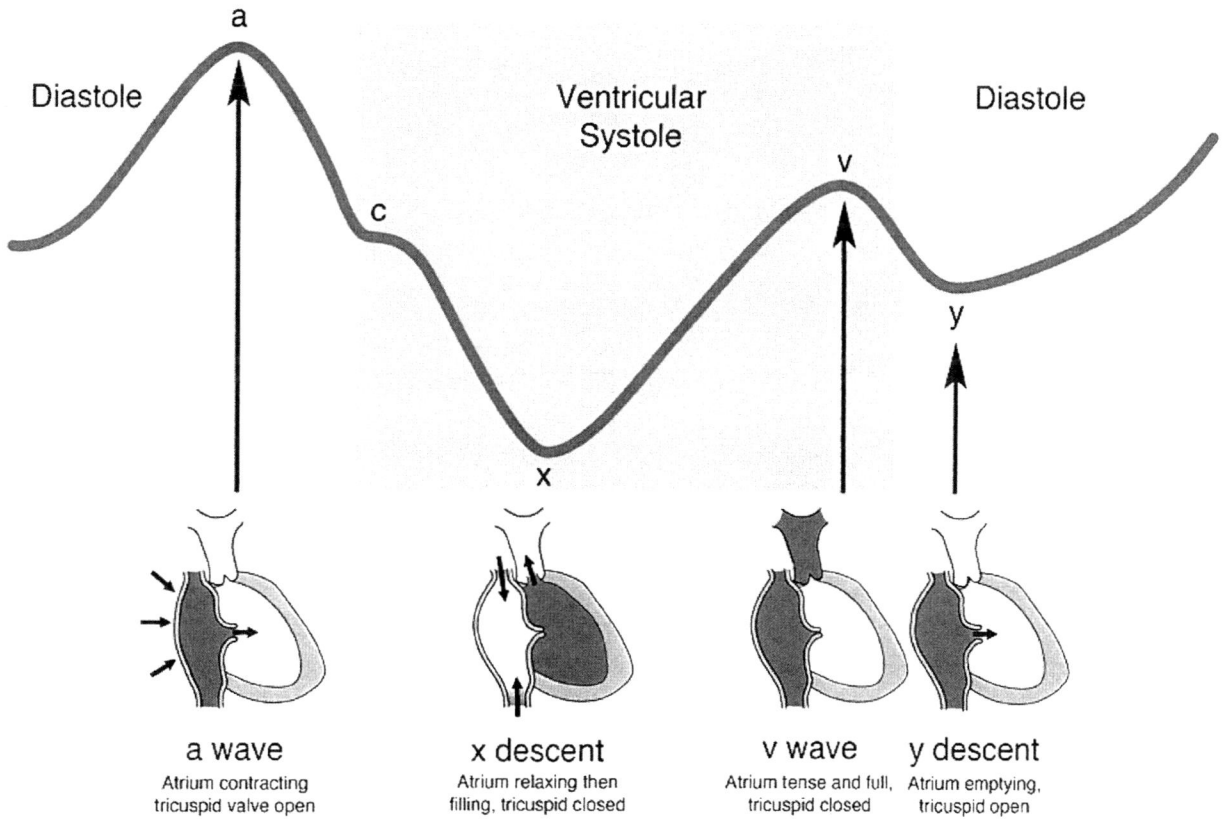

a wave
Atrium contracting
tricuspid valve open

x descent
Atrium relaxing then
filling, tricuspid closed

v wave
Atrium tense and full,
tricuspid closed

y descent
Atrium emptying,
tricuspid open

Normal Hemodynamics
- Normal right atrial filling is bimodal:
  - A surge of blood occurs at the onset of ventricular systole marked by the x descent
  - A 2nd surge occurs when the tricuspid valve opens and the y descent is inscribed

Constriction
- Cardiac volume cannot exceed that enforced by the pericardial scar
- During ventricular systole, volume inside the pericardium decreases sufficiently to allow the x descent to occur
- At the beginning of diastole, volume inside the pericardium is lowest, catastrophic ventricular filling occurs, resulting in a deep y descent

Tamponade (cont.)
- In tamponade, force is exerted on the heart throughout the cardiac cycle
- The pericardial pressure exceeds that of the diastolic atrial pressure, so diastolic filling is obliterated and there is <u>no</u> y descent (!)
- All filling must occur during ventricular systole, during the x descent

Pulsus Paradoxus
- Inspiration enhances venous return, which exacerbates the tension inside the heart by increasing RV volume
- Ventricular filling is already so marginal under tamponade conditions that any preferential filling of the RV occurs at the expense of the LV, resulting in decreased stroke volume

Kussmaul Sign
- Intrathoracic pressure changes cannot affect the intrapericardial volume enforced by the pericardial scar
- Additional venous return during inspiration, therefore, "backs up" behind the right atrium and causes a rise in the jugular venous pressure

AR 83
A 65 yo female undergoing therapy for metastatic breast cancer presents with severe dyspnea, fatigue, vague chest pain, and pre-syncope.
Her BP is 98/60 mmHg, but it drops to 80/50 mmHg on inspiration.
She has JVD that does not change throughout the cardiac cycle.
A single rapid x descent is present in the JVP.
Heart sounds are muffled, but you believe you detect a friction rub.

Which procedure will be needed urgently/emergently?
A. Pericardial stripping.
B. No procedure — restrictive cardiomyopathy is not amenable to invasive treatment.
C. Pericardiocentesis.
D. Pulmonary embolectomy.
E. Invasive coronary angiography.

Answer: _____

Congenital Heart Disease in the Adult

"Great Complexity" Defects
- Cyanotic congenital heart disease
- Eisenmenger syndrome
- Transposition of the great arteries
- Valvular atresia
- Single ventricle
- Truncus arteriosus
- Post-Fontan or conduit procedure

"Moderate Complexity" Defects
- Coarctation
- Ebstein's
- Ostium primum ASD
- Sinus venosus ASD
- Unclosed patent ductus
- Tetralogy of Fallot
- Anomalous pulmonary venous drainage
- Moderate to severe PS/PR
- Subvalvular/Supravalvular AS
- Complex VSDs

"Simple" Defects
- Isolated congenital aortic or mitral disease
- PFO or small ASD
- Small VSD
- Mild PS
- Small patent ductus
- Previously occluded ductus
- Repaired secundum or sinus venosus ASD
- Repaired VSD without residual

Regional Adult Congenital Heart Disease (ACHD) Center
- Cardiologists specializing in ACHD
- Congenital cardiac surgeon
- Cardiac anesthetist
- Diagnostic and interventional catheterization
- Cardiac imaging
- Other specialized personnel

Referral to an ACHD Center
- Every 12–24 months for patients with moderate and complex CHD
- After stabilization, all CHD patients who require urgent or acute care
- All patients who require cardiac imaging, catheterization, or electrophysiology

- Patients with moderate or complex defects who require general anesthesia or moderate sedation
- An ACHD specialist should be notified when a patient with a simple defect is admitted to a non-ACHD center

Pregnancy and ACHD
Patients considering pregnancy must understand the potential risk to mother and baby, including the risk of transmission of heart disease to the infant.

Endocarditis Prophylaxis
- There is a lack of evidence of efficacy of endocarditis prophylaxis, but it seems reasonable in patients with:
  - Previous endocarditis
  - Prosthetic cardiac valve
  - Unrepaired cyanotic heart disease or prior repair with residual leak
  - Cardiac transplant with valvular disease

Atrial Septal Defects

AR 84
A 17 yo woman is having a school physical examination prior to participating in sports.
She is found to have a systolic murmur at the lower left sternal border.
The 2nd heart sound is widely split and does not vary with respiration.
ECG follows.

ECG

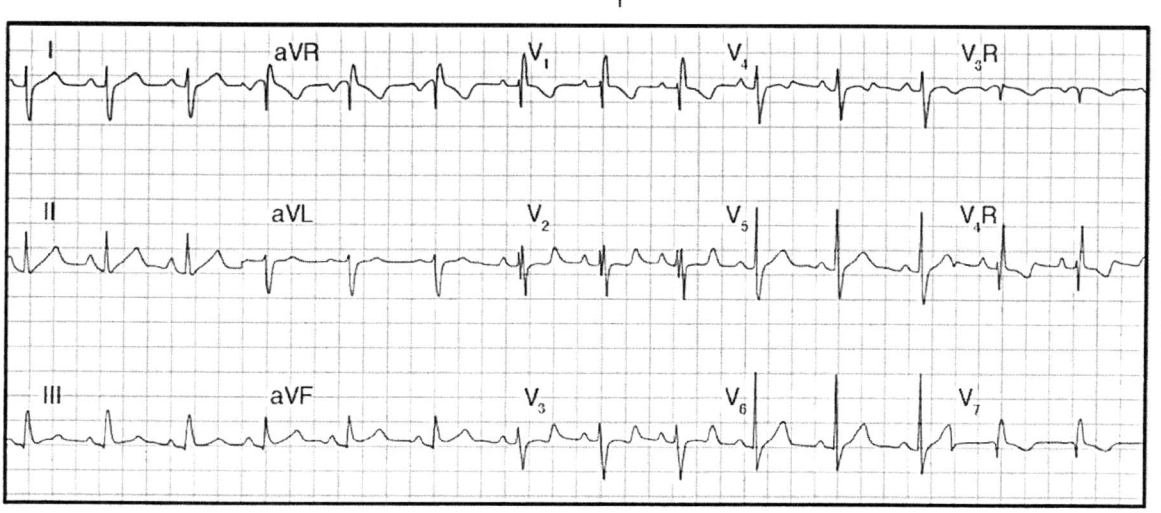

AR 84 (cont.)
What is the likely diagnosis?

A. Membranous VSD
B. Secundum ASD
C. Congenital pulmonic stenosis
D. Congenital aortic stenosis
E. Congenital mitral stenosis

Answer: _____

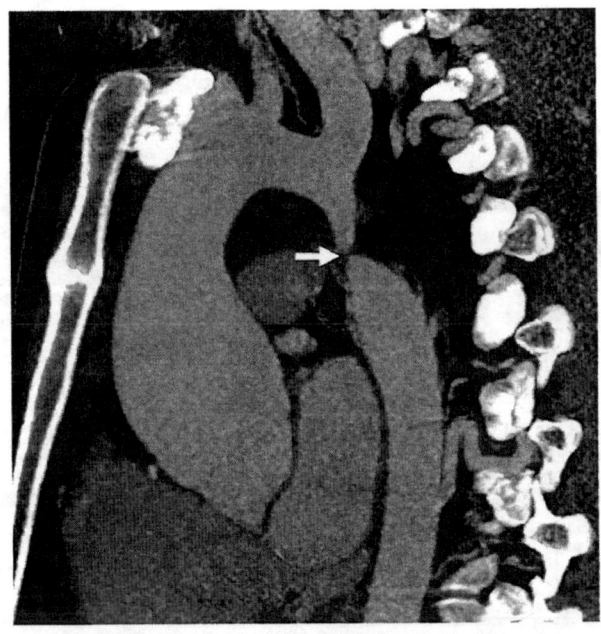

Secundum ASD
- 70% of ASDs
- 2nd most common adult congenital heart disease (after bicuspid aortic valve)
- Atrial fibrillation is common
- Does not require antibiotic prophylaxis

Physical Examination of Secundum ASD
- Systolic ejection murmur at the left sternal border due to increased pulmonary flow
- A diastolic murmur is possible due to increased tricuspid blood flow
- Fixed splitting of the 2nd heart sound

Other Tests for the Diagnosis of Secundum ASD
- ECG shows right axis deviation and/or RBBB
- Chest x-ray shows enlarged RV with shunt vascularity
- Echo is diagnostic (ask for saline study)

Treatment of Secundum ASD
- Surgery is indicated if there is more than a 2:1 left-to-right shunt, even in asymptomatic patients
- If the pulmonary resistance is > 15 U/m², surgery cannot be performed

Patent Ductus
- More common in females
- May have differential cyanosis, with the hands affected but not the feet
- Usually has a continuous, machinery murmur
- Surgical or percutaneous closure should be done in symptomatic patients of any age

Ventricular Septal Defect
- Most common congenital defect in children
- 80% of small defects close spontaneously
- Large VSDs require surgical closure

Coarctation of the Aorta
- Accompanied by a bicuspid aortic valve 70% of the time
- Other left-sided defects are common
- Delay in the femoral pulses
- Upper extremity HTN
- Chest x-ray shows rib notching
- Turner syndrome is associated with coarctation and a bicuspid aortic valve

Coarctation

© 2017 MedStudy Internal Medicine Video Board Review – Cardiology • Matthew Sorrentino, MD

Anomalous Coronary Arteries
- Coronaries that pass between the great vessels can produce sudden death in exercising young people
- Can present with chest pain
- Easily detected by CT angio, but usually found coincidentally

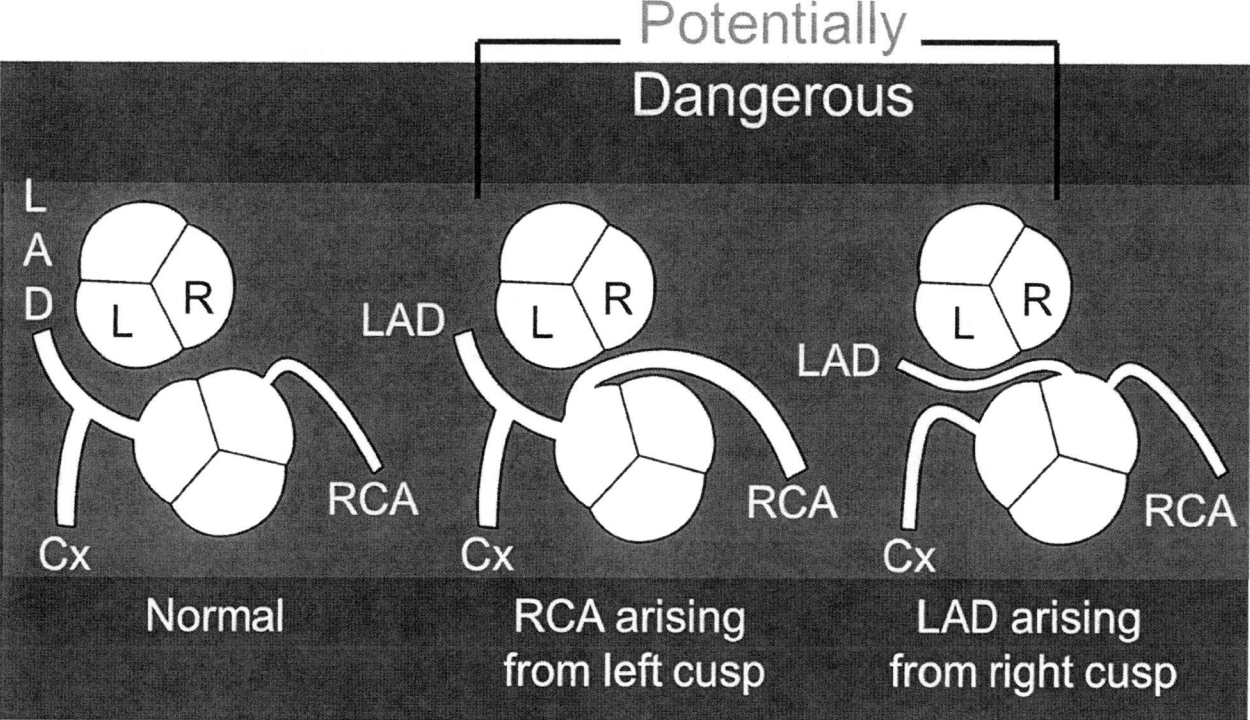

Potentially Dangerous

Normal | RCA arising from left cusp | LAD arising from right cusp

Anomalous Right Coronary

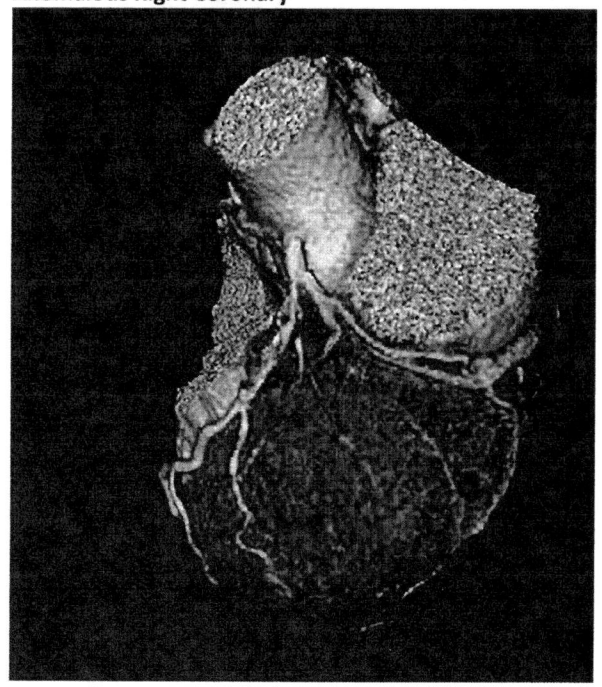

Eisenmenger Syndrome
- A large intracardiac shunt eventually causes pulmonary vascular resistance to exceed systemic resistance
- The shunt becomes right-to-left and causes cyanosis
- All of the intracardiac shunts can cause this, except secundum ASD
- Treatment is heart-lung transplant

Other Congenital Disorders
- Marfan syndrome causes cystic medial necrosis of the aorta and can cause dissection and chronic or acute AR
- Maternal rubella causes congenital pulmonic stenosis, patent ductus, and supravalvular aortic stenosis
- Cystic fibrosis can cause pulmonary HTN

AR 85
A 19 yo male soccer player presents with chest pain on exertion that occurs during soccer practice. Physical exam reveals normal S_1 and physiological splitting of S_2. No murmur, gallop, or rub is detected.

AR 85 (cont.)
Which of the following is associated with sudden cardiac death in young athletes?
A. Concentric LVH
B. Constrictive pericarditis
C. Patent foramen ovale
D. Anomalous coronary artery
E. Uncomplicated secundum ASD

Answer: _____

AR 86

A 38 yo female with a history of unrepaired VSD presents with cyanosis and dyspnea. Lips, fingers, and toes all appear cyanotic. She also complains of lightheadedness. Pregnancy test is negative.

Which of the following complications do you immediately think of?
A. The pregnancy test results are a false negative.
B. She has developed Eisenmenger syndrome.
C. She now has a secundum ASD that has appeared in addition to her known VSD.
D. She has developed Raynaud phenomenon.

Answer: _____

Pulmonary Heart Disease

Multiple Pulmonary Emboli
- Multiple pulmonary emboli, from the right heart or peripheral sources, eventually cause severe pulmonary HTN
- Diagnosis is by CT angio
- If severe, patients require pulmonary thromboendarterectomy, a vena caval filter, and lifelong warfarin

Primary Pulmonary HTN
- Usually occurs in young women
- Fatal in 5–10 years
- Calcium blockers may relieve symptoms
- Only real treatment is heart-lung transplant
- Echo and CT angio are necessary to rule out secondary causes of pulmonary HTN, such as LV failure, multiple pulmonary emboli, etc.

Pregnancy

Contraindications to Pregnancy
- Absolute — cyanotic congenital heart disease, Eisenmenger's, pulmonary HTN
- Relative — secundum ASD, aortic stenosis, and cardiomyopathy

- The latter probably need to be at bed rest throughout the pregnancy
- Secundum ASD is only dangerous if atrial fibrillation develops

Valvular Disease and Pregnancy
- In general, regurgitant lesions are better tolerated than stenotic lesions
- For purposes of exams, warfarin is contraindicated/teratogenic
- Use UFH/LMWH to cover a mechanical prosthetic valve

Medications and Pregnancy
- Warfarin and ACEI/ARB are contraindicated because of teratogenic effects
- Digoxin, beta-blockers, calcium blockers, most diuretics, hydralazine, and electrical cardioversion are safe
- Heparin increases morbidity and mortality in mother and child

The Physical Examination and Pregnancy
- Most pregnant women experience pedal edema
- Flow murmurs, increased jugular venous pressure, and 3rd heart sounds are common
- A pregnant patient who presents with new onset atrial fibrillation and pulmonary edema usually has mitral stenosis or a secundum ASD

Peripartum Cardiomyopathy

Risk Factors
- Age > 30
- Multiparity
- African descent
- Pregnancy with multiple fetuses
- A history of preeclampsia, eclampsia, or postpartum HTN
- Maternal cocaine abuse
- Long-term (> 4 weeks) oral tocolytic therapy with beta-adrenergic agonists such as terbutaline

Diagnosis
- Development of HF in the last month of pregnancy or within 5 months of delivery
- No other obvious causes
- No obvious underlying heart disease
- LVEF < 45%

Management During Pregnancy
- Beta-blockers
- Hydralazine
- Probably digoxin
- Diuretics
- Anticoagulation with heparin?
- May progress to transplantation

Outcome
- Mortality is about 10% in 2 years and transplant rate is about 4%
- Many, however, will recover within 3–6 months of onset
- Patients at higher risk include those with:
  - A worse initial NYHA class
  - African descent
  - Multiparity

Risk During Subsequent Pregnancy
- The risk of worsening heart failure in patients with recovered LV function is mild to moderate
- Patients with persistent LV dysfunction appear to be at very high risk for HF and death during a subsequent pregnancy

AR 87A
A 23 yo African American female presents with increasing dyspnea and intense fatigue 2 weeks after giving birth to her 3rd child.

What do you recommend next?
A. Just go home and rest; having a baby is stressful.
B. Transthoracic echo.
C. Transesophageal echo.
D. Pharmacologic stress nuclear scan.
E. Chest CT.

Answer: _____

AR 87B
What can you advise her about her likely condition?
A. Race or ethnicity does not seem to have any impact on degree of risk.
B. If LV dysfunction persists, she is at greater risk of heart failure and sudden death in any subsequent pregnancy.
C. Mortality is known to be 50% at 2 years.
D. All such patients require heart transplant.

Answer: _____

AR 88
A patient presents with a post viral cardiomyopathy. Coronary angiography is normal.

What is the appropriate treatment?
A. Prednisone
B. Azathioprine
C. An ACE inhibitor
D. Antiretroviral drugs
E. Antiherpes drugs

Answer: _____

AR 89
A patient on no medical therapy presents with a dilated cardiomyopathy (LVEF 30%).
K is 5.3 mg/dL.

What drug would you add?
A. An ACE inhibitor
B. An ARB
C. Nifedipine
D. Carvedilol
E. Amiodarone

Answer: _____

AR 90
In which of the following conditions is BNP not elevated?
A. LV systolic dysfunction
B. LV diastolic dysfunction
C. Acute pulmonary embolism
D. Cor pulmonale
E. Chronic anemia

Answer: _____

AR 91
A 45 yo woman with prior radiation therapy for breast cancer presents with dyspnea and peripheral edema.
On exam, she has elevated neck veins that increase on inspiration and a diastolic knock; BP is 126/80 mmHg on expiration and 122/80 mmHg on inspiration.

What is the diagnosis?
A. Constrictive pericarditis
B. Multiple pulmonary emboli
C. Cardiac tamponade
D. Chronic aortic regurgitation
E. Dilated cardiomyopathy

Answer: _____

AR 92
A 23 yo man presents with worsening dyspnea.
He reports having had a murmur in childhood.
On exam, he has a systolic thrill and a very loud systolic murmur heard widely over the precordium.

What is the diagnosis?
A. ASD
B. VSD
C. Calcific aortic stenosis
D. Rheumatic mitral stenosis
E. Chronic MR from a ruptured chorda

Answer: _____

AR 93

A 62 yo African American woman with a history of severe HTN complains of increasing dyspnea.
Physical exam shows a BP of 180/110 mmHg and a loud 4th heart sound at the apex.
BUN is 31 mg/dL and creatinine 1.9 mg/dL.
Her ECG follows.

ECG

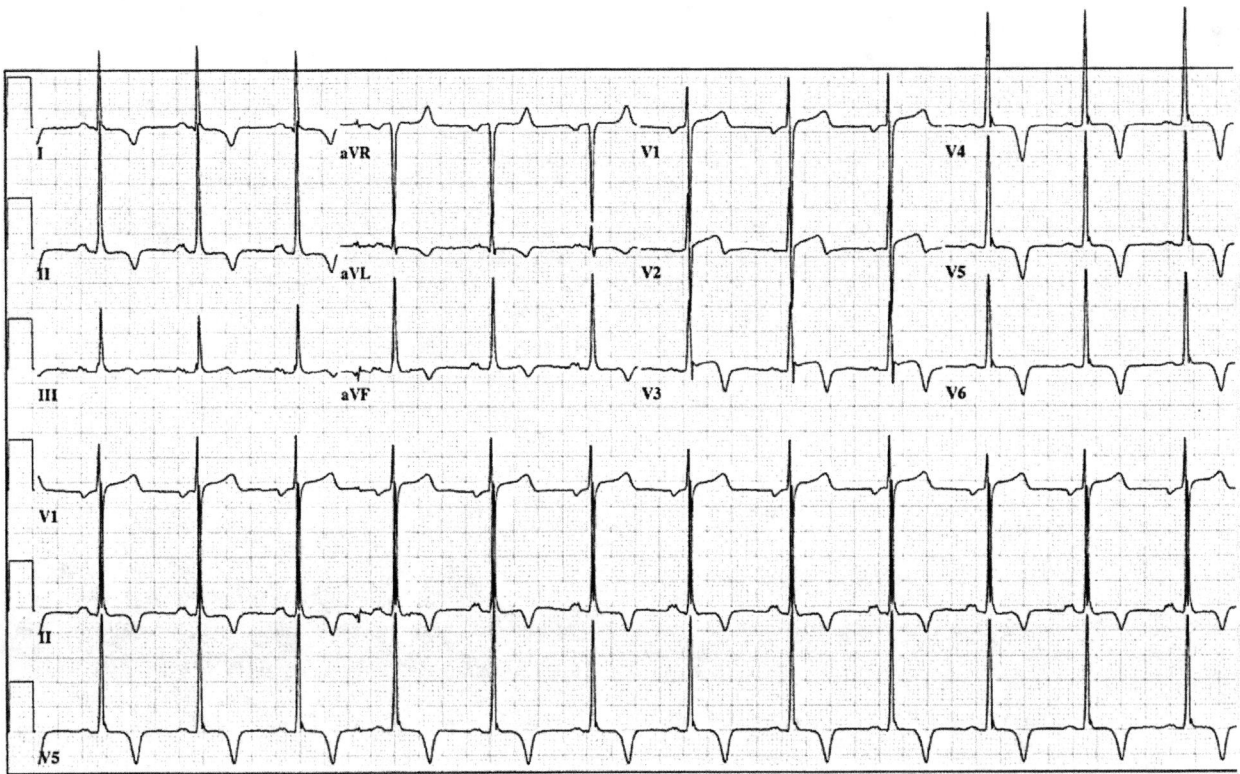

What would an echo be likely to show?

A. Normal findings
B. Critical mitral stenosis
C. Severe aortic regurgitation
D. Severe concentric LVH, LVEF 70%
E. Severe segmental wall motion abnormalities, LVEF 25%

Answer: _____

**Part 7:
ECG Interpretation and
Arrhythmia Management**

Overview
- Usually about 5 ECGs on the exam
- Usually these are included as part of a clinical presentation

AR 94

A patient presents with classical angina.
An exercise stress test shows ST-segment elevation in leads I, aVL, V5–V6.

What coronary lesion would explain this?
A. Left main coronary artery
B. Left anterior descending artery
C. Left circumflex artery
D. Right coronary artery

Answer: _____

Bundle-Branch Blocks

RBBB

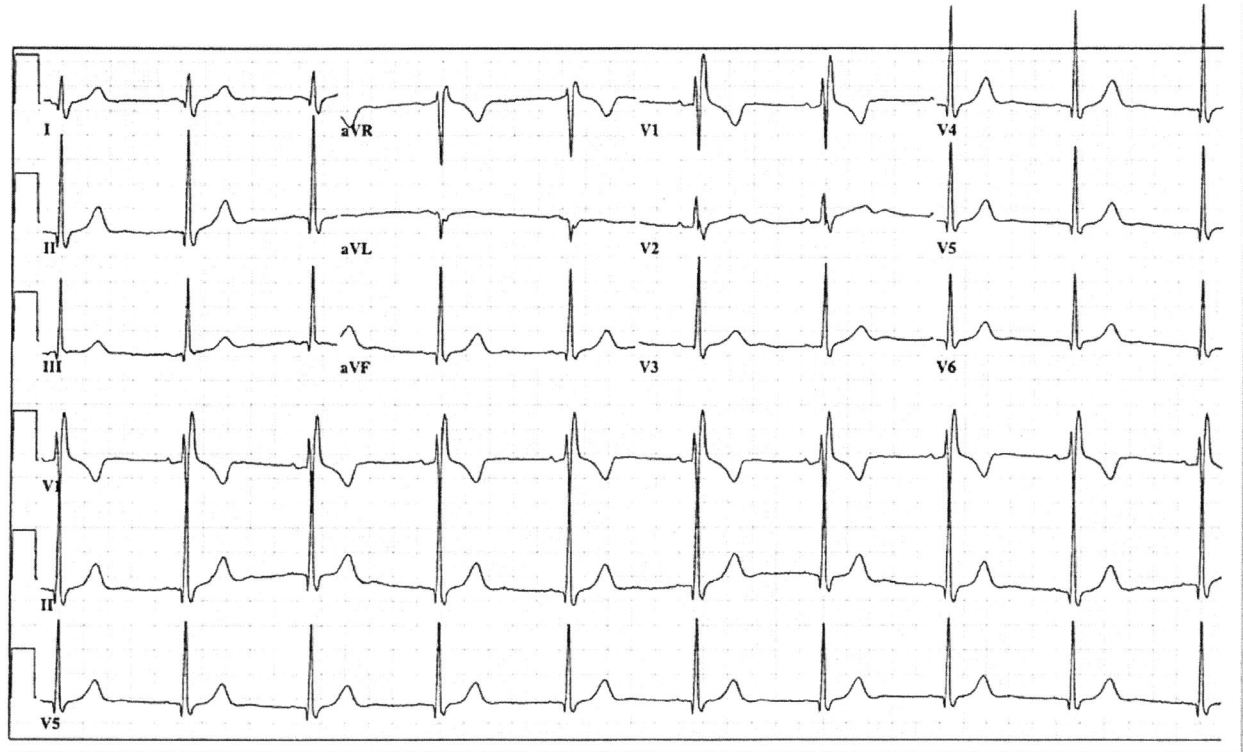

LBBB

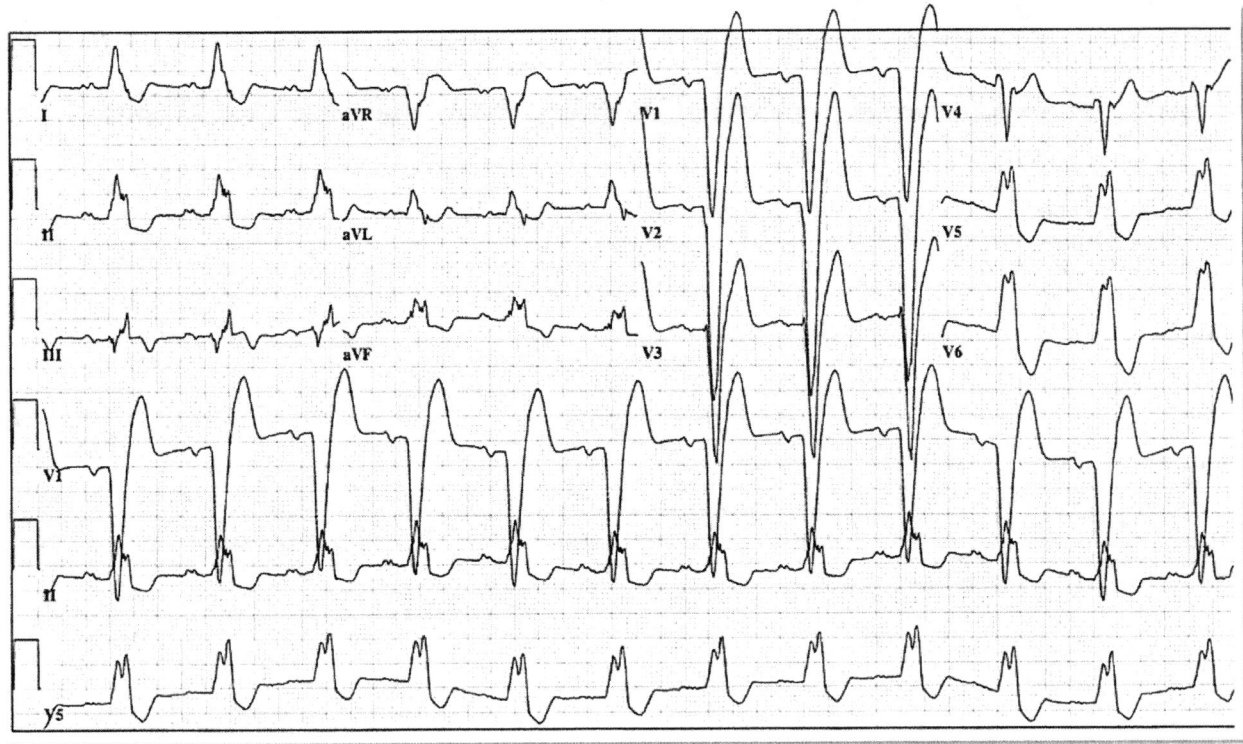

BBB Criteria

	Leads I and V6	Lead V1
RBBB	Wide S wave	Delayed ICT rSR'
LBBB	Delayed ICT Monophasic R wave	rS or Q

ICT = intrinsicoid deflection time (see following slide)

Intrinsicoid Deflection Time: Measured from the onset of the QRS to the peak of the major deflection; Should be < 40 msec

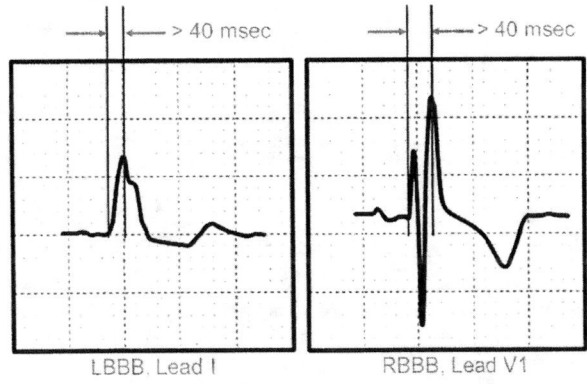

BBB and Infarcts
- Cannot read old MI in LBBB
- Can read old MI in RBBB
- Beware of RBBB and old anteroseptal MI: There is a QR in V1, not an rSR'

© 2017 MedStudy Internal Medicine Video Board Review – Cardiology • Matthew Sorrentino, MD

RBBB and Old Anterior MI

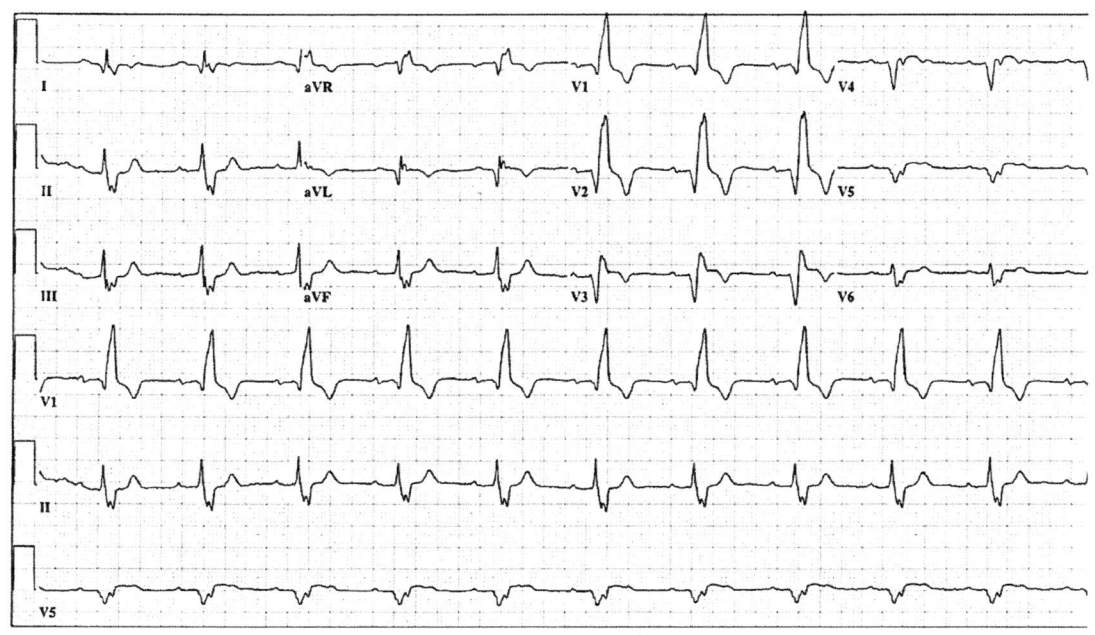

AV Block

2° AV Block Type 1 (Wenckebach)
- Progressive prolongation of the PR interval until there is a dropped QRS
- Produces group beating of QRS complexes
- Always 1 more P wave than QRS complexes in each group
- **Only indication for treatment is symptomatic bradycardia**

2° AV Block Type 1

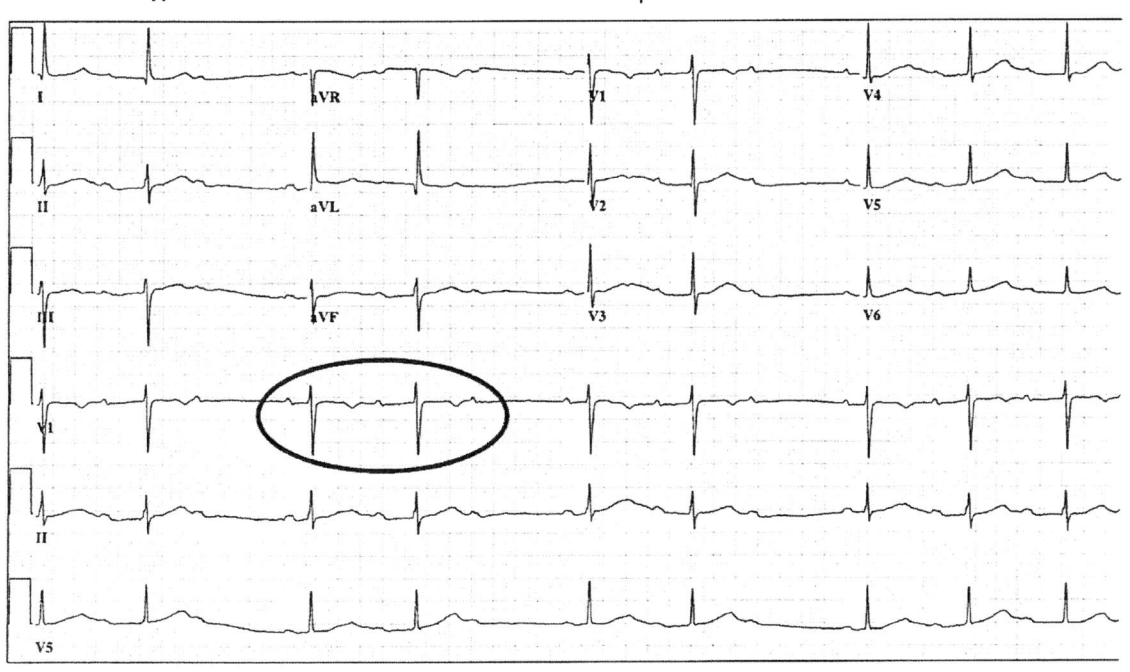

2° AV Block Type 2

- Occasional dropped QRS complexes without progressive PR prolongation
- Group beating is seldom present
- More likely to progress to 3° block
- Pacing is indicated in symptomatic patients

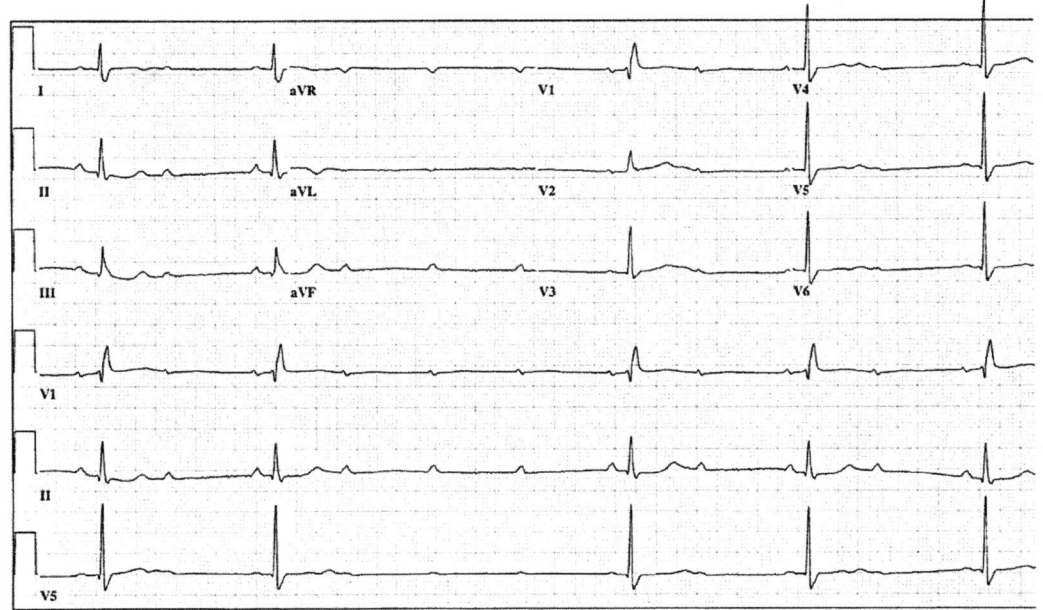

3° AV Block

- No conduction between the atria and ventricles
- An example of AV dissociation
- There is a slow narrow (junctional) or wide (usually ventricular) escape rhythm
- **Permanent pacing is indicated in most patients**

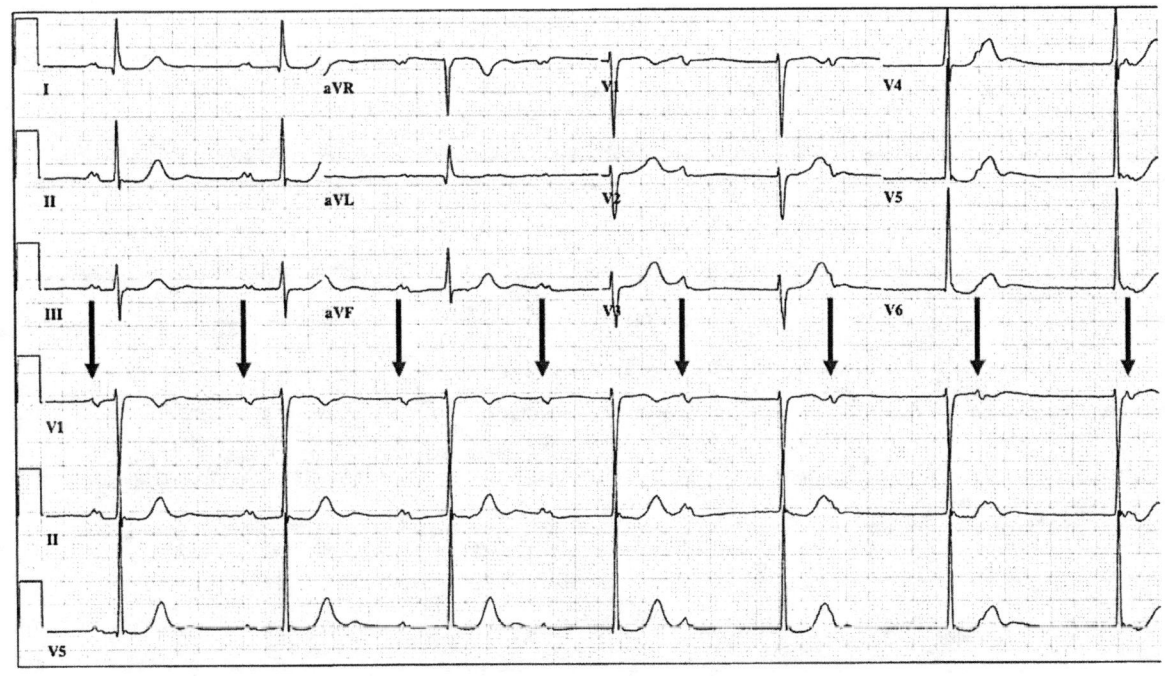

Infarcts and Ischemia

General Considerations
- Distinguish between STEMI and NSTEMI (management is different)
- Know myocardial territories:
  - II, III, aVF = Inferior wall
  - I, aVL, V5, V6 = Lateral
  - V1 & V2 = Septum
  - V3 & V4 = Anterior

Coronary Artery Territories
- RCA: Inferior wall
  - II, III, aVF
- LAD: Anterior wall and septum
  - V1–V4
- LCX: Lateral wall
  - V5–V6, I, aVL

Acute Inferior MI

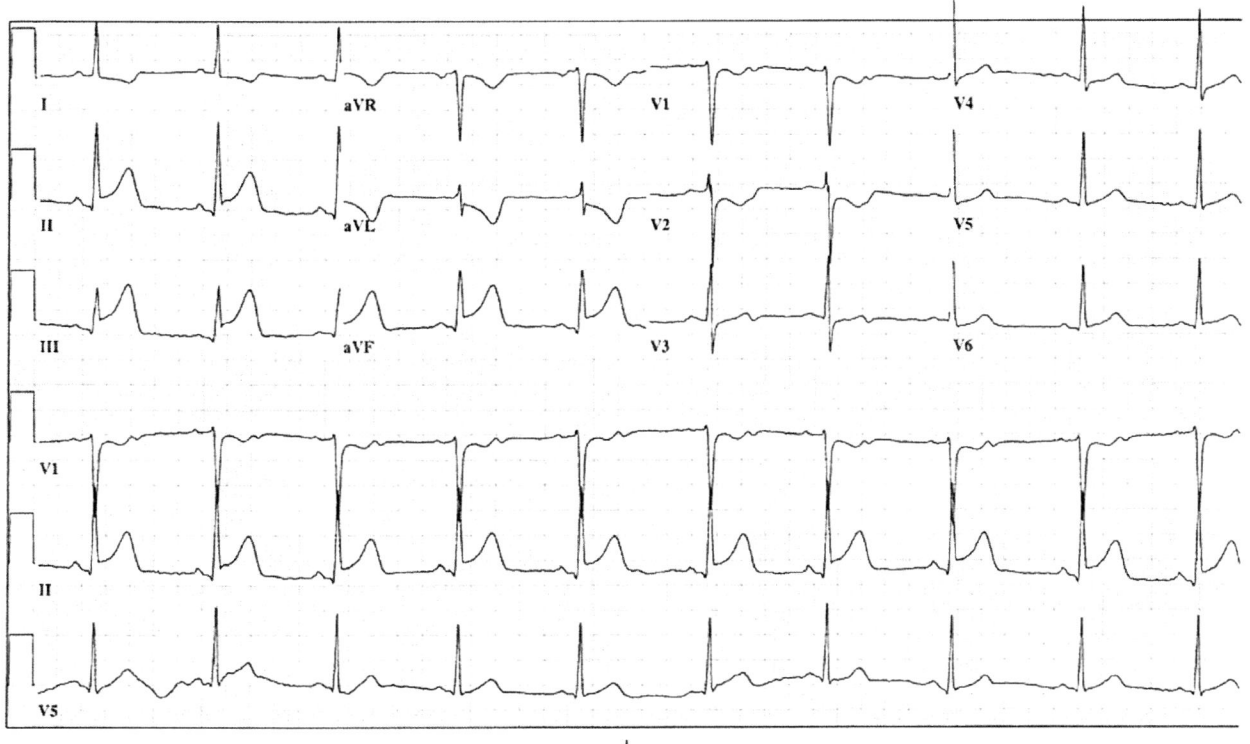

Acute Anterolateral MI

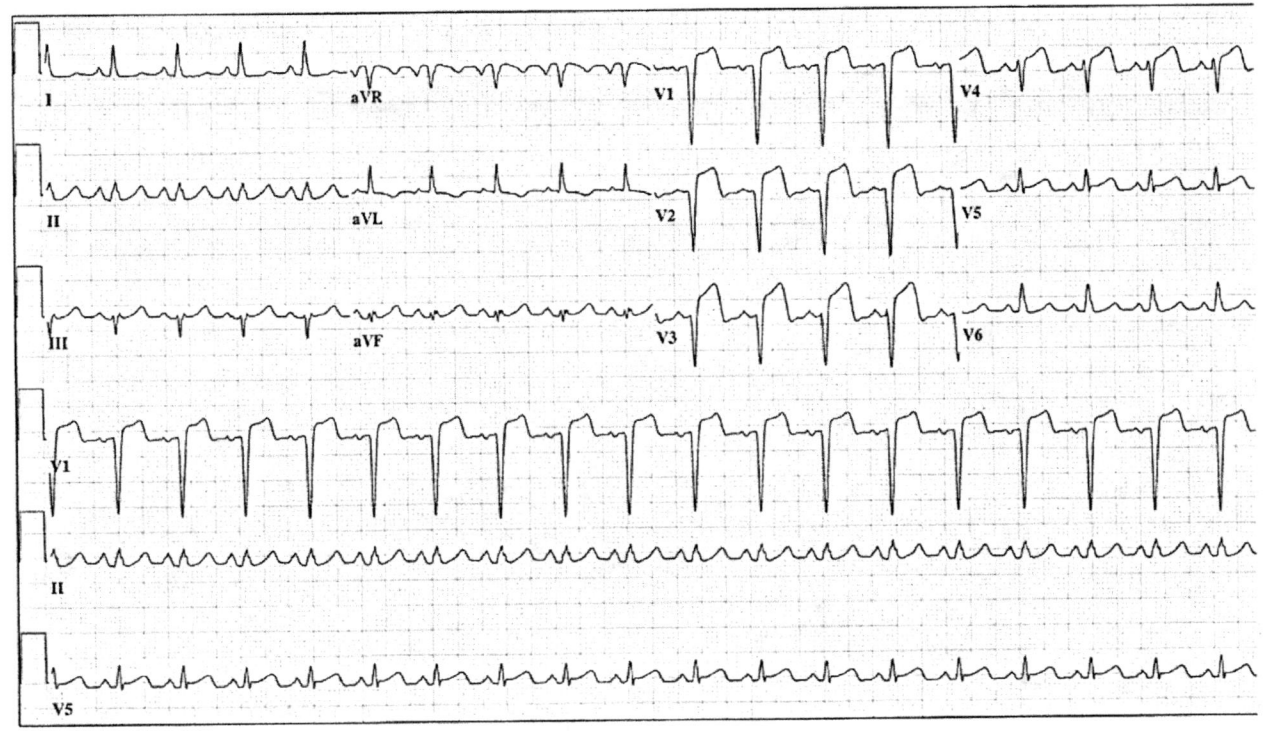

Acute Posterior MI

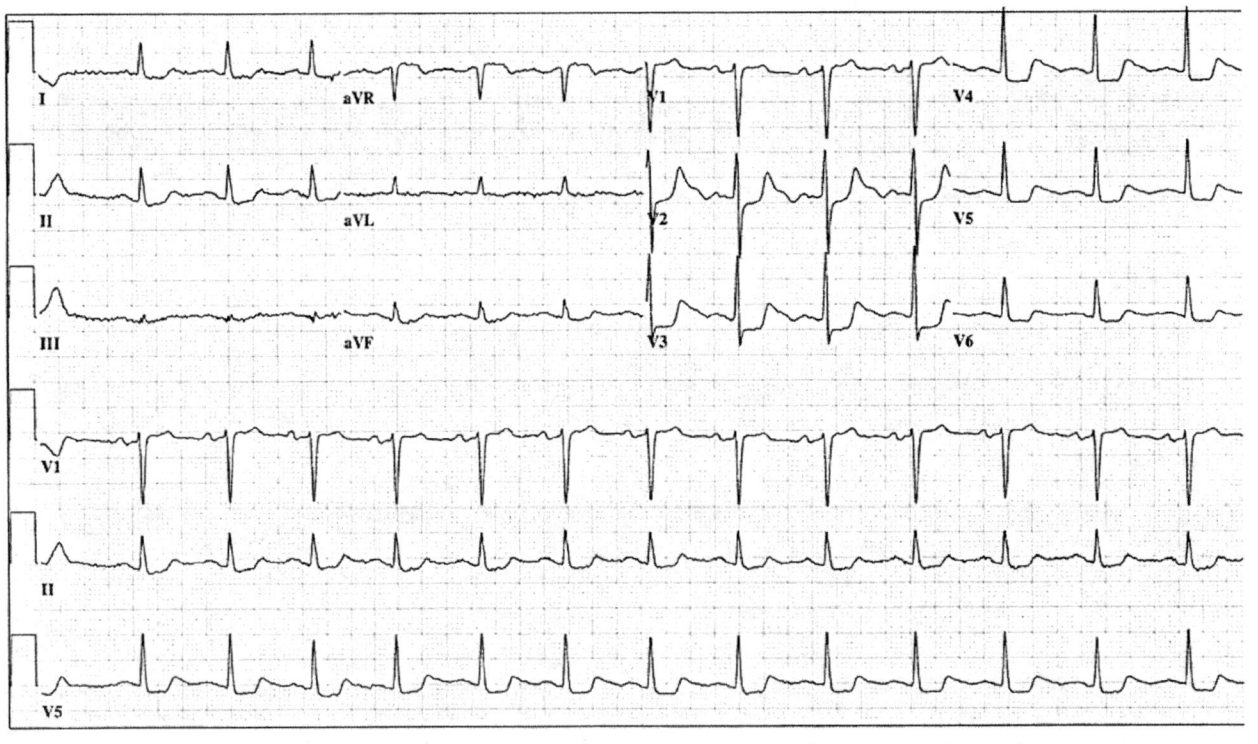

Non–ST-Segment Elevation MI

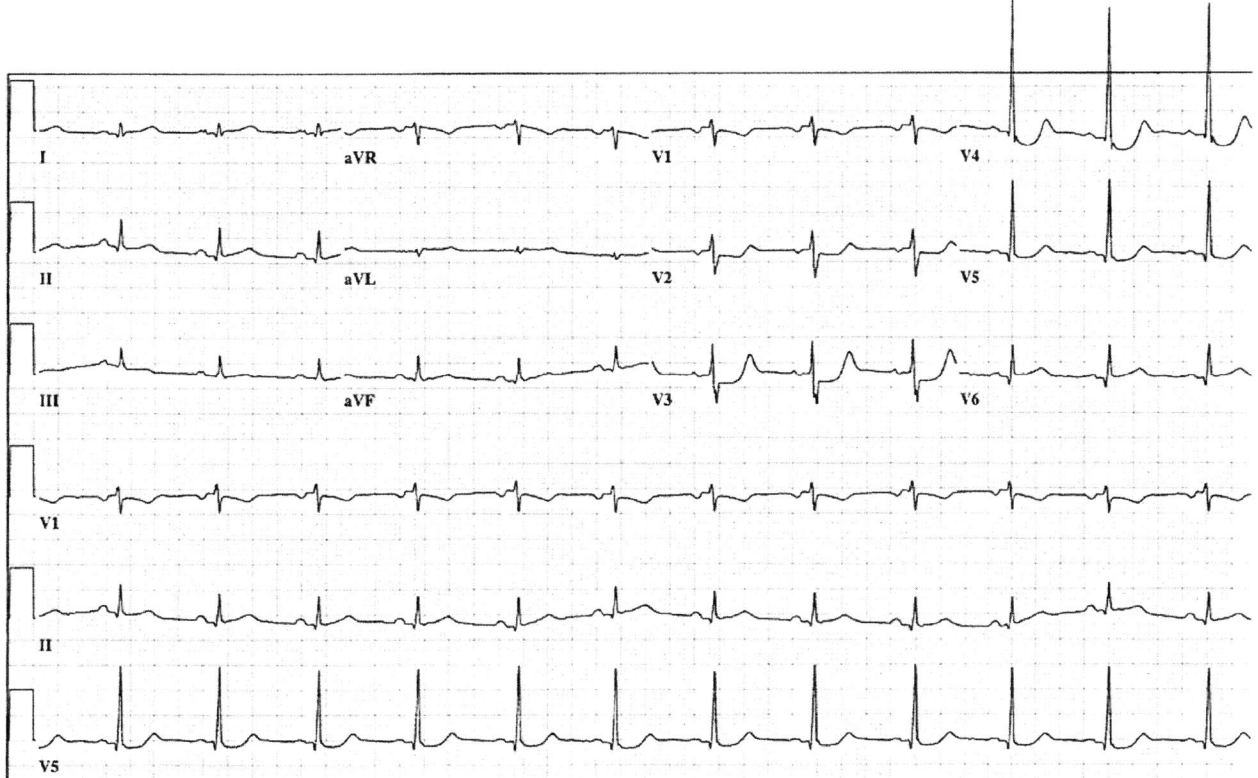

Wolff-Parkinson-White Syndrome

ECG Manifestations
- An accessory pathway allows early depolarization of some part of the ventricle
- ECG has a short PR interval and delta waves
- Cannot call old MIs or LVH
- Can have narrow or wide QRS tachycardias

Management
- Ablation for patients with:
  - Symptomatic arrhythmias
  - Risk for developing atrial fibrillation
- Atrial fibrillation may be life-threatening; Treat with urgent cardioversion

WPW

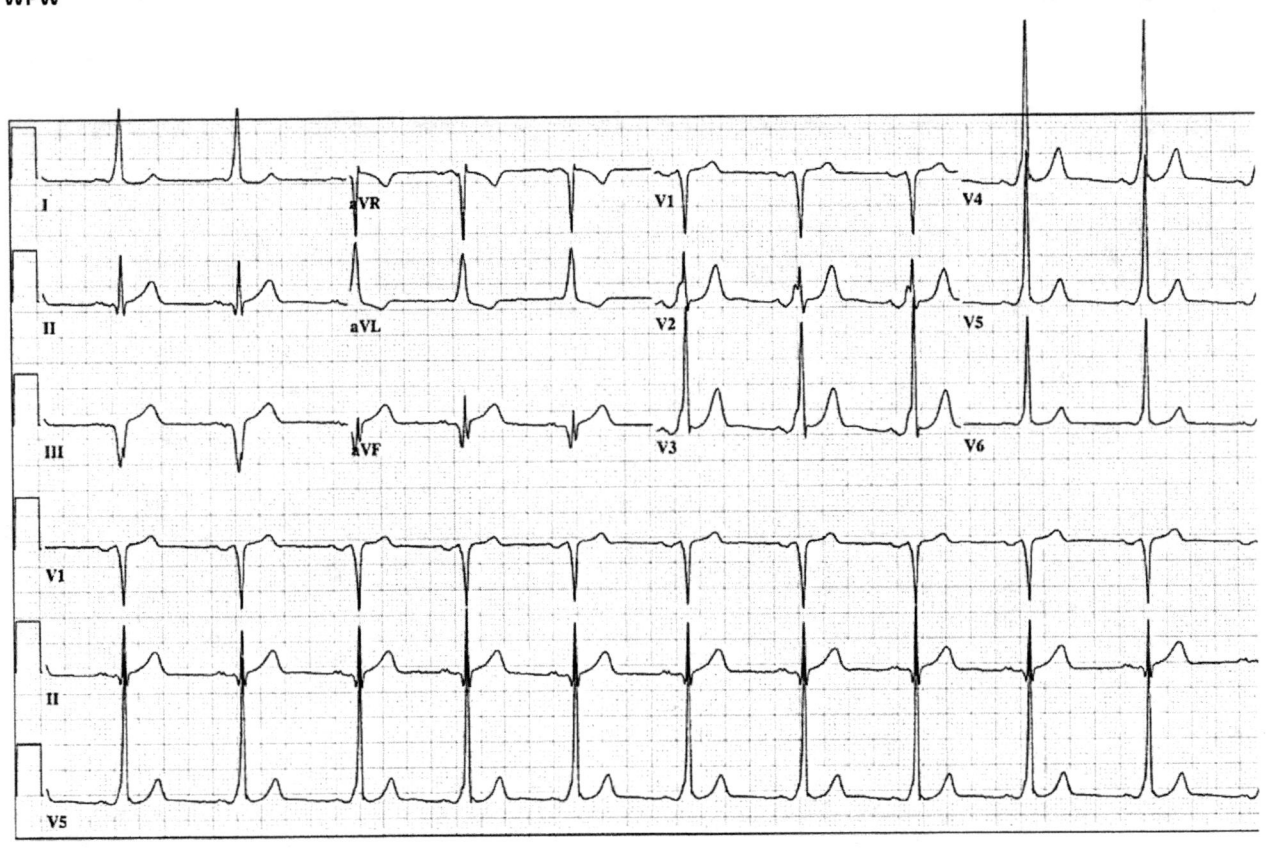

WPW (cont.)

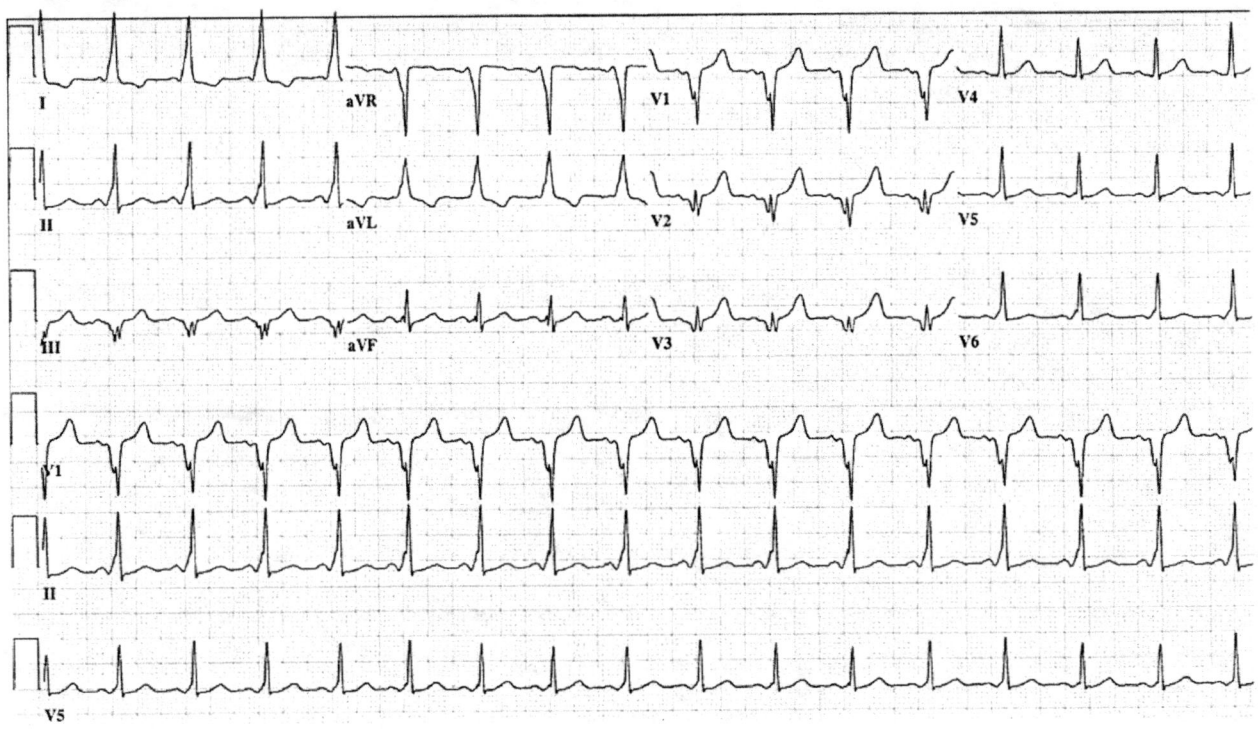

© 2017 MedStudy Internal Medicine Video Board Review – Cardiology • Matthew Sorrentino, MD

Atrial Fibrillation and WPW

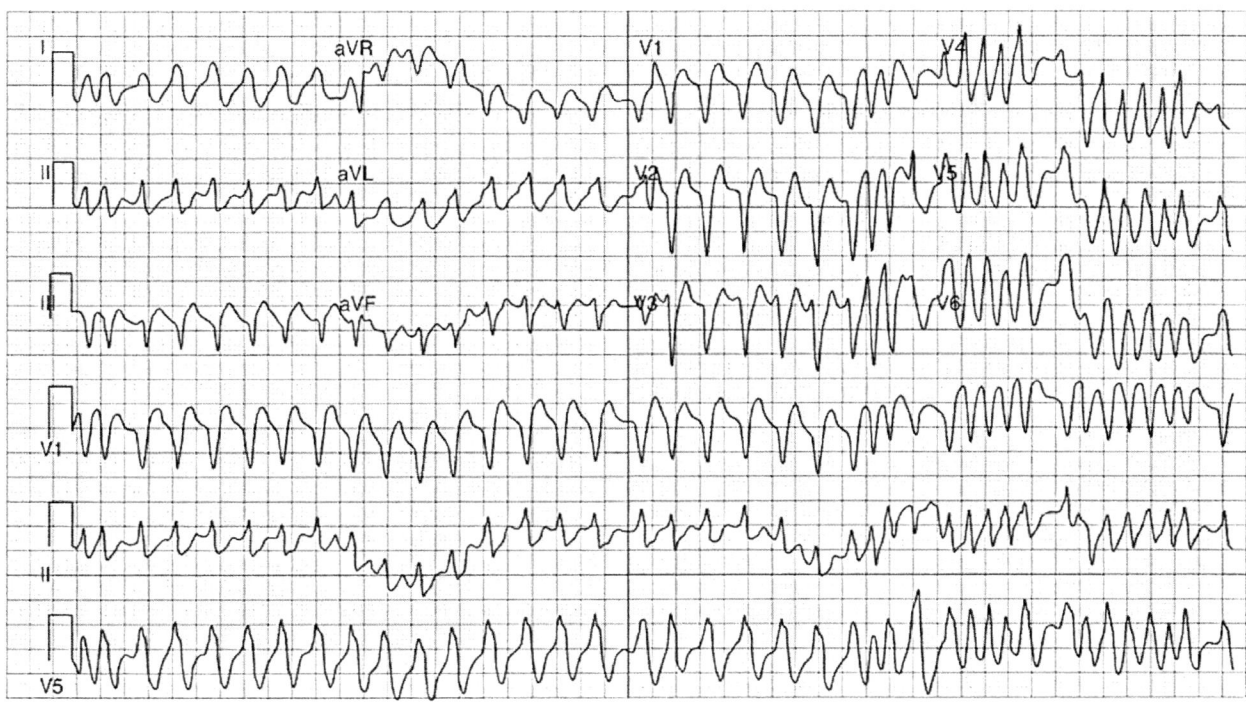

Acute Pericarditis
- Diffuse ST-segment elevation
- PR segment depression, usually most prominent in lead II
- Do not give fibrinolytic therapy
- Treatment is with aspirin plus colchicine

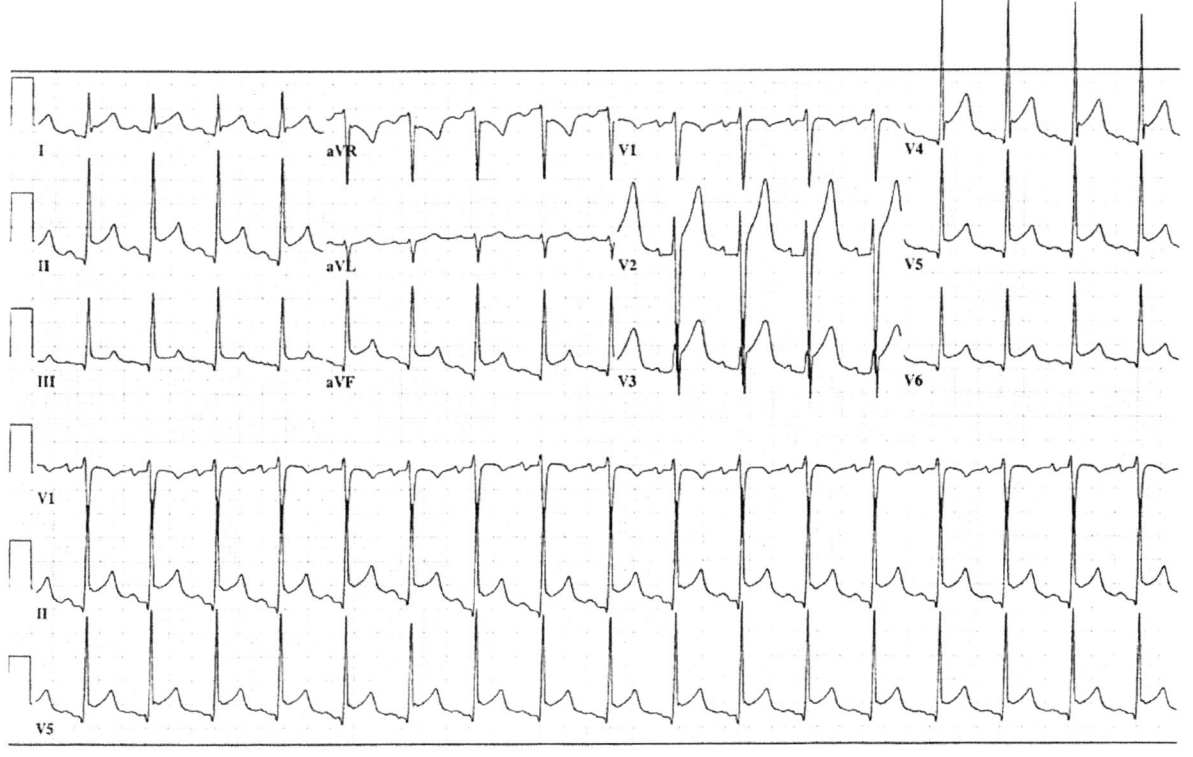

Electrolyte Abnormalities

Moderate Hyperkalemia

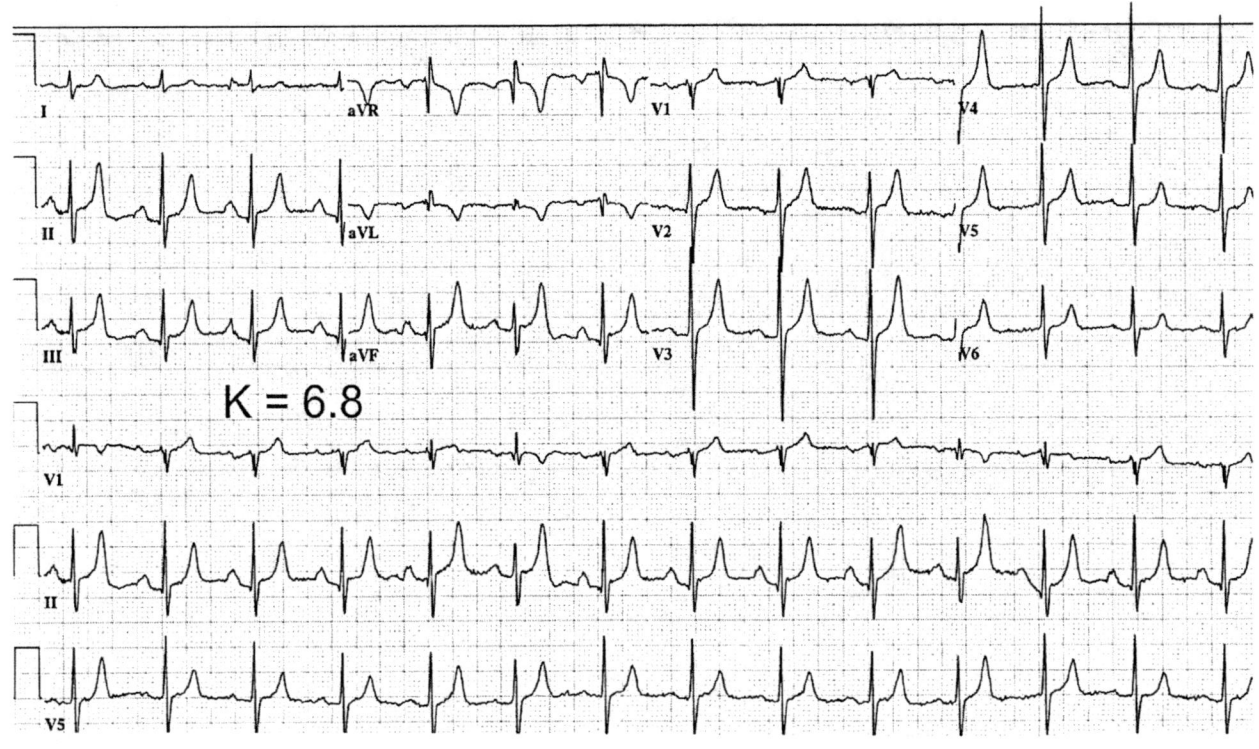

K = 6.8

Severe Hyperkalemia

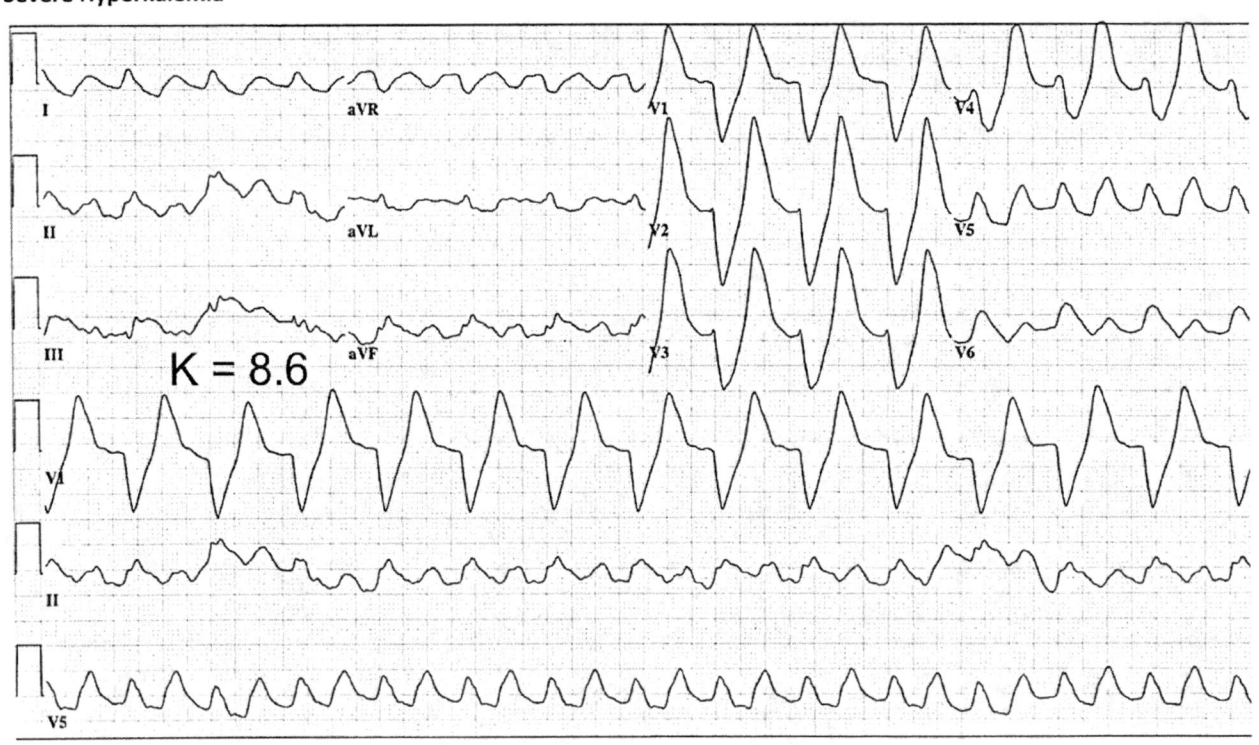

K = 8.6

Arrhythmias

General Principles
- 90% of arrhythmias are reentrant (atrial fib, atrial flutter, AVNRT, VT)
- Narrow QRS tachycardias are supraventricular in origin
- Wide QRS tachycardias could be either supraventricular or ventricular in origin
- Symptomatic arrhythmias should always be treated

Atrial Fibrillation

Patterns of AF

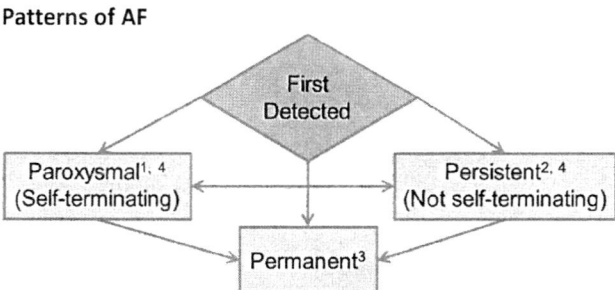

[1]Episodes that generally last ≤ 7 days (most < 24 hours)
[2]Usually > 7 days
[3]Cardioversion failed or not attempted
[4]Both paroxysmal and persistent AF may be recurrent

Mechanism and ECG
- Usually arises from the distal pulmonary veins as they insert into the left atrium
- ECG shows irregular baseline with irregular ventricular response
- Vagal maneuvers or adenosine slow ventricular response

History and Physical Exam
- Associated symptoms
- Clinical type (1st episode, paroxysmal, etc.)
- Date of onset
- Frequency, duration, precipitating, and relieving factors
- Response to medications
- Underlying heart disease or other condition

Possible ECG Findings
- LVH
- Previous P wave morphology
- Preexcitation
- Bundle-branch blocks
- Prior MI
- Other atrial arrhythmias
- Intervals

Echo
- To assess:
  - Chamber size
  - Valvular disease
  - LV function
  - RV pressure
  - LVH
  - Pericardial disease

Blood Tests
- Renal function
- Hepatic function
- Thyroid function

Possible Additional Tests
- Exercise stress testing — for rate control or to check for inducible ischemia
- Holter or event monitoring — to assess rate control or to capture paroxysmal events
- TEE — to guide cardioversion
- Electrophysiology study in selected patients
- Chest x-ray

Evaluation of the Patient
- History and physical examination
- ECG
- Transthoracic echo
- Check thyroid, renal, and hepatic function

Evaluation of the Patient (cont.)

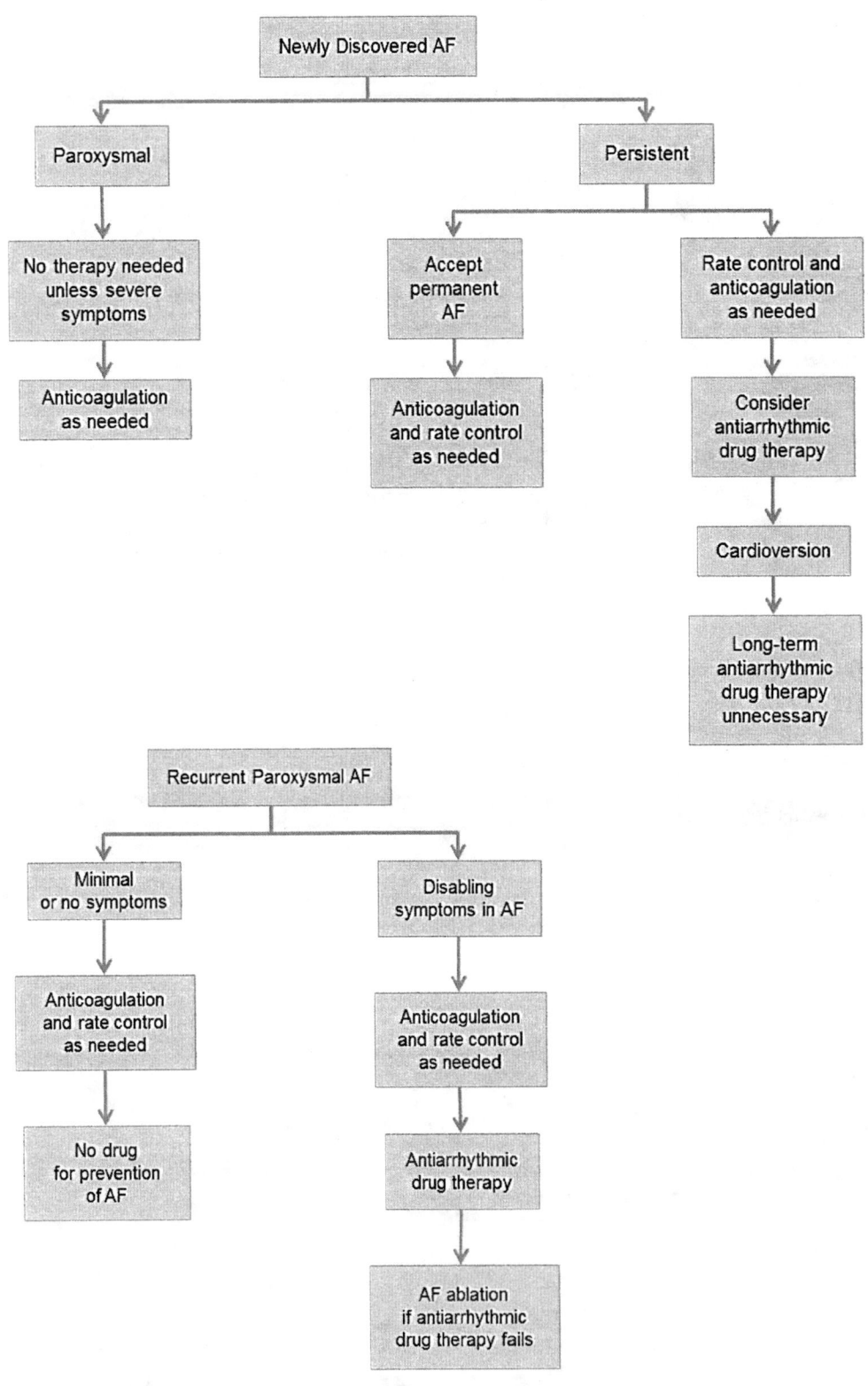

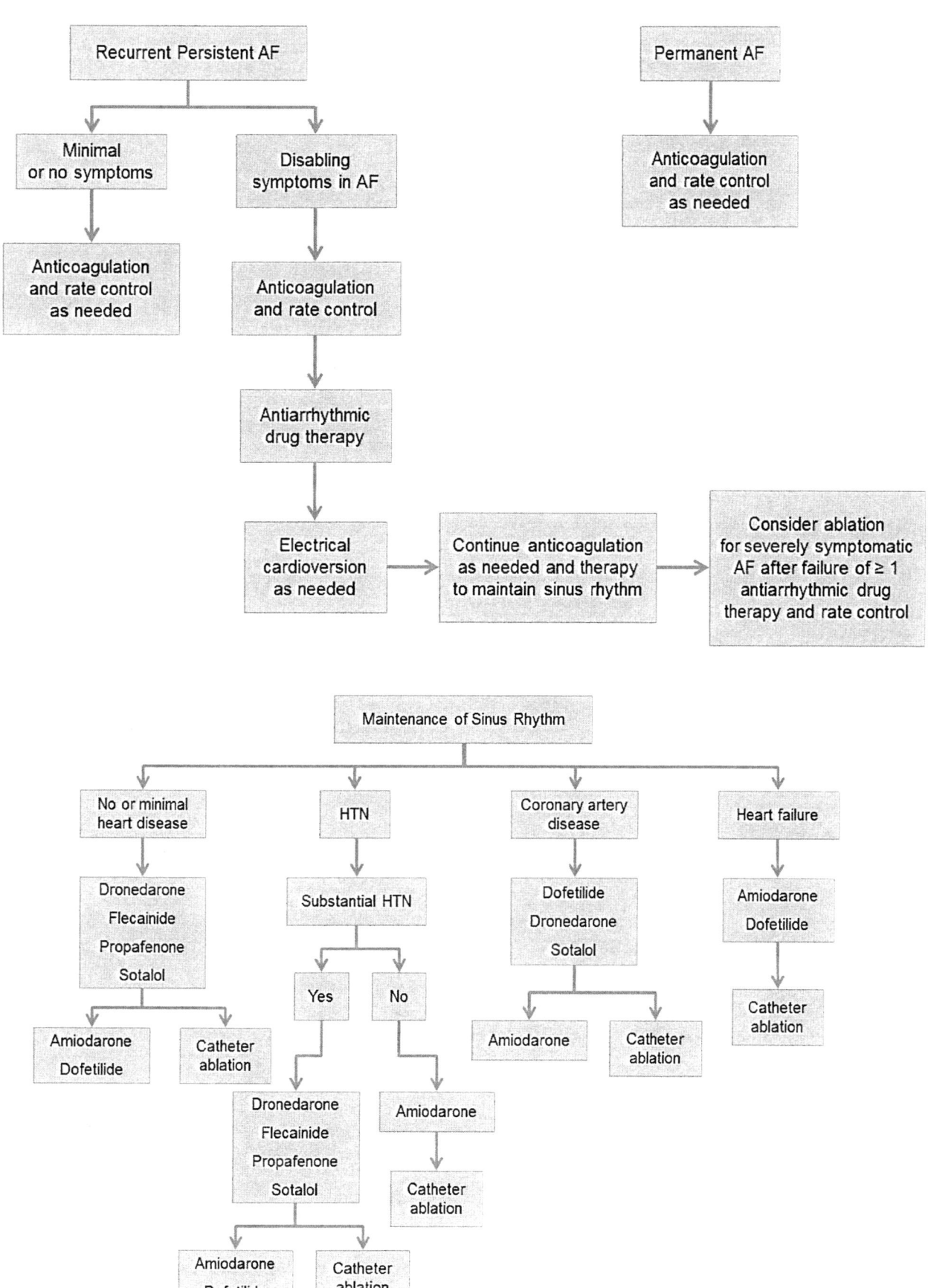

Medications for Rate Control

Medication	Loading Dose	Onset	Maintenance Dose		
Esmolol	500 mcg/kg IV	5 min	60–200 mcg/kg/min IV	I	C
Metoprolol	2.5–5 mg IV up to 3 doses	5 min	25–100 mg twice per day	I	C
Propranolol	0.15 mg/kg IV	5 min	80–240 mg/day in divided doses	I	C
Diltiazem	0.25 mg/kg IV	2–7 min	120–360 mg/day in sustained release	I	B
Verapamil	0.075–0.15 mg/kg IV	3–5 min	120–360 mg/day in sustained release	I	B
Amiodarone (with accessory pathway)	150 mg over 10 min Load: 800 mg/day for 1 week 600 mg/day for 1 week 400 mg/day for 4–6 weeks	Days	200 mg/day	IIa	C
Digoxin (in HF)	0.25 mg IV each 2 hours, up to 1.5 mg	60 min	0.125–0.375 mg/day	I	B
Amiodarone (in HF)	Same as above	Days	200 mg/day	IIa	C

Rate Control vs. Rhythm Control
- Studies comparing rate control with rhythm control have shown no difference in:
  - Quality of life
  - Mortality
  - Cardiac events
- Maintenance of sinus rhythm is indicated in highly symptomatic patients

CHA₂DS₂-VASc Risk Factors for Stroke

C	Congestive heart failure	1
H	Hypertension	1
A	Age ≥ 75	2
D	Diabetes mellitus	1
S	Prior TIA or stroke	2
V	Vascular disease (MI, PAD, carotid stenosis, etc.)	1
A	Age 65–74	1
Sc	Sex category = Female	1

Anticoagulation Strategy

Score	Recommended Therapy
No risk factors (0)	ASA 81–325 mg/day
1 risk factor (1)	ASA 81–325 mg/day or warfarin (INR 2.0–3.0)
2 risk factors (≥ 2)	Warfarin (INR 2.0–3.0; If mechanical valve, INR > 2.5)

Novel Anticoagulants
(Use in place of warfarin)

Dabigatran
- Dabigatran is a direct thrombin inhibitor
- In 1 major trial, dabigatran decreased stroke risk in AF by 34% vs. warfarin
- Dabigatran had a 20% less risk of bleeding compared to warfarin
- Dabigatran dose (150 mg bid) must be adjusted for decreased creatinine clearance

Rivaroxaban
- 20 mg daily with evening meal
- Adjust for CrCl
- Like dabigatran, not recommended in end-stage CKD

Apixaban
- 5 or 2.5 mg bid
- Use 2.5 mg bid if any 2:
  - Cr ≥ 1.5 mg/dL
  - ≥ 80 yo
  - Body weight ≤ 60 kg
- Not recommended in patients with severe hepatic impairment
- No recommendation in severe renal impairment

Edoxaban
- Approved Jan. 2015 for nonvalvular AF
- Once-daily, selective factor Xa inhibitor
- ENGAGE AF-TIMI 48: Edoxaban was not inferior to warfarin
- Do not use if CrCl ≥ 95 mL/min

Valvular Atrial Fibrillation
Only warfarin is approved for anticoagulation of atrial fibrillation due to valvular heart disease (including prosthetic valves).

Atrial Fibrillation

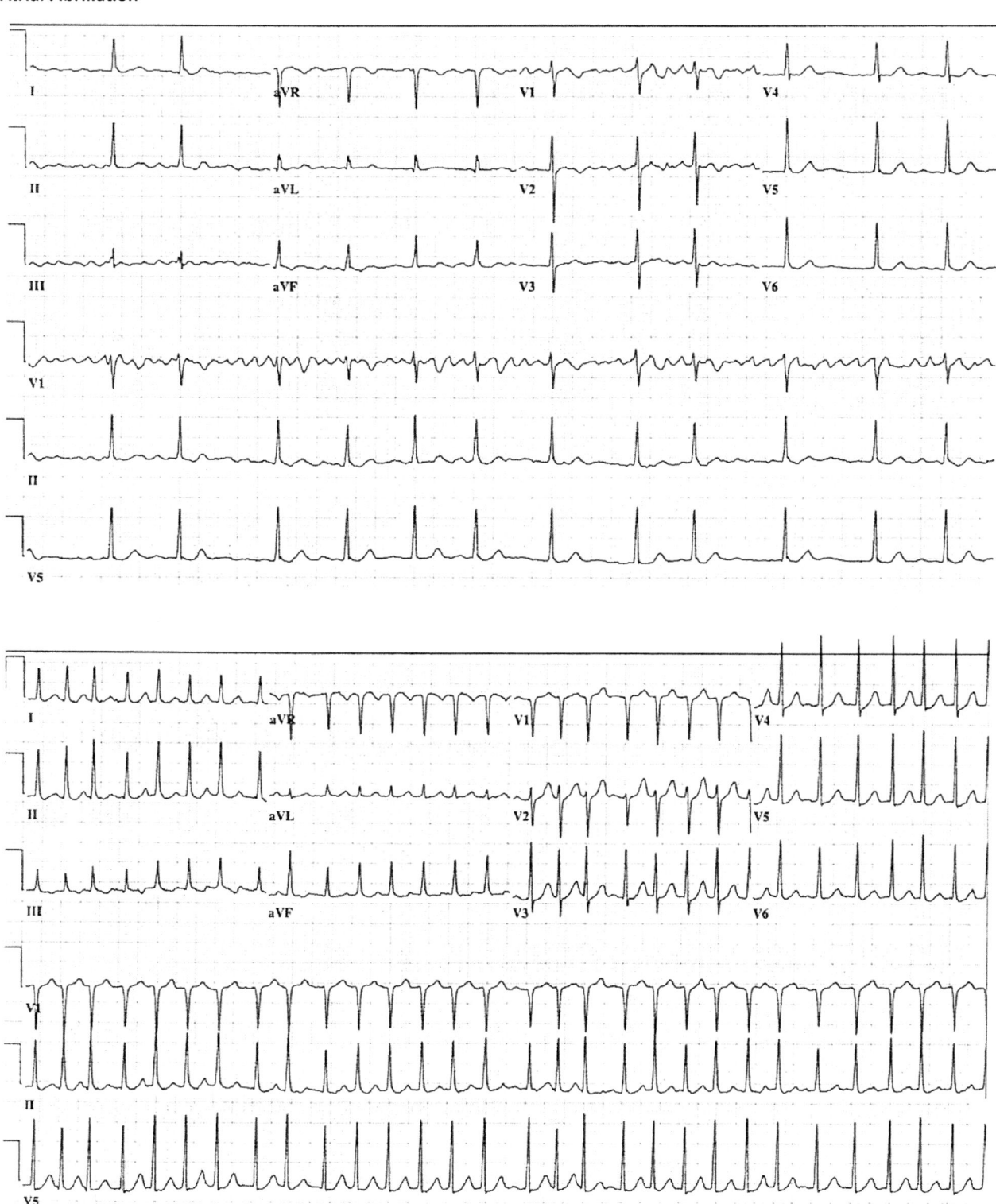

AR 95

An 81 yo female with a history of mechanical MVR presents with persistent atrial fibrillation.

What is your anticoagulation strategy?
A. Switch her from warfarin to dabigatran.
B. Switch her from warfarin to apixaban.
C. Continue her warfarin that she is receiving for her mechanical valve.
D. Discontinue anticoagulation due to her age.

Answer: _____

Atrial Flutter

ECG
- Atrial rate is 220–320
- Ventricular rate is usually an even number division of the atrial rate
- Always consider flutter when HR is 150 bpm
- There is usually a sawtooth pattern in II, III, aVF, and V1

- Every regular SVT with a rate of 150 is AF with 2:1 block until proven otherwise
- Vagal maneuvers and AV nodal blocking medications slow ventricular response

Management
- Rate control strategies similar to atrial fibrillation
- Anticoagulation strategies similar to AF

Atrial Flutter

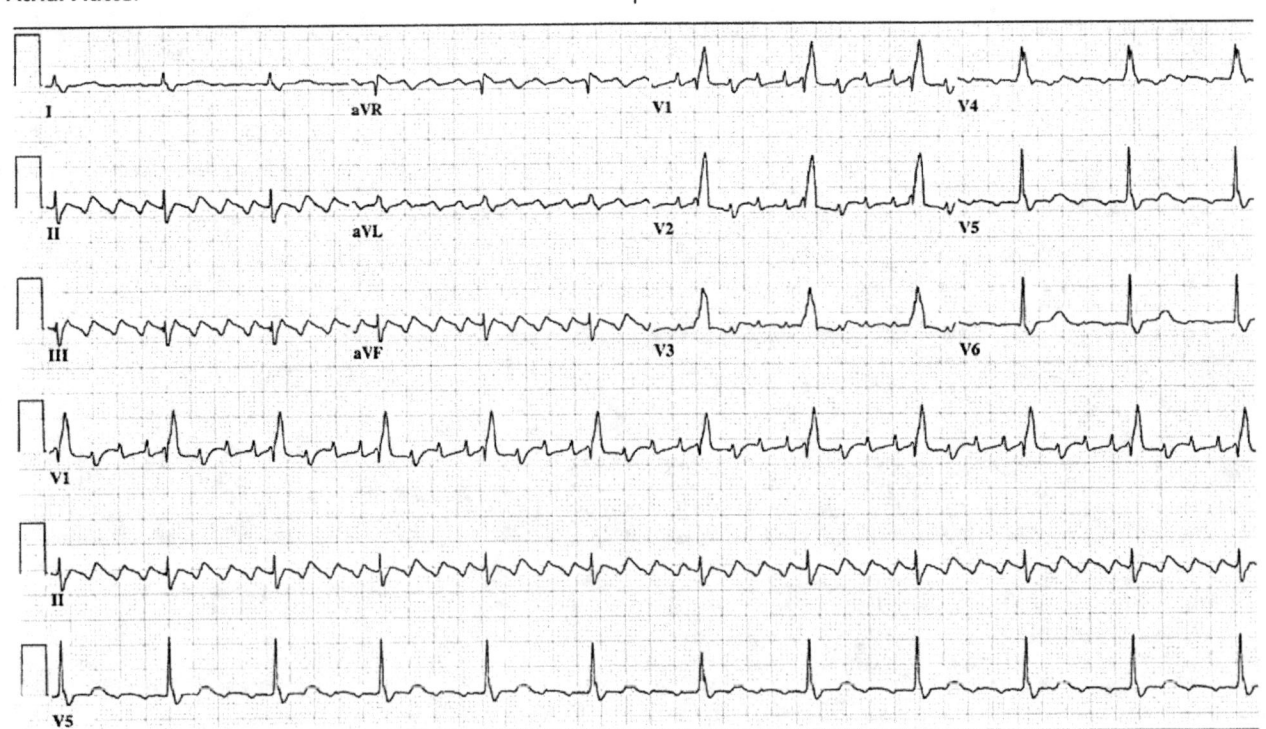

Atrial Flutter (cont.)

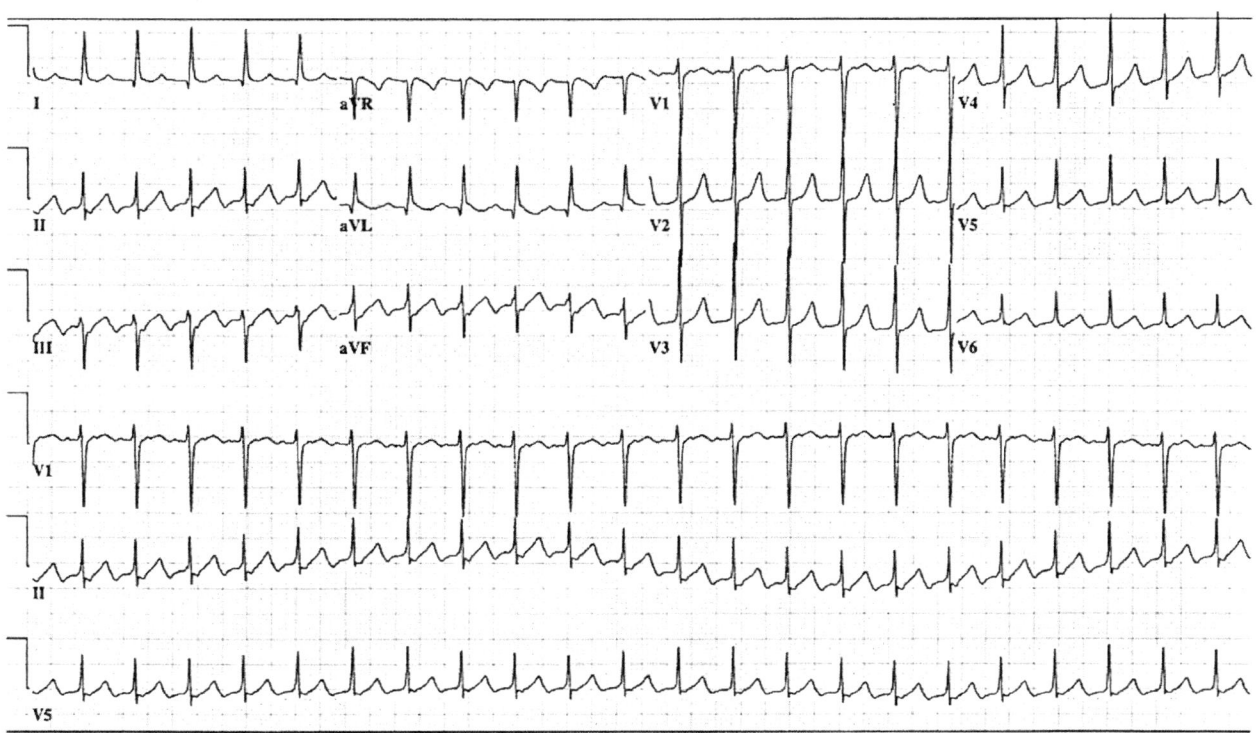

AVNRT

Anatomy of the AV Node

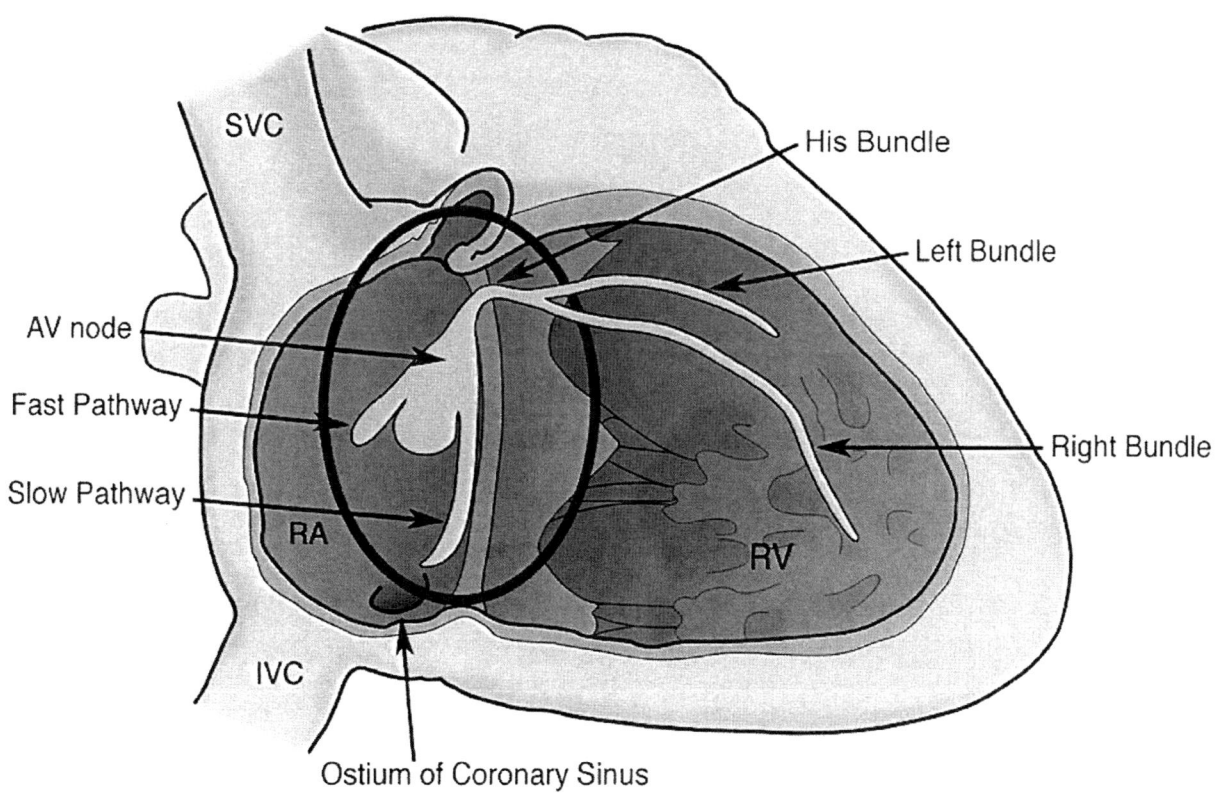

Anatomy of the AV Node (cont.)

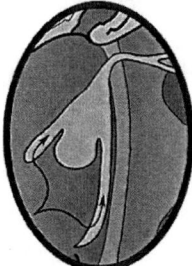

Normal conduction through the AV node

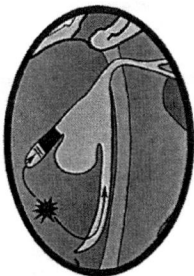

In the situation above, a fortuitously timed PAC is conducted down the slow pathway. The fast pathway, which has a longer repolarization time, is still refractory

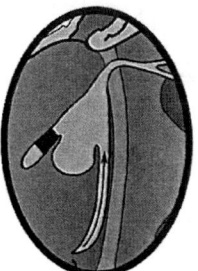

The conduction continues down the slow pathway while the fast pathway completes its repolarization

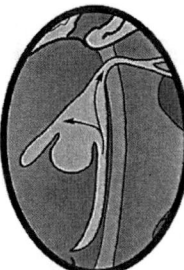

The impulse is free to travel down the His bundle and depolarize the ventricles. Meanwhile, the fast pathway has repolarized

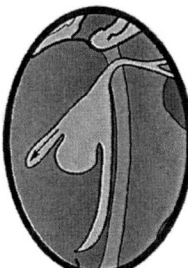

The impulse is free to travel retrograde up the fast pathway

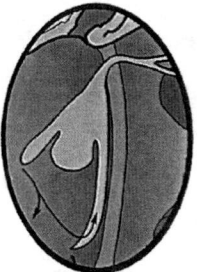

If the impulse arrives at the branch point before the next normal depolarization arrives from above, the reentry loop may sustain itself, resulting in AVNRT

AVNRT

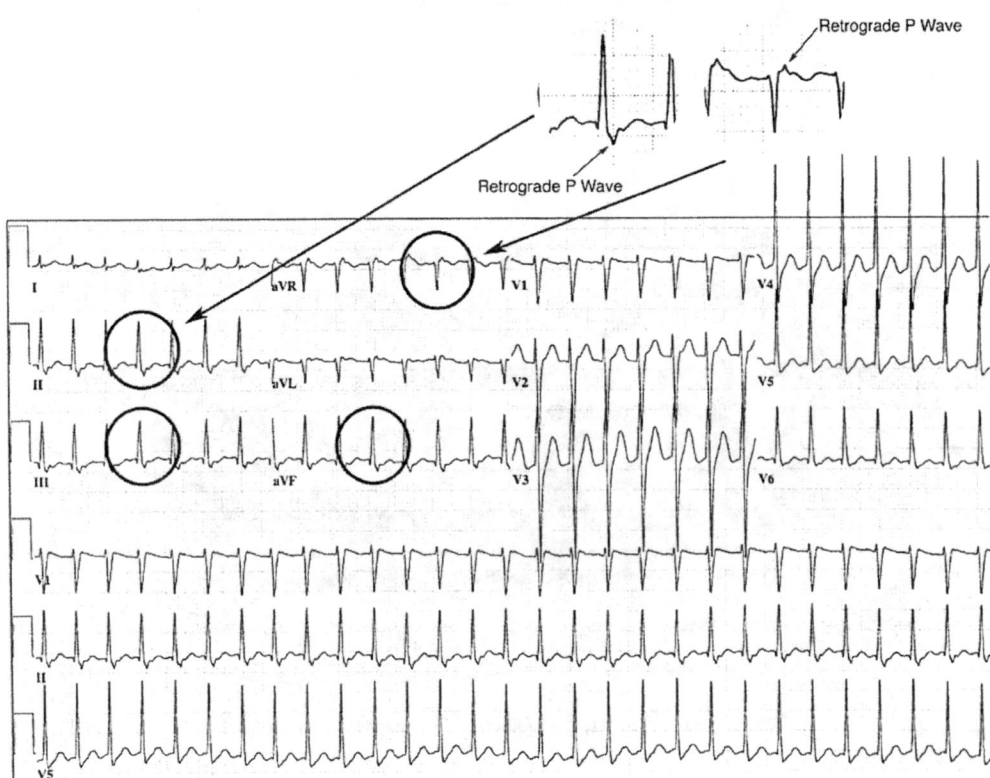

Ventricular Arrhythmias

ECG
- 90% of wide complex (QRS > 120 msec) tachycardias are VT
- The wider and "uglier" the QRS complexes, the more likely they represent VT
- Look for AV dissociation, which proves VT
- Look for capture (Dressler's) beats

Evaluation of the Patient
- History and physical examination
- ECG
- Exercise testing for patients at risk for CAD
- Ambulatory ECG in selected patients
- Transthoracic echo
- Electrophysiology studies in patients with CAD or LV dysfunction

Management
- DC cardioversion for any unstable patient (!!)
- Revascularization of viable myocardium
- Vigorous treatment of heart failure
- Aggressive secondary prevention for CAD
- Maintenance of stable electrolytes

Indications for ICDs
- Prior MI and LVEF < 35%
- Nonischemic dilated cardiomyopathy with LVEF < 35% with at least 1-year survival
- Hypertrophic cardiomyopathy with sustained VT or VF

Antiarrhythmic Drugs

Beta-blockers	Decreases PVCs and VT; Reduces incidence of sudden cardiac death
Amiodarone	Suppresses VT, no survival benefit; Complex drug interactions and side effects
Sotalol	Suppresses VT, no survival benefit, proarrhythmic

Ventricular Tachycardia

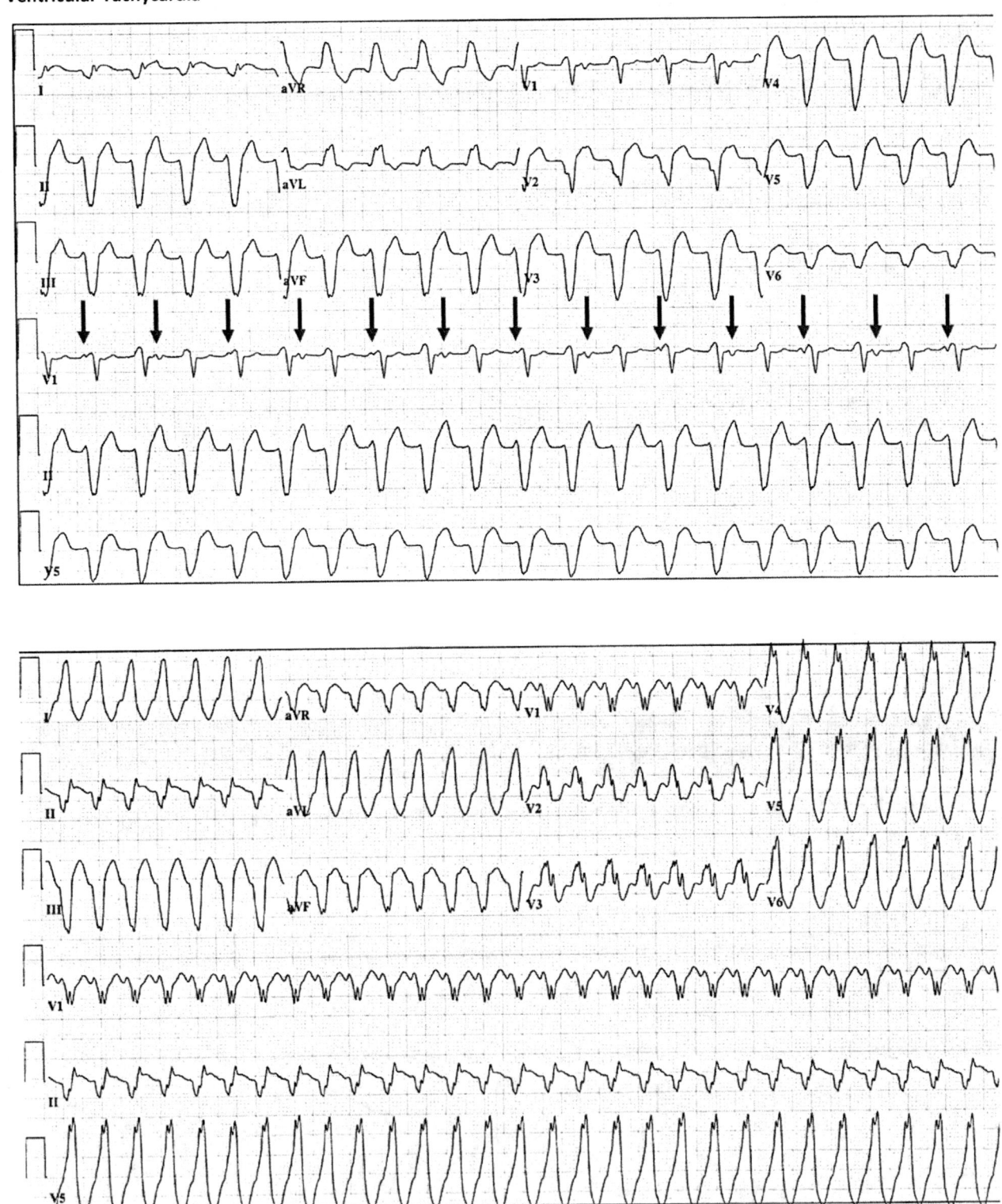

© 2017 MedStudy Internal Medicine Video Board Review – Cardiology • Matthew Sorrentino, MD

AR 96

A young woman presents with 2 episodes of prolonged palpitations while playing basketball.
Her resting ECG follows.

ECG

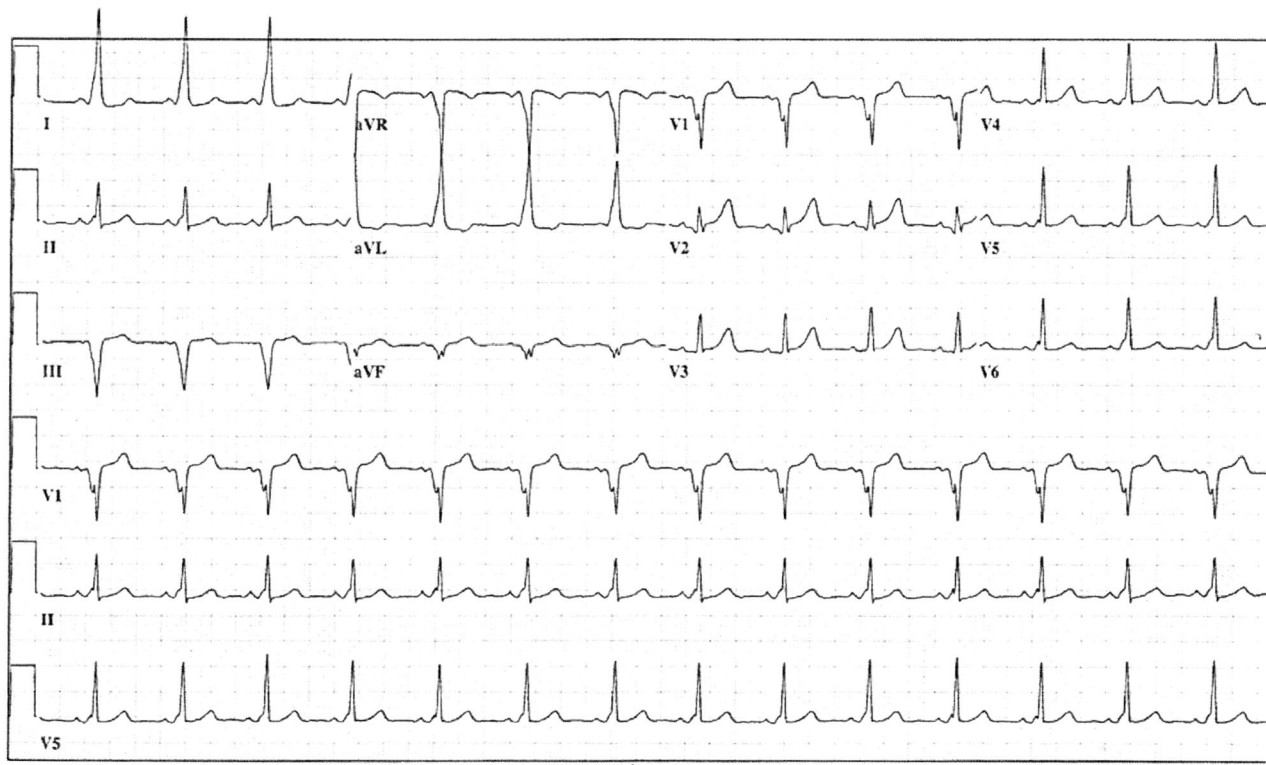

What is the diagnosis?

A. LVH
B. Hypertrophic cardiomyopathy
C. WPW
D. Previous inferior MI
E. Amphetamine abuse

Answer: _____

AR 97

The surgeons have started digoxin in a postoperative patient when you are called because of an arrhythmia.
BP is 120/80 mmHg and the patient is comfortable.
Serum K is 3.1 mg/dL.
His ECG follows.

ECG

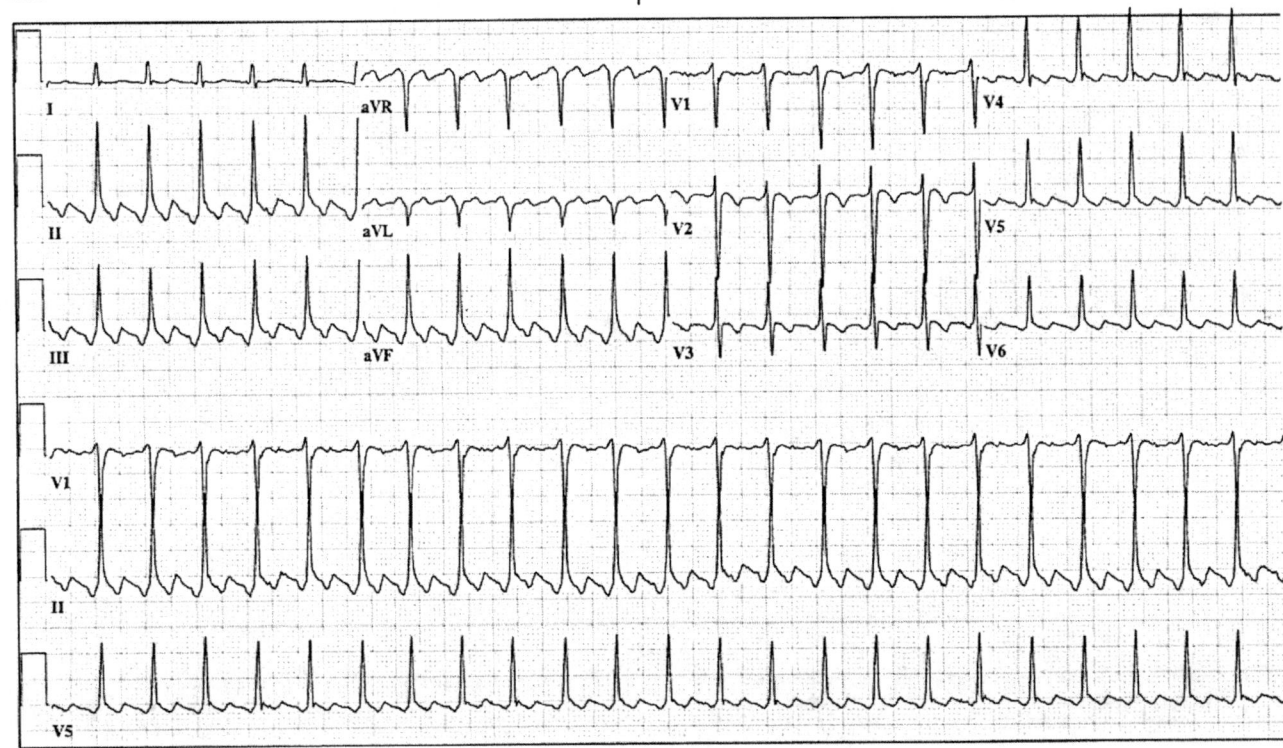

What should you do?
A. Immediate synchronized cardioversion.
B. Give potassium and stop digoxin.
C. Give potassium and increase digoxin.
D. Give potassium and add IV diltiazem.
E. Give potassium and an oral beta-blocker.

Answer: _____

AR 98

A patient presents with his 3rd episode of symptomatic atrial fibrillation in the past 5 years.
His resting ECG shows QT prolongation.

What should be done?
A. Transesophageal echo and cardioversion
B. Ibutilide
C. Amiodarone
D. Verapamil
E. Propafenone

Answer: _____

AR 99

A 20 yo patient presents with a history of sudden death in his 23 yo sister.
His ECG follows.

ECG

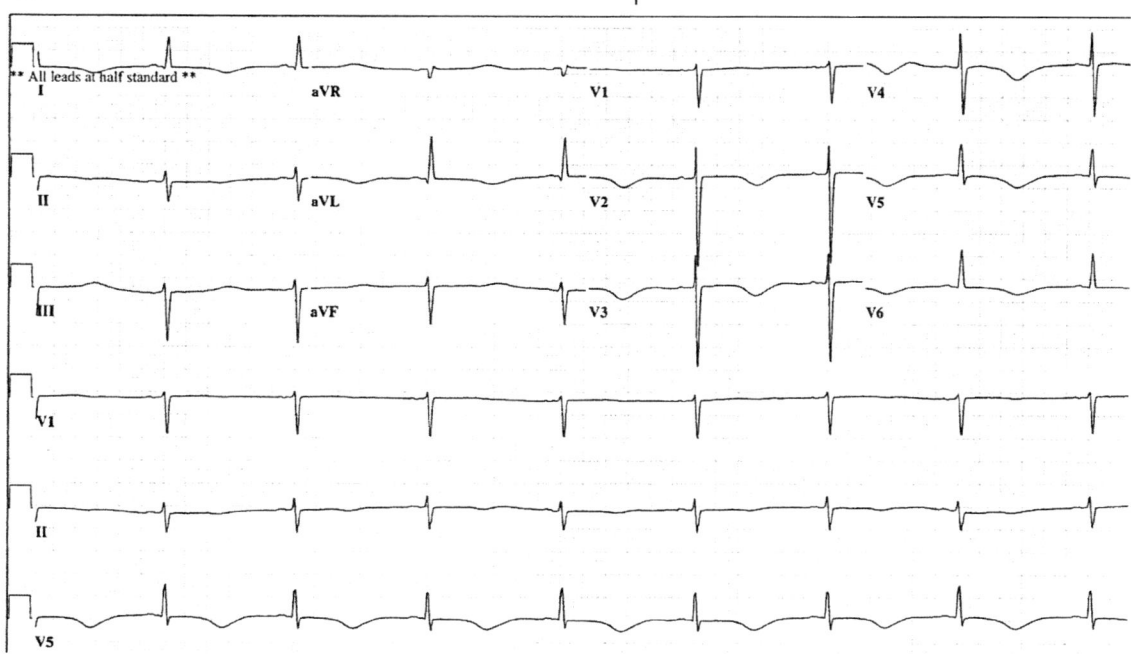

Which of the following statements is true?
A. He should be treated with amiodarone.
B. He should be treated with sotalol.
C. He should be treated with verapamil.
D. He is also at risk for sudden death.
E. No treatment is necessary.

Answer: _____

AR 100

A 25 yo patient who complains of palpitations has the following rhythm strip as part of a 24-hour Holter monitor.
He has no other evidence of cardiac disease.

What should be done?
A. Reassurance
B. An implantable defibrillator
C. Treatment with amiodarone
D. Treatment with verapamil
E. Treatment with an ACE inhibitor

Answer: _____

AR 101

A patient you have not seen previously comes to the ED with the following ECG.
Blood pressure is 70/40 mmHg.

ECG

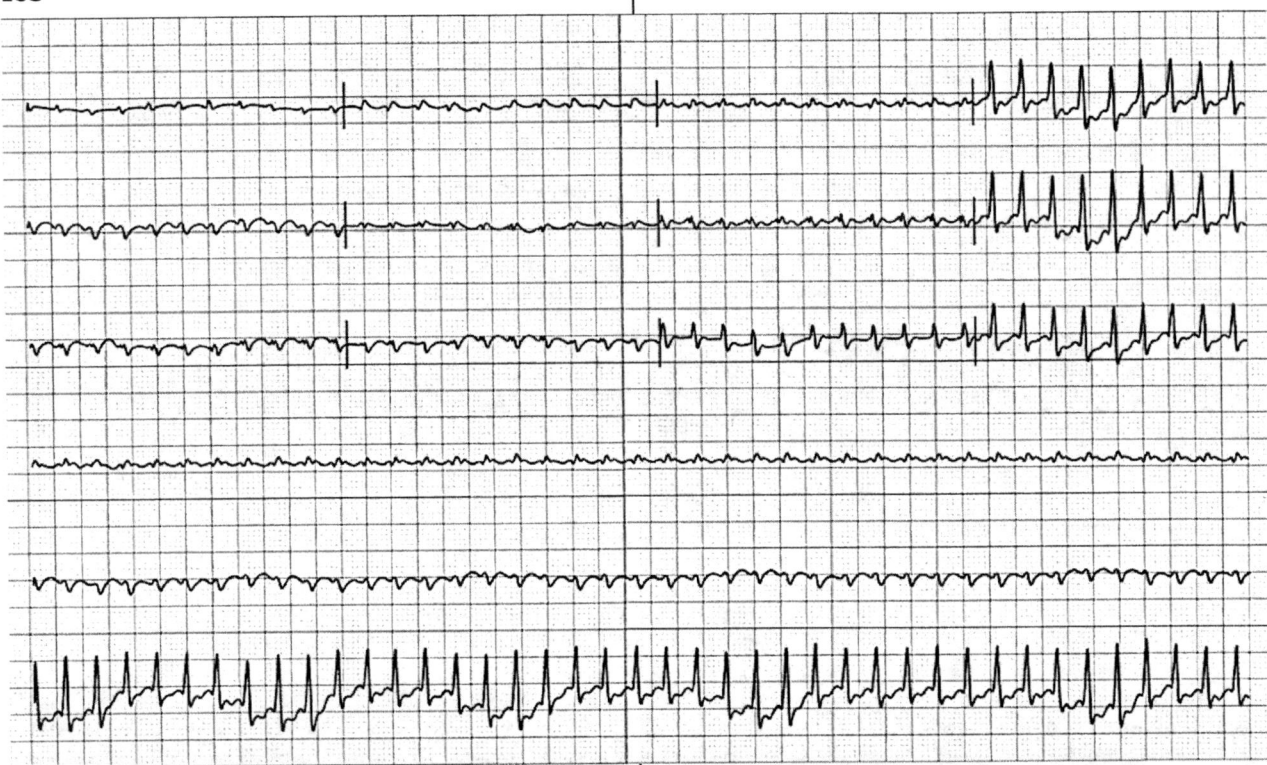

What should you do?
A. Intravenous diltiazem
B. IV amiodarone
C. IV esmolol
D. IV digoxin
E. Immediate synchronized cardioversion

Answer: _____

AR 102

A 72 yo asymptomatic man is noted to have sinus bradycardia at a rate of 50 on a preoperative ECG.
He has no history of cardiac disease and is taking no medications.
He states he can climb 4 flights of stairs with no difficulty.

What should you recommend?
A. Reassurance
B. 24-hour ambulatory ECG (Holter monitor)
C. Exercise stress testing
D. Referral for permanent pacemaker
E. Echocardiography

Answer: _____

AR 103

A 97 yo woman presents with 2 days of nausea and vomiting.

Her other problems include dementia and moderate chronic renal failure.

BP 110/70 mmHg, HR 98 bpm and regularly irregular

Her ECG follows.

ECG

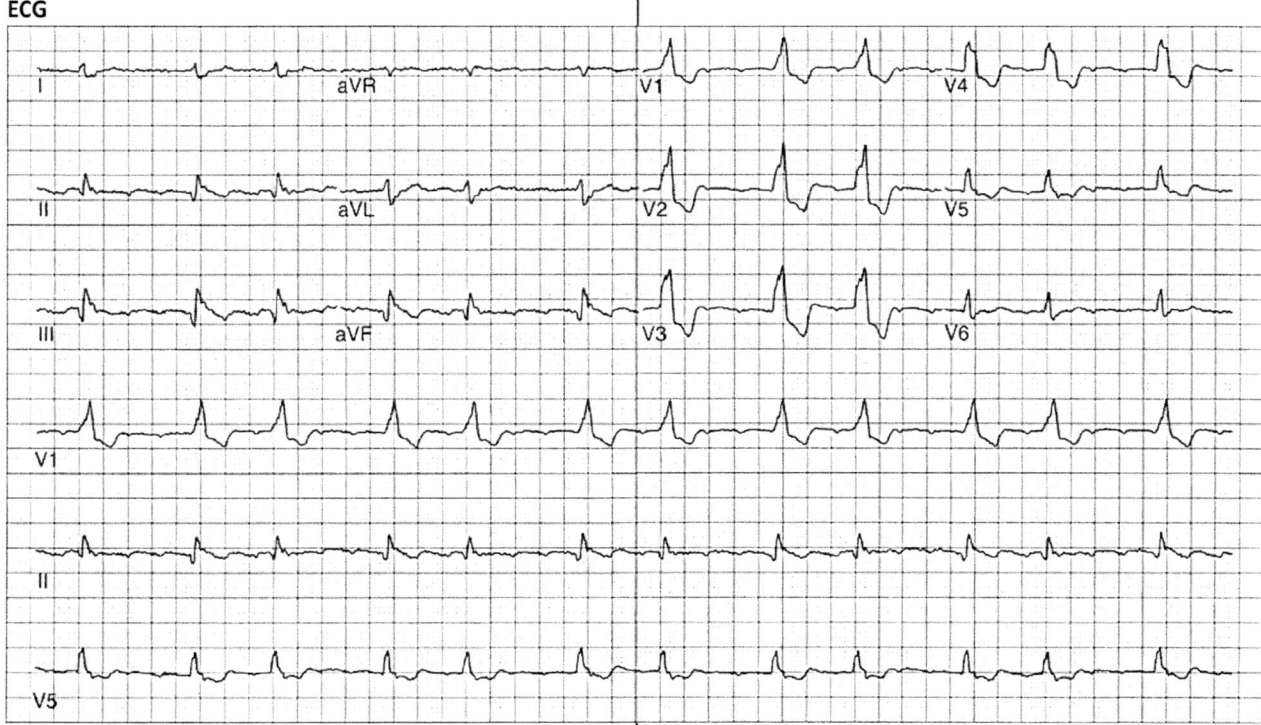

What should you do?

A. Digoxin.

B. Beta-blockers.

C. Diltiazem.

D. Amiodarone.

E. Stop all cardiac medications.

Answer: _____

AR 104

A patient with chest pain presents to the ED.
ECG follows.

ECG

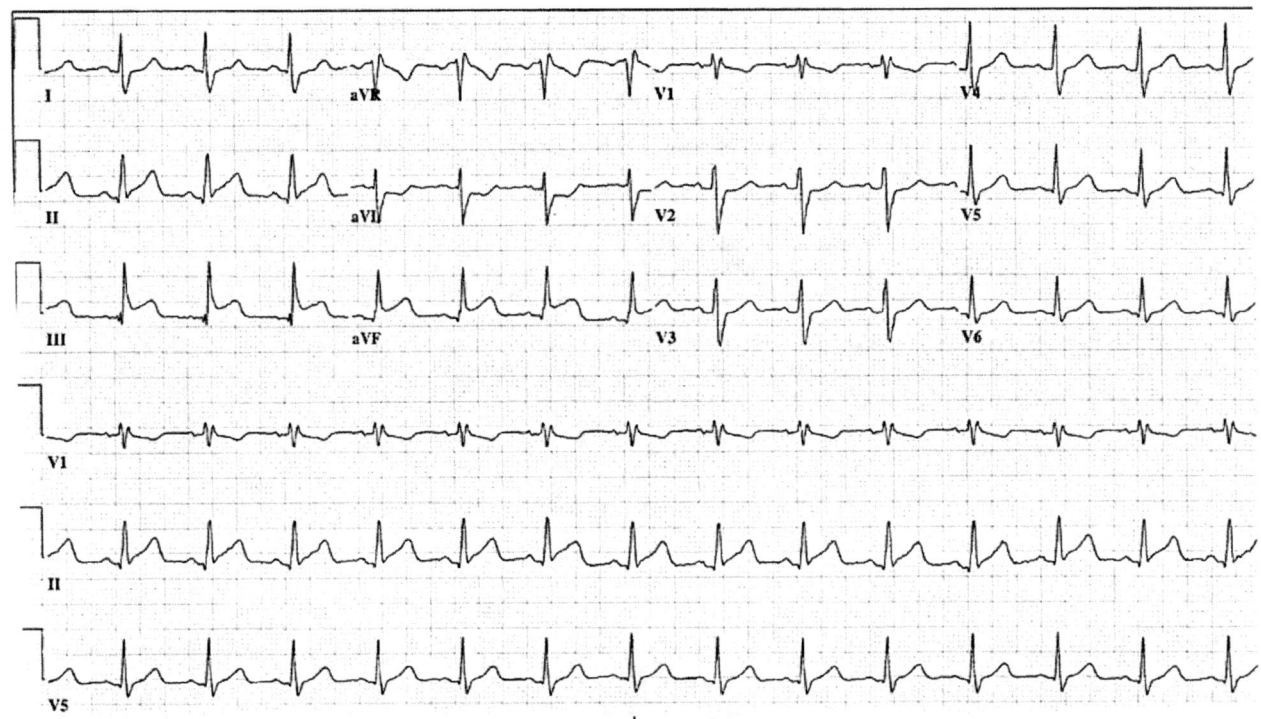

Which coronary artery is most likely to be involved?

A. Left main
B. Right
C. Circumflex
D. Left anterior descending

Answer: _____

Cardiology
Audience Response Answers

Audience Response 1
Answer: E. A large pericardial effusion.

AR 2
Answer: B. Aortic valve surgery.

AR 3
Answer: B. A transthoracic echocardiogram.

AR 4
Answer: C. Transesophageal echo.

AR 5
Answer: B. An exercise stress test
with nuclear perfusion imaging.

AR 6
Answer: D. A dobutamine stress echo.

AR 7
Answer: A. Undergo coronary revascularization
to the anterior wall.

AR 8
Answer: B. Retroperitoneal hemorrhage.

AR 9
Answer: E. Atherosclerotic embolization
to the kidneys and systemically at the time
of catheterization.

AR 10
Answer: D. Nuclear perfusion imaging would improve
the accuracy of the exercise study.

AR 11
Answer: D. Tamponade.

AR 12
Answer: D. Refer her for urgent coronary angiography.

AR 13
Answer: D. Cannon a waves.

AR 14
Answer: C. Moderate-to-severe tricuspid regurgitation
with a vegetation on the tricuspid valve.

AR 15
Answer: D. ASD.

AR 16
Answer: C. Atrial septal defect.

AR 17
Answer: A. An S_3 on examination.

AR 18
Answer: B. A fasting blood glucose of 160 mg/dL.

AR 19
Answer: D. Weight loss counseling.

AR 20
Answer: B. Addition of a statin to his medication
regimen.

AR 21
Answer: C. Addition of lisinopril to her medication
regimen.

AR 22
Answer: B. There is sufficient evidence to recommend
that he begin taking ASA 81 mg daily for primary
prevention.

AR 23
Answer: A. A 12-lead electrocardiogram.

AR 24
Answer: C. Cardiac troponin I.

AR 25
Answer: C. Give ASA 325 mg to chew.

AR 26
Answer: C. Atorvastatin 80 mg.

AR 27
Answer: C. She should be referred for immediate
cardiac catheterization and primary PCI.

AR 28
Answer: A. Immediate coronary angiography.

AR 29
Answer: C. Transfer her to a PCI-capable facility
immediately.

AR 30
Answer: D. Refer for emergent PCI.

AR 31
Answer: B. Due to his age, he is at higher risk
of cardiogenic shock.

AR 32
Answer: D. She should have lisinopril added to her medication list.

AR 33
Answer: D. Perform immediate synchronized electrical cardioversion.

AR 34
Answer: D. RV infarction.

AR 35
Answer: C. Pulmonary congestion on auscultation.

AR 36
Answer: D. Atropine 0.5 mg IV.

AR 37
Answer: C. Acute VSD.

AR 38
Answer: D. Urine drug screen.

AR 39
Answer: C. A 65 yo man with 2 hours of chest pain and new left bundle-branch block.

AR 40
Answer: D. An echo showing an LVEF of 30% would be an indication for coronary angiography.

AR 41
Answer: C. Observe him for 8 hours, draw another set of markers, and obtain another ECG.

AR 42
Answer: E. tPA plus intravenous heparin.

AR 43
Answer: E. Refer him for urgent coronary angiography.

AR 44
Answer: E. ASA, beta-blocker, ACEI, and referral for ICD placement.

AR 45
Answer: C. Referral for catheter-based coronary angiography and possible PCI.

AR 46
Answer: D. Decrease beta-blockers.

AR 47
Answer: D. Slow infusion of normal saline.

AR 48
Answer: C. Cilostazol 100 mg bid can improve his symptoms and increase his walking distance.

AR 49
Answer: A. Buerger disease.

AR 50
Answer: D. Takayasu arteritis.

AR 51
Answer: B. Prinzmetal angina.

AR 52
Answer: E. Dissection can occur in the 3rd trimester of pregnancy without any predisposing factors.

AR 53
Answer: C. TEE.

AR 54A
Answer: A. CT with imaging of the entire aorta.

AR 54B
Answer: C. Immediate cardiothoracic surgery.

AR 55
Answer: C. CT with imaging of the entire aorta.

AR 56
Answer: B. 70 yo male with ascending aortic dissection identified on TEE.

AR 57
Answer: D. Blood cultures.

AR 58
Answer: C. Prosthetic aortic valve.

AR 59
Answer: A. She does not require prophylaxis.

AR 60
Answer: B. Schedule cardiac catheterization in anticipation of aortic valve replacement.

AR 61
Answer: C. This patient will require cardiac catheterization.

AR 62
Answer: B. Chronic aortic regurgitation.

AR 63
Answer: C. Chronic MS.

AR 64
Answer: D. The onset of atrial fibrillation.

AR 65
Answer: A. Chronic MR.

AR 66
Answer: C. Refer for mitral valve replacement.

AR 67
Answer: D. Late systolic murmur at the apex.

AR 68
Answer: C. Obtain an emergent transthoracic echo
and alert cardiac surgery.

AR 69
Answer: D. An ejection sound at the 2nd LICS
that gets softer upon inspiration.

AR 70
Answer: B. Aortic valve replacement for bicuspid
aortic valve.

AR 71
Answer: B. Refer for surgery now.

AR 72
Answer: A. Endocarditis of the tricuspid valve.

AR 73
Answer: C. Acute MR due to chordal rupture.

AR 74
Answer: B. Low-pitched diastolic rumble
at the apex.

AR 75
Answer: A. AR.

AR 76
Answer: A. Sudden death occurs in this condition.

AR 77
Answer: A. He has Stage A heart failure.

AR 78
Answer: C. Class III.

AR 79
Answer: B. Medication combination 2.

AR 80A
Answer: E. Amyloidosis.

AR 80B
Answer: C. Restrictive cardiomyopathy.

AR 81
Answer: A. Beta-blockers.

AR 82
Answer: D. Echocardiogram.

AR 83
Answer: C. Pericardiocentesis.

AR 84
Answer: B. Secundum ASD.

AR 85
Answer: D. Anomalous coronary artery.

AR 86
Answer: B. She has developed
Eisenmenger syndrome.

AR 87A
Answer: B. Transthoracic echo.

AR 87B
Answer: B. If LV dysfunction persists, she is at greater
risk of heart failure and sudden death in any
subsequent pregnancy.

AR 88
Answer: C. An ACE inhibitor.

AR 89
Answer: D. Carvedilol.

AR 90
Answer: E. Chronic anemia.

AR 91
Answer: A. Constrictive pericarditis.

AR 92
Answer: B. VSD.

AR 93
Answer: D. Severe concentric LVH, LVEF 70%.

AR 94
Answer: C. Left circumflex artery.

AR 95
Answer: C. Continue her warfarin that she is receiving
for her mechanical valve.

AR 96
Answer: C. WPW.

AR 97
Answer: B. Give potassium and stop digoxin.

AR 98
Answer: A. Transesophageal echo
and cardioversion.

AR 99
Answer: D. He is also at risk for sudden death.

AR 100
Answer: A. Reassurance.

AR 101
Answer: E. Immediate synchronized cardioversion.

AR 102
Answer: A. Reassurance.

AR 103
Answer: E. Stop all cardiac medications.

AR 104
Answer: B. Right.

MedStudy

Internal Medicine Video Board Review

Dermatology

Presented by

Aaron J. Calderon, MD
Chairman, Department of Medicine
Program Director, Internal Medicine Residency
Saint Joseph Hospital
Clinical Professor of Medicine
University of Colorado School of Medicine
Denver, Colorado

Table of Contents

Dermatology Abbreviations

DFA	Direct fluorescent ab
DH	Dermatitis herpetiformis
DRESS	Drug reaction with eosinophilia and systemic symptoms
ESRD	End-stage renal disease
GFR	Glomerular filtration rate
HAART	Highly active antiviral therapy
HCV	Hepatitis C virus
HPV	Human papilloma virus
HRT	Hormone replacement therapy
IVIG	IV immune globulin
LAV	Live attenuated vaccine
MF	Mycosis fungoides
MRSA	Methicillin-resistant *Staphylococcus aureus*
NBUVB	Narrow band ultraviolet B radiation
OCP	Oral contraceptive pill
PCR	Patient care report; polymerase chain reaction
PUVA	Psoralen and ultraviolet A radiation
RPR	Rapid plasma reagin
SJS	Stevens-Johnson syndrome
TCAs	Tricyclic antidepressants
TEN	Toxic epidermal necrolysis
VDRL	Venereal disease research laboratory
VZV	Varicella zoster virus

Dermatology

Common Skin Disorders

Audience Response 1

A 26 y/o female with asthma presents with numerous rough, weeping, pruritic, erythematous patches in the antecubital and popliteal fossas.

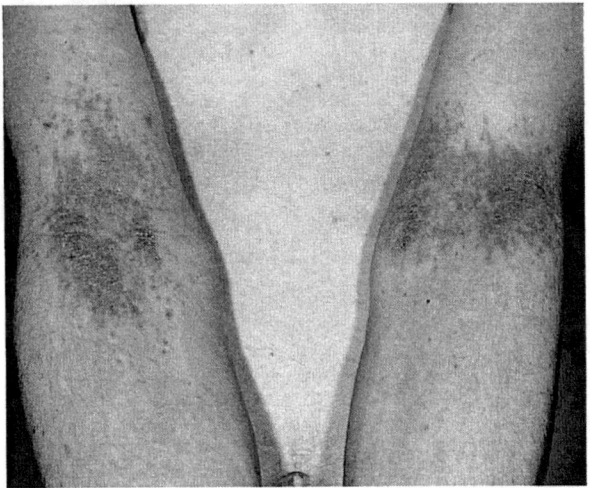

What is the preferred treatment for her condition?
A. Oral antihistamines
B. Topical tacrolimus
C. Oral azathioprine
D. Topical antifungal
E. Topical corticosteroids

Answer: _____

Atopic Dermatitis
- Begins in childhood
- Very pruritic
- Chronic
- Relapsing & remitting
- **Flexural distribution**
  - Antecubital fossa
  - Popliteal fossa
  - Wrists
- Associated with asthma
- Elevated IgE levels

- Susceptibility to cutaneous infections
  - Bacterial (*Staph aureus*)
  - Fungal
  - Viral (warts, molluscum, HSV)

- Flares often precipitated by:
  - Irritants (e.g., wool, pollen)
  - Dry skin
  - Heat, stress
  - Skin infections

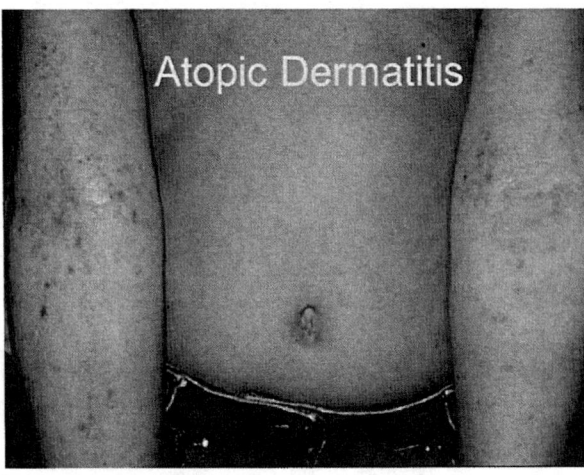

Atopic Dermatitis

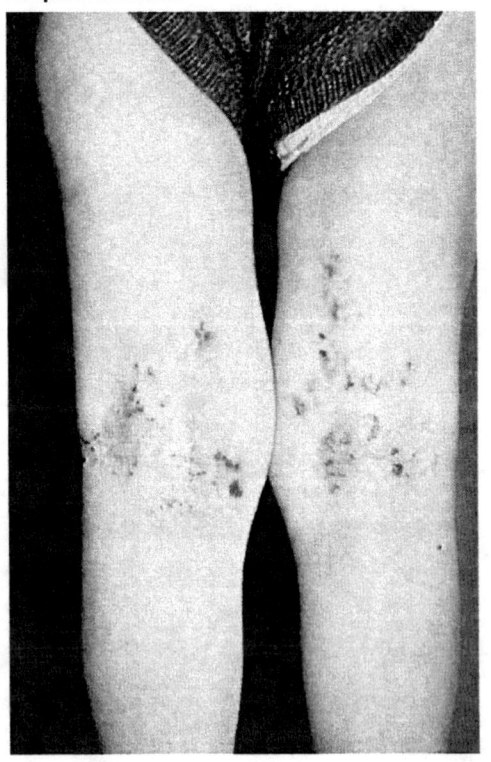

Potential Complications

Atopic Dermatitis — Eczema Herpeticum

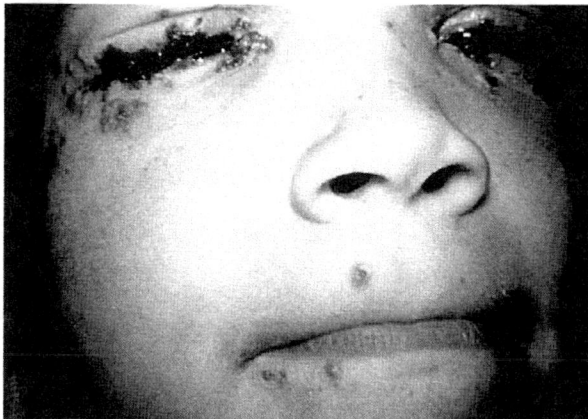

CDC Public Health Image Library

Atopic Dermatitis Treatment
- **Topical corticosteroids**
  - Mainstay Rx for acute flares
  - Use lowest effective dose
  - Use only low-potency on face
- **Topical immunomodulators**
  - Calcineurin inhibitors (tacrolimus, pimecrolimus)
  - Don't cause thin skin or striae (face OK)
  - Risk for T-cell lymphoma?
  - 2nd line; Black Box Warning
- **Systemic immunomodulators**
  - Cyclosporine, azathioprine

Atopic Dermatitis Maintenance
- **Skin hygiene**
  - Tub soaks or showers < 10 minutes
  - Moisturize within 3 minutes
  - Ointment-based emollients best
    - Petroleum jelly is cheap and effective
    - Discourage lotions and oils
  - Gentle cleansers (i.e., nonsoap)
- **Avoid irritants**
  - Wool, fragrances, excessive hand washing
  - Heat, stress

Atopic Dermatitis Treatment Pyramid

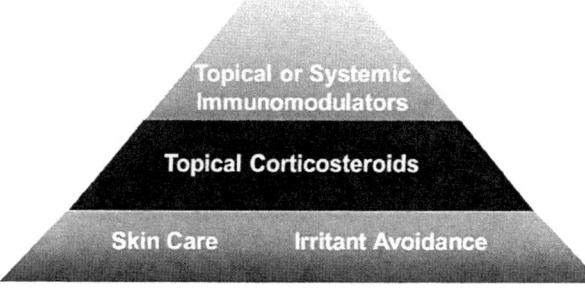

AR 2

This 37 y/o man has not responded to adequate seborrheic dermatitis therapy.

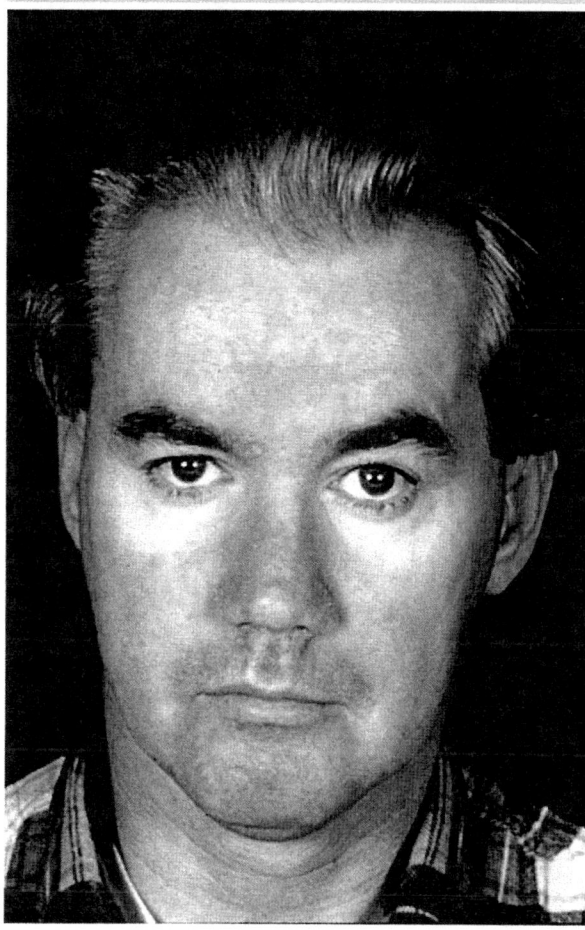

What is the next step in management?
A. Genetic testing.
B. Skin biopsy.
C. CT chest/abdomen/pelvis.
D. Check for HIV.
E. Start oral corticosteroids.

Answer: _____

Seborrheic Dermatitis
- Common, chronic inflammatory condition
- **Greasy, yellow scale ± erythema**
- Typical locations
- Remits and relapses
- ***Malassezia furfur*** yeast thought to play an etiologic role, but unclear
- Higher prevalence in **HIV and Parkinson's**

Seborrheic Dermatitis (cont.)
Distribution
- Scalp
- Eyebrows
- Conchal bowls
- Nasolabial folds
- Chest
- Axilla
- Groin

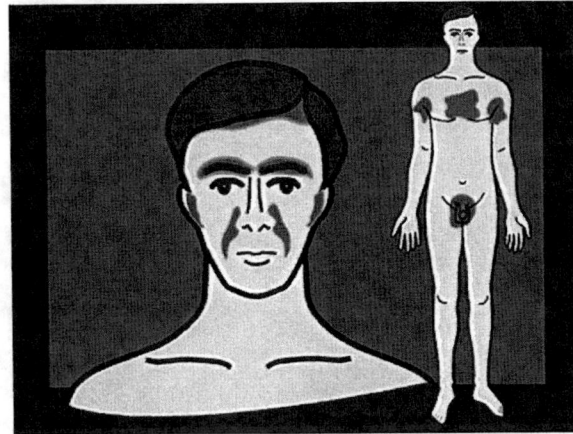

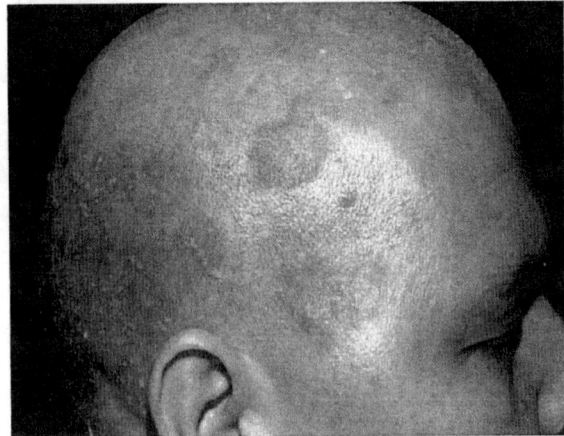

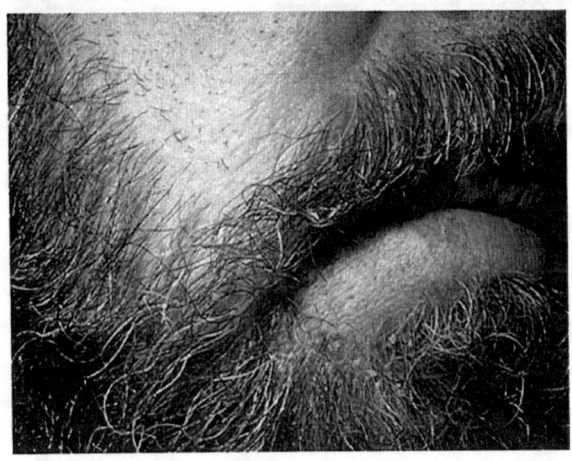

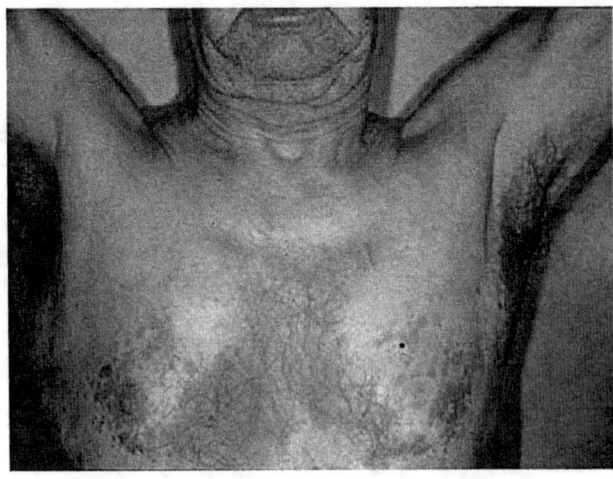

Seborrheic Dermatitis Treatment
- Wash daily to qod: Antidandruff shampoo
  - Zinc pyrithione
  - Selenium sulfide
  - Ketoconazole
  - Ciclopirox
- Ketoconazole cream
- Low-potency topical steroid — but not recommended as maintenance

AR 3
What is the most likely cause of this patient's rash?
A. Poison ivy
B. Penicillin allergy
C. Atopic dermatitis
D. Viral exanthem
E. Seborrheic dermatitis

Answer: _____

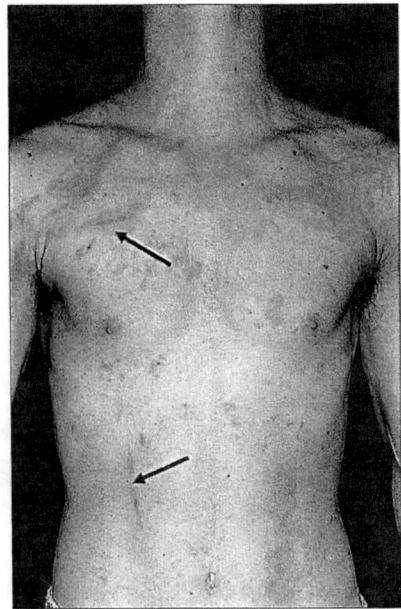

Contact Dermatitis

- **Irritant** (most common)
  - Inherently irritating substance (soap, detergent, hair dyes)
  - No previous exposure necessary
- **Allergic**
  - Latex gloves, nickel, poison ivy/oak, neomycin
  - **Delayed Type IV hypersensitivity response**
  - Sensitization (prior-exposure) required
  - Patch testing gold standard to diagnose allergic contact dermatitis

Patch Testing

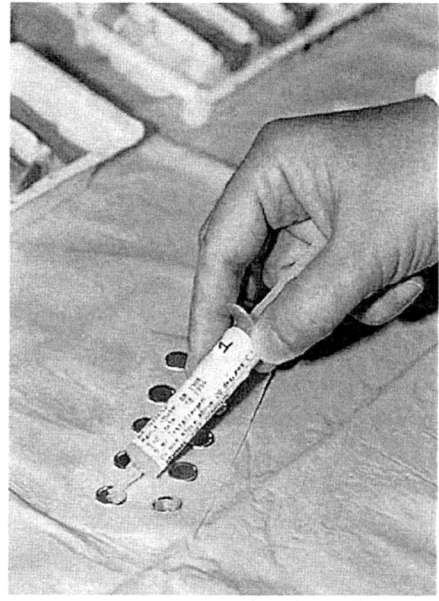

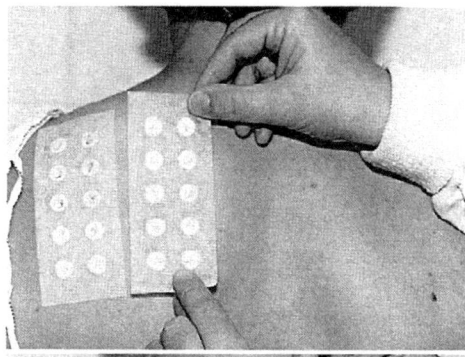

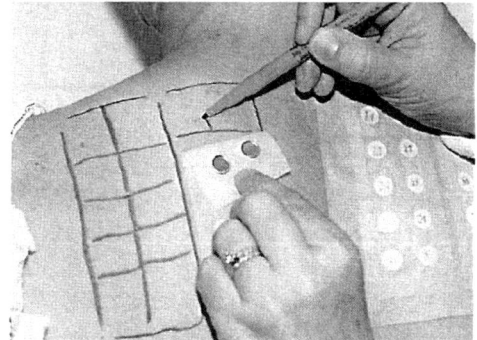

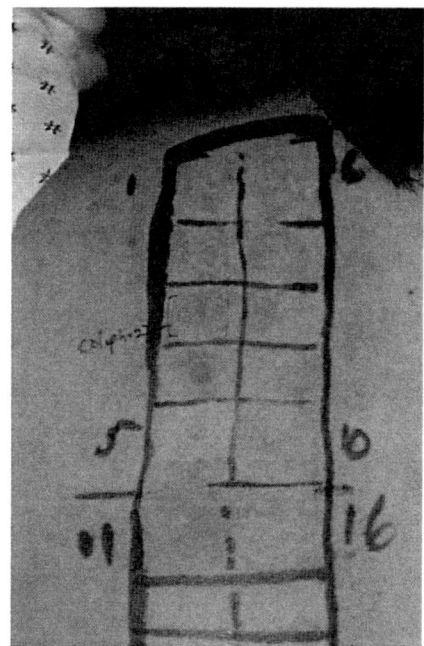

Allergic Contact Dermatitis

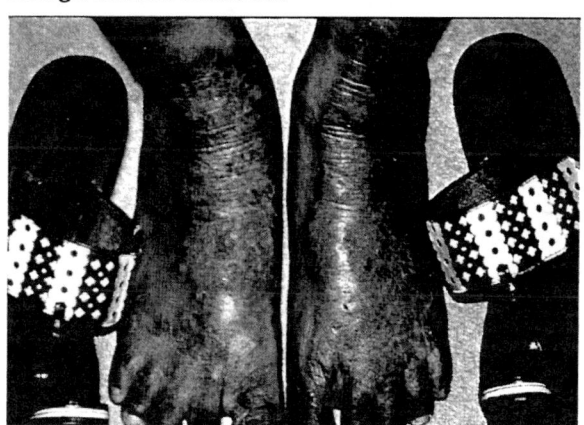

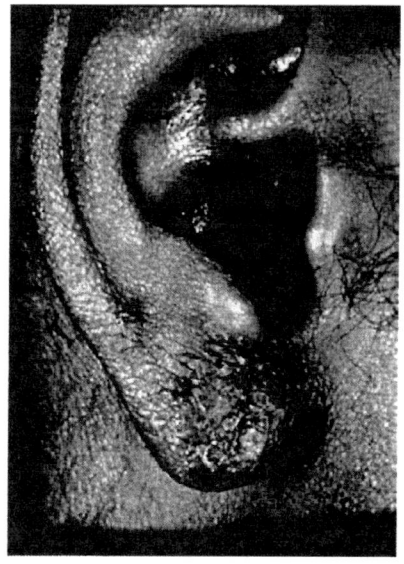

Contact Dermatitis Treatment
- Treatment similar for both (irritant/allergic)
- Identify and remove offending irritant/allergen
- Topical corticosteroids
- Systemic corticosteroids for severe cases
- Aluminum acetate soaks (antiseptic, drying agent)
  - Good for weeping lesions
- Keep affected areas dry

AR 4

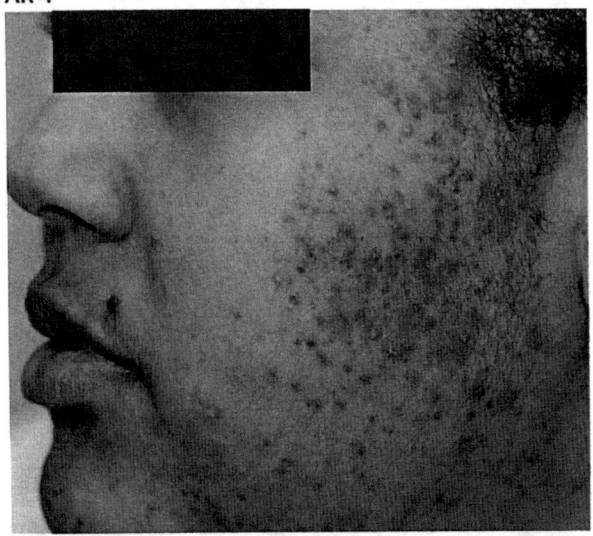

The treatment of choice for this patient's comedonal acne is:

A. Oral tetracycline
B. Isotretinoin
C. Spironolactone
D. Hydrocortisone 2.5% cream
E. Topical retinoid

Answer: _____

AR 5

Which are potential side effects of this oral medication used for severe nodulocystic acne?

A. Pancreatitis
B. Pseudotumor cerebri
C. Hepatotoxicity
D. Choices B. and C.
E. All of the above

Answer: _____

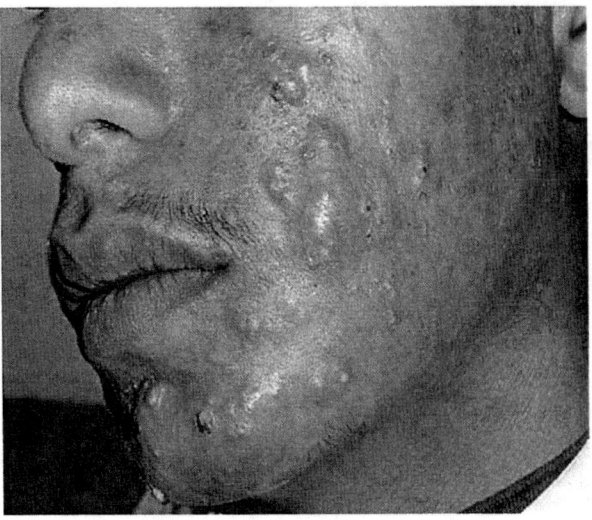

Acne Vulgaris
- Affects 85% of adolescents
- 12% of women continue to get lesions through their 40s
- Predisposing factor is hyperresponsiveness to androgens (e.g., polycystic ovary syndrome)
- **Main types:**
  - **Comedonal** (noninflammatory)
    - Occlusion of follicles
  - **Inflammatory** (papulopustular)
    - Directed against *Propionibacterium acnes*, excess sebum around hair follicle, follicular plugging
  - **Severe nodulocystic** (know isotretinoin)

Acne Vulgaris

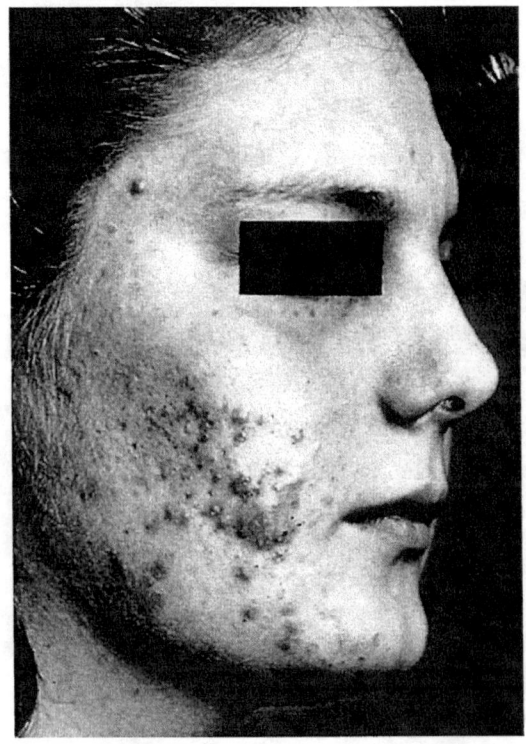

Acne Vulgaris (cont.)

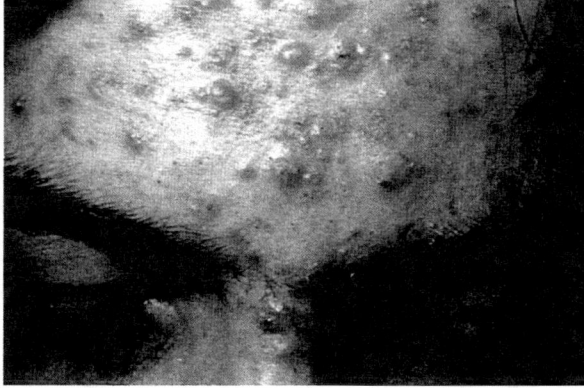

Cystic Acne

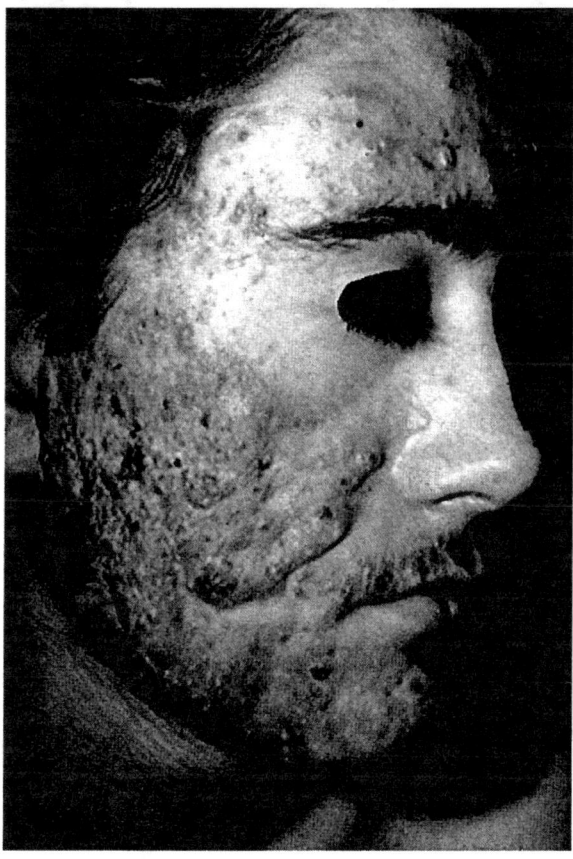

Acne Therapy
- **Comedonal** (noninflammatory)
  - Topical retinoid at night (e.g., tretinoin, adapalene)
- **Mild inflammatory** (papules and pustules)
  - Topical antibiotic (e.g., clindamycin or erythromycin)
  - Benzoyl peroxide
  - Combination decreases resistance
- **Moderate/Severe inflammatory**
  - Oral antibiotics
    (e.g., doxycycline, erythromycin)
- **Severe nodulocystic**
  - Isotretinoin (systemic retinoid)

Isotretinoin
- **Teratogen**
- Must have failed other therapies
- iPLEDGE enrollment required
- Serious side effects include:
  - Depression/psychosis and suicidality
  - Hypertriglyceridemia and pancreatitis
  - Hearing and visual loss
  - Pseudotumor cerebri (esp. with **tetracycline**)
  - Hepatotoxicity

AR 6

A 40 y/o thin woman comes to the office complaining of worsening acne on her central face. She had acne as a child but that resolved. She also complains of facial flushing associated with spicy foods, hot liquids, or alcohol intake.

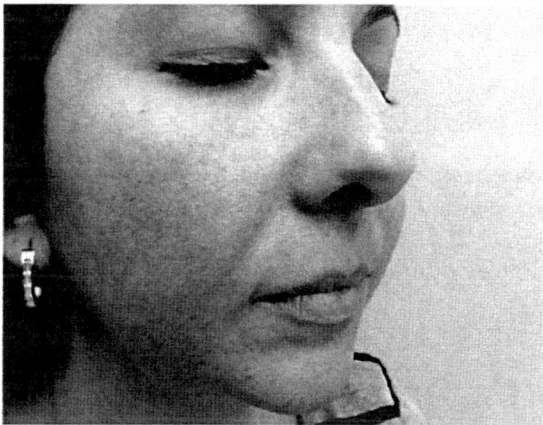

What would you recommend for this patient?
A. Topical steroids.
B. Topical metronidazole.
C. Stop disulfiram use.
D. Carcinoid workup.
E. SLE workup.

Answer: _____

Acne Rosacea

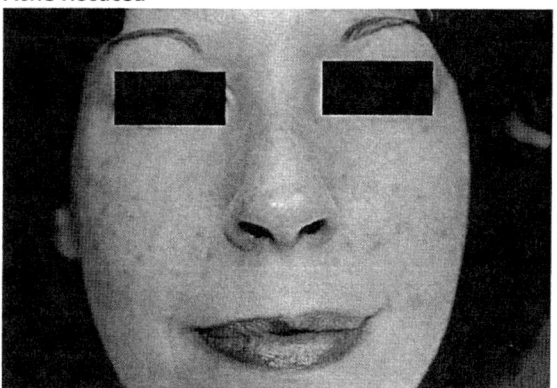

Acne Rosacea (cont.)
- Begins in middle age, "adult acne"
- More common in those of Celtic origin
- Central face involved
- **2 main types:**
  1) Vascular (erythematotelangiectatic)
  2) Inflammatory (papulopustular)
- **No comedones**
- Associated with flushing (spicy foods, alcohol)
- Pathogenesis unknown

Acne Rosacea

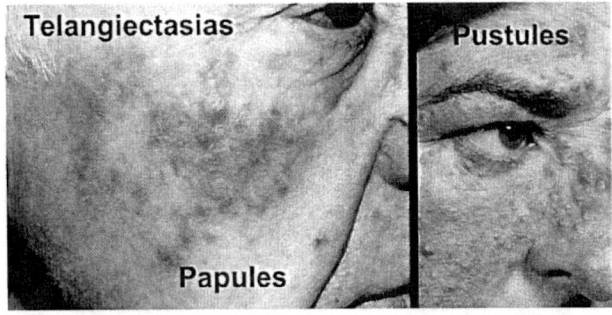

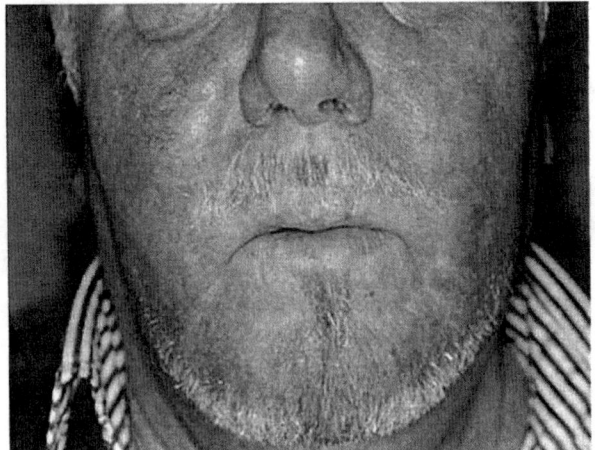

Erythematotelangiectatic

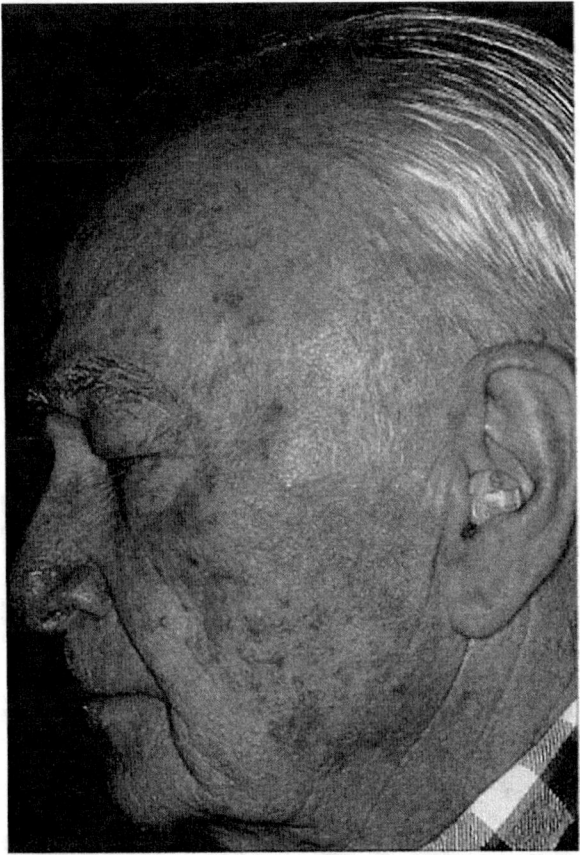

Papulopustular

Acne Rosacea

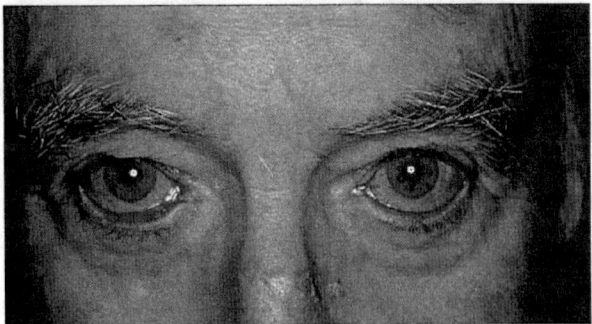

Ocular

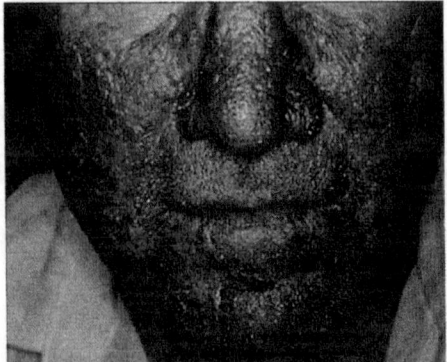

Rhinophyma

© 2017 MedStudy Internal Medicine Video Board Review – Dermatology • Aaron J. Calderon, MD

Acne Rosacea Treatment
- **Topical metronidazole**
- Azelaic acid
- Sulfacetamide preparations
- Low dose doxycycline
  - Pustular inflammatory or ocular type
- Avoid flushing triggers; Use sun protection
- Avoid topical steroids
- Surgical/Laser correction for rhinophyma

Hidradenitis Suppurativa
- Tender nodules/cysts ± sinus tracts
  - Axillae
- Smoking cessation
- Weight loss
- **Treatment**
  - Antibiotics
  - Steroid injections
  - Isotretinoin
  - Surgery
  - Biologics (infliximab, adalimumab)

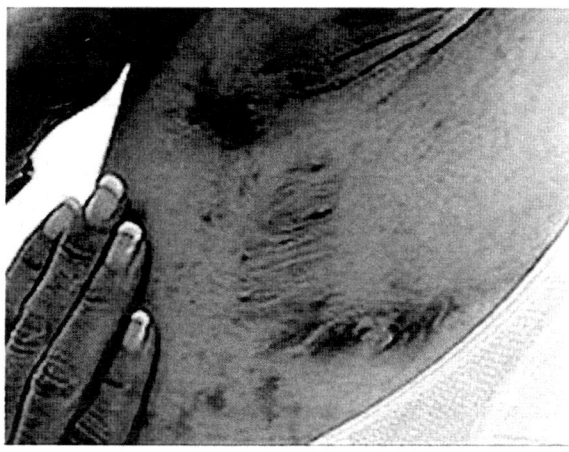

AR 7
A 32 y/o HIV+ male (CD4 count 175) is seen in clinic for whitish plaques on the lateral aspect of his tongue. The lesion is asymptomatic but is of cosmetic concern. You try to scrape it off but it remains adherent.

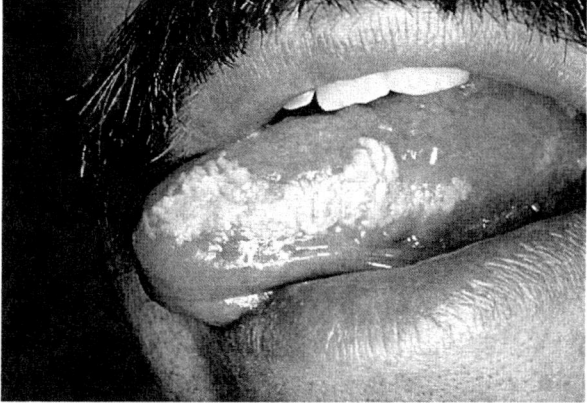

CDC Public Health Image Library

AR 7 (cont.)
The most likely diagnosis is:
A. Candidiasis
B. Oral hairy leukoplakia
C. Geographic tongue
D. Lichen planus
E. Aphthous ulcers

Answer: _____

Oral Hairy Leukoplakia
- Asymptomatic white plaques typically on the lateral aspect of the tongue
- Primarily seen in **HIV+** patients
  - Rare in other immunocompromised patients
- Etiologic agent is **Epstein-Barr virus**
- In contrast to *Candida*, it **can't be scraped off**
- **Rx:**
  - No treatment usually necessary
  - Often spontaneously resolves
  - HAART therapy
  - Cosmetic treatment (antivirals)

Geographic Tongue

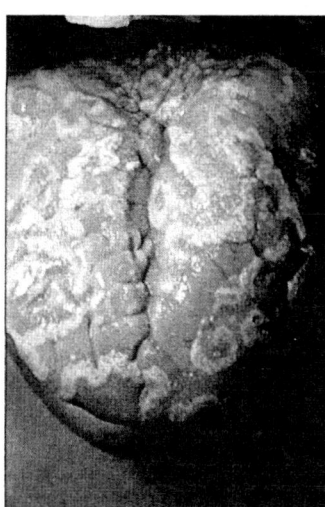

Lichen Planus
- Wickham striae
- Reticulate patches on buccal mucosa

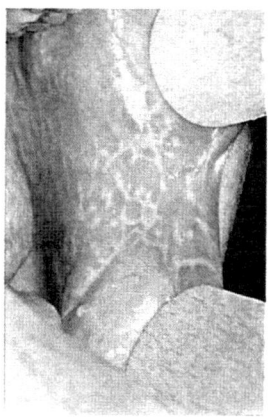

AR 8

A 40 y/o male comes to see you because of striking tongue discoloration. He has no symptoms but is worried about cancer. He is a heavy smoker and drinks 4 cups of coffee daily.

What should you recommend?

A. Topical steroid
B. Tongue biopsy
C. Tongue brushing
D. ENT consult
E. That he join the circus

Answer: _____

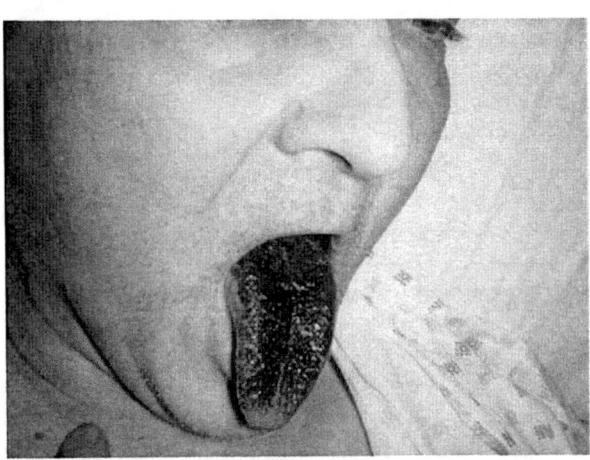

CDC Public Health Image Library

Black Hairy Tongue

- Benign
- Due to hypertrophy of filiform papillae
- Precipitated by coffee, tobacco, antibiotic use
- **Rx:** Tongue brushing/scrubbing

Drug Reactions

AR 9

First-time exposure to a new drug caused this eruption. It was most likely started in the last:

A. 1–2 days
B. 1–2 weeks
C. 1–2 months
D. 1–2 years

Answer: _____

Morbilliform Drug Eruption

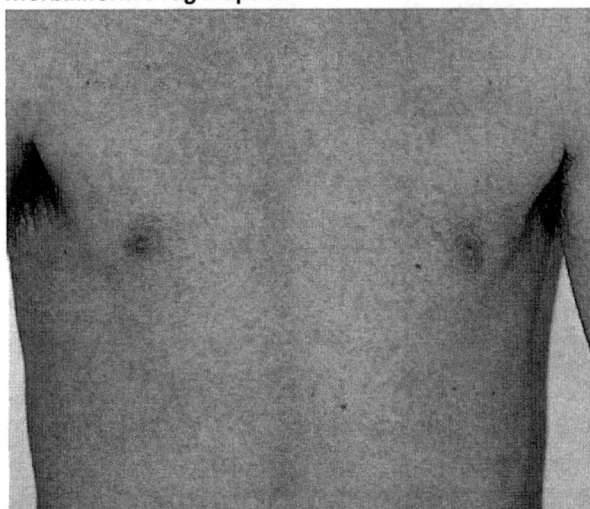

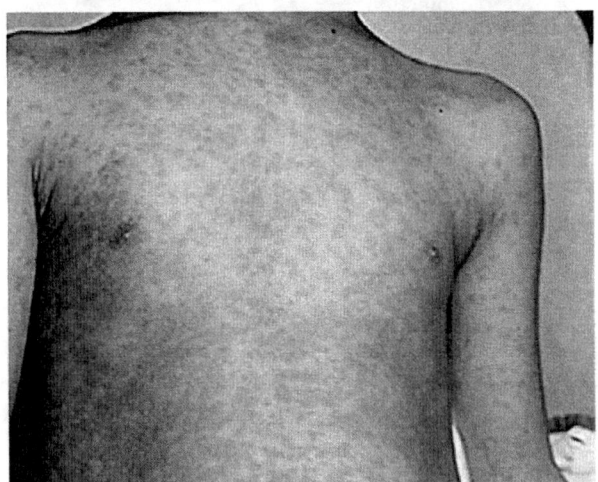

Morbilliform Drug Eruption (cont.)

- Maculopapular
- First 1–2 weeks of treatment
- Delayed Type 4 hypersensitivity reaction
- Begins proximally
- Generalizing in 1–2 days
- Prominent pruritus
- Treatment
  - Supportive
  - Withdrawal of all nonessential medications

AR 10

A 62 y/o woman was started on carbamazepine 2 weeks ago. Yesterday morning, she awoke with red and raw painful skin lesions. Many areas have blisters and sloughed off skin.

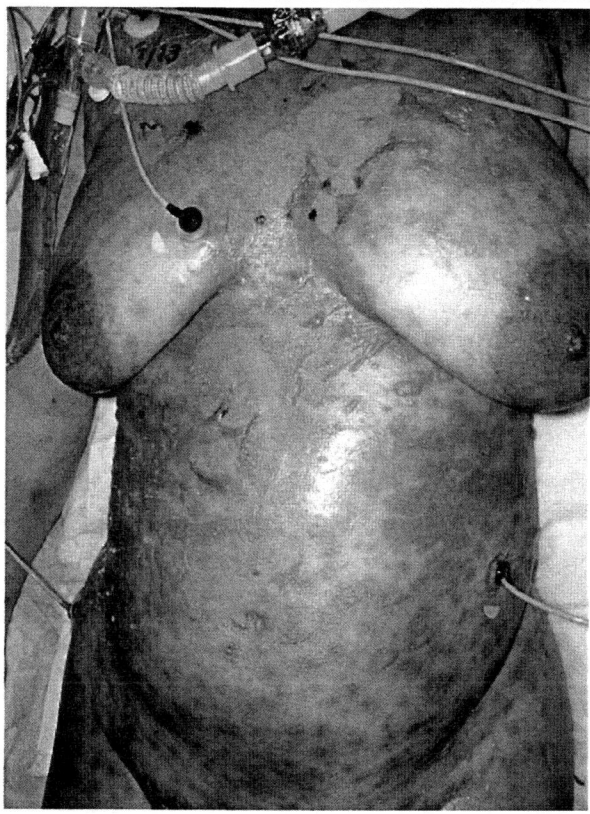

AR 10 (cont.)

Her lesions cover at least 30% of her body. She went to the emergency department where she was also found to have mouth sores and a fever of 102.7° F (39.3° C), BP 100/60, HR 117. She has no lymphadenopathy. Her LFTs and eosinophil count are normal.

What is the patient's most likely diagnosis?
A. Erythema multiforme
B. Stevens-Johnson syndrome
C. Toxic epidermal necrolysis
D. DRESS syndrome
E. Dermatitis herpetiformis

Answer: _____

Toxic Epidermal Necrolysis (TEN)
- Medical emergency
- Mortality rate ~ 40%
- Stop offending drug

- 90% due to drug
  - Sulfa
  - Allopurinol
  - NSAIDs
  - Anticonvulsants
- ICU; Burn care unit
- > 30% body surface area involvement; Mucosa
- IVIG/steroids controversial

DRESS Syndrome
- Drug reaction with eosinophilia and systemic symptoms; typically 2–6 weeks after drug started
- Mortality rate of ~ 10%
- **Facial swelling, lymphadenopathy, ↑ LFTs, hepatomegaly; ≥ 50% have eosinophilia**
- Rash varies but "morbilliform" most common
- **Differs from TEN**
  - Extensive sloughing not seen
  - Mucosal involvement uncommon
- Common offenders:
  - Anticonvulsants and allopurinol
- Steroids typically needed

Drug Reactions

Drug	Reaction
Penicillin	Immediate — anaphylaxis Delayed — vasculitis, morbilliform
Tetracycline	Photosensitivity
NSAIDs	Urticaria, angioedema, asthma, photosensitivity, SJS-TEN
Phenytoin	Gingival hyperplasia
Glucocorticoids	Striae, atrophy, acne
Warfarin	Skin necrosis within 3–10 days of starting
Radio contrast dye	Urticaria, hypersensitivity reaction

Inflammatory Skin Disorders

AR 11
This patient has similar findings on her knees and elbows.

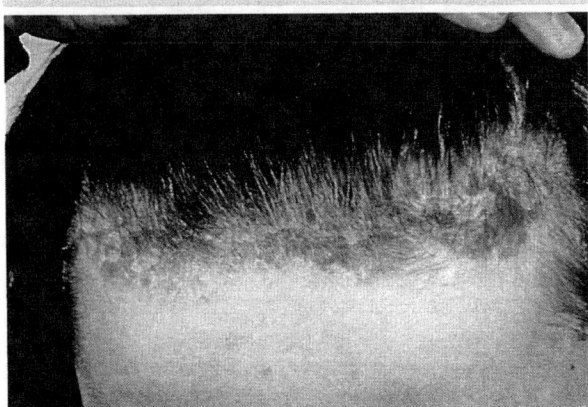

What finding is most likely on her fingernails?
A. Longitudinal ridges and hyperpigmentation
B. Horizontal ridges with white banding
C. Onychorrhexis with grooves
D. Onycholysis and pits
E. Onychogryposis

Answer: _____

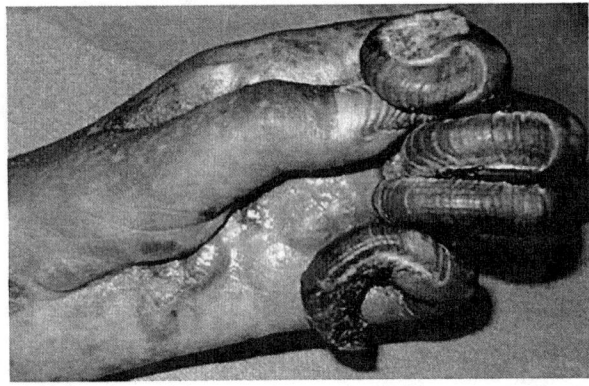

Psoriasis
- Affects 1–3% of the population
- May develop at any age; Genetic predisposition
- **Psoriatic arthritis**
  - Overall incidence ~ 7–10%
  - Usually seen in patients with severe nail/skin disease
- **Plaque psoriasis — most common type**
- May be exacerbated by certain meds
  - Beta-blockers, lithium, antimalarials

Plaque Psoriasis
- Frequent sites:
  - Extensor surfaces
  - Scalp
  - Lumbosacral region
  - Gluteal cleft
  - Glans penis

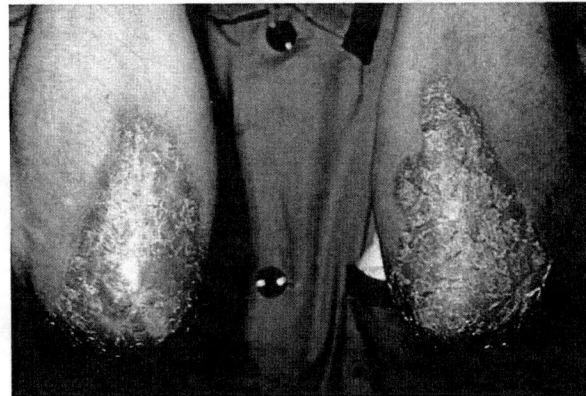

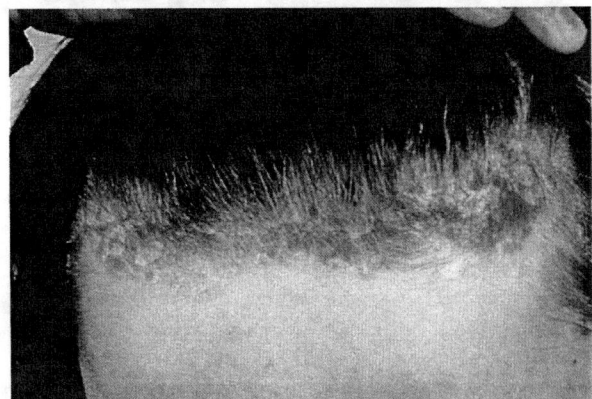

Plaque Psoriasis (cont.)
- Red plaques with loose silvery scale
- Pitted nail
- Oil spot onycholysis

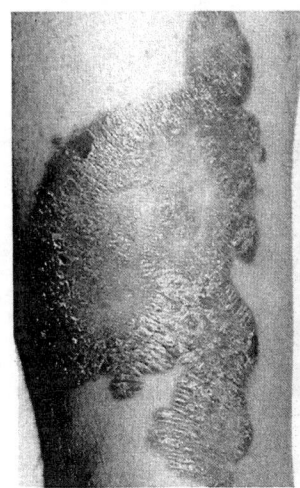
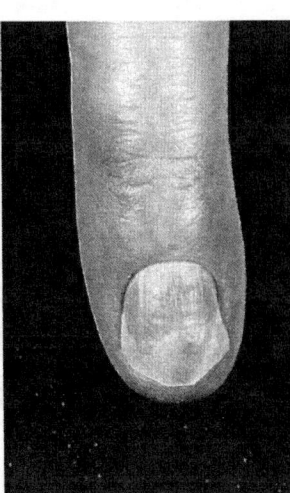

Psoriatic Arthritis

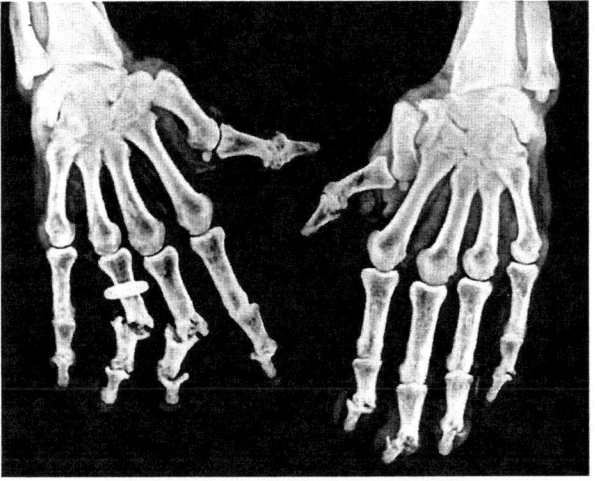

No antimalarials since they may exacerbate skin disease

Psoriatic Arthritis (cont.)
- Nail disease
- Asymmetric oligoarthropathy
- DIP joints
- Sacroiliitis
  - HLA-B27
- Treatment
  - NSAIDs
  - TNF blockers
  - Methotrexate
  - Cyclosporine

Psoriasis Treatment
- **Topical**
  - Emollients
  - Corticosteroids (1st line), vitamin D analogues, calcineurin inhibitors
- **Phototherapy**
  - NBUVB, PUVA
  - No immunosuppression; but doesn't treat arthritis
- Systemic
  - Methotrexate, cyclosporine
- Biologics
  - Infliximab, etc.

Other Psoriasis Associations
- Guttate psoriasis
  - Group A streptococcal infection
- Pustular psoriasis
  - Steroid taper

AR 12

A 50 y/o male patient with discoid lupus asks you how likely it is that he will develop systemic lupus (SLE).

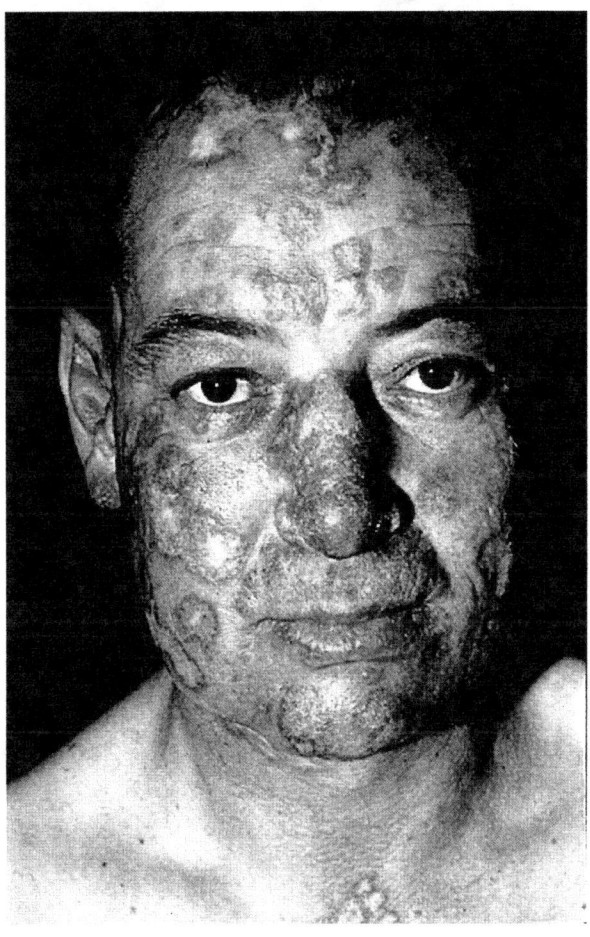

What do you tell him?
A. Almost certain
B. 50% chance
C. 25% chance
D. < 10% chance
E. Never

Answer: _____

Acute Lupus Erythematosus

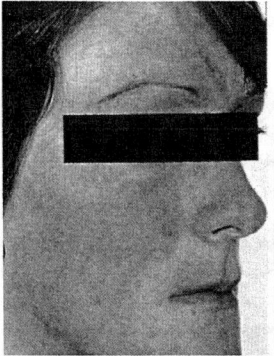
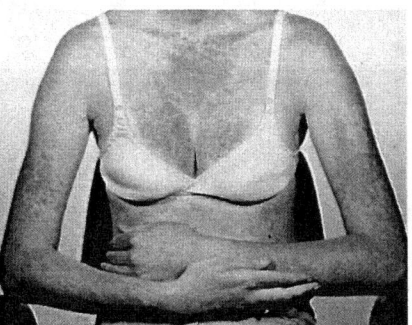

Blanchable erythema
Photo-distribution
Malar rash

Systemic symptoms
Circulating antibodies;
Immunoglobulin deposition
in the skin and other organs

Discoid Lupus
- Photosensitive areas
- Scarring
- Atrophy
- **Rare** to develop SLE
- **Rx:** Avoid sun, topical/intralesional steroids
- Antimalarials

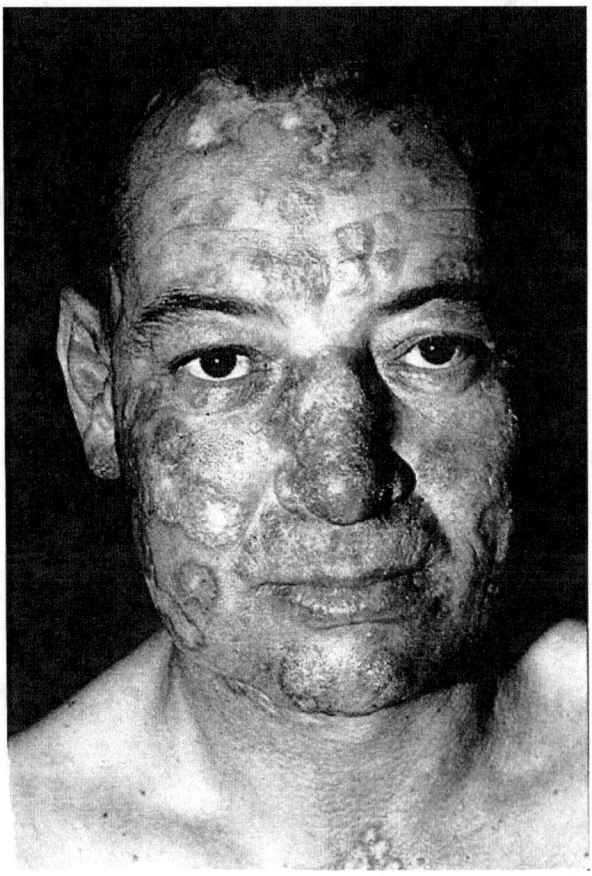

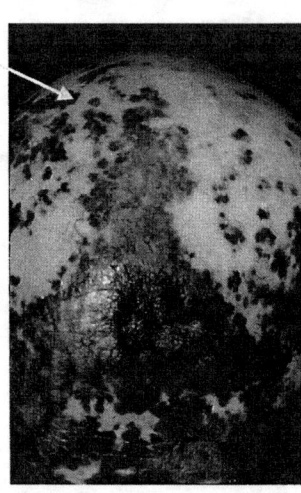

Discoid lupus causes a patchy, scarring alopecia

Systemic lupus causes a patchy, nonscarring alopecia

AR 13

A 30 y/o female presents acutely with fever, polyarthralgias, and painful anterior pretibial nodules. Her CXR reveals bilateral hilar adenopathy.

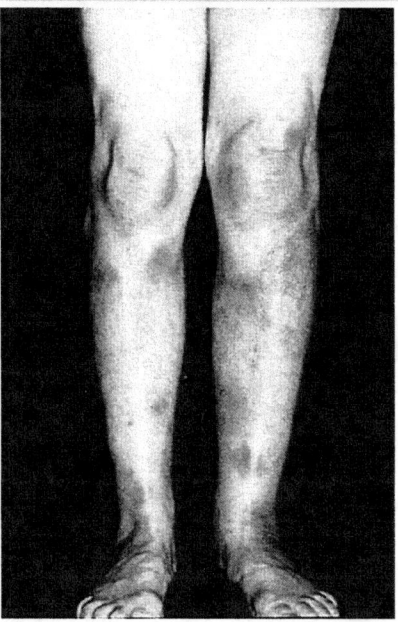

What is the most likely diagnosis?
A. Sweet syndrome
B. Löfgren syndrome
C. Lymphoma
D. Streptococcal infection
E. SLE

Answer: _____

Löfgren Syndrome
- Acute form of sarcoidosis
- Manifests as erythema nodosum, bilateral hilar adenopathy, fever, and arthralgias
- **Excellent prognosis**; Resolves in 2–3 years

Erythema Nodosum
<u>**Differential Diagnosis:**</u>
- Idiopathic
- Streptococcal infection
- Sarcoidosis
- TB/Fungal infections
- HRT, OCP, antibiotics
- Pregnancy
- Inflammatory bowel disease
- Behçet disease
- Lymphoma

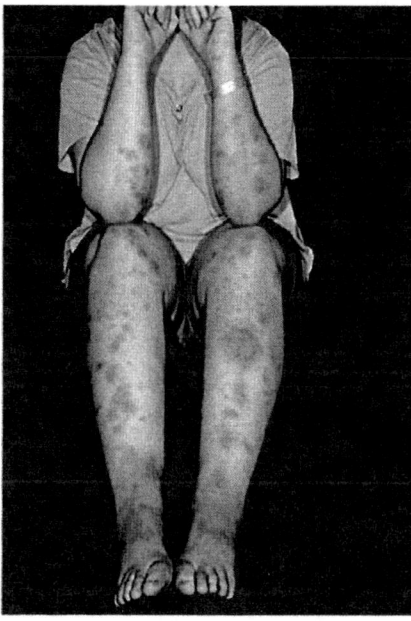

Erythema Nodosum
Treatment:
- Supportive care
- NSAIDs
- Biopsy rarely needed

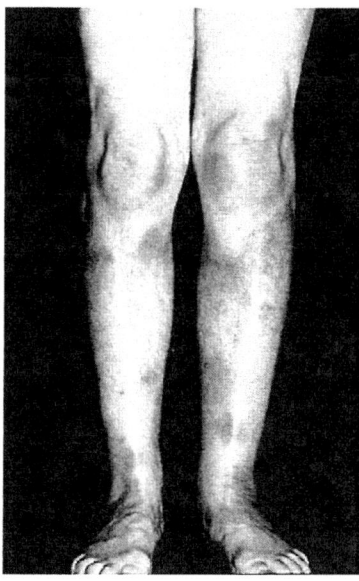

Sarcoidosis (Lupus Pernio)

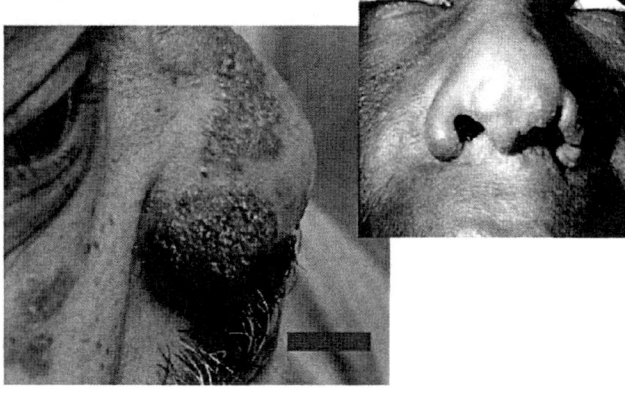

AR 14
What is the most likely diagnosis for this patient with a periorbital heliotropic rash?

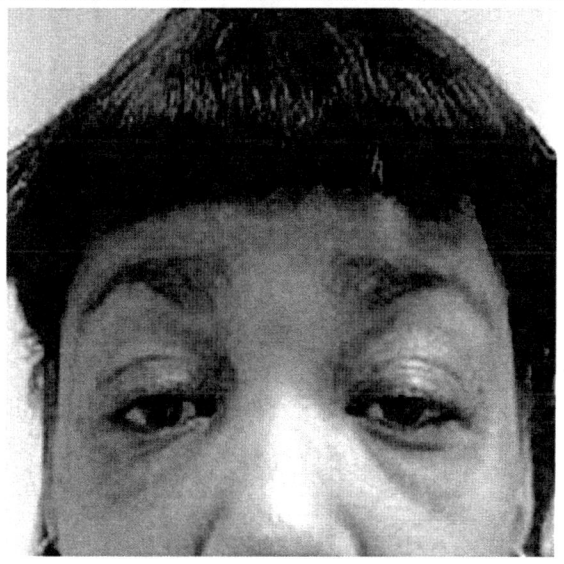

A. Systemic lupus
B. Dermatomyositis
C. Sarcoidosis
D. Scleroderma
E. Contact dermatitis

Answer: _____

Dermatomyositis
- Progressive symmetrical proximal muscle weakness
- Elevated muscle enzymes
- Muscle biopsy consistent with myositis
- Abnormal electromyogram
- Pathognomonic cutaneous disease
  - **Heliotrope rash** (periorbital)
  - **Gottron papules** (bony prominence of hands/fingers)
- Strong association with **malignancy**
  - Age-appropriate cancer screening

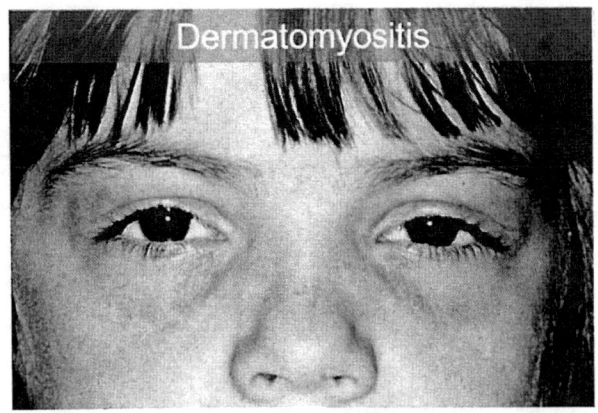

Dermatomyositis

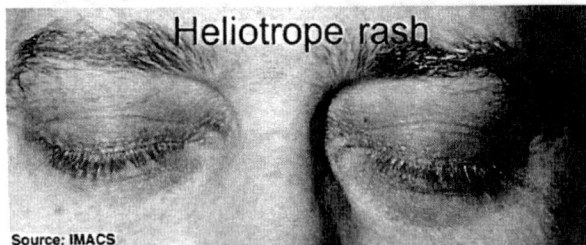

Heliotrope rash

Source: IMACS

Gottron papules

Ragged cuticles

AR 15

An 18 y/o male presents to the emergency department for bloody stools, abdominal pain, and arthritis for several weeks. His urine is remarkable for hematuria and his lower extremities are shown. His platelet count is 94,000.

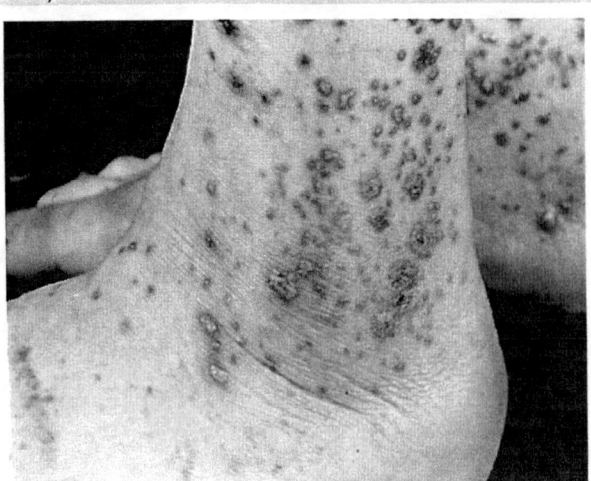

AR 15 (cont.)
The most likely diagnosis is:
A. Temporal arteritis
B. Kawasaki disease
C. Immune thrombocytopenic purpura
D. Henoch-Schönlein purpura
E. Sarcoidosis

Answer: _____

Vasculitis — Palpable Purpura

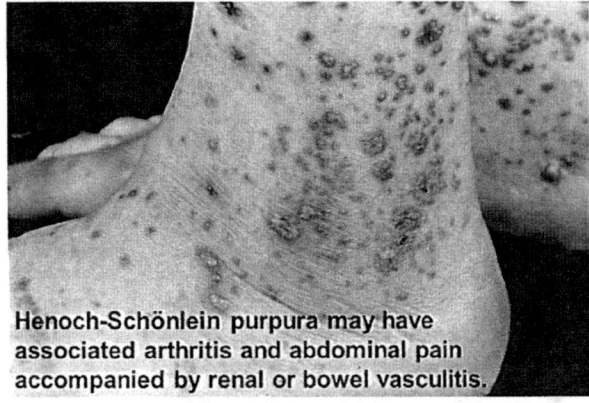

Henoch-Schönlein purpura may have associated arthritis and abdominal pain accompanied by renal or bowel vasculitis.

AR 16

A 55 y/o man developed a pustule which turned into a painful ulcer. The ulcer is deep, has an inflamed border that overhangs the ulcer, and has a violaceous hue. After appropriate testing, no bacteria or fungus was found. He was in good general health except for severe rheumatoid arthritis.

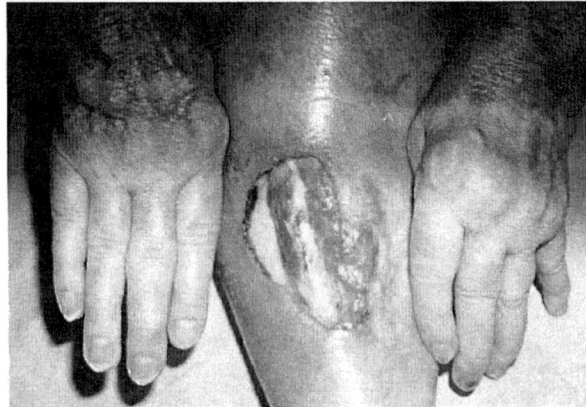

The most likely diagnosis is:
A. Pyoderma gangrenosum
B. "Flesh-eating bacteria"
C. Osteomyelitis
D. Necrotizing fasciitis
E. Vasculitis

Answer: _____

Pyoderma Gangrenosum

- Often associated with an underlying disease, but can be idiopathic
  - **Inflammatory bowel disease**
  - Rheumatoid arthritis
  - Multiple myeloma
- **25% demonstrate pathergy**
- **Biopsy is not diagnostic**
  - Rules out other causes
  - Cultures are negative
- Treat underlying disease
- If idiopathic — systemic steroids

Pyoderma Gangrenosum

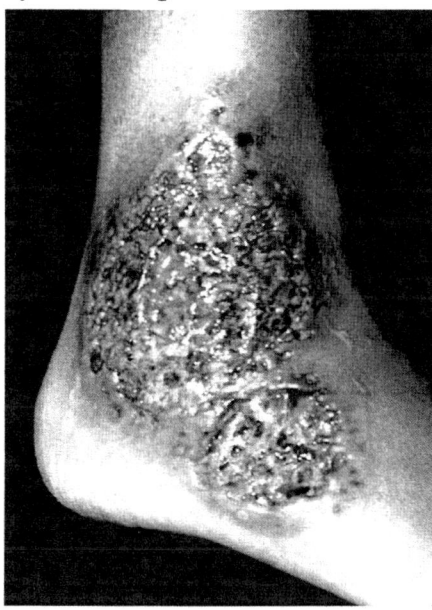

Pyoderma Gangrenosum (cont.)

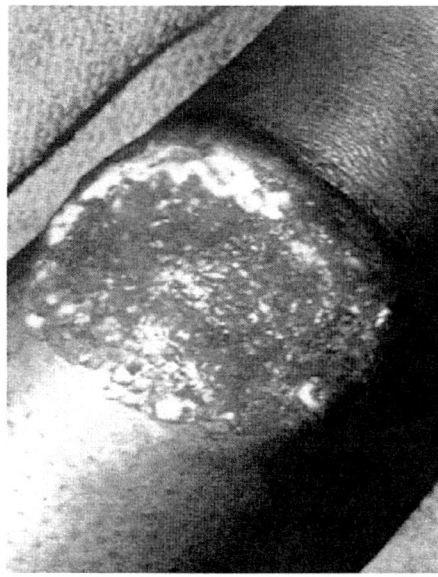

Skin Infections

AR 17
A 42 y/o construction worker presents with an asymptomatic groin rash that he has self-treated with neomycin/polymyxin/bacitracin with no improvement. Wood's lamp examination reveals bright red fluorescence.

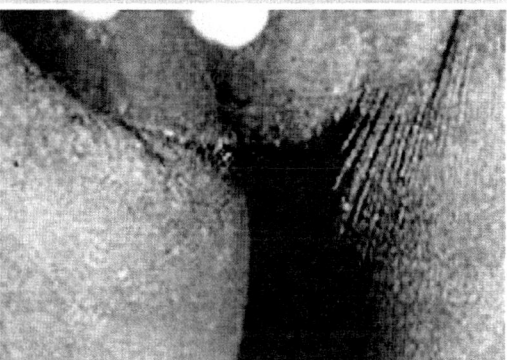

What is the diagnosis?

A. Tinea cruris
B. Contact dermatitis
C. Erythrasma
D. Intertrigo
E. Seborrheic dermatitis

Answer: _____

Erythrasma

- Sharply demarcated, brown, scaly patches
- *Corynebacterium*
- **Wood's lamp diagnostic**
  - **Bright red fluorescence** due to porphyrins
- Treatment
  - **Topical erythromycin** or **clindamycin**
  - Miconazole, clotrimazole
- Main differential is intertrigo or fungal

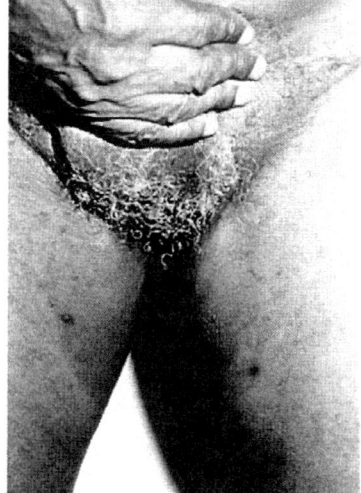

AR 18

A 50 y/o woman with poorly controlled diabetes is admitted to the hospital for cellulitis manifested by fever and a red, painful lower extremity. Two hours later, the nurse wakes you up to say that the infection has spread rapidly despite appropriate antibiotics and is 50% bigger than it was and more painful.

What is the best next step?
A. Add clindamycin to her antibiotic regimen.
B. Order a CT or MRI scan of the leg.
C. Order a plain film to look for gas.
D. Obtain a surgical consultation.
E. Ask the nurse not to call you anymore so you can get some sleep.

Answer: _____

Necrotizing Fasciitis
- A surgical emergency
- Most important is to obtain surgical consultation
- **Imaging and lab studies should not delay surgical evaluation**
- Deep infection can spread very quickly along fascial planes
- Pain often out of proportion to appearance of the infection

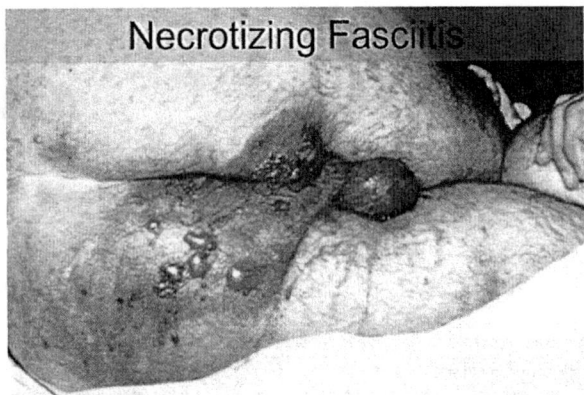
Necrotizing Fasciitis

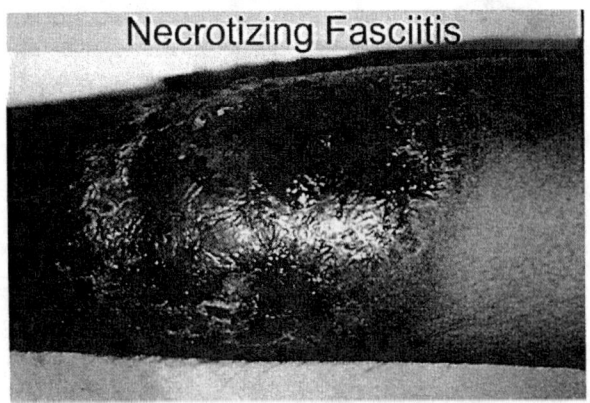
Necrotizing Fasciitis

AR 19

A 19 y/o woman presents to the emergency department because of fever, diarrhea, confusion, myalgias, and dizziness. On exam, she has a painless diffuse "sunburn" rash and conjunctival hyperemia.
BP 80/40, HR 127, fever 103.4° F (39.8° C)
Labs: Hgb 13.0, BUN 50, Cr 3.2
She denies any travel history and takes no medications. Her last menstrual period was 2 days ago.
Blood, urine, and stool cultures remain negative. CXR is negative.

The most likely diagnosis is:
A. Gram-negative sepsis
B. Rocky mountain spotted fever
C. Toxic shock syndrome
D. Disseminated gonococcal infection
E. Too many visits to the tanning salon

Answer: _____

Staph Toxic Shock Syndrome
- Presents with fever, shock, multiorgan system failure
- **Acute phase:** Diffuse macular erythroderma (sunburn)
- Convalescent phase: Desquamation of palms/soles
- Mucous membrane involvement common
- Patient colonized/infected **with toxigenic strain of *S. aureus***
  - Lack antibodies to the toxin (disease of the young)
  - Blood cultures usually negative; Often found in mucosa

- Menstrual (i.e., tampons) and nonmenstrual cases
  - Clinically indistinguishable
- **Rx:** Supportive care, clindamycin + vancomycin or (oxacillin/nafcillin)
- IVIG if hypotension not responding

Toxic Shock Syndrome

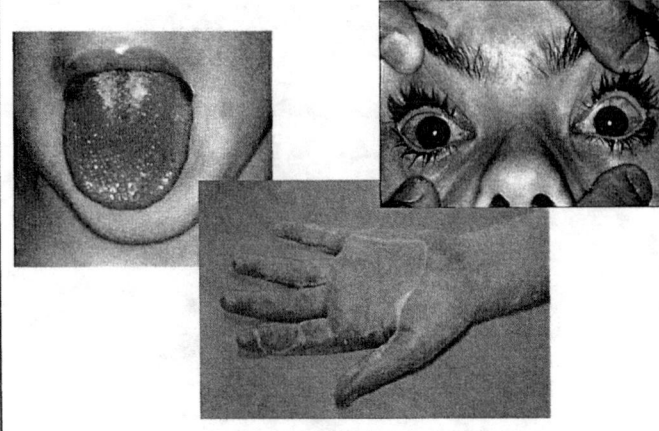

Erysipelas
- Group A strep
- Superficial cellulitis
  - Lymphatics involved
- Sharply demarcated
- Palpable drop off
- Most commonly on the face
- **Rx: Penicillin, amoxicillin**

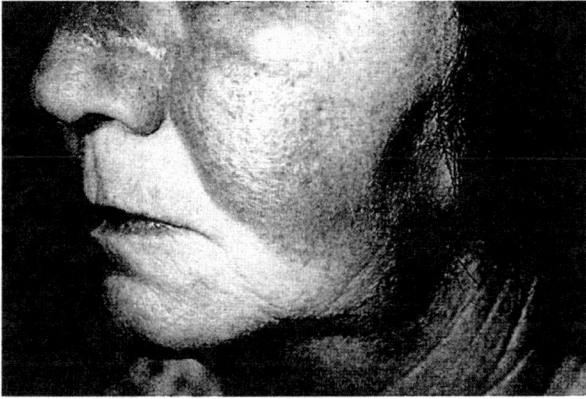

AR 20

A 42 y/o male comes to the office for an exquisitely warm, tender, and fluctuant lesion on his buttock. Pain is worse when sitting.

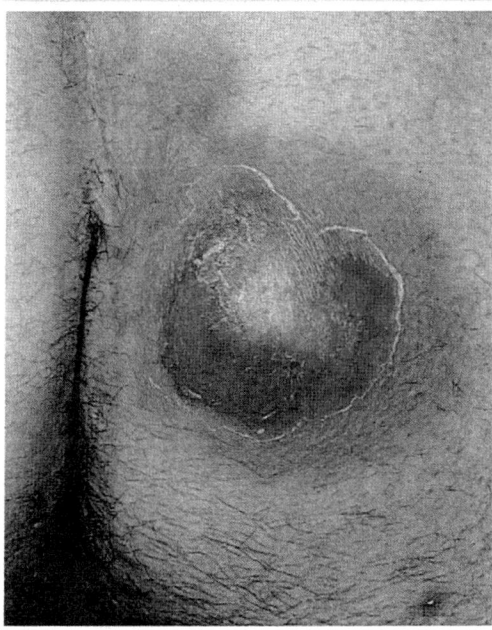

What would you recommend?
A. IV vancomycin.
B. Prednisone 60 mg.
C. Oral antibiotic that covers MRSA.
D. Incision and drainage.
E. "Don't sit for a couple of weeks."

Answer: _____

Abscess and Furuncle / Carbuncle
- Pus-filled nodule in the dermis
- Etiology
  - *Staphylococcus aureus*
  - Other bacteria

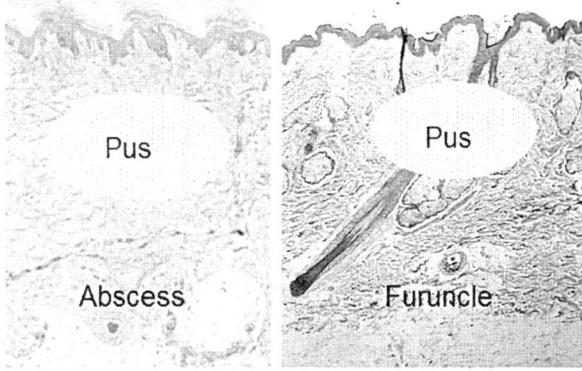

Carbuncle

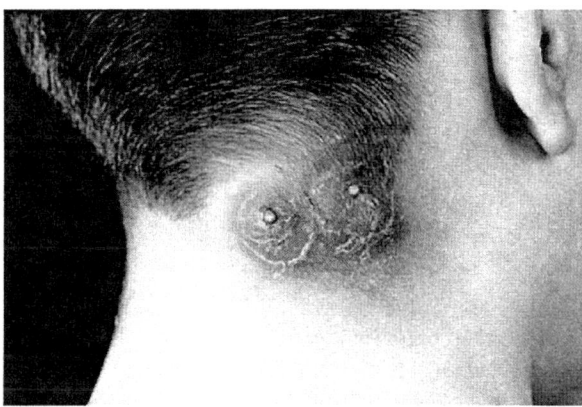

Abscess and Furuncle Treatment
- Warm compresses
- **Incise and drain**
- Gram stain
- Culture
- Antibiotics (MRSA)
  - Only if surrounding erythema or toxic

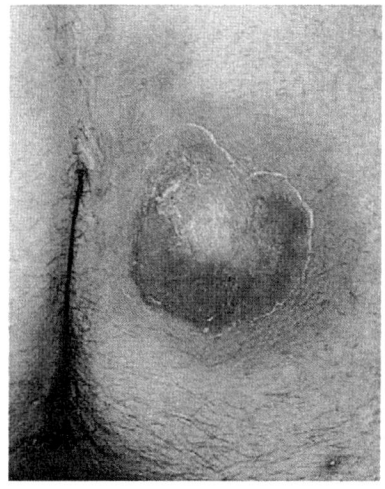

AR 21

A 35 y/o male comes to see you with the following perifollicular lesions. 48 hours ago, he spent some time in a motel with a poorly maintained hot tub. These lesions are mainly in the area of his swimming trunks and cause discomfort.

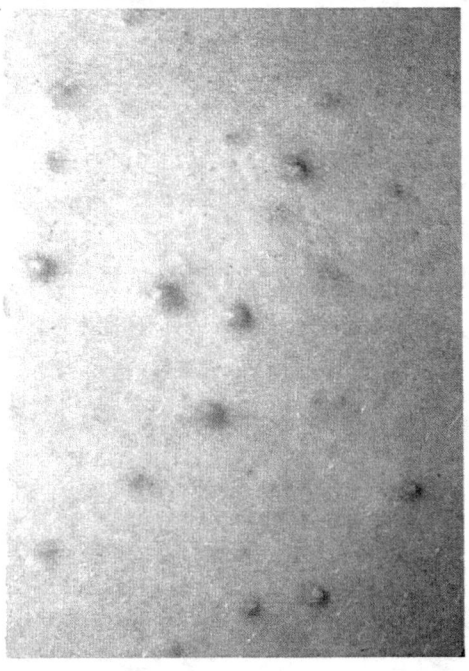

What should you recommend?

A. Topical steroids.
B. Oral fluconazole.
C. 5% acetic acid compresses.
D. Acyclovir.
E. "Avoid cheap motels."

Answer: _____

Folliculitis

- Infection of hair follicle
  - *Staph aureus* most common cause
- **"Hot tub"** folliculitis
  - Due to *Pseudomonas aeruginosa*
  - Exposure to contained contaminated water
  - Spontaneously resolves
  - Oral antibiotics not effective
  - 5% acetic acid compresses

Gonococcemia

- Fever, arthralgia ± asymmetric arthritis
- **Hemorrhagic pustules on extremities**
- Few in number
- Culture is negative from skin but can be positive from source

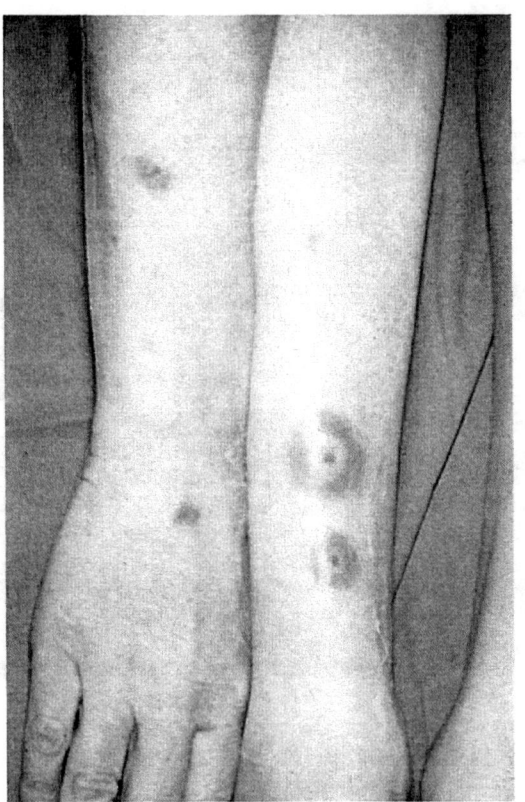

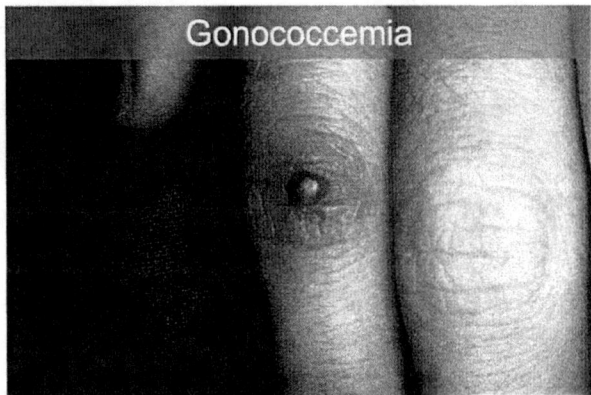
Gonococcemia

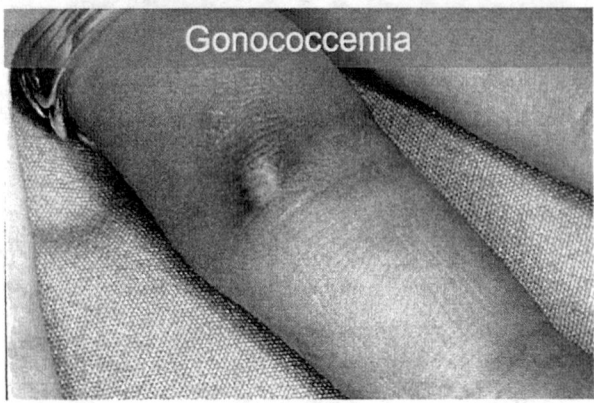
Gonococcemia

AR 22

An otherwise healthy 26 y/o man presents to the emergency department after being bitten by his girlfriend's cat.

What would you recommend?
A. Penicillin.
B. Erythromycin.
C. Tell him to dump his girlfriend.
D. Lavage and suture closed.
E. Amoxicillin/clavulanate.

Answer: _____

Animal Bites
- Dog and cat bites
  - *Pasteurella multocida*
- Human bites
  - Polymicrobial
- Treatment
  - Lavage
  - **Amoxicillin/clavulanate**
- Tetanus if due

AR 23

A 28 y/o school teacher presents with scaly patches of alopecia. Culture confirms tinea capitis.

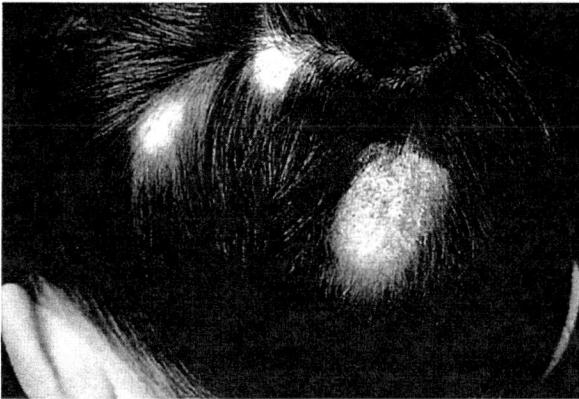

The treatment of choice is:
A. Terbinafine cream
B. Ketoconazole cream
C. Griseofulvin by mouth
D. Selenium sulfide shampoo
E. Ciclopirox gel

Answer: _____

Dermatophytes
- Cause superficial fungal infections (tineas)
- Only infect the outer layer of skin
- **Dx:**
  - KOH — potassium hydroxide wet mount preparation
  - Dissolves keratin but fungal walls remain intact
  - Branching, filamentous hyphae

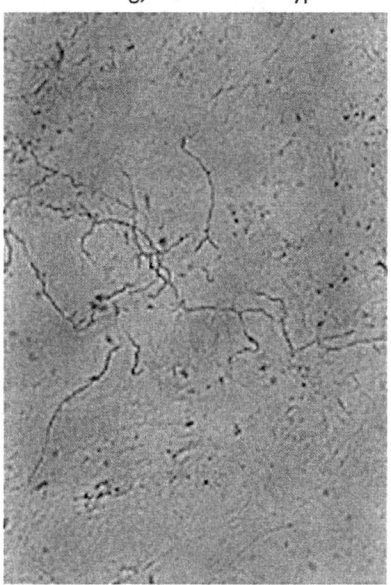

Tinea _____

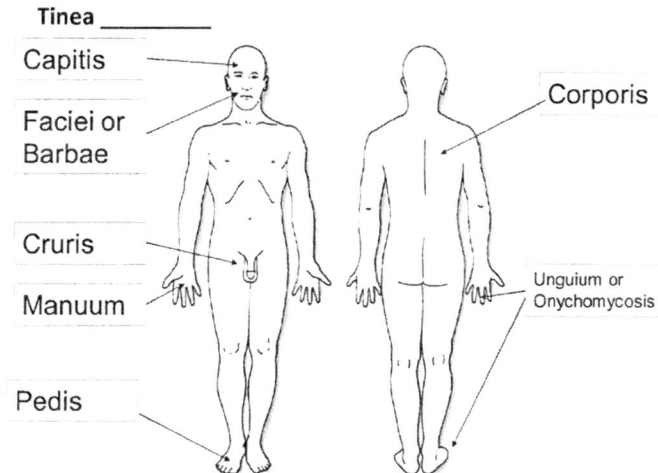

Capitis
Faciei or Barbae
Cruris
Manuum
Pedis
Corporis
Unguium or Onychomycosis

Tinea cruris

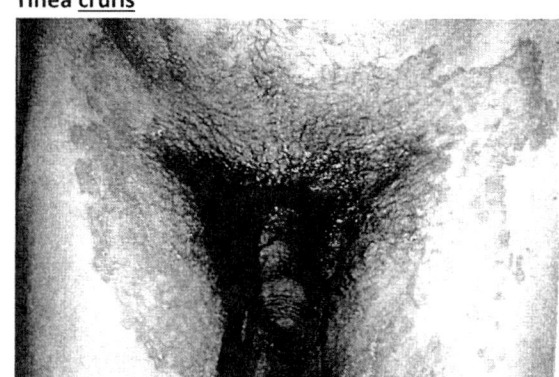

Tinea <u>manuum</u>

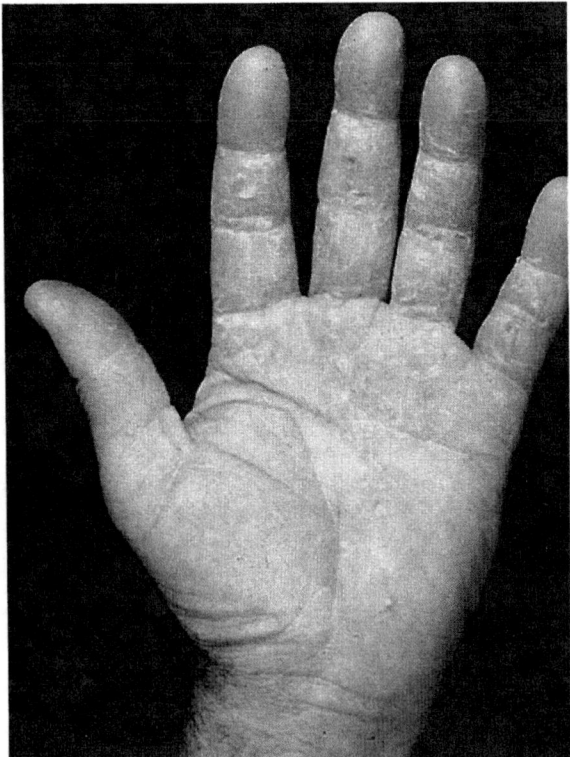

Tinea <u>pedis</u>

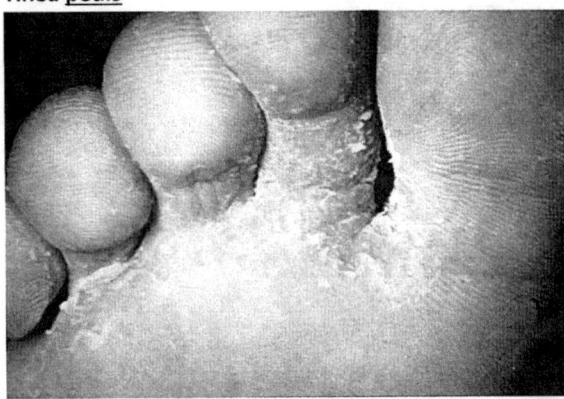

Tinea <u>corporis</u>

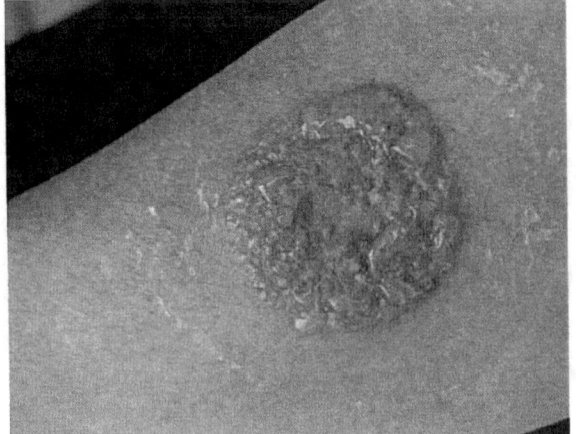

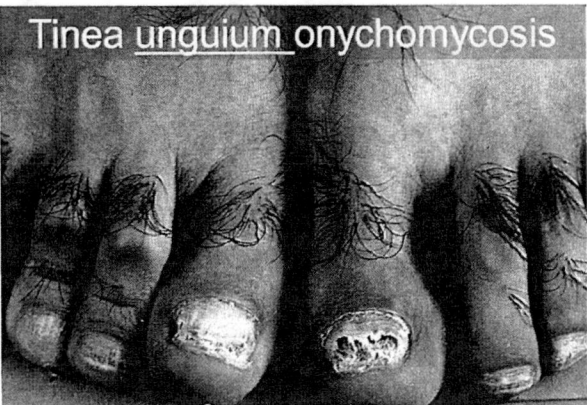

Tinea <u>unguium</u> onychomycosis

Dermatophytosis Treatment
- Most can be treated with topical antifungal creams
  - Imidazoles (clotrimazole, miconazole)
  - Allylamine (terbinafine)
- **Tinea capitis and unguium exceptions**
  - Need oral agents
- Keep moist areas dry

Tinea Capitis Treatment
- Requires oral therapy
- Options include:
  - Griseofulvin
  - **Terbinafine, itraconazole**
- Try to clear fomites from home
  - Asymptomatic carriage is common
  - Remains viable on furniture, combs, brushes, etc.

AR 24
A 30 y/o male comes to see you for a second opinion regarding treatment of his onychomycosis. He was told to take terbinafine for 12 weeks but has concerns about liver toxicity. He has multiple thickened toenails with yellowish, periungual debris.

What is the next best step?
A. Tell him to "man up" and not worry about it.
B. Tell him he can take it for 6 weeks instead.
C. Obtain and send a nail clipping sample to the lab.
D. Prescribe topical terbinafine instead.
E. Prescribe oral ketoconazole instead.

Answer: _____

AR 24 (cont.)
Up to 50% of patients with suspected onychomycosis do not have a fungal infection. Given the potential toxicity of terbinafine, confirmation of the diagnosis is warranted.

Tinea Versicolor
- Pityriasis versicolor
- *Malassezia globosa* or *furfur*
- "Spaghetti and meatballs"
- Light or dark macules and patches with mild pruritus
- **Treatment:**
  - Topical azoles
  - Ketoconazole shampoo
  - Selenium sulfide
  - Oral azole if severe
    - But avoid ketoconazole

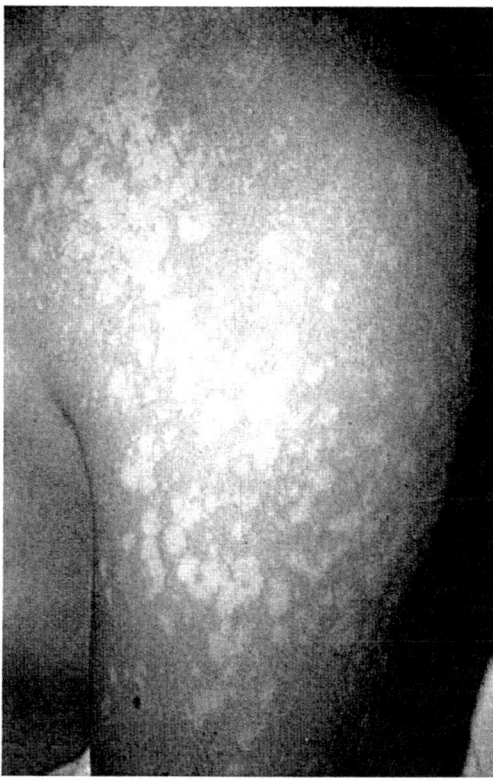

Tinea Versicolor

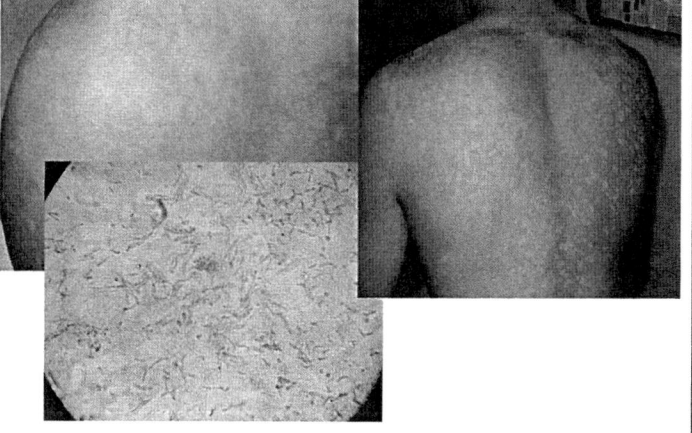

AR 25

A 23 y/o woman comes to your office after spending a week hiking in Maine. She complains of flu-like symptoms and has this rash.

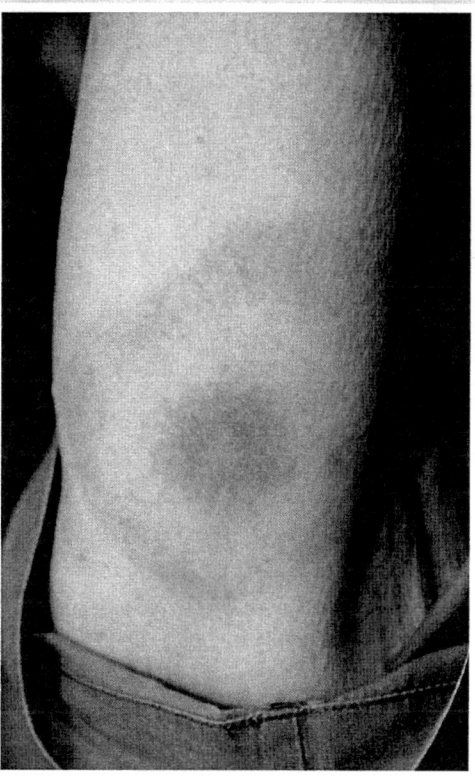

What is the most likely diagnosis?
A. Rocky Mountain spotted fever
B. Lyme disease
C. Ehrlichiosis
D. Spider bite
E. Erythema nodosum

Answer: _____

Lyme Disease
- Borrelia burgdorferi
- Ixodes spp tick
- **Erythema (chronicum) migrans**
  - Bull's-eye; 80%
- NE, Great Lakes, Northern California
- Serology not needed
- Rx:
  - Doxycycline
  - Amoxicillin

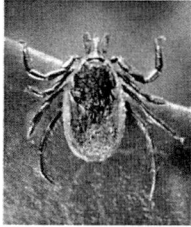

CDC Public Health Image Library

Syphilis

AR 26

A 33 y/o man presents with pink macules on the palms and soles. RPR and VDRL are both positive.

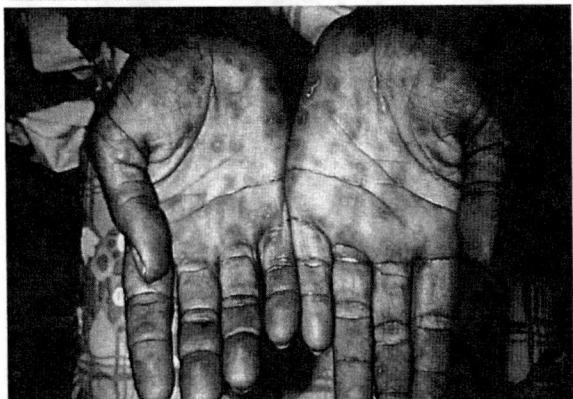

CDC Public Health Image Library

What stage of syphilis does this patient have?

A. Primary
B. Secondary
C. Latent
D. Tertiary
E. Quaternary

Answer: _____

Syphilis — *Treponema pallidum*

- **Primary**
  - Painless chancre (genitals, mouth)
  - Rx: Benzathine PCN G 2.4 M units IM
- **Secondary**
  - All have positive serologies
  - "Palms and soles" rash; Condyloma lata
- **Latent**
  - Positive serologies; Asymptomatic
- **Tertiary**
  - CNS and cardiac involvement
  - Most have gummas

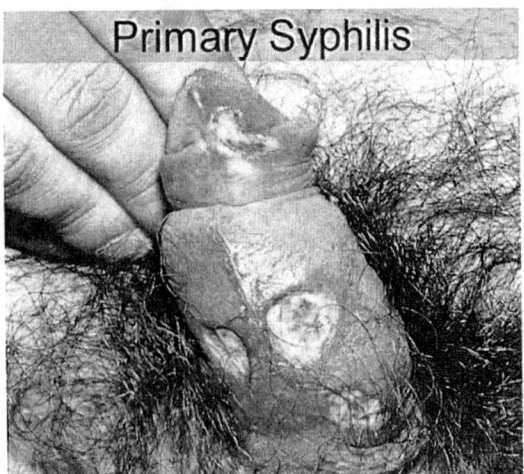

Primary Syphilis

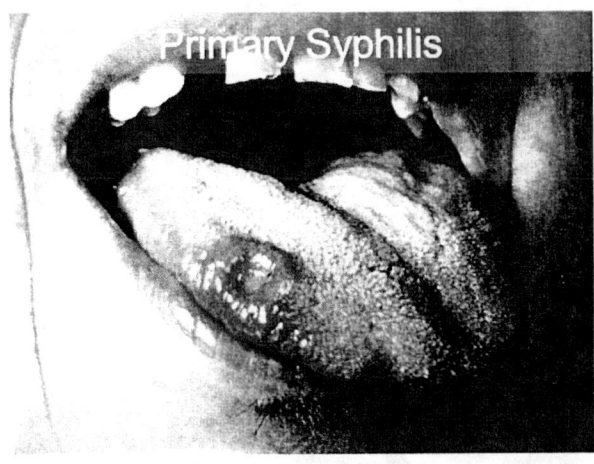

Primary Syphilis

Secondary Syphilis

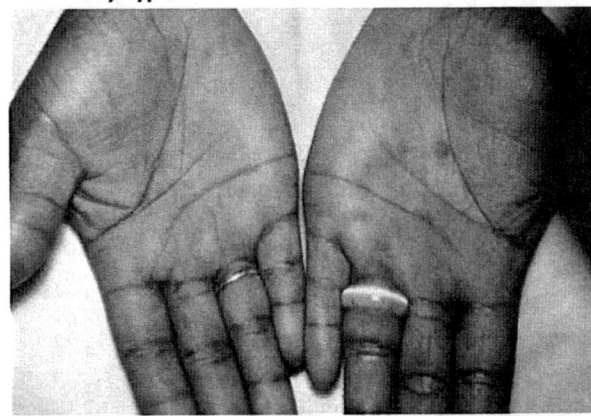

CDC Public Health Image Library

Condyloma Lata — Secondary Syphilis

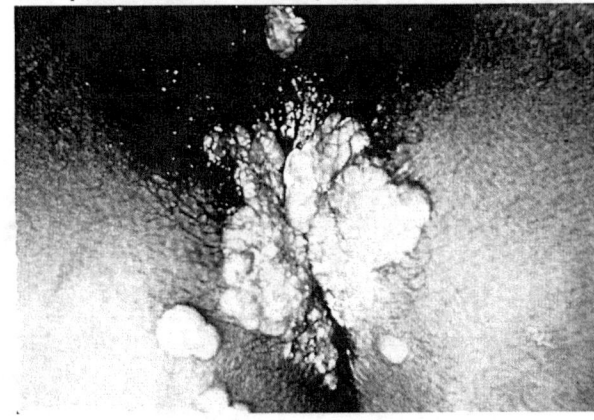

Tertiary Syphilis — Gumma

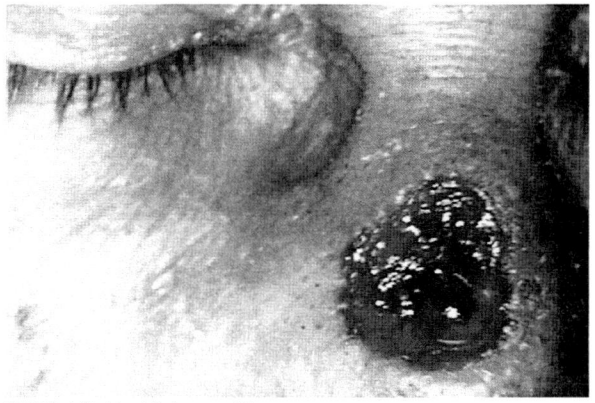

CDC Public Health Image Library

Warts (Verrucae)
- Vulgaris (common wart)
- Plana (flat wart)
- Plantaris (plantar wart)
- Condyloma acuminata (anogenital wart)

Vulgaris (Common Wart)

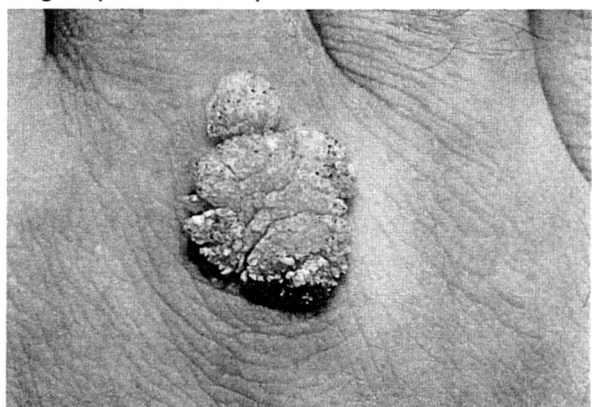

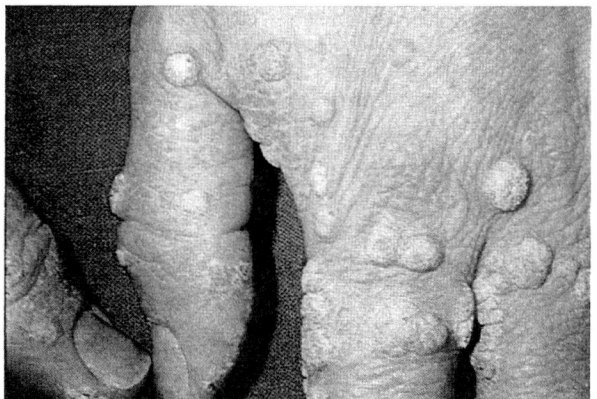

Warts
Plantaris

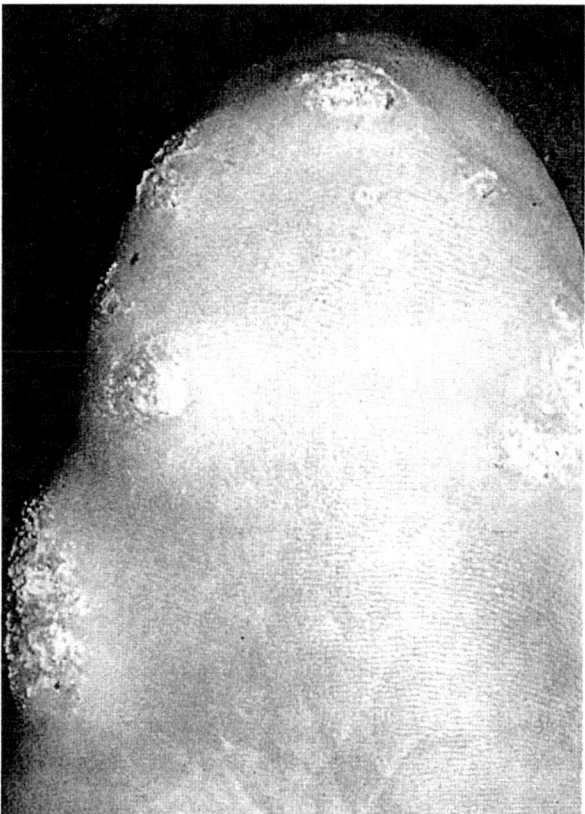

Plana (Flat wart)

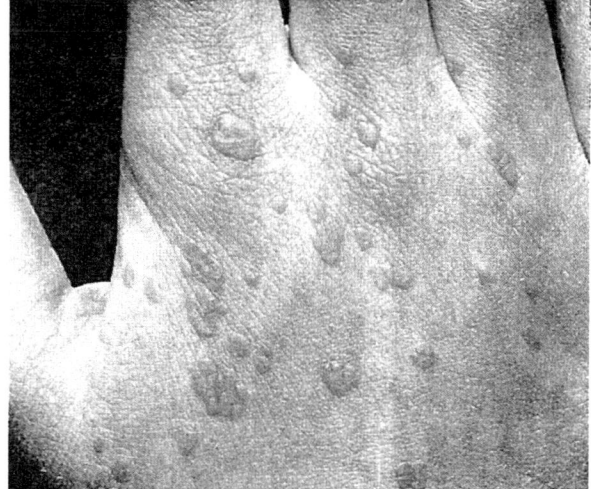

Condyloma Acuminata

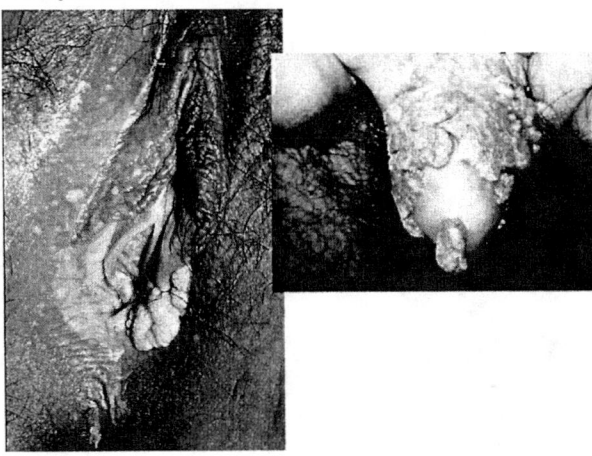

Warts
- Caused by **HPV**
- HPV vaccine can prevent anogenital warts
- Often resolve spontaneously
- Treatment is tissue destruction:
  - Salicylic acid
  - Liquid nitrogen
  - Topical 5% imiquimod (anogenital)

Molluscum Contagiosum
- **Poxvirus**
- Umbilicated pearly papules
- Kids, but can be seen in **sexually active young adults** (pelvic area)
- Often spontaneously resolve except in:
  - **AIDS or immunosuppression**
- Highly contagious > so often treated (cryotherapy, salicylic acid, curettage)

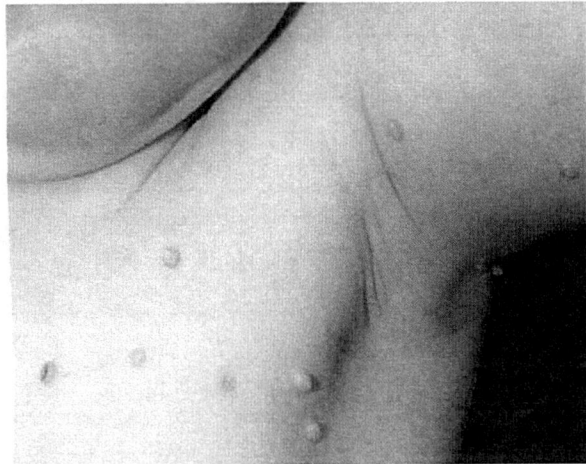

Herpes Infection

AR 27
A 62 y/o man with diabetes presents to the office with unilateral, painful, grouped vesicles on an erythematous base. He also has a lesion on the tip of his nose.

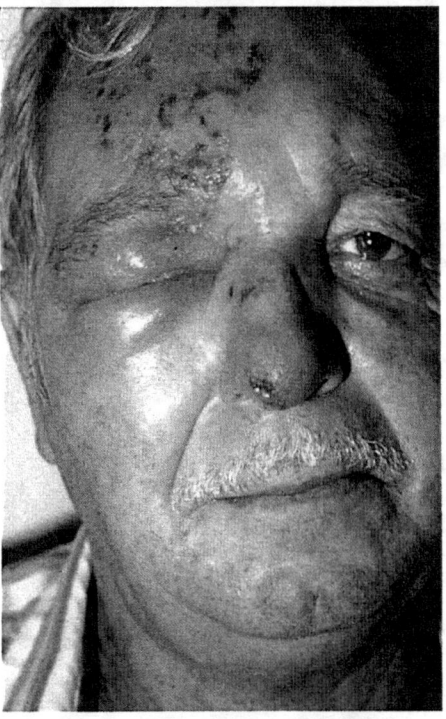

In addition to antiviral therapy, what is the best next step?
A. High-dose oral steroids
B. Gabapentin for pain
C. Herpes-zoster vaccine
D. Ophthalmology consult
E. Steroid eye drops

Answer: _____

Herpes Zoster (Shingles)
- Reactivation of latent varicella-zoster virus
- Older, immunocompromised patients
- Pain grouped vesicles within dermatome(s)
  - HZ ophthalmicus can lead to **vision loss (Hutchinson's sign)**
  - Ramsay Hunt Syndrome
- Treatment:
  - Acyclovir, valacyclovir, famciclovir
  - Most effective within **72 hours**
  - **Steroids typically not used**
- Other
  - **Postherpetic neuralgia** (TCAs, gabapentin, pregabalin)
  - Candidates over 60 should be offered **zoster vaccine** (LAV)

© 2017 MedStudy Internal Medicine Video Board Review – Dermatology • Aaron J. Calderon, MD

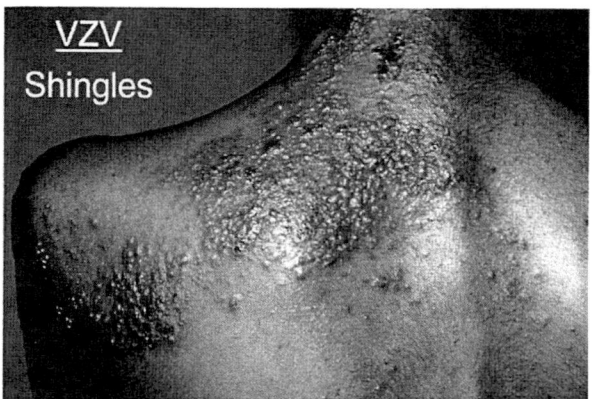

VZV
Shingles

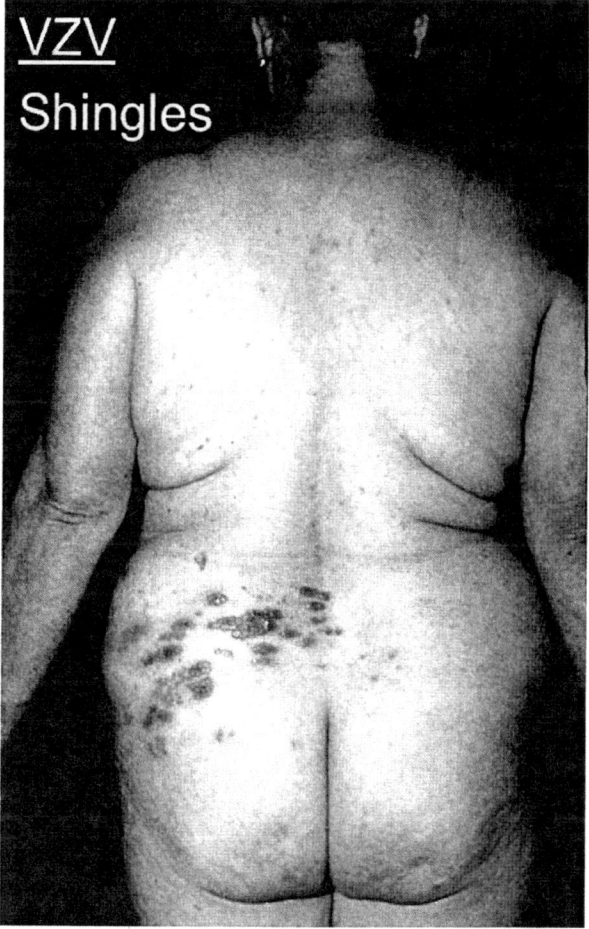

VZV
Shingles

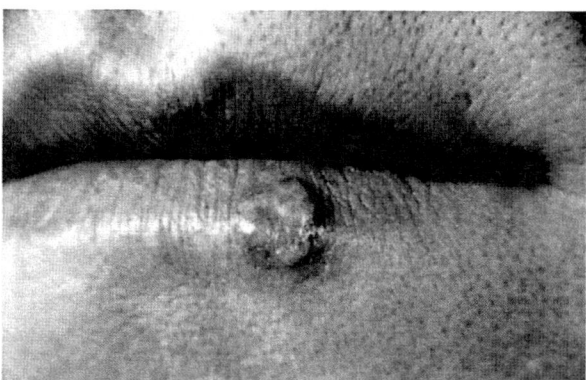

CDC Public Health Image Library

Herpes Simplex Virus

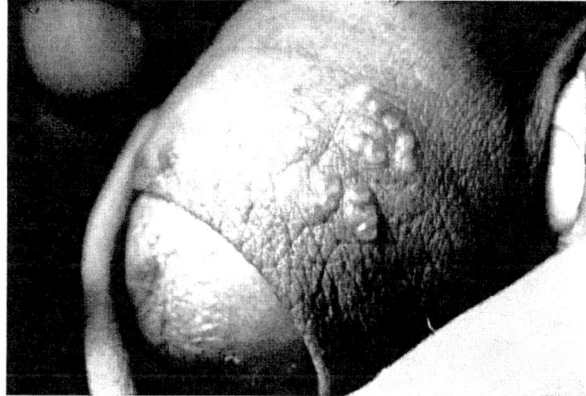

Multinucleated Giant Cell of Herpes Simplex Virus Infection

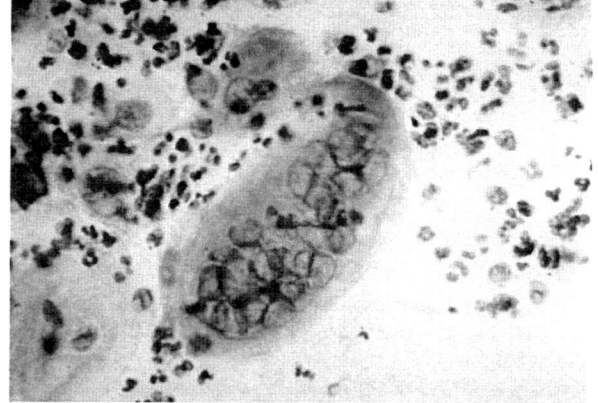

Herpes Simplex Virus (HSV 1 or 2)
- Grouped vesicles on an erythematous base
  - Oral/genital common
- Primary infection can be mild or severe; Systemic symptoms
- Persists in sensory ganglia; Recurs often on lips (prodrome)
- **Dx:** PCR or DFA (direct fluorescent ab); Tzanck smear
- **Rx:** Not usually needed; Use oral antivirals with prodrome

Herpes Simplex Virus

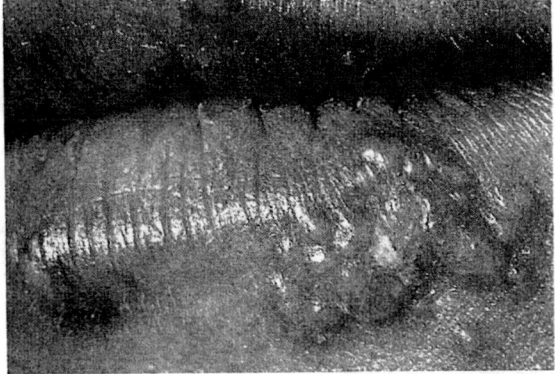

HSV — Herpetic Whitlow

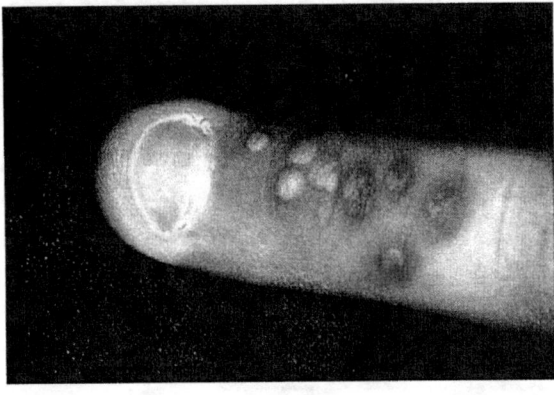

Pityriasis Rosea
- Fine scaling papules and plaques with **collarette of scale**
  - Trunk and proximal extremities
  - Asymptomatic or mild pruritus
  - Unlike syphilis spares palms/soles; **consider RPR**
- Oval, follow skin lines of cleavage
- **Herald patch** appears 1–2 weeks before generalized rash
- Resolves spontaneously
- Low potency steroid if pruritic

Herald Patch — Pityriasis Rosea

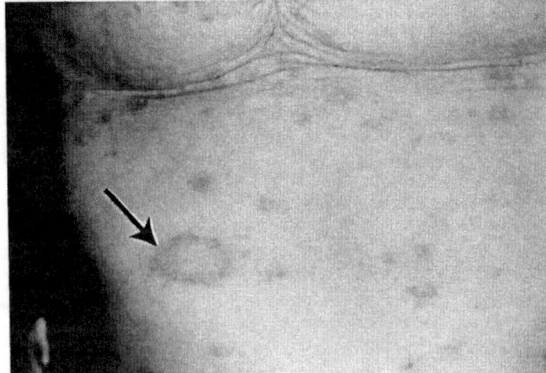

CDC Public Health Image Library

Pityriasis Rosea

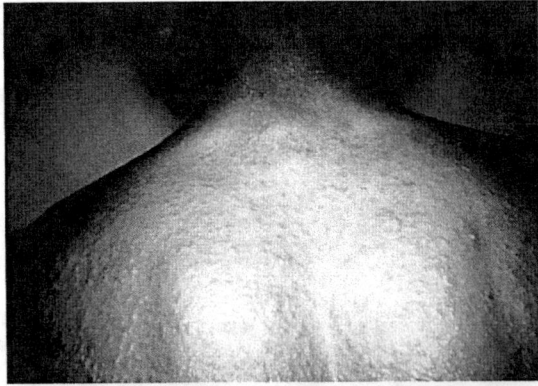

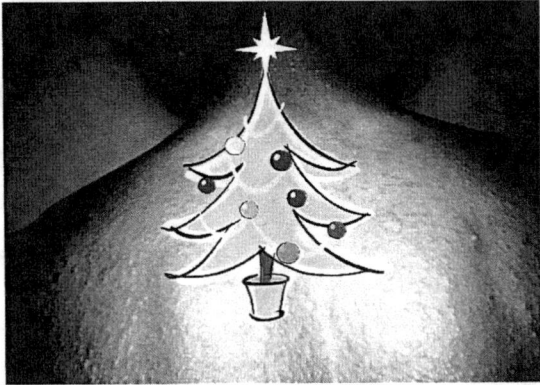

CDC Public Health Image Library

Scabies

AR 28

A 70 y/o nursing home patient is sent to the emergency department for 3 weeks for severe, intense pruritus all over his body. Other tenants have had similar symptoms. Small papules are present on finger web spaces and wrist. Microscopic exam confirmed the diagnosis.

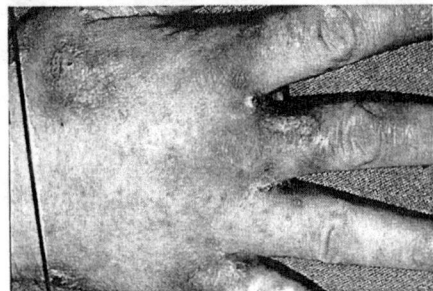

What is the best recommended treatment?
A. Topical steroid
B. Antihistamine
C. Oral ivermectin
D. Lindane 1% lotion
E. Permethrin 5% cream

Answer: _____

 © 2017 MedStudy Internal Medicine Video Board Review – Dermatology • Aaron J. Calderon, MD

Scabies
- Mite — transmitted person to person
- Intense, unexplained itching; Hypersensitivity
- Institutionalized are at higher risk
- **Dx:** Mites, feces, or eggs under microscope
- **Rx:** Permethrin 5%; Repeat dose recommended in a week
- Wash linens used in last 48–72 hrs in hot water

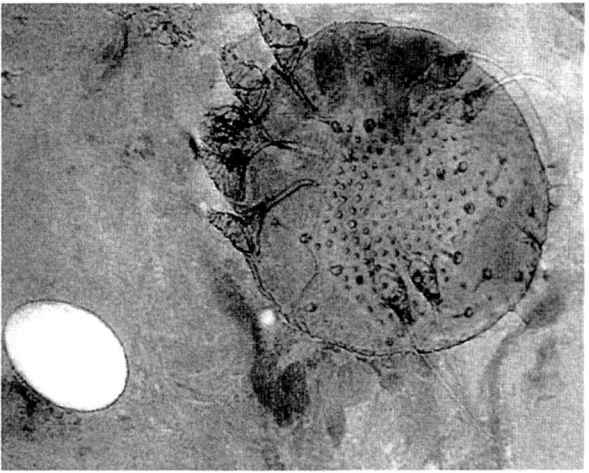

Skin Cancers

AR 29

Which of the following is most important in determining the prognosis of a patient with melanoma?

A. Location of the melanoma
B. Depth of the melanoma
C. Presence or absence of ulceration
D. Duration of the melanoma
E. Surface size of the melanoma

Answer: _____

Melanoma
- **A** – **A**symmetry
- **B** – **B**orders are irregular
- **C** – **C**olor variation
- **D** – **D**iameter > 6 mm is suspicious
- **E** – **E**levation or **E**volution over time

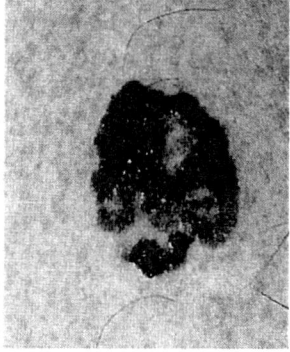

Melanoma Prognosis
- **Depth**
  - < 0.76 mm → 99% five-year survival
  - > 3.6 mm → < 50% five-year survival
- Age
  - Best if < 50 years of age
- Location
  - Best if on trunk

Basal Cell Carcinoma
- **Most common; sun exposed**
- **Rarely metastasizes (< 0.1%)**
- Papules or nodules
- Smooth surface
- Translucent; Pearly
- Telangiectasia
- Central ulcer
  - "Rodent eaten"

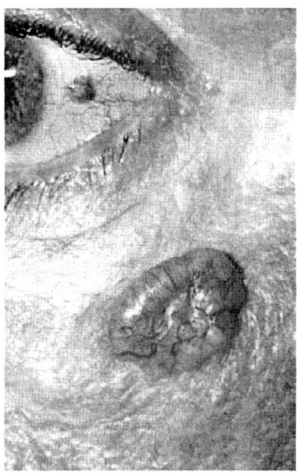

Squamous Cell Carcinoma
- 2nd most common
- May metastasize 0.3–3.7%
- Especially lower lip, ear, and recurring tumors (30%)
- **Most common skin cancer after solid organ transplant**

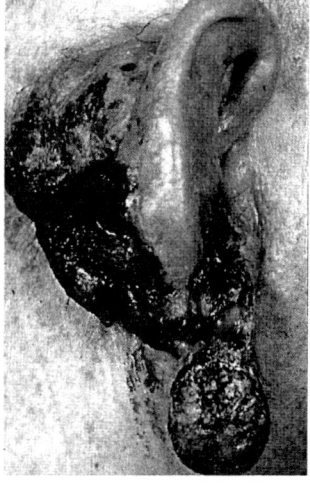

Lentigo Maligna

- Melanoma in situ
- Median age 65 years
- Slowly evolves
- No change in survival if no progression

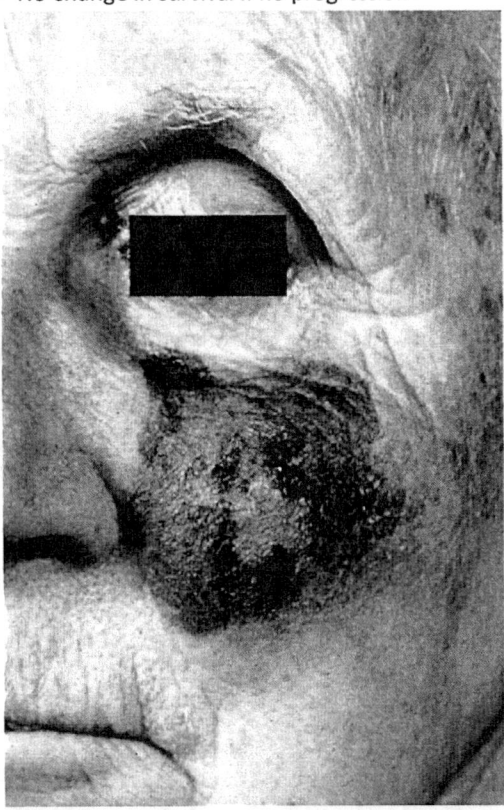

Acral Lentiginous Melanoma

- Palm, sole, or nail bed
- Median age 65 years
- 50–70% of melanomas in African Americans and Asians

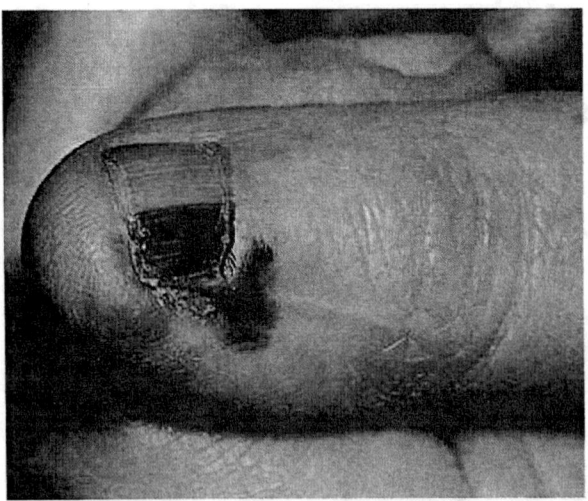

Cutaneous T-Cell Lymphoma

- **Mycosis fungoides**
  - Malignant clonal expansion of CD4+ cells
  - Uncommon (< 1% of all lymphomas)
  - Can be mistaken for psoriasis/eczema
- **Sézary syndrome**
  - 5% of all MF cases
  - Erythroderma
  - Lymphadenopathy
  - Circulating large atypical lymphocytes
    - Cerebriform nuclei

Mycosis Fungoides

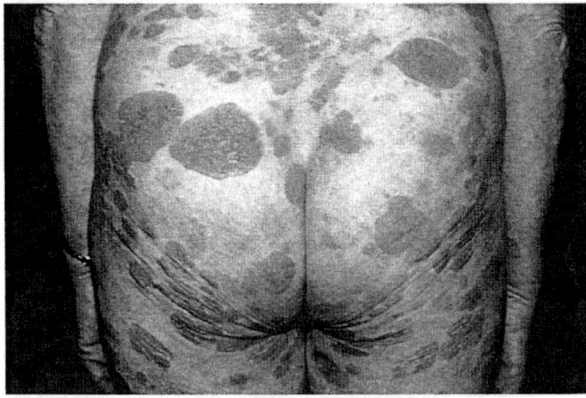

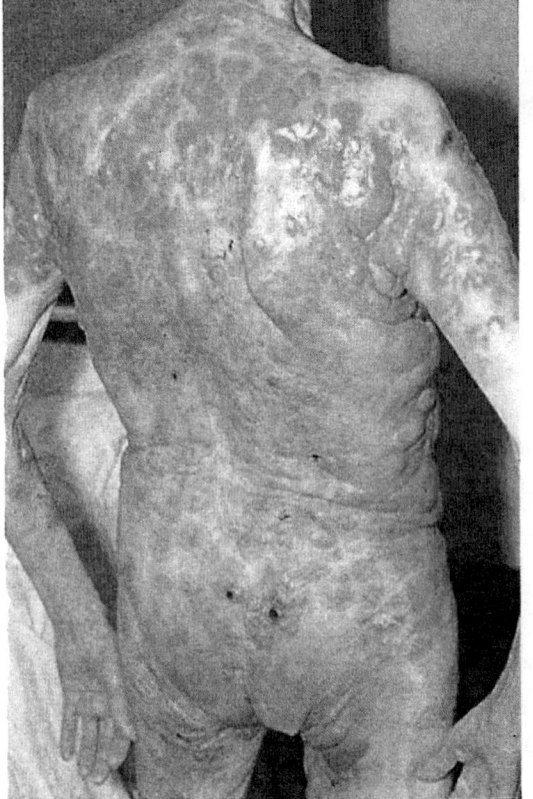

Mycosis Fungoides

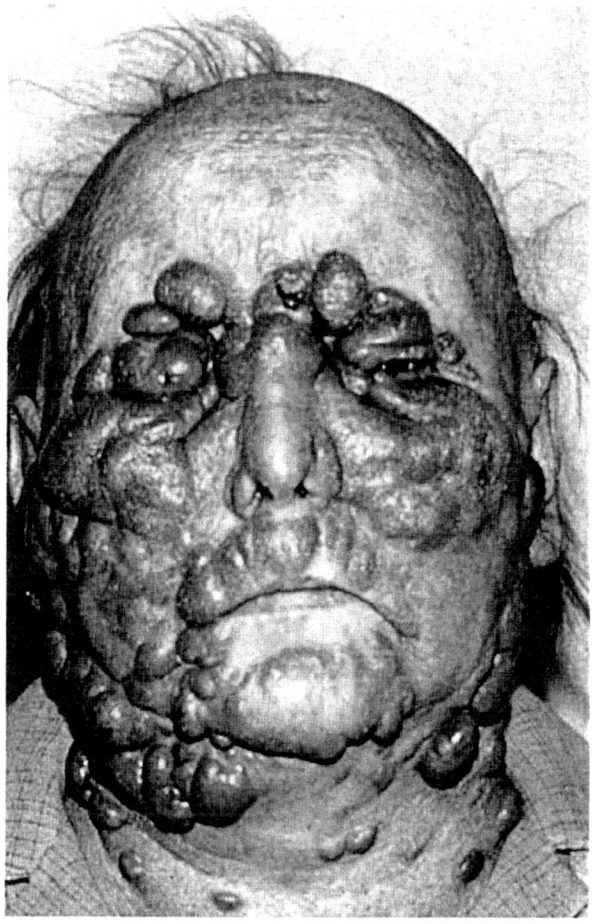

Paget Disease of Breast
- Intraductal breast carcinoma with retrograde extension
- Unilateral eczematous areolar plaque
- **Consider this when there is no response to treatment**

Paget Disease

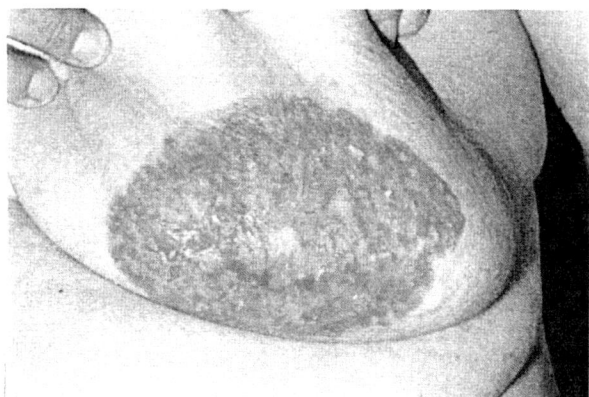

Paget Disease

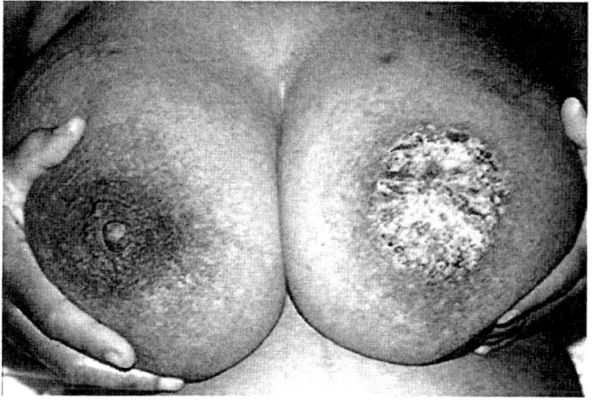

Blistering Lesions

AR 30

A 72 y/o woman is seen for worsening blistering skin lesions. She has no history of hepatitis C or celiac disease and is on no medications. On exam, there are tense blisters on her lower extremities. Nikolsky sign is negative. She has no mucosal involvement.

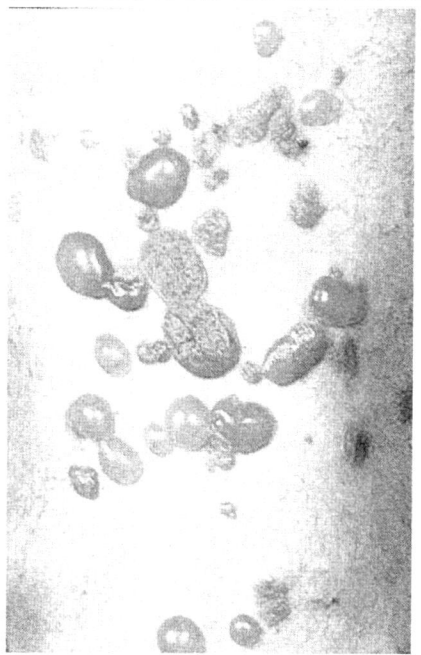

What is the most likely diagnosis?
A. Porphyria cutanea tarda
B. Erythema multiforme
C. Pemphigus vulgaris
D. Dermatitis herpetiformis
E. Bullous pemphigoid

Answer: _____

Bullous Pemphigoid

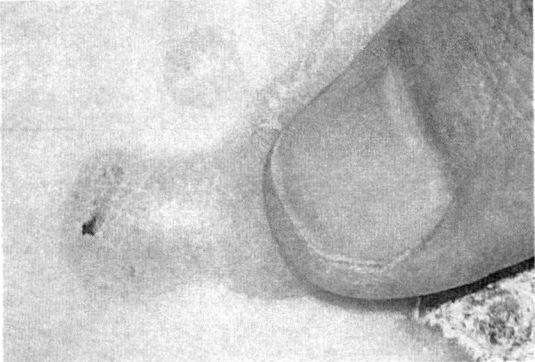

Bullous Pemphigoid (cont.)
- Large tense bullae (intact)
- Nikolsky sign negative
- Mucosal involvement uncommon

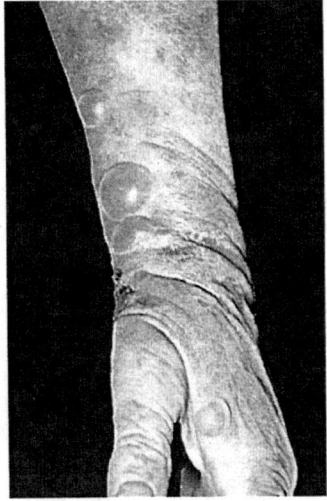

Pemphigus Vulgaris
- Fragile blisters (denuded)
- Nikolsky sign positive
- Mucosal involvement common

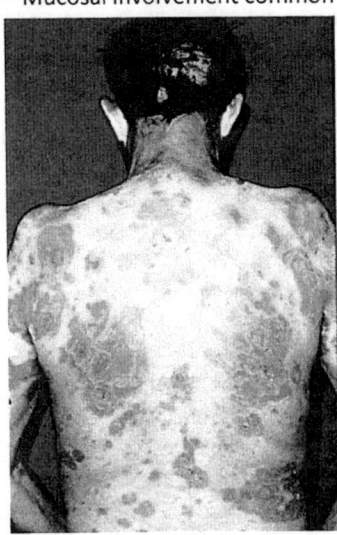

Bullous Pemphigoid
Antibodies to basement membrane (tense and deep)

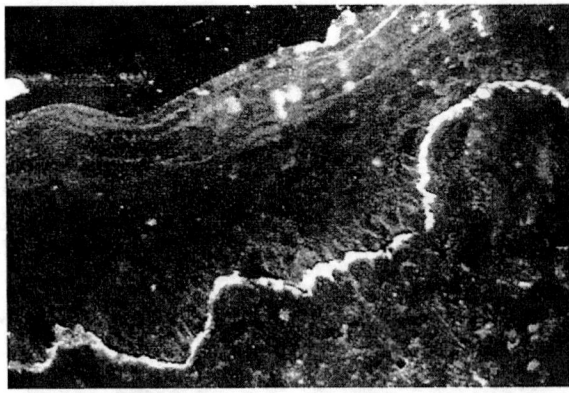

Pemphigus Vulgaris
Intraepidermal antibodies against desmosome (fragile and superficial)

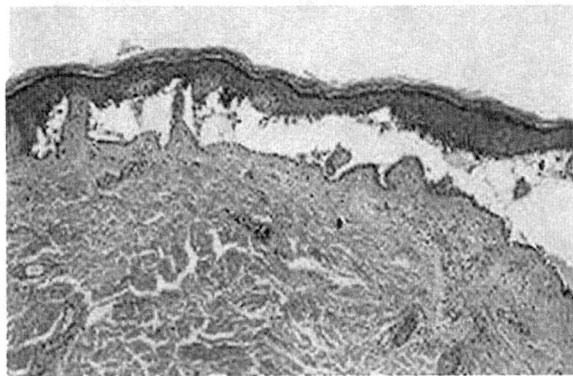

Porphyria Cutanea Tarda
- Deficiency of heme synthetic enzyme uroporphyrinogen decarboxylase
- **Dx:** ↑↑ Urinary copro- and uroporphyrins
- Build-up of phototoxic porphyrins in the skin
- Blisters on sun-exposed skin
- Associated with **hepatitis C**
- Hypertrichosis
- **Rx:** Serial phlebotomy, antimalarials, HCV Rx

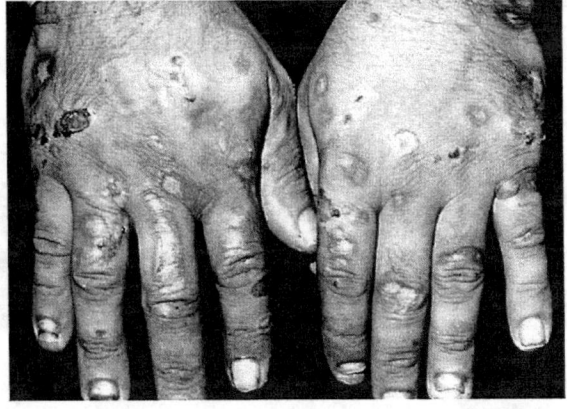

Dermatitis Herpetiformis
- Extremely itchy, symmetric, grouped vesicles most frequently located on extensor surfaces
- Vesicles often broken
- All patients have **celiac disease** (may be asymptomatic)
- **IgA** deposition in dermal papillary tips
- **Gluten-free diet** treats DH and celiac disease
- **Dapsone** will treat DH but not celiac disease
  - Check for G6PD first if at risk

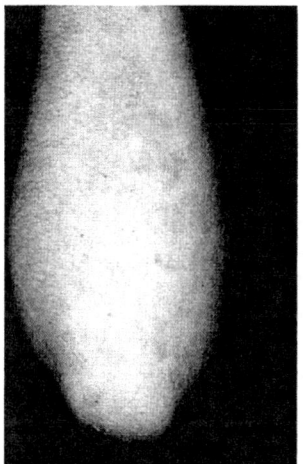
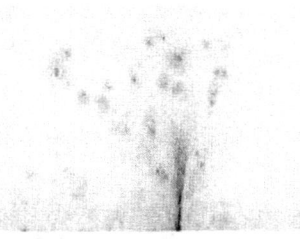
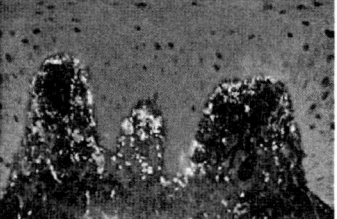

Erythema Multiforme

AR 31

This eruption is most often associated with which virus?

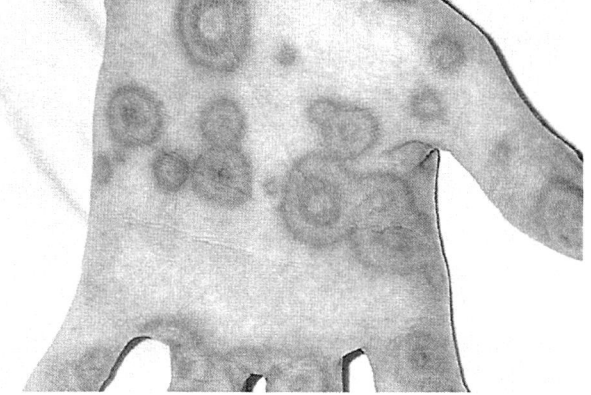

A. Epstein-Barr
B. Cytomegalovirus
C. Herpes simplex
D. Varicella zoster
E. HIV

Answer: _____

Erythema Multiforme
- Acute, target lesions pathognomonic
- Self-limiting (muco) cutaneous disorder
- Infections
  - **HSV** most common cause
  - Often recurrent; May benefit from suppression
  - ***Mycoplasma pneumoniae***
  - Treat active infection if found
- Drugs
  - Sulfonamides, anticonvulsants, penicillins, NSAIDs, allopurinol

Pigment Changes

AR 32

A 45 y/o woman with a BMI of 25 comes to see you because of weight loss and rapid progression of velvety hyperpigmentation on her axilla, neck, and groin. Labs: FBG 80, HbA1c 5.2%, TSH normal.

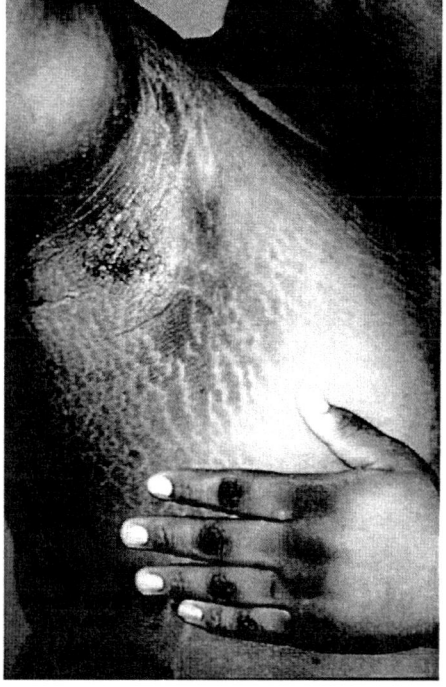

What would be the best next step?
A. Skin biopsy
B. Upper GI endoscopy
C. Chest x-ray
D. Reassurance
E. CT chest/abdomen/pelvis

Answer: _____

Acanthosis Nigricans
- Velvety, hyperpigmented patches
- **Skin folds, esp. axillae**
- Obese patients
- Endocrinopathy (diabetes)
- **Gastric adenocarcinoma**
- Niacin overuse

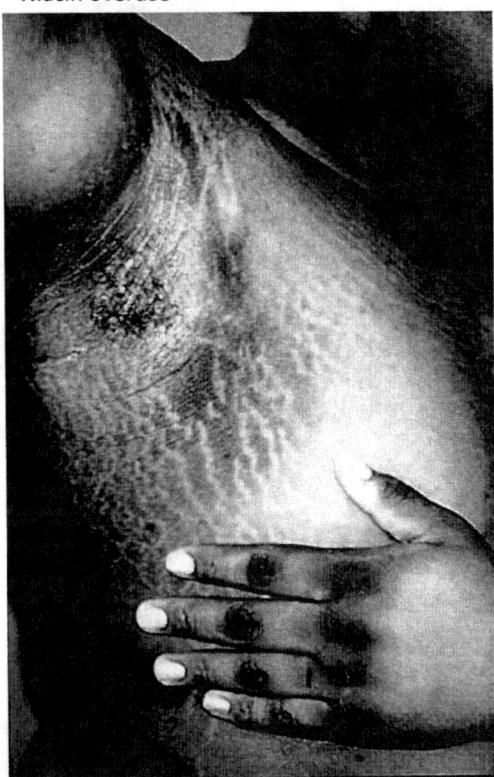

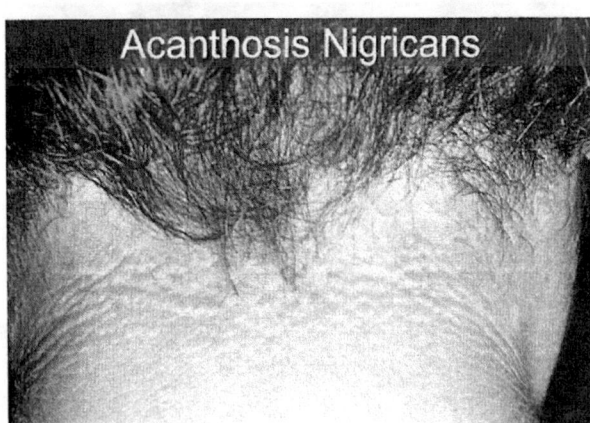

Acanthosis Nigricans

AR 33
A 40 y/o woman with Type 1 diabetes, hypothyroidism, and this skin disorder is found to have gingival hyperpigmentation upon examination for unintentional weight loss.

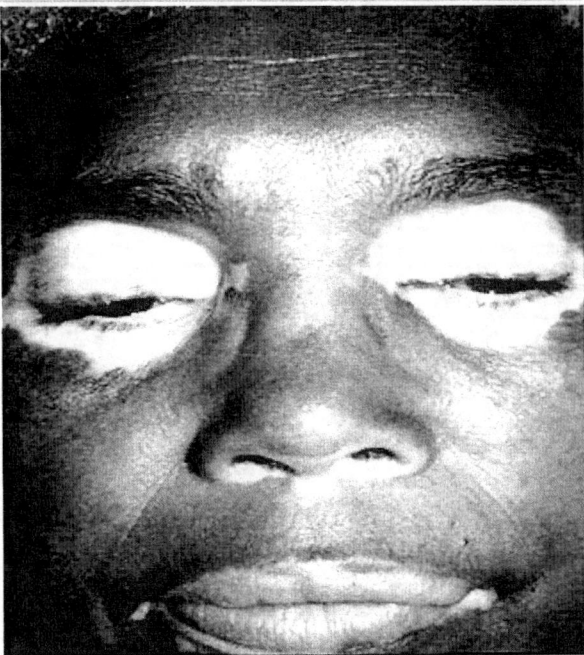

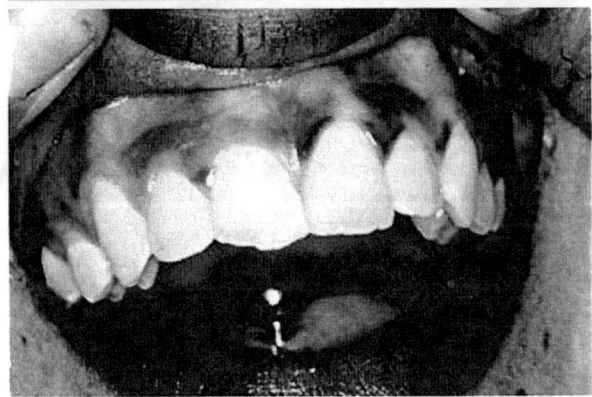

Which diagnosis is most likely?
A. Acanthosis nigricans
B. Melanoma
C. Peutz-Jeghers syndrome
D. Addison's disease
E. Hemochromatosis

Answer: _____

Vitiligo
- Depigmented macules and patches
- Usually healthy patients
- Rarely part of the polyglandular autoimmune deficiency syndromes

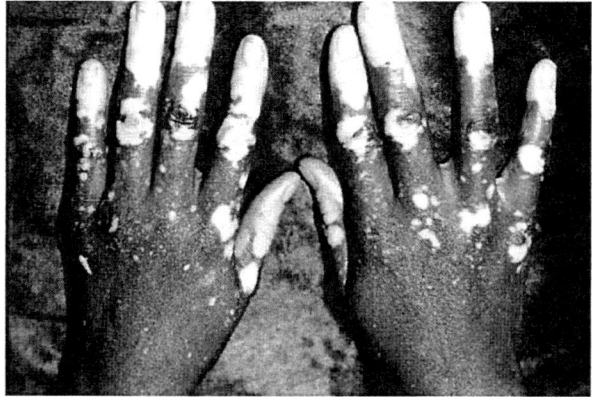

Calciphylaxis

AR 34

A 72 y/o woman with a history of ESRD and secondary hyperparathyroidism presents with painful, violaceous, symmetric lesions on the legs which then developed into nonhealing necrotic ulcers.
Labs: Ca^{2+} 10.0, Phos 8.1, Bun 82, Cr 5.3.

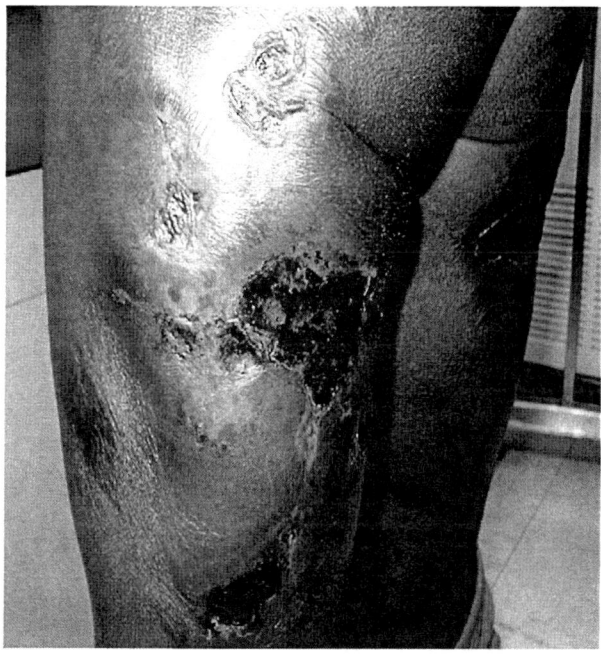

The most likely diagnosis is:
A. Nephrogenic systemic fibrosis
B. Calciphylaxis
C. Pyoderma gangrenosum
D. Necrotizing fasciitis
E. Multiple bites from a brown recluse spider gone rogue

Answer: _____

Calciphylaxis
- Most commonly seen in **ESRD** patients
- Associated with **secondary hyperparathyroidism**
  - Ca^{2+} **x Phos product > 55 to 70**
- Medial calcification of **arterial** wall with intimal proliferation → ischemia and tissue necrosis
- Painful, symmetric, violaceous nodules → ulcerate
  - Areas of greatest adiposity (thighs, buttocks, abd)
- Poor prognosis, especially proximal lesions
- **Rx:**
  - Wound care
  - Lower Ca^{2+} x Phos product
  - Thiosulfate

Nephrogenic Systemic Fibrosis
- Fibrosing disease similar to scleroderma
  - Face spared
- Associated with **gadolinium**
  - Contrast used for MRI
- Typically occurs in patients with ESRD or GFR < 30
- No proven therapy (transplant?)
- Prevention is key
  - **Do not give gadolinium to patient with GFR < 30**

Spider Bite

Spider Bite — Brown Recluse
- Brown recluse can cause **skin necrosis and ulceration**
- Located primarily in the Midwest and Southeast U.S.
- **Violin**-shaped marking behind its head; 6 eyes
- Dapsone?
- **Mistaken for spider bites**
  - MRSA
  - Pyoderma gangrenosum

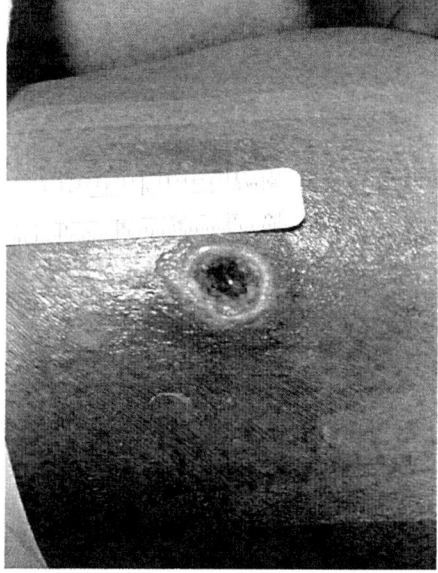

Bibliography

- Fitzpatrick, et al. *Color Atlas and Synopsis of Clinical Dermatology,* 7th Ed., 2013.
- Habif TP. *Clinical Dermatology: A Color Guide to Diagnosis and Therapy,* 5th Ed., 2010.
- Usantine RP. Interactive Dermatology Atlas. Department of Family and Community Medicine of the University of Texas Health Science Center. [Online] **http://www.dermatlas.net/**
- Fleischer AB Jr., Feldman SR, McConnell RC. The most common dermatologic problems identified by family physicians, 1990–1994. *Fam Med.* 1997;29:648.
- Federman DG, Kirsner RS. The patient with skin disease: an approach for nondermatologists. *Ostomy Wound Manage.* 2002;48:22.

Dermatology
Audience Response Answers

Audience Response 1
Answer: E. Topical corticosteroids.

AR 2
Answer: D. Check for HIV.

AR 3
Answer: A. Poison ivy.

AR 4
Answer: E. Topical retinoid.

AR 5
Answer: E. All of the above.

AR 6
Answer: B. Topical metronidazole.

AR 7
Answer: B. Oral hairy leukoplakia.

AR 8
Answer: C. Tongue brushing.

AR 9
Answer: B. 1–2 weeks.

AR 10
Answer: C. Toxic epidermal necrolysis.

AR 11
Answer: D. Onycholysis and pits.

AR 12
Answer: D. < 10% chance.

AR 13
Answer: B. Löfgren syndrome.

AR 14
Answer: B. Dermatomyositis.

AR 15
Answer: D. Henoch-Schönlein purpura.

AR 16
Answer: A. Pyoderma gangrenosum.

AR 17
Answer: C. Erythrasma.

AR 18
Answer: D. Obtain a surgical consultation.

AR 19
Answer: C. Toxic shock syndrome.

AR 20
Answer: D. Incision and drainage.

AR 21
Answer: C. 5% acetic acid compresses.

AR 22
Answer: E. Amoxicillin/clavulanate.

AR 23
Answer: C. Griseofulvin by mouth.

AR 24
Answer: C. Obtain and send a nail clipping
sample to the lab.

AR 25
Answer: B. Lyme disease.

AR 26
Answer: B. Secondary.

AR 27
Answer: D. Ophthalmology consult.

AR 28
Answer: E. Permethrin 5% cream.

AR 29
Answer: B. Depth of the melanoma.

AR 30
Answer: E. Bullous pemphigoid.

AR 31
Answer: C. Herpes simplex.

AR 32
Answer: B. Upper GI endoscopy.

AR 33
Answer: D. Addison's disease.

AR 34
Answer: B. Calciphylaxis.

MedStudy

Internal Medicine Video Board Review

Endocrinology

Presented by

Janet Schlechte, MD
Professor of Medicine
Department of Internal Medicine
University of Iowa Carver College of Medicine
Iowa City, Iowa

Table of Contents

Endocrinology Abbreviations

ACEI	Angiotensin-converting enzyme inhibitor
ACTH	Adrenocorticotropic hormone
ADH	Antidiuretic hormone
ARB	Angiotensin II receptor antagonist
BMD	Bone mineral density
BMI	Body mass index
BUN	Blood urea nitrogen
CVD	Cardiovascular disease
DHEA-S	Dehydroepiandrosterone sulfate
DI	Diabetes insipidus
DM	Diabetes mellitus
DST	Dexamethasone suppression test
ESR	Erythrocyte sedimentation rate
FBG	Fasting blood glucose
FNA	Fine needle aspiration
FPG	Fasting plasma glucose
FRAX	Fracture risk assessment tool
FSH	Follicle stimulating hormone
FT_4	Free T_4
GFR	Glomerular filtration rate
GH	Growth hormone
GHRH	Growth hormone-releasing hormone
GLP	Glucagon-like peptide
GnRH	Gonadotropin releasing hormone
IGF-1	Insulin-like growth factor 1
LH	Luteinizing hormone
MEN 1	Multiple endocrine neoplasia Type 1
MEN 2	Multiple endocrine neoplasia Type 2
NPH	Neutral protamine Hagedorn insulin
NS	Normal saline
OGTT	Oral glucose tolerance test
PCOS	Polycystic ovarian syndrome
POF	Premature ovarian failure
PRL	Prolactin
PTH	Parathyroid hormone
PTU	Propylthiouracil
QOL	Quality of life
RAI	Radioactive iodine
SIADH	Syndrome of inappropriate antidiuretic hormone
SSRI	Selective serotonin reuptake inhibitor
TBG	Thyroid-binding globulin
TG	Triglycerides
TPO	Thyroid peroxidase
TSH	Thyroid stimulating hormone
UACR	Urine albumin to creatinine ratio
UFC	Urine free cortisol

Endocrinology

Pituitary

Pituitary Tumors
- Anterior pituitary dysfunction
- Headache, visual loss
- Nonfunctioning tumor
  - No recognizable clinical syndrome
- Functioning tumor
  - PRL, ACTH, GH
  - Prolactinoma most common

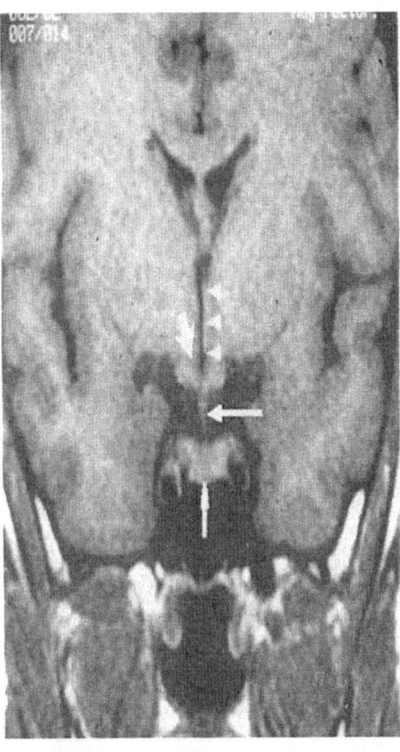

Management of Hyperprolactinemia

$\uparrow$ PRL $\rightarrow$ Galactorrhea
$\downarrow$
$\downarrow$ LH, FSH
$\downarrow$
Estradiol/Testosterone
$\downarrow$
Amenorrhea
Hypogonadism
Infertility
Low libido

DDX of Hyperprolactinemia
- Medications
- Prolactinoma
- Hypothyroidism
- Pregnancy
- Renal insufficiency
- Chest trauma
- Pituitary stalk compression
- Hypothalamic tumor

Medication-Induced Hyperprolactinemia
- **Metoclopramide**
- **Phenothiazines**
- **Risperidone**
- Butyrophenones
- Any interference with dopaminergic activity will increase PRL
- Tricyclics
- Opiates
- Verapamil
- Estrogen
- SSRI

Audience Response 1
A 22 yo has had milky breast discharge and amenorrhea for 9 months. She takes no medications, and thyroid and renal function tests are normal. Prolactin is 75 ($\uparrow$), and a pituitary MRI reveals a 4-mm mass. A pregnancy test is negative.

Which of the following is most consistent with this clinical picture?
A. $\uparrow$ Estradiol
B. $\downarrow$ FSH
C. $\downarrow$ Cortisol and free T_4
D. Abnormal visual fields

Answer: _____

Typical PRL Secreting Microadenoma
- 31 yo female
- PRL 60 ($\uparrow$)
- Amenorrhea, galactorrhea, infertility
- Normal pituitary function
- No neurologic dysfunction
- **Microadenoma, rare tumor growth**

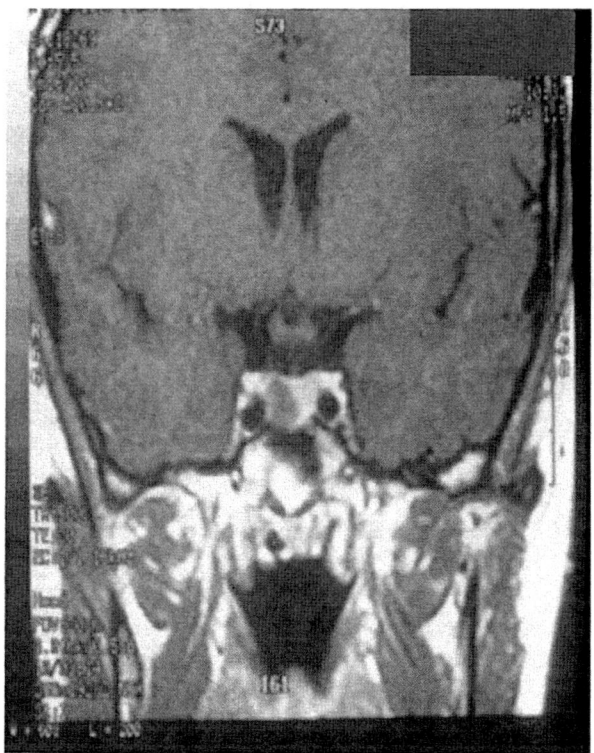

Typical PRL Secreting Macroadenoma
- 52 yo male
- PRL 2,000 ($\uparrow\uparrow$)
- Diplopia/Headache
- Erectile dysfunction
- Infertility
- Hypopituitarism
- Macroadenoma
- May increase in size

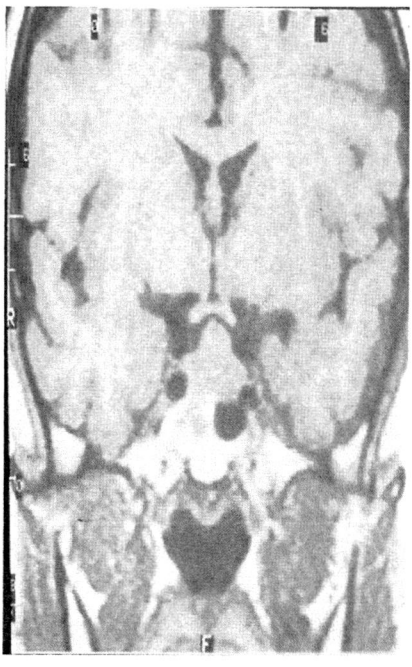

Prolactinoma Treatment
- Treatment indications — fertility, hypogonadism, and macroadenoma
- **Dopamine agonist treatment of choice even for large tumors — normalizes PRL and $\downarrow$ tumor size**
- **Cabergoline/Bromocriptine, neither is teratogenic — drug is stopped when pregnancy is achieved**
- Low doses of dopamine agonist used chronically no major side effects

AR 2

A 27 yo was found to have a 4-mm pituitary tumor 3 months ago. Her prolactin was 195 ($\uparrow$), and she was started on bromocriptine. Today, she reports a positive pregnancy test.

What advice should you give?
A. Stop bromocriptine; continue follow-up with an obstetrician.
B. Stop bromocriptine; switch to an equivalent dose of cabergoline.
C. Continue bromocriptine and repeat prolactin level monthly until delivery.
D. Continue bromocriptine and schedule MRI and formal visual field testing.

Answer: _____

AR 3

As part of an evaluation for headaches and visual loss, a 46 yo man has a 13-mm pituitary mass which does not impinge on the optic chiasm.
His prolactin is 1,500 ($\uparrow\uparrow$), free T_4 0.6 ($\downarrow$), cortisol 2 ($\downarrow$), and testosterone 80 ($\downarrow$).

In addition to starting thyroid and adrenal replacement, what do you recommend?
A. Transsphenoidal surgery
B. Cabergoline
C. Radiation therapy
D. Testosterone

Answer: _____

Acromegaly

Clinical Features
- Coarse facial features
- "Spade-like" hands
- Excessive sweating
- Macroglossia
- Colonic polyps
- Hypertension
- Diabetes
- Sleep apnea
- Impaired glucose tolerance
- $\uparrow$ Mortality

AR 4

A 35 yo farmer has diabetes, carpal tunnel syndrome, sweating, and he snores a lot. On exam he has large hands. His lab evaluation has included an A1c of 9% and an elevated fasting growth hormone.

Does he have acromegaly?

A. Yes

B. No

Answer: _____

Regulation of Growth Hormone

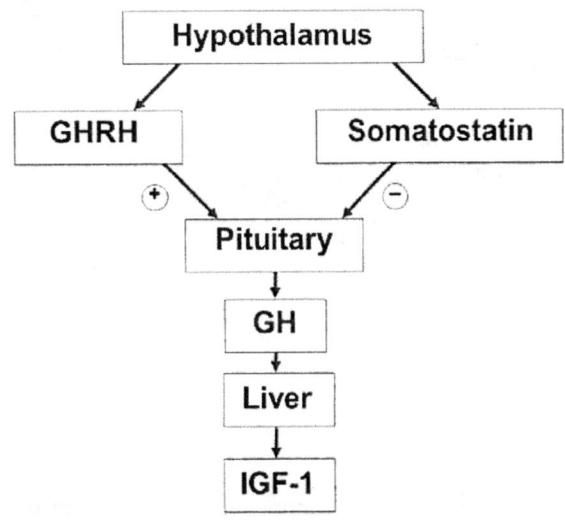

Making the Diagnosis of Acromegaly

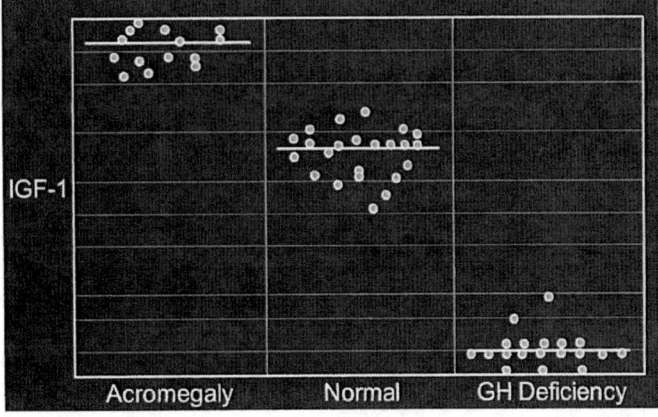

GH Suppression Test in the Diagnosis of Acromegaly

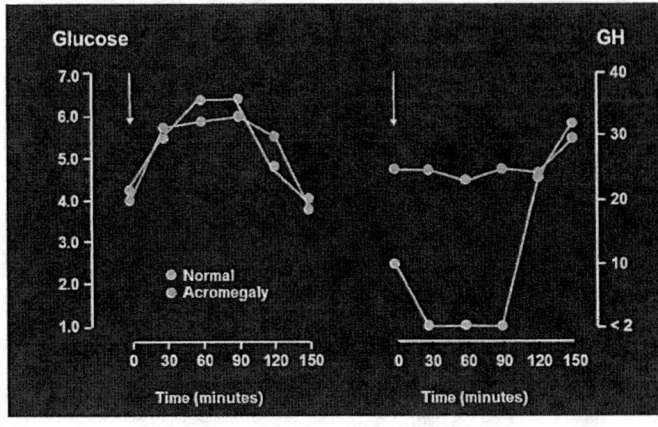

Treatment of Acromegaly
- Macroadenoma usually
- Hypopituitarism uncommon
- Transsphenoidal surgery: 70–80% success rate
- Medical therapy if surgery fails
  - Somatostatin
  - Cabergoline
  - GH receptor antagonist
- Radiation therapy

Nonfunctioning Tumors and Hypopituitarism

AR 5
- A 75 yo presents with visual loss and a massive tumor; He has cold intolerance, fatigue, weight gain, and headaches
- Blood pressure 110/60, pale skin, ↓ beard growth, breast enlargement; Labs: Prolactin 20 (nl), cortisol 2 (↓), testosterone 50 (↓), FT$_4$ 0.4 (↓)
- Thyroid hormone and hydrocortisone are initiated, and he is sent for formal visual field testing

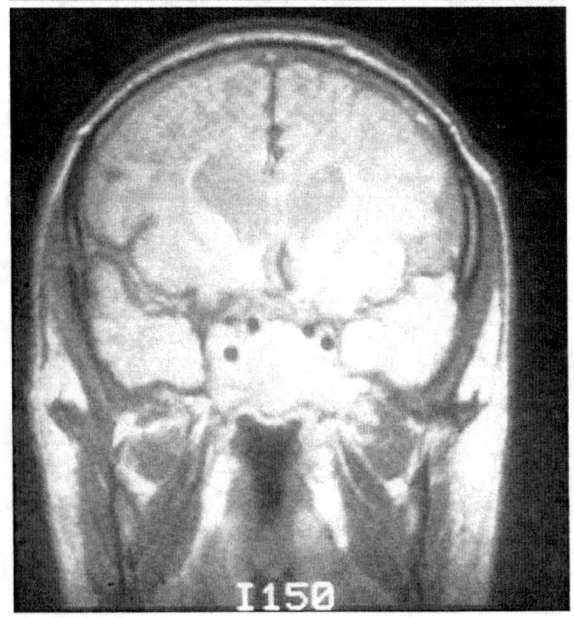

AR 5 (cont.)
What is the next step?
A. Neurosurgery consult.
B. Radiation therapy consult.
C. Testosterone replacement.
D. Measure GH and IGF-1.

Answer: _____

Nonfunctioning Pituitary Tumors
- Large tumors
  - Visual loss, headaches common
  - Hypopituitarism
- No clinically evident hormone production
- α subunit glycoprotein hormone may be elevated
- Do not respond to medical therapy
- Transsphenoidal surgery
- Radiation therapy

AR 6
A 75 yo presents with a severe headache.
An MRI shows suprasellar and lateral extension of a large pituitary tumor. He has also noted fatigue, low libido, cold intolerance, and weight gain.

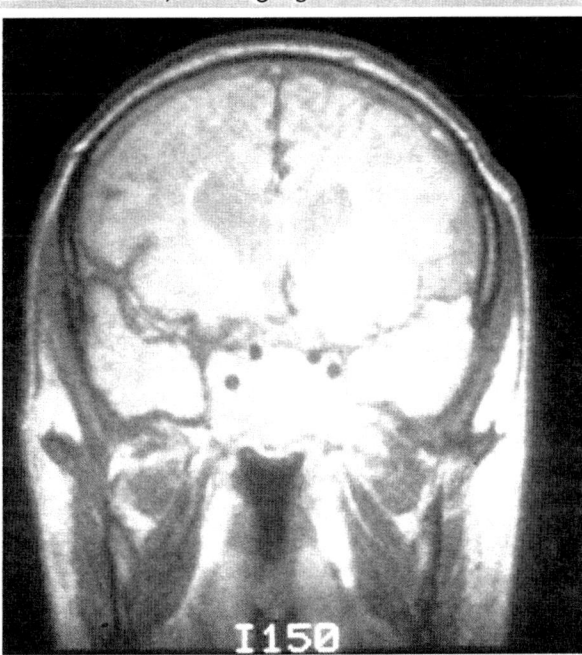

Which of the following are the most likely hormonal abnormalities?
A. $\downarrow$ Cortisol, $\uparrow$ ACTH
B. $\downarrow$ FT_4, $\uparrow$ TSH
C. $\downarrow$ Testosterone, $\downarrow$ FSH
D. $\downarrow$ GH, $\uparrow$ IGF-1

Answer: _____

Hypopituitarism
- Pituitary thyroid axis
  - $\downarrow$ FT_4, $\downarrow$ TSH
- Pituitary adrenal axis
  - $\downarrow$ Cortisol, $\downarrow$ ACTH
- Pituitary gonadal axis
  - $\downarrow$ Testosterone/estradiol
  - $\downarrow$ LH, FSH
- PRL normal unless the tumor is a prolactinoma

Clinical Features of Hypopituitarism
- Hypothyroidism
  - Symptoms same as in primary
- Hypoadrenalism
  - Fatigue
  - Loss of axillary and groin hair
  - No hyperpigmentation
- Hypogonadism
  - Amenorrhea
  - Erectile dysfunction
  - Infertility
  - Symptoms same as in primary
- GH deficiency

Less Common Causes of Hypopituitarism
- Pituitary apoplexy
  - Severe headache
  - ACTH deficiency common
- Sheehan syndrome
  - Enlarged pituitary and tenuous blood supply
  - Failure to lactate (PRL)
  - Amenorrhea (LH, FSH)
  - Loss of axillary/pubic hair (ACTH)
  - Weight gain (TSH)
- Sarcoidosis
- Hemochromatosis
- Metastases

AR 7
After an extremely difficult delivery of her 2nd child, a 26 yo has developed amenorrhea, fatigue, dry skin, and abdominal pain. FT_4 0.6 (0.8–1.9) and TSH 0.6 (0.2–4.2).

In addition to starting levothyroxine, what is the most appropriate next step?
A. Measure prolactin.
B. Measure estradiol.
C. Measure IGF-1.
D. Measure serum cortisol.

Answer: _____

Treatment of Hypopituitarism

- Thyroid
  - Levothyroxine
  - **Monitor therapy with FT$_4$**
  - **Don't use TSH to monitor thyroid hormone therapy**
- Adrenal
  - Prednisone
  - Hydrocortisone
- Gonadal
  - Oral contraceptive
  - Topical or injectable androgen

Empty Sella

A 55 yo woman had this MRI as part of an evaluation for headaches. She is treated for benign intracranial hypertension.

Usually normal pituitary function.

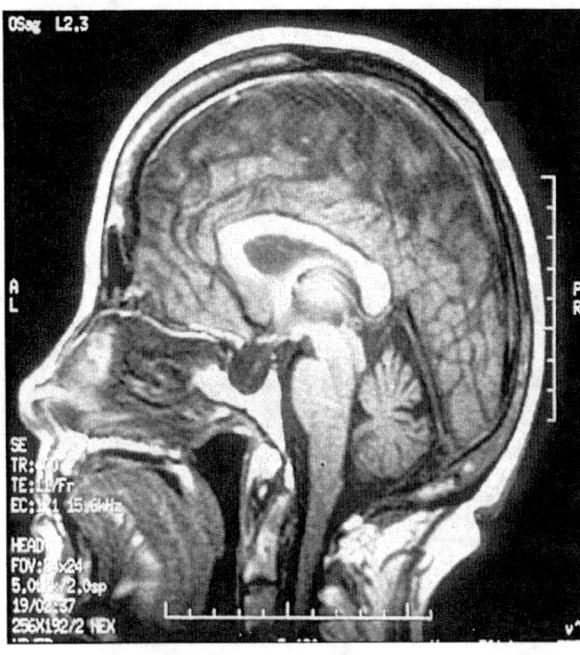

Pituitary Incidentaloma

A healthy 25 yo had an MRI after a car accident. There is a 4-mm mass in the pituitary. She has regular menses, her weight is stable and her exam is normal.

- 10% of healthy individuals
- Usually microadenoma
- Clinical symptoms guide workup and radiographic follow-up

Posterior Pituitary

- Source of antidiuretic hormone (ADH) and oxytocin
- Both are synthesized in brain, transported to posterior pituitary and released directly
- Loss of ADH leads to central diabetes insipidus, which causes polyuria and nocturia along with dilute urine and increased serum osmolality

Workup and Management of Polyuria

AR 8

A 30 yo complains of increased thirst and nocturia for 3 months. She has a normal exam, and electrolytes, calcium, and glucose are normal. Following an overnight fast, her urine specific gravity was 1.020 and her urine osmolality was 700.

What should you do now?

A. Formal H$_2$O deprivation test.
B. Begin amiloride.
C. Begin desmopressin.
D. No additional testing.

Answer: _____

Workup of Polyuria

- Withholding H$_2$O in a healthy subject will lead to ↑ plasma osmolality, ↑ ADH, and ↑ urine osmolality
- With H$_2$O restriction a healthy person will concentrate urine and osmolality should reach 700–800
- If urine remains dilute after H$_2$O restriction, need additional testing to confirm the presence of diabetes insipidus

Confirmation of DI in a Patient with Polyuria

- Withhold water and serially monitor weight, sodium, and blood pressure
- When plasma osmolality reaches 295–300, give desmopressin (DDAVP, Stimate)
- **Central DI**
  - **50% increase in urine osmolality after desmopressin**
- **Nephrogenic DI**
  - **No increase in urine osmolality after desmopressin**

AR 9

A 30 yo noted recent onset of increased thirst and frequent urination. She takes no medications and has normal calcium, glucose, and electrolytes. She has been NPO for 12 hours and her urine osmolality is 300. She is given desmopressin, and her urine osmolality increases to 650.

The most likely cause of the polyuria is:

A. Central diabetes insipidus
B. Nephrogenic diabetes insipidus
C. Primary polydipsia
D. She surreptitiously obtained H$_2$O during the test

Answer: _____

Central (Neurogenic) Diabetes Insipidus
- ADH deficiency
  - Partial or complete
  - Genetic
  - Acquired
  - Trauma, sarcoid, pituitary surgery
  - Idiopathic
  - Polyuria, nocturia
  - $\uparrow$ Serum osmolality, $\downarrow$ urine osmolality
- Treatment: Intranasal or oral desmopressin

Nephrogenic Diabetes Insipidus
- Normal ADH levels but kidneys are resistant to water-retaining effect of ADH
- Genetic
  - Mutation in ADH receptor
- Acquired
  - Lithium, hypercalcemia, Sjögren syndrome
  - Sickle cell disease
- Treatment
  - Low-sodium diet
  - Thiazides
  - Amiodarone

AR 10

A 65 yo female is recovering from a hip fracture. She is taking an opiate, levothyroxine, and sertraline. Her blood pressure is 120/80, she is alert and oriented, has no edema, and her neurologic exam is normal.
Sodium 126, potassium 3.9, chloride 98, and CO_2 24. Her TSH is 2.2 (nl), urine osmolality 600, and urine sodium 42. An 8 a.m. cortisol is 13 (nl).

Which of the following should you recommend for treatment of the hyponatremia?
A. Hypertonic saline
B. Vasopressin receptor antagonist
C. Fluid restriction
D. NaCl tablets
E. Hydrocortisone

Answer: _____

Criteria for Diagnosis of SIADH
- $\downarrow$ Plasma osmolality
- $\uparrow$ Urine osmolality
- Urine sodium > 40 mEq/L
- Normal creatinine
- Normal adrenal and thyroid function
- $\downarrow$ Uric acid
- $\downarrow$ BUN

SIADH
- CNS disorders
- Malignancy (small cell lung)
- SSRI (especially in elderly) — <u>pearl</u>!
- Chemotherapeutic agents
- Surgery
- Pulmonary disease
- Fluid restriction effective for most

Disorders of Thyroid Function

AR 11

A 40 yo has gained 10 pounds, has cold intolerance, fatigue, and constipation. Her exam is normal except for a diffusely enlarged thyroid. Her TSH is 25 (0.2–4.2).

Which of the following lab tests must be completed to confirm the diagnosis and before initiating therapy?
A. TPO antibodies
B. Free T_3
C. Reverse T_3
D. Thyroglobulin
E. None

Answer: _____

Primary Hypothyroidism
- $\downarrow$ FT_4, $\uparrow$ TSH
- Autoimmune — antibodies to thyroid microsomes and thyroglobulin
- With or without goiter
- More common in women
- **Look for other autoimmune disease (diabetes, adrenal insufficiency)**
- Lithium, amiodarone, interferon

Hypothyroidism Features
- Menorrhagia
- Fatigue/Constipation
- Weight gain
- Muscle cramps
- Cold intolerance
- Hyponatremia
- Hyperlipidemia

Thyroid Hormone Replacement
- Levothyroxine best
- **Start full replacement dose (1.6 µg/kg), except in elderly and in patients with CV disease**
- Repeat TFTs in 8–10 weeks, then annual measurement after levels are normal
- Take on empty stomach separated by 2 hours from food and other medications
- Keep TSH in normal range
- Calcium, fibrates, iron, sucralfate can impair absorption

AR 12

A 50 yo with coronary artery disease and hyperlipidemia has a free T_4 of 0.3 ($\downarrow$), a TSH of 80 ($\uparrow$), and LDL of 140. He has muscle pain, cold intolerance, and bradycardia.

Which regimen should you recommend?
A. Combination levothyroxine (T_4) and liothyronine (T_3)
B. Liothyronine (T_3)
C. Thyroid extract
D. Levothyroxine (T_4)

Answer: _____

AR 13

A 75 yo has been taking 1 grain (60 mg) of thyroid extract daily. She feels fatigued. Today her FT_4 is 0.5 (0.9–1.5), TSH 1.2 (0.2–4.2), T_3 2.1 (0.8–2). Her exam (including the thyroid exam) is normal.

Which of the following should you recommend?
A. Increase dose to 1½ grains (90 mg).
B. Make no changes.
C. Measure free T_3.
D. Measure antithyroid antibodies (TPO).

Answer: _____

Thyroid Replacement
- **Avoid T_3 and combination T_4– T_3 replacement especially in elderly and those with heart disease**
- T_3 short half-life, rapid onset of action, could precipitate arrhythmia especially in elderly
- If T_3 or combination therapy is only option, monitor efficacy of therapy with TSH

Thyroid Replacement in the Elderly
- Hypothyroidism occurs in at least 5% of women over 65 years of age
- Signs and symptoms are similar to common symptoms of aging, making the diagnosis easy to overlook
- Coronary disease is common in the elderly, so replacement in elderly patients with hypothyroidism should start with low (25 µg) doses of levothyroxine

Thyroid Replacement in Pregnancy
- Need for thyroxine increases by about 50%
- Increased need persists throughout pregnancy
- TSH may return to normal after delivery
- Use trimester specific TSH and monthly check of thyroid hormone

Myxedema Coma
- Rare
- Extreme hypothyroidism
- Preexisting thyroid disease likely
- Stroke, infection may precipitate
- Mental status changes, hypoventilation, hypothermia, hyponatremia
- High mortality
- IV levothyroxine
- IV liothyronine risky in elderly and benefit not proven
- IV glucocorticoid therapy

AR 14

Which of these patients needs therapy for hypothyroidism?
A. 40 yo with menorrhagia, weight gain, fatigue, cold intolerance, and constipation; FT_4 0.6 ($\downarrow$), TSH 26 ($\uparrow$)
B. 30 yo with constipation, fatigue, cold intolerance, dry skin, and weight gain; FT_4 0.7 ($\downarrow$), TSH 2.1 (nl)
C. Both

Answer: _____

Secondary Hypothyroidism
- Pituitary/Hypothalamic disease
- $FT_4 \downarrow$, TSH $\downarrow$
- Look for other signs of pituitary hypofunction especially ACTH deficiency
- Symptoms are the same as in primary
- **Monitor therapy with free T_4**

Hyperthyroidism

Clinical Features
- Weight loss
- Tremor
- Fatigue
- Amenorrhea
- Palpitations
- Heat intolerance
- Hyperdefecation
- Impaired concentration
- Lid lag, proptosis
- Apathetic thyrotoxicosis in elderly

Causes of Hyperthyroidism

	FT_4	TSH
Graves'	$\uparrow$	$\downarrow$
Hot nodule	$\uparrow$	$\downarrow$
Subacute thyroiditis	$\uparrow$	$\downarrow$
Surreptitious use of T_4	$\uparrow$	$\downarrow$

Graves Disease

- Autoimmune
- Thyroid-stimulating antibodies bind to TSH receptors
- Diffuse smooth thyroid enlargement
- Orbitopathy in 5–10%
- ↑ RAI uptake

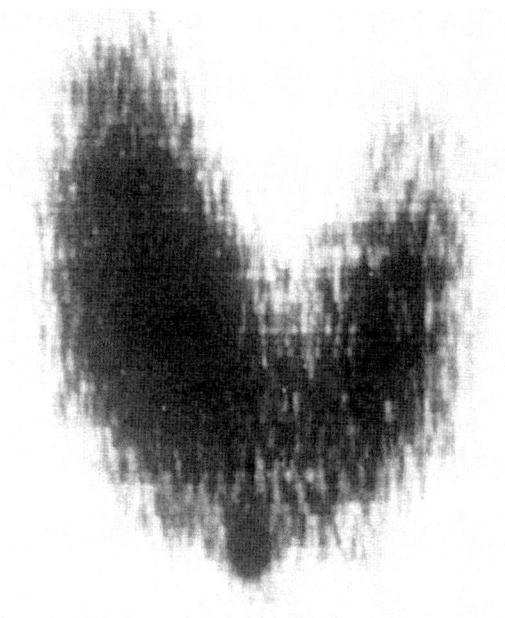

Hyperfunctioning Nodule

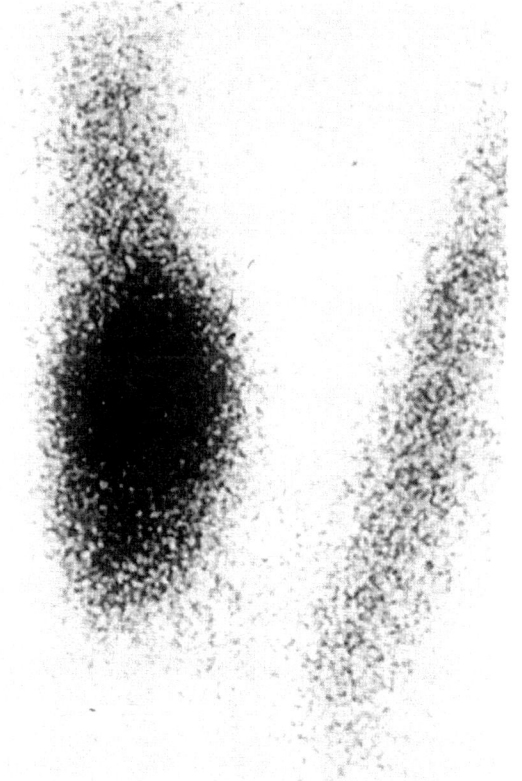

- Palpable nodule on exam
- ↑ RAI uptake in nodule

Toxic Nodular Goiter

- Common in elderly
- Enlarged gland with irregular nodular features on palpation

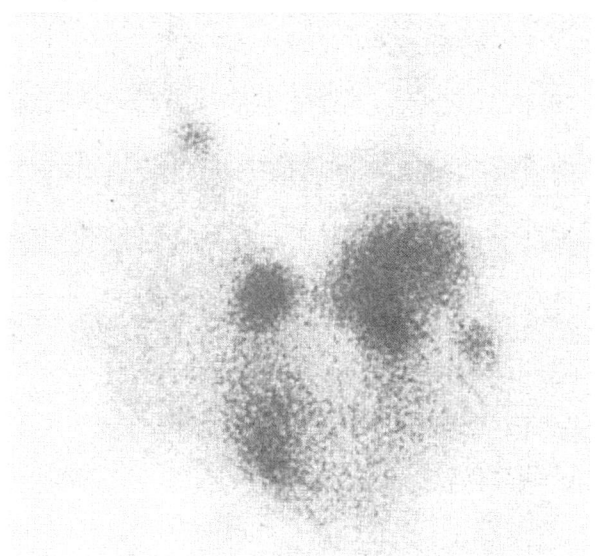

Graves'	Thyroiditis
TSIG	Inflammation
↓	↓
Thyroid Hormone Synthesis	Release of Thyroid Hormone
↓	↓
↑ T_4 ↑ T_3	↑ T_4 ↑ T_3
↓	↓
Suppressed TSH	Suppressed TSH
	↓
	↓ Thyroid Hormone Synthesis

Normal

Thyroiditis

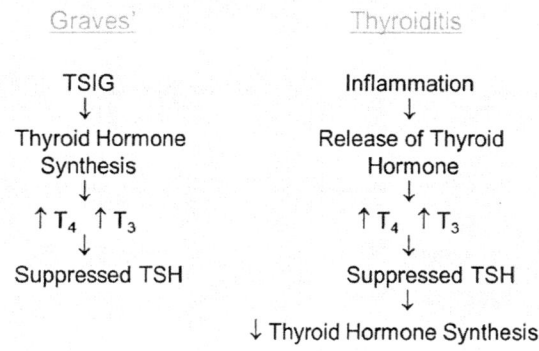

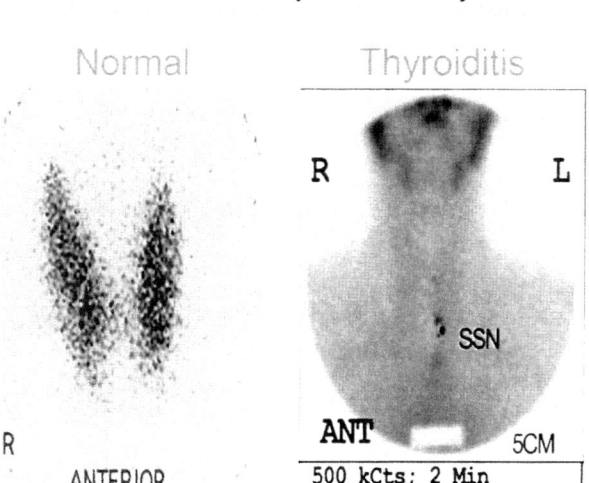

R

ANTERIOR

R   L

SSN

ANT   5CM

500 kCts; 2 Min

Subacute Thyroiditis
- Painful gland, ear pain
- Elevated ESR
- Mild hyperthyroidism
- **Hyperthyroid phase followed by transient hypothyroidism before return to normal**
- Occurs postpartum too

AR 15

For the last 6 months, a 25 yo has maintained a voracious appetite but has not gained weight. She has proptosis, palpitations, and is nervous and irritable; she feels hot all of the time. On exam, her BP is 125/86, pulse 100; she is diaphoretic; her thyroid is enlarged and smooth, and her DTRs are 3+ throughout.
Labs today: Free T_4 2.1 (0.9–1.7), TSH < 0.01 (0.2–4.2)

What is the most likely cause of the ↑ free T_4?
A. Graves'
B. Hyperfunctioning nodule
C. Subacute thyroiditis
D. Toxic multinodular goiter

Answer: _____

AR 16

A 76-year-old male has been increasingly fatigued, anorexic, and confused. He has not had any nausea or GI symptoms.
On exam: BP 160/60, P 100 (irregular)
Cardiac: No murmurs or gallops
Ext: No clubbing or cyanosis
Thyroid: Not enlarged
Lab: Hct 39, Na^+ 140, K^+ 4, Bun 18, Cr 1.1, Ca^{2+} 10.7

What is the most likely cause of his symptoms?
A. Adrenal insufficiency
B. Hypothyroidism
C. Hyperthyroidism
D. Hyperparathyroidism

Answer: _____

Hyperthyroidism in the Elderly
- 1/3 of elderly patients with hyperthyroidism have **"apathetic hyperthyroidism"**
  - Anorexia
  - Weight loss
  - Constipation
  - 40% have heart rates < 100
  - Absence of "typical" symptoms

AR 17

A 25 yo nursing assistant has a 1-month history of palpitations. She is trying to lose weight. On exam, her thyroid is not palpable, she has a fine tremor, and her pulse is 96. FT_4 2.1, TSH 0.01. You are concerned that she might be surreptitiously using thyroid hormone.

Which test would help answer this question?
A. T_3
B. Reverse T_3
C. Thyroglobulin
D. TPO antibodies

Answer: _____

AR 18

A 50 yo has a 1-month history of tremor, palpitations, and heat intolerance. His pulse is 100, the thyroid is smooth and tender, and he has no proptosis. He has no family history of thyroid disease.
FT_4 2.1 (↑)
TSH 0.01 (↓)

Based on this information, which is the most likely?
A. Graves disease
B. Hot nodule
C. Subacute thyroiditis
D. Toxic multinodular goiter

Answer: _____

Treatment of Hyperthyroidism
- Antithyroid drugs
  - Methimazole
  - Propylthiouracil
- Radioactive iodine
- Thyroidectomy

Radioactive Iodine
- Gland destruction
- TSH receptor antibodies persist after treatment
- Avoid RAI in patient with severe Graves' ophthalmopathy
- Single dose effective in 90%
- Most become hypothyroid after 2–3 months but time course variable

Antithyroid Agents
- Methimazole
  - Decreases thyroid-stimulating immunoglobulin levels and blocks T_4 synthesis
  - 30–50% have spontaneous remission after 1 year of therapy—remission more likely with mild disease and small gland
  - Agranulocytosis and hepatitis are very rare side effects

- Propylthiouracil
  - Use only in 1st trimester of pregnancy and in thyroid storm
- Higher likelihood of hepatic dysfunction

Hyperthyroidism in Pregnancy
- **Use PTU in 1st trimester, then methimazole**
- **Keep FT_4 at upper limit of normal range**
- Too much of the antithyroid agent could lead to fetal hypothyroidism
- Radioactive iodine contraindicated
- Both PTU and methimazole cross placenta

AR 19
A 70 yo with steroid-dependent asthma is admitted with HF, atrial fibrillation, fever, and confusion. She has an enlarged thyroid, and her free T_4 is 7 ($\uparrow\uparrow$). Her ventricular rate is 120. She has received an IV β-blocker and 100 mg hydrocortisone in the ICU.

What should be done next?
A. Radioactive iodine
B. Propylthiouracil
C. Cold iodine (nonradioactive)
D. Technetium scan
E. TSH receptor antibodies

Answer: _____

Thyroid Storm
- Exaggerated symptoms of hyperthyroidism
- Surgery, infection, iodine load may precipitate
- First, block T_4 synthesis with PTU, then block T_4 release with nonradioactive iodine
- High mortality
- Glucocorticoids and PTU decrease $T_4 \rightarrow T_3$ conversion
- Glucocorticoids to treat relative adrenal insufficiency

AR 20
An 84 yo woman presents with lower extremity edema. BP is 130/70, P 70 (regular). Other medical problems include depression and CRI. The only lab abnormality is a TSH of 0.15 (0.4–4.5) with a normal free T_4 and a normal T_3.

What do you recommend?
A. Repeat TSH in 3–6 months.
B. Check reverse T_3 level.
C. Thyroid scan.
D. Start β-blocker.

Answer: _____

Subclinical Hyperthyroidism
- Definition—low TSH with normal FT_4 and T_3
- Most common cause is overreplacement with thyroid hormone
- Progression to overt hyperthyroidism 6% first year, and rare after that (about 0.5%)
- More common to progress in patients with Graves disease or nodular goiter
- Progression < 1% per year if TSH is 0.1–0.4
- If TSH is < 0.1, likelihood of progression is higher

- Increased risk of atrial fibrillation
- Low bone density
- Elderly patients with TSH < 0.1 should be treated
- For patients with TSH 0.1–0.4, observation with repeat testing is reasonable
- Assessment of cause can help with decision; If a radionuclide scan shows increased areas of uptake, then treatment is appropriate

Thyroid Nodules

This morning, a 24 yo found this lump in her neck. Her thyroid function tests 2 months ago were normal. She has no dysphagia, cold intolerance, or menorrhagia.

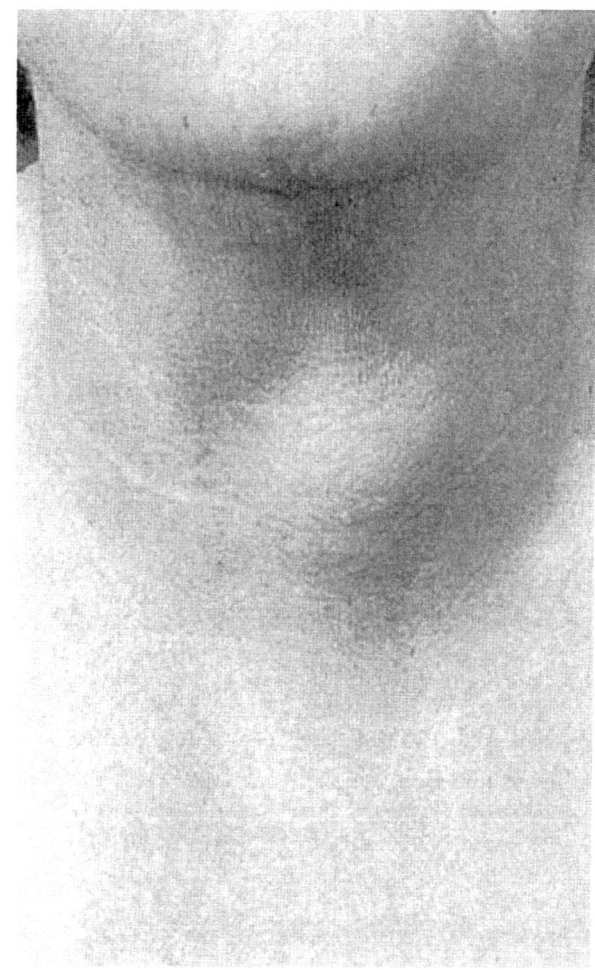

Thyroid Nodule Risk Factors
- History of radiation exposure
- Family history
- Male
- Nodule increasing in size
- Age < 20 or > 70
- Cancer risk 5–10%

Evaluation of a Nodule in a Euthyroid Patient

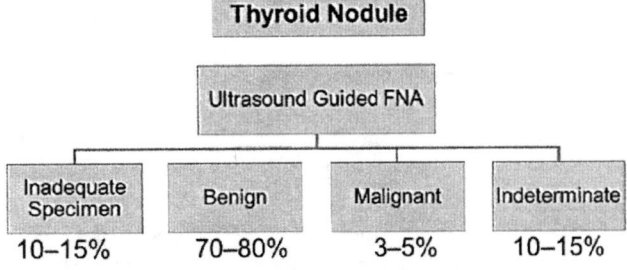

Reasons to Consider Fine-Needle Aspiration of a Thyroid Nodule
- Calcifications
- High intravascular flow
- Hypoechogenicity Irregular borders
- False negative rate of 1–11%; 90–95% sensitivity

Thyroid Cancer
- Papillary and follicular
  - Indolent course
  - Surgery ± radioactive iodine
- Medullary
  - Calcitonin biomarker
  - Surgery
  - MEN association
- Anaplastic
  - Rare and poor prognosis

Thyroid Hormone Replacement in Thyroid Cancer
- No clear evidence that TSH suppression improves survival
- With stage 1 and 2 disease and no evidence of metastasis, keep TSH between 0.1 and 2

AR 21

A 68 yo has lost 15 lbs and is fatigued. On exam, there is a 2-cm nodule in her thyroid. Her pulse is 90, and her skin is dry. Free T_4 is 1.9 (↑), and TSH is < 0.05 (↓).

Which is the best next step in evaluating the nodule?
A. Technetium scan.
B. Ultrasound-guided FNA.
C. TSH receptor antibodies.
D. Measure thyroglobulin.

Answer: _____

Hyperfunctioning Nodule
- Rarely malignant
- Many are euthyroid
- FNA usually not necessary

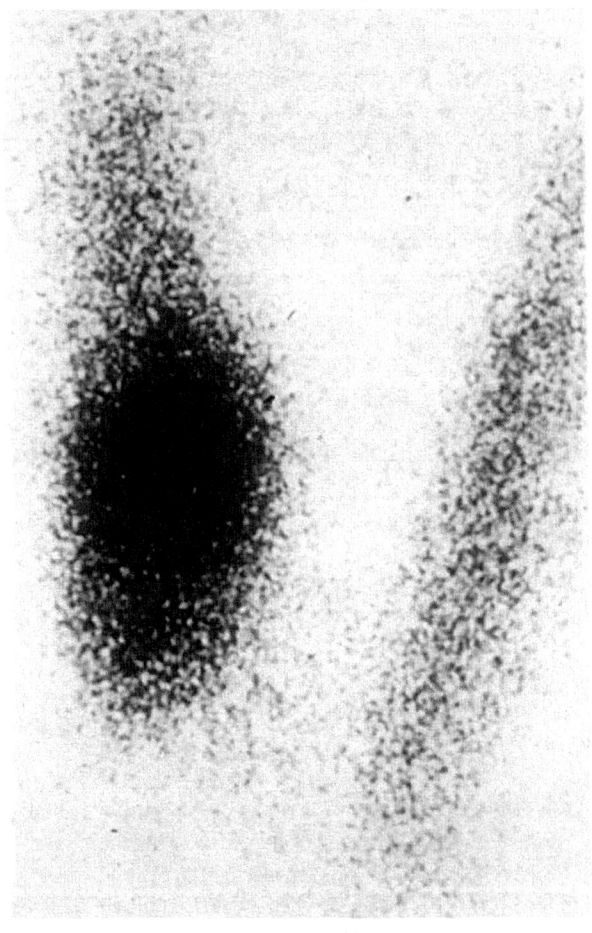

T_3 **Toxicosis**

AR 22

An 80 yo has noted increasing fatigue and she is slowly losing weight.
On exam, her pulse is 90, she has dry skin, and her thyroid is not palpable. Lab included a free T_4 of 1.2 (nl) and a TSH of < 0.01.

What is the next step?
A. T_3
B. Reverse T_3
C. Ultrasound
D. Thyroid scan

Answer: _____

© 2017 MedStudy Internal Medicine Video Board Review – Endocrinology • Janet Schlechte, MD

Thyroid Incidentaloma

AR 23

On a neck CT scan, a 70 yo is found to have osteoarthritis and an enlarged right lobe of the thyroid. She has no complaints. Her exam and TSH are normal. A thyroid ultrasound shows a 6-mm nodule in the right lobe.

What should be done now?
A. Ultrasound-guided FNA.
B. Technetium scan.
C. Measure TPO antibodies.
D. Repeat ultrasound in 1 year.

Answer: _____

Thyroid Incidentaloma
- Nodules noted on MRI or CT need to be evaluated by ultrasound
  - Cystic vs. solid
  - Number and size of nodules
- Refer for ultrasound-guided FNA if nodule(s) > 1 cm or has suspicious characteristics

AR 24

An 80 yo has been hospitalized for 2 months after treatment of a perforated ulcer. He has no history of thyroid disease. Over the last week, he has noted cold intolerance, dry skin, and periorbital puffiness. His surgeons obtained these tests:
$FT_4 \downarrow$, $TSH \downarrow$, $T_3 \downarrow$.
You are asked to treat the hypothyroidism.

What do you recommend?
A. 25 µg levothyroxine.
B. 10 µg liothyronine.
C. Repeat levels in 1 week.
D. No intervention.

Answer: _____

Euthyroid Sick Syndrome
- $\downarrow FT_4$, $\downarrow TSH$, $\downarrow T_3$
- **Reverse T_3 $\uparrow$ but rarely measured**
- May be adaptive mechanism to counter catabolic state of illness
- Levels normalize after recovery
- **Avoid checking thyroid function in hospitalized patients**

Effect of Drugs on Thyroid Function
- Glucocorticoids, androgen
  - Low TBG
- Estrogen, raloxifene
  - High TBG
- Salicylates
  - Decrease binding to TBG
- Dilantin, phenobarbital
  - Increase T_4 clearance
- Glucocorticoids
  - Decrease T_4–T_3 conversion

Drug-Induced Hypothyroidism
- Lithium
- Amiodarone
  - High iodine content of drug
  - Those with autoimmune disease and nodular goiter at highest risk
  - Treat same as other cases of hypothyroidism

Drug-Induced Hyperthyroidism
- Lithium
- Interferon
- Amiodarone
  - Type 1 increased T_4 synthesis
  - Type 2 destructive thyroiditis
  - Type 1 methimazole
  - Type 2 glucocorticoid

Adrenal Disorders

General Concepts
- ACTH and cortisol are secreted episodically and in a diurnal fashion, so single values rarely diagnostic
- Mineralocorticoids $\uparrow$ Na^+ absorption and K^+ excretion
- Glucocorticoids stimulate lipolysis and $\uparrow$ gluconeogenesis
- Adrenal androgens — hirsutism, virilization

The Rationale for the 1-mg (Overnight) Dexamethasone Suppression Test

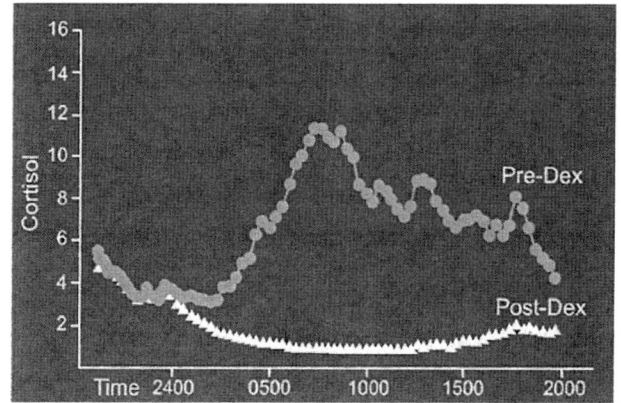

Glucocorticoid Excess

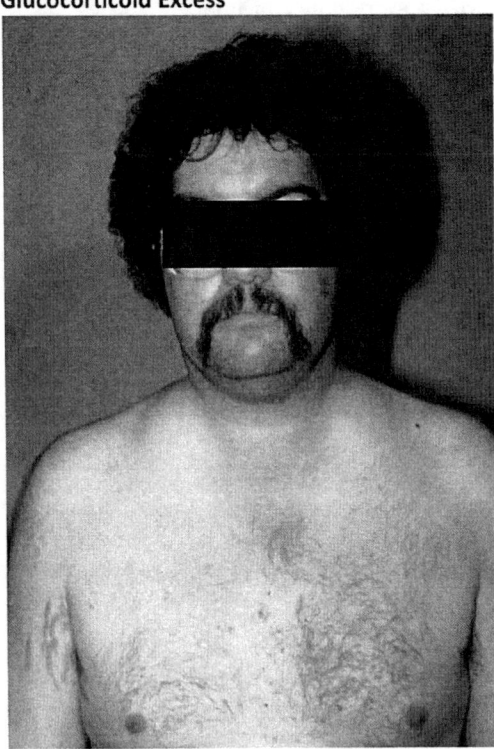

Clinical Features
- Weight gain
- Glucose intolerance
- Hypertension
- Hypokalemia
- Edema

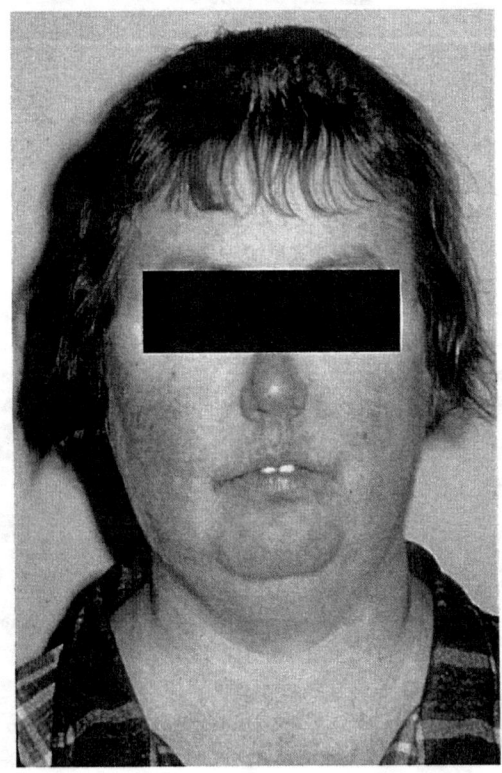

Classic Features
- Centripetal obesity
- Violaceous striae
- Proximal muscle weakness
- Amenorrhea
- Thin skin
- Bruising

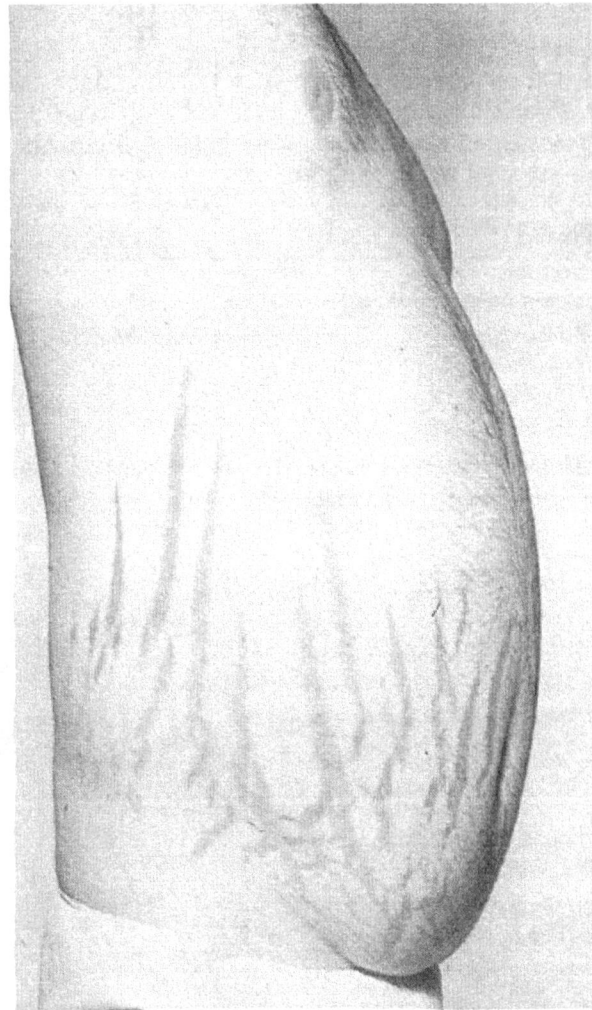

Causes of Cortisol Excess
- ACTH-secreting pituitary tumor
- Adrenal adenoma/carcinoma
- Ectopic ACTH production
- Exogenous glucocorticoid
- Except for ectopic ACTH due to malignancy, it is difficult to distinguish between causes of Cushing's clinically

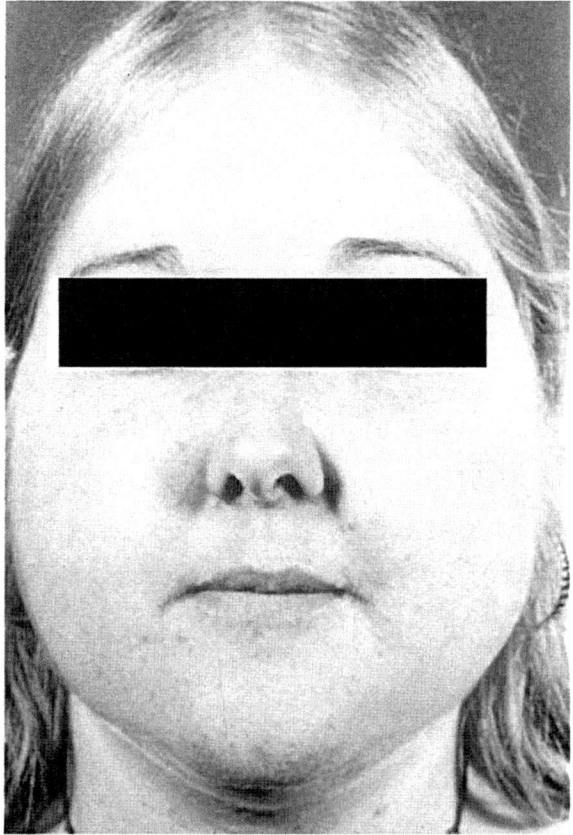

How to Screen for Cushing Syndrome

Common Clinical Characteristics Associated with Glucocorticoid Excess
- A 50 yo has gained 20 pounds in the last year and also complains of muscle weakness, bruising, and a "buffalo hump"
- These are incredibly common complaints, yet Cushing's is a rare disease

Tests to Screen for Cortisol Excess
- **Urine-free cortisol (UFC)**
  - 24-hour collection
  - Most sensitive
  - Few false positives
- **1-mg DST**
  - 1 mg of dexamethasone at 11 p.m., followed by 8 a.m. cortisol
  - If cortisol < 2 μg after Dex, Cushing's is excluded
  - False positives include phenytoin (Dilantin, Phenytek), estrogen, obesity, stress, depression
- 11 p.m. salivary cortisol

AR 25
A 50 yo woman has gained 50 lbs in the last year and bruises easily. She has a buffalo hump, proximal muscle weakness, and pale striae on her abdomen. Her BMI is 40. A 24-hour urine cortisol is 25 μg (< 50).

Which of the following is correct?
A. She likely has pituitary Cushing's.
B. She likely has an adrenal adenoma.
C. The next step is to measure ACTH.
D. Cushing's has been excluded.

Answer: _____

When You Suspect Cushing's
Step 1
- Do screening test
- If screening test is negative, Cushing's is ruled out
- If screen is positive, do a confirmatory test — repeat UFC or 1-mg DST

Step 2
- If confirmatory test is positive, measure an ACTH
  - ↑ ACTH suggests pituitary or ectopic
  - ↓ ACTH suggests adrenal adenoma or carcinoma

Step 3
- Test for dexamethasone; Give 8 mg of dexamethasone at 11 p.m. followed by an 8 a.m. cortisol
- If cortisol falls < 5, pituitary disease is likely diagnosis; Get pituitary MRI
- If cortisol does not fall after Dex, ectopic ACTH is likely diagnosis
- Pancreatic or lung carcinoid possible; Some benign bronchial adenomas hypersecrete ACTH

Pituitary Cushing's
- ACTH secreting tumor
- Usually microadenoma
- Hypopituitarism rare
- **MRI is negative in 50%**
- Transsphenoidal surgery ~ 80% successful
- Cortisol levels will suppress after high dose dexamethasone

Ectopic ACTH
- Small cell lung cancer
- Bronchial carcinoid
- Lack classic stigmata of Cushing's
- **Severe hypokalemia**
- **Metabolic alkalosis**
- **Muscle weakness**
- Hyperpigmentation
- Chest/Abdominal CT may be necessary
- Cortisol levels will not suppress after dexamethasone

AR 26

A 36 yo has gained 20 lbs in 6 months and has developed high blood pressure, bruising, and muscle weakness. Her BMI is 30. Her only medication is a BCP. She thinks she has Cushing's.

Which test should you recommend?

A. 24-hour urine cortisol
B. 8 a.m. and 4 p.m. cortisol levels
C. Overnight 1-mg dexamethasone suppression test
D. 8 a.m. ACTH

Answer: _____

AR 27

A 36 yo has gained 20 pounds, has high blood pressure, and many bruises. Her BMI is 40.
A serum cortisol drawn at 8 a.m. after 1 mg of dexamethasone at 11 p.m. the night before was 6 ($\uparrow$).

What should you do next?

A. Adrenal CT.
B. Pituitary MRI.
C. Measure ACTH.
D. 24-hour urine cortisol.

Answer: _____

AR 28

A 30 yo taking no medications has gained 30 lbs, has muscle weakness, amenorrhea, and hirsutism.
A 1-mg dexamethasone test showed an 8 a.m. cortisol of 15 (< 2). One week later, a 24-hour urine cortisol was 1,400 ($\uparrow$) and an 8 a.m. ACTH was 2 ($\downarrow$).

The most likely etiology of the cortisol excess is:

A. ACTH-secreting pituitary tumor
B. Adrenal adenoma
C. Ectopic ACTH

Answer: _____

AR 29

A 40 yo has gained weight and developed bruising, elevated blood pressure, and proximal muscle weakness.
A 24-hour urine cortisol on 2 occasions was > 300 μg/dL (< 45) and an ACTH is 960 (10–60).
After an overnight 8-mg dexamethasone suppression test, a cortisol was 2 ($\downarrow$).

Which is the most likely cause of this patient's Cushing's?

A. Pituitary tumor
B. Ectopic ACTH
C. Surreptitious cortisol use
D. Adrenal adenoma

Answer: _____

Treatment of Cushing's

- Pituitary tumor
  - Transsphenoidal surgery success rate 70–80%
- Adrenal adenoma/carcinoma
  - Adrenalectomy
- Medical therapy
  - Ketoconazole, aminoglutethimide for ectopic ACTH or if surgery not feasible

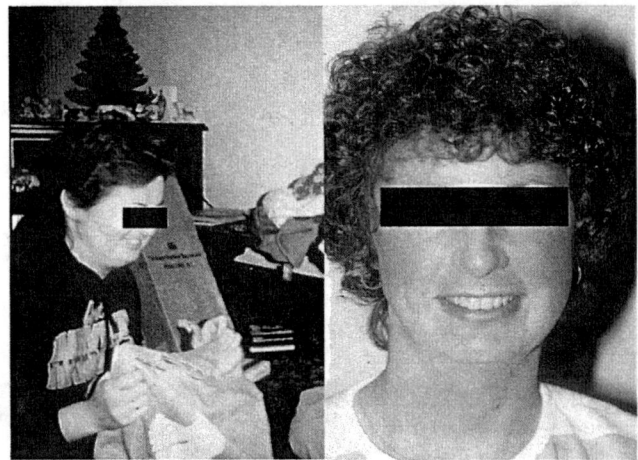

Adrenal Insufficiency

AR 30

A 41 yo male collapsed on the golf course in August. For 6 months, he has had fatigue, dizziness, nausea, and abdominal pain.
Now his blood pressure is 60/– and pulse is 130.
He has a deep tan, hyperpigmented buccal mucosa, a normal neurologic exam, and his BMI is 21.
His sodium is 125, potassium 6.4, chloride 98, and CO_2 18.

Which of the following is the cause of his electrolyte abnormality?

A. Primary adrenal insufficiency
B. Secondary adrenal insufficiency
C. SIADH
D. Severe dehydration

Answer: _____

Clinical Features of Primary Adrenal Insufficiency
- Fatigue and weakness
- Hyperpigmentation
- Hypotension
- Postural dizziness
- Abdominal pain
- Weight loss
- Hypoglycemia

Causes of Primary Adrenal Insufficiency
- Autoimmune disease
- Adrenal hemorrhage
- Granulomatous disease
- HIV associated
- Medications
  - Ketoconazole, etomidate

Polyendocrine Failure
- Autoimmune hypothyroidism
- Primary adrenal insufficiency
- Diabetes
- Hypogonadism
- Hypoparathyroidism
- Pernicious anemia
- Vitiligo
- Premature ovary failure

Laboratory Features of Primary Adrenal Insufficiency
- $\downarrow Na^+$, $\uparrow K^+$, $\downarrow CO_2$, $\downarrow$ glucose
- $\downarrow$ Cortisol, $\uparrow$ ACTH
- Use cosyntropin (Cortrosyn, Synacthen) stimulation test to confirm diagnosis

Short Cosyntropin Stimulation Test

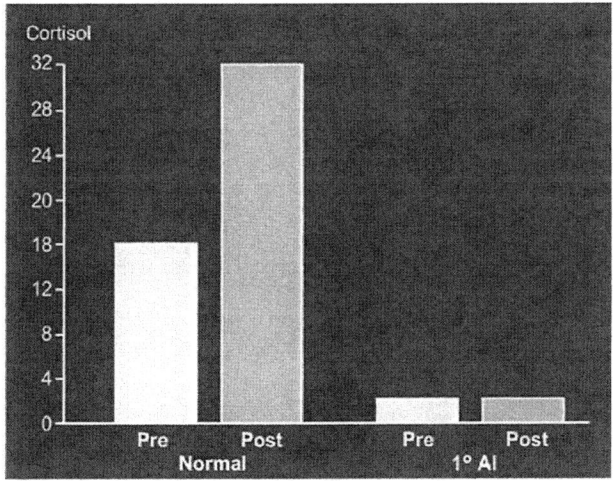

Therapy of Primary Adrenal Insufficiency
- **Hydrocortisone ± fludrocortisone**
- Prednisone and dexamethasone have little or no mineralocorticoid activity and are not a good choice
- Monitor therapy clinically and with electrolytes
- Add mineralocorticoid if K^+ remains elevated or CO_2 not improved
- Screen for other autoimmune disease

Secondary Adrenal Insufficiency

AR 31
A 60 yo has noted headaches, fatigue, weight loss, abdominal pain, and loss of axillary hair. An a.m. cortisol was 1.2 and only increased to 3 mg after cosyntropin. An ACTH was 2 ($\downarrow$). You start 5 mg of prednisone, but his symptoms do not improve, and he develops cold intolerance and constipation. His TSH is 0.9 (nl).

What should you do?
A. Increase prednisone to 10 mg daily.
B. Add fludrocortisone.
C. Measure testosterone.
D. Measure free T_4.

Answer: _____

A 60 yo man has had fatigue and headaches.
He has lost weight and has noted decreasing axillary and groin hair. His electrolytes and blood sugar are normal; his blood pressure is 120/70.
He had this MRI because of headaches.
Why is this case in the adrenal section?

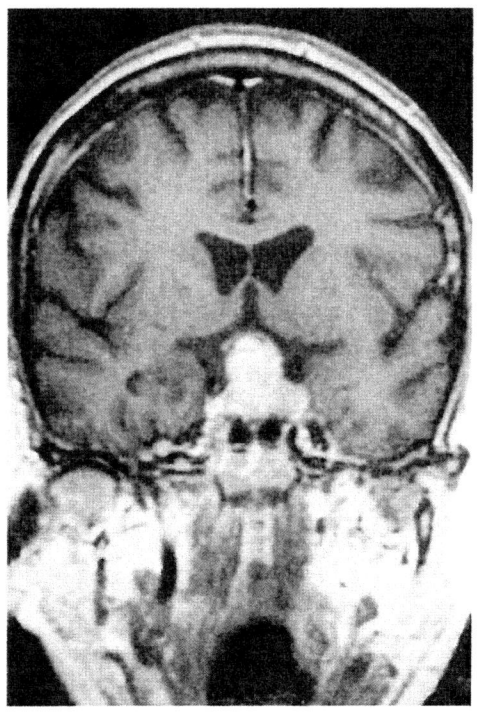

Secondary Adrenal Insufficiency
- Cortisol deficiency is due to absent ACTH, not to adrenal failure
- Symptoms nonspecific
  - Fatigue, weight loss, absent axillary and groin hair
- No hyperpigmentation
- Normal electrolytes and BP usually
- **Cortisol ↓, ACTH ↓**
- **Remember that other pituitary hormones may be affected**

Causes of Secondary Adrenal Insufficiency
- Pituitary or hypothalamic tumor
- Sarcoidosis
- Hemochromatosis
- Glucocorticoid therapy
- Megestrol acetate (suppresses ACTH)

Cosyntropin Stimulation in 1° and 2° AI

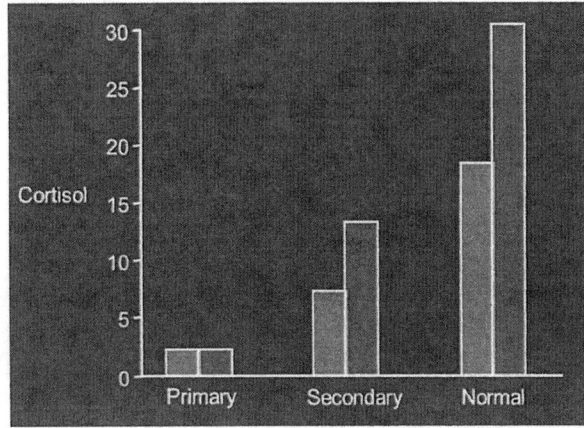

Secondary Adrenal Insufficiency
- **May be accompanied by global pituitary dysfunction**
- 2° hypothyroidism
  - ↓ FT_4, ↓ TSH
- 2° hypogonadism
  - ↓ Testosterone, ↓ estradiol, ↓ FSH

Treatment of Secondary Adrenal Insufficiency
- Glucocorticoid only (like prednisone) usually okay
- Can't monitor efficacy of treatment with cortisol or ACTH levels
- Be sure to monitor thyroid and gonadal function

Primary Aldosteronism
- Poorly controlled or hard-to-control hypertension on multiple agents
- Hypokalemia (not in all)
- ↓ Renin, ↑ aldosterone
- **Aldo/renin ratio > 20, but be sure the aldosterone is > 15 before applying the ratio**

- PRA ratio > 20 and aldosterone > 15 suggest primary aldosteronism
- Salt suppression test is next step
- **Persistent elevation of aldosterone after salt load confirms hyperaldosteronism**
- Abdominal CT scan to delineate bilateral hyperplasia from single adenoma
- Bilateral hyperplasia
  - Spironolactone or eplerenone
- Adenoma
  - Surgery

AR 32
A 32 yo was recently diagnosed with primary adrenal insufficiency. For 1 month, she has taken 5 mg of prednisone daily and feels better. Her only other medication is levothyroxine. Labs today showed sodium 130, potassium 5.0 (3.5–4.5), and CO_2 18 (24–32).

What should you do now?
A. Check cortisol and ACTH.
B. Stop prednisone; change to hydrocortisone.
C. Do adrenal CT scan.
D. Increase dose of prednisone.

Answer: _____

Adrenal Incidentaloma

A 45 yo man had this CT as part of an evaluation for abdominal pain. There is a 2.5-cm mass in the left adrenal. His BP is 130/80.
What tests should be done on all incidentally discovered adrenal nodules?

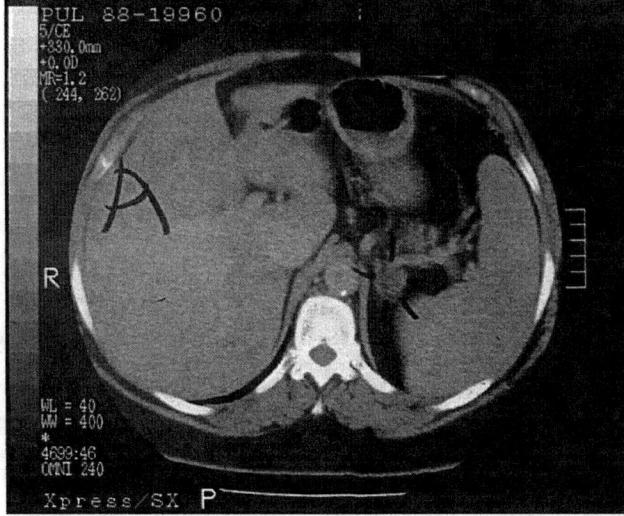

Adrenal Incidentaloma (cont.)
- **Screen for pheochromocytoma in all incidentalomas**
  - Plasma metanephrines
  - Urine catecholamines/metanephrines
- **Screen for subclinical Cushing's in all**
  - 1-mg dexamethasone suppression test
  - 8 a.m. cortisol < 5 μg normal
- > 4 cm send to surgery
- Potassium, plasma renin, aldosterone to rule out hyperaldosteronism
- Adrenal androgens (DHEA) in presence of hirsutism or virilization

- Repeat CT in 12 months
- Surgery if mass increases in size
- No consensus on need or timing of repeat hormone testing

Pheochromocytoma
- Most secrete norepinephrine
- 90% arise in adrenal medulla
- 90% of patients have sustained hypertension
- Triad of headache, diaphoresis, palpitations

Diagnosis
- Plasma-free metanephrines or fractionated urine metanephrines and catecholamines
- CT scan with contrast
- May be hyperintense on T2-weighted MRI
- Surgery definitive treatment, pretreat with phenoxybenzamine
- Avoid β-blocker until adequate α blockade

Female Hypogonadism

Gonadal Disorders — General Concepts
- Hypothalamic GnRH stimulates release of LH and FSH
- LH stimulates production of testosterone and estradiol
- FSH matures sperm and oocytes
- Negative feedback of estradiol and testosterone on GnRH

Amenorrhea
- Primary — no menses by age 16 years
  - Rare
  - Uterine outflow tract abnormality
  - Genetic absence of uterus
  - Androgen insensitivity
- Secondary — absence of periods for 6 months

Diagnostic Workup
First, do pregnancy test, then measure gonadotrophins to distinguish between pituitary/hypothalamic central and ovarian causes.

Pituitary $\downarrow$ LH, FSH
             $\downarrow$ Estradiol

Ovarian $\uparrow$ LH, FSH
             $\downarrow$ Estradiol

Progesterone Challenge Test
- To assess whether tissue has been exposed to estrogen do progesterone challenge test
- Oral progesterone for 10 days
- If menses occur, there is adequate estrogen and normal outflow tract
- No menses means low estrogen or abnormal anatomy

Central Causes
- Pituitary tumors
  - Nonfunctioning tumor
  - Prolactinoma
  - Hypopituitarism
  - Sheehan's syndrome
- Hypothalamic disorders
  - Craniopharyngioma
  - Eating disorder
  - Severe weight loss
  - Anorexia

Ovarian Causes
- Premature ovary failure (autoimmune)
- Polycystic ovary syndrome
- Turner syndrome
- Chemotherapy
- Radiation

AR 33
An 18 yo is referred for evaluation of primary amenorrhea. She has had no headaches or changes in her vision. She takes no medications. Her weight is stable, and she has no complaints except for the absent menses.
On exam, she is 4' 1" tall, has a BMI of 25, absent breast tissue, a mildly enlarged thyroid, and no bruises.

Labs:
       Estradiol < 5 (12–166)
       TSH 4.8 (0.2–4.2)
       FSH 100 (3.5–12.5)
       Prolactin 21 (4.8–23.2)

AR 33 (cont.)
Which of the following is the most likely cause of the primary amenorrhea?
A. Craniopharyngioma
B. Prolactinoma
C. Primary hypothyroidism
D. Turner syndrome
E. Late-onset congenital adrenal hyperplasia

Answer: _____

Turner Syndrome
• XO gonadal dysgenesis
• Bicuspid aortic valve
• Hypertension
• 1° hypothyroidism, glucose intolerance
• Short stature
• Webbed neck
• Widely spaced nipples

AR 34
A 30 yo with Type 1 diabetes has had amenorrhea since the birth of her last child 3 years ago. Her exam is normal except for peripheral neuropathy. In addition to insulin, she takes metoclopramide and levothyroxine.

Prolactin	120 ($\uparrow$)
TSH	7.2 ($\uparrow$)
FSH	40 ($\uparrow$)
Estradiol	1 ($\downarrow$)
A1c	8.9%

What is the most likely cause of her amenorrhea?
A. Poorly controlled diabetes
B. Sheehan syndrome
C. Premature ovary failure
D. Prolactinoma

Answer: _____

Premature Ovary Failure (POF)
• Autoimmune effect on ovary
• Secondary amenorrhea before menopause
• Generalized ovary sclerosis and decreased follicles
• **Look for other autoimmune disease — thyroid/adrenal**
• Irradiation, chemotherapy may also cause POF

AR 35
An 18 yo developed amenorrhea 9 months ago when she started college. She has joined the track team and is having trouble keeping up with her classes.
A pregnancy test is negative. Her exam is normal. BMI is 19.

Which of the following is most consistent with this clinical picture?
A. $\downarrow$ FSH
B. $\uparrow$ TSH
C. $\uparrow$ DHEA-S
D. $\uparrow$ LH/FSH ratio

Answer: _____

Hypothalamic Amenorrhea
• Low body weight/fat
• $\downarrow$ GnRH secretion from hypothalamus
• Athlete
• Stress
• Eating disorder

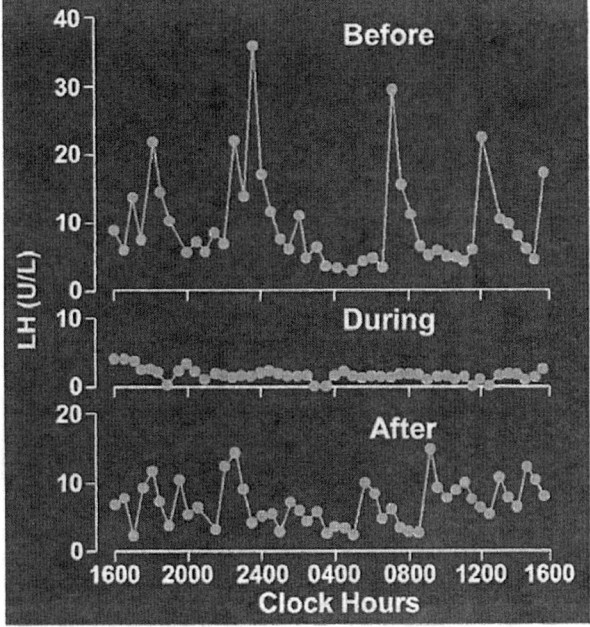

Kallmann Syndrome
• Rare hypothalamic disorder
• Isolated GnRH deficiency
• Midline defects
• Anosmia
• $\downarrow$ Estradiol, $\downarrow$ LH, $\downarrow$ FSH

AR 36
A 40 yo with Type 2 diabetes has severe gastroparesis. After starting metoclopramide, she developed amenorrhea. When she stops the metoclopramide, her menses return, but the nausea and vomiting are intolerable. Lab: Prolactin 110 ($\uparrow$), A1c 9%, TSH 2 (nl), FSH 3 ($\downarrow$).
She can't tolerate bromocriptine.

Which of the following is the best approach to treat the amenorrhea?
A. Cabergoline.
B. Oral contraceptive.
C. Improve blood sugar control.

Answer: _____

Causes of Androgen Excess
- Polycystic ovary disease
- Ovarian tumor
- Congenital adrenal hyperplasia
- Danazol, cyclosporine
- Adrenal tumor

Hirsutism
- Excessive growth of hormone-dependent pubic, axillary, abdominal, chest, and facial hair
- Ethnic background
- Age of onset
- Rate of progression
- Virilization: Hirsutism plus clitoromegaly, temporal balding, and ↑ muscle mass
- Dehydroepiandrosterone sulfate (DHEA-S)
- Testosterone
  - Total and free

Polycystic Ovary Syndrome (PCOS)
- Ovaries and adrenals make androgen, which is aromatized to estrogen
- Estrogen leads to ↓ FSH and ↑ LH
- ↑ LH leads to hyperplasia of ovarian stroma and more androgen
- Vicious cycle

- Amenorrhea/Oligomenorrhea
- Hirsutism
- Acne
- Obesity
- Insulin resistance
- Starts at puberty
- Not associated with virilization

PCOS Diagnosis
- Ovulatory dysfunction
- Clinical and/or biochemical evidence of androgen excess
- Cystic ovaries on ultrasound
- ↑ LH:FSH ratio (2–3:1)
- Mildly ↑ testosterone
- Mildly ↑ DHEA-S

Treatment Options
- Weight loss
- Oral contraceptive
  - Low-androgen progestin
- Spironolactone
- Metformin
  - Off-label indication
- Medroxyprogesterone
  - Endometrial protection

Spironolactone
- ↓ Testosterone synthesis
- Competes with testosterone at receptor on hair follicles
- 9–12 months to see an effect
- Contraindicated in pregnancy, as it may feminize a male fetus

AR 37
A 20 yo has noted dark facial hair since she entered puberty. Her only medication is a BCP. Her BMI is 25, and she has dark hair on her upper lip and areole. A pelvic exam is normal. A1c is 5% and testosterone 10 (6–82).
DHEA-S is normal.

What should you recommend now?
A. Measure 17-OH progesterone.
B. Transvaginal ultrasound.
C. Metformin.
D. Spironolactone.

Answer: _____

AR 38
A 24 yo has had amenorrhea for 15 months.
She acutely developed dark hair on her face, breasts, and lower abdomen. Her pelvic exam shows an enlarged clitoris. Her BMI is 30.
Testosterone 220 (↑), DHEA-S 180 (200–335), A1c 9.0%

The most likely cause of this clinical picture is:
A. PCOS
B. Ovarian tumor
C. Idiopathic hirsutism
D. Congenital adrenal hyperplasia (late onset)
E. Adrenal adenoma

Answer: _____

In a Virilized Patient
- Ovarian tumor will be associated with ↑↑ testosterone
- Adrenal tumor will be associated with ↑↑ DHEA-S
- Use transvaginal ultrasound and/or abdominal CT to look at adrenals and ovaries

Late Onset Congenital Adrenal Hyperplasia
- Late onset 21-hydroxylase deficiency
- Rare: 0.1–1% of women
- Hirsutism at menarche, oligo, or amenorrhea in early adulthood
- Measure 17-OH progesterone before and after ACTH
- Treat with dexamethasone to suppress ACTH stimulation of adrenal

AR 39
A 58 yo woman complains of hot flashes and difficulty sleeping. She has been amenorrheic for 1 year and has severe migraine headaches.

Which of the following should you recommend to treat hot flashes?
A. Phytoestrogen (isoflavones)
B. SSRI
C. Black cohosh
D. Clonidine

Answer: _____

Menopausal Issues
- Hot flashes occur in 75%
- Sleep and mood disturbances
- Short-term estrogen is treatment of choice
- SSRI effective
- Gabapentin
- Progesterone
- Efficacy of alternative therapy not established

Male Hypogonadism

Clinical Features
- Low libido
- Erectile dysfunction
- Infertility
- Gynecomastia
- Delayed development
- ↓ Facial hair
- Hot flashes
- Azoospermia

Male Hypogonadism Diagnostic Workup
- Morning total testosterone
- If level is low, confirm with 3 subsequent a.m. values
- LH, FSH
- Prolactin
- FT_4/TSH

Male Hypogonadism
- Primary
  - Chemotherapy
  - Testicular injury
  - Klinefelter's
  - Usually associated with infertility
- Secondary
  - Hypothalamic
  - Pituitary tumor
  - Craniopharyngioma
  - Kallmann syndrome

Gynecomastia

AR 40
An 18 yo army recruit has noted breast enlargement for 1 year. His exam is normal with 5-cm testes. His workup has included normal PRL, testosterone, estradiol, β-HCG, FSH, and TSH.

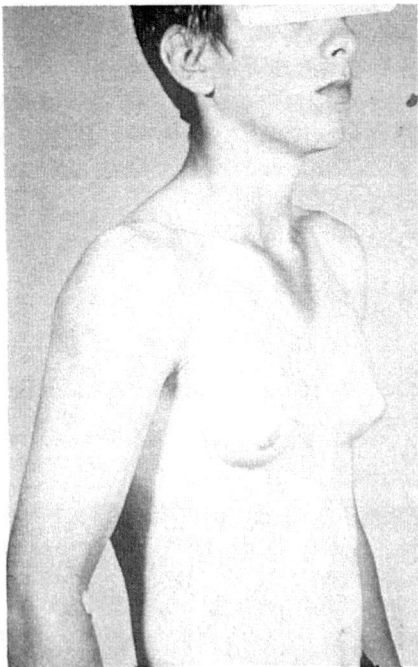

What is the most likely cause of the gynecomastia?
A. Testicular tumor
B. Pituitary tumor
C. Puberty
D. Klinefelter's

Answer: _____

Gynecomastia Etiology
- Puberty
- Old age
- Estrogen therapy
- Hyperthyroidism
- Testicular tumor
- Klinefelter syndrome
- Androgen therapy
- Spironolactone
- Digoxin

Workup and Treatment
- Testicular exam
- β-HCG
- Estradiol
- Prolactin
- Testosterone
- Thyroid function
- Reassurance for most
- Pubertal gynecomastia is transient
- Anti-estrogens are not uniformly effective
- Surgery may be necessary for serious cosmetic issues

AR 41

A 35 yo salesman complains of decreased libido and is undergoing an infertility evaluation. He is 5' 9" tall, 180 lbs, testes 4 cm in length, and he has normal secondary sex characteristics. He has no other complaints, and exam is normal.
LH 38 ($\uparrow$), FSH 52 ($\uparrow$),
FT_4 1.2 (nl), cortisol 25 (nl),
testosterone 130 ($\downarrow$)

These findings are most consistent with which of the following?
A. Nonfunctioning pituitary tumor
B. Craniopharyngioma (hypothalamic tumor)
C. Klinefelter's
D. Testicular injury

Answer: _____

Klinefelter Syndrome

AR 42

A healthy 17 yo is referred because of breast enlargement. He is 5' 11" tall, 170 lbs; testes 1 cm, and thyroid not palpable. Testosterone 190 ($\downarrow$), β-HCG neg, FSH 30 ($\uparrow$), estradiol 10 ($\downarrow$)

What is the most likely cause of the breast enlargement?
A. Puberty
B. Klinefelter's
C. Testicular tumor
D. Anabolic steroids

Answer: _____

AR 42 (cont.)
- $\downarrow$ Testosterone, $\uparrow$ LH, $\uparrow$ FSH
- XXY karyotype
- Arm span > height
- Eunuchoid habitus
- Atrophic testicles
- Infertility
- Gynecomastia

AR 43

A 70 yo presents with a large, nonfunctioning pituitary adenoma and has been started on thyroid and adrenal replacement. Today, his total testosterone is 150 ($\downarrow$) and prolactin is 15 (nl). His FT_4 is 1.4 (nl).

Which test will tell you whether the low testosterone is due to hypopituitarism or is age-related?
A. Free testosterone
B. FSH
C. Pituitary MRI
D. DHEA-S

Answer: _____

Testosterone Replacement Options
- Testosterone enanthate/cypionate
  – Injection q 2–3 weeks
- Daily topical androgen
- Buccal tablet
- Testosterone pellets
- Human chorionic gonadotrophin
- Injectable more likely to be associated with erythrocytosis

AR 44

Men using chronic androgen therapy are at risk for which of the following?
A. Increased LDL cholesterol
B. Erythrocytosis
C. Prostate cancer
D. Anemia

Answer: _____

AR 45

A 50 yo developed hypogonadism after pituitary tumor surgery and is using q 2-week injections of testosterone. Labs this week showed hematocrit 58 (40–52), FT_4 1.2 (0.9–1.5), and PSA 0.1.

What should you recommend?

A. Stop testosterone.
B. Continue current dose and monitor therapy using free testosterone.
C. Change to a topical androgen preparation.
D. Change to an oral androgen preparation.

Answer: _____

Side Effects of Testosterone Replacement

- Gynecomastia
- ↑ PSA
- Erythrocytosis
- Prostatic enlargement
- ↓ HDL
- Use with caution in elderly, those with heart disease, and individuals with untreated obstructive sleep apnea and history of deep venous thrombosis

---

Calcium, Bone, and Vitamin D

Regulation of Calcium and Vitamin D

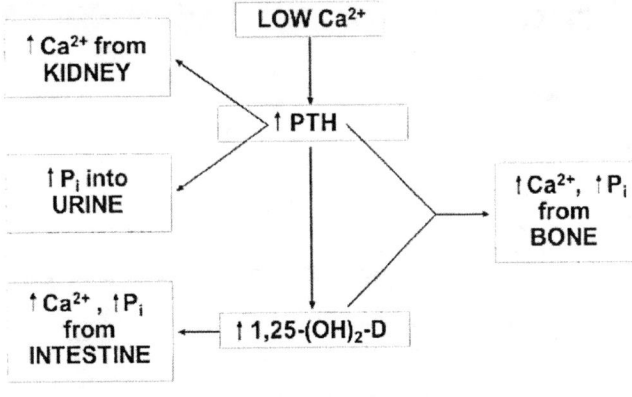

Hypercalcemia

Clinical Manifestations

- Asymptomatic
- Polyuria
- Constipation
- Anorexia
- Abdominal pain
- Lethargy
- Stupor, coma

Causes

- Primary hyperparathyroidism
- Malignancy
- Lithium, thiazides
- Vitamin D excess
- Hyperthyroidism
- Sarcoidosis
- Multiple myeloma

1° Hyperparathyroidism

- ↑ Ca^{2+}, ↓ PO_4, ↑ PTH, ↑ urine calcium
- Common in elderly women
- 85% single parathyroid adenoma
- 15% diffuse hyperplasia
- Usually asymptomatic

AR 46

A healthy 65 yo was noted to have hypercalcemia 2 years ago. She takes 1,000 IU of vitamin D daily, but no other medications. A DXA scan shows T-scores of −2.2 in the radius, −2.0 in the hip, and −2.1 in the spine. Her exam is unremarkable.

Calcium 11.0 (8.5–10.5),
PO_4 2.7, PTH 86 (↑), creatinine 0.9,
25-OH-vitamin D 30 (nl)

Which of the following do you recommend for management of the hypercalcemia?

A. Monitor calcium and PTH yearly.
B. Refer for parathyroidectomy.
C. Stop vitamin D.
D. Start bisphosphonate therapy.

Answer: _____

Criteria for Therapy of Primary Hyperparathyroidism

- Calcium > 1 mg/dL above normal
- GFR < 60 mL/min
- Age < 50 years
- T-score less than −2.5 in hip, spine, or forearm
- 24-hour urine calcium > 400 mg
- Symptoms

Hypercalcemia of Malignancy

- **Clinical Presentation**
- Obtundation, coma, lethargy
- ↑ Ca^{2+}, ↓ PO_4, ↓ PTH, ↑ PTHrP
- Treat volume depletion
- IV bisphosphonate
- Response in 2–4 days

- Some solid tumors like breast, renal cell, squamous cell make PTHrP
- Lymphoma, leukemia associated with $\uparrow$ 1,25-(OH)$_2$-vitamin D
- Multiple myeloma — osteoclast activating factor
- Metastatic disease
- PTHrP not picked up in PTH assay

Other Causes of Hypercalcemia
- **Granulomatous disease**
  - **Macrophages make 1,25-(OH)$_2$-vitamin D**
  - $\uparrow$ **Ca^{2+}, $\downarrow$ PO$_4$, $\downarrow$ PTH**
- B-cell lymphoma can make 1,25-(OH)$_2$-vitamin D
- Vitamin D toxicity
- Vitamin A toxicity

AR 47

A 70 yo with a history of lung cancer is brought to the ED because of confusion and somnolence. On arrival, her calcium was 16 ($\uparrow\uparrow$). She has received 3 liters of IV saline and a repeat calcium is 15.8. Her creatinine is 2.0.

In addition to continuing fluid replacement, what should be ordered next to treat the elevated calcium?
A. Calcitonin
B. Zoledronic acid
C. Prednisone
D. Loop diuretic

Answer: _____

AR 48

A 55 yo was treated 5 years ago for squamous cell lung cancer. She has done well and has no complaints. She takes calcium and vitamin D.
Her exam is normal.

Labs today:
Calcium 11.4 ($\uparrow$)   PO$_4$ 2.1 ($\downarrow$)
Alk phos 180 ($\uparrow$)   PTH 108 ($\uparrow$)
Vitamin D 15 ($\downarrow$)   Creatinine 1.2 (nl)

What is the most likely cause of the hypercalcemia?
A. Recurrent lung cancer
B. 1° hyperparathyroidism
C. Vitamin D deficiency
D. Excessive calcium intake

Answer: _____

Hypocalcemia

Causes
- Hypoparathyroidism (autoimmune)
- Vitamin D deficiency
- **Hypomagnesemia**
- **Anticonvulsants**
- Malabsorption
- **Gastric bypass**
- Neck surgery

Symptoms
- Many will be asymptomatic
- Paresthesias
- Perioral numbness
- Chvostek/Trousseau signs
- Tetany
- Laryngeal spasm

Treatment
- Calcium carbonate and vitamin D for maintenance therapy
- IV calcium gluconate — emergency
- Maintain Ca^{2+} 8–8.5, as over-replacement can lead to hypercalciuria

AR 49

A 60 yo woman has occasional numbness and tingling in her fingers and toes and has noted numbness around her mouth, especially when she is stressed. She had thyroid surgery 2 years ago and takes levothyroxine and 1 tablet of calcium daily. On exam, her blood pressure is 130/80 and she has cramping in her right forearm and fingers when the blood pressure cuff is inflated.

Based on this history and exam, which of the following is most likely?
A. Calcium 6.0 (8.5–10.5), PTH 2 (10–65), PO$_4$ 6.0 (2.7–4.5)
B. Calcium 8.0, PTH 98, PO$_4$ 2.1
C. Calcium 10.8, PTH 108, PO$_4$ 2.3

Answer: _____

Vitamin D Deficiency

AR 50

An 80 yo resident of a nursing home has been complaining of bone pain; last week, she fractured her wrist. She takes levothyroxine, phenytoin, and a multivitamin. Ca^{2+} 8.2 ($\downarrow$), PTH 80 ($\uparrow$), alk phos 250 ($\uparrow$), PO_4 2 ($\downarrow$).

What is the most likely cause of this clinical picture?
A. 1° hyperparathyroidism
B. Vitamin D deficiency
C. Autoimmune hypoparathyroidism
D. Hypomagnesemia

Answer: _____

Vitamin D Deficiency
- Measure 25-OH not 1,25-(OH)$_2$
- Obese
- Liver disease
- Elderly
- Lack of sun exposure
- Celiac disease
- Anticonvulsants

Secondary Hyperparathyroidism
- Vitamin D deficiency stimulates PTH production
- Vitamin D replacement should restore PTH to normal
- Also seen in elderly and those with kidney disease and declining GFR
- Calcium remains normal
- May lead to bone pain if severe

Osteomalacia
- Inadequate bone mineralization
- Another consequence of vitamin D deficiency
- Malabsorption
- Anticonvulsant therapy
- Renal tubular acidosis
- Chronic renal failure
- Hypophosphatemia
- Celiac disease

Clinical and Biochemical Changes Seen in Osteomalacia
- Bone pain
- Proximal myopathy
- $\downarrow Ca^{2+}$
- $\downarrow PO_4$
- $\uparrow$ PTH
- $\downarrow$ Vitamin D

AR 51

A 70 yo had a recent DXA scan with T-scores of −2.7 in the total hip and −1.1 in L1–L4.

What is the correct interpretation of the scan?
A. Osteoporosis
B. Osteopenia
C. Osteoporosis in hip and osteopenia in spine

Answer: _____

WHO Criteria

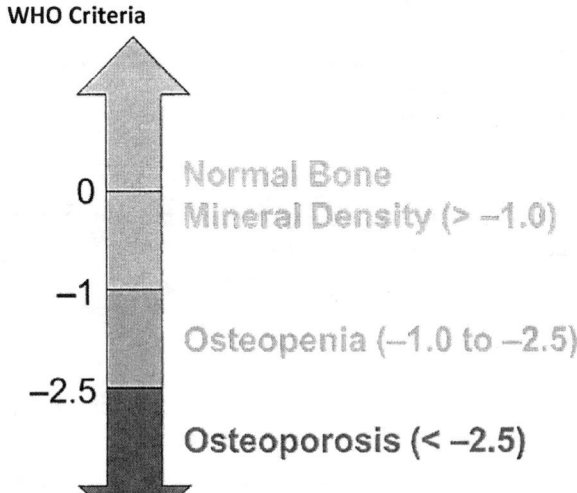

AR 52

A 56-year-old woman is concerned about osteoporosis because a 69-year-old friend just fractured her hip. The patient has never been on HRT. She is an obese, nonsmoking woman without underlying medical problems.
She has no FH of osteoporosis.

What would you recommend?
A. DXA scan.
B. Begin HRT.
C. Begin bisphosphonate.
D. Begin calcium and vitamin D.

Answer: _____

When to Order a DXA Scan?
- USPHS task force recommendations
- **A woman should get a DXA at age 65 unless she has 1 risk factor in addition to menopause**
- Some guidelines suggest men get first DXA at 70; Other guidelines suggest first DXA in men over 50 who have risk factors

© 2017 MedStudy Internal Medicine Video Board Review – Endocrinology • Janet Schlechte, MD

In Conjunction with a Scan, Assess Risk Factors for Bone Loss
- Age
- **Fragility fx**
- Falls
- **Fam hx hip fx**
- Low body weight
- **Smoking**
- **Alcohol**
- Primary HPT
- Eating disorders
- Glucocorticoids
- Celiac disease
- Anticonvulsants

Who to Treat
Postmenopausal women and men > 50 who have:
- Hip or spine fracture
- Spine or femoral neck T score < −2.5

- Using FRAX tool and WHO algorithm
  - Osteopenia and 10-year probability of hip fracture > 3%
  - Osteopenia and 10-year probability of major osteoporotic fracture > 20%

Efficacy of Antiresorptive Agents on Reducing Hip and Spine Fractures

	Spine	Hip
Bisphosphonate	Y	Y
Denosumab	Y	Y
Estrogen	Y	Y
Raloxifene	Y	N
Calcitonin	N	N

NNT to Prevent Fracture

T < −2.5	15
T < −2.0q	20
T < −1.6 to −2.0	> 500
One prior vertebral Fx	40
Two or more vertebral Fx	10

Treatment of Osteoporosis
- Calcium 1,200 mg/day
- Vitamin D 800 IU/day
- Exercise
- Choose an antiresorptive agent which will decrease risk of both hip and spine fractures
- Examine drug side effects and mode of administration

- Bisphosphonates
  - Decrease hip and spine fractures by 40–60%
  - May cause GI upset and muscle pain
  - Long-term therapy — osteonecrosis of jaw and subtrochanteric fracture
- Denosumab
  - Decrease hip and spine fractures by 40–60%
  - Twice yearly therapy — subcutaneously
  - Skin infection
  - Hypocalcemia
  - More expensive

Osteoporosis Therapy
- Raloxifene
  - No decrease in hip fracture
  - Hot flashes
  - 40% reduction in spine fracture
- Estrogen
  - Decreases hip and spine fracture
  - Not ideal for chronic therapy

Anabolic Therapy
- Recombinant PTH (teriparatide) increases BMD and decreases spine fractures
- Rarely used as primary therapy
- Daily injection
- Expensive
- Only 2 years of therapy, followed by an antiresorptive agent
- Use when antiresorptive agent fails

AR 53
A 65-year-old woman wants to start therapy for osteoporosis. She has no family history of osteoporosis. She drinks alcohol occasionally and does not smoke.
Meds: HCTZ 25 mg daily, omeprazole 20 mg daily
Exam: BP 140/86, Wt 177 lbs
T score in hip −1.6
T score in spine −1.8

In addition to starting calcium and vitamin D what would you recommend?
A. No additional therapy.
B. Add a bisphosphonate.
C. Add raloxifene.
D. Add denosumab.

Answer: _____

AR 54

A 78-year-old woman is healthy except for osteoporosis and GERD. She had a DXA scan 6 years ago with T-scores of −1.7 at the hip and −1.6 at the spine. She was started on alendronate. Last year a DXA scan showed T-scores of −1.7 at the hip and −1.7 at the spine.

In addition to daily calcium and vitamin D replacement what would you recommend?

A. Stop alendronate.
B. Begin teriparatide.
C. Begin calcitonin.
D. Begin denosumab.

Answer: _____

AR 55

A 63-year-old woman with a strong family history of osteoporosis presents with a hip fracture.
She has no complicating causes other than osteoporosis. She has a history of breast cancer in her mother and 2 sisters. Other history includes Type 2 DM and reflux esophagitis with stricture. Her exam is unremarkable except for paraspinous tenderness. She takes calcium and vitamin D daily.

What would you recommend?

A. IV bisphosphonate
B. Estrogen
C. Teriparatide
D. Raloxifene

Answer: _____

AR 56

A 77-year-old man who lives in a nursing home is evaluated for recent fall. He has neuropathy and decreased quad strength. A DXA scan shows a T-score at the spine of < −0.8 and < −0.6 at the hip. He has a Hx of HTN and GERD. He takes calcium and vitamin D occasionally.

What would you recommend as the next step?

A. Begin teriparatide.
B. Begin bisphosphonate.
C. Begin hydrochlorothiazide.
D. Check vitamin D level.

Answer: _____

Therapeutic Approach to Falls

- Start with H & P, "get up and go" test, observe walking
- If evidence of lower extremity weakness:
  – Strength training of LE
- If evidence of balance problems: Gait and balance training
- If medication risks: Drug withdrawal/substitution
- If orthostatic hypotension: Drug reduction or withdrawal, drug/meal separation, stockings
- Home safety eval — get rid of throw rugs!!

Paget Disease of Bone

AR 57

After a fall, x-rays in a 75 yo showed radiographic changes of Paget disease in her sacrum. She has no complaints and walks ~ 2 miles daily.

Labs drawn last week revealed:

Ca^{2+}	9.4 (nl)
Alkaline phosphatase	125 (35–104)
Vitamin D	40 (nl)
PO_4	2.9 (nl)

What do you recommend for the Paget disease?

A. Bisphosphonate
B. No therapy
C. Calcitonin
D. Nonsteroidal antiinflammatory agent

Answer: _____

Paget Disease of Bone

- Usually asymptomatic
- ↑ Bone turnover → structurally weak bone
- ↑↑ Alkaline phosphatase
- Treat with bisphosphonate if pain is severe, if pagetic lesions are in weight-bearing areas, or there are lytic lesions

Familial Hypocalciuric Hypercalcemia (FHH)

- **Rare**
- **↓ Sensitivity of Ca^{2+}-sensing receptor**
- Higher Ca^{2+} levels are needed to suppress PTH
- Familial autosomal dominant
- Asymptomatic
- Low urine calcium (< 100 mg/24 hr)
- Calcium/creatinine clearance of < 0.01
- ↑ Mg^{2+}
- ↑ or normal PTH
- **Parathyroid surgery not indicated**

AR 58

A 68 yo had a DXA scan 2 years ago with a hip T score of -3.6. She has been taking an oral bisphosphonate and a repeat DXA today shows a hip T score of -4.2. She has been taking calcium and vitamin D regularly.

What should you recommend?
A. Change from oral to IV bisphosphonate
B. Add denosumab
C. Increase the dose of the bisphosphonate
D. Start teriparatide

Answer: _____

AR 59

A 65 yo with a history of venous thromboembolism had a DXA scan last week. The spine T-score was -0.2, and the hip T-score was -2.7. She smokes, and her mother had a hip fracture.

In addition to calcium and vitamin D, which of the following should you recommend to prevent bone loss?
A. Estrogen/Progesterone
B. Bisphosphonate
C. Raloxifene
D. No additional therapy

Answer: _____

AR 60

A 66-year-old man presents with severe back pain in the thoracic region, which developed suddenly after a sneezing fit. An x-ray shows a compression fracture at T5 and an older compression at T8. He has no history of trauma. DXA scan shows a T-score of -2.9 vertebral and -2.7 at the hip.

What would be the most useful test in this patient?
A. Chest CT scan
B. Bone scan
C. SPEP
D. Testosterone level
E. LFTs

Answer: _____

Osteoporosis in Men
- Advancing age
- Low testosterone levels
- Alcoholism
- Glucocorticoid treatment

Multiple Endocrine Neoplasia

MEN1
- 1° HPT (parathyroid hyperplasia)
- Pituitary tumor
- Pancreatic tumor (gastrin, insulin)
- Gene maps to chromosome 11q13
- Autosomal dominant

MEN2
- 1° HPT (parathyroid hyperplasia)
- Medullary thyroid cancer
- Pheochromocytoma
- Chromosome 10
- RET proto oncogene
- Genetic testing for presymptomatic individuals

Pressure Sores
- Location: Sacrum, trochanter, heels, iliac crest
  - Stage 1: Nonblanching erythema
  - Stage 2: Partial-thickness skin loss (superficial ulcer)
  - Stage 3: Full-thickness skin loss
  - Stage 4: Tissue loss to muscle, tendon, or bone

Pressure Sores Therapy
- Early stage, noninfected: Hydrocolloid dressing
- Avoid pressure on the sore and optimize nutrition
- Necrotic tissue should be removed
  - Wet-to-dry dressings
  - Surgical debridement

Diabetes Mellitus

Testing for Diabetes in Asymptomatic Adults
- ADA
  - Adults with BMI > 25 and 1 other risk factor
  - Test at 45 years of age and then at 3-year intervals if normal
- AACE
  - Test annually beginning at 30 years of age

Risk Factors
- 1st degree relative
- BMI > 25, ≥ 23 in Asians
- History of impaired glucose tolerance
- Hypertension
- Hyperlipidemia (HDL < 35; TG > 250)
- Gestational DM
- PCOS
- High-risk ethnicity
- History of CVD

Prediabetes
- Increased risk for future DM
- FPG 100–125
  or
- A1c 5.7–6.4%
  or
- 2-hr glucose 140–199 on 75-g OGTT
- OGTT more sensitive than FPG but impractical

Diagnosis of Diabetes
- A1c > 6.5%
  or
- FPG ≥ 126
  or
- 2-hr glucose > 200 on 75-g OGTT
  or
- Random glucose ≥ 200 and symptoms

- To confirm the diagnosis, use same test as used initially
- If 2 different tests are both above threshold, the diagnosis is confirmed
- If there are discordant results between 2 tests, the result above the diagnostic cut off should be repeated and the diagnosis made on the basis of the confirmed test

- Concordance between tests imperfect
- **Problems with A1c**
  - Hemoglobinopathy
  - Thalassemia
  - Increased red-cell turnover (pregnancy)
  - Blood loss
  - Transfusions
  - Erythropoietin

AR 61
Which of the following individuals has prediabetes?
A. 50 yo woman with a HbA1c of 6.8%
B. 50 yo man with fasting plasma glucose of 113 mg/dL
C. 50 yo man with plasma glucose of 232 two hours after receiving 75 g of oral glucose
D. 50 yo woman with a plasma glucose of 130 two hours after receiving 75 g of oral glucose

Answer: _____

Type 1 Diabetes
- 5–10% of diabetics
- Absolute insulin deficiency
- Autoimmune destruction of beta cells
- One or more autoimmune markers
  - Glutamic acid decarboxylase antibody
  - Islet cell antibody
  - Anti-insulin antibody
- Associated with other autoimmune disease
- Can occur at any age

Type 2 Diabetes
- 90–95% of diabetes cases
- Insulin resistance and eventually insulin deficiency
- Ketoacidosis rare
- Strongly hereditary
- Risk increases with age, obesity, and lack of physical activity
- Increased in some racial/ethnic subgroups

Glycemic Goals for Nonpregnant Adults
- Aim for A1c ~ 7%
- Fasting 80–130
- Postprandial 140–180
- Bedtime 110–140

Glycemic Goals
- Individualize therapy
- ~ 7% in nonpregnant adults
- Good glycemic control reduces microvascular and neuropathic complications
- The elderly, those with hypoglycemia, and those with advanced microvascular disease warrant less stringent control

Glycemic Control and Complications
- DCCT
  - 60% reduction in retinopathy, nephropathy, neuropathy with persistent benefits
- UKPDS
  - 25% reduction in microvascular complications with enduring effect
- ACCORD
  - Increased mortality, no macrovascular benefit, and no reduction in CVD outcome
- ADVANCE and VADT
  - No macrovascular benefit and no reduction in CVD outcome

AR 62
An 80 yo with coronary artery disease and Type 1 diabetes uses insulin glargine 20 units daily and 3–6 units of lispro premeal. This is her blood sugar record:

	F	L	S	HS
Day 1	90	130	115	90
Day 2	80	112	100	112

BP 126/82, LDL 96,
BMI 22; A1c 6.9%

What do you recommend with respect to her insulin management?
A. Continue current regimen.
B. Decrease glargine.
C. Check postprandial sugars.
D. Increase dose of supper lispro.

Answer: _____

Other Targets
- Blood pressure
  - < 140/90
  - When Rx necessary, use ACE inhibitor or ARB, then diuretic, then beta-blocker
  - Pregnant patients 110/65–129/79
  - No ACE or ARB in pregnancy, can use labetalol, diltiazem, prazosin, and clonidine

Aspirin (75–162 mg/day)
- Primary prevention in those with ↑ CV risk (10-yr risk > 10%)
- Risk of bleeding may offset beneficial effects for those with DM and low CVD risk
- Not recommended for CVD prevention with low CVD risk
- Secondary prevention in those with DM and history of CVD
- For ASA allergy, use clopidogrel

Nephropathy
- Urine albumin to creatinine ratio (UACR) annually
  - Type 1 after 5 years
  - Type 2 at diagnosis
- Serum creatinine and estimated GFR annually
- ACEI and ARBs delay progression of nephropathy by decreasing intraglomerular pressure
- Low-protein diet (0.8–1.0 g/kg/d) may slow progression of albuminuria

Retinopathy Screening
- Adults with Type 1 within 5 years after onset
- Type 2 shortly after diagnosis
- Retinal photography not a substitute for comprehensive eye exam
- Dot hemorrhage early finding
- Neovascularization late finding
- Usually precedes nephropathy

Neuropathy
- Screen annually with simple clinical tests
- Electrophysiologic testing rarely needed
- Optimize sugar control, use medication to improve QOL
- Mononeuropathy usually affects 3rd and 6th cranial nerves, peroneal and radial nerves
- Strict control improves nerve conduction

Yearly Monitoring
- Urine albumin to creatinine ratio
- GFR
- Ophthalmology
- No routine screening for CAD for asymptomatic patients
- No ACE or ARB for primary prevention with normal BP and normal UACR

AR 63
A 50 yo woman has Type 2 diabetes treated with 1,200 mg of metformin bid. Her BMI is 39 kg/m^2, and her A1c last week was 9.2%.

Which of the following approaches will be the most effective in reducing weight and improving A1c?
A. Exenatide
B. Liraglutide
C. Lorcaserin
D. A very low-calorie diet

Answer: _____

Efficacy of Different Approaches to Weight Reduction
- VLCD leads to 17% weight loss in 3 months and almost as good as gastric banding
- Exenatide and liraglutide will lead to 3% weight loss
- Lorcaserin FDA approved, but only 3–4% weight loss

AR 64
You have just diagnosed a 66 yo with Type 2 diabetes. She has no complaints, and her exam is normal except for a BMI of 30. Her fasting blood sugar is 252, and this morning her A1c is 7.9%. She has normal renal and thyroid function.

In addition to therapeutic lifestyle changes, what would you recommend?
A. Pioglitazone
B. Glyburide
C. Metformin
D. Insulin glargine
E. No other intervention now

Answer: _____

Metformin ($)
- Reduces hepatic glucose production
- No weight gain or hypoglycemia
- Start 500 mg daily, increase slowly to 2,500 mg maximum
- Takes 8–12 weeks to see effect
- Don't use with poor tissue perfusion, HF, radiographic contrast
- Check vitamin B_{12} occasionally
- Low cost

Metformin and Renal Disease
- Get GFR before starting therapy then yearly
- Don't use if GFR < 30 mL/min
- Don't start if GFR between 30 and 45 mL/min
- Reassess benefits when GFR falls to < 45 mL/min
- Stop before contrast in patient with GRF 30–60 mL/min

When Single-Agent Metformin is Not Effective
If A1c target is not achieved after 3 months, continue metformin and proceed to 2-drug combination adding one of these drugs:
- Sulfonylurea
- Thiazolidinedione
- DPP-4 inhibitor
- SGLT2 inhibitor
- GLP-1 agonist
- Insulin

When Deciding Which Drug to Use, Consider:
- Mechanism of action
- Efficacy in lowering A1c
- Cost
- Side effects
- Likelihood of hypoglycemia
- Patient preference

Sulfonylureas ($)
- Insulin secretagogues
- Effectiveness decreases over time
- All cause hypoglycemia
- Use short-acting (glipizide) to reduce hypoglycemia
- Potential weight gain
- Low cost
- Highly effective

Thiazolidinediones ($$)
- Highly effective
- Improve hepatic and peripheral insulin sensitivity
- Weight gain, edema
- HF (FDA warning)
- Myocardial ischemia
- ? Increase risk of bladder cancer — pioglitazone, fractures?
- No hypoglycemia

GLP-1 Agonists ($$$)
- Effective
- ↓ Weight
- ↑ Insulin secretion
- ↓ Gastric emptying
- ↓ Glucagon
- Pancreatitis?
- Thyroid C-cell tumors?
- Slow nutrient absorption and ↑ satiety
- Low risk of hypoglycemia

DPP-4 Inhibitors ($$$)
- Intermediate efficacy
- Raise endogenous GLP-1
- No weight change
- Nasopharyngitis
- ? Effect on β-cell apoptosis
- Decrease postprandial glucose
- ? Pancreatitis
- No hypoglycemia
- Weight neutral
- Expensive

SGLT2 Inhibitors ($$$)
- Intermediate efficacy
- Sodium glucose cotransport inhibitor
- Reduces glucose reabsorption and increases renal excretion of glucose
- Vulvovaginal infection, dehydration, UTI, ketoacidosis, ? fractures
- Low risk of hypoglycemia
- ↓ Weight
- High cost

AR 65
A 50 yo is seen in your clinic complaining of recurrent vaginal infections, blurry vision, and thirst. Her family history is positive for diabetes. Her BMI is 35; she has dry buccal mucosa; a random sugar is 450; and her kidney function is normal. Today her A1c is 11%.
One month ago she was given a prescription for metformin.

What should you recommend now?
A. Insulin
B. DPP-4 inhibitor
C. GLP-1 agonist
D. SGLT2 inhibitor

Answer: _____

Comparison of Glargine, Detemir, and NPH Insulin

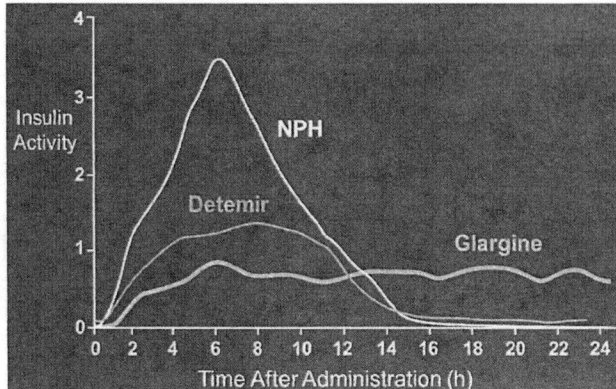

Diabetes. 2000;49:2142.

Adding Insulin
- Start with a single daily dose of a long-acting insulin
- Glargine, NPH, or detemir at bedtime
- More hypoglycemia with NPH
- Check fasting sugar daily
- Increase by 2–3 units every 3 days if FBG > 130

AR 66

Three months after starting glargine and progressively increasing the dose, your patient has this blood sugar record and is taking 30 units of glargine daily. Her new job requires long car trips. Her weight is stable, and she continues to take metformin 2,500 mg daily. She is very worried about hypoglycemia.
Her A1c is 9%, and her creatinine is 1.2.

	Fast	PM	HS
12/1	190	180	200
12/2	210	190	180

Which of the following do you recommend?
A. Stop metformin.
B. Add sulfonylurea.
C. Add premeal lispro insulin.
D. Increase glargine to 40 units.
E. Add a GLP-1 agonist.

Answer: _____

What would you recommend if she preferred insulin and her job was entirely sedentary?
- If/When basal insulin alone is ineffective, add premeal short-acting insulin
- Fast-acting or regular insulin
  - Consider cost
  - Start with 4–5 units premeal and increase by 2–3 units every 3 days until target is reached

AR 67

A 46 yo with Type 2 diabetes uses metformin, 15 units of glargine bid, and 5 units of lispro before each meal. An A1c 3 months ago was 8% and today is 9%. His blood sugar record is shown below.

	F	L	S	HS
Day 1	120	146	138	142
Day 2	136	148	128	136

What should you do next?
A. Make no changes in his insulin doses.
B. Increase morning glargine to 18 units.
C. Check postprandial sugars.
D. Increase premeal lispro insulin to 7 units.

Answer: _____

AR 68

A 40 yo with Type 1 diabetes is scheduled for laparoscopic hysterectomy. Her insulin regimen is 20 units of glargine each morning and 6–7 units of lispro insulin before meals.
Her A1c is 9.5%. You are asked to write her insulin orders for the morning of surgery.

Which of the following should you recommend?
A. Give 20 units of glargine and hold lispro.
B. Hold glargine and lispro and use sliding scale regular insulin.
C. Hold lispro and give 10 units of NPH insulin.
D. Administer usual doses of lispro and glargine.

Answer: _____

AR 69

A 40 yo with Type 1 diabetes is admitted to the ICU because of sepsis. His insulin regimen at home is 30 units of glargine daily and 6 units of lispro before meals. He is on ventilator support and is receiving IV antibiotics and pressors.

Which of the following would be the optimal insulin regimen while he is in the ICU?
A. Continuous insulin infusion to keep sugars 100–140
B. Continuous insulin infusion to keep sugars 140–180
C. Glargine insulin twice daily plus sliding scale
D. Sliding scale insulin

Answer: _____

Intensive Therapy in Critically Ill Patients
- Higher 90-day mortality compared to conventional therapy
- Severe hypoglycemia more common with intensive control
- Current guidelines suggest maintaining sugar in 140–180 range for all hospitalized patients

Sugar Control in Hospitalized Non-ICU Patients
- Scheduled long-acting insulin
- Scheduled prandial insulin
- Correction premeal insulin
- Glucose goals 140–180
- **Avoid Sliding Scale**

Sliding Scale Insulin
- Not effective in the majority of patients
- Increases risk of hypoglycemia
- Increases risk of hyperglycemia
- Adverse outcomes in general surgery patients

AR 70

You are treating a 35 yo male with diabetic ketoacidosis. On admission, his glucose was 600, Na^+ 129, K^+ 5.9, Cl^- 90, and his anion gap was 21. His pH was 7.2. After an IV bolus of 10 units of insulin, followed by 3 U/hr and vigorous IV hydration, he is feeling better. The table below shows the course of treatment thus far.

Time		Glucose	AG	K^+	PO_4
10 U → 3 U	midnight	600	21	5.9	4.0
3 U	1 a.m.	550	—	—	—
3 U	2 a.m.	430	—	—	—
3 U	3 a.m.	200	14	4.3	3.9

It is 3 a.m. Which of the following would be the most appropriate intervention now?
A. Decrease the insulin to 2 U/hr and change blood sugar checks to q 2 hr.
B. Maintain the current dose of insulin and change to D10 1/2 NS.
C. Increase the insulin rate to 5 U/hr.
D. Increase the insulin to 5 U/hr and change the IV to D10 1/2 NS.

Answer: _____

AR 71

A 21 yo with Type 1 diabetes mellitus has just learned she is pregnant. She is using a programmable insulin pump.

Which of the following is an appropriate target during pregnancy?
A. A1c 7%
B. Premeal glucose 60–90
C. Postmeal glucose < 100

Answer: _____

Glycemic Control in Pregnancy
- Preconception aim for A1c < 7% to prevent birth defects, preeclampsia, and macrosomia
- During pregnancy sugars
  - 60–99 premeal and hs
  - 100–129 peak postprandial
  - A1c < 6%
- Increased RBC production with short life span so can check A1c monthly

AR 72

A 27 yo with Type 1 diabetes takes 15 units of NPH and 10 units of regular insulin at breakfast and supper. She has a limited budget and cannot afford more expensive insulins. Her BMI is 22, and her exam is normal. This is a record of her blood sugars recorded at home.

	3 a.m.	F	L	S	HS
Day 1	90	240	140	110	120
Day 2	100	220	130	120	140

Which of the following should you recommend to improve her control?
A. Increase regular to 15 units at breakfast.
B. Increase supper NPH to 20 units.
C. Move p.m. NPH to bedtime.
D. Move p.m. regular to bedtime.

Answer: _____

AR 73

A 20 yo with Type 1 diabetes mellitus is treated with 12 units of glargine at bedtime and 6–10 units of lispro insulin before each meal. Her A1c 3 months ago was 7%. Her recent blood sugar log looks like this:

	F	L	D	HS
Day 1	70	126	140	120
Day 2	90	110	120	100
Day 3	90	132	120	130

Her only complaint is persistent morning headaches.

What should you recommend related to her insulin regimen?
A. Make no changes.
B. Take glargine before breakfast.
C. Decrease breakfast dose of lispro.
D. A bigger bedtime snack.

Answer: _____

AR 74

A 24 yo is referred for evaluation of almost daily spells that are associated with diaphoresis and tachycardia. Her weight is stable, and she takes no medications. Using her sister's glucometer, she has noted sugars varying from 40–50 most days.
After an overnight fast, her blood sugar is 65 and a total insulin level is 4 (< 20).

These findings are most consistent with:
A. Insulinoma
B. Surreptitious use of insulin
C. Surreptitious use of glipizide
D. Normal pancreatic insulin secretion

Answer: _____

AR 75

An 80 yo man with Type 2 diabetes treated with glyburide was brought to the ED because of obtundation. On exam, his BP is 80/–, pulse 102, and he is severely dehydrated.
Labs:
Sodium 156 ($\uparrow$), potassium 4.2, chloride 110, bicarbonate 23, creatinine 2.3, glucose 1,500

What should you recommend as initial therapy?
A. D_5W 500 mL/hr and 0.1 U/kg regular insulin/hr
B. D_5W 1 liter/hr and 0.5 U/kg regular insulin/hr
C. 0.9% NS 1 liter/hr and 0.1 U/kg regular insulin/hr
D. 0.9% NS 1 liter/hr and 0.5 U/kg regular insulin/hr

Answer: _____

Hyperosmolar Nonketotic State
- Glucose > 600
- pH > 7.3, CO_2 > 15
- Minimal ketonemia/ketonuria
- Correct Na^+ for hyperglycemia (for each 100 mg/dL glucose > 100 add 1.6 mg to serum sodium)
- If K^+ is < 3.3, give K^+ before insulin

Hyperosmolar Syndrome
- Restore plasma volume
- Calculate total body H_2O deficit and replace 1/2 of deficit in first 24 hours and remainder over 3 days
- Start insulin after fluid therapy underway at rate ~ 0.1 U/kg/hr

AR 76

A patient with no history of diabetes had a CABG. His sugars have been elevated in the ICU, and he has received continuous infusion of insulin. In the last 24 hours, he has needed 40 units of insulin to maintain blood sugars between 140 and 180. He is ready to transfer to the floor.
You are called to write insulin orders.

What should you recommend?
A. Stop insulin, sugars will normalize within 24 hours.
B. Give 40 units of glargine q a.m.
C. Give 20 units of glargine q a.m. and start metformin.
D. Give 20 units of glargine q a.m. and 6 units of lispro before each meal.

Answer: _____

Basal / Bolus Insulin
- Most physiologic regimen
- Total daily dose = 40 units
- 1/2 basal (glargine)
- 1/2 bolus (lispro) split into thirds to be given premeal

AR 77

A 30 yo medical technician has had recurring episodes of anxiety and shakiness. The symptoms are worse if he misses a meal, but may also occur after eating. His wife has Type 2 diabetes. He has had a number of finger stick glucose levels < 50. During a 48-hour fast, he had these levels drawn before the fast was stopped.
Glucose 20
Insulin 30 (< 20)
C-peptide 6.1 (1.1–4.4)

What is the next step?
A. Abdominal CT.
B. Psych consult to address surreptitious use of insulin.
C. Urine sulfonylurea screen.
D. Repeat fast, making it at least 72 hours.

Answer: _____

Hypoglycemia

	Glucose	Insulin	C-peptide
Insulinoma	$\downarrow$	$\uparrow$	$\uparrow$
Surreptitious insulin	$\downarrow$	$\uparrow$	$\downarrow$
Surreptitious	$\downarrow$	$\uparrow$	$\uparrow$ sulfonylurea

AR 78

You are treating a 35 yo male with diabetic ketoacidosis. On admission, his glucose was 600, Na^+ 129, K^+ 5.9, Cl^- 90, and his anion gap was 21. His pH was 7.2.
After an IV bolus of 10 units of insulin, followed by 3 U/hr and vigorous IV hydration, he is feeling better. The table below shows the course of treatment thus far.

Time	Glucose	AG	K^+	PO_4
10 U → 3 U midnight	600	21	5.9	4.0
3 U 1 a.m.	550	—	—	—
3 U 2 a.m.	430	—	—	—
3 U 3 a.m.	200	21	5.8	3.9

AR 78 (cont.)

It is 3 a.m. Which of the following would be the most appropriate intervention now?

A. Decrease the insulin to 2 U/hr and change blood sugar checks to q 2 hr.

B. Maintain the current dose of insulin and change to D10 1/2 NS.

C. Increase the insulin rate to 5 U/hr.

D. Increase the insulin to 5 U/hr and change the IV to D10 1/2 NS.

Answer: _____

AR 79

An 80 yo man who lives alone was found confused and disoriented this a.m. In the ED, he is somnolent, his BP is 90/60, pulse 120, and his skin and oral mucosa are dry. He weighs 70 kg.
Labs: Sodium 159, potassium 4.9, chloride 120, bicarbonate 21, creatinine 2.5, and glucose 250

What is his free H_2O deficit?

A. 5.6 liters

B. 4.2 liters

C. 1.2 liters

D. 7.2 liters

Answer: _____

To Determine Free H_2O Deficit:

0.6 x (weight) x $\frac{(sodium - 140)}{140}$

0.6 (70) x $\frac{159 - 140}{140}$

42 x $\frac{19}{140}$ = 5.6 liters

Give free H_2O slowly to decrease sodium by 10–12 mEq/L/day.

AR 80

A 75 yo has Type 2 DM and CAD. On glimepiride, his A1c three months ago was 6.4%. Today, he complains of headaches and confusion, especially in the morning. His A1c today is 6% and his creatinine is 1.9.

What should you recommend?

A. Continue current therapy.

B. Stop glimepiride and start glipizide.

C. Continue glimepiride and start metformin.

D. Stop glimepiride and add SGLT2 inhibitor.

E. Stop glimepiride.

Answer: _____

AR 81

Which of the following agents is contraindicated in a diabetic with gastroparesis?

A. GLP-1 agonist

B. SGLT2 inhibitor

C. Sulfonylurea

D. Metformin

Answer: _____

AR 82

An 85-year-old man with a history of HF, stroke, and Type 2 DM presents to the ED with altered mental status and a blood sugar of 34. He has an 8-year history of Type 2 diabetes treated with glyburide.
Labs at his ED visit: Na^+ 136, K^+ 4, Cl^- 103, HCO_3^- 26, BUN 20, Cr 1.9. The glyburide is stopped, and he is treated for 24 hours with D10 drip.
When he returns for follow-up in 2 weeks, he has had blood sugars of 140–180.
His A1c is 8.4%.

What would you recommend?

A. Metformin

B. Thiazolidinedione

C. Glipizide

D. GLP-1 agonist

E. No therapy

Answer: _____

A1c Targets in the Elderly (ADA)

• Healthy	< 7.5%
• Frail with chronic illness Mild/moderate cognitive impairment	< 8.5%
• Frail with poor health/ Long-term care facility	< 8.5%

Med Clin NA. 2015;99:351-377.

AR 83

A 74-year-old man with Type 2 diabetes and hypertension presents for evaluation. He was previously treated with metformin and glyburide but had hypoglycemic episodes. Glyburide was stopped.

Medications: Amlodipine, lisinopril, metformin, atorvastatin, aspirin

BP 150/94, p 60
Labs: HbA1c 8.8, BUN 14, Cr 1.1

© 2017 MedStudy Internal Medicine Video Board Review – Endocrinology • Janet Schlechte, MD

What would you recommend?
A. Glipizide
B. Pioglitazone
C. SGLT2 inhibitor
D. No treatment

Answer: _____

Diabetes Treatment in The Elderly
- Hypoglycemia related to sulfonylureas can last 24–48 hours
- Pioglitazone should not be used in patients with HF
- GLP-1 agonists and DPP-4 inhibitors
  - Advantage — no hypoglycemia
  - Disadvantage — cost, GI side effects
- SGLT2 inhibitor
  - Avoids hypoglycemia, lowers BP (helpful in patient with hypertension)
  - Okay with mild renal insufficiency; Avoid with severe CKD
  - UTI/yeast infections — especially in women

Med Clin NA. 2015;99:351-377.

AR 84
A 35-year-old Hispanic woman has done 2 home pregnancy tests, both positive. She has a rapid pregnancy test confirmed in the office today.
On exam, her BMI is 30, BP 120/70, P 70.
Fasting Labs: HbA1c 7.7%, Glu 140, Na^+ 140, HCO_3^- 28, Hct 36, TC 200, LDL 140

What is her diagnosis?
A. Impaired glucose tolerance
B. Gestational diabetes
C. Type 2 diabetes
D. Type 1 diabetes

Answer: _____

Gestational Diabetes
- Fasting BS ≥ 92
              or
- 1-hour BS ≥ 180 after 75 g OGTT
              or
- 2-hour BS ≥ 153 after 75 g OGTT

AR 85
A 24-year-old woman with Type 1 diabetes wishes to become pregnant. She has been using glargine insulin once a day and fast acting insulin with meals. Her last 3 glycated hemoglobins were 7.0, 7.2, and 7.3. She is currently on an oral contraceptive.

What should you advise her?
A. Stop the OCP; keep glycated Hb no greater than 7.0.
B. Stop the OCP; keep glycated Hb no greater than 7.5.
C. Continue on the OCP; intensify insulin regimen for target glycated Hb < 6%.
D. Continue on the OCP; keep glycated Hb no greater than 7.0.

Answer: _____

Diabetes and Pregnancy
- Tight control (A1c < 6%) before conception x 1–2 months before stopping birth control
- Keep A1c ~ 6% throughout pregnancy
- 1st trimester more insulin-sensitive; 2nd/3rd trimester more insulin-resistant

- Preconception counseling
- Increased risk of embryopathy and spontaneous abortion with uncontrolled DM
- Aim for A1c < 7% prior to conception and < 6% during pregnancy
- Target blood pressure 110–129/65–79

Endocrinology
Audience Response Answers

Audience Response 1
Answer: B. ↓ FSH.

AR 2
Answer: A. Stop bromocriptine; continue follow-up
with an obstetrician.

AR 3
Answer: B. Cabergoline.

AR 4
Answer: B. No.

AR 5
Answer: A. Neurosurgery consult.

AR 6
Answer C. ↓ Testosterone, ↓ FSH.

AR 7
Answer: D. Measure serum cortisol.

AR 8
Answer: D. No additional testing.

AR 9
Answer: A. Central diabetes insipidus.

AR 10
Answer: C. Fluid restriction.

AR 11
Answer: E. None.

AR 12
Answer: D. Levothyroxine (T_4).

AR 13
Answer: B. Make no changes.

AR 14
Answer: C. Both.

AR 15
Answer: A. Graves'.

AR 16
Answer: C. Hyperthyroidism.

AR 17
Answer: C. Thyroglobulin.

AR 18
Answer: C. Subacute thyroiditis.

AR 19
Answer: B. Propylthiouracil.

AR 20
Answer: A. Repeat TSH in 3–6 months.

AR 21
Answer: A. Technetium scan.

AR 22
Answer: A. T_3.

AR 23
Answer: D. Repeat ultrasound in 1 year.

AR 24
Answer: D. No intervention.

AR 25
Answer: D. Cushing's has been excluded.

AR 26
Answer: A. 24-hour urine cortisol.

AR 27
Answer: D. 24-hour urine cortisol.

AR 28
Answer: B. Adrenal adenoma.

AR 29
Answer: A. Pituitary tumor.

AR 30
Answer: A. Primary adrenal insufficiency.

AR 31
Answer: D. Measure free T_4.

AR 32
Answer: B. Stop prednisone; change to hydrocortisone.

AR 33
Answer: D. Turner syndrome.

AR 34
Answer: C. Premature ovarian failure.

AR 35
Answer: A. ↓FSH.

AR 36
Answer: B. Oral contraceptive.

AR 37
Answer: D. Spironolactone.

AR 38
Answer: B. Ovarian tumor.

AR 39
Answer: B. SSRI.

AR 40
Answer: C. Puberty.

AR 41
Answer: D. Testicular injury.

AR 42
Answer: B. Klinefelter's.

AR 43
Answer: B. FSH.

AR 44
Answer: B. Erythrocytosis.

AR 45
Answer: C. Change to a topical
androgen preparation.

AR 46
Answer: A. Monitor Calcium and PTH yearly.

AR 47
Answer: B. Zoledronic acid.

AR 48
Answer: B. 1° hyperparathyroidism.

AR 49
Answer: A. Calcium 6.0 (8.5–10.5),
PTH 2 (10–65), PO_4 6.0 (2.7–4.5).

AR 50
Answer: B. Vitamin D deficiency.

AR 51
Answer: A. Osteoporosis.

AR 52
Answer: D. Begin calcium and vitamin D.

AR 53
Answer: A. No additional therapy.

AR 54
Answer: A. Stop alendronate.

AR 55
Answer: A. IV bisphosphonate.

AR 56
Answer: D. Check vitamin D level.

AR 57
Answer: B. No therapy.

AR 58
Answer: D. Start teriparatide.

AR 59
Answer: B. Bisphosphonate.

AR 60
Answer: D. Testosterone level.

AR 61
Answer: B. 50 yo man with fasting plasma glucose
of 113 mg/dL.

AR 62
Answer: B. Decrease glargine.

AR 63
Answer: D. A very low-calorie diet.

AR 64
Answer: C. Metformin.

AR 65
Answer: A. Insulin.

AR 66
Answer: E. Add a GLP-1 agonist.

AR 67
Answer: C. Check postprandial sugars.

AR 68
Answer: A. Give 20 units of glargine
and hold lispro.

AR 69
Answer: B. Continuous insulin infusion
to keep sugars 140–180.

AR 70
Answer: B. Maintain the current dose
of insulin and change to D10 1/2 NS.

AR 71
Answer: B. Premeal glucose 60–90.

AR 72
Answer: C. Move p.m. NPH to bedtime.

AR 73
Answer: B. Take glargine before breakfast.

AR 74
Answer: D. Normal pancreatic
insulin secretion.

AR 75
Answer: C. 0.9% NS 1 liter/hr and 0.1 U/kg regular
insulin/hr.

AR 76
Answer: D. Give 20 units of glargine q a.m. and 6 units
of lispro before each meal.

AR 77
Answer: C. Urine sulfonylurea screen.

AR 78
Answer: D. Increase the insulin to 5 U/hr and change
the IV to D10 1/2 NS.

AR 79
Answer: A. 5.6 liters.

AR 80
Answer: E. Stop glimepiride.

AR 81
Answer: A. GLP-1 agonist.

AR 82
Answer: E. No therapy.

AR 83
Answer: C. SGLT2 inhibitor.

AR 84
Answer: B. Gestational diabetes.

AR 85
Answer: C. Continue on the OCP; intensify insulin
regimen for target glycated Hb < 6%.

MedStudy

Internal Medicine Video Board Review

Gastroenterology

Presented by

Nimisha K. Parekh, MD, MPH
Clinical Professor of Medicine
Program Director of Gastroenterology Fellowship
UC Irvine Health
Orange, California

Table of Contents

© 2017 MedStudy Internal Medicine Video Board Review – Gastroenterology • Nimisha K. Parekh, MD

Gastroenterology Abbreviations

AAA	Abdominal aortic aneurysm
AFP	Alpha-fetoprotein
AIH	Autoimmune hepatitis
AVM	Arteriovenous malformation
CBD	Common bile duct
CEA	Carcinoembryonic antigen
CMV	Cytomegalovirus
DAAD	Direct-acting antiviral drug
DES	Diffuse esophageal spasm
DKA	Diabetic ketoacidosis
EAEC	Enteroadherent *E. coli*
EGD	Esophagogastroduodenoscopy
ELISA	Enzyme-linked immunosorbent assay
EMR	Endoscopic mucosa (mucosal) resection
EOE	Eosinophilic esophagitis
ERCP	Endoscopic retrograde cholangiopancreatography
ETEC	Enterotoxigenic *E. coli*
EUS	Endoscopic ultrasound
FAP	Familial adenomatous polyposis
GEJ	Gastroesophageal junction
GER	Gastroesophageal reflux
GERD	Gastroesophageal reflux disease
GDH	Glutamate dehydrogenase
GGT	Gamma glutamyl transferase
GIST	Gastrointestinal stromal tumor
HCC	Hepatocellular carcinoma
HELLP	Hemolysis, elevated liver enzymes, low platelets
HGD	High-grade dysplasia
HIDA	Hepatobiliary imaging
HNPCC	Hereditary nonpolyposis colon cancer
IBD	Inflammatory bowel disease
IBS	Irritable bowel syndrome
IPMN	Intraductal papillary mucinous neoplasm
LES	Lower esophageal sphincter
MALT	Mucosa-associated lymphoid tissue
MELD	Model for end-stage liver disease
MEN	Multiple endocrine neoplasia
MRCP	Magnetic resonance cholangiopancreatography
MYH	Heavy-chain myosin
NAFLD	Nonalcoholic fatty liver disease
NASH	Nonalcoholic steatohepatitis
NET	Neuroendocrine tumor
NGL	Nasogastric lavage
NGT	Nasogastric tube
OCP	Oral contraceptive pill; ova, cyst, and parasite (test)
PBC	Primary biliary cirrhosis
PDT	Pancreatic duodenal transplantation
PPI	Proton pump inhibitor
PSC	Primary sclerosing cholangitis
PUD	Peptic ulcer disease
RF	Rheumatoid factor
RFA	Radiofrequency ablation therapy
SBP	Spontaneous bacterial peritonitis
SMA	Superior mesenteric artery
TACE	Transarterial chemoembolization
TCA	Tricyclic antidepressant
TIPS	Transjugular intrahepatic portal systemic shunt
TNF	Tumor necrosis factor
TPN	Total parenteral nutrition
TTG	Tissue transglutaminase
TTP	Thrombotic thrombocytopenic purpura
UC	Ulcerative colitis
UGI	Upper gastrointestinal; upper gastrointestinal x-ray series
ZE	Zollinger-Ellison syndrome

Speaker Disclosure
Nimisha K. Parekh, MD, MPH, has documented that she
has no commercial relationships to disclose.

Gastroenterology in a Nutshell
or
Everything you ever wanted to know about poop
but were afraid to ask ...

Outline
- Esophagus
- Stomach
- IBD
- Diarrhea
- Celiac Sprue
- Malabsorption
- Constipation
- IBS
- Colon Cancer
- Acute Diverticulitis
- GI Bleeding
- Pancreas
- Liver

GI Procedures
- EGD
- Colonoscopy
- ERCP
- EUS

Esophagus — Anatomy

Esophagus — Physiology
- Deglutition — voluntary
  - Relaxation of upper sphincter; epiglottis closure
- Peristalsis in esophageal body
  - Involuntary; propels food
  - Smooth muscle
- Relaxation of LES
- Know, since this relates to dysphagia and reflux

Symptoms of Esophageal Disorders
- Dysphagia
- Globus
- Odynophagia
- Reflux/Chest pain
Emphasis should be on the history:
This should assist in determining workup

Swallowing
Swallowing mechanism with 2 components:
1) Oropharyngeal process: Food goes from mouth
   to hypopharynx
2) Esophageal process: Food bolus through the
   esophagus into the stomach

History
- Choking, coughing, nasal regurgitation with swallowing
  — oropharyngeal or neurologic
- Pain with swallowing — odynophagia:
  Pill esophagitis or infection
- Liquids (cold) and solids — motility
- Intermittent solid food — lower esophageal ring
- Progressive solid food — stricture or malignancy

Dysphagia
Patients report "feeling of food getting stuck."

Dysphagia Causes
- Oropharyngeal
  - Neurologic deficits
- Esophageal
  - Physical obstruction of the esophageal lumen
- Motility disorders (esophageal)
  - Trouble with transporting food from the upper
    esophagus to stomach

Options for Workup
- Empiric treatment of reflux with PPI
- Esophagram: More for oropharyngeal dysphagia
- EGD
- Motility Studies

Audience Response 1
A 50-year-old male
Dysphagia for solid and liquid foods for 3 years
Not extremely progressive 5-lb weight loss
Nocturnal regurgitation

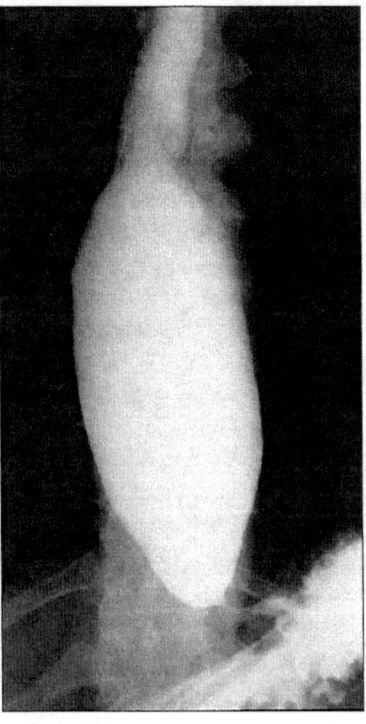

What is the most likely diagnosis?
A. Achalasia
B. Diffuse esophageal spasm
C. Esophageal stricture
D. Esophageal cancer

Answer: _____

Motility Disorders
- Achalasia
- DES/Nutcracker esophagus
- Systemic sclerosis/Scleroderma

Achalasia
- Pathogenesis — ganglion cell degeneration of myenteric plexus
- Pathophysiology
  - No peristalsis in smooth muscle
  - Elevated LES pressure
  - Failure of LES to relax completely, thus unable to open up completely
  - Simultaneous, low-amplitude contractions

- Symptoms: Usually longstanding
  - Dysphagia for solids and liquids
  - Regurgitation (delayed)
  - Nocturnal cough, aspiration
  - Occasional chest pain

Achalasia — Diagnosis
- Barium swallow
- EGD
- Motility/Manometry
- Barium swallow
  - Dilated esophagus — degree of dilation correlating with duration
  - "Bird-beak" distal esophagus
  - Delay in emptying
  - Retained food in esophagus

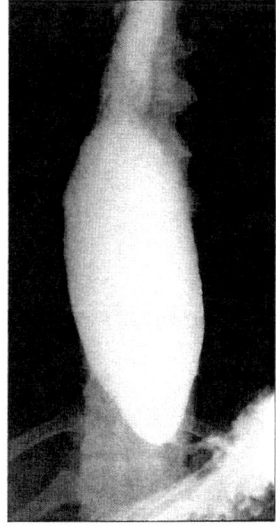

Achalasia — Diagnosis (cont.)
- EGD
  - Dilated esophagus/Retained food
  - Performed to rule out tumor at gastroesophageal junction
- Motility
  - Showing no organized peristalsis
  - Nonrelaxing, high-pressure LES
  - Low-amplitude, simultaneous contractions

Pseudoachalasia
- Also known as secondary achalasia
- The presentation of achalasia due to malignancy
- Clinical features: Age > 60 years, short duration of symptoms, profound weight loss
- Barium swallow and manometry may be exactly the same
- Dx: Endoscopy — view GEJ on retroflexion

Achalasia — Treatment
- No effective medical treatment
- Standard would be pneumatic dilation (this is different from regular dilations; A much larger balloon)
- Surgical — laparoscopic myotomy
- Endoscopic BOTOX for high-risk patient — reserve for the very old or very frail

- Patients will have heartburn — **from lactic acid produced by fermentation of esophageal contents — doesn't respond to PPI**
- Pancreatic enzymes have no role in treatment

Achalasia — Summary
- Know based on history
- Recognize barium swallow
- Order EGD and manometry

Diffuse Esophageal Spasm (DES)
- Intermittent dysphagia for solids and liquids (especially cold liquids)
- Chest pain — atypical for angina
- Barium swallow; Usually normal but can show "corkscrew"

DES Esophagram

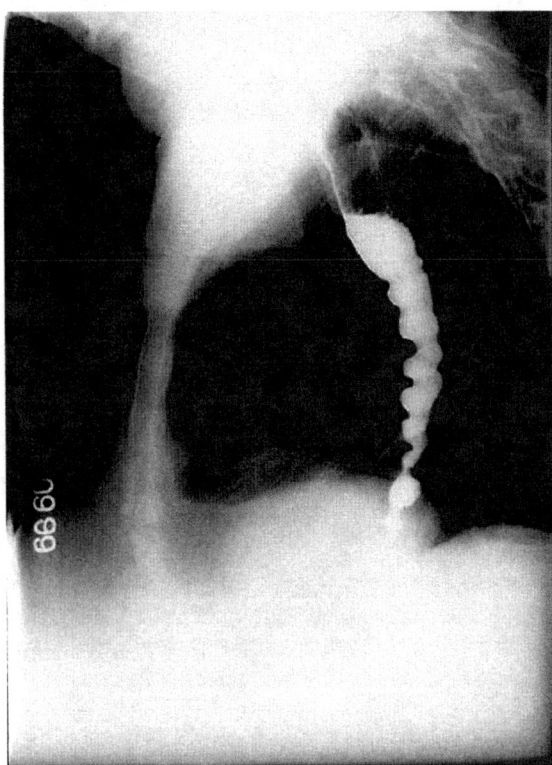

Possible Exam Question
- Shows classic x-ray
- Clearly DES — diffuse esophageal spasm
- But is the question just to recognize x-ray and know diagnosis?
- Or is it how to treat medically?

DES — Workup
- EGD — very low yield
- 24-hr pH probe — some cases are due to atypical reflux
- Motility — diagnostic criteria for DES, Most of time, no additional workup needed

DES Treatment
- Trial proton pump inhibitor (PPI)
- Antispasm agents
- Antianxiety
- Calcium channel antagonists (best evidence)
- Just reassurance
- Nothing works really well …

Scleroderma / Systemic Sclerosis
- Incompetent LES, poor peristalsis
- At risk for severe GERD
- Dysphagia can be due to esophagitis, stricture, or just poor motility
- Work up if dysphagia: Barium swallow and EGD
- Important to assess for GERD complications
- Only treatment is PPI; Dilate if stricture

Dysphagia — The Mechanical or Structural Causes
- Lower esophageal ring
- Esophageal stricture
- Esophageal webs
- Neoplasm

Lower Esophageal Ring
- Also known as Schatzki ring
- Intermittent solid food dysphagia
- Often for steak, **chicken**
- Often regurgitates for relief
- May have hiatal hernia; Unknown if reflux plays a role, but it is becoming common, if not standard, to put on PPI after dilation
- Treatment: Dilation

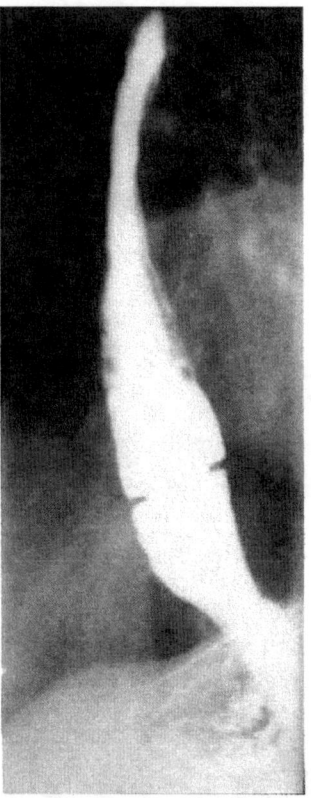

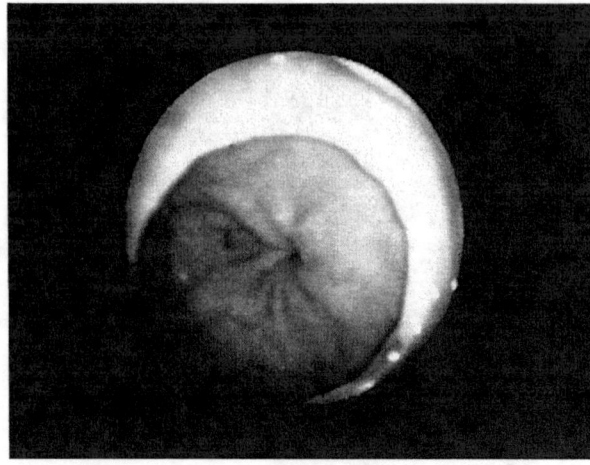

Esophageal Strictures
- Most common cause: Reflux
- Treatment: Various types of dilation
- Other causes: Radiation, lye ingestion, nasogastric tube trauma, pill-induced
- Malignant obstruction: Adenocarcinoma or squamous cell carcinoma

Benign Esophageal Stricture
- Dilation can be accomplished safely
- Peptic strictures will require long-term medication use
- PPI provides better relief than standard dose histamine-2 receptor antagonists

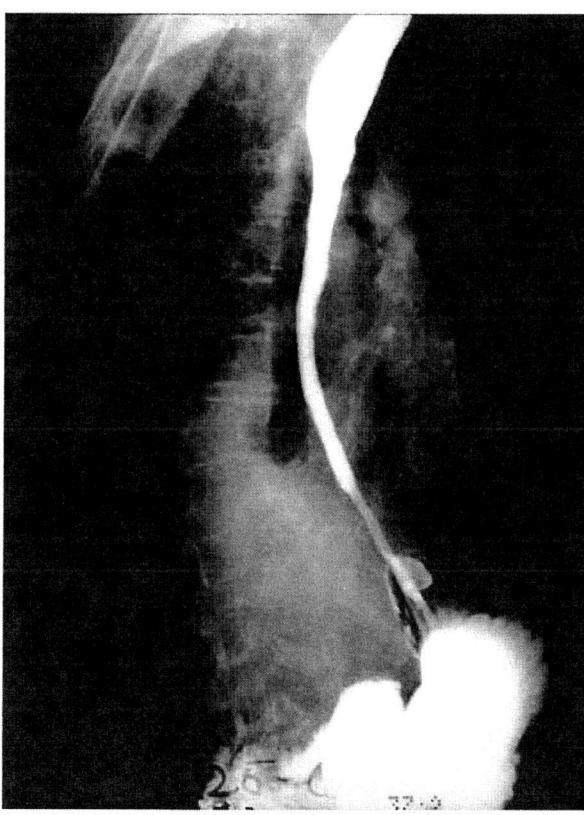

Esophagus
- Zenker's diverticulum
- Esophageal web

AR 2
A 24-year-old male presents to the ED with symptoms of salivation, spitting up frothy secretions 6 hours after eating chicken. He can't drink water without regurgitating. This is the 4th episode of this. He denies heartburn.
PE is normal.
Labs and CXR are okay.

What is the next appropriate step?
A. GI consult for EGD to remove food bolus
B. Barium swallow
C. CT of chest
D. Surgery consult

Answer: _____

AR 2 (cont.)
For an acute food impaction, you can go straight to EGD. Any ingested contrast, (e.g., barium) may pose a risk of aspiration and make the scope more difficult.

Esophagitis
- Infections
- Pill-induced
- Eosinophilic esophagitis (EOS)

Infections — Esophagitis
- *Candida*
- CMV
- HSV
- AIDS-induced ulcers

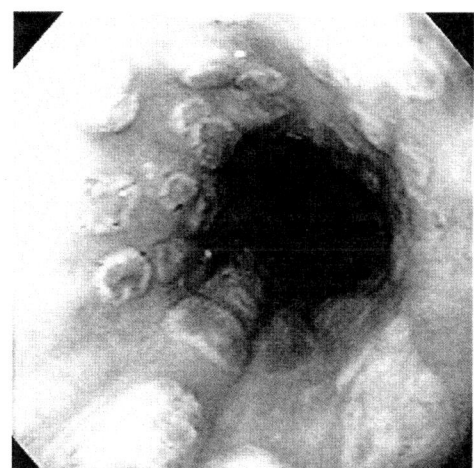

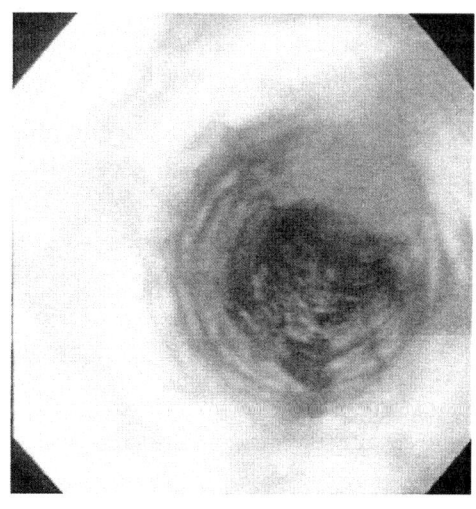

Infections — Esophagitis (cont.)

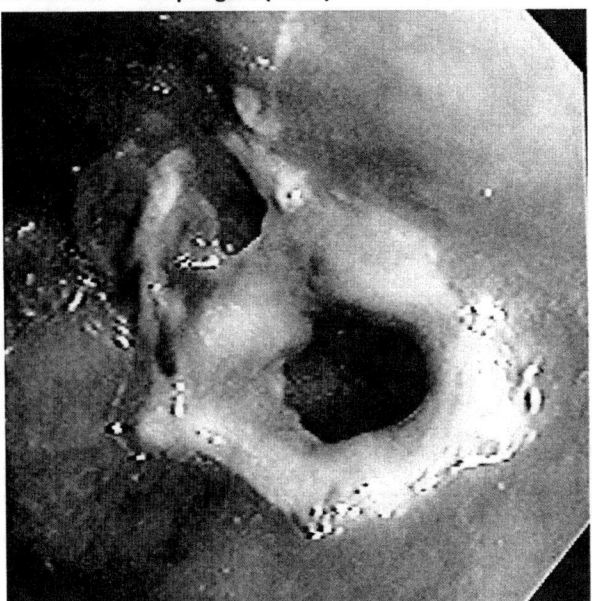

AR 3

An 18-year-old male presents to the acute care portion of the emergency department with the sudden onset of pain with any attempts to swallow either solid or liquid items. He points to the mid-chest as the area where he hurts. This started just this morning.
He denies any prior history of dysphagia or reflux.
His past medical history is negative.
He is taking some medicine for acne but can't remember the name of it.

What is the most likely diagnosis?

A. Esophageal stricture
B. Doxycycline-induced esophageal ulceration
C. An opportunistic infection like *Candida* esophagitis
D. Diffuse esophageal spasm

Answer: _____

AR 3 (cont.)
- The most likely culprit is doxycycline or tetracycline for acne, a.k.a. pill esophagitis
- Very common question on exams

Odynophagia
- Rare for common entities of stricture, Schatzki ring
- Infections: CMV, *Candida* esophagitis, herpes
- Medication-induced: ASA, NSAIDs, doxycycline, KCl, $FeSO_4$, alendronate, quinidine

Eosinophilic Esophagitis (EOE)
- Solid food dysphagia — especially food impaction
- Young males
- Often history of allergy, asthma

- EGD shows "ringed" esophagus/trachealization of esophagus
- Biopsy reveals infiltrate of eosinophils (> 15 eos/HPF)
- Must rule out PPI-responsive esophagitis

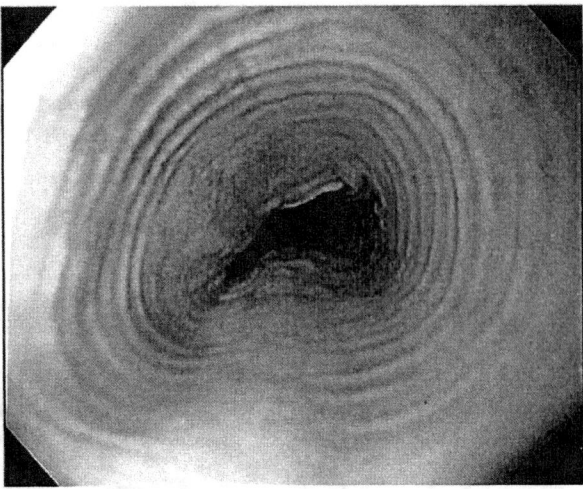

Eosinophilic Esophagitis (EOE) (cont.)
- Treat: PPI and ingested fluticasone or budesonide, allergy testing
- Food elimination diet

AR 4

A 40-year-old female comes to see you for a 5-week history of heartburn occurring several times per week and occasionally waking her up at night. She denies abdominal pain, change in appetite, weight loss, or change in bowel habits. She denies any new medications. She denies any food triggers. She has tried OTC antacids with partial relief.
Physical exam is normal.
Labs are normal.

What is the next appropriate step in management?

A. Just give patient reassurance.
B. EGD.
C. Trial of PPI therapy.
D. Manometry.

Answer: _____

© 2017 MedStudy Internal Medicine Video Board Review – Gastroenterology • Nimisha K. Parekh, MD

GERD Physiology

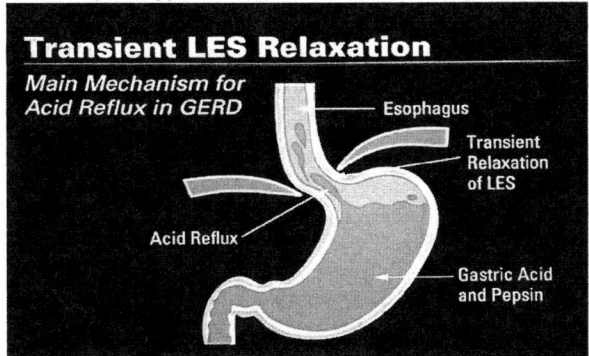

Transient LES Relaxation
Main Mechanism for Acid Reflux in GERD
- Esophagus
- Transient Relaxation of LES
- Acid Reflux
- Gastric Acid and Pepsin

GERD Symptoms
- Typical heartburn
- Atypical chest pain
- Hoarseness, sore throat; throat clearing
- Chronic cough, especially nocturnal
- Asthma

GERD History
- Simple or complicated?
- Typical symptoms or atypical?
- Any alarm symptoms?
- If simple, typical, and no alarms, treat with proton pump inhibitor (PPI)
- Age of onset of symptoms

Workup of Suspected GERD

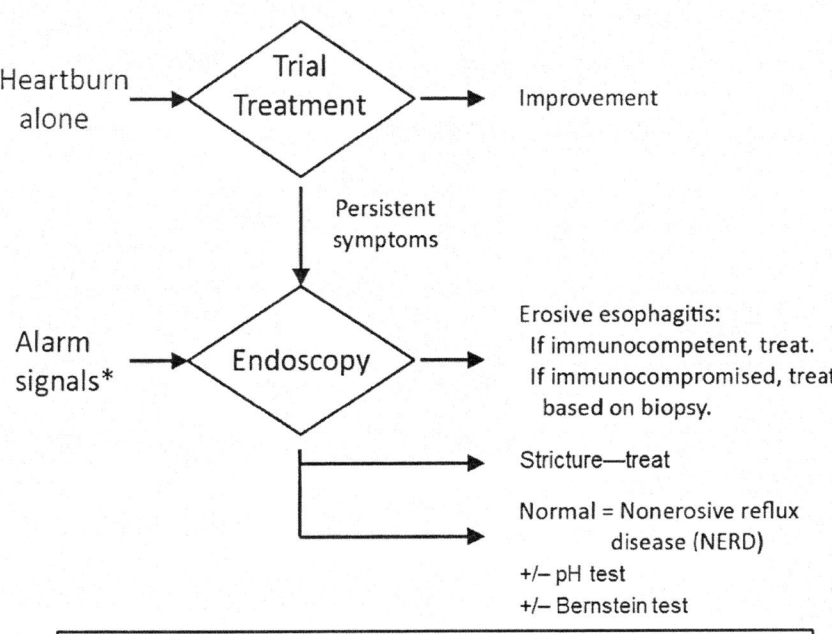

Heartburn alone → Trial Treatment → Improvement

Persistent symptoms

Alarm signals* → Endoscopy →

Erosive esophagitis:
  If immunocompetent, treat.
  If immunocompromised, treat based on biopsy.

Stricture—treat

Normal = Nonerosive reflux disease (NERD)
+/– pH test
+/– Bernstein test

*Note: If a patient has dysphagia and symptoms of obstruction, a barium swallow may precede endoscopy.

Alarm Signals in GERD Indicating the Need for EGD
- Nausea/Emesis
- Blood in the stool
- Family history of PUD
- Weight loss
- Anorexia
- Iron deficiency anemia
- Long duration of frequent symptoms, especially in Caucasian males > 50 years of age
- Failure to respond to full doses of a PPI
- Dysphagia/Odynophagia
- Barrett's confirmation, follow-up
- **Everyone with reflux needn't get an upper endoscopy**

How can a 24-hour pH study help?
- 60-year-old with 3 years of cough
- EGD shows small hiatal hernia but no esophagitis
- PPI bid doesn't help
- 24-hour pH study — helpful in atypical cases, like refractory symptoms and normal EGD, or atypical symptoms like cough, hoarseness

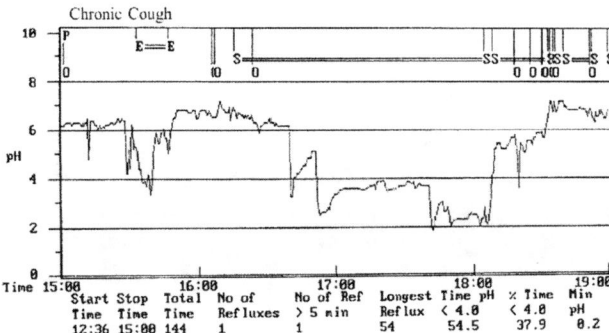

GERD Complications
- Complications:
  - Ulcerative esophagitis
  - Bleeding
  - Stricture
  - Barrett esophagus

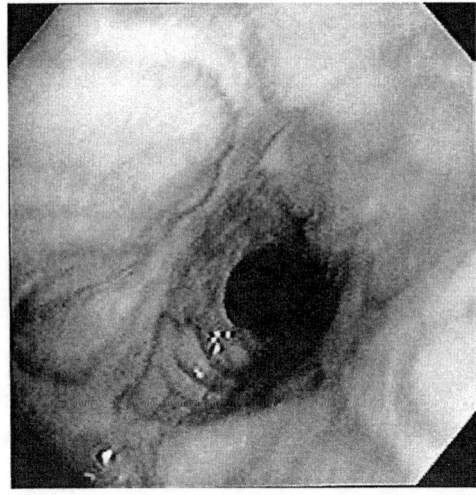

Patient with Ulcerative Esophagitis
- Start with PPI daily
- Rescope to assess healing and exclude Barrett esophagitis
- If persistent esophagitis: Change PPI to bid
- Indefinite maintenance treatment — up to 80% recur off meds

GERD Treatment
- Lifestyle modifications: raise head of bed, weight loss, smoking cessation
- H_2 blockers (heal 50% of reflux esophagitis)
- PPIs (heal 80–95% of reflux esophagitis)

Let's Blame Everything on PPIs
- Very likely to be on exams:
  - Osteoporosis (?)
  - Vitamin D deficiency
  - Hypomagnesemia
  - B_{12} deficiency
  - *C. difficile* infection
  - Clopidogrel interaction debunked

GERD Treatment
- Antireflux surgery
- Nissen fundoplication

GERD Surgery
- Long-term follow-up study (10 years) — *JAMA* 01
- 62% of surgical patients on acid-reducing meds
- Doesn't cure Barrett esophagus

GERD Surgery — Fundoplication
- Real world — can be overutilized, other times quite appropriate
- Possible exam topics:
  - Young patient, definite GERD, intolerant of PPIs but effective when taken
  - Any patient — refractory regurgitation leading to cough, asthma, aspiration pneumonia

GERD Treatment
- Endoscopic therapies
- They are emerging therapies
- To date have not shown long-term benefit

GERD Pearls
- Patients with atypical Sxs take longer to respond to Tx; Require more aggressive Tx
- For example — hoarseness from reflux: Treat with PPI bid for 3 months
- *H. pylori* does not cause reflux
- Sucralfate doesn't do anything

AR 5

A 66-year-old male presents with a 20-year history of heartburn that has been controlled with once daily PPI therapy. Over the past 6 months, he notes some breakthrough symptoms at night. Denies change in appetite, weight loss, nausea or vomiting. Physical exam is normal.
EGD shows a 4-cm segment of salmon-colored mucosa. Pathology shows Barrett esophagus with no dysplasia.

What is the next step?
A. Surgical fundoplication.
B. Repeat endoscopy in 3 years.
C. Do nothing.
D. Endoscopic therapy for GERD.

Answer: _____

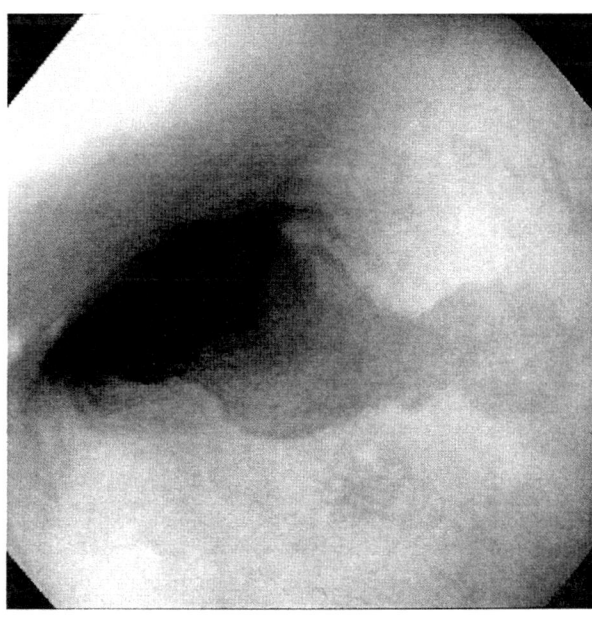

Barrett Esophagus
- Change in cell type of esophagus in response to chronic injury from GER
- Biopsy: Specialized intestinal epithelium

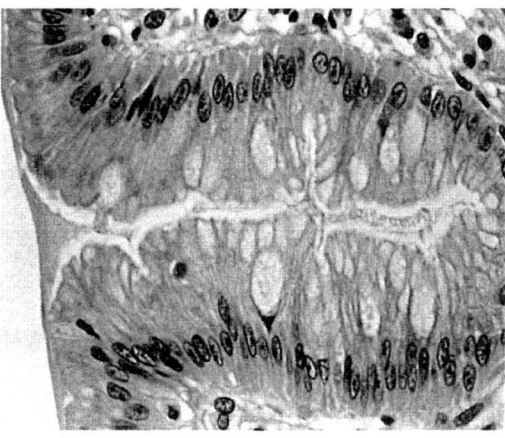

Barrett Esophagus (cont.)
- Symptoms of reflux may not be prominent
- Symptoms are 2° complications like stricture, esophagitis

- How common?
- 60-year-old Caucasian male with GER symptoms: 10–20%
- Women: 2%
- Associated with adenocarcinoma of esophagus
- 0.5% per year risk

- Endoscopic surveillance
- No dysplasia: 3–5 years
- Low-grade dysplasia: 6–12 months
- High-grade dysplasia in the absence of eradication therapy: 3 months

- Endoscopic treatments for HGD
- RFA
- PDT
- EMR

Barrett's and Possible Exam Questions
- Patient with long history of reflux. First EGD shows Barrett's, biopsy confirms, but no dysplasia
- What do you do next?
- Answer: Repeat EGD in 1 year with biopsies:
  - If no dysplasia, then can go to every 3 years
  - If dysplasia, can either do intense surveillance, ablation (RF – *NEJM* 2009), or surgery

Barrett's and Other Possible Questions
- Other issue would be low-grade dysplasia — bring back in 6 months
- If high-grade dysplasia — can a lesion or small mass be removed?
- Treat all these patients as if reflux medically

AR 6

A 70-year-old Asian male who hasn't seen a doctor in 20 years presents. No significant history; brought in by family who report that patient is not eating and is losing weight. Patient says he has progressive difficulty swallowing. Six months ago, he could swallow soft foods, but now it is slow even getting liquids down. There is a long history of cigarettes and alcohol.

Exam shows muscle wasting.
Labs are significant for Hgb of 10 and MCV of 72.
A barium swallow shows a 3-cm segment of severe narrowing of the proximal esophagus.

AR 6 (cont.)
What is the most effective next step?
A. Samples of PPI.
B. Esophageal motility.
C. Refer to GI for EGD.
D. Calcium channel antagonist.

Answer: _____

There is high likelihood that this is esophageal cancer, most likely squamous cell cancer. The next step would be EGD to confirm the diagnosis with biopsies.

Squamous Cell Esophageal Cancer
- Location: Proximal 2/3 of esophagus
- Smoking and alcohol are risk factors
- Other risk factors: Lye stricture, other head and neck malignancy

Adenocarcinoma of Esophagus
- Location: Distal 1/3 of esophagus
- Related to reflux and Barrett's
- Increasing incidence
- Caucasian males

Esophageal Cancer
- Workup: EGD and biopsy, endoscopic ultrasound, CT abdomen and chest
- Treat: Surgery, if localized
- XRT + cisplatin + 5FU
- Neoadjuvant Tx before surgery

The Stomach
- Anatomy and physiology
- PUD
- Complications of PUD
- Dyspepsia
- *H. pylori*
- Gastroparesis
- Gastric lesions and malignancies

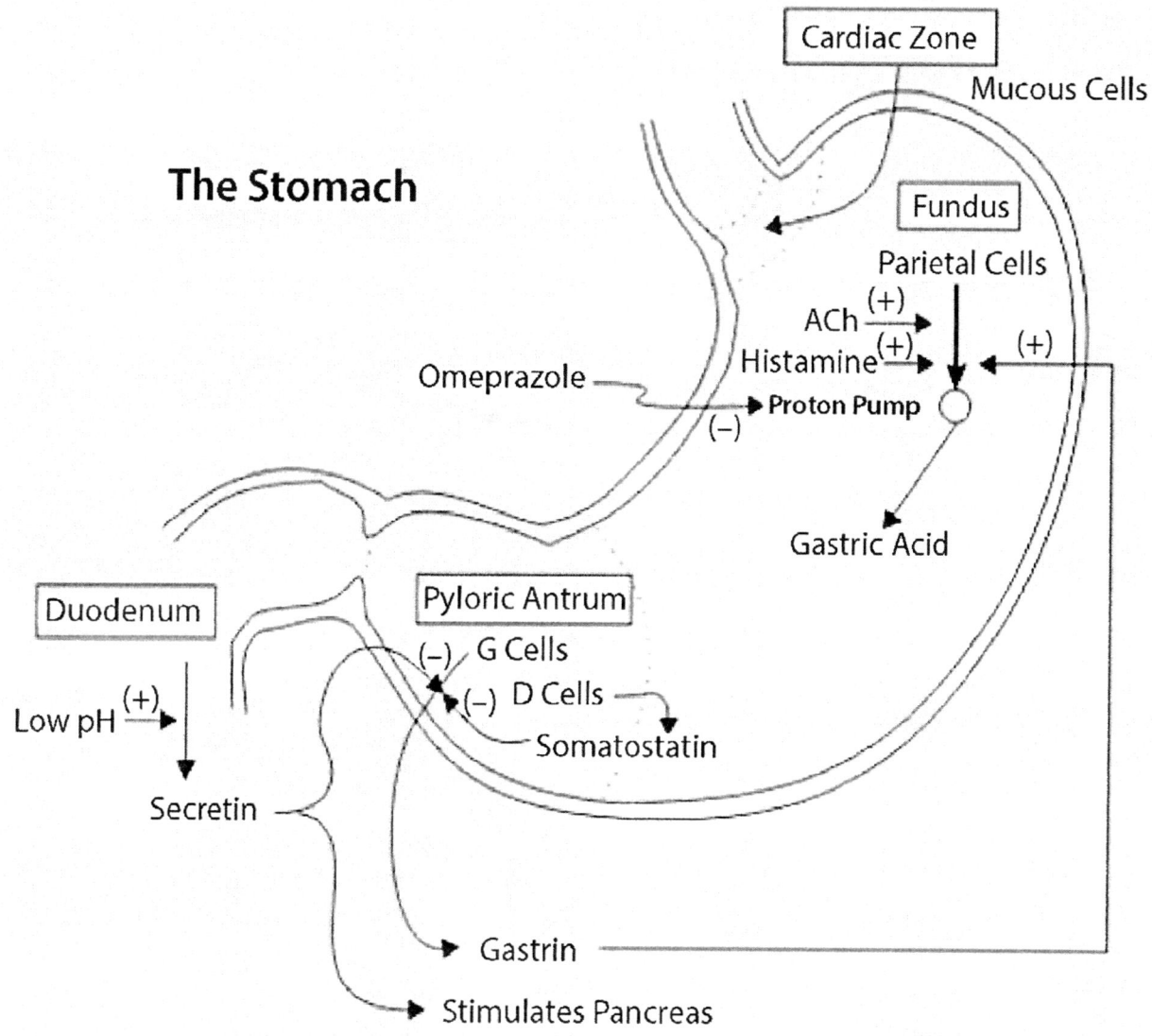

The Stomach

Note: low pH decreases gastrin by stimulating the D cells to produce somatostatin and the duodenum to produce secretin.

Secretion of Gastric Acid (Parietal Cells)
- Histamine-2 receptor
  - Histamine released from enterochromaffin-like cells
  - Blocked by H2RA; e.g., cimetidine
- Gastrin receptor
  - Gastrin principal mediator
  - From antral G cells
  - Stimulated by amino acids and amines
  - Negative feedback pH < 3
- M-1 cholinergic receptor
- Ultimate secretion via "proton pump" mechanism involving H-K-ATPase
  - Blocked by proton pump inhibitor

AR 7

A 45-year-old female presents to ED with 3-day history of epigastric pain, nausea, and black stools. She does report taking ibuprofen for 3 weeks for a sprained ankle. She has no other medical or surgical history.
On exam: HR 115, BP 80/65, RR 14, epigastric pain noted on exam without rebound or guarding.
Rectal exam shows melena.
Labs show Hgb 6.1, BUN of 55, CR of 1.3.

What is the next appropriate step?
A. Blood transfusion and PPI drip
B. Octreotide infusion
C. IV fluids and PPI drip
D. Send straight to GI lab for endoscopy

Answer: _____

Peptic Ulcer Disease
- Causes:
  - *H. pylori*
  - NSAIDs
    - Prevalence in patients on NSAIDs 10–30%
  - Zollinger-Ellison syndrome
  - Crohn's disease
- Types/Location:
  - Gastric: NSAIDs, *H. pylori*
  - Rule out malignancy
  - Duodenal: NSAIDs, *H. pylori*
  - Uncomplicated vs. complicated

Uncomplicated
- Symptoms
  - Epigastric pain, relief with eating, early satiety, bloating, abd fullness

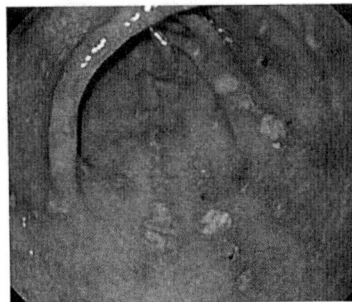

Complicated
- Presentation
  - GI bleeding
  - Perforation
  - Obstruction
- Alarm signs
  - Age > 55 years
  - Weight loss
  - GI bleeding
  - Anemia
  - Recurrent vomiting

Peptic Ulcer Disease — Diagnosis
- EGD
- Rarely is UGI used
- If severe pain: Consider perforated ulcer
  - Patient may be on steroids
  - Abd films before any study
  - Do not order EGD/UGI

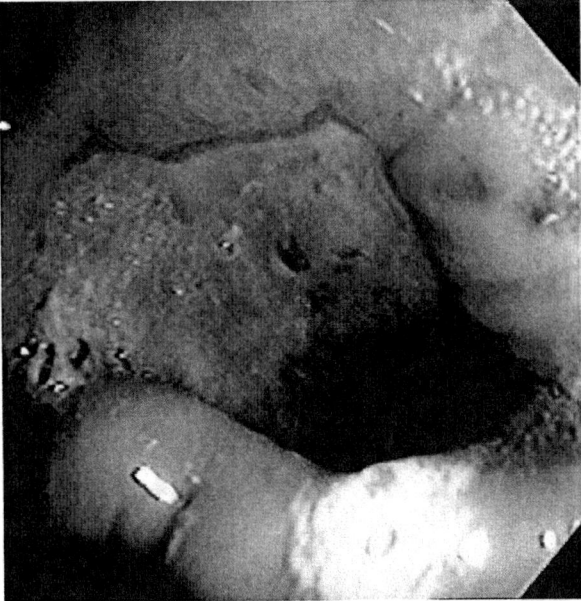

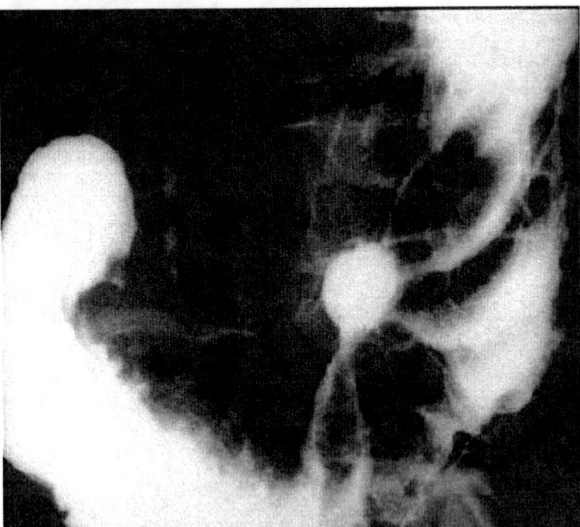

Indications for Endoscopy in PUD
- New onset epigastric pain in age > 55 years
- GI bleeding (overt or occult)
- Anemia, iron deficiency (start workup from below, usually colonoscopy)
- Recurrent vomiting
- Weight loss
- Abnormal upper GI series or CT
- Follow-up healing of gastric ulcer (maybe not all cases; e.g., young patient and due to NSAIDs)

Peptic Ulcer Disease — Treatment
- Decrease acid secretion (PPI, H_2 receptor antagonists)
- Stop exacerbating process (NSAIDs, smoking, alcohol)
- *H. pylori* treatment

NSAID Complications — Highest Risk
- Higher doses
- First 3 months of administration
- Advanced age
- History of ulcer disease (most important)
- Concomitant corticosteroids
- Serious medical illness
- Less risk: COX-2, misoprostol, PPI
- Lowest risk: COX-2 + PPI
- But: COX-2 plus ASA has same ulcer risk

Indications for Surgery in PUD
- UGI bleed unable to be stopped by endoscopic therapy or IR (5%)
- Perforation
- Gastric outlet obstruction
- Zollinger-Ellison Syndrome: Surgery for underlying gastrinoma

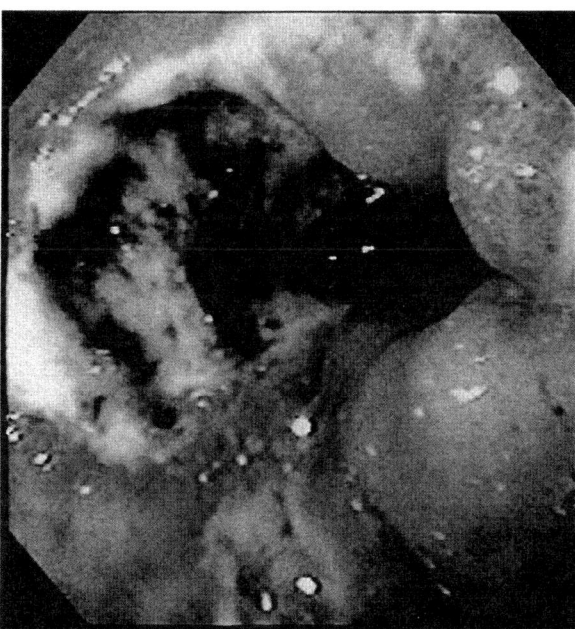

AR 8
A 65-year-old woman has moved to the U.S. from Korea. Her chief complaint is of upper abdominal discomfort — postprandial, not severe.
It has led to her eating less than usual and, therefore, to weight loss.
She has dyspepsia with some bloating and belching.

Past medical history is otherwise negative. She is on no medications. She denies taking any NSAIDs.
Review of systems: Pertinent for a 5-lb weight loss
Physical exam: Reveals no abnormalities

Which of the following do you recommend to initiate the workup on this patient?
A. *H. pylori* ELISA and treat if positive
B. EGD
C. CT of the abdomen
D. Upper GI x-ray

Answer: _____

Teaching Point
- *H. pylori* test-and-treat strategy is fine, but you have to make sure it is young patient without red flags
- This patient is high risk, needs an endoscopy

Dyspepsia
- Symptoms: Epigastric pain, abdominal fullness, bloating, belching, nausea, vomiting
- Requires workup, especially if recent onset or age > 50 years, exclude other causes
- Differential diagnosis: *H. pylori*, PUD, gastroparesis, celiac, biliary disease, carbohydrate malabsorption, pancreas issues, IBD, medications, abdominal wall pain, thyroid disease, DM, malignancy

Dyspepsia Workup
- Test and treat *H. pylori*
- DC NSAIDs
- Trial PPI
- Referral to GI if above does not work
- Diagnostic criteria:
  One or more of the following for 3 months:
  − Postprandial fullness
  − Early satiety
  − Epigastric pain
  − No evidence of structural disease

Dyspepsia — Treatment
- Dietary modification, lifestyle modifications, trial of PPI
- Referral to GI if above does not work
- CAM: STW 5 (herbal supplement)
- Psychological treatments:
  Hypnotherapy, relaxation therapy, imagery

AR 9

Treatment of *H. pylori* may cause regression of which malignancy?

A. MALT lymphoma of the stomach
B. Gastric adenocarcinoma
C. Pancreatic adenocarcinoma
D. Adenocarcinoma of the esophagus

Answer: _____

Helicobacter pylori

- Epidemiology
  - Childhood — underdeveloped countries
  - U.S. — 50% by age 60 years
  - Increased in lower socioeconomic class
  - Transmission uncertain
  - Present in many asymptomatic persons
- Histology
  - Spiral, flagellated GNR
  - Lives in mucous layer
  - Mucosal invasion rare
  - <u>Chronic</u>, <u>active</u>, nonspecific gastritis
  - Infiltration PMN + lymphocytes

H. pylori

- One of most common human bacterial infections
- Causally linked: Gastritis, PUD, gastric adenocarcinoma, gastric B-cell lymphoma
- Mucosa-associated lymphoid tissue/MALT
- Infected patients: 15% lifetime PUD risk
- But chronic gastritis in all patients

- Natural history
- Chronic superficial gastritis to atrophic
- Antral predominant: Tendency duodenal ulcer
- Body predominant: Cancer
- Multifocal atrophic gastritis to intestinal metaplasia
- Severity of body gastritis inversely related to acid secretion

When do you look for *H. pylori*?

- Any prior history of peptic ulcer disease
- The EGD shows gastritis, or ulcer in stomach or duodenum
- MALT lymphoma
- Maybe family history of gastric cancer
- Dyspeptic symptoms: To test and treat, if age < 50 years and no alarm symptoms

Tests for *H. pylori*

Endoscopic Testing	Advantages	Disadvantages
*1. Histology	Excellent sensitivity and specificity	Expensive and requires infrastructure and trained personnel
*2. Rapid urease testing	Inexpensive and provides rapid results. Excellent specificity and very good sensitivity in properly selected patients	Sensitivity significantly reduced in the posttreatment setting
*3. Culture	Excellent specificity. Allows determination of antibiotic sensitivities	Expensive, difficult to perform, and not widely available. Only marginal sensitivity
*4. Polymerase chain reaction	Excellent sensitivity and specificity. Allows determination of antibiotic sensitivities	Methodology not standardized across laboratories and not widely available

Nonendoscopic Testing	Advantages	Disadvantages
1. Antibody testing (quantitative and qualitative)	Inexpensive, widely available, very good NPV	PPV dependent upon background *H. pylori* prevalence. Not recommended after *H. pylori* therapy
*2. Urea breath tests (^{13}C and ^{14}C)	Identifies active *H. pylori* infection. Excellent PPV and NPV regardless of *H. pylori* prevalence. Useful before and after *H. pylori* therapy	Reimbursement and availability remain inconsistent. PPI affects results.
*3. Fecal antigen test	Identifies active *H. pylori* infection. Excellent positive and negative predictive values regardless of *H. pylori* prevalence. Useful before and after *H. pylori* therapy	Polyclonal test less well validated than the UBT in the posttreatment setting. Monoclonal test appears reliable before and after antibiotic therapy. Unpleasantness associated with collecting stool. PPI affects results.

H. pylori — Treatment
- Multidrug regimens; Generally 10–14 days
  - PPI + bismuth + metronidazole + tetracycline: 95%
  - PPI + amoxicillin + clarithromycin
  - PPI + metronidazole + clarithromycin
  - PPI should be bid
  - Sequential therapy

H. pylori (cont.)
- Testing to confirm eradication of *H. pylori* recommended
- Perform no earlier than 4 weeks after completing therapy
- PPI should be stopped 2 weeks prior to testing (PPI Tx suppresses the bacteria)

AR 10
A 30-year-old male has a 3-month history of epigastric pain. He was found to have an *H. pylori* ELISA that was positive. You treated him at that time with a 10-day course of omeprazole, amoxicillin, and clarithromycin. He comes back for follow-up after the antibiotics, and he now feels fine. The symptoms have completely resolved. But he wants to make sure that the *H. pylori* has been eradicated.

You offer which of the following as the best test to determine the eradication of *H. pylori*?
A. EGD with rapid urease test
B. EGD with mucosal biopsy to look for chronic gastritis
C. *H. pylori* ELISA
D. Stool antigen test for *H. pylori*

Answer: _____

Teaching Point
For confirmation of *H. pylori* eradication, use either stool antigen test or urease breath test.

Other Gastropathy
- Intestinal metaplasia
- Atrophic gastritis
- Eosinophilic gastritis
- Lymphocytic gastritis
- IBD

Gastroparesis
- Associated symptoms: Nausea, vomiting, abdominal pain, satiety, fullness
- Diagnosis confirmed by gastric-emptying scan
- But always exclude obstruction with EGD
  - EGD may show retained food or bezoar

Causes of Gastroparesis
- Diabetes
- Scleroderma
- Idiopathic
- Post-vagotomy
- Opioids
- Anticholinergic medications
- L-dopA
- Glucagon
- Calcium channel blockers
- TCAs
- Octreotide

Diabetic Gastroparesis
- More prevalent in DM Type 1
- Usually long-standing with other complications, esp. autonomic neuropathy
- High blood sugar exacerbates symptoms
- Likewise, gastroparesis leads to poor glycemic control
- Variable Sxs: N, V, distention, fullness, abdominal pain

AR 11
A 50-year-old with long-standing Type 1 diabetes mellitus complains of nausea, postprandial fullness, and epigastric discomfort. EGD shows retained food in stomach. A nuclear medicine gastric emptying scan is abnormal with 1/2 emptying at 3 hours.

You recommend:
A. Omeprazole 20 mg PO daily
B. Erythromycin 125 mg PO qid
C. Dicyclomine 10 mg PO qid
D. Metoclopramide 10 mg before meals

Answer: _____

AR 11 (cont.)
Omeprazole may help symptoms, but the only available promotility agent is metoclopramide.

Treatment of Gastroparesis
- Improve diabetes control
- Small frequent meals, low fiber, low residue
- Metoclopramide (dopamine antagonist) useful, except for side effects such as tardive dyskinesia
- Erythromycin (motilin agonist): Not indicated but does cause strong gastric contractions and tachyphylaxis
- Domperidone (not approved in U.S.)
- Gastric pacemakers

AR 12
A 40-year-old woman has suffered with chronic heartburn and diarrhea for 2 years. She takes over-the-counter omeprazole, which gives some relief of the heartburn. She also complains of chronic diarrhea, with 5–6 loose bowel movements a day and some epigastric discomfort. EGD is done and shows grade III esophagitis. Multiple shallow ulcers are seen in the duodenal bulb and 2nd portion of the duodenum.

You recommend:
A. Continue omeprazole, but add sucralfate qid.
B. Continue omeprazole, but add metoclopramide before meals.
C. Order *H. pylori* ELISA.
D. Order fasting serum gastrin after stopping the omeprazole for 7 days.

Answer: _____

Teaching Points
- Remember Zollinger-Ellison syndrome, especially if chronic diarrhea accompanies either bad esophagitis or peptic ulcer disease
- **Order fasting serum gastrin after stopping the omeprazole for 7 days**

Gastrinoma — Zollinger-Ellison Syndrome
- Ulcer disease of upper GI tract
- 30% have diarrhea
- Non-beta islet cell tumor of pancreas or duodenal wall
- Marked increase gastric acid and elevated serum gastrin

- 20% MEN1
- Workup: Somatostatin-receptor scintigraphy and endoscopic ultrasound (EUS)
- Surgical exploration
  - Remember: Most common cause of increased gastrin is achlorhydria ("no acid" means no inhibition of gastrin secretion) atrophic gastritis/PPI/chronic gastritis

Zollinger-Ellison Syndrome
- Be suspicious if:
  - Recurrent ulcers: No other factors
  - Recurrent complicated ulcer
  - Duodenal ulcer and big folds in stomach
  - Duodenal ulcer and diarrhea
  - Chronic diarrhea and severe esophagitis

Lesions in the Stomach
- Gastric polyps
- Gastric subepithelial lesions
- GIST — stromal tumor
- Malignancy
  - Carcinoid
  - Lymphoma
  - Adenocarcinoma

Gastric Polyps
- 90% of polyps found are fundic gland polyps (associated with PPI use) or hyperplastic
  - Usually less than 10 polyps
- Can be associated with FAP or MYH-associated polyposis syndromes (usually > 30 polyps)

Gastric Subepithelial Lesions
- Usually patients are asymptomatic
- Found during EGD or radiologic imaging
- Benign lesions: Lipoma, pancreatic rest, duplication cysts
- Potentially malignant: GIST, lymphoma, carcinoid

Gastrointestinal Stromal Tumors (GIST)
- Less than 1% of all tumors of stomach
- Diagnosis by EUS
- Mesenchymal tumors arising from interstitial cell of Cajal
- 95% of GIST have a *KIT* mutation, CD 117 stain positive
- Prognosis based on mitotic index, size and location

Gastric Carcinoid
- Also known as gastric neuroendocrine tumor (NET)
- Gastrin is usually elevated
- Derived from enterochromaffin cells of stomach
- Endoscopic polypectomy is curative if polyp < 1 cm in size
- Rarely causes carcinoid syndrome
- Three subtypes
  - Type I: 80% of lesions, associated with autoimmune gastritis, hypergastrinemia
  - Type II: MEN1 syndrome and ZE syndrome
  - Type III: Gastrin independent, poorer prognosis

Gastric Lymphoma
- Diffuse histiocytic lymphoma
- Better prognosis than adenocarcinoma
- MALT — *H. pylori*
- Possible exam question — treat MALT with omeprazole/amoxicillin/clarithromycin and F/U

Gastric Adenocarcinoma
- Usually diagnosed after symptoms
- Most with symptoms are advanced
- Abdominal pain, nausea, satiety, weight loss
- Most common of the gastric neoplasms — with recent trend of increase in proximal stomach near junction of esophagus and stomach

Cancer of the Stomach
- Risk factors, associations
  - Chronic *H. pylori* leads to chronic inflammation and hypochlorhydria
- Chronic atrophic gastritis and intestinal metaplasia
- Ménétrier disease
- Adenomatous gastric polyps

Diagnosis and Staging
- Endoscopy, brush, and biopsy
  - CT and EUS for staging
  - Most have regional nodes or direct invasion
- Treatment and survival
  - Surgical resection if possible Node-negative: 5-year survival 85–90%
    Node-positive: 5–10%
  - Chemotherapy — adjuvant post-op chemoradiation 5FU based with leucovorin

Don't Forget Rare Diseases with Diagnostic Physical Findings
- Osler-Weber-Rendu (hereditary hemorrhagic telangiectasia): Telangiectasia of fingers and nasal and oral mucosa; history of nosebleeds; familial
- Peutz-Jeghers: Perioral pigmentation; hamartomas of GI tract can bleed

Complications of Gastric Surgery
- Bariatric surgery
- Afferent loop syndrome
- Dumping syndrome
- Nutritional deficiencies

The Colon

Inflammatory Bowel Disease (IBD)
- Crohn's and ulcerative colitis
- Diagnosis, treatment, extraintestinal complications

Case
- 28-year-old Jewish female presents to clinic with diarrhea (6x/daily), intermittent rectal bleeding and cramping for 3 weeks, 10-pound weight loss
- Traveled to Africa 2 months ago. Patient had GI distress and diarrhea, took metronidazole (Flagyl) for 10 days, partial relief
- PMH: None
- Family history: Sister with psoriasis, brother with Crohn's disease, father with colon cancer at age 52
- Social history: Quit smoking 6 months ago, smoked for 10 years, 1 ppd, engaged, IT specialist
- ROS: Occasional knee pain
- PE: VSS, mild RLQ tenderness, no rebound or guarding, rectal brown stool, heme+, 2 skin tags

Differential Diagnosis
- Infectious diarrhea
- Medication induced colitis
- Celiac disease
- Irritable bowel syndrome
- Lactose intolerance
- Malignancy
- Ischemic colitis
- Diverticulitis
- Radiation colitis
- Microscopic colitis
- Neuroendocrine tumors

Diagnosis

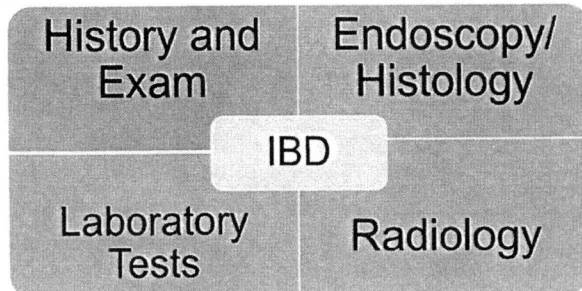

Clinical Symptoms
- Diarrhea
- Fecal urgency
- Hematochezia
- Anal pain
- Abdominal pain
- Fevers
- Fatigue
- Weight loss
- Growth failure
- Extraintestinal manifestations
- Stunted growth in children

Symptoms
- Crohn's disease
- Can be variable
- Abdominal pain, diarrhea, weight loss
- UC
- Bloody diarrhea, tenesmus, abdominal discomfort and incontinence

Crohn's Disease — Diagnosis
- Colonoscopy
  - Findings: Patchy disease, aphthous and deep ulcers, strictures, fistula
  - Colonic disease: Rectal sparing, skip lesions, perirectal disease
  - Ileal disease
- Radiology:
  - MRI or CT scan: Shows small bowel or colonic inflammation or thickening
  - UGI with small bowel
  - String sign: Ileal disease
- Colon only: 30%; SB only: 30%; Colon and small intestine: 40%

Crohn's Disease

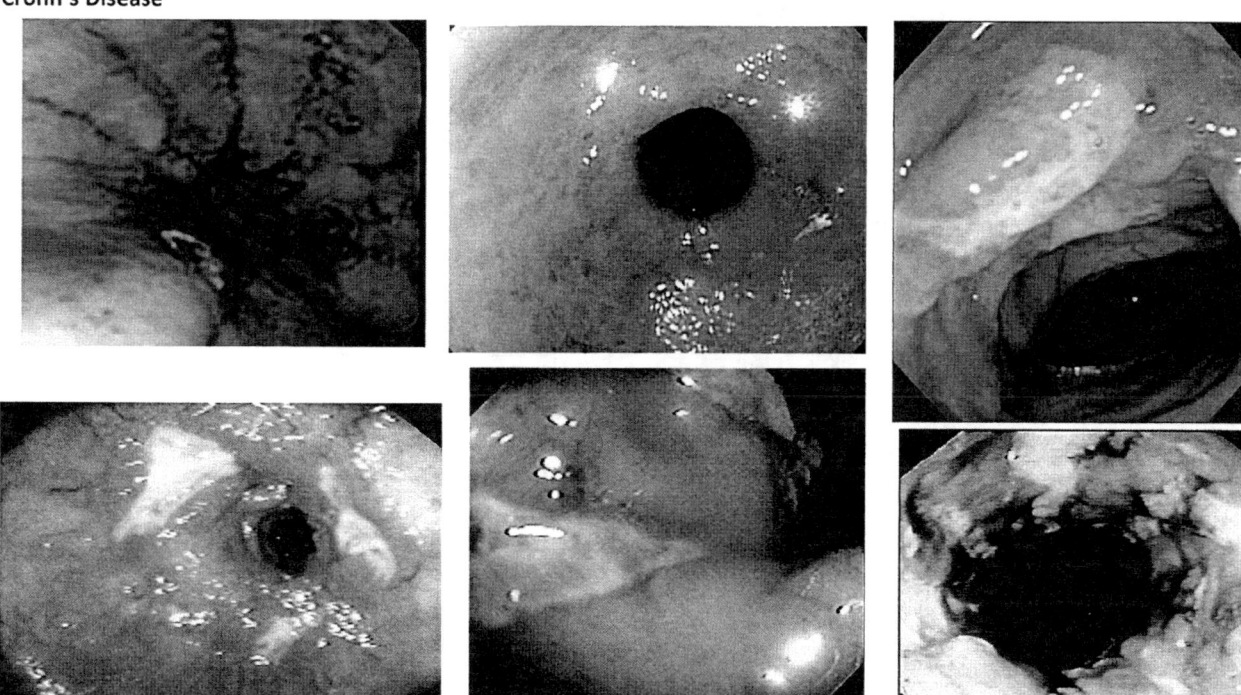

Crohn's Disease — Radiology

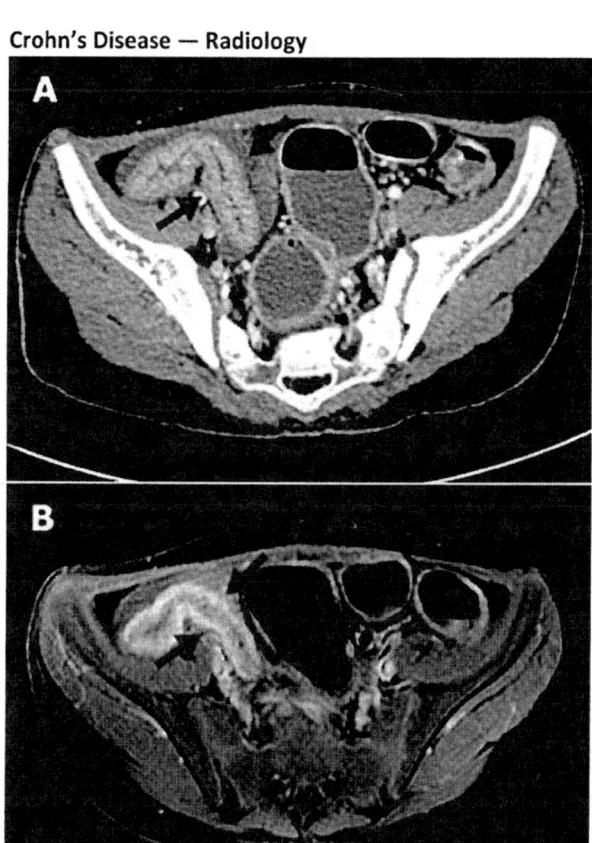

Ulcerative Colitis (UC)
- Colonoscopy findings
  - Uniform, continuous, mucosal inflammation; May be shallow ulcers, never deep
  - Starts in rectum, variable extent
    - Proctitis: Rectum only
    - Proctosigmoiditis
    - Extensive colitis (pancolitis)
    - Radiology may show loss of haustral folds

Endoscopic Spectrum of Severity

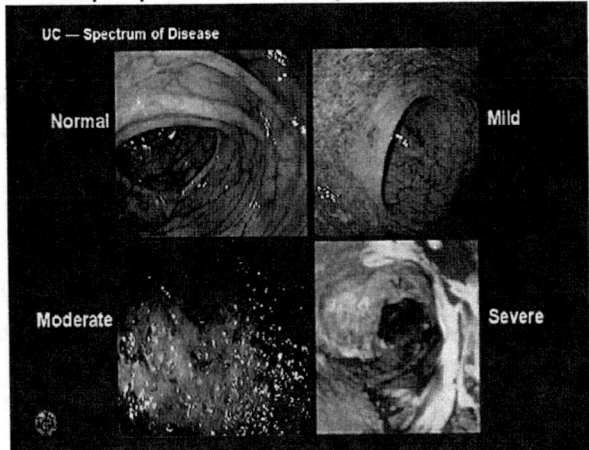

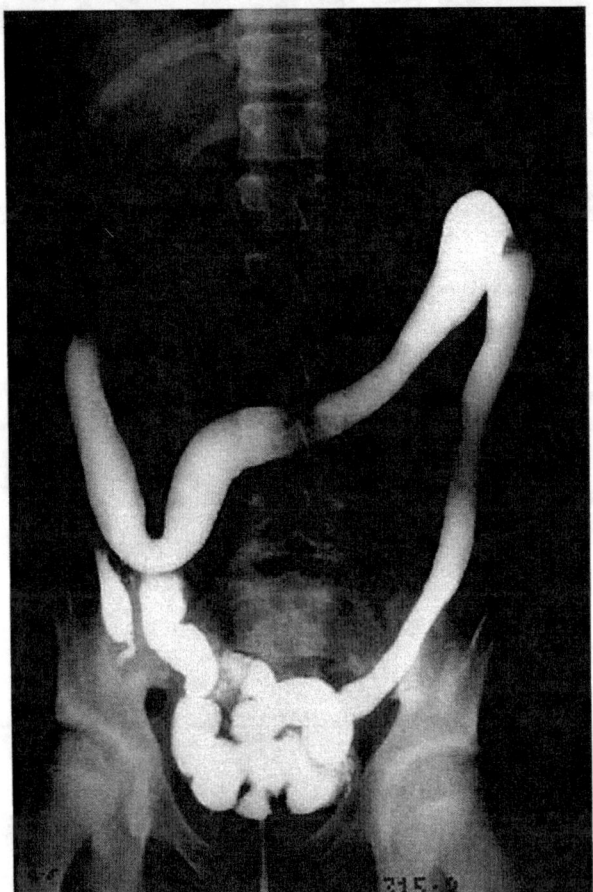

IBD — Diagnosis
- Histology
  - Granulomas found in Crohn's, but diagnostic
  - Architectural disarray
- Labs: Inflammatory markers can be elevated; Serologies are present
  - ASCA positive in Crohn's
  - ANCA positive in UC

- Anemia is common
  - Iron deficiency
  - B_{12} deficiency in Crohn's

Inflammatory Bowel Disease (IBD) (cont.)

	Crohn's	UC
Lesions	Focal, skip, deep	Shallow, continuous
Granulomas	Pathognomonic	None
Rectal involve	Sparing	Always
Perianal disease	Abscess, fistula	None

Our Patient
- WBC 6.9
- Hgb 11.2
- CMP: WNL
- CRP: 2.2
- Stool studies negative for O&P, positive for WBC, RBC
- EGD: Mild gastritis
- Colonoscopy: Patchy moderate colonic disease, unable to get into terminal ileum due to stenosis of IC valve
- 5 days later, develops a skin rash on legs, red coin like lesions

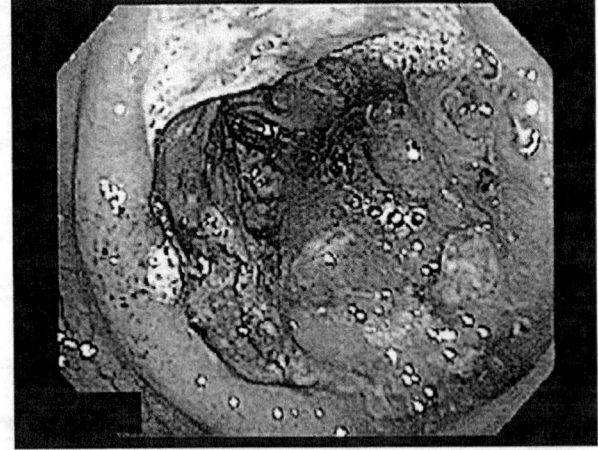

IBD — Systemic Manifestations

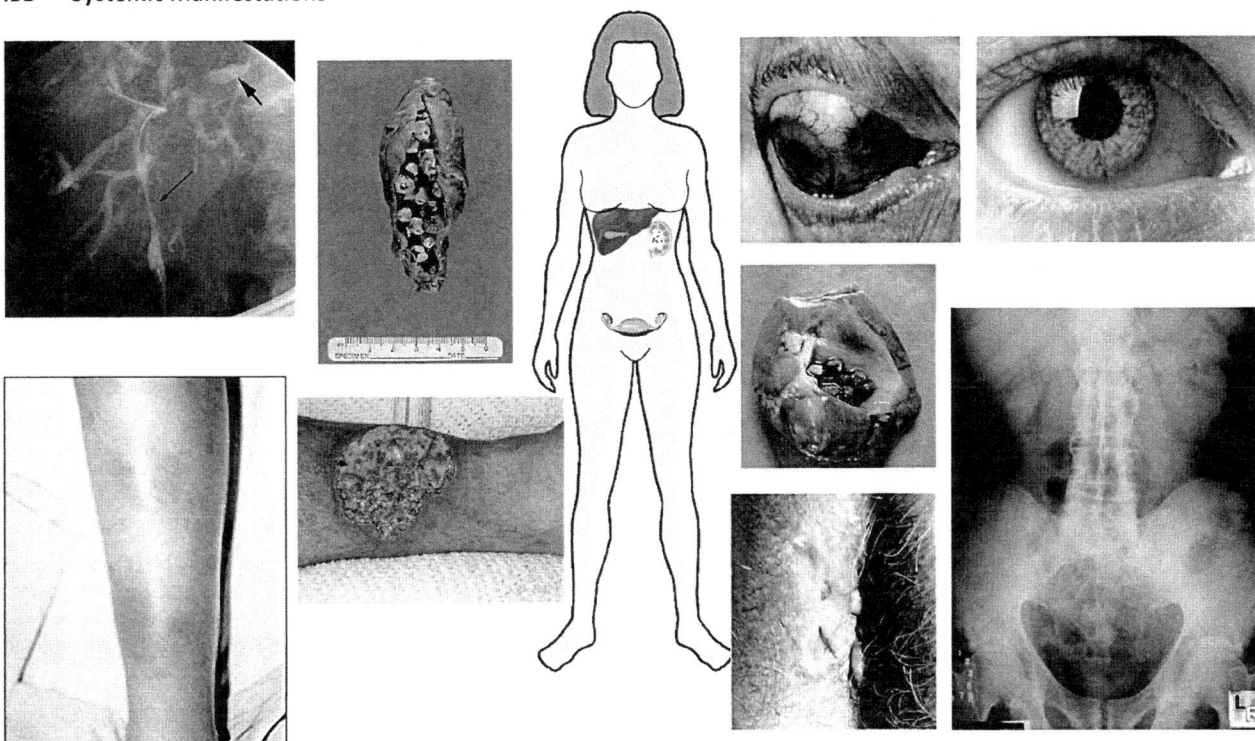

IBD
- Extraintestinal manifestations:
  - Relates to colonic disease
  - Peripheral polyarthritis (RF negative)
  - Ankylosing spondylitis (HLA-B27)
  - Skin lesions (*E. nodosum*, pyoderma)
  - Eye: Iritis, episcleritis, uveitis
  - HLA association tends not to improve with colitis Tx
  - Not unique to UC; Seen with Crohn's
  - PSC, uveitis, axial arthropathy — no improvement with colitis treatment

IBD and Primary Sclerosing Cholangitis (PSC)
- Know association of PSC with both Crohn's and UC
- Always consider if increased liver enzymes
- First test: Either ultrasound or MRCP
- Can occur after colectomy
- Increased risk for colon cancer, will require yearly screening colonoscopy

Our Patient
- Serology: +ASCA IgG, +Omp-C, +C Bir
- Had a MRE because afraid of radiation exposure
- MRE shows ileal inflammation/narrowing of 6 cm in length
- One week after the MRE patient reports that she has some drainage from her perineum
- In addition, she notes a red spot on her right leg

- She has ileocolonic Crohn's disease with ileal inflammation (possible stricture), perianal fistula, and possible erythema nodosum
- How should we proceed with her treatment?

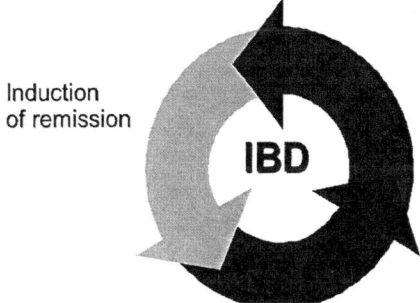

Induction of remission

Maintenance of remission off steroids and/or mucosal healing (histology)

IBD

Maintenance of remission

Picking Therapy Based on Patient

Symptoms	Severity of Inflammation	Location
	Superficial ulcerations	Limited ileal disease
Mild—bothered but functions at a normal capacity	Deep ulcerations/ inflammatory stricture	Extensive small bowel involvement
Moderate (affects daily life)	Fibrotic stricture	
	Internal perforating disease (± abscess)	Extensive colonic involvement
Severe (close to or needing hospitalization)	Perianal perforating	Rectal disease

IBD Therapy in 2017

Antibiotics	Ciprofloxacin Metronidazole	Immunomodulator	6 MP Azathioprine Methotrexate Tacrolimus Thalidomide
Mesalamine	Apriso Pentasa Asacol Sulfasalazine Lialda Colazal Rowasa Canasa	Anti-TNF	Infliximab Adalimumab Certolizumab Golimumab
		Antiintegrin	Natalizumab Vedolizumab
Steroids	Entocort/Uceris Prednisone Hydrocortisone enemas Cortifoam	Anti-Il 12/23	

IBD Treatment Mesalamine (5-ASA)
Site of delivery

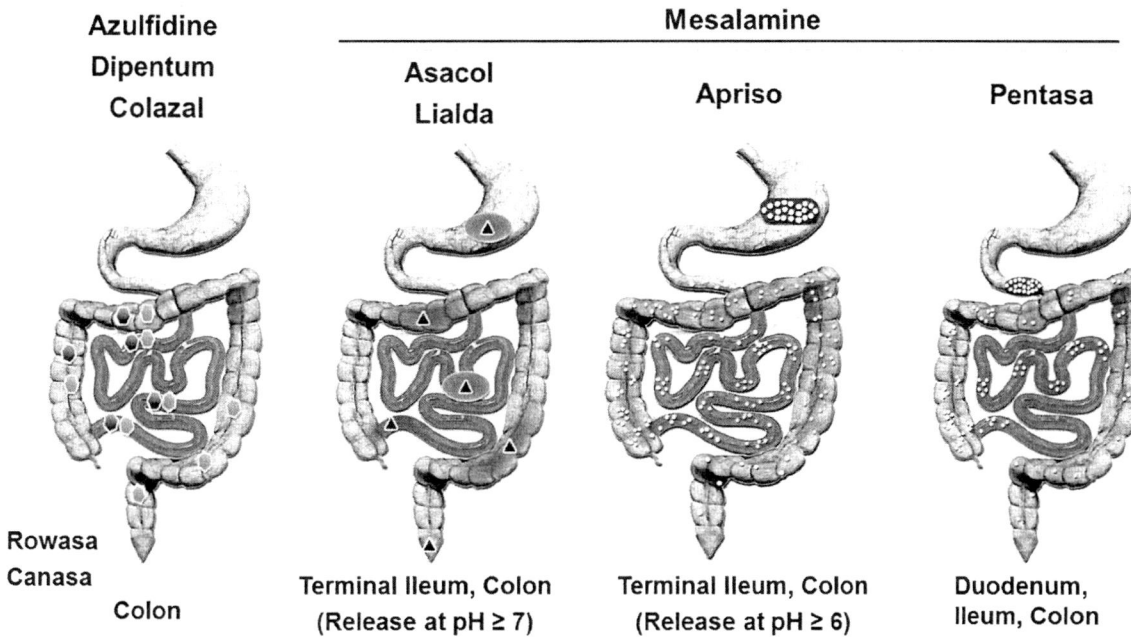

Azulfidine Dipentum Colazal

Mesalamine

Asacol Lialda

Apriso

Pentasa

Rowasa Canasa

Colon

Terminal Ileum, Colon (Release at pH ≥ 7)

Terminal Ileum, Colon (Release at pH ≥ 6)

Duodenum, Ileum, Colon

Adapted from Baumgart DC, Sandborn WJ. *Lancet.* 2007;369:1641–1657.
Adapted from Sandborn WJ. *J Clin Gastroenterol.* 2008;42:338–344.

Adverse Effects Associated with Oral 5-ASAs

Sulfasalazine		Olsalazine, Balsalazide, Mesalamine
Headache	Pancreatitis	Headache
Nausea/vomiting	Pericarditis	Nausea
Dyspepsia	Hepatitis	Rash
Anorexia	Paradoxical exacerbation of colitis	Hair loss
Rash		Interstitial nephritis
Bone marrow suppression		Pericarditis
Interstitial nephritis		Pneumonitis
Megaloblastic anemia		Hepatitis
Apparently reversible oligospermia		Pancreatitis
		Paradoxical exacerbation of colitis
Folate malabsorption		Secretory diarrhea (olsalazine)
Connective tissue disease		

Kornbluth A, Sachar DB. *Am J Gastroenterol.* 2010;105:501.
Sands B. *Gastroenterology.* 2000;118:S68.
Azulfidine (sulfasalazine) [package insert]. New York, NY: Pfizer; August 2006.

IBD Treatment — Steroids
- Budesonide
  - Enteric-coated
  - Ileal Crohn's
  - New formulation that releases in colon
  - Mild-to-moderate disease
- Prednisone
  - Oral or IV
- Topical steroids
  - Enema
  - Suppository

Steroid Side Effects

Event	Estimated Frequency
Any side effect leading to the d/c of prednisone	55%
Ankle swelling	11%
Facial swelling	35%
Easy bruising	7%
Acne	50%
Memory problems	7%
Psychosis	1%
Infections	13%
Cataracts	9%
Increased intraocular pressure	22%
HTN	13%
Osteoporosis	33%
Diabetes	10x increased risk

When to Introduce Other Medications?
- Tipping point is usually steroids
- Steroid dependent disease?
  - Immunomodulators/Biologics
- Steroid refractory disease?
  - Immunomodulators/Biologics?

IBD Treatment — Immunomodulators
- Azathioprine and 6-MP and methotrexate
- Takes 3–4 months to start working
- Bone marrow suppression, esp. WBC — monthly CBC first year
- Pancreatitis in 1 to 5% of patients
- Raises risk of lymphoma
- Use for Crohn's or UC

IBD Treatment — Biologic Therapies
- Tumor necrosis factor (TNF) antagonists
  - Certolizumab, golimumab, infliximab, adalimumab
  - Indications:

	Mod–severe active Crohn's	Refractory ulcerative colitis
Certolizumab pegol	Yes	No
Golimumab	No	Yes
Infliximab	Yes	Yes
Adalimumab	Yes	Yes

  - Generally requires ongoing treatment
  - Screen for TB before treating
  - Screen for hepatitis B before treating
  - Lymphoma risk

- Vedolizumab: Antiintegrin
  - Humanized monoclonal antibody that blocks the interaction between alpha 4 beta 7 integrin and mucosal address in cell adhesion molecule-1 (MAdCAM-1), thereby inhibiting the migration of memory T-lymphocytes across the inflamed intestinal wall in Crohn's and UC
  - Indications: Crohn's disease or ulcerative colitis that is steroid dependent or refractory to treatment

- Ustekinumab (approved Nov. 2016)
  - Anti-IL12/23
  - Indications: Crohn's disease is steroid dependent or refractory to treatment (likely not to be on exam)

IBD Treatment — Antibiotics
- Metronidazole
  - Crohn's: Perianal abscess, fistula
    - Occasional maintenance use
  - Ulcerative colitis: Only if peritonitis, toxic megacolon, pouchitis
  - Side effects, esp. neuropathy, limit long-term use
  - Ciprofloxacin also used

Back to our Patient
- She has ileocolonic Crohn's disease with ileal inflammation, perianal fistula, and possible erythema nodosum
- How should we proceed with her treatment?

Our Patient
- Started Budesonide
- Plan to start anti-TNF agent after her wedding and honeymoon that was in 1 week
- 1 week after honeymoon, had worsening and increasing RLQ pain worse after eating, and had abdominal distention with nausea/vomiting and inability to pass gas or bowel movement
- Admitted to hospital for SBO

Indications for Surgery
- Exsanguinating hemorrhage
- Fibrostenotic stricture with obstruction
- Abscess
- Perforation
- Toxic megacolon
- Failure of medical therapy
- Cancer/Dysplasia

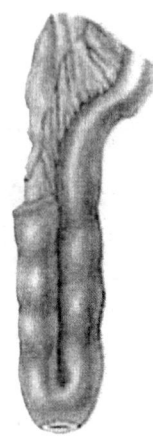

Crohn's Obstruction
Surgical options are generally resection vs. stricturoplasty (repair)

UC Surgery
Total proctocolectomy with option of
- Ileal pouch anal anastomosis/J-pouch: A "neo-reservoir" is fashioned from small intestine

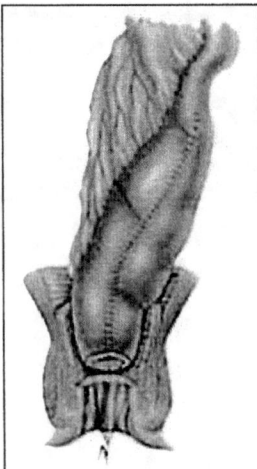

- Permanent ileostomy: Attaches terminal ileum to skin and allows patient to wear bag to collect stool

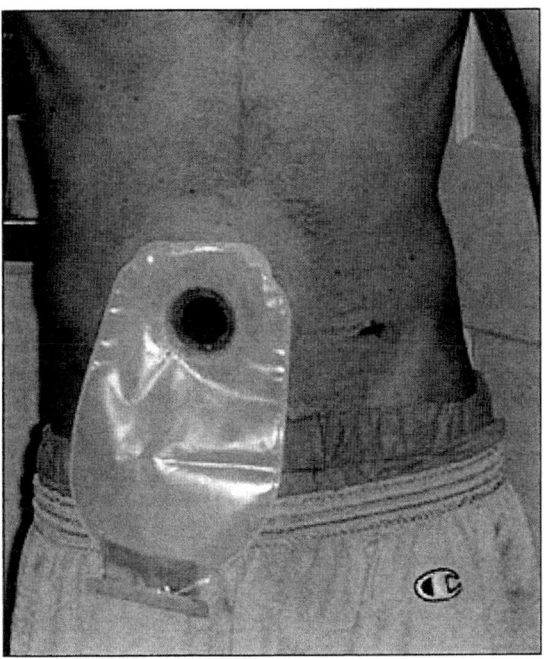

Our Patient
- She underwent a laparoscopic ileocecectomy for an ileal stricture
- Small perianal fistula noted during surgery, seton was placed
- Post-operatively did well
- Placed on post-operative maintenance therapy of anti-TNF

Crohn's Disease — Treatment Scenarios
- Colon only: Mesalamine, also sulfasalazine
- Small bowel involvement: Mesalamine and budesonide (if mild/very mild)
- Fistula or perianal: Metronidazole, 6-MP, anti-TNF (infliximab/adalimumab/**certo**lizumab)
- Steroid-dependent or refractory: 6-MP/azathioprine, anti-TNF (infliximab/adalimumab/**certo**lizumab), or vedolizumab
- Acute small bowel obstruction: Corticosteroids, possible surgery

Ulcerative Colitis — Treatment
- Mild disease: Sulfasalazine, 5-ASA, topical
  - Treatment by extent
    - Proctitis: Suppository mesalamine
    - Proctosigmoiditis: Enema (hydrocortisone or mesalamine
- Moderate to severe: Steroids for Induction, then immunomodulators or anti-TNF agents or antiintegrin therapy
- Fulminant: Hospital, IV fluids, cyclosporine or anti-TNF agents or surgery

AR 13
25-year-old female presents with diagnosis of UC for 3 years, previously maintained on mesalamine 2.4 g daily. She had flare up of symptoms 2 weeks ago. Infections ruled out, started on prednisone 40 mg daily with no improvement in symptoms. Reports 8–9 bloody bowel movements daily, abdominal pain, and decreased appetite.
Physical exam: HR 99, BP 110/70, afebrile, abdomen with mild LLQ tenderness, no rebound or guarding
Labs: Hgb 11. 5, CRP 5.6, stool studies negative for *C. difficile*

What is the next appropriate therapy?
A. Increase prednisone to 60 mg daily.
B. Initiate infliximab.
C. Start metronidazole.
D. Refer to surgery.

Answer: _____

AR 14
A 30-year-old woman has long-standing Crohn's disease. She had one prior surgery 3 years ago, at which time 24 inches of the ileum and cecum were removed. She has had no other surgeries and takes mesalamine 1.6 g each day. There has been no evaluation in the past 3 years. She comes into the office with 2 months of intermittent RLQ pain and loose stools. She denies fever, nausea, or vomiting. Exam reveals tenderness in RLQ but without mass.
CBC and LFTs are normal.

What is the most likely diagnosis for this patient?
A. Primary sclerosing cholangitis
B. Gallstones
C. Kidney stones
D. An exacerbation of Crohn's disease

Answer: _____

AR 14 (cont.)
Gallstones, kidney stones, and PSC can all be seen in Crohn's disease. However, most patients — after a resection — will have a recurrence of the Crohn's, and the presentation of chronic diarrhea and abdominal pain in the RLQ would favor this.

What is the most common side effect from infliximab?

A. Reactivate tuberculosis
B. Arthralgias
C. Small bowel perforation
D. Anaphylaxis

Answer: _____

AR 15 (cont.)
They can be very severe.

AR 16
A 27-year-old male has been newly diagnosed with mild-to-moderate ulcerative colitis that has not been treated yet.

He presented with 2 months of bleeding and urgency with his bowel movements. You referred him for colonoscopy, which demonstrated typical ulcerative colitis with disease extending to the splenic flexure. Above the splenic flexure is normal all the way around through the colon and into a normal-appearing terminal ileum.

What would you recommend as the initial treatment for this patient?

A. Oral mesalamine 800 mg PO tid
B. Mesalamine suppositories 1 g qhs
C. Azathioprine 100 mg/day to start and then advance the dosage to 2.5 mg/kg after following his CBC
D. Infliximab 5 mg/kg infusion

Answer: _____

AR 17
An upper GI shows the following:

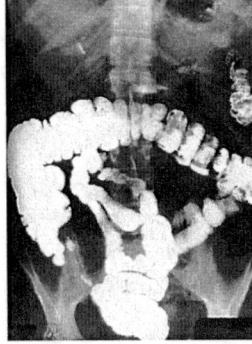 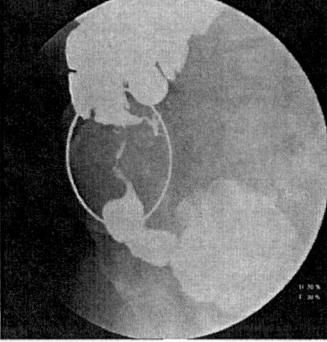

AR 17 (cont.)
What do you recommend?

A. Surgery consult.
B. Course of steroids.
C. Do nothing.
D. Start infliximab.

Answer: _____

Crohn's Disease
- Complications related to ileal disease/resection
  - Calcium oxalate kidney stones
  - Cholesterol gallstones
  - B_{12} deficiency
  - Hypocalcemia (vitamin D malabsorption)
  - Bile acid–induced diarrhea (< 100 cm resected, cholestyramine)
- Steatorrhea 2° depleted bile acids (> 100 cm resected, low-fat diet, and medium-chain triglycerides)

Ulcerative Colitis — Cancer Risk
- 2 key factors: Duration of disease and extent of disease (PSC most serious)
- Duration of disease: 2% — 10 years, 15% — 20 years
- Disease extent: Pancolitis obviously greater risk than proctitis
- Screening: Colonoscopy q 1–2 years after 8 years after onset of symptoms in pancolitis, 15 years if left-sided colitis, start immediately if PSC
- High-grade dysplasia: Colectomy
- Any mass lesion or stricture or cancer: Colectomy
- Remember that incidental adenomas happen too

Possible Exam Question
- Crohn's and osteoporosis
- May or may not have prior history of steroid use
- Only 30% have normal bone density
- IBD and increased risk of DVT

Ulcerative Colitis
- Pearls
  - If flare: R/O *C. difficile*, and also remember the other bacterial infections
  - Biopsies for CMV/HSV, esp. if immune suppressed
  - Loperamide (Imodium) is okay

IBD — Miscellaneous
- Colonoscopy: Usual method to assess
- Very little role for barium enema
- Never BE in acute illness
- Crohn's patients should quit smoking
- Most UC patients are nonsmokers — can even use nicotine patches for extra "push" in fulminant UC

Diarrhea
- Definition: More than 200–250 g/day
  - Normal is 150–180 g/day
  - Normal frequency 3–21 stools/week
- Mechanism: Osmotic, secretory, increased motility
- Timing: Acute vs. chronic

Acute Diarrhea
- Acute is up to 14 days
- 14–30 days is persistent
- More than 30 days is chronic
- Check diet and travel history

- Work up with stool cultures, rule out parasites (O&P) if appropriate history, *Giardia* and *Crypto* antigen, *C. difficile* toxin
- Very rarely is endoscopy needed
- Oral rehydration or IV fluids

Infectious Diarrhea
- Viral
  - Rotavirus: Most common
  - Norovirus: Cruise ship
- Bacterial
- Protozoal: Consider if prolonged; *Giardia* and *Cryptosporidium*
- Viral most common of all diarrhea
- Bacterial most common if severe

AR 18
A 24-year-old female is back from spring break in Cancun. She was there for nearly a week. Three days into the trip, she developed watery diarrhea — up to 6 bowel movements a day. She has mild abdominal cramps, but no bleeding or fever. The symptoms lasted 3 days, and then she had no bowel movements for 2 days. It is now 6 days later, and her bowel movements are back to normal.

At this point, which of the following do you recommend?
A. Rifaximin 400 mg PO bid for 5 days
B. Ciprofloxacin 500 mg bid for 5 days
C. Metronidazole 500 mg tid for 5 days
D. No treatment

Answer: _____

Traveler's Diarrhea
- Definition: Occurs during or within 10 days of travel
- Attack rate: Up to 40%
- Most common: Enterotoxigenic and enteroadherent *E. coli* (ETEC and EAEC)
- Lasts 3–5 days
- Prevention is key

- Prevent with bismuth subsalicylate (Pepto-Bismol, Kaopectate) or *Lactobacillus* or rifaximin (overkill)
- Treat: TMP/SMX, doxycycline, fluoroquinolone, rifaximin

Acute Diarrhea (cont.)
- Infectious: Invasive
  - *Salmonella* (sickle cell, achlorhydria)
  - *Campylobacter* (most common)
  - *Shigella*
  - *Yersinia* (joint pains, rash)
  - *E. coli* O157:H7
  - Does cause histologic damage
  - Stool WBC positive, ± for RBCs
  - Patient may be febrile

Acute Diarrhea — When to Admit for Evaluation
- Profuse diarrhea
- Hypovolemia
- Bloody diarrhea, fever
- Significant abdominal pain
- Immunocompromised or elderly patient
- Recent antibiotics or hospitalization

Campylobacter jejuni
- Most common bacterial colitis
- 90%: Diarrhea and fever
- Abdominal pain and bloody stools common
- Assoc with Guillain-Barré
- Erythromycin and azithromycin preferred; Ciprofloxacin works, but increasing resistance
- No treatment if mild

Salmonella
- Same symptoms
- Treat if severe, sepsis, or underlying medical or immune disorder
- Resistance ampicillin and TMP/SMX (okay to use if sensitive)
- Ciprofloxacin effective, higher relapse
- Levofloxacin for 5–7 days

Shigella
- Small inoculum
- Treat with ampicillin unless PCN-allergic or community has resistance
- TMP/SMX effective
- Fluoroquinolone good choice if acquired in developing country

Hemorrhagic *E. coli* (O157:H7)
- Contaminated beef
  - Inadequate cooking
- Sporadic and epidemic disease
- Bloody diarrhea, often nausea and vomiting
- Right colon involved
- Complicated hemolytic uremic syndrome and TTP (elderly and children)
- Don't treat with antibiotics

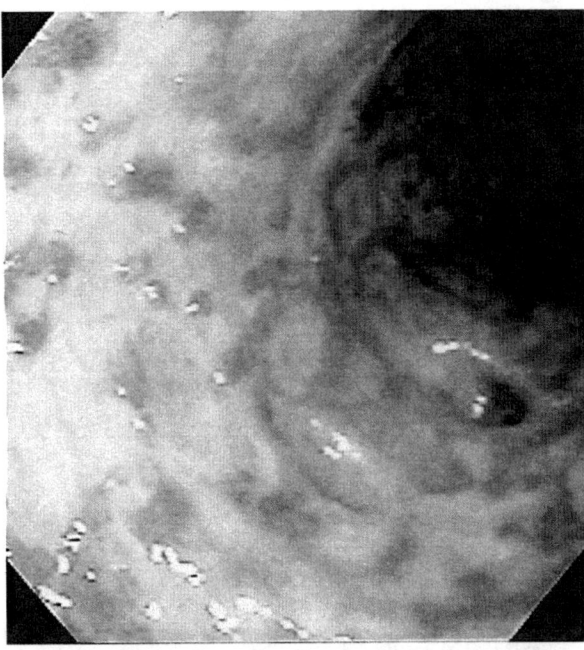

Issues in Infectious Diarrhea
- Can you use diphenoxylate hydrochloride and atropine sulfate (Lomotil)/loperamide?
- Empiric antibiotic treatment if severe: > 8 stools per day, bloody, fever, volume depletion, severe enough for admit, immunocompromised
- Empiric Tx — fluoroquinolone
- Postinflammatory irritable bowel syndrome

Amoebiasis
Travelers and immigrants. Most are asymptomatic; or symptoms can be prolonged or subacute. 1% fulminant.
- Diarrhea can be bloody, abdominal pain, constitutional symptoms
- Dx: Stool trophozoites, PMNs, serologic tests
- Stool antigen by ELISA is best
- Tx: Metronidazole + iodoquinol
- And paromomycin

Computerized tomography of amebic liver abscess in the right lobe of the liver.

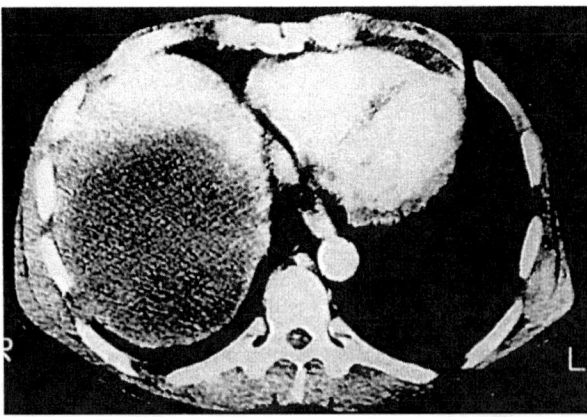

Amebic Liver Abscess
- Most common extraintestinal manifestation
- Fever, RUQ pain, WBC > 10,000
- Concurrent diarrhea in approx 1/3
- Abnormal LFTs common; alk phos in 75%
- Rare increase in bili
- Multiple abscesses
- Complications: Rupture into chest, peritoneum

AR 19
A 51-year-old male returns from a Montana fishing and camping trip complaining of the sudden onset of diarrhea, abdominal distention, and foul-smelling flatus. He denies any prior history of bowel complaints before this.

The empiric use of which of the following antibiotics would be most likely to give this person relief?
A. Metronidazole
B. Vancomycin
C. Ciprofloxacin
D. Amoxicillin/clavulanate

Answer: _____

Parasitic Infections
- Giardiasis
  - Scenarios: Travel (mountain streams — anywhere in the world), day care workers
  - Presentation: Acute, subacute, and chronic; Foul-smelling diarrhea, bloating, cramps, malabsorption, weight loss
  - *Giardia* is hardy in cold water and resistant to chlorine at the levels used in water treatment facilities

Giardiasis
- How to treat?
  - Metronidazole and tinidazole
- How to diagnose?
  - Stool antigen
- Is there eosinophilia? **No**
- Is there fever? **Rarely**
- Are there fecal leukocytes? **No**
- Consider empiric treatment if history/geography suggestive

C. difficile Colitis
- Pseudomembranous colitis
- Caused by many antibiotics — 1–8 weeks
- Other risk factors: GI surgery, elderly, enteral feeding
- Is PPI use a risk factor?
- Hospital- or community-acquired

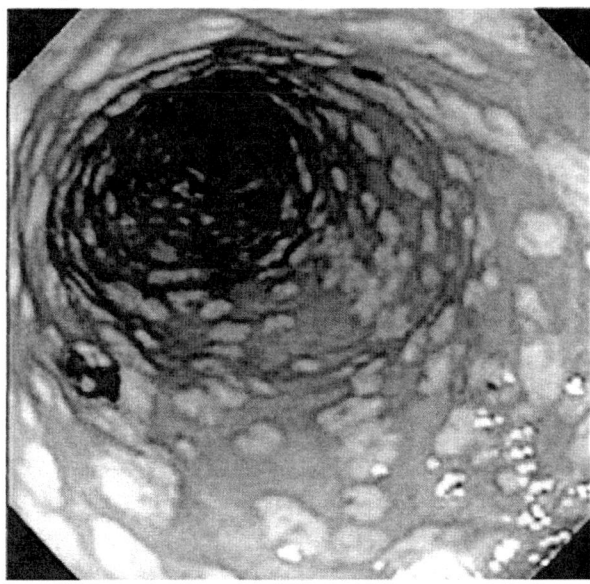

C. difficile Colitis (cont.)
- Symptoms
  - Increasing frequency
  - Diarrhea may have blood
  - Abdominal pain, fever
  - Leukocytosis is common

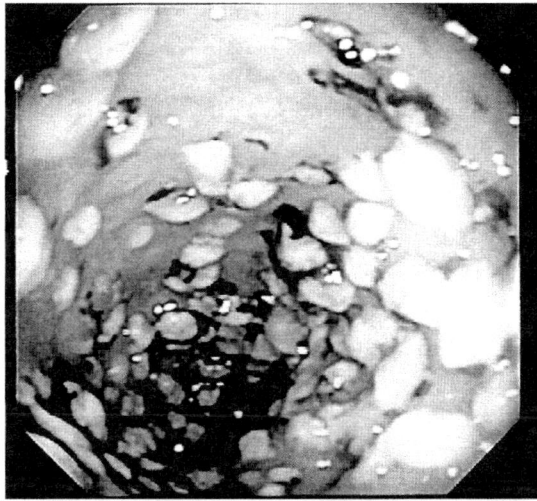

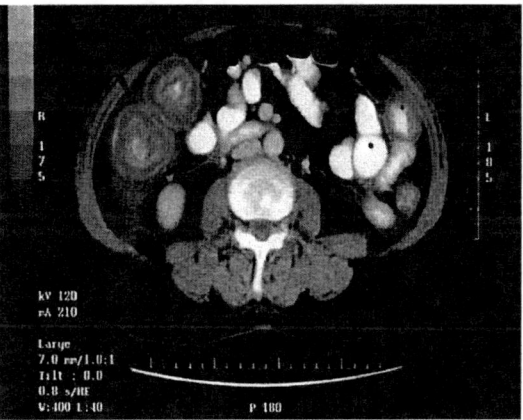

C. difficile Colitis (cont.)
- Diagnosis
  - Stool PCR**: Tests for gene encoding toxin B, preferred test
  - Stool toxin, enzyme immunoassay: Sensitivity 90% if 3 stools sent
  - Stool culture
  - Sigmoidoscopy — pseudomembranes not always seen

Testing for *Clostridium difficile*
- PCR assay
  - Tests for gene encoding toxin B
  - Preferred test by ACG[1]
- Enzyme immunoassay
  - Detects toxin A or B
  - Previously most widely used, however reduced sensitivity (toxins degrade in environment)
- Glutamate dehydrogenase (GDH) screening
  - Sensitive (high NPV) but not specific, therefore need confirmatory test (PCR or EIA)

Surawicz et al. *The American Journal of Gastroenterology*. April 2013.

CDC: Frequently Asked Questions about *Clostridium difficile* for Healthcare Providers.

Testing for *Clostridium difficile* (cont.)
- Stool culture
  - Most sensitive, but no diagnostic use; false positives due to nontoxigenic *Clostridium difficile* strains
  - Can reduce false positive by testing isolates for toxin production
- Antigen detection for *Clostridium difficile*
  - Similar to stool culture, not specific for toxigenic strains and requires confirmatory test
- Tissue culture cytotoxicity assay
  - Detects toxin B
  - Historical gold standard, but costly and timely; now less sensitive than PCR

Surawicz et al. *The American Journal of Gastroenterology.* April 2013.
CDC: Frequently Asked Questions about *Clostridium difficile* for Healthcare Providers.

C. difficile Colitis
- Treatment
- Based on severity of disease
  - Metronidazole
  - Vancomycin
  - Fidaxomicin
  - Fecal microbiota transplant
  - Surgery

Current Approach to Therapy

Initial episode

Mild-to-moderate infection	Metronidazole 500 mg orally tid x 10 days *consider switching to vancomycin if no improvement in 5-7 days
Severe infection (or intolerance of metronidazole)	Vancomycin 125 mg orally qid x 10 days
Severe and complicated	Vancomycin 500 mg orally qid and metronidazole 500 mg IV q 8 hr and vancomycin 500 mg per rectum qid

First recurrence

Mild-to-moderate infection	Metronidazole 500 mg tid x 10 days *consider switching to vancomycin if no improvement in 5-7 days **Alternative: Fidaxomicin 200 mg bid x 10 days
Severe infection (or intolerance of metronidazole)	Vancomycin 125 mg qid x 10 days

Second recurrence

	Vancomycin pulse: 125 mg qid x 10 days 125 mg daily q 3 days for 30 more days
	Alternative: Fidaxomicin 200 mg bid x 10 days

Third recurrence

	Fecal microbiota transplant

Surawicz et al. *The American Journal of Gastroenterology,* April 2013

Possible Exam Topics
- Initial treatment — metronidazole or vancomycin for 10–14 days
- 1st Relapse — confirm & treat the same
- 2nd Relapse — confirm & tapering vancomycin or fidaxomicin
- Complications — acute abdomen and toxic megacolon then surgery
- Recurrent *C. difficile*, consider fecal transplant

What is Chronic Diarrhea?
- **Dictionary:**
  "Abnormal frequency and liquidity of fecal evacuations"
- **Research:**
  a) > 3 bowel movements per day
  b) Stool weight > 200 g/day
- **Patients:**
  a) Generally do not weigh stools
  b) Inc liquidity (<u>consistency</u>)

Classification of Chronic Diarrhea

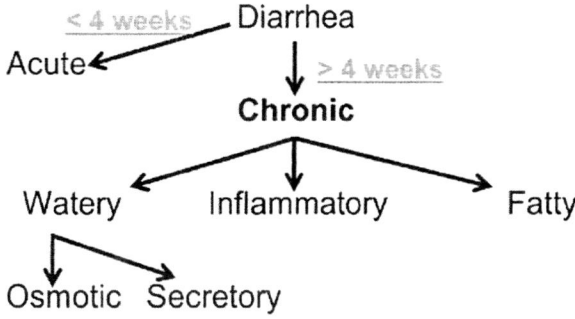

Bristol Stool Chart

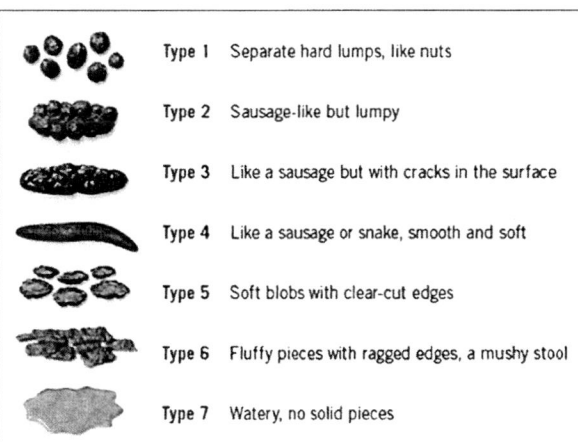

	Type 1	Separate hard lumps, like nuts
	Type 2	Sausage-like but lumpy
	Type 3	Like a sausage but with cracks in the surface
	Type 4	Like a sausage or snake, smooth and soft
	Type 5	Soft blobs with clear-cut edges
	Type 6	Fluffy pieces with ragged edges, a mushy stool
	Type 7	Watery, no solid pieces

Pathophysiology
- Normally SB and colon absorb 99% of both oral intake and endogenous secretions from salivary glands, stomach, liver, pancreas (9–10 L/day)
- Water is not actively transported; moves across intestinal mucosa secondary to osmotic forces generated by the transport of solutes
- Diarrhea results from disruption of this normally fine-tuned mechanism

McNally. *GI/Liver Secrets*. 2001.

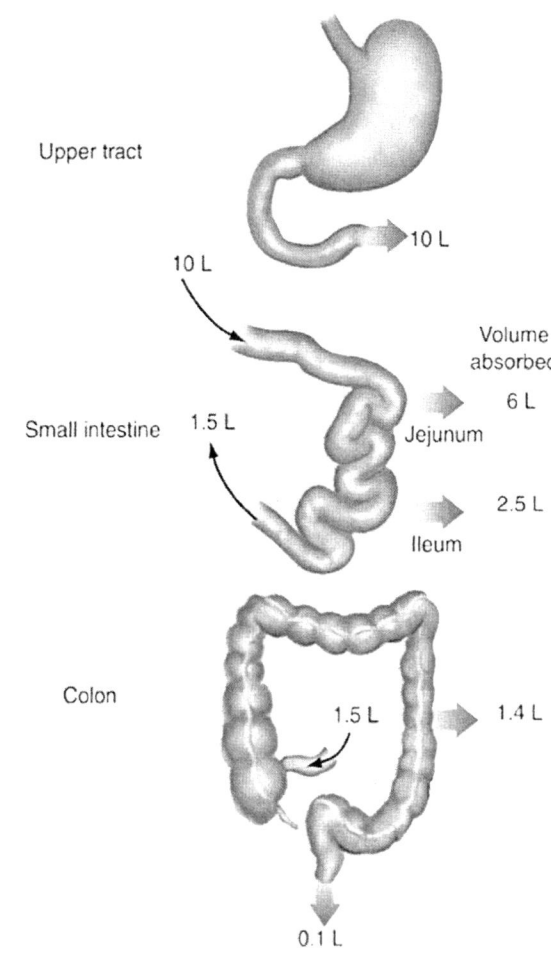

Major Pathophysiologic Mechanisms for Diarrhea
1) Osmotic load within the intestine resulting in retention of water within the lumen
2) Excessive secretion of electrolytes and water into the intestinal lumen
3) Exudation of fluid and protein from the intestinal mucosa
4) Altered intestinal motility resulting in rapid transit through the colon

Osmotic Diarrhea
- Ingestion of poorly absorbed, osmotically active substances
  - Retains fluid in intestinal lumen → diarrhea
- **Ions:** Magnesium, sulfate, phosphate
- Lactose intolerance common cause
- Poorly absorbed carbohydrates: Sorbitol, fructose
- Malabsorption: Mucosal defects, bacterial overgrowth
- **Example:**
  - Lactulose — synthetic disaccharide — can't be hydrolyzed → not absorbed → osmotic diarrhea when quantity overwhelms colonic bacteria metabolic capacity

Secretory Diarrhea
- Results from net secretion of anions (chloride or bicarbonate) or net inhibition of sodium absorption
- Infection: Enterotoxin inhibit Na^+–H exchange → inhibits electrolyte/fluid absorption
- Peptides (VIP), neurotransmitters (Ach, serotonin): Alter intracellular messengers ▢ stimulate secretion by intestinal epithelial cells
- Epithelial injury: Shift in balance of absorptive and secretory pathways
  - e.g., viral gastroenteritis
- Dec. intestinal blood flow: Dec. fluid transport?
  - e.g., mesenteric ischemia, radiation enteritis

Fecal Osmotic Gap
- Osmolality of colonic fluid in equilibrium with body fluid (290 mOsm/kg)
- Calculation of osmotic gap
  - Stool Osm = $2(Na^+ + K^+)$ + unmeasured osmotically active molecules
  - **< 50 = secretory**
  - **> 100 = osmotic**

Secretory vs. Osmotic Diarrhea
Secretory
- Large volume
- Persists with fasting
- Osmotic gap < 50
Osmotic
- Stool volume < 1 L
- Decreases with fasting
- Osmotic gap > 100

Chronic Diarrhea Osmotic vs. Secretory		
	Osmotic	Secretory
Volume/day	< 1 L	> 1 L
Effect of Fasting on Diarrhea	Decreases volume > 50%	Decreases volume < 20%
Serum Osmolality (~ stool osmolality)	290	290
Example $[Na^+]$ $[K^+]$ $[Na^+]+[K^+]$ $2([Na^+]+[K^+])$	40 20 60 120	105 40 145 280
Osmolal gap (criteria)	170 (> 50)	10 (< 25)

Inflammatory Diarrhea
Presentation
- Mucoid, bloody stools
- Tenesmus, fever
- Small volume, frequent bowel movements
- Dehydration unusual
- + WBCs, occult blood
Examples
- Intestinal infections
  - *Campylobacter, Salmonella, Shigella, E. coli*
- *C. difficile* colitis
- IBD (UC or Crohn's)
- Radiation, ischemia
- Neoplasm (lymphoma, colon Ca)

Fatty Diarrhea
Presentation
- Greasy, malodorous stools that may float
- Consistency and volume of stools vary
- Fecal fat positive
Examples
- Celiac disease
- Pancreatic insufficiency
- SIBO
- Short bowel syndrome, postresection diarrhea

Chronic Diarrhea — Workup
- History
- Look for alarm signs
- Physical exam
- Diagnostic testing

Helpful History
- FH: IBD, celiac disease, MEN
- Dietary Hx: "Sugar free foods" (sorbitol, mannitol)
- Travel History: *Giardia*, amoeba, *Crypto*
- Weight loss: Malabsorption, panc exocrine insufficiency, neoplasm
- Secondary gain: Laxative abuse
- Systemic illness: Hyperthyroidism, DM, vasculitis, IBD, TB, mastocytosis
- IVDU, sexual promiscuity: AIDS
- Excessive flatus: Carbohydrate malabsorption
- Prior intervention: Radiation enteritis, postsurgical diarrhea
- Leakage of stool: Fecal incontinence
- Hx refractory PUD: Gastrin

Diagnostic Evaluation for Chronic Diarrhea
- Fecal occult blood
- Fecal WBC
- Stool pH
- Stool weight/fat analysis
- Stool culture
- Stool [Na^+], [K^+], osmotic gap
- Biopsy samples of upper/lower GI tract
- Visualization of small bowel (barium vs. capsule)
- Abdominal imaging
- Gut secretory hormones
  - Gastrin, calcitonin, VIP, somatostatin, Urine 5 HIAA (carcinoid syndrome)
- Breath tests
  - Bacterial overgrowth
  - Carbohydrate malabsorption

Helpful PE Findings
- Urticaria pigmentosa → **mastocytosis**
- Macroglossia, waxy papules → **amyloidosis**
- Increased pigmentation → **Addison's disease**
- Migratory necrotizing erythema → **glucagonoma**
- Dermatitis herpetiformis → **celiac disease**
- Flushing, right-sided heart murmur, HM → **carcinoid syndrome**

AR 20
A 51-year-old female presents for evaluation of diarrhea. She reports 4 loose stools daily for the past 2 months. She describes the stools as watery. She reports some crampy mid-abdominal pain. She denies travel, fevers, or blood in stool. She reports taking intermittent ibuprofen for low back pain a few times a week.
Physical exam shows normal vital signs and normal exam. Labs show normal CBC, CMP, lipase, and negative stool cultures.

What is next appropriate step?
A. Abdominal CT scan
B. Dairy- and gluten-free diet
C. Colonoscopy with biopsy
D. Stool electrolytes

Answer: _____

Selected Diarrheal Syndromes

Medications and Toxins Causing Diarrhea
- Acid-suppressing agents (H2RA, PPI)
- Antacids (e.g., those that contain Mg^{2+})
- Antiarrhythmics (e.g., quinidine)
- Antibiotics (most)
- Antiinflammatory agents (e.g., 5ASA, NSAIDs)
- Antihypertensives (e.g., beta-blockers)
- Antineoplastic agents (many)
- Antiretroviral agents
- Colchicine
- Prostaglandin analogs (e.g., misoprostol)
- Theophylline
- Vitamin and mineral supplements, herbal products

Diarrhea in Diabetes
- Occurs in ~ 3.7% of diabetics[1]
- Usually Type 1 with autonomic neuropathy and other complications
  - (5.2% DM1 vs. 0.4% DM2, $p < 0.01$)[1]
  - Correlates with duration of DM and HbA1c
- Course can alternate with diabetic constipation
- Most common cause: Metformin
- Other mechanisms: Enteric neuropathy of SB and colon, SIBO, celiac disease, panc exocrine insufficiency

[1]Goldin. Am J Gastroenterol. 1999.

Lactase Deficiency
- Usually due to delayed loss of lactase activity
- Norm for many populations
- Can be a temporary, secondary feature of infection
- Distention, pain, flatulence, diarrhea
- Diagnosis: Trial vs. tolerance test
- Consider for any IBS patient
- There is a diagnostic test, but of limited utility

AR 21
A 30-year-old female has a long history of loose bowel movements. This has been present for 3–4 years.
On review of systems, it is noted that she has minimal menstrual bleeding each month. She does complain of slight fatigue. She denies any history of overt rectal bleeding. She does say that she has had an itchy rash on the extremities for several months.

AR 21 (cont.)

On physical exam, she is slightly pale but otherwise normal.

With routine lab testing, she is found to have a hemoglobin of 8 g with an MCV of 64. The rest of the CBC and comprehensive metabolic panel are normal.

Which of the following do you recommend?

A. Administer trial of antispasm medicine, like dicyclomine.
B. PRN use of antidiarrheal agents.
C. Increase fiber in the diet.
D. Order tissue transglutaminase (TTG).

Answer: _____

Celiac Sprue
- Malabsorption due to small bowel atrophy of villi
- Clinical spectrum:
  - Variable presentation
  - Rash: Dermatitis herpetiformis
  - Iron deficiency
  - From decreased absorption; Diarrhea, weight loss, malabsorption, osteoporosis, infertility, unexplained increased LFTs

- Genetics: HLA DQ2 — must be present to have it
- Pathogenesis: Immune-mediated gluten sensitivity leads to atrophy of villi and inflammatory infiltrate; Crypt hypertrophy
- Diagnosis:
  - Antigliadin Ab
  - Antiendomysial Ab
  - **Tissue transglutaminase IgA**
- Treatment: Gluten-free diet
- Remember gluten is in wheat, barley, and rye; May be present in oats from cross-contamination
- Most common cause of refractory disease: Noncompliance with diet

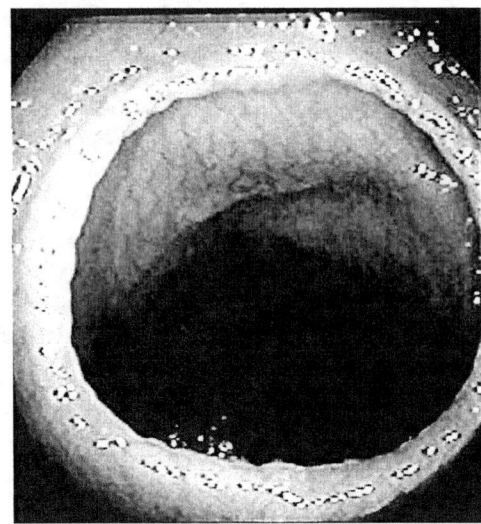

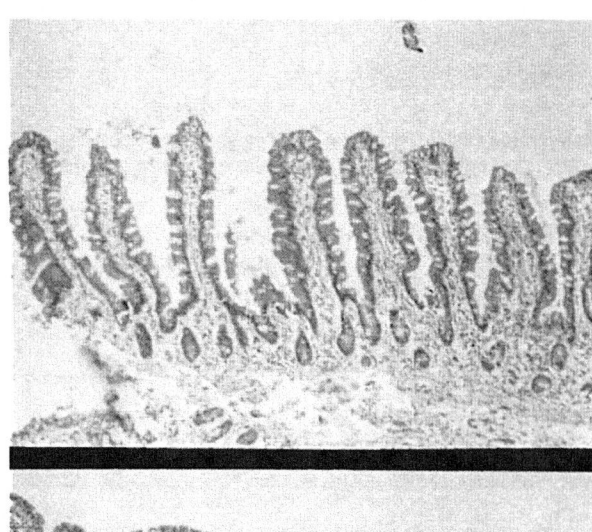

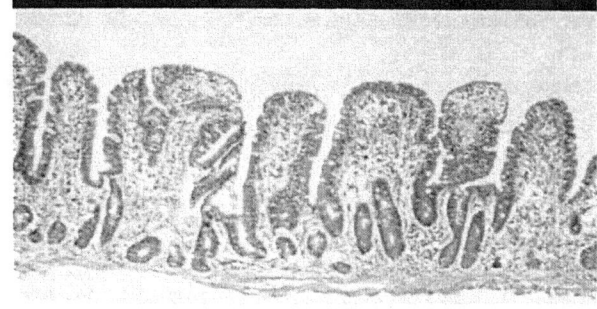

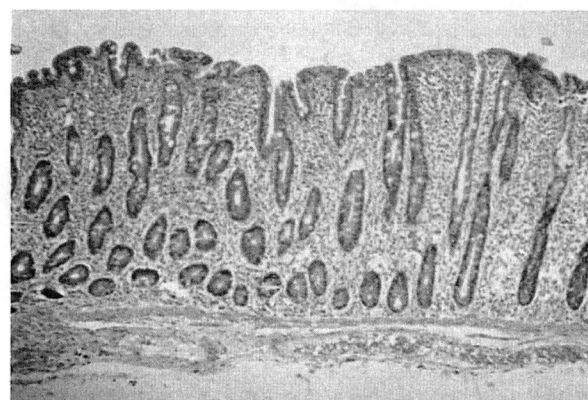

Other Types of Sprue
- Collagenous sprue
- Tropical sprue

Possible Exam Topics
- Association with dermatitis herpetiformis
- Histology of the dermatitis — vesicles, neutrophils, microabscesses
- **Patient with abdominal pain, low ferritin, low calcium, positive serology**
- Sounds like irritable bowel, but anemic or low ferritin
- Associated with osteoporosis

Remember that olmesartan can cause a sprue-like enteropathy!

FDA issued an advisory in 2013, so it's the right time for this to show up on exams!

Whipple Disease
- Tropheryma whipplei
- Symptoms: Weight loss, arthralgias, abdominal pain, diarrhea
- Older male patients
- Diagnosis: Endoscopy with small bowel biopsy
- Bx: Foamy macrophages, bacterial remnants stain with PAS stain
- Ceftriaxone, then TMP for 1 year
- CNS or relapse — long-term ceftriaxone

- Male, chronic diarrhea, malabsorption, and arthralgias
- Dx: Whipple's
- Significance of PAS-positive

How about diarrhea with eosinophilia?
- Eosinophilic gastroenteritis: Yes
- *Strongyloides*: Yes
- *Giardia*: No

Malabsorption — Decreased Digestion
- Pancreatic insufficiency
  - Chronic pancreatitis, pancreatic cancer, cystic fibrosis
- Bile acid deficiency
  - Ileal resection or disease
  - Severe liver disease
  - Bacterial overgrowth

Malabsorption
- Steatorrhea: Best indicator
- Sudan stain: Best screening test
- Serum carotene: Less specific
- Quantitative fecal fat (> 14 g per day)
- Pancreatic insufficiency — the most fecal fat

- Most exam questions: Clear history; e.g., chronic diarrhea described as "oily"
- But there could be no diarrhea and a specific deficiency
  - Iron: Think celiac
  - B_{12}: Think Crohn's

AR 22
A 55-year-old male describes a 1-year history of diarrhea. He has multiple loose stools every day. He denies any abdominal pain or weight loss.
Past medical history: Negative; No medications
Social history: He has not had any alcohol in 5 years but implies that he may have once had a problem with alcohol.
Family history: Negative

Physical exam: Unrevealing
Colonoscopy result is normal.
The initial workup shows a 24-hour fecal fat of 15 g.
You order a D-xylose test, and this is normal. CBC, iron, TIBC, B_{12}, and folate are all normal.

What is the most likely diagnosis in this case?
A. Celiac disease
B. Whipple disease
C. Chronic pancreatitis
D. Carcinoid syndrome

Answer: _____

Malabsorption — Workup
- Steatorrhea; Next step: D-xylose
- NL D-xylose excludes small bowel disease (urine > 5 g after 25-g oral dose)
- Low D-xylose: Small bowel disease, poor gastric emptying, bacterial overgrowth, ascites, renal insufficiency, old age
- Low D-xylose:
  Q: What is next step?
  A: Prob small bowel Bx

Malabsorption — Pearls
- Normal D-xylose:
  - Trial pancreatic enzymes
  - Remember: Normal D-xylose = normal small bowel
- Mucosal malabsorption:
  - Low serum carotene
  - Hypocalcemia
  - Increased prothrombin time (ProTime)
  - Iron deficiency

AR 23
A 50-year-old female has a long history of scleroderma.
For the past year, she has had abdominal distention.
She also has chronic diarrhea, although her weight is stable.
She denies any severe abdominal pain.
Physical examination shows typical scleroderma changes on the face and hands.
The abdomen seems slightly distended and tympanic.
There is no tenderness.

AR 23 (cont.)
Upper GI series done:

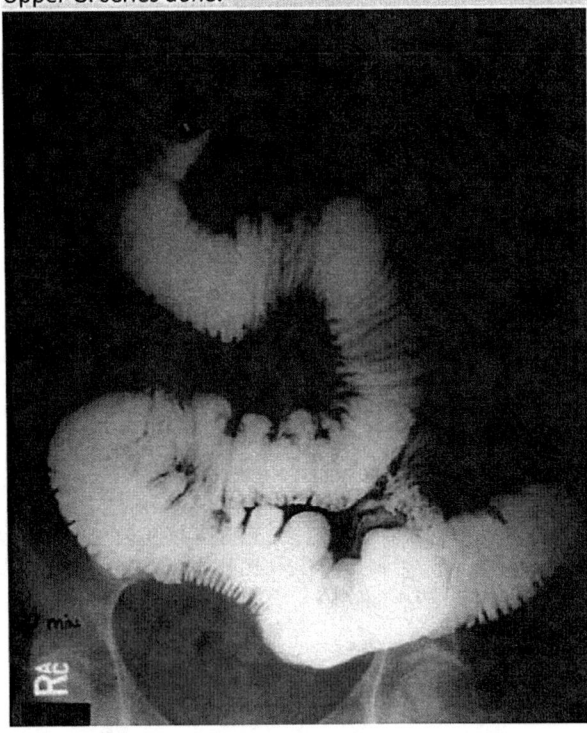

Which of the following treatments is most likely to benefit this patient?
A. A 2-week course of amoxicillin/clavulanate
B. Dicyclomine 10 mg tid
C. Amitriptyline 50 mg qhs
D. Cholestyramine bid

Answer: _____

Bacterial Overgrowth
- Causes:
  - Structural abnormalities: Diverticula, prior surgery
  - Motility disorders: Diabetes, scleroderma
  - Drugs — especially PPI
  - Symptoms: Diarrhea, steatorrhea, abdominal distention, weight loss

- Creates osmotic diarrhea, steatorrhea
  - Bile acid deconjugation by bacteria
  - Destruction brush-border disaccharidases
- Diagnosis
  - Lactulose breath test
  - Empiric trial: Tetracycline, amoxicillin/clavulanate, or rifaximin 550mg bid for 7 to 10 days
- Pearl: Increased folic acid, but high MCV from B_{12} deficiency

Possible Exam Topics
- Chronic diarrhea with flushing episodes:
  - Know diagnosis of carcinoid syndrome
  - Make Dx with urine for 5-HIAA
  - Will an abdominal CT be abnormal — probably with liver mets
  - Syndrome means the tumor is metastatic to liver

Constipation
- Commonly due to medications
- Sudden onset of symptoms implies some obstruction
- Evaluation: If anywhere close to 50 years of age, then colonoscopy
- Complications: Fecal impaction
- Treatment:
  - Dietary fiber, water, exercise
  - Oral polyethylene glycol or lubiprostone
  - Opioids — daily laxatives, consider methylnaltrexone (*NEJM* 2008)
  - Linaclotide (Linzess) is now available

AR 24
An 85-year-old nursing home patient has dementia but has been active enough to ambulate and go to the dining room. She likes watching "Wheel of Fortune" every evening. She also has a long history of constipation, which has been treated with stool softeners.
Today, the patient's daughter calls you. The patient has a new onset of diarrhea. The patient is incontinent of small volume, watery stools. The patient is expressing discomfort, although it is difficult to determine where the discomfort is. The nurse at the nursing home thinks that maybe some of the other residents have been suffering from viral syndromes lately.

What is the most likely diagnosis?
A. *Shigella*
B. Fecal impaction
C. *Giardia*
D. *E. coli* O157:H7

Irritable Bowel Syndrome (IBS)
- Pathophysiology: Increased motor reactivity to various stimuli — meals, CCK balloon distention, stress
- Patient characteristics:
  - Most probably do not seek medical attention
  - Western world: Female-predominant
  - Asia: Male-predominant
  - Increased perception of stress
  - Possible childhood abuse

© 2017 *MedStudy* Internal Medicine Video Board Review – Gastroenterology • Nimisha K. Parekh, MD

- Clinical characteristics:
  - Abdominal pain relieved by defecation
  - Altered stool frequency
  - Altered stool form (hard or loose/watery)
  - Altered stool passage — strain, urgency, incomplete evacuation
  - Abdominal distention
  - No organic symptoms
  - No nocturnal symptoms
  - Chronicity: Symptoms more than 3 months

AR 25

A 24-year-old male, currently in his 6th year of college, describes intermittent diarrhea for 3 years.
The loose stools can alternate with constipation.
He never has nocturnal stools, and suffers with mild abdominal cramps.
PMH negative.
Review of systems: Negative for weight loss, fever, joint pain, and skin rash.
Social history: Beer on weekends, 2 glasses of milk each day, and sugar-free gum constantly.
No travel.

You recommend:
A. 72-hour fecal fat collection
B. Colonoscopy
C. CT of abdomen and pelvis
D. Trial of lactose-free, sorbitol-free diet

Answer: _____

AR 25 (cont.)

This is probably IBS. There are no red flags to prompt an aggressive workup.
Remember that lactose and sorbitol can always be factors.

Irritable Bowel Syndrome (IBS)
- Evaluation
  1) Avoid unneeded tests
  2) Diagnosis of exclusion
  3) Stool tests
  4) R/O lactose intolerance, sorbitol use
  5) Role of invasive test, like sigmoidoscopy or colonoscopy
  6) Always be on the lookout for "red flags": Bleeding, weight loss, anemia
  7) Always keep celiac disease in back of mind

IBS — Possible Exam Topics
- Fiber 1st step
- Dicyclomine
- TCA for refractory symptoms
- Sexual abuse history
- Diagnosis in a patient with bloating and alternating diarrhea and constipation

IBS
- IBS is the most common cause of chronic diarrhea
- But if weight loss, increased inflammatory markers, anemia, you should think other disease, such as celiac or inflammatory bowel disease
- If late onset (e.g., age 45), order colonoscopy with biopsy

Microscopic Colitis
- Chronic, watery diarrhea (500–1,000 g/day)
- Middle-aged-to-elderly female
- Associations: NSAIDs, autoimmune disease
- Know how to make diagnosis: Need colonoscopy or sigmoidoscopy with biopsy of normal-looking mucosa
- Many options for treatment
- Does not evolve into ulcerative colitis or Crohn's (though case reports)

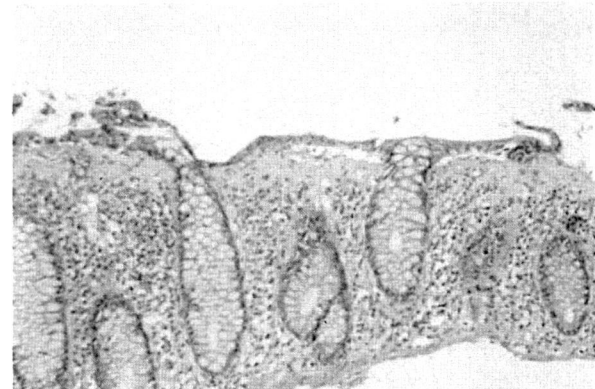

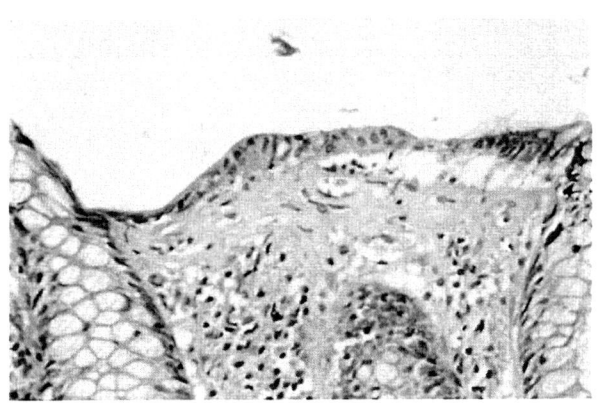

Colon Polyps
- Most colon cancers arise from adenomas
- Risk of cancer: Size > 2 cm, sessile base, multiple polyps, villous
- Present in 25% of Americans > 50 years
- No malignant potential: Hyperplastic polyps
- Treatment: Remove at colonoscopy and follow closely

Polyp-Cancer Sequence

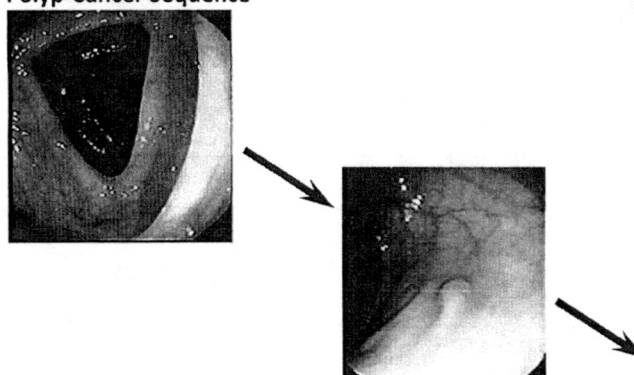
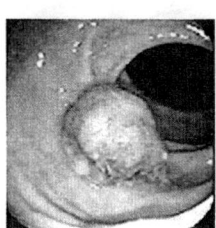
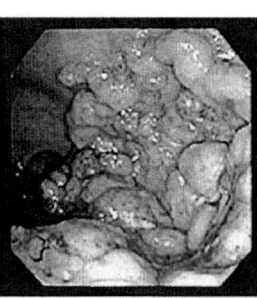

AR 26

A 55-year-old male is in for an executive health check. He has no specific complaints and is not taking any medications. He doesn't have any family history of colon cancer. As part of the exam, you recommend screening colonoscopy, and this is performed.
On this exam, a pedunculated 5-mm polyp in the ascending colon was removed with snare technique.
The pathology of the polyp showed a tubular adenoma.
The patient now asks you when he should have a follow-up colonoscopy.

Which of the following recommendations do you give the patient regarding follow-up colonoscopy?
A. 1 year.
B. 5 years.
C. 10 years.
D. No follow-up is needed.

Answer: _____

AR 26 (cont.)

Know the appropriate intervals for colonoscopy:
- If no polyp or hyperplastic, can f/u in 10 years
- 1 or 2 small (≤ 5 mm) adenomas, then 5 years
- 3–10 adenomas or 1 adenoma > 1 cm, then 3 years
- 10 adenomas, repeat colonoscopy < 3 years
Polyps that are removed piecemeal require repeat colonoscopy in 2–6 months

Polyp Surveillance
- Repeat colonoscopy in 3 years for any of the following:
  - 3–10 adenomas found
  - Any adenoma > 10 mm
  - Any adenoma with villous features
  - Any adenoma with high-grade dysplasia

Screening/Surveillance

Baseline colonoscopy: Most advanced finding(s)	Recommended interval (y)
No polyps	10
Small HPs in rectum or sigmoid	10
1–2 small (< 10 mm) adenomas	5–10
3–10 adenomas	3
> 10 adenomas	< 3
Any adenoma > 10 mm	3
Any adenoma with villous elements (villous or tubulovillous) **or** with high-grade dysplasia	3

Adapted from U.S. Multi-Society Task Force on Colorectal Cancer, 2012.

Serrated Polyp Surveillance

Baseline colonoscopy: Most advanced finding(s)	Recommended interval (y)
SSA(s) < 10 mm with no dysplasia	5
SSA(s) ≥ 10 mm	3
SSA with dysplasia	3
Traditional serrated adenoma	3
Serrated polyposis syndrome*	1

*Data from WHO Classification of Tumors of the Digestive System
At least 5 serrated polyps proximal to the sigmoid colon, with 2 or more being > 10 mm, OR
Any number of serrated polyps proximal to the sigmoid colon in an individual who has a first-degree relative with serrated polyposis, OR
> 20 serrated polyps of any size, distributed throughout the colon
Adapted from U.S. Multi-Society Task Force on Colorectal Cancer, 2012.

Familial Adenomatous Polyposis (FAP)
- Autosomal dominant
- FAP: Hundreds of adenomas, 100% Ca risk
  - Scope to confirm diagnosis
  - Elective proctocolectomy age 20 years
- Gardner syndrome: Same as FAP except bone lesions — osteomas, soft tissue tumors

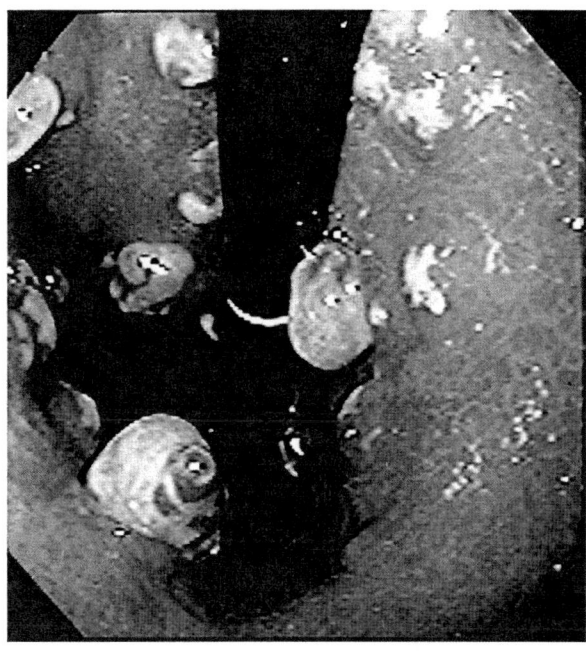

Keys to FAP
- Suspect diagnosis based on family history
- Make diagnosis
- Offer colectomy
- Later, screen upper GI tract with EGD
  - Gastric polyps — not a factor
  - Duodenal polyps — a big deal
- Screen family members

Familial Polyposis Syndromes
- Peutz-Jeghers Syndrome
  - Hamartomatous polyps GI tract
  - Pigmentation on lips
  - Can bleed or obstruct
  - Main clinical problem early: Small bowel obstruction from intussusception
  - Clinical problem later: At risk for different malignancies

Hereditary Nonpolyposis Colon Ca
- HNPCC or Lynch syndrome
- Colon Ca in three 1st degree relatives over 2 generations, one with Dx < 50 years of age (3-2-1)
- Right-sided colon cancers
- Other malignancies: Endometrial, ovarian, renal, ureteral, gastric, pancreas, biliary tree
- Start screening early
  - Colonoscopy at 25

AR 27

A 30-year-old man comes to your office to establish health care. He has no specific complaints and feels well and healthy. He does relate that his father was diagnosed with colon cancer at the age of 45. His father was part of a family with 5 siblings, and none of them have had colon cancer. Likewise, neither of the father's parents had colon cancer.

The patient asks if he would be at increased risk for colon cancer and if there is any screening test that would be appropriate.

Which of the following would be recommended?

A. Colonoscopy at age 35 years
B. Colonoscopy at age 45 years
C. Colonoscopy at age 50 years
D. CT colonography (virtual colonoscopy) now

Answer: _____

Colon Cancer Risk Factors

- Age > 50 years
- History of adenomas
- 1st degree relative
- Familial polyposis
- Ulcerative colitis or Crohn's
- Hereditary nonpolyposis: HNPCC
  - GI tract, brain, endometrium, urinary tract, ovaries
  - Misnomer — they do get polyps but not always
- Diet: High fat, low fiber

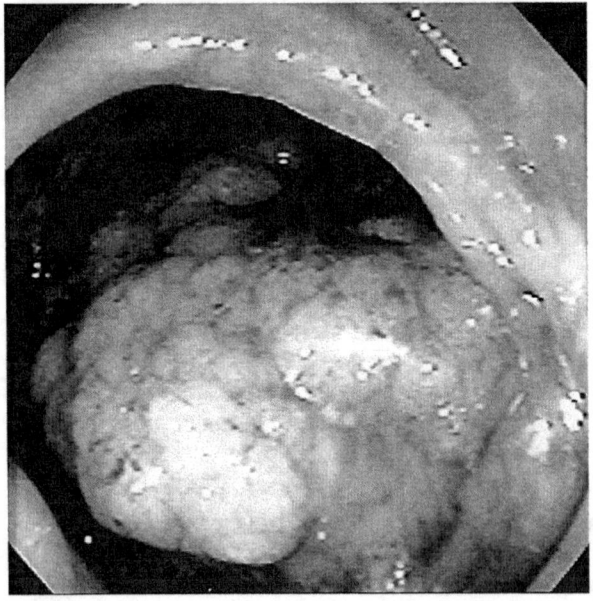

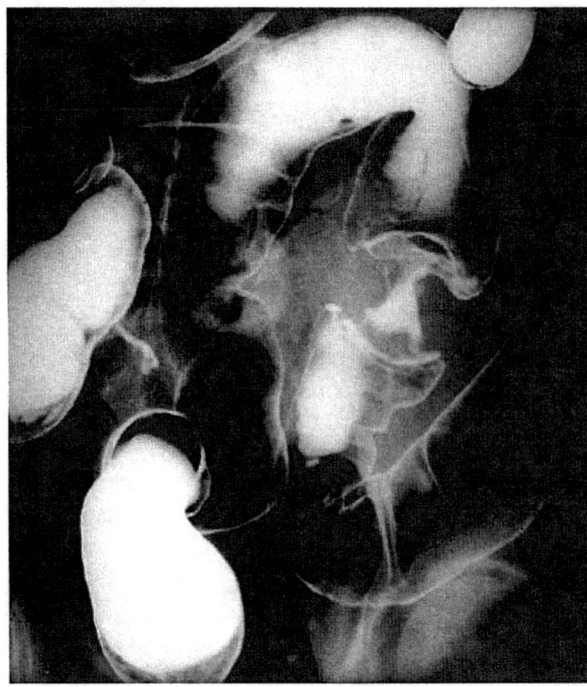

Colon Cancer Screenings

4 options:
1) Fecal occult blood test q 1 year
2) Flexible sigmoidoscopy q 4–5 years
3) Double contrast barium enema q 5 years
4) Colonoscopy q 10 years

How about virtual colonoscopy?
   Maybe best use is incomplete scope to evaluate rest of colon or patient who can't tolerate sedation. Still requires prep.

Withdrawal times? *NEJM* 2008 — 6 minutes

AR 28

A 60-year-old patient comes in for a general checkup. She has no specific complaints. Past medical history is negative. She is on no medications. She has mild, untreated hyperlipidemia. She is not taking any antiinflammatory drugs at all.

Her family history is negative for GI malignancies. On review of systems, she denies any changes in bowel habits.

As part of her routine check, you recommend a screening colonoscopy, but she declines this exam.

She has heard that it is painful, but she does agree to do 3 stools for occult blood. She mails these back to you, and one of the 3 stools is positive for blood.

You now recommend which of the following?
A. Repeat 3 more stools for occult blood.
B. Encourage her to get a colonoscopy.
C. Recommend a flexible sigmoidoscopy.
D. No further treatment, but simply recheck next year.

Answer: _____

Colon Cancer Screening
- Positive fecal occult blood: 2%
  Significance: Ca 10%, polyp 30%
- Positive test mandates workup: Colonoscopy ideally
- Limitations: Test is negative in more than half of proven cancer patients

- Positive family history
- Single 1st degree family member doubles risk of cancer from 3% to 6% lifetime risk
- Start screening at age 10 years before

Colon Cancer — CEA
- Not a screening test — stands for "carcinoembryonic antigen"
- Can check for recurrence of cancer after resection

Colon Cancer
- TNM I, Dukes A
- Cancer confined to the mucosa and submucosa
- About a quarter of cases
- 5-year survival: 93%
- No treatment after resection, but careful follow-up
- TNM II, Dukes B
- Cancer extends into or through the muscularis, but no lymph node involvement
- About 30% of cases
- 5-year survival: 72–85%
- Chemo if locally advanced

- TNM III, Dukes C
- Cancer extends into lymph nodes
- 26% of cases
- 5-year survival: 44–83%
- Treat with FOLFOX: 5FU + leucovorin + oxaliplatin
- TNM IV, Dukes D
- Distant metastases
- 20% of cases
- 5-year survival: 5%, though higher at some centers

- Radiation helpful for rectal lesions: Reduces local recurrence; Give before surgery
- Metastatic disease: Probably now FOLFOX (leucovorin, 5FU, oxaliplatin)
- Aspirin may reduce risk of death after diagnosis — *JAMA* 2009

Colonoscopy Indications
- Occult bleeding
- Iron deficiency anemia
- Gross lower GI bleeding
  - Not rectal bleeding (bright red) in young
- Abnormal barium enema
- Adenomatous polyp on flexible sigmoidoscopy or in past
- History of colon cancer
- Family history of colon cancer

- FAP, HNPCC
- IBD: Suspicion, follow-up, surveillance
- Bacteremia: *Strep bovis, Clostridium septicum*
- Ischemic colitis
- Decompression
- After an acute attack of diverticulitis: 4–8 weeks later

AR 29
A 72-year-old female with no prior GI history presents to the ED with one day of LLQ pain. This has been constant but not severe. There is no diarrhea or rectal bleeding. She does feel distended. Overnight, she had a fever of 101.0° F (38.3° C). PMH is significant for mild hyperlipidemia.
Family history is negative for GI disease.
She has never had a colonoscopy.
PE: Abdomen slightly distended, and there is tenderness in the LLQ
CBC: WBC 17,000 and Hgb 15 g

You recommend:
A. CT of abdomen and pelvis
B. Colonoscopy
C. Barium enema
D. Mesenteric angiogram

Answer: _____

AR 29 (cont.)
The diagnosis is likely acute diverticulitis, and a CT would help confirm the diagnosis and establish whether a complication, like an abscess, has occurred.
The other tests would not be helpful, and colonoscopy could even be harmful.

Acute Diverticulitis

- LLQ pain, tenderness, mass
- Fever, increased WBC
- Obstipation
- No bleeding!
- CT scan defines abscess
- Avoid endoscopic studies
- Treatment: Fluoroquinolones + metronidazole, or 2nd or 3rd generation cephalosporin
- Complications: Abscess, peritonitis, fistula, obstruction
- When to have surgery

Diverticular Bleeding

- Painless maroon stool
- Diagnosis: Colonoscopy, tagged RBC scan, angiography
- Treatment: Supportive
- Remember: Different from diverticulitis

Oh nooooo!

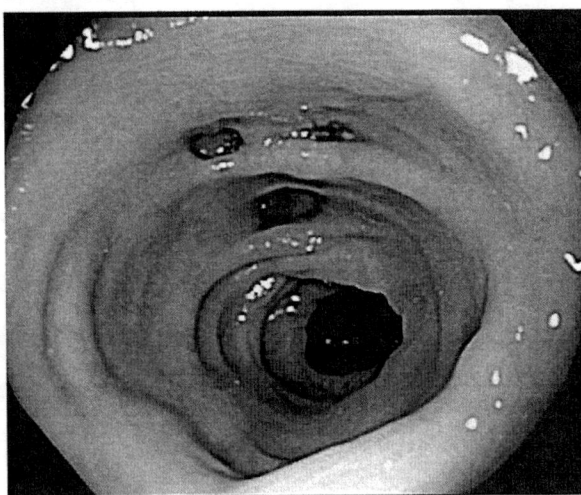

Meckel Diverticulum

- Most frequent congenital GI anomaly
- Cause of half of GI bleeds in children
- Can cause obstruction, intussusception
- Not seen on barium enema, rarely on upper GI series
- Dx with technetium scan

GI Bleeding

- Upper GI bleeding
- Lower GI bleeding
- Obscure GI bleeding
- GI ischemia

AR 30

A 72-year-old man is evaluated in the ED for a 2-week history of gnawing epigastric pain followed by one episode of coffee-ground emesis 6 hours ago. He has a history of prosthetic mitral valve replacement and chronic A-fib, and he had a TIA 1 year ago.
No history of liver disease. His current medications are warfarin and metoprolol. He is started on IV PPI.
On physical exam, BP is 120/85 mmHg, HR 90, RR 16. The abdomen is tender to palpation in the epigastrium. 1There are no stigmata of liver disease.
Labs: Hg 12.5, INR 2.3, BUN 46, Cr 1.0

Which of the following is the most appropriate management?

A. Fresh frozen plasma
B. IV vitamin K
C. PO vitamin K
D. Upper endoscopy

Answer: _____

Types / Location of GI Bleeding

- Hematemesis
  - Suggests source proximal to ligament of Treitz
- Melena
  - Seen with as little as 50 mL of blood
  - 90% proximal to ligament of Treitz
  - Can be small bowel or right colon
- Hematochezia
  - Suggests colonic bleeding
  - **But** could be **rapid** upper GI bleeding

Jensen DM. *Gastroenterology*. 1988 Dec;95(6):1569–74.

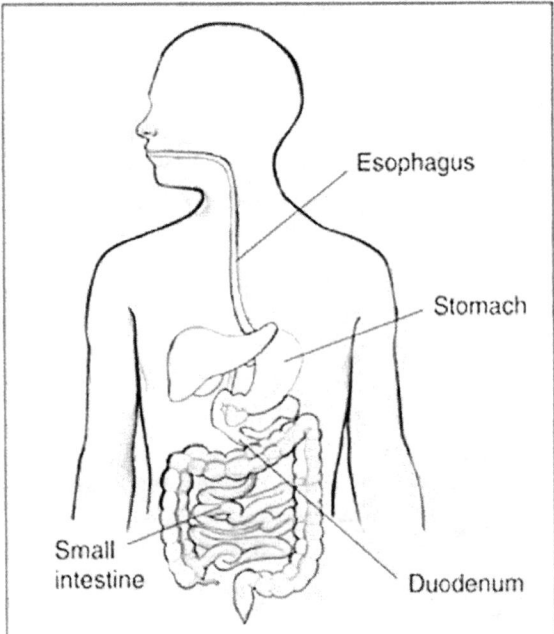

Importance of Vital Signs

Finding	Volume Status
Resting Tachycardia	Mild to Mod Hypovolemia
Orthostatic Hypotension	Blood loss of 15%
Supine Hypotension	Blood loss of > 40%

Resuscitation!
- Resuscitation is the **most** important thing to do for an acute GI bleed
- First step is to obtain appropriate access: Two large bore peripheral IVs or a central line
- Next step is to expand patient's intravascular volume with both crystalloid and, if needed, PRBC
- Transfuse PRBC when Hg < 7 g/dL
- Goal should be Hg > 7–8 g/dL
- Consider higher Hg goal of 9–10 g/dL in patients with significant coronary artery disease

Barkun, et al. *Ann. Int. Med.* 2010.

AR 31
A 40-year-old woman presents to the emergency department after passing a dark, tarry stool this morning. This was followed by the passage of dark red blood. She experienced some lightheadedness but did not pass out, and her family brought her to the emergency department promptly. This woman is otherwise healthy except for arthritis pain, for which she takes ibuprofen on a daily basis. Her only other medicine is 81 mg of aspirin, which she takes because of a family history of coronary artery disease. She has never been told that she has any heart problems.

While in the emergency department, IV fluids are started, and the patient has stable blood pressure and heart rate. A nasogastric tube is passed and lavage of the stomach is negative for any blood.

At this point, which of the following diagnostic studies do you recommend?
A. EGD
B. Tagged RBC bleeding scan
C. Colonoscopy
D. Video capsule

Answer: _____

Teaching Point
- NG tube can be helpful but is not definite; Only determines if blood is in stomach at that point in time — and is only negative if you aspirate bile
- Bleeding could have stopped for past couple of hours or duodenal ulcer could be the cause
- If positive, it helps
- If negative, still could be upper bleed
- Just get an EGD

AR 31 (cont.)
- EGD is done
- A duodenal ulcer with a spurting vessel is detected; Endoscopic therapy includes injection and thermal therapy

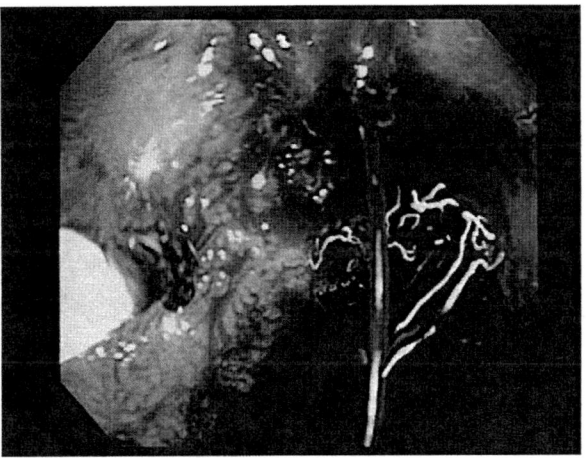

AR 31 (cont.)
How long should this patient remain on PPI therapy?

Treatment of Bleeding PUD
- Current role for IV PPI
- Use for 72 hours in any patient with endoscopic therapy (injection therapy with thermal coagulation or hemoclip)
- Start oral PPI after EGD unless reason to keep NPO
- High dose?

Goals of Endoscopy
- Determine the cause of bleeding
- Assess the risk of rebleeding
- Administer endoscopic therapy
- Injection: Epinephrine
- Thermal
  - Heater probe
  - Bipolar probe
  - Argon plasma coagulator
- Mechanical
  - Hemoclips
  - Banding

Endoscopic Lesions — Things We Definitely Treat

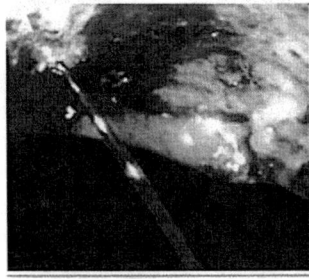 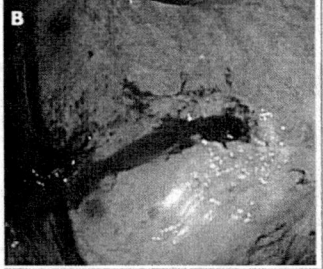

Arterial spurt
95% risk of rebleeding

Oozing
55% risk of rebleeding

ASGE Guideline on the Role of Endoscopy in Non-Variceal Upper GI Hemorrhage 2004.

Endoscopic Lesions — Things We Treat

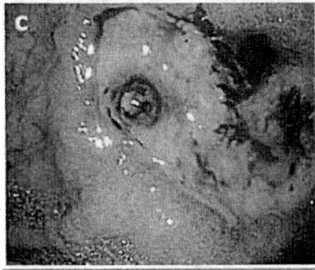

Visible vessel
50% risk of rebleeding

Adherent clot
30–35% risk of rebleeding

Endoscopic Lesions — Things We Do Not Treat

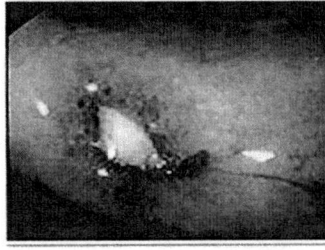 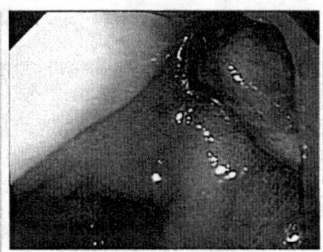

Red spot
7–10% risk of rebleeding

Clean based
5% risk of rebleeding

EGD in PUD Bleeding
- EGD-based risk (spurting vessel, visible vessel 50%, adherent clot 30%, flat red spot)
- EGD-based endoscopic treatment
- EGD-based triage — discharge (clean base = little risk — early discharge)
- Surgery for endoscopic Tx failure

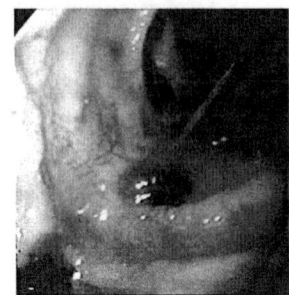

GI Bleeding
- Other causes:
  - Mallory-Weiss tear
  - Esophageal varices or gastric varices
  - Aorto-enteric fistula — always remember this if the patient has a history of abdominal aortic aneurysm (AAA) repair, presents with melena, then severe hemorrhage
  - Dieulafoy lesions

Blood Transfusions in Variceal Bleeds
- Cause of variceal bleeding is portal hypertension
- Over-aggressive transfusion can lead to an increase in portal pressures, which can lead to increased bleeding
- Guidelines suggest transfusion to hemodynamic stability and a Hgb of 8 g/dL

Garcia-Tsao, et al. *Hepatology.* 2007.

Upper GI Bleeding — Take Home Points
- Early aggressive resuscitation is very important
- Adequate peripheral access and admission to appropriate level of care is essential
- Airway protection
- Start PPI IV drip if you suspect upper GI bleeding
- No need to correct mild coagulopathy (INR < 2.5)
- NGT not necessary in most cases
- Timing of endoscopy between 12–24 hrs in most cases
- PPI drip to be continued for 72 hrs if endoscopic intervention is employed for PUD or high risk ulcer is seen
- Octreotide and antibiotics for cirrhotic bleeders

AR 32

A 65-year-old man is evaluated in the ED for painless bright red blood per rectum that began 6 hours ago. He has no other medical conditions and takes no medications.
BP 130/78, HR 96. Abdominal exam is normal. Rectal examination discloses no external hemorrhoids; bright red blood is noted in the rectal vault.
Hg 10.4, Plt 380.

Which of the following is the most likely cause of this patient's bleeding?
A. Colon cancer
B. Diverticulosis
C. Duodenal ulcer
D. Ischemic colitis

Answer: _____

Lower GI Hemorrhage
- Diverticulosis — most common, painless
- Arteriovenous malformation (AVM)
- Colon cancer or polyp (and post-polypectomy)
- Ischemic colitis — always with pain
- Upper source; e.g., duodenal ulcer
- Meckel diverticulum — young patient
- Anorectal source; e.g., hemorrhoids

Nasogastric Lavage
- NGL should be considered in cases of hemodynamic compromise to rule out a brisk upper GI source of bleeding
- NGL Results:
  - If **bloody** → EGD
  - If **bilious** → Unlikely UGI Bleed
  - If no bile or blood → Cannot rule out UGI Bleed
- Can be helpful for delivery of an oral purgative for rapid purge prior to colonoscopy

Wilcox et al. *Am J Gastroenterol.* 1997.
ASGE Guideline on the Role of Endoscopy in the patient with lower GI bleeding 2005.

Colonoscopy in LGIB

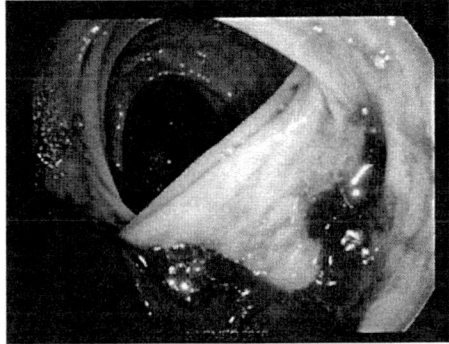

Advantages
- Potential localization
- Potential therapeutic intervention

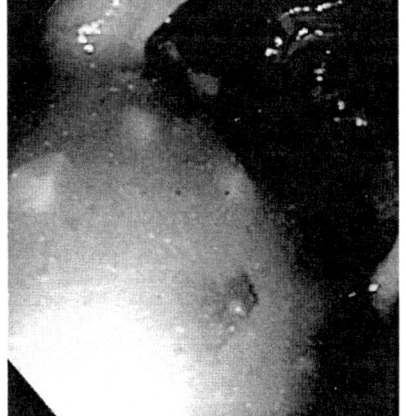

Disadvantages
- Poor visualization in unprepared colon
- Risks of sedation
- Variable sensitivity

Rapid Purge Urgent Colonoscopy
- Colo performed within 6–12 hours of hospitalization
- 4- to 11-liter purge
- Requires patient to consume 1 L q 30–45 minutes
- Consider metoclopramide 10 mg IV prior to purge
- NGT if unable to tolerate PO

Management
- Stabilization
- Nasogastric aspirate, even EGD!
- Ongoing bleeding (tagged scan/angio)
- Colonoscopy — timing?

Tagged RBC Scan
Scintography
- Rate of bleeding has to be > 0.1 mL per minute
- Technetium sulfur Colloid (99mTc)
  - Rapidly cleared — Imaging over a few minutes
- Pertechnetate-labeled RBCs
  - Permit multiple scanning over 24 hours

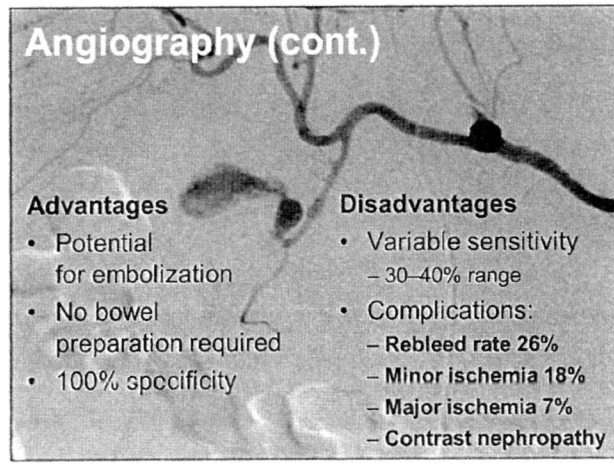

Advantages
- Potential to pick up a slow bleed
- May help "select" patients for angiography

Disadvantages
- Wide-range sensitivity
  - 32–87%
- Poor localization
  - Usually < 50%
  - Blood peristaltic/Antiperist

Early · Late

Angiography
- Rate of bleeding > 1 mL per minute
- Allow for super-selective embolization of bleeding site
- SMA is examined first
  - 50–80% of diverticular bleeds are supplied by SMA

Angiography (cont.)

Advantages
- Potential for embolization
- No bowel preparation required
- 100% specificity

Disadvantages
- Variable sensitivity
  - 30–40% range
- Complications:
  - Rebleed rate 26%
  - Minor ischemia 18%
  - Major ischemia 7%
  - Contrast nephropathy

AR 33

60-year-old man in emergency department
with 3rd episode of melena
Negative workup 3 years ago for 1st episode
No GI Sxs, feels weak
Fam Hx: Positive for GI bleeding
ROS: Epistaxis
PE: Telangiectasias on lips, fingertips
EGD: Gastric and duodenal AVMs

Which of the following is the most likely diagnosis?
A. Peutz-Jeghers syndrome
B. Familial polyposis
C. Hereditary hemorrhagic telangiectasia
D. Diverticular bleeding
E. Celiac sprue

Answer: _____

Hereditary Hemorrhagic Telangiectasia
• Characteristic physical exam
• History: Epistaxis
• Family history of GI bleeding or epistaxis
• AVMs (multiple) of GI tract — more upper than lower

Angiodysplasia
1) Also called AVM, vascular ectasia
2) Cause of acute or occult bleeding
3) Elderly
4) In colon: Cecum, ascending endoscopic therapy
   may be appropriate

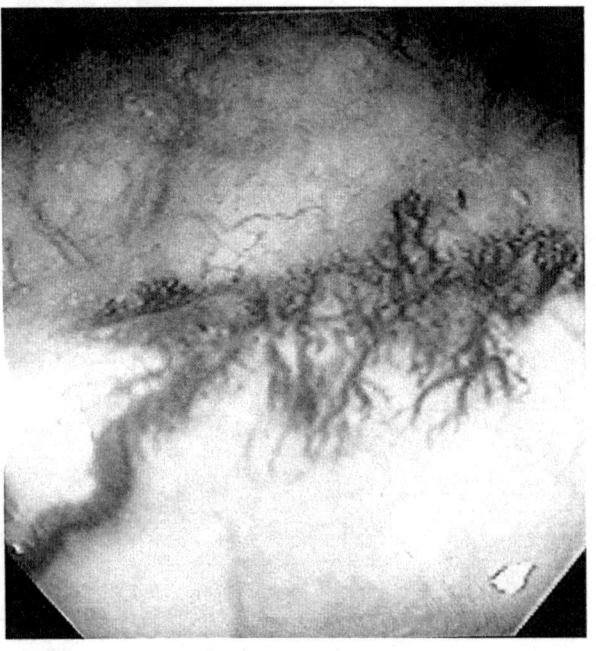

Acute Lower GI Bleeding — Take Home Points
• Early aggressive resuscitation is very important
• Adequate peripheral access and admission to
  appropriate level of care is essential
• Most common cause of lower GI bleed is diverticulosis
• NGT can be helpful if you suspect brisk upper
  GI bleeding
• Urgent rapid prep vs. elective (nonurgent) prep:
  No difference in early/late rebleed rates or mortality …
  so typically not necessary to do rapid prep
• Consider angiography, RBC scan, surgical consult
  in massive GI bleeding

AR 34

A 65-year-old man: Recurrent melena
4 admissions in the past year
Required 15 units of RBCs
Bleeding will spontaneously cease
Never abdominal pain
Past medical history: Severe coronary artery disease,
2 stents in place, 1 recent. He is on aspirin (81 mg)
and clopidogrel.

His past workup has included 2 upper endoscopies and
2 colonoscopies, which were both normal. There has also
been an upper GI bowel series, which was normal.
The patient is now admitted with his 5th hospitalization,
again presenting with melena.
The Hgb is 8. A tagged RBC scan is done when the patient
arrives, but this is negative for showing a bleeding
source.

What is the best diagnostic test in this situation?
A. Video capsule
B. CT abdomen
C. A repeat of EGD and colonoscopy
D. Mesenteric angiogram

Answer: _____

AR 34 (cont.)
Video capsule is best test for obscure GI bleeding,
meaning that upper and lower causes have been
excluded.
An angiogram would only be helpful if very active
bleeding; for instance, a positive tagged RBC scan.

GI Ischemia
• Ischemic colitis
• Chronic mesenteric ischemia
• Acute intestinal infarction

Ischemic Colitis
- Bloody diarrhea associated with severe abdominal pain
- Involves watershed area — splenic flexure
- Low-flow state, not embolic
- At risk: HF, hypovolemic
- Treatment: Bowel rest, IV fluid, possible antibiotics
- Usual resolution > 50%
- Dx: Colonoscopy
- No angiogram

- Young patients: Protein C def., antithrombin III def.
- Females: Oral contraceptives
- Cocaine use
- Pseudoephedrine use
- Long-distance runners

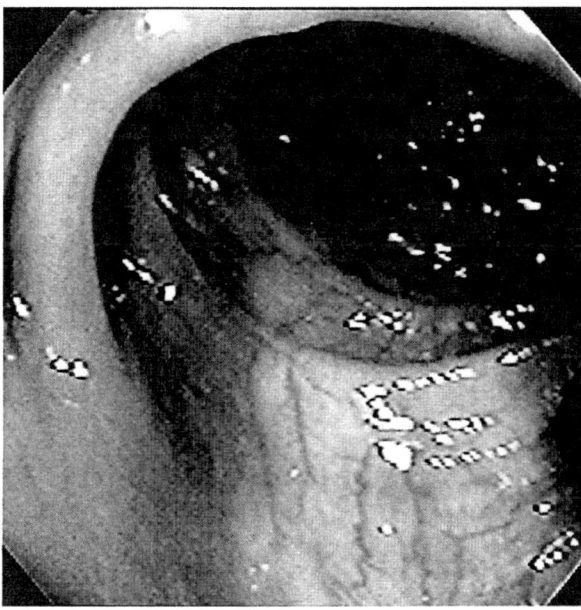

Chronic Mesenteric Ischemia
- Classic Triad:
  1) Abdominal pain after meals — intestinal angina
  2) Decreased pain with smaller meals and weight loss
  3) Abdominal bruit

Smoking Hx, PVD, CAD

Dx: CT angiogram or MR angiogram
   Doppler U/S can help,
   Mesenteric angiography (definitive)

Tx: Surgical bypass or angioplasty

Acute Mesenteric Ischemia
- Acute, severe abdominal pain, symptoms out of proportion to exam
- Vomiting, diarrhea, occult blood (not gross)
- Atrial fib., valvular disease, post-MI
- Acidosis, elevated amylase
- Typical Sxs — make diagnosis with angiogram
- Diagnosis made by CT Angiography
- Treatment: Angioplasty, surgery, embolectomy

AR 35
Which of the following are poor clinical prognostic indicators for acute pancreatitis?
A. Rising lipase
B. Elevated creatinine level
C. Hematocrit > 44
D. All of the above
E. B. and C.

Answer: _____

Pancreas

Acute Pancreatitis — Etiology
- Gallstones and alcohol (#1 and #2 causes in U.S.)
- Metabolic: Triglycerides, hypercalcemia
- Duct obstruction: Tumor, trauma
- Meds: Sulfa, estrogen, thiazides, tetracyclines
- Iatrogenic: ERCP

Acute Pancreatitis
- Idiopathic pancreatitis:
  - May have biliary crystals or sludge (negative ultrasound)
  - Cholecystectomy or sphincterotomy if recurrent
  - Recurrent pancreatitis, sludge only on ultrasound — know to do cholecystectomy (before discharge if possible)

- Presentation: Abdominal pain
- Pain radiates to back
- Nausea and vomiting

Acute Pancreatitis — Labs
- Amylase 3x normal
- Lipase: Later peak
- Hemoconcentration
- Leukocytosis
- Bili > 3 and increased ALT suggest common bile duct stone
- Do not need serial measurements of pancreatic enzymes

- First test: Ultrasound to R/O gallstones
  - Shows gallbladder stones, but not good for common duct stones
- Even if negative; possible CBD stones
- Some idiopathic cases: Microlithiasis

2012 Atlanta Criteria
- 2 of 3 must be present
  1) Upper abdominal pain radiating through to the back
  2) Serum amylase or lipase 3x the upper limit of normal
  3) Cross-sectional imaging consistent with acute pancreatitis

Acute Pancreatitis — Severity
- Dynamic CT assesses pancreatic necrosis
- Pancreatic necrosis (25% of acute panc)
- Other organ failure
- Cardiovascular; e.g., hypotension
- Pulmonary: Decreased O_2
- Renal insufficiency
- Metabolic abnormality; e.g., hypocalcemia
- Altered mental status

Acute Pancreatitis (Severity Scoring)
Ranson Criteria

Age > 55	Hct fall > 10%
Glucose > 200	BUN rise > 5
WBC > 16	Base deficit > 4
AST > 250	Calcium < 8
LDH > 350	PO_2 < 60
Fluid sequest > 6 L	

Newer Scoring systems: APACHE II, BISAP

Acute Pancreatitis — Management
- NPO, aggressive IV fluids
- Nasogastric tube if ileus or vomiting
- Abs: Imipenem if necrosis on CT
- Feed: TPN vs. nasojejunal — jejunal feeding is superior and safe, but access can be difficult
- Gastric feeding might be okay, but **feed the patient ASAP**

AR 36
A 40-year-old male presents to the emergency department with severe epigastric pain for the past 16 hours. The pain radiates to the back and is associated with vomiting. The patient neither smokes cigarettes nor drinks alcohol. He takes ibuprofen occasionally for lower back pain.
Physical exam: He is in moderate distress with a heart rate of 105 bpm.
The epigastric region of his abdomen is tender.

On initial labs, hemoglobin is 16 g; his white blood cell count is 17,000. The amylase is 150, and this was within normal limits for this lab. His liver enzymes are normal, but his triglyceride level is 2,000. Abdominal flat-plate x-ray is performed, and this reveals no free air in the diaphragm.

Which of the following is the most likely diagnosis?
A. Acute pancreatitis
B. Duodenal ulcer
C. Acute intestinal infarct
D. Ischemic colitis

Answer: _____

Acute Pancreatitis — Pearls
- Cullen sign: Periumbilical discoloration
- Turner sign: Flank discoloration indicates retroperitoneal bleeding
- Hypocalcemia may cause muscle cramps
- Hypertriglyceridemia masks increased amylase
- Differentiate from DKA

Pancreatic Pseudocyst
- Can be seen in acute (10–15%) or chronic
- Usually 2–4 weeks after acute episode
- Can spontaneously resolve
- Size > 5 cm unlikely to resolve
- Can be complicated: Infection, hemorrhage
- How to manage 5-cm cyst in acute setting: Observe rather than surgery, drainage, etc.
- Consider if delayed recurrence of pain with another elevation of amylase

Pancreatic Abscess
- Late complication: Severe acute pancreatitis
- Fever, shock, mass
- CT scan with needle aspiration

Acute Pancreatitis
- Timing of ERCP
  - Early only if ongoing biliary sepsis, biliary obstruction, cholangitis, rising bilirubin
  - Later for other cases; suspected due to CBD stone, unknown cause, Ca of pancreas
- Timing of lap. cholecystectomy: Can/Should be early; e.g., same admission, just wait until pancreatitis has subsided; High risk of recurrence if not done

Pancreatitis
- Remember the differential diagnosis of abdominal pain and elevated amylase:
  - Acute pancreatitis
  - Acute cholecystitis
  - Salpingitis
  - Perforated ulcer
  - DKA
  - Ectopic pregnancy

Autoimmune Pancreatitis
- Rare cause of pancreatitis
- Characterized by painless obstructive jaundice and cross-sectional imaging with "sausage shaped pancreas"
- Two types
  - Type 1 AIP, systemic, elevated IgG4,
  - Type 2 AIP, IgG4 not always elevated

AR 37

55-year-old male presents for evaluation of diarrhea. He reports 5 loose stools daily without blood for the past 3 months. He also reports intermittent epigastric pain and weight loss. No other past medical history.

On social history, he drinks a 12 pack of beer daily and smokes 2 packs per day for the past 30 years. He uses no other medications.

Physical exam: He is thin and has mild tenderness in epigastrium, but is otherwise normal.

Labs show lipase of 30, albumin 3.1, hemoglobin of 13.3. Stool cultures are negative.

Colonoscopy was normal.

Which of the following diagnostic tests is the next step in management?

A. Serum for IgG4
B. CT scan
C. Gastrin level
D. Glycated hemoglobin A1c

Answer: _____

Chronic Pancreatitis
- Causes
  - Alcohol abuse (70%) usually > 10 years
  - Idiopathic (30%)
  - Cystic fibrosis
  - Hereditary disorders
  - Pancreas Divisum
  - Autoimmune Pancreatitis

- Clinical features
- Early: Recurrent pain episodes
- Late: Steatorrhea and diabetes (80–90% function lost)
- Fecal fat can be very high (40–100 g/day)
- Increased risk of cancer

- Diagnosis: Calcification on KUB — not usually seen, but significant if present
- CT and EUS: Best second step
- Classic diagnostic triad: Pancreatic calcifications, diabetes, steatorrhea
- MRCP: Visualizes pancreatic and bile ducts; Order before the invasive ERCP
- Secretin test: Most sensitive, but complicated
  - Measures direct duodenal secretions: Bicarb, volume

Chronic Pancreatitis — Therapy
- If persistent pain
  - Rule out continued alcohol
  - Rule out pseudocyst
  - Define ductal anatomy: EUS and/or MRCP
  - High-dose pancreatic enzyme supplementation
  - Quit smoking
- Steatorrhea: Treated with oral pancreatic enzyme supplementation

Pancreas Cyst
- Mucinous cystic neoplasm and intraductal papillary mucinous neoplasm (IPMN) most common
  - Can involve main or branch ducts
  - Most IPMNs are branch ducts
- Prevalence of cysts is 10% in patients > 70 years of age, majority are asymptomatic
- Surveillance recommended by AGA if cyst is > 3 cm, pancreatic duct dilation, solid component to the cyst

For those that are interested, the AGA has guidelines on management of pancreas cysts.

Pancreatic Neoplasms
- Adenocarcinoma:
  - Risk factors: Smoking, chronic pancreatitis, diabetes mellitus
  - 5th leading cause of cancer death in U.S.
  - Presentation: Jaundice, abdominal or back pain, and weight loss
  - Most located at head of pancreas
  - Elevated CA 19-9
  - Advanced disease: Poor survival
  - If mass: CT-guided biopsy, or needle biopsy at EUS

- If no mets: Consider eval for surgery
  - Most still not resectable
  - Most common reasons for nonresectable: Distant mets (liver), encasement of vessels
- If mets or local vascular invasion: ERCP + stent
- Gemcitabine: Improves survival, reduces pain and improves quality of life
- Preoperative biliary drainage increases risk of complications in jaundiced patients (*NEJM* 2010)

- Glucagonoma
  - Necrolytic erythema, weight loss, diarrhea, hyperglycemia
- Insulinoma
- Gastrinoma
  - Serum gastrin > 500, 50% found in duodenum, 24% in pancreas
- VIPoma
  - Profuse secretory diarrhea, increased serum VIP, hypokalemia

"Double Duct Sign"

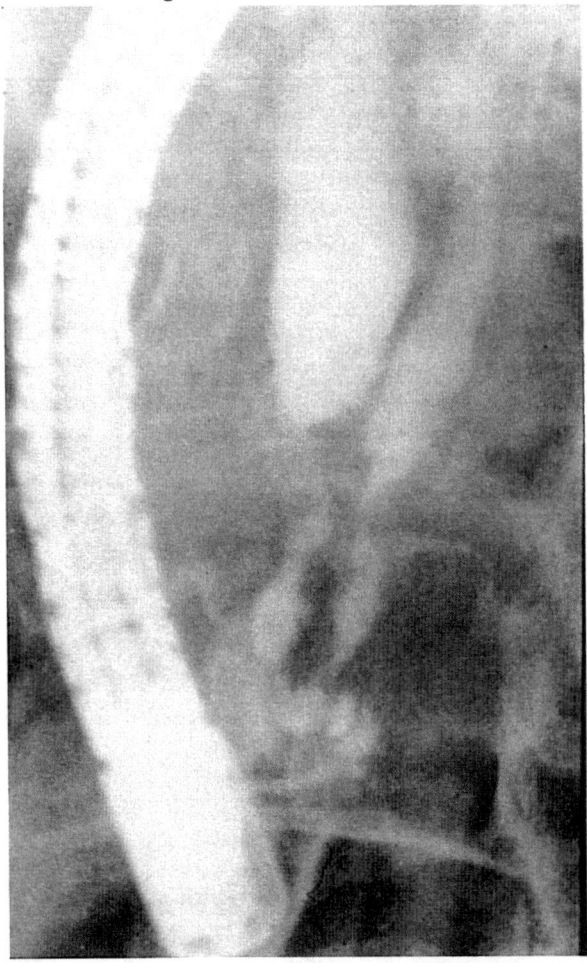

Gallbladder

AR 38
A 33-year-old male with no past medical history presents to the ED with 12 hours of severe RUQ pain with fevers, nausea, and one episode of vomiting. He takes no medications. Temp 99.9° F (37.7° C), HR 95, BP 100/70, and abdominal exam reveals positive Murphy's sign. Labs show WBC of 14, TB 1.5, ALT 55, AST 60, Alk phos normal.
Abdominal sonogram shows thickened gallbladder wall with pericholecystic fluid with some gallstones and normal size CBD.

What is the next step in management after antibiotics?
A. ERCP with biliary sphincterotomy
B. CCK HIDA scan
C. EGD
D. Cholecystectomy

Answer: _____

Biliary Colic vs. Cholecystitis
Biliary Colic
- Acute upper abdominal pain with nausea and vomiting
- Fatty food intolerance is a nonspecific symptom
Cholecystitis
- Acute severe abdominal pain with nausea, vomiting, fevers, elevated WBC, elevated LFTS

Cholecystitis
- 90% of cases occur due to gallstone obstruction
- Murphy's sign positive
- Thickened gallbladder wall, presence of pericholecystic fluid
- Management is IV antibiotics and cholecystectomy (usually laparoscopic)
- Some cases may require percutaneous or endoscopic drainage

Acalculous Cholecystitis
- Patients who are sick can have cholecystitis without having gallstones
- Etiology is bacterial seeding of gallbladder wall or gallbladder wall ischemia
- Diagnosis by abdominal sonogram or radionuclide imaging
- Management: Cholecystectomy if possible or percutaneous or endoscopic drainage

Cholelithiasis
- Clinical features:
  - More common in females
  - Often asymptomatic
  - Males catch up later in life
  - Most are cholesterol (other kind: Pigment)

Cholesterol Stones — Most Common
- Risk factors
  - Certain ethnic groups (e.g., Native American)
  - Family history
  - Obesity
  - Rapid weight reduction
  - Diabetes
  - Bowel rest and TPN
  - Hypertriglyceridemia
  - Estrogen, incl. OCP
  - Pregnancy

Pigment Stones
- Can occur in bile duct with chronic infection: *Clonorchis*, strictures, cholangitis
- Can occur in gallbladder with hemolysis
- Can occur in Crohn's patients, with ileal disease or ileal resection
- 50% radio-opaque

Cholelithiasis (cont.)
- Symptoms: Pain is epigastric or RUQ; Constant for 20–60 minutes; Nausea and vomiting; (Dyspepsia, heartburn, and fatty food intolerance are not Sxs)
- Ultrasound: 90% sensitive
- HIDA for acute cystic duct obstruction

- Treatment if symptomatic: Cholecystectomy
- If asymptomatic: Only 20% develop Sxs
- Bile acid treatment: For cholesterol stones, < 1 cm, few in number, 25% benefit; therefore, almost never used
- Common bile duct stones: ERCP

AR 39
A 60-year-old woman had a CT scan of the abdomen ordered for some mild upper abdominal discomfort, which did not improve with 2 weeks of omeprazole. This exam showed calcification of the gallbladder wall.

Which of the following do you recommend?
A. Cholecystectomy.
B. ERCP.
C. Simply observe and repeat the scan in 1 year.
D. Ultrasound of the abdomen.

Answer: _____

Porcelain Gallbladder
Imaging that shows a gallbladder with a calcified outline ("porcelain gallbladder") suggests the possibility of cancer and is an indication for laparoscopic cholecystectomy.

AR 40
A 60-year-old woman presents with acute onset RUQ pain and fever. She has had prior episodes of self-limited pain that never lasted more than 30 minutes. Now in pain for 2 hours. PMH negative. No medications.
ROS: Slight darkening of urine.
PE: Temp 100° F (37.8° C), HR 100, BP 130/80
Tender RUQ without peritoneal signs

Labs: Hgb 15, WBC 16,000, T bili 3.0
      AST 120, ALT 110, Alk Phos 400
      Amylase and lipase NL
Ultrasound: Gallbladder has many stones;
      No gallbladder wall thickening
Dilated common bile duct with several apparent stones
Antibiotics started

What do you recommend?
A. ERCP
B. MRCP
C. EGD
D. Abdominal CT scan

Answer: _____

AR 40 (cont.)
We have enough evidence from the labs, presentation, and the ultrasound that she has cholangitis from the common duct stones to proceed directly with the ERCP.

Cholelithiasis — Exam Questions
- Treatment with asymptomatic patient
- Treatment of CBD stones
- Acalculous cholecystitis:
  - Occurs in ill, hospitalized patient
  - Atypical presentation, late Dx
  - Dx: Ultrasound — thickened gallbladder wall, no stones, HIDA scan
  - Tx: Cholecystectomy

Common Bile Duct Gallstones
- Cholangitis: Charcot's triad, abdominal pain, fever and chills, jaundice
- Pigmented stones or cholesterol
- Management: Antibiotics, ERCP with sphincterotomy, surgery

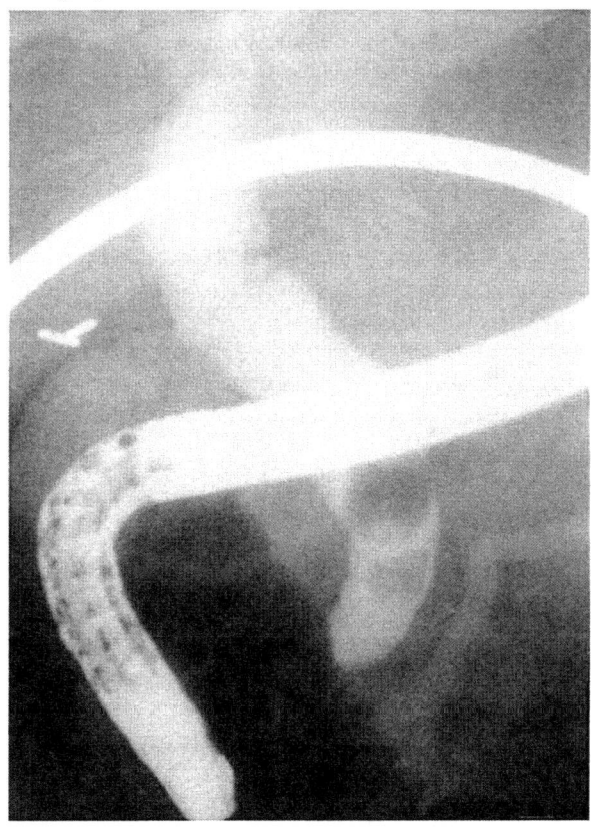

After Cholecystectomy
- Pain and increased LFTs
- Immediate post-op: Bile duct leak
- Any delay: Choledocholithiasis; for example, months to years later

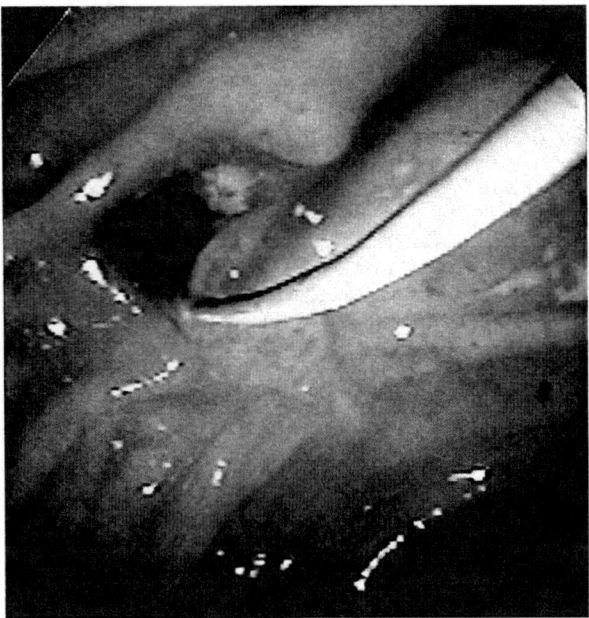

MRCP
- MR cholangiography: Sensitivity for CBD stones about same as ERCP
- Use when index of suspicion is low to moderate
- Examples: Case of pancreatitis where U/S shows slightly dilated CBD, but bili is normal
- If high index, go straight to ERCP

Gallbladder Cancer
- Less than 5,000 cases per year, usually diagnosed at late stage
- Risk Factors: Cholelithiasis, gallbladder polyps, porcelain gallbladder, obesity, anomalous pancreas/biliary junction
- Symptoms: RUQ pain, N/V, weight loss, jaundice
- Diagnosis: Cross-sectional imaging
- Treatment: Surgery if resectable, chemo/XRT if not resectable

Cholangiocarcinoma
- Associated PSC: More commonly men
  - Lifetime risk of cancer: 10%
  - Time with PSC before Ca: Variable 1–25 years, (1/3 within 2 years)
- Other associations: Choledochal cysts, *Clonorchis sinensis*

- Painless jaundice, pruritus
- Alk phos, GGT > transaminases
- CA 19-9 > 100 in 80%
- ERCP: Brush cytology 50% yield
- CT, MRI, EUS
- Surgery if found early
- Consider transplant in a patient with a history of PSC who has developed cholangiocarcinoma
  - Percutaneous biopsy may disqualify for transplant

Questions??

Liver

AR 41

A 55-year-old woman presents for a routine checkup. She complains of mild fatigue, but she is otherwise healthy. She is on no medications. Her family history is negative for any gastrointestinal or liver disease. On physical examination, you notice the presence of both xanthomas and xanthelasma as well as a liver that is slightly enlarged.
She had laboratory tests done at her workplace recently, and, although she had a normal AST, she had an alkaline phosphatase that was 2x normal.

Which of the following do you recommend?
A. Antismooth muscle antibody
B. Antimitochondrial antibody
C. An evaluation for hemochromatosis with iron, TIBC, and *HFE* gene
D. TTG to rule out celiac disease

Answer: _____

Primary Biliary Cirrhosis (PBC)
- Middle-aged women: (Age at Dx 55 years, > 90% female)
- Main symptoms: Fatigue, pruritus, often suspected based on symptoms alone
- Often asymptomatic
- Autoimmune disorders are common (Sjögren's, CREST, thyroiditis)
- PE: Xanthelasma, skin hyperpigmentation, hepatomegaly, other signs of liver disease

- Diagnosis
  - Increased alk phos (can be marked) and GGT
  - Antimitochondrial Ab
    - Level no relation to severity
  - Increased cholesterol: This is HDL
  - Increased IgM
  - Bili usually normal
  - Liver biopsy required

- Nonsuppurative destruction of small bile ducts
- Reduced biliary excretion
- Accumulation of bile acids and copper
- Early stage: (I) chronic inflammatory cells and granulomas adjacent to damaged bile ducts

PBC — Natural History
- Asymptomatic: Survival 10–16 years
- Symptomatic: Survival 7 years
- Symptom treatment:
  - Pruritus: Cholestyramine
  - Metabolic bone disease: Calcium, vitamin D, estrogen, bisphosphonates
  - Malabsorption: Restrict dietary fat, medium-chain triglycerides

PBC Possible Exam Questions
- Treatment: Ursodeoxycholic acid
- Bili increasing > 2: Poor prognosis
- Know to transplant
- Best test for diagnosis — AMA

PBC Complications
- Steatorrhea: Can treat by reducing dietary fat
- Weight loss
- At risk for deficiency of fat-soluble vitamins: A, D, E, and K; Most important clinically is D
- Liver failure

Serum Markers in Certain Disease

	Primary Biliary Cirrhosis	Drug-induced AIH	Autoimmune AIH
Anti-mitochondrial Ab	90% pos	+occ	+occ (low titers)
Anti-smooth muscle Ab	- neg -	- neg -	pos

One Last Note
Remember drug history when approaching patient with cholestatic liver disease: Phenothiazine, steroids, trimethoprim/sulfa.

Primary Sclerosing Cholangitis (PSC)
- Male to female — 2:1
- Average age: 45
- 75% of PSC patients have IBD, especially ulcerative colitis
- No relation to severity of colitis
- Often asymptomatic at first
- Later symptoms: Weakness, fatigue, itching, jaundice, cholangitis

PSC — Diagnosis
- Increased alk phos and bilirubin
- Mild increase in AST and ALT
- Positive p-ANCA
- MRCP and ERCP show multiple strictures of intra- and extrahepatic bile ducts, beaded appearance
- MRCP is first test appropriate in suspected PSC
- Liver biopsy: onion skin fibrosis in portal triad
- Just suspect diagnosis — liver tests

PSC — Management and Course
- Slow, indolent course
- 5-year survival: 60–70%
- Most will progress to liver failure
- Cholangiocarcinoma in 10%
- Liver transplant for end-stage disease
- Ursodeoxycholic acid may help pruritus
- Stricture dilation

- 80% of patients with PSC will have IBD; Only 20% of patients with IBD will have PSC
- Patients with IBD and PSC have significant colon cancer risk, more than just colitis
- UC + PSC — start annual screening colonoscopy at time of diagnosis

PSC

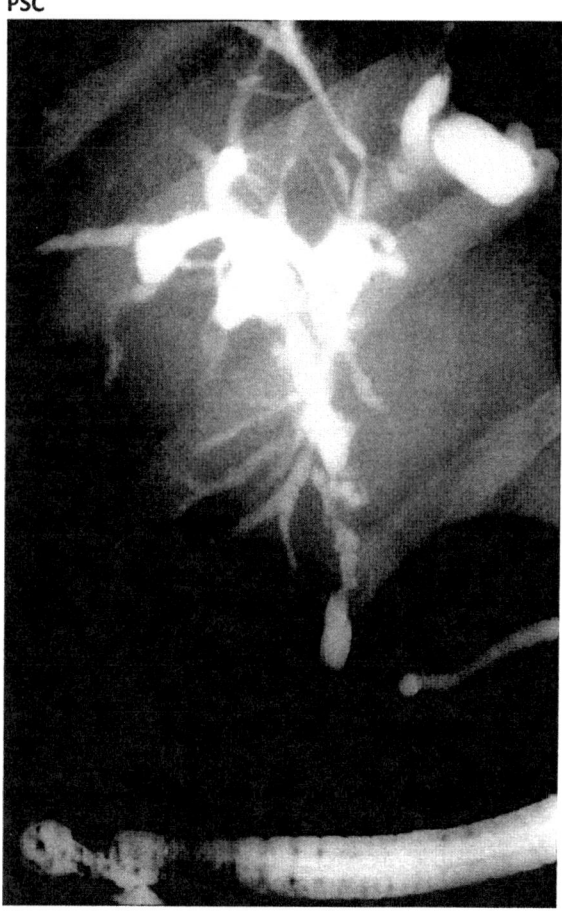

The Liver — Prelude to Hepatitis
- ALT more liver-specific than AST
- Alcohol AST:ALT 3:1
- Viral hepatitis ALT > AST
- Workup for (persistently) increased ALT:
  Full set biochemical — alk phos, direct and indirect bili, albumin, ProTime, CBC
- Persistent increase: Hep A, B, C; Fe; TIBC; ferritin

Hepatitis A (HAV)
- RNA virus
- Transmission fecal-oral, food, or water; Incubation 15–50 days
- Acute infection: Anti-HAV IgM
- No carrier state, rarely fulminant
- Vaccine available

HAV — Clinical Spectrum
- Developing countries: Childhood Dz
- Small children: Rare Sxs
- Infected adults: 70% have Sxs
- Prolonged cholestasis: Rare complication
- Nonspecific symptoms: Fatigue, nausea, headache, myalgias
- Later, RUQ pain and jaundice
- Rare cases — fulminant hepatitis

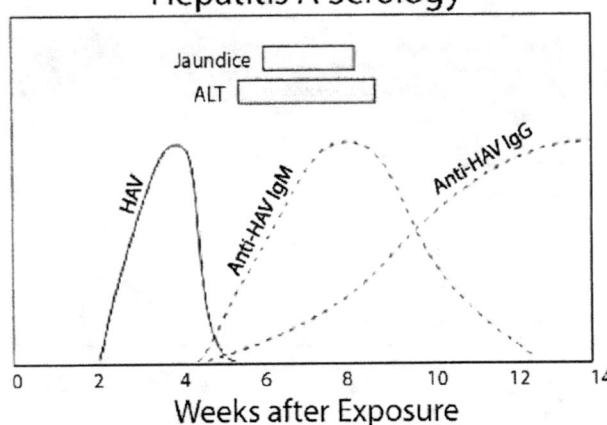

Hepatitis A Serology

HAV — Vaccine (2 doses)
1) Travel or working in high-risk countries
2) Children in communities with high rates of Dz (> 2 years)
3) Individuals with high-risk behavior
4) Patients with chronic liver disease

Hepatitis B (HBV)
- Only hepatitis DNA virus
- Incubation 1–6 months
- Transmission: Sexual contact, IV drugs, vertical mother to newborn
- Activates cellular immune system
- Vigor of immune response determines course

HBV — Presentation
- Acute HBV:
  1) Usually acute infection asymptomatic
  2) Can present as serum sickness due to immune complex disease with fever, urticaria, arthralgias
  3) Glomerulonephritis, vasculitis, PAN
- Chronic HBV nonspecific Sxs: Malaise, fatigue, anorexia

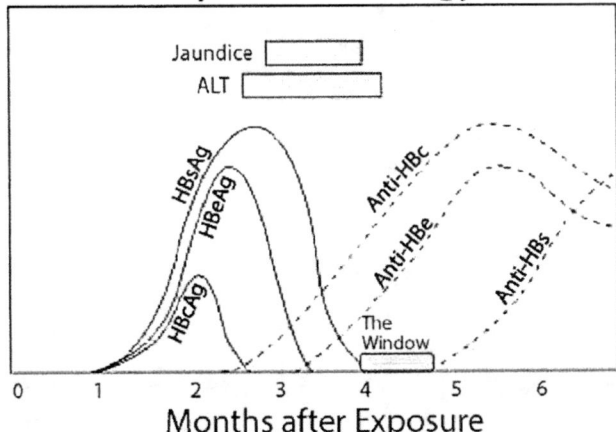

Hepatitis B Serology

HBV
- Initial rise HBsAg
- Later anti-HBc
- HBsAg usually becomes undetectable
- Window period: Anti-HBc IgM
- HBeAg correlates with intact virus and infectivity

Confused??
HBsAg+ means patient is making hepatitis B virus. Levels may be low or very high; it can be acute or chronic.

HBsAb+ almost always means the patient is "cured" of previous hepatitis B infection or, if this is the only marker (specifically no IgG HBcAb), then the patient was vaccinated.

HBeAg+ means the patient is highly infectious and actively making hepatitis B virus.

HBV
- Risk of chronic HBV inversely related to age:
  - 90% infants infected at birth
  - 25–50% children aged 1–5
  - 1–5% older children and adults
- Development of clinical disease relates to age:
  - 10% of children have Sxs
  - 30% adults over 30 have Sxs

Hepatitis B Scenarios

HBsAg	HBcAb	HBsAb	Interpretation
+	−	−	Acute infection
+	+	−	Acute infxn, chronic hep B, inactive carrier
−	−	+	Remote infxn, immunized

Hepatitis B Scenarios (cont.)

HBsAg	HBcAb	HBsAb	Interpretation
−	+	+	Remote infection
−	+	−	Window, remote infxn, false positive
+	+	+	More than one infection

Chronic Active Hepatitis B
- Most have HBsAg
- Usually HBeAg (in the U.S.)
- Positive HBcAb IgG
- High levels of HBV DNA

HBV — Chronic Carrier
- Termed nonreplicative state
- HBsAg persists
- HBcAb present
- HBV DNA present low levels
- Inflammatory response minimal

Hepatitis B Vaccines
- Recombinant vaccines
- Universal neonatal and high-risk groups
- Indicated pre- and postexposure: Prophylaxis
- Postexposure: Give HBIG too
- Check HBsAb for effect
- Reduced response in cirrhosis, chronic renal failure, immunosuppressed

HBV — Vaccine
- Immunocompetent patients: 90–95% develop ab
- Chronic hemodialysis patients: 50–60% develop ab

Sample Question — What Do You Do?
HBsAg-positive mother gives birth:
A. Give newborn HBIG and vaccine.
B. Wait 2 months for vaccine.
C. Wait 2 months to give both.
D. No need for either.

Answer: _____

HBV — Treatment
- Whom to treat:
  - Consider for any HBeAg+
  - HBeAg — with HBV DNA > 20,000 and ALT > 2x ULN
  - Compensated cirrhosis with HBV DNA > 2,000

- Options for treatment:
  - 1st line therapy: Interferon, **entecavir**, **tenofovir**
  - Telbivudine, lamivudine, adefovir (not used)
- What could be on exams?
  That lamivudine has highest risk of developing resistance

HBV and Liver Transplantation
- Indication for OLT:
  - High rate of recurrent infection (up to 100%)
  - Give long-term HBIG, lamivudine

HBV — HCC screening
- Lifetime risk HCC around 20%
- Risk of HCC varies with viral load:
  Increased risk with HBV DNA level
- Therefore, screen with ultrasound q 6 months
  - Asian men > 40 years of age, Asian women > 50 years of age
  - All patients with cirrhosis
  - Family history of HCC
  - Africans > 20 years of age
  - > 40 years of age, ALT elevation and/or high HBV DNA level

AR 42
A 37-year-old Vietnamese male tried to donate blood but was denied and recommended to see his physician. He denies any medical history, any history of alcohol, new medications, or IV drug use. He does not know his family history.
Physical exam is normal.
Labs show the following: ALT normal, AST normal, total bilirubin is normal. Hep BsAG positive, Hep B S antibody negative, Hep Be antibody positive, Hepatitis Be antigen negative, HBV DNA is 50 IU/mL.

AR 42 (cont.)
What are your recommendations?
A. Start entecavir.
B. Check AFP every 2 years.
C. HCC screening with ultrasound every 6 months starting now.
D. HCC screening with ultrasound every 6 months starting at age 40 years.

Answer: _____

Hepatitis C (HCV) — Molecular Biology
- Single-stranded RNA
- Genotype 1: 70% U.S. infections
- Prone to mutation — genetic diversity

Hepatitis B and Hepatitis C
- Both parenterally transmitted
- Both cause acute and chronic hepatitis
- B: Self-limited 90–95%
- C: Self-limited 10–15%
- B: Virus level in blood and body fluids high
- C: Virus level low

HCV — Background
- Most common cause of chronic viral hepatitis in U.S.
- Probably 4 million Americans +HCVAB (1.5%)
- Complications: Cirrhosis, liver failure, HCC
- Leading cause for liver transplantation in U.S.

HCV — Increased Risk
- IV drug abuse
- High-risk sexual behavior
- Blood transfusion before 1990
- Tattoos, piercing
- Prisoners
- Snorting cocaine

HCV — Epidemiology
- Peak incidence in 1989: 175,000 new cases
- Bloodborne for transfusion before 1992
- Current risk of HCV after transfusion 0.001%
- 60% of new infections relate to IV drug use

HCV — Transmission
- Sexual transmission is low:
  - Monogamous relationship 10–20 years: 5%
- Household contact: Extremely low
- Maternal infant transmission: < 5%
- Health care worker needlestick: 5–10% from known infected patient
- No treatment after needlestick

HCV — Clinical Spectrum
- Acute infection: Only 25–35% have Sxs
- Rare, fulminant liver failure
- Incubation period: 7 weeks (range 3–20)
- Chronic phase:
  - 30% carriers: No Sxs and NL LFTs
  - 50% no Sxs and abnormal LFTs
  - 20% clinical liver Dz with Sxs

HCV — Extrahepatic Disease
- Small vessel vasculitis
- Most common cause: Essential mixed cryo
  - Skin rash: Purpura, vasculitis, urticaria
  - Joint, muscle aches
- Porphyria cutanea tarda:
  Know what this looks like — blisters on hands
- Neuropathy, glomerulonephritis: With cryo

HCV — Natural History
- 20% develop cirrhosis within 20 years
- Risk of cirrhosis increases with EtOH consumption
- Other risk factors: Age > 40 years; Male sex
- After cirrhosis established: 5-year survival 90%
- If liver failure Sxs, complications: 5-year survival 50%

HCV — Testing
- If positive in low-risk patient:
  Confirm with Recombinant Immunoblot Assay or HCV-RNA
- HCV-RNA by PCR: Useful in response to Tx, confirm diagnosis
- Liver Bx: Assess severity, presence cirrhosis
- ALT usually > AST

HCV — Treatment
- Rapidly evolving!
- IFN-free therapy is now standard
- RBV-free therapy is available
- Protease inhibitors are **dead**
- Indications: Abnormal LFTs, moderate fibrosis on Bx or noninvasive fibrosis testing;
  Lack of abnormal LFTs does not mean no cirrhosis

Available DAAD
- Sofosbuvir — FDA approved for genotypes 1 and 4 with IFN/RBV and genotypes 2 and 3 with RBV (no IFN):
  12 weeks for everyone except genotype 3
- Ledipasvir/sofosbuvir combo (Harvoni) is FDA approved for genotype 1 only:
  - 24 weeks for treatment experienced cirrhotic patients
  - 12 weeks for everyone else

- Ombitasvir, paritaprevir, and ritonavir tablets; Dasabuvir tablets with or without RBV (Viekira Pak):
  - Genotype 1 only
  - G1A with cirrhosis 24 weeks; Everyone else 12 weeks
  - G1B without cirrhosis: No RBV
- Simeprevir plus sofosbuvir:
  - Genotype 1 only
  - In general, 12 weeks
  - 24 weeks if cirrhosis

HCV — Treatment
- Genotype 1:
  - Most common in U.S.
  - Typically high viral load
  - Lowest response to treatment
- Genotypes 2 and 3:
  - Better response
- Treatment response now 90% or greater, as measured by SVR

- Overweight patient: Poor response
- Best response: Female, less than 40, less fibrosis on biopsy
- Ribavirin side effect: Hemolytic anemia
- Vaccinate for HBV and HAV

HCV and HIV
- PEG interferon and ribavirin
- 27% sustained virologic response at 72 weeks
- No coadministration of didanosine
- But this is all going to change in coming years with new drugs

HCV and Hepatocellular Ca
- Known complication
- Median interval: 30 years
- Surveillance: Ultrasound/CT — AFP no longer recommended
- HCV incidence is decreasing but picking up old cases will continue, as will cancer cases

Hepatitis D (HDV)
- RNA virus, requires HBV
- Found IVDA, high-risk HBsAg carriers
- Can be severe if superinfects HBV carrier
- Diagnosis: Anti-HDV IgM

Hepatitis E (HEV)
- Fecal-oral spread like HAV
- Far East, Africa, Central America
- Contamination of water supply
- No chronic state
- High-risk fulminant in pregnancy (mortality 20%)

Autoimmune Hepatitis (AIH)
- Young women; 50% autoimmune disease
- Acute, fulminant, or indolent
- Can be asymptomatic or nonspecific Sx
- Anti-smooth muscle antibody 80%
- Low-titer AMA, ANA
- Elevation of gamma globulin
- How to diagnose

AR 43
A 24-year-old woman presents with several months of fatigue. She denies abdominal pain, jaundice, or itching. She is not taking any medications, including no OTC preparations and no herbals/supplements.
Social: No EtOH, travel, or high-risk behavior
PE: NL, no hepatomegaly
Initial lab: ALT 120, AST 90, NL Alk Phos and Bili
Subsequent testing: NL Fe, TIBC, ferritin, and ceruloplasmin, –HCV, –HBV
Elevated anti-smooth muscle antibody

Which therapy is likely to help?
A. Pegylated interferon
B. Prednisone and azathioprine
C. Ursodeoxycholic acid
D. Cholestyramine

Answer: _____

AR 43 (cont.)
This is a case of autoimmune hepatitis, and the standard therapy would be prednisone and azathioprine.

Indications for Treatment of AIH
- AST greater than 10x ULN
- ALT greater than 5x ULN and elevated gamma-glob (2x ULN)
- Fibrosis on biopsy
- Relative:
  - Symptoms
  - Lower elevations
  - Interface hepatitis

Drug-Related Liver Disease
- Hepatitis: Methyldopa, nitrofurantoin, phenytoin
- Cholestasis: Oral contraceptives, anabolic steroids, chlorpromazine, erythromycin
- Fulminant hepatitis: Ketoconazole, INH
- Indolent cirrhosis: Methotrexate (lifetime dose)

- Acetaminophen:
  - Glutathione reduces toxic metabolite
  - Glutathione depletion: Toxin accumulates
  - Treat with N-acetylcysteine acutely after checking acetaminophen level

More on Acetaminophen
- Chronic, moderate-to-heavy alcohol induces cytochrome p 450 and depletes glutathione
- At risk for toxicity at relatively low levels of acetaminophen; e.g., dose < 4 g a day
- Other risks: Dieting, Weight loss, Gastric bypass, Malnutrition

Alcoholic Liver Disease
- **Macro**vesicular fat accumulation
- Women more susceptible
- GGT disproportionately high
- AST – ALT 3:1
- AST less than 300

One drink = 1.5 oz spirits, 4 oz wine, or 8 oz beer

Possible Exam Question
- 28-year-old on oral contraceptives
- Has RUQ pain and the following CT:

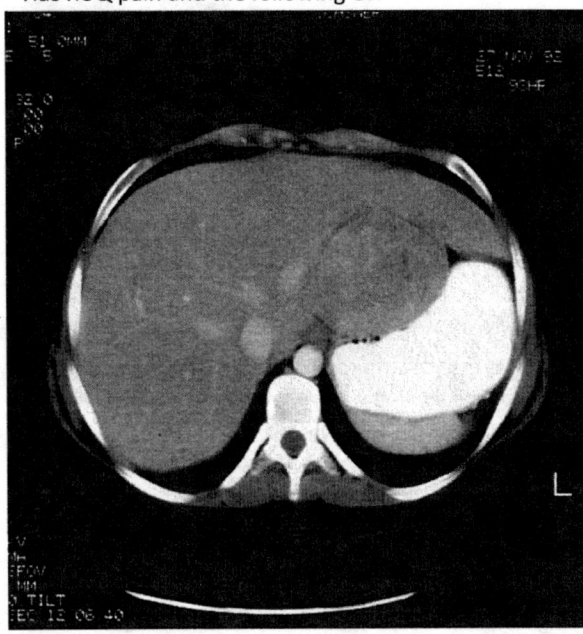

Hepatic Adenoma
- Young women
- Typically, solitary lesion
- Oral contraceptives and glycogen storage disease
- Can cause pain and rare complications like rupture/hemoperitoneum

NAFLD
- Nonalcoholic steatohepatitis (NASH)
- Typical patient: Obese, diabetic female, hyperlipidemia
- Can cause hepatomegaly, RUQ pain
- Mild increase: ALT > AST
- Ultrasound: Fat, diffuse
- Can cause fibrosis, cirrhosis
- Can have abnormal ASMA

Hepatocellular Ca
- Hepatomegaly, RUQ bruit
- High alk phos, calcium, alpha-fetoprotein
- 75% prior cirrhosis — any type
- Developing countries: HBV acquired at birth

Hepatocellular Carcinoma
- Highest risk: Non-Caucasian
- Rising incidence overall
- Leading U.S. causes: HCV, HBV, EtOH
- HCV with cirrhosis: Cancer develops 1–4% per year
- IFN Tx may decrease risk of HCC
- Surveillance: Ultrasound q 6 months
- Criteria for liver transplant

Milan Criteria
- 1 lesion < 5 cm, or up to 3 lesions all < 3 cm
- No macrovascular invasion
- No lymphatic spread
- **Biopsy not mandatory!**
- "Down-staging" is allowed — i.e., TACE then reevaluate

Cirrhosis
- Common causes: Alcohol, HBV, HCV
- Uncommon causes:
  - Postnecrotic (drug)
  - Biliary disease
  - R-sided HF
  - A1AT
  - Hemochromatosis
  - Wilson's
  - Schistosomiasis

AR 44
A 50-year-old patient has cirrhosis due to hepatitis C and alcohol. He has now been abstinent from alcohol for 5 years. As part of routine screening, an EGD found large varices in the distal esophagus. He has never had any episodes of variceal bleeding, nor has he had any other complications like spontaneous bacterial peritonitis.

Which of the following would you recommend?
A. EGD with sclerotherapy of the varices.
B. Initiate beta-blocker therapy with propranolol.
C. Refer to radiology for a TIPS procedure.
D. No treatment for now, just repeat EGD in 6 months.

Answer: _____

Cirrhosis — Complications
Variceal hemorrhage
- 30% mortality (older data), 30% cirrhotics bleed
- Risk of bleeding higher for large varices
- Primary prevention: Beta-blockers
- Acute treatment: Banding (or sclero) and octreotide infusion
- Treatment failure: TIPS

Bands

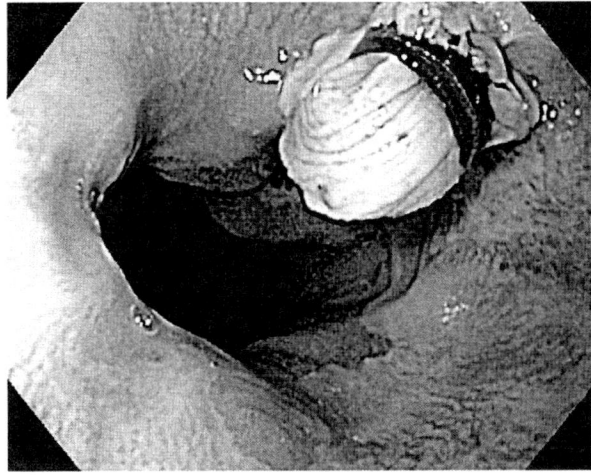

Possible Exam Question
- Cirrhotic patient with variceal bleed
- On octreotide, had variceal banding
- What else for you to do?
- Answer: Antibiotics to prevent SBP
  (patient has tense ascites)

Cirrhosis — Complications (cont.)
Hepatic encephalopathy
- Many precipitating factors: GI bleed, pneumonia, protein intake, low K, sedatives, alkalosis
- Hyperreflexia, asterixis
- Treat: Lactulose, antibiotics — neomycin or metronidazole or rifaximin

Hepatorenal syndrome
- Oliguric renal failure
- Renal vasoconstriction
- Often iatrogenic, poor survival (older data)
- Urinary $Na^+ < 10$
- Attempt volume expansion
- Midodrine and octreotide

Ascites
- Appearance:
  - Bloody: Ca; Cloudy: Infection;
  - Milky: Lymphatic obstruction
- Serum albumin — ascitic albumin
  - Difference > 1.1: Portal hypertension
  - Difference < 1.1: TBC, nephrotic, pancreatitis, peritoneal carcinomatosis
  - Know for ascites with low A-A

Protein and Albumin in Ascites

Causes	Serum/Ascites Albumin	Ascites T. Protein
Cirrhosis, liver failure, Budd-Chiari synd., and myxedema	> 1.1	< 2.5
Right heart failure	> 1.1	> 2.5
TB peritonitis, nephrotic synd., pancreatitis, and peritoneal carcinomatosis	< 1.1	> 2.5

Key Concepts — Ascites
- Dietary Na^+ restriction is vital
- Cirrhosis is most common cause
- Combination furosemide and spironolactone is first-line diuretic therapy
- Refractory: Transplant or TIPS
- Avoid NSAIDs, ASA, aminoglycosides

Speaking of TIPS
- Contraindications to TIPS:
  - No: Low platelets, transplant candidate
  - Yes: HF, encephalopathic
- Not used for primary prophylaxis of bleeding
- Main indications: Variceal hemorrhage and ascites

Spontaneous Bacterial Peritonitis
- Risk factors: Prior SBP, bili > 2.5, fluid protein < 1, UGI hemorrhage
- Paracentesis: > 250 neutrophils
- *E. coli, S. pneum, Klebsiella*
- Initial treatment: Cefotaxime
- Give IV albumin: Less renal impairment and lower mortality

When to Suspect SBP
- Fever
- Unexplained leukocytosis
- Unexplained renal failure
- Hepatic encephalopathy
- SBP with confusion as only symptom

Gilbert Syndrome
- Unconjugated hyperbilirubinemia (indirect, without bilirubinuria)
- Jaundice after physical stress, fasting
- Common, hereditary condition
- Autosomal dominant
- Know for exams

Hemochromatosis
- Genetic or acquired
- *C282Y* mutation 0.44% of U.S. non-Hispanic Caucasian population
- Autosomal recessive
- Abnormal increased intestinal iron (Fe) absorption
- Fe deposition: Liver, heart, pancreas, pituitary
- Association with arthritis

- Hepatomegaly 95%; Hyperpigmentation 90%; Diabetes 65%; Arthropathy 40%; Cardiac 15%
- Diagnosis:
  - High iron saturation (> 45%)
  - High ferritin
  - *HFE* gene
- Screen family members
- Treat with phlebotomy; Try to get ferritin level around 50

Wilson Disease
- Autosomal recessive
- Impaired excretion of copper into bile resulting in excess copper in body
- Presents: Adolescents with liver, neuro, psych
- Young girl with personality change and increased LFTs
- Hemolysis

- Serum ceruloplasmin is low (<u>very</u> low in my 2-patient experience)
- Urinary copper is high
- Slit-lamp exam shows Kayser-Fleischer ring
- Liver biopsy: High copper, but this is also seen in PBC and PSC
- Liver biopsy can also look like NAFLD

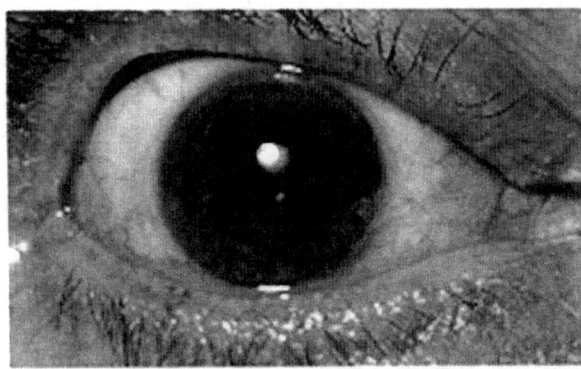

Liver Disease During Pregnancy
- First trimester
  - Hyperemesis gravidarum: Mild increase AST/ALT
  - Acute viral hepatitis: Viral hepatitis E can be severe
  - Gallstones: Pain, abnormal U/S, 2nd trimester is best time for surgery

- Second trimester
  - Intrahepatic cholestasis of pregnancy: Itching, late in pregnancy, increased ALT/AST, alk phos, and bili
  - Acute viral hepatitis/Gallstones

- Third trimester
  - Fatty liver of pregnancy
  - HELLP
  - Preeclampsia
  - Intrahepatic cholestasis of pregnancy

Fatty Liver of Pregnancy
- Microvesicular fat deposition
- Occurs in last trimester
- Abdominal pain, nausea, vomiting
- Encephalopathy, hypoglycemia
- Pruritus is rare
- Complications: Fulminant liver failure, encephalopathy, jaundice, hypoglycemia, coagulopathy
- Modest elevation of AST/ALT/bili
- Treatment: Prompt delivery

Liver Transplant
- Consider for any patient with end-stage, acute/chronic disease or with HCC
- End-stage disease: Bili > 10; Alb < 2.5; INR 2
- Refractory Sxs: Pruritus, Encephalopathy, Ascites
- Assess with MELD: Includes bili, INR, and creatinine
- New scoring system MELD-Na may be coming — includes serum sodium

AR 45

What is the most common cause of acute liver failure in the U.S.?
A. Drug hepatotoxicity
B. Wilson's
C. HBV
D. Amanita mushrooms

Answer: _____

Drug Hepatotoxicity
- Drug hepatotoxicity, including acetaminophen
  - Can be suicide attempt or accidental
  - Several days of taking 3–5 per day
  - Alcoholics at increased risk
  - Better prognosis for the suicide attempts
  - Some lead to transplant

Questions??

Gastroenterology
Audience Response Answers

Audience Response 1
Answer: A. Achalasia.

AR 2
Answer: A. GI consult for EGD to remove food bolus.

AR 3
Answer: B. Doxycycline-induced esophageal ulceration.

AR 4
Answer: B. EGD.

AR 5
Answer: B. Repeat endoscopy in 3 years.

AR 6
Answer: C. Refer to GI for EGD.

AR 7
Answer: A. Blood transfusion and PPI drip.

AR 8
Answer: A. *H. pylori* ELISA and treat if positive.

AR 9
Answer: A. MALT lymphoma of the stomach.

AR 10
Answer: D. Stool antigen test for *H. pylori*.

AR 11
Answer: D. Metoclopramide 10 mg before meals.

AR 12
Answer: D. Order fasting serum gastrin
after stopping the omeprazole for 7 days.

AR 13
Answer: B. Initiate infliximab.

AR 14
Answer: D. An exacerbation of Crohn's disease.

AR 15
Answer: B. Arthralgias.

AR 16
Answer: A. Oral mesalamine 800 mg PO tid.

AR 17
Answer: A. Surgery consult.

AR 18
Answer: D. No treatment.

AR 19
Answer: A. Metronidazole.

AR 20
Answer: C. Colonoscopy with biopsy.

AR 21
Answer: D. Order tissue transglutaminase (TTG).

AR 22
Answer: C. Chronic pancreatitis.

AR 23
Answer: A. A 2-week course of amoxicillin/clavulanate.

AR 24
Answer: B. Fecal impaction.

AR 25
Answer: D. Trial of lactose-free, sorbitol-free diet.

AR 26
Answer: B. 5 years.

AR 27
Answer: A. Colonoscopy at age 35 years.

AR 28
Answer: B. Encourage her to get a colonoscopy.

AR 29
Answer: A. CT of abdomen and pelvis.

AR 30
Answer: D. Upper endoscopy.

AR 31
Answer: A. EGD.

AR 32
Answer: B. Diverticulosis.

AR 33
Answer: C. Hereditary hemorrhagic telangiectasia.

AR 34
Answer: A. Video capsule.

AR 35
Answer: E. B and C.

AR 36
Answer: A. Acute pancreatitis.

AR 37
Answer: B. CT scan.

AR 38
Answer: D. Cholecystectomy.

AR 39
Answer: A. Cholecystectomy.

AR 40
Answer: A. ERCP.

AR 41
Answer: B. Antimitochondrial antibody.

AR 42
Answer: D. HCC screening with ultrasound every 6 months starting at age 40 years.

AR 43
Answer: B. Prednisone and azathioprine.

AR 44
Answer: B. Initiate beta-blocker therapy with propranolol.

AR 45
Answer: A. Drug hepatotoxicity.

MedStudy

Internal Medicine Video Board Review

General Internal Medicine

Presented by

Doug Paauw, MD
Professor, Medicine
Director, Internal Medicine Medical Student Programs
University of Washington School of Medicine
Department of Medicine
Seattle, Washington

General Internal Medicine

Table of Contents

General Internal Medicine Abbreviations

AAA	Abdominal aortic aneurysm
ABG	Arterial blood gas
ACE	Angiotensin-converting enzyme
ACEI	Angiotensin-converting enzyme inhibitor
AD	Alzheimer disease
ALT	Alanine aminotransferase test
ARB	Angiotensin receptor blocker
AST	Aspartate aminotransferase (formerly serum glutamic oxaloacetic transaminase [SGOT])
BMP	Basic metabolic panel
BNP	B-type natriuretic peptide
BPV	Benign positional vertigo
BUN	Blood urea nitrogen
Ca	Cancer
CAD	Coronary artery disease
CBC	Complete blood count
CBT	Cognitive behavioral therapy
ChE-I	Cholinesterase inhibitor
CI	Confidence interval
COPD	Chronic obstructive pulmonary disease
CPK	Creatine phosphokinase
CRI	Chronic renal insufficiency
DBP	Diastolic blood pressure
DM	Diabetes mellitus
DVT	Deep vein thrombosis
ECG-NSR	Echocardiogram normal sinus rhythm
ED	Emergency department; Erectile dysfunction
EOM	Extraocular muscle
ESRD	End-stage renal disease
EtOH	Ethanol alcohol
FEV_1	Forced expiratory volume in 1 second
FOBT	Fecal occult blood test
G_1P_0	Gravida 1 (first pregnancy), Para 0 (no births)
GERD	Gastroesophageal reflux disease
HAART	Highly active antiretroviral treatment
HCTZ	Hydrochlorothiazide
HIV	Human immunodeficiency virus
HPV	Human papilloma virus
HSV	Herpes simplex virus
JVP	Jugular venous pressure
LVH	Left ventricular hypertrophy
MAOI	Monoamine oxidase inhibitor
MCV	Mean cell volume
METs	Metabolic equivalents
MI	Myocardial infarction
MRI	Magnetic resonance imaging
NAC	N-acetylcysteine
NNH	Number needed to harm
NNT	Number needed to treat
NPH	Neutral protamine Hagedorn
NVD	Neovascularization of the optic disc
NVE	Native valve endocarditis
OCP	Oral contraceptive pill
PPI	Proton pump inhibitor
PT	Prothrombin time
PTT	Partial thromboplastin time
PUD	Peptic ulcer disease
PVC	Premature ventricular contraction
PVD	Pulmonary vascular disease
RUQ	Right upper quadrant
$S_1S_2 + S_4$	Heart sounds 1, 2, and 4
S_3	Heart sound 3
SBP	Systolic blood pressure
SEM	Systolic ejection murmur
SLE	Systemic lupus erythematosus
T&C	Type and cross-match (blood)
TB	Tuberculosis
TSH	Thyroid-stimulating hormone
TTE	Transthoracic echocardiogram
TURP	Transurethral resection of the prostate
UGI	Upper gastrointestinal
V/Q scan	Ventilation perfusion lung scan
VA	Visual acuity

Speaker Disclosure
Doug Paauw, MD, has documented that he has no commercial relationships to disclose.

General Internal Medicine

Drug Interactions and Important Side Effects

Audience Response 1
A 55-year-old woman with a Hx of hypothyroidism presents with increasing fatigue and bradycardia. Her TSH has risen from 4 mU/L a year ago to 45. Her meds are simvastatin, verapamil, warfarin, citalopram, calcium, and an MVI.

An interaction with which of these is the most likely cause of her increased TSH?
A. Simvastatin
B. Verapamil
C. Warfarin
D. Citalopram
E. Calcium

Answer: _____

Absorption — Thyroid Hormone / Quinolones
- These drugs are easily bound by cations and binders:
  - Iron
  - Antacids
  - Calcium
  - Cholestyramine
  - Sucralfate
- PPIs can decrease thyroid absorption by as much as 33%
- When a patient has had a stable TSH on thyroid replacement and now has an increase in TSH, look for an absorption problem

What should you do with a patient on thyroxine with a rising TSH?
- Assess compliance
- Taking $FeSO_4$?
- Taking $CaCO_3$?
- Taking sucralfate/cholestyramine?
- Taking PPI or H_2 blocker?
- Could the patient have achlorhydria?
- Could the patient have sprue?

AR 2
A 70-year-old male S/P AV replacement 2 years ago for aortic stenosis presents with widespread ecchymosis on his back/legs and some bruising on the back of both hands. His last INR was 3 weeks ago and was 3.0. He states he saw an MD 6 days ago for a cough and was put on a medication described as a "white tablet."

His chronic medications include warfarin 5 mg daily, albuterol inhaler 2 puffs 4x/day, and nortriptyline 25 mg q hs.

What medication was he placed on?
A. Codeine
B. Cephalexin
C. Azithromycin
D. TMP/SMX
E. Amoxicillin

Answer: _____

Warfarin Interactions Decrease Metabolism (Increase PT)

Most Severe	Possible*
TMP/SMX	Ciprofloxacin
Erythromycin	Omeprazole
Amiodarone	Clarithromycin
Propafenone	Azithromycin
Ketoconazole/Fluconazole	*especially elderly
Itraconazole	and polypharmacy
Metronidazole	

AR 3
A 39-year-old woman with a prosthetic aortic valve presents with bruising.
Her last INR 6 weeks ago was 2.4; today's INR is 6.5. She has not taken any extra warfarin.

Which of the following, when taken on a daily basis, could explain her increased INR?
A. Acetaminophen
B. Calcium carbonate
C. OCP
D. Ranitidine
E. DOSS

Answer: _____

Warfarin and Acetaminophen
- 3 studies suggest increased INR with acetaminophen + warfarin
  - > 9,100 mg/week led to 10x risk of having INR > 6*
  - In double-blind crossover trial, patients on warfarin plus 4 g/day of acetaminophen had PT 1.75x control[+]
  - In a double-blind crossover study, patients on warfarin therapy received 1 g of acetaminophen 4x/day or a placebo; Mean INR at 1 week was 3.45 with acetaminophen vs. 2.66 with the placebo ($p = 0.03$)[#]

*JAMA. 1998;279:657–662.
[+] Clin Res. 1984;32:698a.
[#] Haematologica. 2006;91:1621–1627.

Antibiotics for UTI in Patients on Warfarin
- Penicillins/Cephalosporins — okay
- Nitrofurantoin — okay
- Quinolones — be worried
- TMP/SMX — don't use

Problems with Statins

AR 4
A 65-year-old man presents with cough and fever. He has had severe diarrhea for 2 days. He was on a cruise with a friend who was diagnosed with *Legionella* yesterday.
PMH: Diabetes, hyperlipidemia, hypertension
Meds: Lisinopril, simvastatin, amlodipine, gemfibrozil, metformin
Chest x-ray shows patchy bilateral infiltrates
WBC 17,000, Na^+ 125

What is the most appropriate treatment?
A. Amoxicillin/clavulanate
B. Clarithromycin
C. Levofloxacin
D. Cefuroxime
E. TMP/SMX

Answer: _____

Drugs That Increase Risk of Statin Toxicity
- Fibrates (gemfibrozil 15x >> fenofibrate)
- Azole antifungals
- Amiodarone
- Erythromycin/Clarithromycin
- Protease inhibitors
- Verapamil/Diltiazem
- Fewest drug interactions with pravastatin

Side Effects of Statins
- Rhabdomyolysis (rare) 0.01%
- Hepatotoxicity (rare)
- Liver failure 0.0001%
- Myalgias 5–18%

Myalgias and Statins
- Appears to be dose- and possibly drug-related
- Check TSH level
- More common in patients with low body mass
- More common in Asian patients
- ? Role of vitamin D
- ? Benefit of coenzyme Q10 (low ubiquinone levels?)
- Biopsies of muscle in statin-treated patients with myalgia and normal CPK levels have shown myopathy
- Biopsies of muscle in statin-treated patients with no symptoms have shown muscle cell damage

AR 5
A 68-year-old man has questions about his medications. He is concerned about interactions with his meds. He is on omeprazole, nifedipine, citalopram, and testosterone.

What beverage should he avoid taking on a daily basis?
A. Orange juice
B. Green tea
C. Apple juice
D. Grapefruit juice
E. Lemonade

Answer: _____

Grapefruit Juice and Statins
- Statins metabolized via CYP3A4 are most affected (simvastatin/lovastatin > atorvastatin)
- Small amounts of grapefruit juice (half a grapefruit/small glass) or low doses of statin are unlikely to be clinically important
- Pravastatin/fluvastatin/rosuvastatin do not rely on CYP3A4 metabolism

- 200 mg double-strength grapefruit juice and lovastatin 80 mg or simvastatin 60 mg
- Lovastatin and simvastatin AUC increased 15x
Clin Pharmacol Ther. 1998;63:397–402.

**What Should You Worry About
When Prescribing Simvastatin?**
- Major interaction with grapefruit juice
- Mild interaction with warfarin
- Major interaction with amiodarone
- Usual statin concern with fibrates/clarithromycin/azoles
- Red flags should go off when prescribing for patients with A-fib, where they might be on both warfarin and amiodarone (and a Ca^{2+} channel blocker)

AR 6
A 38-year-old woman with RA presents with a skin lesion that is painful and has developed over the past 24 hours (see image). She has had fevers.
Meds: Prednisone 10 mg daily, hydroxychloroquine 200 mg daily, methotrexate 25 mg/week, omeprazole 20 mg/day, and naproxen 500 mg bid

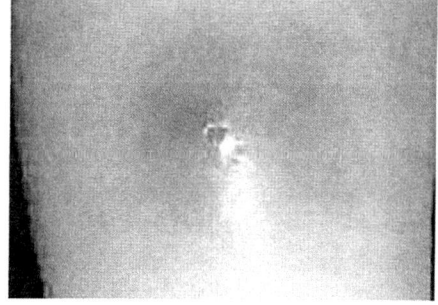

AR 6 (cont.)
What is the most appropriate treatment?
A. Doxycycline
B. TMP/SMX
C. Dicloxacillin
D. Levofloxacin

Answer: _____

AR 7
An 85-year-old man is brought to the emergency department for evaluation of weakness and nausea. He was diagnosed 10 days ago with prostatitis. His other problems include hypertension, CHF, and CRI.
Meds: Carvedilol, furosemide, TMP/SMX, verapamil, digoxin
Exam: BP 100/60, P 100, T 98.4° F (36.9° C) cardiac — grade 2/6 SEM, lower extremity edema present
Labs: Na^+ 132, K^+ 6.8, Bun 37, Cr 2.3

What is the most likely cause of his hyperkalemia?
A. Chronic renal insufficiency
B. Carvedilol
C. TMP/SMX
D. Verapamil
E. Digoxin

Answer: _____

Trimethoprim / Sulfa-Induced Hyperkalemia
- Risk greatest in patients with CKD, patients taking ACEI or ARBS
- Hyperkalemia has been reported in elderly patients receiving oral TMP/SMX
- The elevation may be severe
- Mechanism is due to trimethoprim blockage of amiloride-sensitive Na^+/K^+ channels

Hyperkalemia — Drug-Induced
- ACE inhibitors/ARB
- K^+-sparing diuretics
- TMP/SMX
- NSAIDs
- Salt substitute

When Not to Use TMP/SMX
- Patient taking warfarin
- Patient taking methotrexate
- Allergy
- Elderly patients with renal insufficiency

AR 8
A 60-year-old man presents with peripheral edema. He has been bothered by this for the past 6 months, but it has become a bit worse in the past 3 weeks. He recently (3 weeks ago) returned from a trip to Thailand. He has no dyspnea or leg pain.

PMH: Depression, hypertension, GERD
Meds: Ranitidine, fluoxetine, nifedipine, hydrochlorothiazide, ginkgo
Exam: BP 120/70, P 70; No elevated JVP; Normal cardiac exam; Extremities 2+ bilateral edema
Labs: Na^+ 135, K^+ 3.4, Cl^- 98, Bun 10, Cr 1.0, D-dimer 0.2 (normal = < 0.4)

What is the most likely cause for his edema?
A. DVT
B. CHF
C. Cirrhosis
D. Fluoxetine
E. Ranitidine
F. Nifedipine
G. Ginkgo

Answer: _____

Drug-Induced Edema
- Dihydropyridines (nifedipine, felodipine, amlodipine)
- Pioglitazone
- NSAIDs
- Estrogen and testosterone
- Pramipexole
- Gabapentin and pregabalin (7–8%)
- Omeprazole

NSAIDs and CHF in the Elderly
- 365 cases of patients admitted with CHF compared to 658 control patients admitted without CHF
- NSAID users had an odds ratio of 2.1 for admission for CHF
- Odds ratio of 10.5 for first admit for CHF if patient had heart disease and used NSAIDs
- Risk of admission for CHF correlates with dose of NSAID and long-acting drug
Arch Intern Med. 2000;160:777–784.

Drugs That Increase Serum Uric Acid
- Diuretics
- Niacin
- Cyclosporine
- Ethambutol/Pyrazinamide
- Topiramate

AR 9

An 80-year-old man presents to the ED following a seizure. He has a history of hypertension and chronic neck pain. Medications include: Amitriptyline, hydrochlorothiazide, tramadol, benazepril, and DOSS. His exam is unremarkable except for postictal confusion.
Labs: Bun 20, Cr 1.2, Na^+ 140, K^+ 4.2, Ca^{2+} 9.8
Head CT with contrast: No abnormalities

What would you recommend?
A. Stop benazepril.
B. Stop tramadol.
C. Obtain lumbar puncture.
D. Obtain MRI.
E. Begin phenytoin.

Answer: _____

AR 10

A 46-year-old woman with diabetes and seizure disorder presents with nausea and fatigue. Physical exam is unremarkable.
Meds: Glyburide 5 mg daily, metformin 850 mg bid, phenytoin 300 mg daily, topiramate 400 mg daily, pantoprazole 40 mg daily
Labs: Na^+ 133, K^+ 3.9, Cl^- 112, HCO_3^- 13, Glu 158, Bun 18, Cr 1.0

What is the most likely cause of this patient's acidosis?
A. Phenytoin
B. Topiramate
C. Metformin
D. Pantoprazole

Answer: _____

Topiramate and Acidosis
- Topiramate acts as a carbonic anhydrase inhibitor
- Metabolic nonanion gap hyperchloremic acidosis can occur
- Average drop in bicarbonate is 4, but can be severe, especially in the setting of surgery
- Also raises serum uric acid levels

AR 11

A 66-year-old woman presents with hypotension and confusion. She was in her usual state of health until 4 hours prior when she felt ill and vomited a small amount of bloody material. She did not seek medical attention for 2 additional hours. She had another episode of emesis, this time of a large amount of bloody material. She has also had 1 episode of maroon stool.

PMH: HTN, osteoporosis, and depression
Meds: Fluoxetine, benazepril, hydrochlorothiazide, acetaminophen, and estrogen/progestin

Which medication has the strongest association with UGI bleeding?
A. Fluoxetine
B. Benazepril
C. Hydrochlorothiazide
D. Acetaminophen
E. Estrogen

Answer: _____

SSRIs and GI Bleeding
- Multiple retrospective studies show relative risk for UGI bleeding of 3–4 with the use of SSRIs
- Risk is further increased with concurrent use of a nonsteroidal; Odds ratio 6.33 if SSRI combined with NSAID
- Risk is highest in the elderly
- Strongly consider gastroprotection if combination used in patients with history of UGI bleeding, in patients taking NSAIDs, or the elderly
Arch Intern Med. 2003;163:59–64.
BMJ. 1999;319 (7217):1106–1109.
Aliment Pharmacol Ther. 2008;27:31–40.

AR 12

A 69-year-old woman presents with symptoms of severe muscle pain and joint pain. This has been present for the past 3 weeks. She has had no fevers, chills, or trauma. She has a past history of HTN, hypothyroidism, CAD, osteoporosis, GERD, and depression.
Meds: Omeprazole, metoprolol, alendronate, citalopram, levothyroxine

What is the most likely cause of her pain?
A. Citalopram
B. Omeprazole
C. Alendronate
D. Metoprolol
E. Hypothyroidism

FDA Advisory on Bisphosphonates and Musculoskeletal Pain
- Strongly consider bisphosphonate as cause for musculoskeletal pain in patients who are taking them and have severe pain
- Strongly consider temporarily or permanently stopping the medication
- Much more likely with weekly or monthly dosing

AR 13

A 66-year-old woman presents with fatigue.
She has a history of bipolar disorder and reflux disease.
She has felt well the past few months up until the recent several weeks.
Medications: Rabeprazole, lithium, paroxetine, calcium
Physical exam is normal.
As part of her workup, she is found to have the following labs: Na^+ 120, K^+ 3.6, Bun 3, Cr 0.7

What is the most likely cause of her low sodium?
A. Hyperlipidemia
B. Lithium
C. Acute psychosis
D. Rabeprazole
E. Paroxetine

Answer: _____

SSRIs and Hyponatremia
- Older age
- Female
- Concomitant diuretic use
- Low body weight

Most Important Drug Causes of Hyponatremia
- Hydrochlorothiazide (30% risk)
- SSRIs
- Carbamazepine

Think Before Putting SSRIs in the Drinking Water
- Probable increased risk of UGI bleed
- Often overlooked cause of hyponatremia
- Sexual dysfunction (20–50%)

Lab Abnormalities Caused by Hydrochlorothiazide
- Hyponatremia
- Hypokalemia
- Hyperuricemia
- Hypercalcemia
- Increased lipids
- Slight glucose increase

Statistics
- Sensitivity and specificity
- Positive predictive value
- Negative predictive value
- *P* value
- NNT

Interpretation of Test Results

	Disease Present	Not Present
+	True Positive	False Positive
−	False Negative	True Negative

AR 14

A new blood test is developed to screen for pancreatic cancer. The sensitivity of the test is 75%.

Which of the following is correct?
A. Patients with a negative test result have a 75% chance of not having the disease.
B. Patients with a positive test result have a 75% chance of having the disease.
C. In patients who have the disease, 25% have a negative test result.
D. In patients with negative test results, 75% do not have the disease.

Answer: _____

Sensitivity
- Proportion of diseased population with positive test results
- $TP/(TP + FN)$

AR 15

In a study of 3,000 patients with a history of colon cancer, fecal occult blood testing (FOBT) is done to screen for recurrent colon cancer. 300 patients have positive FOBT and 2,700 patients have negative FOBT. Colonoscopy is done on all the patients, finding 40 cancers. 10 patients with positive FOBT have colon cancer, and 30 with negative tests have colon cancer.

What is the sensitivity for FOBT?
A. 90%
B. 95%
C. 33%
D. 25%

Answer: _____

Sensitivity

$$\text{Sensitivity} = 10/(10 + 30)$$
$$= 25\%$$

AR 16
A new test for bladder cancer has a specificity of 85%.

Which of the following is correct?
A. 15% of patients who do have bladder cancer are missed by this test.
B. 85% of patients with bladder cancer test positive for this test.
C. 15% of patients without bladder cancer test positive for this test.
D. 85% of patients with bladder cancer test positive for this test.

Answer: _____

SPIN and SNOUT
- Sensitivity: A highly sensitive test rules a disease <u>out</u> (**SNOUT**) — people with the disease should have a positive test, so if they don't have a positive test they don't have the disease
- Specificity: a highly specific test should rule a disease <u>in</u> (**SPIN**) — that is, no one who does not have the disease should test positive

AR 17
Which point would have the highest positive predictive value for a disease?

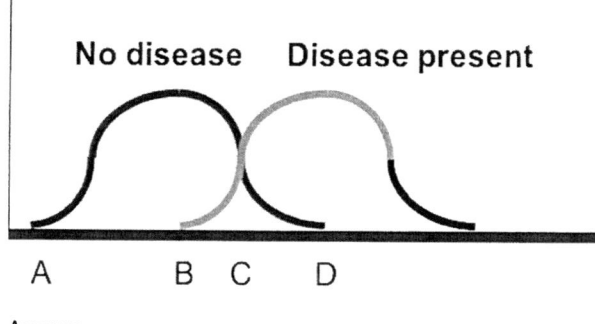

Answer: _____

Positive Predictive Value
- Positive predictive value is the proportion of those with positive tests who have the disease
- TP/(TP + FP)

AR 18
Which point would have the highest negative predictive value for a disease?

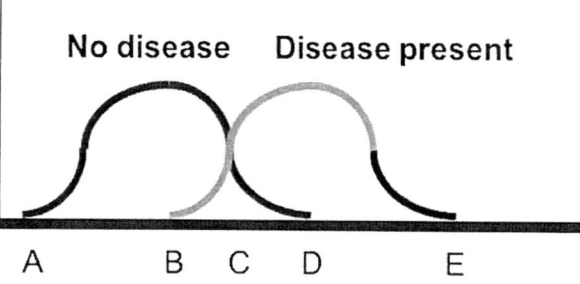

Negative Predictive Value
- Negative predictive value is the proportion of patients with a negative test result who are disease-free
- NPV = TN/(FN + TN)

AR 19
A study is done to evaluate mammography as a screening tool for women between the ages of 40 and 45. 1,100 mammograms are obtained. 25 women have a positive mammogram and turn out to have breast cancer. 175 women have positive mammograms and do not have cancer. 890 women have negative mammograms and do not have cancer, while 10 women with negative mammograms end up having breast cancer.

What is the NPV for mammography?
A. 20%
B. 90%
C. 93%
D. 96%
E. 99%

Answer: _____

Negative Predictive Value (cont.)
- NPV = TN/(FN + TN)
- NPV = 890/(10 + 890) = 98.9%

AR 20
In many labs, the cutoff for a normal PSA is 4.0.

What would happen if the cutoff for normal PSA was changed to 2.5?
A. Sensitivity and specificity would increase.
B. Positive predictive value would increase, but negative predictive value would decrease.
C. Positive and negative predictive value would increase.
D. Sensitivity would increase; specificity would decrease.

Answer: _____

Changing Normal limits
If you make the normal limit less (e.g., reduce upper limit of normal on PSA from 4.0 to 2.5) you will have more false positives, which will decrease specificity; You will have fewer false negatives, which will increase sensitivity

AR 21
A new therapy for lung cancer is extremely successful, prolonging life by an average of 3 years. This treatment becomes standard of care for lung cancer patients.

What effect does this have on lung cancer statistics?
A. Increases the incidence
B. Increases the prevalence
C. Increases the sensitivity of screening tests
D. Deceases the specificity of screening tests
E. Reduces the positive predictive value of screening tests

Answer: _____

Incidence and Prevalence
- Incidence — The incidence is the number of newly diagnosed cases during a specific time period
- Prevalence — The prevalence is the number of cases alive at a certain date

Influence of Disease Prevalence on PPV and NPV
- Prevalence of a disease within a screening population greatly influences the performance of a screening test
- As prevalence of a disease falls, PPV drops and NPV rises
- The less common a disease, the more likely a positive test represents a false positive

AR 22
A researcher wants to study the effects of exposure to high doses of aspartame and the development of renal cancer. He wishes to complete his study within 15 months.

What would be the most appropriate study design?
A. Case series
B. Case-control trial
C. Randomized-control trial
D. Cohort study

Answer: _____

Case-Control Study
- Used to identify factors that may contribute to a medical condition
- The starting point of a case-control study is subjects with the disease or condition under study (cases)
- A control group is selected from patients without the disease but otherwise similar characteristics

AR 23
Which of the following is the best example of key medical information derived from a case-control study?
A. ACEIs delay progression of diabetic nephropathy.
B. Tricyclic antidepressants decrease the pain of post-herpetic neuralgia.
C. Triple therapy against *H. pylori* can cure PUD.
D. Cigarette smoking can cause lung cancer.

Answer: _____

AR 24
An average normal platelet count is 225,000 with a standard deviation of 50,000 platelets.

What percent of normal individuals would have a platelet count < 125,000?
A. 1%
B. 2.5%
C. 5%
D. 10%
E. 15%

Answer: _____

P Value
- P value is used to express a study's statistical significance
- A p value of 0.10 means the likelihood that the results are due to chance is 10%
- P values < 0.05 are generally considered statistically significant; The lower the p value the better ($p < 0.001$ better than $p < 0.01$)

AR 25
A meta-analysis is done to see if blood glucose monitoring leads to lower glycohemoglobin levels. Several studies are chosen for the meta-analysis:

© 2017 MedStudy Internal Medicine Video Board Review – General Internal Medicine • Doug Paauw, MD

AR 25 (cont.)

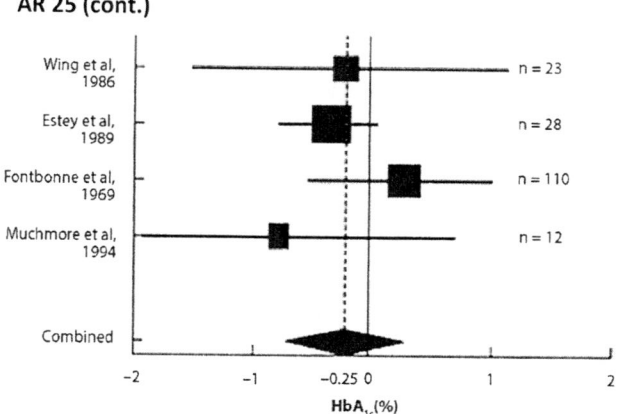

What is a correct interpretation?
A. Blood glucose monitoring has a small, statistically significant improvement in HbA1c.
B. Blood glucose monitoring leads to a small, statistically significant worsening in HbA1c.
C. Blood glucose monitoring leads to a moderately statistically significant improvement in HbA1c.
D. Blood glucose monitoring is not associated with a statistically significant change in HbA1c.

Answer: _____

AR 26
A study looks to see if there is an association between use of methylphenidate in childhood and depression during adulthood. A relative risk of 2.3 was found with a p value of < 0.05.

Which of the following would be a possible 95% confidence interval for this study?
A. 0.8–4.6
B. 0.8–3.8
C. 0.6–4.2
D. 1.2–4.0
E. 2.3–5.6

Answer: _____

Confidence Intervals
- If the 95% confidence interval crosses zero for a treatment, then it is <u>not</u> significant
- If a 95% confidence interval crosses 1 for a relative risk or odds ratio, then it is <u>not</u> significant
  - Example: CI for breast self-exam and death from breast cancer RR 0.8 with CI 0.6–1.2; This <u>would not</u> be statistically significant

Lead-Time Bias
- Early diagnosis falsely appears to prolong survival
- Overestimation of survival duration among screen-detected cases (relative to those detected by signs and symptoms) when survival is measured from diagnosis

AR 27
A study is done to test a new treatment for heart failure. Patients received usual CHF treatment plus Drug X or usual treatment plus a placebo. 10/50 patients who received the drug died, and 20/50 patients who received the placebo died.

What is the number needed to treat (NNT) for this new drug?
A. 2
B. 5
C. 10
D. 15
E. 50

Answer: _____

Number Needed to Treat (NNT)
- Number of people needed to treat to prevent 1 bad outcome
- 1/(absolute risk reduction) = 1/(rate in placebo group minus rate in treatment group)
- Example:
  For placebo 20/50 and drug 10/50,
  $1/(0.4 - 0.2) = 1/0.2 = 5$

Number Needed to Harm
The number needed to harm (NNH) is the number of patients who get a drug or intervention for each patient harmed.

AR 28
If the presence of peripheral edema has a sensitivity of 80% and a specificity of 40% for the presence of cirrhosis, what is the likelihood ratio if a patient has edema?
A. 3
B. 2.4
C. 2
D. 1.33
E. 0.75

Answer: _____

Positive Likelihood Ratio
- To calculate: Sensitivity/(1 – Specificity)
- The positive likelihood ratio is used with positive test results (the probability of a patient who has the disease testing positive divided by the probability of a person not having the disease testing positive)

AR 29
If the absence of peripheral pulses has a sensitivity of 90% for PAD and a specificity of 95%, what is the negative likelihood ratio for PAD if a patient has peripheral pulses?
A. 1.0
B. 0.5
C. 0.3
D. 0.1
E. 0.05

Answer: _____

Negative Likelihood Ratio
- Calculated as: (1 – Sensitivity)/Specificity
- Use this when you have a negative test result and you are looking to see how much less likely something is with a negative test

Geriatrics
- Falls
- Pressure ulcers
- Depression/Delirium
- Infections in the elderly
- Erectile dysfunction
- Incontinence/Prostate disease

Falls
- Increasing age increases fall risk (25% in 70-year-olds, 50% in 80-year-olds)
- Risks for falls
  - Poor vision
  - Neuropathy and loss of proprioception
  - Lower extremity weakness
  - Medications
  - Past falls
  - Cognitive impairment
  - Arthritis

Medications and Fall Risk
- Tricyclics (orthostatic hypotension)
- Benzodiazepines
- Vasodilators
- Antipsychotics

AR 30
A 76-year-old woman is brought in for evaluation of several recent falls. She lives in a nearby nursing home. She spends much of her day in bed, getting up for lunch and dinner. She has Type 2 diabetes, hypertension, coronary disease, and reflux.
Meds: Omeprazole, nortriptyline, hydrochlorothiazide, acarbose, and estrogen

What would you recommend?
A. 24-hour Holter monitor.
B. Event recorder monitor.
C. Stop nortriptyline.
D. Begin alendronate.

Answer: _____

Rule #1
for Geriatrics Exam Questions
If you can stop a medication, do it!

Rule #2
for Geriatrics Exam Questions
If you can't stop a med,
then order physical therapy.

AR 31
A 77-year-old man who is a NH resident is evaluated for a recent fall. He has some neuropathy and some decreased quad strength. He has a DXA scan done with a T-score at the spine of < –0.8 and < –0.6 at the hip. He has a Hx of HTN and GERD.

What would you recommend as an appropriate next step?
A. Begin teriparatide.
B. Begin alendronate.
C. Begin hydrochlorothiazide.
D. Recommend special shoes.
E. Check vitamin D level.

Answer: _____

Vitamin D Deficiency
- Extremely common in NH patients
- Higher fall risk
- Also possible cause of LE pain

Therapeutic Approach to Falls
- Start with H & P, "Get up and go" test, observe walking
- If evidence of lower extremity weakness: Strength training of LE
- If evidence of balance problems: Gait and balance training
- If medication risks: Drug withdrawal/substitution

- If orthostatic hypotension: Drug reduction or withdrawal, drug/meal separation, stockings
- Home safety eval — get rid of throw rugs!!

Pressure Sores
Location: Sacrum, trochanter, heels, iliac crest
- Stage 1: Nonblanching erythema
- Stage 2: Partial-thickness skin loss (superficial ulcer)
- Stage 3: Full-thickness skin loss
- Stage 4: Tissue loss to muscle, tendon, or bone

Pressure Sores Therapy
- Early stage, noninfected: Hydrocolloid dressing
- Avoid pressure on the sore and optimize nutrition
- Necrotic tissue should be removed
  - Wet-to-dry dressings
  - Surgical debridement

Geriatric Psychiatry

AR 32

A 70-year-old man is brought to the ED by his family because he has been "talking nonsense" for the past 3 days. He believes his family wants to kill him and that his wife is a paid assassin. He also believes he is continually being transported all night long against his will. He has been feeling poorly for 2 weeks with fatigue, lethargy, and confusion. His medical problems include Parkinson disease, hypertension, recurrent urinary tract infections, and atrial fibrillation.

Medications: Warfarin, diltiazem, ciprofloxacin, selegiline, hydrochlorothiazide, and lisinopril
Physical exam: BP 140/90, P 80 (irregular), T 99.1° F (37.3° C); Nonfocal exam
Labs: HB 13, Hct 39, WBC 8,000, Na^+ 135, K^+ 3.9, HCO_3^- 26, Bun 30, Cr 2.1, INR 1.9

What is the most likely cause of his symptoms?
A. Paranoid schizophrenia
B. Paranoid personality disorder
C. Delirium due to infection
D. Drug side effect of ciprofloxacin
E. Stroke due to atrial fibrillation

Answer: _____

Delirium
- Confusion with altered consciousness
- Features include:
  - Abnormal attention span
  - Disorganized thinking (hallucinations)
  - Altered consciousness (increased or decreased)

CNS Effects of Quinolones
- Insomnia
- Nightmares
- Psychosis
- Hallucinations

AR 33

A 78-year-old woman is admitted with a perforated duodenal ulcer. She has surgery and is moved to the ICU. After removal from the ventilator, she is extremely confused. She does not know where she is or who she is. She keeps trying to get out of bed.

What would be the best way to manage this patient?
A. 2-point restraints.
B. 4-point restraints.
C. Keep a sitter at the bedside.
D. Treatment with haloperidol.
E. Treatment with meperidine.

Answer: _____

AR 34

An 84-year-old man fractures his hip. He is on no medications. On day 2 of hospitalization, he becomes confused and is diagnosed with delirium.
BP 180/100, P 130, tremor present
Admission labs: Hct 36, MCV 103, Na^+ 136, K^+ 3.1, Mg^{2+} 0.8

What do you recommend?
A. Haloperidol
B. Olanzapine
C. Chlordiazepoxide
D. Zolpidem
E. Nitroprusside drip

Answer: _____

Delirium Causes
- Infection
- Medications
- Bladder catheter
- Restraints
- Decreased sleep
- New surroundings
- Alcohol withdrawal!!!

Delirium Medication Causes
- Anticholinergic meds
  - Tricyclic antidepressants
  - Antipsychotics
  - Antihistamines
  - Antiemetics
  - Antiparkinsonian drugs

Delirium Medication Causes (cont.)
- Analgesics
  - Narcotics
  - NSAIDs
- Steroids
- Quinolones
- Sedatives/Hypnotics

Delirium Don'ts
- Avoid restraints if possible (especially 4-point)
- Don't miss alcohol withdrawal
- Don't use meperidine
- Avoid jumping to medication treatment

Alcohol in the Elderly
- Safe drinking guidelines recommend no more than 7 drinks/week in those > 65
- Many over the age of 65 drink much more than this, often 2–4 drinks daily and are at risk for EtOH withdrawal when hospitalized

Delirium Do's
- Provide orienting stimuli (clocks, calendars, windows)
- Put glasses on patients who wear them
- Hearing aids, if used
- Remove catheters and lines ASAP
- Reassurance, touch

AR 35

An 85-year-old woman is brought to the ED after a syncopal episode. Her caregivers report a similar episode 2 weeks ago, but she recovered so quickly they did not seek evaluation for her.
Meds: Omeprazole 20 mg, pravastatin 40 mg, citalopram 10 mg, albuterol, donepezil 10 mg, isosorbide mononitrate 60 mg, and calcium
On exam: BP 100/60, P 55
ECG bradycardia with normal intervals

What drug most likely caused her syncope?
A. Citalopram
B. Pravastatin
C. Donepezil
D. Isosorbide
E. Calcium

Answer: _____

Cholinesterase Inhibitors and Syncope
- Cholinesterase inhibitors and bradycardia
  - ChE-I → RR bradycardia ↑ 1.4 (95% CI, 1.1–1.6)
  - Dose effect: Donepezil > 10 mg → 2.1 ↑ risk
  J Am Geriatr Soc. 2009;57:1997.

- Clinical significance: ChE-I use associated with:
  - Syncope: HR ↑ 1.76 (95% CI, 1.57–1.98)
  - ED visits for bradycardia: HR ↑ 1.69
  - Pacemaker placement: HR ↑ 1.49
  - Hip Fx: HR ↑ 1.18 (95% CI, 1.03–1.34)
  Arch Intern Med. 2009;169:867.

Dementia
- Decrease in level of cognition, including memory
- Behavioral disturbance
- Interference with daily function and independence

Dementia Syndromes
- Alzheimer disease (most common)
- Vascular (multi-infarct) dementia
- Parkinson disease/Lewy body/progressive supranuclear palsy
- Frontal lobe dementia
- Reversible dementias

Reversible Dementias
- Medication-induced: Analgesics, sedatives, psychotropics, anticholinergics
- Depression
- Normal pressure hydrocephalus
- Alcohol-related
- Metabolic disorders: Thyroid, B_{12}, hypercalcemia, hepatic dysfunction

AR 36

A 76-year-old man is evaluated for memory loss. He scores 20/30 on MMSE. Workup for reversible causes of dementia is negative. He is otherwise healthy, with his only medical problem being knee osteoarthritis.

What do you recommend?
A. Memantine
B. Donepezil
C. Vitamin E (2,000 units)
D. Selegiline
E. No therapy

Answer: _____

Dementia Therapy
- Medications work best when treating mild-to-moderate AD — slows progression
- Does not usually significantly improve cognition
- Mild-to-moderate AD, use cholinesterase inhibitor; For moderate-to-severe AD, consider adding:
  - Memantine
  - Therapy may help neuropsychiatric symptoms

AR 37

A 78-year-old woman is brought in for evaluation of visual hallucinations. She describes seeing cats and cockroaches running across her floor. She was diagnosed with dementia last year, after getting lost driving. Her MMSE score was 20, losing points for inability to spell "world" backwards, copy figures, and inability to do calculations.
She has done fairly well this past year, with only several episodes of getting suddenly confused. She has had 2 falls in the past 3 months.

What would be the most appropriate therapy for her symptoms?
A. Donepezil
B. Haloperidol
C. Risperidone
D. Lorazepam
E. Cataract surgery

Answer: _____

Lewy Body Dementia
- Fluctuating levels of consciousness
- Visual spatial difficulties
- Hallucinations at onset has 83% PPV
- Falls more common (coexistent PD)
- Difficulty on MMSE with copying, calculations, and spelling "world" backwards
- Increased danger with use of neuroleptics

Beware Prescribing Neuroleptics to Patients with Dementia
- Will unlikely be the correct answer, as there is a higher mortality rate due to increased sudden death risk in this population
- In patients with LBD, potential for severe neuroleptic sensitivity reactions, including exacerbation of parkinsonism, confusion, or autonomic dysfunction

AR 38

An 83-year-old man presents to clinic to discuss his insomnia. He has problems falling asleep, usually falling asleep 2 hours after his wife goes to sleep. He has tried exercising in the late afternoon, reading in bed, and watching unstimulating TV at bedtime without benefit.

What do you recommend?
A. Exercise 2 hours before bedtime on his exercise bike.
B. Do not go to the bedroom until he is tired.
C. Trial of diphenhydramine at bedtime.
D. Trial of trazodone at bedtime.
E. Trial of lorazepam at bedtime.

Answer: _____

Treatment of Insomnia in the Elderly
- Get a good history; See if they actually have insomnia
- Check med list for drugs that could be causing insomnia — steroids, SSRIs, beta-agonists, quinolones
- **Sleep Hygiene**! Avoid caffeine; Go to bed only when sleepy; Set a schedule; Daily exercise, but not before bedtime; No bright lights, TV, computer right before bedtime
- CBT and sleep restriction
- Meds: Avoid benzos, antihistamines, trazodone, antipsychotics

AR 39A

A 72-year-old woman reports discomfort in both of her lower extremities. The discomfort is present when she is seated, occurring in both calves. It does not bother her when she is walking. She describes it as a deep ache, sometimes with an itching or pulling feeling.
She has increased symptoms at nighttime when she is in bed. She has a history of DM and HTN.
Meds: Hydrochlorothiazide, lisinopril, metformin
Exam is unremarkable.

What is the most appropriate test?
A. Ankle brachial indices
B. Serum potassium level
C. Ferritin level
D. CPK
E. CT scan

Answer: _____

AR 39B

The patient's labs return normal (ferritin 80, renal function normal).

What is the most appropriate pharmacologic therapy?
A. Ibuprofen
B. Pramipexole
C. Felodipine
D. Oxycodone
E. Topiramate

Answer: _____

Restless Leg Syndrome
- Occurs more frequently with advancing age, up to 19% in those > 80
- Symptoms at rest, especially in bed, usually below the knees
- Symptoms relieved by movement
- Check for Fe^{2+} deficiency in all patients
- Treatment: Stretching, dopaminergic agents, gabapentin, $FeSO_4$ if Fe^{2+} deficient (treat if ferritin < 50)

AR 40

An 83-year-old woman comes to the clinic with concerns about worsening dizziness. She has had an increase in disequilibrium recently, including a recent fall. She has no history of CAD or seizure disorder. Her symptoms begin when she stands up and starts to walk. They are improved when she stops for a minute and touches the wall.
Meds: Sertraline, nizatidine, estrogen, and $CaCO_3$

What is the most likely diagnosis?
A. Benign positional vertigo
B. Vestibular neuronitis
C. Orthostatic hypotension
D. Panic attacks
E. Multiple sensory deficits

Answer: _____

Types of Dizziness
- Vertigo
- Presyncope
- Disequilibrium
- "Ill-defined lightheadedness"

Multiple Sensory Deficits
- Combination of decreased vision and hearing sensation and orthopedic problems can cause disequilibrium
- Symptoms improve when patient uses their hands (holds on to someone's arm, uses a cane or walker)

Ill-Defined Lightheadedness
- Panic disorder
- Anxiety disorder with hyperventilation

AR 41

A 66-year-old male presents for routine clinic visit with complaints of dizziness. He states episodes are particularly common at night when he rolls over in bed. They last for 15–30 seconds and then resolve.
The sensation is that of the room spinning around him. The symptoms have been occurring for the past 3 weeks.

What is the appropriate treatment?
A. Meclizine
B. Prednisone
C. Diazepam
D. Epley maneuver
E. Hydrochlorothiazide

Answer: _____

Treatment of BPV
- Epley maneuver (repositioning maneuver) symptom resolution at 10 days: 50% for Epley vs. 17% for sham
- Drugs: Not useful, given the brevity of attacks; Consider only in patients who do not respond to Epley and have very frequent attacks

AR 42

A 72-year-old man presents for evaluation of dizziness. He reports the acute onset of dizziness occurring yesterday. The symptoms have been persistent and bothersome to the point of his not leaving his house. He reports feeling like his head is spinning around. On exam, he has vertical nystagmus. A Dix-Hallpike maneuver increases the vertigo. The vertigo persists when the maneuver is repeated.

What is the most likely cause of his vertigo?
A. Orthostatic hypotension
B. Vestibular neuronitis
C. Benign positional vertigo
D. Acoustic neuroma
E. Brainstem ischemia

Answer: _____

Sorting Out Vertigo
- Vertical nystagmus suggests central cause
- If repeat Dix-Hallpike maneuvers decrease the symptoms, then fatigability is present, which suggests the patient has benign positional vertigo
- Most patients with central vertigo are older, with atherosclerosis, and often have other brainstem symptoms or cerebellar symptoms (dysarthria, diplopia, or motor symptoms)

Vertigo
- Benign positional vertigo
  - Brief vertigo with positional change
- Vestibular neuronitis
  - Sudden, severe vertigo x days
- Ménière syndrome
  - Ear fullness, vertigo, tinnitus, hearing loss
- Central vertigo (15%)
  - Associated symptoms universal

AR 43

A 76-year-old man is seen for hypertension. He has had 6 outside BP readings (166/80, 160/80, 156/78, 180/77, 174/60, and 178/66). He has a history of GERD, depression, and gout.

What would you recommend?
A. No drug treatment
B. Hydrochlorothiazide
C. Atenolol
D. Amlodipine
E. Clonidine

Answer: _____

Treatment of Hypertension in the Elderly
- Appropriate to treat isolated systolic hypertension; Definitely treat SBP > 160, JNC 8 recommends BP > 150/90
- Avoid β-blockers — not as effective as other agents; Especially avoid atenolol, not as effective as other β-blockers
- Avoid clonidine — increased CNS effects especially bad in the elderly
- Preferred drugs — low-dose diuretics (chlorthalidone > hydrochlorothiazide), dihydropyridines (e.g., amlodipine), ACEIs

AR 44
A 68-year-old man with HTN and DM presents with increasing dyspnea. He has been having problems with dyspnea when sleeping recumbent for the past 3 weeks.
On exam, he has rales and an S_3.
Chest x-ray shows pleural effusions and Kerley B lines
Labs: BNP 790, Bun 20, Cr 1.3, K^+ 3.9
Current meds: Glipizide, metformin, and enalapril

What medication will offer possible mortality benefit?
A. Furosemide
B. Digoxin
C. Long-acting nitroglycerin
D. Spironolactone
E. Hydrochlorothiazide

Answer: _____

Drugs That Affect Mortality in CHF
- β-blockers
- ACEI
- Spironolactone
- Hydralazine plus nitrates

AR 45
An 88-year-old woman has been having frequent episodes of fecal incontinence over the past week. She has had a small amount of liquid seepage several times a day. She has also had abdominal pain. Abdominal film as shown.

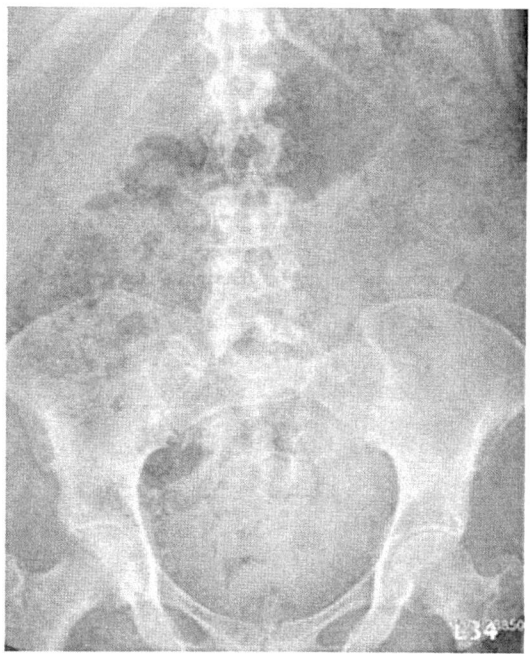

What is the most appropriate treatment?
A. Loperamide 1 tablet a day
B. Diphenoxylate/atropine 1 tablet daily
C. Fecal disimpaction
D. Amoxicillin/clavulanate
E. Lactulose twice a day

Answer: _____

Fecal Incontinence
- Definition: Minor — partial soiling of undergarments with liquid stool; Major — involuntary excretion of feces
- 15% in patients older than 70, and up to 50% in NH residents
- Etiology
  - Fecal impaction (common) causes constant inhibition of internal anal sphincter tone, allowing seepage of liquid stool
  - Trauma (surgery/childbirth injury)

AR 46
An 84-year-old man is brought to the physician by his daughter for evaluation of weight loss. He has lost 15 lbs over the past 6 months.
His weight has declined from 200 lbs to 185.
He has also had 2 falls during those 6 months.
PMH: CAD, HTN, gout
Meds: Atorvastatin, ASA, lisinopril
PE: BP 130/70, P 78, BMI 20

AR 46 (cont.)
What is the most likely cause for his weight loss?
A. Depression
B. Hyperthyroidism
C. Malignancy
D. Diabetes
E. Malabsorption

Answer: _____

Weight Loss in the Elderly
- Depression (#1)
- Dentition, dysgeusia, diarrhea, dysphagia (#2)
- Disease (cancer) (#3)
- Drugs
- Dementia
- Don't know (25%)

AR 47
An elderly nursing home patient has lost 15 pounds in the past 6 months. Complete evaluation shows the cause of his weight loss is depression.

What would be the most appropriate treatment?
A. Bupropion
B. Buspirone
C. Fluoxetine
D. Mirtazapine
E. Methylphenidate

Answer: _____

Weight Gain with Antidepressants
- MAOI (very likely)
- TCA (very likely)
- Paroxetine (more likely than other SSRIs)
- Mirtazapine (likely)

Geriatric Urology

Urinary Incontinence
Normal micturition requires appropriate cerebral cortex function, sacral nerve function (S2–S4), and bladder muscle function (detrusor and sphincter muscles).

- Urge incontinence: Detrusor overactivity
- Stress incontinence: Outlet incompetence
- Overflow incontinence: Outlet obstruction, anticholinergic drugs, detrusor underactivity

AR 48
A 79-year-old woman reports problems with urinary incontinence on a daily basis. She has to void many times during the day, yet leaks urine frequently before she can get to the restroom. She has not had hematuria or dysuria.
Meds: Omeprazole, sertraline, and enalapril
U/A is normal.

What is the most likely cause of the incontinence?
A. Detrusor underactivity
B. Sphincter dysfunction
C. Detrusor overactivity
D. Side effect of sertraline
E. Side effect of enalapril

Answer: _____

Urinary Incontinence — Reversible Causes
Drugs: Diuretics, anticholinergic drugs
Restricted mobility
Infection, impaction
Polyuric states: Hyperglycemia, CHF

Urinary Incontinence Symptoms
- Urge incontinence: Not being able to reach restroom in time, small-volume voiding
- Stress incontinence: Incontinence with cough, sneezing, jumping, laughing, standing
- Overflow incontinence: Risk factors — large prostate, diabetic
- Neuropathy, MS, psych medications

AR 49
A 76-year-old woman is evaluated for urinary incontinence. She reports a 6-year history of incontinence occurring when she laughs, coughs, or sneezes. Recently, she has had incontinence with standing.
U/A is normal.
Bun 14, Cr 1.1, Glu 111

What would you recommend?
A. Begin oxybutynin 2.5 mg PO bid.
B. Begin doxazosin 2 mg PO bid.
C. Recommend Kegel exercises.
D. Begin imipramine 25 mg PO q hs.

Answer: _____

Urinary Incontinence Therapy
- Urge incontinence: Oxybutynin, imipramine, bladder training
- Stress incontinence: Kegel exercises (PT referral if needed), alpha-adrenergic agonist (pseudoephedrine)
- Overflow incontinence: Remove offending meds, alpha-blockers for BPH

AR 50
A 76-year-old man presents for evaluation of urinary frequency and decreased urinary stream. The symptoms have been present for the past 3 years but have worsened in the last 6 months. He is now getting up 4 times a night to urinate. On exam, his prostate is 3+ enlarged without nodularity. PSA is 3.0.

© 2017 MedStudy Internal Medicine Video Board Review – General Internal Medicine • Doug Paauw, MD

What do you recommend?
A. Terazosin
B. Finasteride
C. TURP
D. Prostate ultrasound
E. Prostate biopsy

Answer: _____

Benign Prostatic Hypertrophy Therapy
- 1st line: Alpha-blockers
  - Terazosin
  - Doxazosin
  - Tamsulosin (alpha-1a-blocker)
- 2nd line
  - Finasteride (5-alpha-reductase inhibitor)
- 3rd line
  - TURP

Alpha-Blockers and
5-Alpha-Reductase Inhibitors for BPH
- Short-term therapy (1 year or less): Better response with alpha-blocker, no benefit by adding 5-alpha-reductase inhibitor
- Long-term therapy (over 4 years): Alpha-blocker + finasteride better than alpha-blocker or finasteride alone; Risk of acute urinary retention and need for invasive therapy was reduced by combination therapy or finasteride alone, but not by alpha-blocker alone

Alpha-Blockers for BPH
- Tamsulosin: Fewest side effects
- Prazosin: Greatest side effects, should be avoided
- Doxazosin/terazosin both available for $4/month

AR 51
An 84-year-old man presents with hematuria. He had an episode last week but has had hematuria for the past 4 days. He has had some hesitancy, frequency, and nocturia for several years.
Meds: ASA, MVI, omeprazole.
A urinalysis is done which just shows RBCs, no WBCs. Cystoscopy shows no bladder malignancy.
CT scan of the abdomen shows no renal lesions.

What do you recommend to help stop
future hematuria?
A. Tamsulosin.
B. Weekly dose of norfloxacin.
C. Finasteride.
D. Pyridium.
E. Stop his aspirin.

Answer: _____

Finasteride Treatment of Hematuria
in Patients with BPH
- Meta-analysis of multiple small studies for using finasteride for treatment of BPH-associated hematuria
- Use of finasteride resulted in decreased hematuria (OR 0.11, 95% CI [0.06–0.21], $p < 0.05$) over 12 months
Zhonghua Nan Ke Xua. Effects of finasteride on hematuria associated with benign prostatic hyperplasia: a meta-analysis. 2010 Aug:16(8):726–729.

What is finasteride good for?
- Symptoms of BPH — marginal
- Decreasing risk of acute urinary obstruction
- BPH-related hematuria

Erectile Dysfunction

Erectile Dysfunction (ED) Etiology
- Vascular: Diabetes, other PVD
- Neurogenic: Diabetes, Shy-Drager, peripheral neuropathy
- Hypogonadism: Low libido along with ED
- Medications: β-blockers, diuretics most common
- Psychogenic: Associated with acute onset, may be partner specific, depression

AR 52
A 67-year-old man presents for treatment of erectile dysfunction. He has had problems sustaining erections for the past year. He has a normal libido.
Meds: Pravastatin, omeprazole, isosorbide mononitrate, lisinopril, aspirin

What would you recommend for therapy?
A. Intraurethral alprostadil (Muse)
B. Sildenafil (Viagra, Revatio)
C. Testosterone patch (Androderm, Testoderm TTS)
D. Referral for penile implant

Answer: _____

Erectile Dysfunction Therapy
- Sildenafil/vardenafil (Levitra, Staxyn)/tadalafil (Cialis, Adcirca): Phosphodiesterase-5 inhibitor; Contraindicated with nitrates
- Penile injections: Alprostadil and/or papaverine
- Vacuum device: Safe but time-consuming
- Intraurethral alprostadil: Safe but can be uncomfortable and costly
- Penile implants: Use only after other therapies

Other Sexual Dysfunction
- Dyspareunia: Usually due to atrophic vaginitis in the elderly; Treat with oral/topical estrogen or lubricant
- Decreased libido: In men, due to hypogonadism or meds, often SSRIs
- Delayed orgasm: Occurs in up to 30% of patients on SSRIs

Geriatrics Review
- Order lots of physical therapy
- Stop medications
- Don't give NSAIDs!
- Try to treat delirium with TLC and not drugs

Ethics

Ethics
- Patient preferences: Respect for patient autonomy
- Beneficence: To act in the best interests and welfare of the patient and the health of society
- Nonmaleficence: The duty to do no harm to the patient

Respect for Patient Autonomy
- Religious differences
  - Cannot force adults to receive care if contrary to religious preferences
- Pregnancy
  - Pregnant women usually cannot be forced to have care for the fetus (C-section, internal monitoring)
- Paternalism
  - Practice of overriding or ignoring a patient's preferences in order to enhance welfare — usually ethically unsound

AR 53
A 29-year-old woman presents with hematemesis. She is found to have a Hct of 20. She receives IVF and is T&C for transfusion. A repeat Hct 2 hours later is 14. The patient refuses the blood transfusion when it is brought in because of religious convictions. Her husband, who is in the room with her, supports her stance. She has another episode of hematemesis while you wait for the surgeons to arrive.

What would you do?
A. Obtain a court-appointed representative.
B. Get a hospital ethics consult.
C. Give blood because this is a life-threatening emergency.
D. Give blood because of the principle of beneficence.
E. Do not give blood products.

Answer: _____

AR 54
A 21-year-old college student is brought to the ED by her roommate for symptoms of headache and fever with stiff neck over the past 18 hours.
On exam, she is somnolent but able to be aroused, with a temp of 102.2° F (39.0° C), BP 100/52, P 112. Nuchal rigidity is present. The remainder of her exam is unremarkable. WBC is 24,000. The patient gives consent for a lumbar puncture. You order a stat dose of IV antibiotics, which the patient overhears. She becomes agitated and refuses the antibiotics.

You carefully explain the high risk of death from untreated meningitis. The patient continues to refuse antibiotics and is more agitated.

What should you do?
A. Treat with IV fluids only because antibiotics carry a risk and shouldn't be given without patient consent.
B. Treat with antibiotics because the patient has a life-threatening condition.
C. Obtain a court order urgently for treatment.
D. Obtain consent from the patient's roommate and give antibiotics.

Answer: _____

Patient Competency for Decision-Making
- If patient is incapacitated by illness to make a prudent decision, another person can intervene
- Decision-making capacity refers to act of comprehending, evaluating, and choosing among realistic options
- Surrogate decision maker:
  Spouse > parents > children > siblings
- Durable power of attorney for medical affairs supersedes family

AR 55
A 76-year-old man with end-stage COPD (FEV_1 0.30) presents unconscious. He is found to have a pCO_2 of 110. He has stated in several clinic visits his desire not to be intubated.
His children, who brought him in, request everything be done, including intubation.

What is the most appropriate care?
A. Do not intubate patient; keep him comfortable.
B. Intubate patient.
C. Obtain a court-appointed representative.
D. Obtain an ethics consult.

Answer: _____

Living Will
- Allows persons to express their wishes for care when they are incapable of expressing preference
- Gives guidance in terminal and irreversible states
- Problems: Management when a condition is potentially reversible; Terms often vague — artificial means and heroic measures

An Approach to Ethical Dilemmas
- Clarify ethical issues:
  - Patient autonomy issue?
  - Competency issue?
- If dilemma can't be solved, consider ethics consult (useless in urgent situations)
- Court decision: Last resort

AR 56
An 86-year-old woman who lives in a nursing home is admitted with a severe aspiration pneumonia. She is unconscious with a fever of 104.0° F (40.0° C). ABG 7.22/52/66. She has been started on IV antibiotics and fluids. Her nephew has the durable power of attorney for health care. The patient has never completed a living will or advance directives. The nephew meets with you, stating that his aunt has become demented over the past few years, and the nephew would like IV fluids and antibiotics discontinued, with comfort care only.

Which of the following statements about the nephew is true?
A. Because the patient has not left specific advance directives, instructions to discontinue IVF and antibiotics should not be carried out.
B. The patient has a son who is next of kin, and therefore the nephew can't make medical decisions for her.
C. The nephew's instructions can be carried out only if it is determined that he had discussed this issue with his aunt and is carrying out substituted judgment.
D. The nephew's request to discontinue IVF and antibiotics is within his capacity to act with the patient's durable power of attorney.

Answer: _____

AR 57
A 66-year-old man who is a patient of yours dies after a protracted illness. It is not clear what the diagnosis was that caused his decline. His spouse wishes to get an autopsy. His daughter who had DPA for medical affairs does not wish to get an autopsy.
He has 2 other children who have not expressed their opinion.

What should you do?
A. Obtain an autopsy.
B. Do not obtain an autopsy.
C. Hold a meeting with all three children to see if they all agree.
D. Contact the patient's brother for permission for an autopsy.

Answer: _____

Durable Power of Attorney for Health Care
- Authorizes individuals to appoint another person to act as their agent to make all health care decisions after they become incapacitated
- Obligation of durable power of attorney: Carry out wishes of patient or, if such wishes are unknown, to act in best interest of the patient
- Durable power of attorney supersedes wishes of family members; But remember, it ends when the patient dies (not useful in gaining permission for autopsies)

AR 58
An 80-year-old Cambodian woman is brought to the emergency department with abdominal pain and nausea. A CT scan is done that shows multiple lesions in the liver and a large pancreatic mass. Her children ask that you do not tell her what the diagnosis is, as in their culture it isn't appropriate to tell the patient they have terminal cancer and that they are dying.

What do you do?
A. Ask the patient if she would like to designate a family member to help make decisions about her care.
B. Tell the patient that she has cancer and that it is serious.
C. Tell the patient that she has cancer and that it is terminal.

Answer: _____

Cultural Differences
- In patients from Southeast Asia especially, there is a strong desire to protect elders from hearing a terminal diagnosis
- There is also a goal of not dying in the hospital
- Important to respect cultural differences, which may change some of our approaches

AR 59
A 50-year-old man returns for follow-up CT for staging of a recently diagnosed lung cancer. The CT scan shows multiple enlarged nodes in the mediastinum and numerous liver lesions consistent with mets. He does not want his family to know. The patient requests you do not tell his wife or children.

AR 59 (cont.)
What should you do?
A. Tell the patient you want to meet with the family and the patient to discuss the diagnosis.
B. Tell the patient he must tell his spouse.
C. Tell the patient you will inform the spouse.
D. Tell the patient you understand his feelings and that you will be available to talk to the family if he wants you to.

Answer: _____

Confidentiality
- Doctor-patient relationship not absolute
- If patient confides plan to harm
- If patient conveys plans to harm named individual, these plans must be reported
- Request to withhold medical info from person at risk (HIV, TB, STI exposures); Must make sure person at risk is notified (usually by contacting public health)

AR 60
Your practice partner confides in you that he is very much attracted to one of his patients, and he believes the patient feels the same way. He asks you for advice.

What is the most appropriate statement regarding intimate interactions between a physician and his or her patient?
A. The physician should terminate the professional relationship and wait a period of time before pursuing personal contacts with the patient.
B. The physician should terminate the professional relationship and then may have personal contact with the patient.
C. The physician can never have an intimate relationship with this patient.
D. The physician may have an intimate relationship with the patient as long as it is initiated by the patient.

Answer: _____

Physician-Patient Sexual Relationships
- Any intimate relationship between patient and physician is inappropriate
- A physician needs to terminate the professional relationship with a patient and wait a period of time before pursuing a personal relationship with a former patient

AR 61
A 56-year-old man with Type 2 diabetes is hospitalized for treatment of cellulitis. He is given 100 units of NPH insulin instead of the 10 units that he usually takes. This is discovered 15 minutes after he receives the dose. He is placed on a D10 drip.

What should the physician tell the patient?
A. He is at risk for low blood sugar, so he will be receiving a drip with glucose in it.
B. A dosage error was made, and he received 10x the insulin dose he was supposed to receive. He is receiving glucose to help prevent low blood sugar.
C. He may have too much insulin right now, so he is being put on a glucose drip to avoid low blood sugar.
D. You are concerned that he could develop low blood sugar today, so you will be monitoring him closely and will have him on a glucose drip to prevent low blood sugar.
E. You will discuss this if he asks about it.

Answer: _____

Disclosure of Medical Errors
- A medical error should be disclosed if a physician suspects or knows that it has an actual or potential impact on the patient's health, well-being, or medical decision-making
- Disclosure is not conditioned by the likelihood that the error will be otherwise recognized
- Errors do not necessarily imply negligent or unethical behavior, but failure to disclose them may
- Health care professionals are ethically obligated to be forthcoming about health care injuries and errors
- Virtually all patients want physicians to acknowledge even minor errors
Jacobson, JA. Disclosing a medical error. *PIER ACP*. 2006.

Best Resource for Ethics
ACP Ethics Manual (free online)
http://www.acponline.org/running_practice/ethics/manual/

AR 62
A 57-year-old man with metastatic lung cancer is admitted for weakness and pain. He has been taking two 5-mg tablets of hydromorphone 4x a day at home for pain.

What would be an appropriate starting daily dose for pain treatment in the hospital?
A. 60 mg of oral morphine
B. 60 mg of oral hydrocodone
C. 40 mg of oral oxycodone
D. 40 mg of IV morphine

Answer: _____

Narcotic Equivalent Doses
- Morphine (oral) 1
- Morphine IV/SQ 1/3
- Oxycodone (oral) 2/3
- Oxymorphone (oral) 1/3
- Methadone 1/3
- Hydromorphone (oral) 1/4
- Hydromorphone (IV) 1/50

AR 63

A 50-year-old man presents for management of leg pain. He reports that he hurt his leg 4 months ago when his bicycle was hit by a car (ED note shows negative leg x-ray at the initial visit). His pain is rated 7/10. He has been seeing an orthopedist for the past 2 months and has been participating in physical therapy regularly.

Medications: Gabapentin, oxycodone, naproxen
Exam: Pain with extension of right leg
MRI R leg: No joint damage/fractures

What do you recommend for treatment?
A. Refill gabapentin/naproxen.
B. Refill gabapentin/naproxen/oxycodone.
C. Refill gabapentin/naproxen/taper oxycodone and start duloxetine.
D. Refill gabapentin/switch to oxycodone/start duloxetine.

Answer: _____

CDC Opioid Guidelines
- 3/2016 guidelines for prescribing opioids were released by CDC
- Bottom line — if you use opioids for acute pain, keep duration short (less than a week if possible)
- Always weigh risk/benefit of continuing

High chance this is on exam
JAMA 2016; April 19; 315(15):1624-45.

Evaluation and Treatment of Lipids

AR 64

A 48-year-old man with hypertension presents for annual follow-up. His last lipids were checked 5 years ago (TC 190, LDL 125, HDL 45, Tri 100).
Meds: Nifedipine and chlorthalidone
Exam: BP 140/60, P 80, chest — clear
Cardiac: nl S_1S_2, no M. Ext — 2+ edema
Labs: TC 255, LDL 190, HDL 40, Tri 160

What is the appropriate next step?
A. Start pravastatin.
B. Start atorvastatin.
C. Start ezetimibe.
D. Check CMP, U/A, and TSH.
E. Check BMP, testosterone.

Answer: _____

Secondary Hyperlipidemia
- Increased LDL
  - Hypothyroidism
  - Nephrotic Syndrome
  - Cholestatic liver disease
- Increased Triglycerides
  - Diabetes
  - Alcohol
  - Estrogen

Current Lipid Management
- AHA/ACC guidelines (2013)
- NCEP guidelines (NCEP 3 /ATP 3) 2001
AHA guidelines are all about risk, with cholesterol level factored in
No treat to target

NCEP Approach — Treatment for Primary Prevention

Risk	Goal LDL	Start TLC	Start Drug
High (10 yr > 20%) CAD or CADE	< 100	≥ 100	≥ 130
Moderate High (10 yr 10–20%) ≥ 2 risk factors	< 130	≥ 130	≥ 130
Moderate (10 yr < 10%) ≥ 2 risk factor	< 130	≥ 130	≥ 160
Low 0–1 risk factor	< 160	≥ 160	≥ 190

From ATP III Executive Summary

Treatment for Secondary Prevention
- In those with CHD or CHD equivalent, treat more aggressively than for those with 2 risk factors:
  - If LDL > 100, start TLC
  - If LDL > 130, start TLC + drug
- Goal LDL is < 70 or < 100
- Statins 1st line because they improve mortality

ACC / AHA Approach
4 statin benefit groups:
1) Clinical atherosclerotic CV disease
2) Familial hypercholesterolemia
3) Diabetics 40–75 with LDL 70–189 and no atherosclerotic CV disease
4) Diabetics with low lipids but a 10-year risk of CV disease > 7.5%

ACC / AHA

Heart Risk Calculator

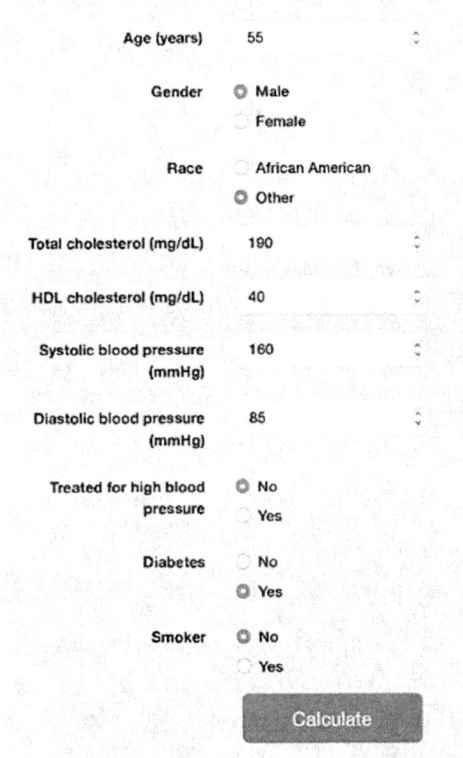

AR 65
A 61-year-old woman with hyperlipidemia, Type 2 DM, and a family history of early MI had coronary artery stenting. She is taking 40 mg of pravastatin and metformin.
Labs: A1c 6.5%, TC 210, HDL 45, LDL 119, TG 183

What is the most appropriate treatment?
A. Pravastatin 80 mg
B. Atorvastatin 80 mg
C. Atorvastatin 80 mg + niacin 1,000 mg
D. Niacin 1,000 mg

Answer: _____

AR 66
A 65-year-old man presents for primary care visit.
He has no symptoms.
PMH: Hypertension, GERD, nonsmoker
PE: BP 120/70, P 66
Labs: HbA1c 5.2, Bun 10, Cr 1.1, TC 190, LDL 135, HDL 42

What do you recommend?
A. Diet and exercise, recheck cholesterol
B. Fenofibrate
C. Pravastatin 40 mg
D. Atorvastatin 80 mg
E. No intervention

Answer: _____

Using AHA Cardiac Risk Calculator
- Risk of MI/stroke 14.3% over next 10 years
- Recommendation: Low- to moderate-intensity statin (pravastatin 40 mg/atorvastatin 20 mg)
- In general, if 65 with 1 or more risk factors, will have > 7.5% risk over 10 years

2013 ACC/AHA Guidelines

High-dose statin
- Atorvastatin 40–80 mg
- Rosuvastatin 20–40 mg

Mod-dose statin
- Atorvastatin 10–20 mg
- Rosuvastatin 5–10 mg
- Simvastatin 20–40 mg
- Pravastatin 40–80 mg

With few exceptions, use of lipid-modifying drugs other than statins is discouraged

USPSTF Has Weighed In
The USPSTF recommends initiating use of low- to moderate-dose statins in adults age 40 to 75 years without a history of CVD who have 1 or more CVD risk factors (dyslipidemia, diabetes, hypertension, or smoking) and a calculated 10-year CVD event risk of 10% or greater (B recommendation)
JAMA. 2016 Nov 15;316(19):1997–2007.

AR 67

While undergoing evaluation following a hysterectomy, a 50-year-old is noted to have TC 245, HDL 56, TG 645. She has an A1c of 5.6%. Her exam is normal and her medications include atenolol, hydrochlorothiazide, and oral estrogen.

What do you recommend now?
A. No change in therapy.
B. Add niacin.
C. Add gemfibrozil.
D. Stop atenolol and oral estrogen.

Answer: _____

Ezetimibe
- 2nd line lowering
- Inhibits cholesterol absorption at brush border
- Lowers LDL by 15–25%
- Approved for use alone or with statin or fenofibrate
- Increased risk of statin induced myopathy
- Avoid use with gemfibrozil

Bile Acid Sequestrants (Resins)
- Cholestyramine, colestipol
- 2nd line LDL lowering
- May increase TG
- Slightly $\uparrow$ HDL
- Lower LDL by 10–25%
- Adjuvant in combination with statins
- Side effects: Nausea, vomiting, bloating

Nicotinic Acid
- Blocks LDL synthesis
- $\downarrow$ LDL by 5–25%
- $\uparrow$ HDL by 15–35%
- $\downarrow$ TG by 20–50%
- Flushing, hyperuricemia, hepatotoxicity
- $\downarrow$ Cardiac events
- ? Effect on mortality
- No benefit when added to statin

Fibrates
- Gemfibrozil
  - $\downarrow$ TG by 50%
  - $\uparrow$ HDL by 15%
  - $\downarrow$ LDL
- Fenofibrate best combination with a statin (less drug interactions)
  - $\downarrow$ VLDL

AR 68

A 78-year-old man with a history of hypertension and DM falls and fractures his hip. He will require hip surgery.
Exam: BP 150/90, P 90; Chest clear, cardiac nl S_1S_2 +S_4, no murmur; Ext: No edema; ECG-NSR, LVH HB 11, Hct 33, Glu 148

What would you recommend?
A. Dipyridamole (Persantine) thallium stress test.
B. Echocardiogram.
C. Transfuse 2 units of blood.
D. Okay for immediate surgery.

Answer: _____

AR 69

A 72-year-old man with Type 2 DM and history of MI 6 years ago is found to have a pulsatile abdominal mass on exam.
Ultrasound reveals a 7-cm aortic aneurysm.
He walks 8–10 blocks every day without symptoms.
Exam: BP 120/70, P 105; Chest: Clear;
Cardiac: Nl S_1S_2 with no murmur;
ECG: Atrial fibrillation with PVCs, Hct 38, Glu 160

What would you recommend?
A. Proceed with surgery.
B. Obtain TTE before surgery.
C. Risk-assess with dipyridamole thallium test.
D. Risk-assess with cardiac catheterization.
E. No surgery.

Answer: _____

AR 70

An 86-year-old man with CHF, Hx of 2 MIs in the past 2 years (most recent 6 months ago) and CKD (GFR 25) is evaluated for upcoming cataract surgery. He is currently asymptomatic at rest, but he rarely ambulates more than 30 steps because of fatigue.
BP 120/80, P 80
Chest: Dull to percussion at the bases
Cardiac: Nl S_1S_2, grade 2/6 SEM at the LSB into axilla
ECG unchanged from ECG 3 months ago

What is the pre-op recommendation?
A. Echocardiogram.
B. Dipyridamole/Thallium stress test.
C. 24-hour Holter monitor.
D. No further testing needed.
E. Patient cannot undergo surgery.

Answer: _____

Key Points for Pre-Op Assessment
- Emergency surgery — don't waste time with pre-op assessment
- Active cardiac disease — uncompensated heart failure/unstable coronary syndrome/significant arrhythmia/severe valvular disease — workup needed pre-op
- Low-risk surgery — proceed to surgery
- Good functional capacity — can go to surgery (> 4 METs)

AR 71

A 66-year-old man presents for pre-op assessment. He has a history of stroke 4 years ago. He hasn't had any subsequent cerebrovascular problems. He has a history of HTN treated with lisinopril and HCTZ. PE is unremarkable. He will be having a right knee replacement.
Labs: Cr 0.8, Bun 6, Glu 88, Na^+ 140, K^+ 4.5

What would you recommend?
A. Baseline chest x-ray.
B. Carotid duplex.
C. Perioperative β-blockers.
D. Thallium stress test.
E. None of the above.

Answer: _____

Perioperative β-Blockers
- AHA Guidelines (2014) — Who to give them to:
  - Class 1 recommendations
    - Continue in patients already receiving for angina, arrhythmia, or hypertension
  - Class 2b recommendations
    - Vascular surgery patients with positive pre-op stress test
    - 3 or more revised cardiac risk index factors
  - Could possibly cause harm in lower-risk cardiac patients

Circulation. 2014;130:2215–2245.

Preoperative Cardiac Evaluation
- Young patients with no risk history can have minor surgery without evaluation
- Low- to moderate-risk patients having low- to medium-risk surgery usually do not need stress testing
- Preoperative coronary revascularization does not appear to reduce perioperative risk in patients with significant but stable coronary artery disease; Medical therapy should be optimized for these patients, including the application of β-blockers in high-risk vascular surgery patients with positive stress tests
- Red flags for needing cardiac testing: Major vascular surgery, unstable angina, decompensated CHF, recent MI, severe valvular disease

AR 72

A 75-year-old man with atrial fibrillation will be having an elective cholecystectomy.
Medications: Warfarin, metoprolol, amlodipine
PMH: Hypertension
Labs: INR 2.2, Na^+ 137, K^+ 4.0, Bun 10, Cr 1.0, Glu 80

What do you recommend for anticoagulation management?
A. Stop warfarin 5 days before surgery, bridge with enoxaparin, restart 1st day post-op.
B. Stop warfarin 5 days before surgery, restart 1st post-op day.
C. Stop warfarin 5 days before surgery, bridge with rivaroxaban, stop day before, restart warfarin post-op day 1.
D. Stop warfarin 1 week before surgery, bridge with enoxaparin, restart warfarin post-op day 1.

Answer: _____

Management of Warfarin Pre-op
- For A-fib and CHADS2 four or less, no need to use enoxaparin bridge
- Stop warfarin 5–7 days before procedure
- Okay to continue warfarin for minor procedures (like cataracts)

AR 73

A 74-year-old man comes in for pre-op assessment before a right knee replacement for OA.
PMH: CAD, DES stent placement 8 months ago; HTN; Hx colon Ca 8 years ago
Medications: Lisinopril, chlorthalidone, clopidogrel, aspirin
BP 130/70, P 70

What do you recommend?
A. Stop ASA 1 week before procedure.
B. Stop ASA 1 week before procedure, clopidogrel 5 days before procedure.
C. Start perioperative β-blocker.
D. Delay surgery at least 4 months.

Answer: _____

Management ASA/Clopidogrel
- Stop ASA 1 week prior to surgery
- Stop clopidogrel 5 days prior to surgery
- Do not do elective surgery that requires cessation of clopidogrel within 1 year of placement of DES

Pre-Op Evaluation — Labs
- Generally, order as few as possible
- **Hct** — Patients > 65 undergoing major surgery or any patient with major anticipated blood loss
- **Cr** — Patients > 50 undergoing intermediate- to high-risk surgery, younger patients at risk for renal disease
- **ECG** — Patients having vascular surgery or patients with Hx cardiac disease
- **Chest x-ray** — Not routinely!!! In patients with significant lung disease or having AAA surgery, or upper abdominal/thoracic surgery
- **PT/PTT** — No, unless a bleeding history

Preventive Medicine

It is All About the USPSTF Recommendations
All the rest is fluff.

Important Screening Exams to Know
- **Blood pressure:** Check every 2 years and at every clinic visit
- **Smoking counseling:** Each visit in smokers
- **Cholesterol:** Men 35–65, women 45–65, every 5 years
- **FOBT:** Annually after 50
- **DXA scan:** For women > 65
- **Flex sig:** Every 3–5 years after age 50 or colonoscopy every 10 years (no FOBT if choose colonoscopy)
- **Mammography:** Every 2 years after age 50 (USPSTF); Discuss between 40–50, but no recommendation to routinely screen in this age group (USPSTF)

AR 74
A 38-year-old woman with a 5-year history of hypertension presents for primary care. Her last Pap smear was normal 2 years ago, and she has never had abnormal Paps. She has never had mammography, colonoscopy, or lipids checked.
Meds: Lisinopril, chlorthalidone

What do you recommend?
A. Pap smear, mammogram
B. Pap smear, mammogram, lipids
C. Mammogram, lipids
D. Lipids
E. No testing

Answer: _____

Lipid Screening Recommendations
- Men age 35 and older (Grade A)
- Men 20–35 with risk factor (Grade B)
- Women age 45 and older at increased risk for CHD (Grade A)
- Women 20–45 at increased risk for CHD (Grade B)
- Men 20–35 no risk, women 20–45 no risk (Grade C)

AR 75
A woman makes an appointment for a physical exam when she turns 65. She has not seen a physician for 12 years. Her last visit was for a skin rash. She has not had a regular doctor because she lacked insurance. She has a 60-pack-year smoking history, but she quit smoking 10 years ago.

Appropriate preventive care should include:
A. Mammogram, Pap smear
B. Mammogram, CBC, colonoscopy, U/S of aorta
C. Mammogram, CBC, colonoscopy
D. Mammogram, Pap smear, colonoscopy
E. Breast exam, mammogram, colonoscopy

Answer: _____

Pap Smear Screening
- Start at age 21 or within 3 years of onset of sexual activity
- After 3 negative annual Pap tests, can screen every 3 years; after age 30 if HPV negative, can lengthen to q 5 years
- If patient has dysplastic Pap, should do annual screening
- If normal q 3-yr Paps, can stop screening at age 65 (USPSTF)
- No Pap smears in women who have had hysterectomy for benign disease

Pap Smear Screening — No Need to Screen
- After hysterectomy for benign disease
- After age 65 with repeatedly normal smears

AR 76
A 74-year-old man with CAD and Parkinson disease presents for primary care. His exam is remarkable for seborrheic dermatitis, some cogwheel rigidity, and a slightly enlarged prostate.

What testing would you recommend?
A. Cholesterol
B. Cholesterol, PSA
C. PSA
D. Cholesterol, PSA, CBC

Answer: _____

PSA Screening
- USPSTF and Canadian TF do not recommend screening
- ACP recommends discussing benefits and harms with patients age 50–69
- ACS and AUA recommend annual PSA age 50–69 (start at age 40 in African American men and those with FH of early prostate CA)

Colorectal Cancer Screening
- USPSTF recommends annual FOBT or flex sig every 5 years or both in adults age > 50 or colonoscopy every 10 years
- USPSTF does not recommend CT colography
- Medicare now pays for screening colonoscopy, making it an appropriate choice
- AGA recommends annual FOBT and flex sig every 5 years starting at age 50 (age 40 if FH in a 1st degree relative)

Breast Cancer Screening
- Mammogram every 2 years after age 50 (USPSTF), upper age limit not clear — should be based on comorbid conditions
- Mammograms for age 40–50 are controversial; ACS recommends yearly, USPSTF recommends against
- **Very Important**: Know the high false-positive risk in this age group — estimated 30% chance of breast biopsy if woman has annual exams from ages 40–50

AR 77
A 58-year-old man comes for a routine primary care visit. He was last seen 3 years ago. He has hypertension (treated with lisinopril), a Hx of depression, and a 50-pack-year smoking history (currently smoking 1 ppd). His last colonoscopy was at age 50 (no polyps).

What do you recommend?
A. Lipid panel
B. Lipid panel and abdominal ultrasound
C. Lipid panel and chest x-ray
D. Lipid panel and chest CT
E. Lipid panel and colonoscopy

Answer: _____

Lung Cancer Screening in Smokers
- 20% lung cancer mortality benefit with annual low-dose chest CT screening in smokers compared to chest x-ray
- Ages 55–79
- Current smoker or quit within 15 years
- More than 30-pack-year Hx

AR 78
Which patient would be appropriate to screen for AAA?
A. 50-year-old man who presents with chest pain
B. 55-year-old woman who presents with a stroke
C. 60-year-old woman with a 100-pack-year Hx of smoking
D. 75-year-old woman with 100-pack-year Hx of smoking
E. 66-year-old man with 60-pack-year Hx of smoking, quit 10 years ago

Answer: _____

Screening Guidelines for AAA
- USPSTF and ACC/AHA recommend one-time screening (ultrasound) for AAA in men ages 65–75 if they have a Hx of ever smoking
- No recommendation for screening in women

Toxins and Overdoses

AR 79
A 39-year-old man with a history of alcoholism presents with nausea, vomiting, ataxia, and confusion.
Physical exam: BP 80/60, P 120, RR 24;
      Neuro exam — oriented only to person
Labs: Na^+ 133, Glu 80, K^+ 5.0, Cl^- 96, HCO_3^- 10, Bun 14, Cr 1.5, serum osmolality 295

What is the most likely diagnosis?
A. Lactic acidosis
B. Isopropyl alcohol ingestion
C. Salicylate ingestion
D. Ethylene glycol ingestion
E. Renal tubular acidosis

Answer: _____

Anion Gap Acidosis Differential Diagnosis
M ethanol
U remia
L actate
E thylene glycol

P araldehyde
A spirin
K etoacidosis

Osmolar Gap and Gap Acidosis
Methanol
Ethylene glycol

Ethylene Glycol and Methanol — Clinical Findings
Ethylene Glycol
Inebriation
Headache
Nausea/vomiting
Anion & osmolar gap
Renal dysfunction
Urinary oxalate crystals

Methanol
Mild inebriation
Headache, dizziness
Nausea/vomiting
Anion & osmolar gap
Pancreatitis
Visual disturbances

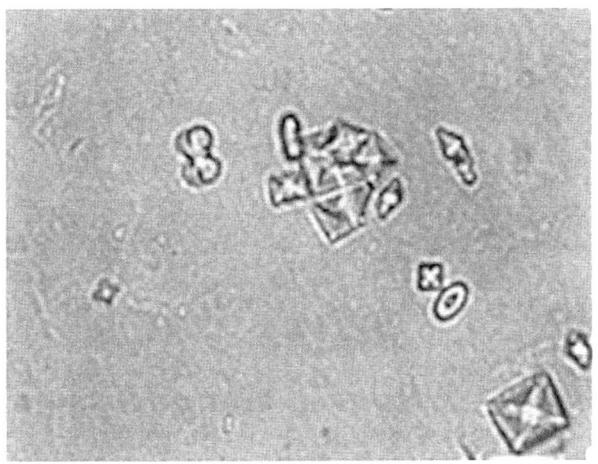

Pearls about Ethylene Glycol Poisoning
- Oxalate crystals in urine
- Renal insufficiency
- Urine may fluoresce with Woods lamp
- Fomepizole is an appropriate therapy

AR 80
A 29-year-old woman presents with abdominal pain and nausea without vomiting. She reports taking several over-the-counter pain relievers today to treat her abdominal pain. She has been drinking alcohol for the past week (she reports 8–10 beers/day). Her last drink was 1 hour ago.
Her exam reveals: BP 100/60, P 100, RR 22
Abd: Soft, tender in RUQ
Chest: Clear
Labs: Hb 12, Hct 36, MCV 104,
        Na^+ 135, K^+ 3.5, Cl^- 100, HCO_3^- 14,
        Bun 20, Cr 1.0, Glu 90, AST 60,
        ALT 30, EtOH 170,
        ABG 7.42/PO_2 120/PCO_2 18

What is the most serious problem with this patient?
A. Pulmonary embolism
B. Acetaminophen overdose
C. Salicylate overdose
D. Alcoholic ketoacidosis
E. Pancreatitis with lactic acidosis

Answer: _____

Aspirin
- Early manifestations: N/V, tinnitus, listlessness, and hyperventilation
- Respiratory alkalosis is followed by severe metabolic acidosis, hypokalemia, and hypoglycemia
- Seizures, hyperpyrexia, and coma

- Look for subacute toxicity in the elderly or chronically ill: Manifested by dehydration, obtundation, and acidosis
- Cerebral and pulmonary edema and death are more common in patients with subacute toxicity

Salicylate Overdose Treatment
- Lavage (beware of bezoars)
- Check serial salicylate levels
- Activated charcoal
- Forced alkalize diuresis
- Occasionally — charcoal hemoperfusion or dialysis

Overdose — Cyclic Antidepressants
- Effects: Cardiovascular toxicity, CNS effects, anticholinergic effects
- Protect that **airway**!!
- Block absorption: Charcoal, lavage, charcoal
- Antidote: Sodium bicarbonate (**not** physostigmine!!)
- Drug levels **do not** rule out significant toxicity

Charcoal <u>Not</u> Effective for the Following
- Caustics
- Cyanide
- Electrolytes
- Alcohols (ethanol, ethylene glycol, methanol)
- Hydrocarbons
- Heavy metals (iron, lead, mercury)

Contraindications for Activated Charcoal Administration
Caustic <u>acid</u> or <u>alkali</u> ingestions

The Stages of Poisoning with Acetaminophen
- **Stage 1: (0–24 hrs)**
  - Asymptomatic or flu-like (nausea, vomiting, malaise)
- **Stage 2: (24–48 hrs)**
  - Asymptomatic
  - Liver enzymes may start to rise
- **Stage 3: (49–96 hrs)**
  - Peak symptoms
  - Peak liver abnormalities
  - Death may occur from coagulopathy or liver failure
- **Stage 4:**
  - Recovery

Acetaminophen Overdose
- > 7.5 g ingestion in a healthy adult can cause liver damage
- Toxic dose less if patient has underlying liver disease or chronic alcohol use

Management of Acetaminophen Overdose
- Gastric emptying if within 2 hours of ingestion
- Activated charcoal if within 4 hours of ingestion
- N-acetylcysteine (17 doses) orally maximally effective if given within 16 hours of ingestion, **or** IV NAC for 21 hours
- Administration of NAC even late appears to be helpful in patients with acute liver failure

AR 81

A 29-year-old man is brought to the ED by friends. The patient was at a party with his friends when he became confused and then unresponsive.
On exam: BP 60/30, P 140, T 97.0° F (36.1° C),
O_2 saturation 88%; Extremities with marked cyanosis; Mouth — cyanosis of lips
Labs: Hb 14; Hct 42; WBC 1,000;
ABG–pH 7.32; PO_2 46; PCO_2 44;
Na^+ 136; K^+ 4.0; Cl^- 105; HCO_3^- 20
The patient is placed on 100% O_2 by mask without improvement in his cyanosis.

What therapy should he receive?
A. Amyl nitrite
B. Methylene blue
C. Bicarbonate drip
D. Naloxone
E. IV alcohol

Answer: _____

Clinical Features of Nitrite Abuse
- Tachypnea
- Tachycardia
- Headache
- Hypotension
- Cyanosis unresponsive to oxygen

Therapy for Amyl Nitrite Overdose
- High-dose oxygen
- Treatment for methemoglobinemia (methylene blue)

AR 82

A 50-year-old with a history of bipolar disorder presents with ataxia and severe tremor. He has had nausea and diarrhea for the past 48 hours.
Current medications: Amlodipine, aripiprazole, lisinopril, lithium, zolpidem.
On exam he has BP 140/90, P 100, a course tremor is present, and fasciculations.
Labs: Na^+ 148, Bun 28, Cr 2.2

What are the symptoms in the case most likely due to?
A. Aripiprazole-lithium interaction
B. Zolpidem-lithium interaction
C. Lisinopril-lithium interaction
D. Amlodipine-aripiprazole interaction
E. Amlodipine-lithium interaction

Answer: _____

Lithium Toxicity
- Lithium is the most common cause of nephrogenic DI (Know this!!!)
- Symptoms of lithium toxicity — ataxia, coarse tremors, fasciculations, mental status changes, seizures, nausea, vomiting, diarrhea
- Drug interactions — ACEI, diuretics, NSAIDs

Cyanide Poisoning
- Clinical features:
  - Headache, confusion, coma, seizures
  - Bright red color to skin (blush)
  - Vomiting, abdominal pain
- Treatment
  - Step 1 — treat with amyl nitrite or sodium nitrite to induce methemoglobinemia
  - Step 2 — give sodium thiosulfate
  - Other option is to give hydroxocobalamin and sodium thiosulfate

Carbon Monoxide Poisoning — Clinical Features
- Dyspnea
- Tachypnea
- Headache
- Emotional lability
- Confusion/Impaired judgment
- Syncope
- Nausea/Vomiting/Diarrhea

Poisonings and Overdoses Antidotes

Toxin	Antidote
Acetaminophen	N-acetylcysteine
Narcotics	Naloxone
Benzodiazepines	Flumazenil
Nitrates	Methylene blue
Iron	Deferoxamine
Ethylene glycol/meth	Alcohol
Organophosphates	Atropine/pralidoxime (2-Protopam)

AR 83

An anxious 19-year-old with marked diaphoresis is brought to the emergency department. She was at a party and took some drugs orally and smoked something as well.

On exam, she has pronounced bruxism.

BP 180/110, P 110

Labs: Bun 16, Cr 1.0, Na$^+$ 124

What drug is most consistent with all these findings?

A. Heroin

B. Crack

C. LSD

D. Ecstasy

E. Ingested cocaine

Answer: _____

Features of MDMA (Ecstasy) Intoxication

- Common features
  - Euphoria
  - Bruxism
  - Tachycardia
- Serious side effects
  - Severe hypertension
  - Hyperthermia
  - Hyponatremia
- Distinguishing features
  - Bruxism
  - Hyponatremia

Methamphetamine Abuse

- Important clinical features:
  - Hypertension/Tachycardia
  - Meth mouth with chronic use (less saliva/bruxism leads to dental cracking and severe caries)
  - Skin excoriations

HEENT: The Eye

AR 84

An obese, 36-year-old woman presents for evaluation of headaches. She has had increasing problems with headaches over the past 6 months. She has had no visual symptoms. She has occasional nausea but no focal neurologic symptoms.

On physical exam: BP 120/70, P 80

Skin: Without lesions

Fundi: As shown

Neurologic exam: Normal

Medications: CaCO₃, OCP, fluoxetine

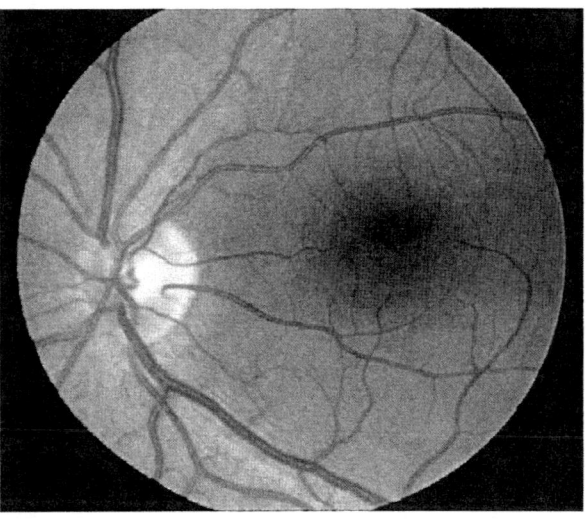

What is the most likely diagnosis?

A. Glioblastoma.

B. Pseudotumor cerebri.

C. Tuberous sclerosis.

D. Prader-Willi syndrome.

E. None of the above.

Answer: _____

Headaches in Reproductive-Age Women

- Incidence of OCP-associated HA: 600/100,000
- Incidence of pseudotumor cerebri: 3.3/100,000

Pseudotumor Cerebri — Clinical Features

- Headaches (94%) — worse in a.m.
- Visual disturbances
- Papilledema

Sample Question

An obese, 26-year-old woman presents for evaluation of headaches. She has had severe headaches for the past 6 months. She also reports short, 15–30 second episodes of transient visual loss occurring several times a week. She has frequent nausea but no vomiting.

On physical exam: BP 140/90, P 80

Skin: Acne on back and face

Fundi: As shown

Neurologic exam: Nonfocal

Medications: CaCO₃, isotretinoin, fluoxetine

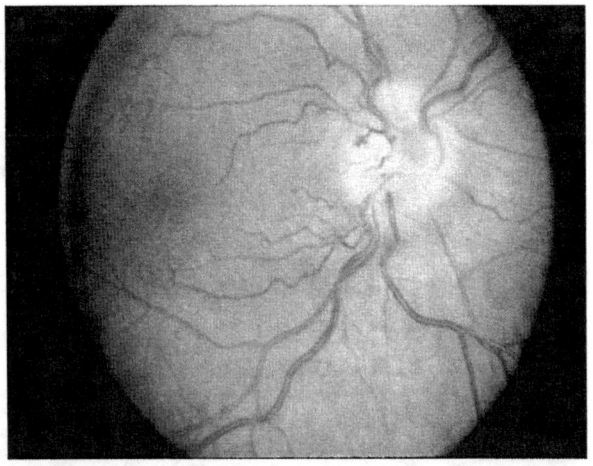

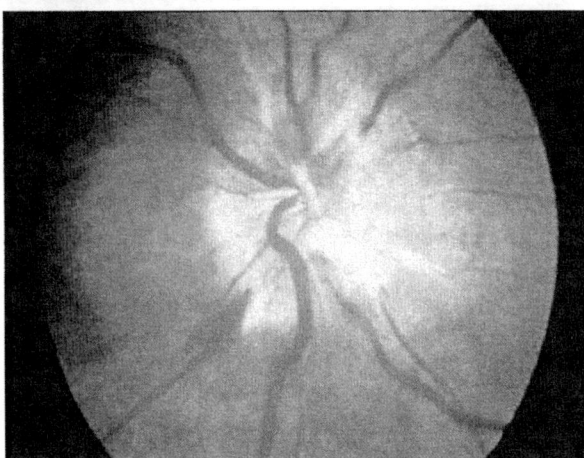

Key Features of Pseudotumor Cerebri
- Female
- Obesity
- Isotretinoin*
- Transient visual obstructions*
- Headache

*Most discriminating features

AR 85

A 58-year-old woman comes in for follow-up of HTN. She notes that her vision has gradually become more blurred, R > L. She failed the screening eye exam to renew her driver's license last week.

Eye exam as shown.

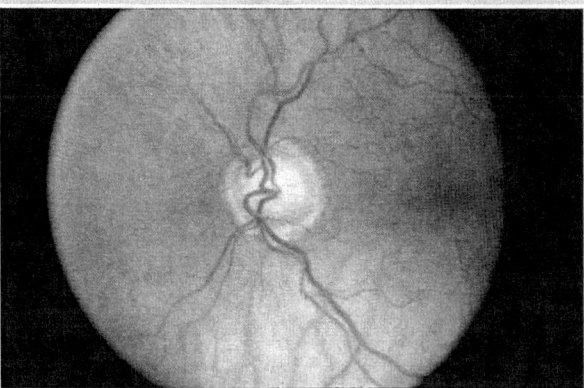

Her eye exam (as shown) is most consistent with:
A. Cataracts
B. Hypertensive retinopathy
C. Glaucoma
D. Macular degeneration

Answer: _____

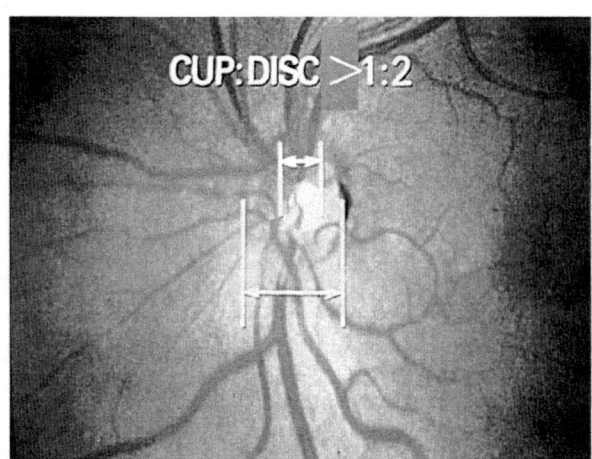

CUP:DISC >1:2

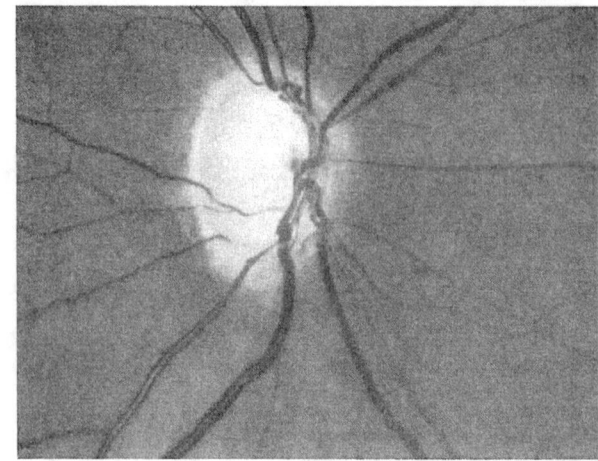

AR 86

A 70-year-old man with Type 2 diabetes presents with sudden right eye visual loss.
He has no other symptoms (no headache or weakness, no history of head injury). He has no history of diabetic retinopathy.

Eye exam as shown.

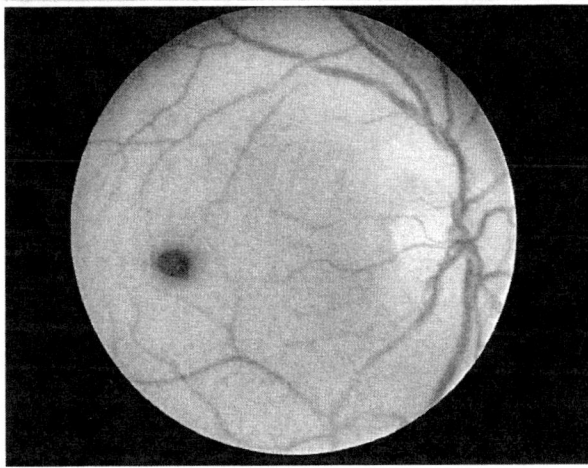

What is the most appropriate workup?

A. Head CT scan.
B. Cerebral angiography.
C. Head MRI.
D. Carotid duplex.
E. Measure intraocular pressure.

Answer: _____

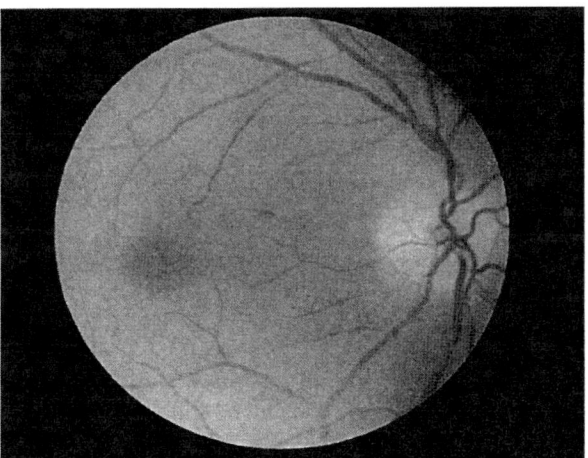

AR 87

A 34-year-old male notices a visual disturbance in his right eye while playing soccer. He has decreased vision in his right lateral visual field which he describes as a waving curtain.

The symptom has been persistent for 3 hours. He has no headache history. He does wear glasses for nearsightedness.
Exam: BP 150/80, P 88
Eye exam: Normal

What do you recommend?

A. Sumatriptan 100 mg oral
B. Sumatriptan 6 mg IM
C. Metoclopramide 10 mg IV
D. Carotid ultrasound
E. Ophthalmologic consultation

Answer: _____

Sudden Visual Loss

Condition	Pain	Ophthalmologic Findings
Retinal detachment	No	Retinal separation
Retinal artery occlusion	No	Cherry-red spot
Retinal vein occlusion	No	Retinal hemorrhage
Endophthalmitis	Yes	Decreased red reflex
Occipital cortex infarct	No	None

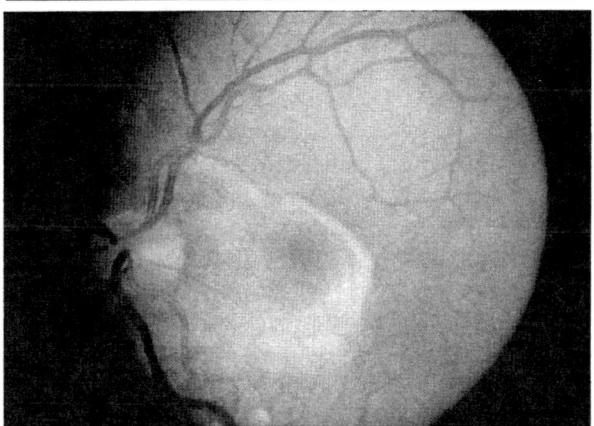

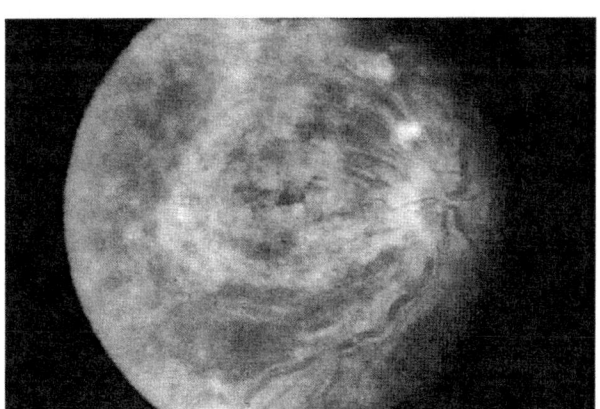

AR 88

A 44-year-old woman with diabetes comes in for routine follow-up. She feels well but has noted decrease in vision without diplopia.

Exam: BP 168/102, P 72

VA 20/30 OS, 20/40 OD with her usual lenses; EOM function normal

Funduscopic examination is shown.

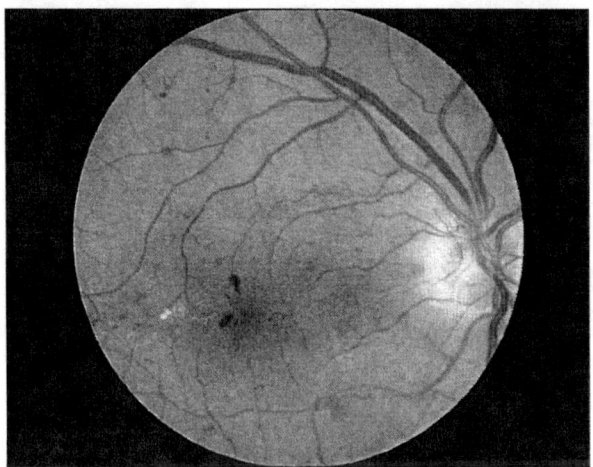

This patient should receive which of the following?

A. Immediate referral to ophthalmology because laser therapy in the macular region may be beneficial in protecting vision.

B. Immediate referral to ophthalmology for laser therapy of new vessel disease.

C. Referral to ophthalmology within the next several months for routine examination.

D. Review medication list for those that increase intraocular pressure.

E. Emphasize to patient that treatment of systemic hypertension may delay progression of her existing hypertensive retinopathy.

Answer: _____

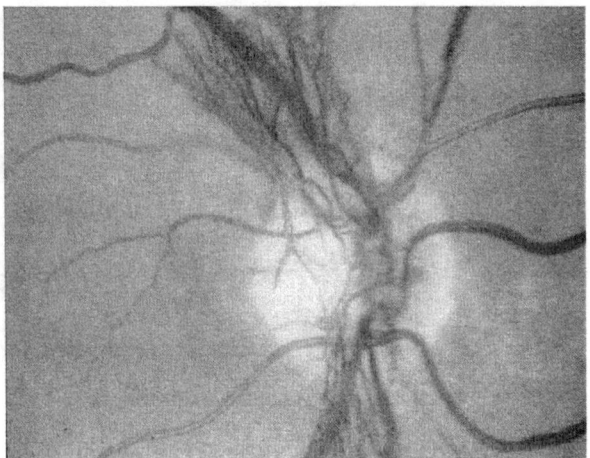

Proliferative Diabetic Retinopathy

- New vessels (NVE, NVD)
- Fibrous strands/scar (retinitis proliferans)
- Vitreous hemorrhage
- Retinal detachment

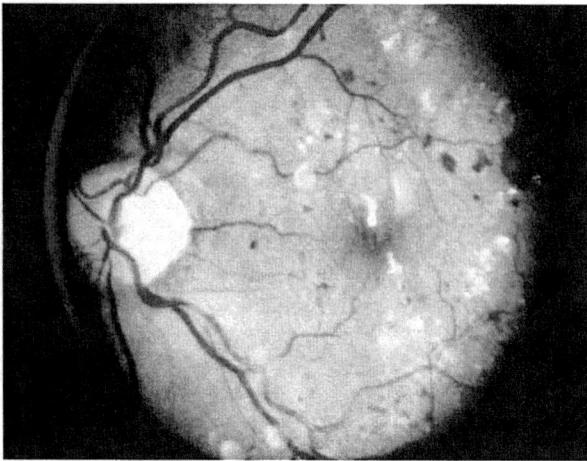

Nonproliferative (Background) DM Retinopathy

- Increased capillary permeability
- Capillary closure and dilation
- Microaneurysms
- Arteriovenous shunt
- Dilated veins
- Hemorrhages (dot and blot, flame)

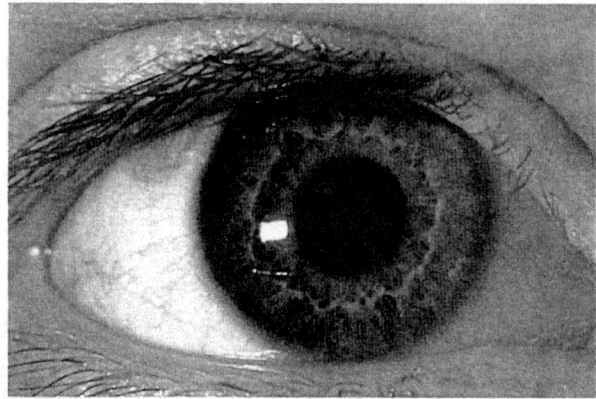

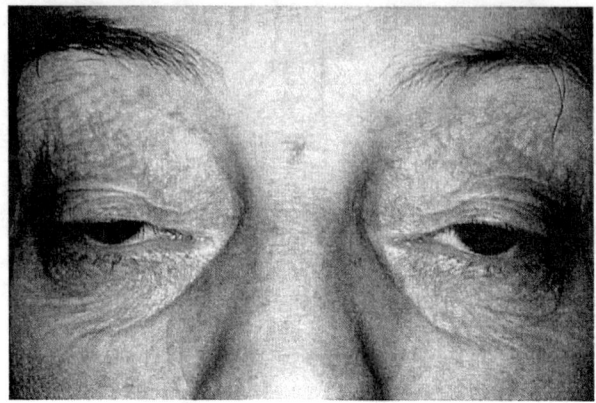

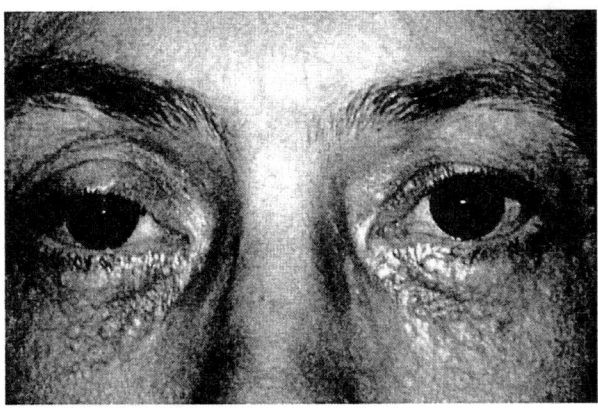

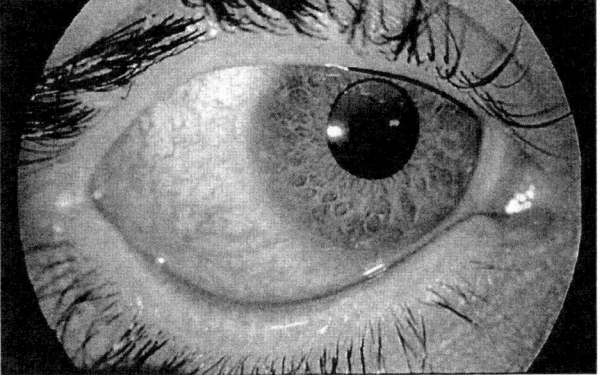

Red Eye Pearls

- Most infectious causes do not cause pain
- Viral conjunctivitis (adenovirus) is the most common cause of acute red eye
- If eye is red and painful, think iritis, keratitis, or acute glaucoma
- Visual acuity isn't affected with viral and bacterial conjunctivitis; Think iritis or acute glaucoma
- Photophobia suggests iritis
- Subconjunctival hemorrhage causes confluent blood, no pain, no visual disturbance; Looks bad but doesn't feel bad

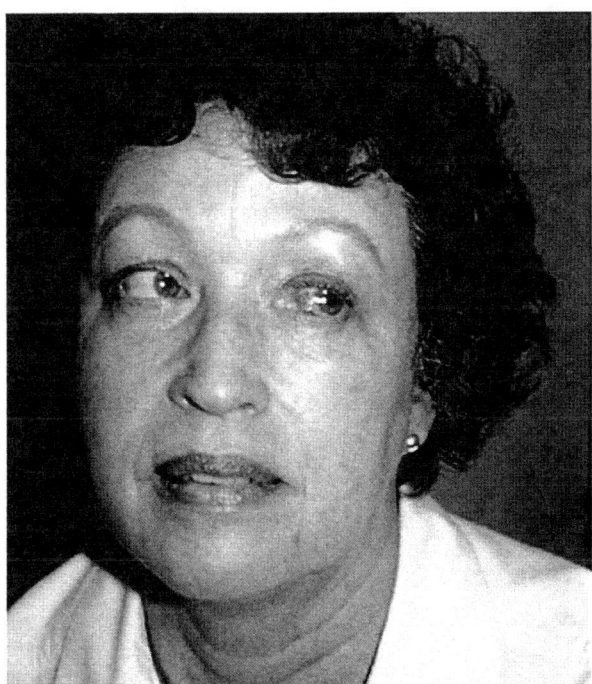

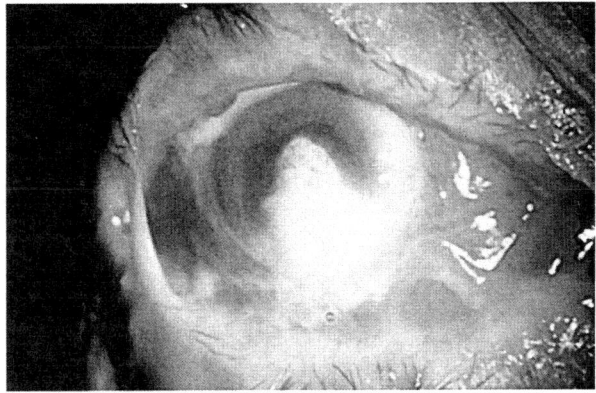

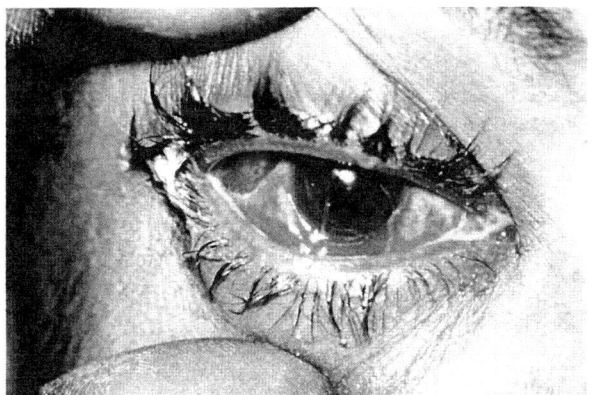

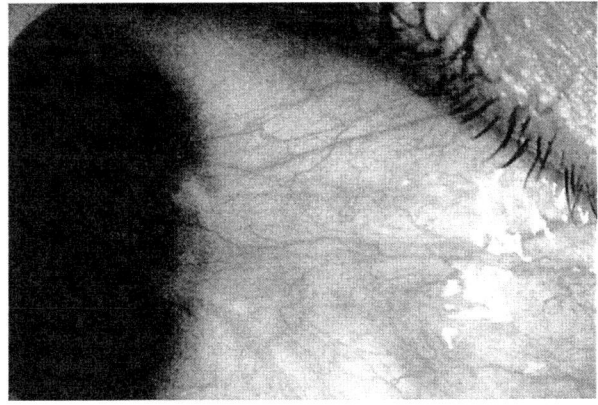

AR 89

A 78-year-old man presents with 3 days of burning pain on the forehead and has noticed a blister on the tip of his nose and on his forehead. He has no eye pain or visual changes. On exam he has 3 blisters on the left forehead and one on the tip of the nose. Sclera/conjunctiva are not injected.

In addition to starting an antiviral, what do you recommend?
A. Emergent referral to the ophthalmologist
B. Evaluation by ophthalmologist within 24–48 hours
C. Evaluation by ophthalmologist within 1–2 weeks
D. No evaluation by ophthalmologist needed

Answer: _____

When Do You Need an Ophthalmologic Eval in Patients with Zoster?
- Red eye and reduced vision — same day
- Red eye without visual complaints — 24–48 hours
- Hutchinson sign with no red eye or visual complaints — 1–2 weeks

BMJ. 2009;339:b2624.
Med Clin N Am. 2013;97:503–522.

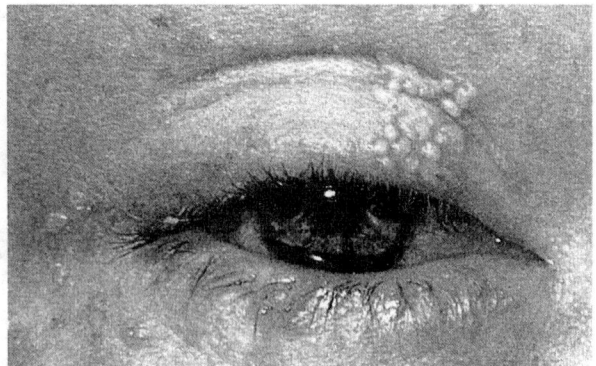

AR 90

You are evaluating a 30-year-old woman in the emergency department who c/o red-eye discomfort bilaterally for 2 days. She wears contact lenses.
Exam: WD/WN individual in moderate distress.
    BP 132/90; Pupils 4 mm bilaterally, no nystagmus, full EOMs, VA 20/30 OU
Eye exam is shown
Skin with flesh-colored papules on back and extremities

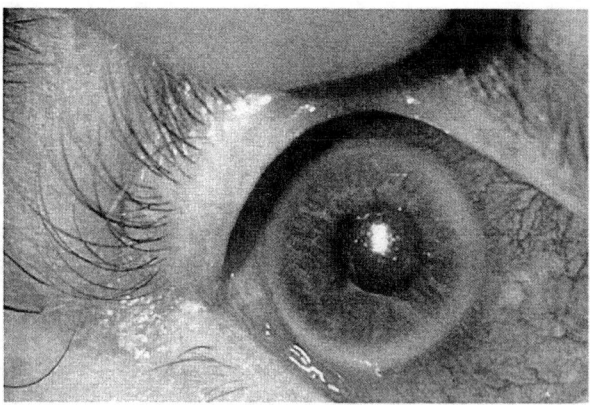

The most appropriate care of this patient includes:
A. Treatment with steroid ophthalmic preparation.
B. Treatment with sulfacetamide 10% ophthalmic drops until redness clears.
C. Avoid contact lens use; treat with oral ciprofloxacin.
D. Chest x-ray and immediate referral to ophthalmology.
E. Treatment with oral acyclovir for 10 days.

Answer: _____

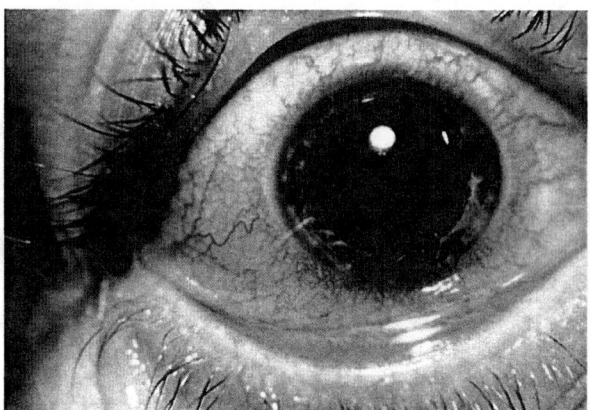

Uveitis Disease Associations
- Ankylosing spondylitis
- Reactive arthritis (Reiter syndrome)
- Sarcoidosis
- Granulomatous infection

Ophthalmologic Emergencies (Emergent Consultation)
- Alkali burn
- Retinal artery occlusion
- Angle-closure glaucoma
- Penetrating injury
- Endophthalmitis
- Retinal detachment

HEENT: The Ear

Hearing Loss

AR 91

A 66-year-old male presents with decreased hearing in his right ear. He was recently diagnosed with prostate cancer. He had presented with urosepsis because of urinary tract obstruction.

He was successfully treated with gentamicin and ceftazidime.

On exam, he has cerumen in both ear canals.

The Weber test lateralizes to his right ear. A Rinne test shows air conduction louder in the left ear and bone conduction louder in the right ear.

What is the most likely cause of the hearing loss?
A. Gentamicin toxicity
B. Cochlear osteosclerosis
C. Ménière disease
D. Cerumen impaction
E. Acoustic neuroma

Answer: _____

Hearing Loss Physical Exam
- Rinne test: Conductive hearing loss; Bone conduction > air conduction
- Weber test: Sound perceived in middle = normal hearing or symmetrical hearing loss; Sound lateralizes = conductive hearing loss in ipsilateral ear or sensorineural loss in opposite ear

Conductive Hearing Loss
- External canal obstruction
- Otitis externa and media
- Cholesteatoma
- Otosclerosis
- Trauma
- Middle ear masses

AR 92

A 57-year-old man calls to report sudden hearing loss in his left ear. He comes into clinic and has a normal exam except for minimal hearing present in his left ear. His ear canals are clear.

PMH: HTN, GERD, BPH

Meds: Omeprazole, terazosin, hydrochlorothiazide, and spironolactone

What do you recommend?
A. Stop hydrochlorothiazide.
B. Stop spironolactone.
C. Stop terazosin.
D. Acyclovir.
E. Prednisone.

Answer: _____

Sudden Sensorineural Hearing Loss

Patients should receive immediate treatment with corticosteroids, usually prednisone 60 mg x 10 days.

Sensorineural Hearing Loss
- Presbycusis
- Infectious/Inflammatory
- Vascular
- Trauma
- Neoplasm
- Medications

HEENT: The Head

AR 93

A 29-year-old woman presents for treatment of a headache. She reports that she has had frequent headaches over the past 12 months that include pressure pain on her forehead, under her eyes, and over her cheeks. She usually has nasal congestion as well. She has not had any fevers or purulent nasal discharge.

What is the most appropriate treatment?
A. Amoxicillin
B. Levofloxacin
C. Amoxicillin/clavulanate
D. Oral decongestants
E. Sumatriptan

Answer: _____

"Sinus" Headaches are Usually Migraine Headaches
- 2,991 patients screened who reported at least 6 headaches during the previous 6 months self-diagnosed or physician-diagnosed as sinus headaches
- 88% of these patients met IHS criteria for migraine HA (80%) or migrainous criteria (8%); Most common Sxs patients reported were sinus pressure (84%), sinus pain (82%), and nasal congestion (63%)

Arch Intern Med. 2004;164(16):1769–1772.

Psychiatry

Bulimia Nervosa
- Epidemiology: Usually women ages 20–30 (older than anorexia patients)
- Clinical features
  - Erosion of dental enamel
  - Reflux symptoms
  - Mallory-Weiss tears
- Lab abnormalities
  - Hypokalemia
  - Hypochloremia, low urinary chloride

Anorexia Nervosa
- Epidemiology: Onset usually in adolescent girls
- Clinical features:
  - Weight loss of 15% under ideal
  - Preoccupation with food
  - Intense fear of becoming fat
  - Distorted self-image
  - Loss of menstrual cycles
  - Bradycardia, anemia, low albumin

Panic Disorder — Epidemiology
- Prevalence 3.8%
- Onset usually between ages 20 and 40
- Often familial
- Cocaine use may be a precipitant
- Major depression occurs in half of the patients with panic disorder

Panic Disorder Presentation
- 75% of patients seek care for their worst attack
- 50% present for care at time of first attack
- 40% of ED patients with atypical chest pain have panic attacks
- 33% of cardiology patients with chest pain and normal coronary arteries have panic disorder
- Of newly diagnosed patients with panic disorder at a tertiary care facility, 70% had seen at least 10 physicians

Panic Disorder — Treatment
- SSRI is the mainstay
- Okay to use short-term benzodiazepine when starting treatment or longer-term use in patients who are not adequately treated with SSRI; Longer-acting drug like clonazepam is preferable to short-acting alprazolam
- Cognitive behavioral therapy can be a good option

AR 94
A 27-year-old woman presents for evaluation. She demands thyroid medication to make her stronger as she is now "Senator for the State of California." She reports she has been sleeping about 2–3 hours a night for the past 2 weeks and feels well. She has not been hungry. She tells you she left her last medical provider because he was reporting information to the election canvassing board that was damaging her election hopes.

What is her most likely diagnosis?
A. Bipolar disorder
B. Paranoid schizophrenia
C. Paranoid personality disorder
D. Histrionic personality disorder
E. Frontal lobe brain tumor

Answer: _____

Bipolar Disorder — Clinical Features
- Excited, emotional lability
- Demanding, egocentric
- Elevated self-esteem
- Flight of ideas
- Poor judgment
- Paranoia
- Delusions, hallucinations
- Insomnia, little need for sleep

Bipolar Disorder — Common Issues
- Multiple sexual partners
- Credit card debt
- Call friends in middle of night

AR 95
A 33-year-old woman presents to establish primary care. She has had 3 primary care physicians over the past year. She reports all of them were not good listeners, but it is obvious that you are a superb listener and an outstanding doctor. She discusses how her best friend was unreliable, and she can't be trusted.

What is the most likely diagnosis?
A. Paranoid personality disorder
B. Bipolar disorder
C. Antisocial personality disorder
D. Borderline personality disorder
E. Schizophrenia

Answer: _____

AR 96
A 30-year-old man is diagnosed with an anxiety disorder. He is started on a medication, which he finds helpful, except he has sexual side effects of delayed orgasm.

What medication was he started on?
A. Citalopram
B. Buspirone
C. Bupropion
D. Clonazepam
E. Imipramine

Answer: _____

AR 97
A 38-year-old man with a diagnosis of depression presents for follow-up. He has had a good response to treatment with sertraline (Zoloft) but would like to stop treatment because of sexual side effects. He has been on antidepressant therapy for 6 weeks.

 © 2017 MedStudy Internal Medicine Video Board Review – General Internal Medicine • Doug Paauw, MD

What would you recommend?
A. Stop sertraline.
B. Stop sertraline; begin paroxetine.
C. Stop sertraline; begin fluoxetine.
D. Stop sertraline; begin bupropion.
E. Stop sertraline; begin amitriptyline.

Answer: _____

Antidepressants with Fewer Sexual Side Effects
- Bupropion
- Mirtazapine?

Depression SSRIs
- Less drowsiness as a class
- No orthostatic hypotension/minimal anticholinergic symptoms
- Sexual side effects in 30–50%
- Cause of hyponatremia!
  (Remember this, especially in the elderly.)

AR 98
A 45-year-old woman is seen for treatment of depression. You suggest an SSRI, but she is reluctant to take it. She says that the last time she was treated with an SSRI, she got really sick when she stopped it.

With this history, which SSRI would you avoid and which would be preferred?
A. Avoid citalopram; prefer sertraline.
B. Avoid paroxetine; prefer fluoxetine.
C. Avoid sertraline; prefer paroxetine.
D. Avoid fluoxetine; prefer citalopram.
E. Avoid any SSRI.

Answer: _____

Serotonin Discontinuation Syndrome
- Symptoms of dizziness, headaches, chills, insomnia, fatigue, anxiety
- Paroxetine is by far the most likely to cause this, due to very short half-life
- Fluoxetine least likely due to long half-life
- Tapering of SSRI decreases this
- If problems tapering, can switch patient to fluoxetine (10–20 mg/day) and taper

AR 99
A 67-year-old man, 3 months following myocardial infarction, reports problems with severe insomnia. He cannot fall asleep easily and wakes up at about 4.30 a.m. each morning. He has had increased fatigue since his MI and is more forgetful with increased problems concentrating.
Other medical problems include: GERD, BPH, and Hx of stroke with related seizure disorder

What would you recommend?
A. Zolpidem (Ambien)
B. Amitriptyline
C. Nortriptyline
D. Paroxetine (Paxil)
E. Bupropion (Wellbutrin)

Answer: _____

Side Effect Question!
- When there appear to be several okay choices, it is a side effect question
- All but one of the choices are contraindicated or ineffective

Contraindications for Antidepressants
- Tricyclic antidepressants: Arrhythmias, Hx MI, BPH
- Bupropion: Seizure disorder, eating disorders, alcoholism

AR 100
A 30-year-old woman presents with symptoms of depression. She has successfully been treated for depression in the past but gained 20 lbs on therapy. She is reluctant to take medications because of fear of weight gain.

What antidepressant would be the best option for her in regard to weight gain?
A. Amitriptyline
B. Paroxetine
C. Mirtazapine
D. Bupropion
E. Nortriptyline

Answer: _____

Antidepressants That Don't Cause Weight Gain
- Bupropion
- Venlafaxine
- SSRIs (other than paroxetine)?

AR 101
A 45-year-old woman comes to her clinic appointment with increasing symptoms of confusion over the past day, sweating, and increasing anxiety. She fell while roller-skating yesterday and severely injured her shoulder (her R arm is in a sling).
She has a history of depression, GERD, hypertension, and headaches.
Meds: Omeprazole, lisinopril, metoprolol, citalopram, tramadol, and sumatriptan prn
PE:
  Vitals: BP 160/100, P 100, tremor present, muscle rigidity

AR 101 (cont.)
What is the most appropriate treatment?
A. Dantrolene.
B. IVF.
C. Mannitol.
D. Discontinue metoprolol.
E. Discontinue citalopram and tramadol.

Answer: _____

Serotonin Syndrome
- Symptoms: Confusion, sweating, agitation, anxiety, vomiting, diarrhea
- Signs: Tachycardia, hypertension, fever, muscle rigidity, hyperreflexia, tremor
- Usually caused by several serotonergic drugs combined: SSRIs, tramadol, linezolid, meperidine, dextromethorphan, TCA, MAOI, buspirone, trazodone

AR 102
A 63-year-old man with Parkinson disease is brought to the ED by his wife for evaluation of high fever.
He has been experiencing increasing confusion over the past 48 hours. He has developed marked diaphoresis.
Medications include: Omeprazole, lorazepam, and benazepril.
He stopped taking his levodopa-carbidopa and bromocriptine 1 week ago.
Exam: T 104.8° F (40.4° C), BP 80/60, P 150
Ext: Marked muscle rigidity
Labs: HB 13, Hct 39, WBC 13,000, Ca^{2+} 8.6, CPK 605

What is the most likely cause of his symptoms?
A. Parkinson disease
B. Meningitis
C. Catatonia
D. Neuroleptic malignant syndrome
E. Thalamic stroke

Answer: _____

Neuroleptic Malignant Syndrome — Clinical Features
- Fever
- Mental status changes
- Muscle rigidity
- Autonomic dysfunction

Neuroleptic Malignant Syndrome — Etiology
- Discontinuation of anti-Parkinson meds
- Neuroleptics
  - Haloperidol
  - Chlorpromazine
  - Clozapine

Genetics

AR 103
A man and his wife have a child with cystic fibrosis. His wife dies, and he gets remarried.

If the prevalence of CF in the population is 1/1,600, what is the probability that the first child that he and his new wife have will have cystic fibrosis?
A. 25%
B. 20%
C. 5%
D. 2.5%
E. 1.25%

Answer: _____

Risk of 1st Child Having CF
- Father's risk of carrying = 1
- Mother's risk is population risk (0.05); This number is derived from population prevalence of 1/1,600; This means the average carrier risk is 1/20, so the risk of a couple both carrying is 1/20 x 1/20 (1/400) and of those pregnancies 1/4 will have CF (1/20 x 1/20 x 1/4 = 1/1,600)
- Risk of 1st child having CF in this case = 1 (father's risk) x 0.05 (mother's risk) x 0.25 (risk of a CF child if both parents are carriers) = 0.0125 or 1.25%

AR 104
A 27-year-old female whose brother died of cystic fibrosis is married to a 25-year-old whose sister (age 16) has cystic fibrosis.

What is the risk their first child will have CF?
A. 1/4
B. 1/9
C. 1/12
D. 1/16
E. 1/64

Answer: _____

Risk of Child Having CF if Both Parents Have Sibs with CF
- Each parent does not have CF; So their risk of carrying the gene is 2/3
- 2/3 x 2/3 x 1/4 = 4/36 = 1/9

Hallmarks of Autosomal Recessive Inheritance
- Usually seen only in sibship of proband
- Recurrence risk for future sibs = 1/4
- Male-female incidence equal
- Carrier risk is 2/3 for any unaffected child

Hallmarks of Autosomal Dominant Disease
- Vertical transmission (involving several generations)
- Risk to each child of an affected individual is 50%
- Male-male transmission observed
- Normal parents don't transmit trait*
  *Exceptions
  - Reduced penetrance
  - New mutations
  - Gonadal mosaicism
  - Non-paternity

Hallmarks of X-Linked Inheritance
- Inheritance of trait is male >>> female
- All daughters of affected male will be carriers
- Males never pass gene on to sons
- Heterozygotes will usually be unaffected

Penetrance
- A measure of how often one sees a characteristic phenotype in an individual who possesses the gene that causes the phenotype
- A penetrance of 1 (100%) means all gene carriers will show phenotype
- Age-related penetrance; e.g., Huntington disease, neurofibromatosis, tuberous sclerosis

Polycystic Kidney Disease
- Autosomal dominant inheritance
- Accounts for 10% of ESRD
Clinical Features
- Onset $3^{rd}/4^{th}$ decades
- Flank pain
- Gross and microscopic hematuria
- Palpable kidneys
- Hypertension (75%)
- Hepatic cysts (30%)
- Cerebral aneurysm rupture (10%)

Pregnancy

AR 105
A 24-year-old woman G_1P_0 presents 20 weeks of gestation for follow-up. Her BP at work yesterday was 145/90. Today in the office, the BP is 146/93. She feels fine. U/A is done and is normal.

What do you recommend?
A. Begin hydrochlorothiazide 12.5 mg daily.
B. Begin chlorthalidone 25 mg daily.
C. Begin losartan 100 mg daily.
D. Begin metoprolol 100 mg daily.
E. No treatment.

Answer: _____

Hypertension in Pregnancy
- In patients with chronic hypertension, goal is higher BP; Do not want BP < 120/80, and most antihypertensives are bad news in pregnancy
- Make sure the patient does not have preeclampsia (always look for protein)
- Don't need to treat hypertension in pregnancy, if not preeclampsia, unless SBP > 150 or DBP > 95

AR 106
A 29-year-old G_2P_1 female with Type 1 DM presents at 16 weeks with increasing pedal edema. Her BP is 170/110.
A U/A reveals 3+ proteinuria. She has no headaches or neurologic symptoms.

What treatment would you recommend?
A. Valsartan
B. Lisinopril
C. Labetalol
D. Nitroprusside drip

Answer: _____

Preeclampsia / Eclampsia —Clinical Features
- Increased BP
- Edema
- Headache, visual disturbances
- Hyperreflexia

Preeclampsia / Eclampsia — Lab Abnormalities
- Proteinuria
- Increased Cr
- Increased uric acid
- Increased transaminases
- Decreased platelets
- Decreased antithrombin III

Drugs to Absolutely Avoid During Pregnancy
- Isotretinoin
- ACE inhibitors
- ARBs
- Benzodiazepines
- Quinolones
- Tetracyclines
- Nitroprusside
- Warfarin

AR 107

A 25-year-old female G_1P_0 presents at 15 weeks of pregnancy for evaluation. She is asymptomatic.
Labs: HB 12, Hct 36, urine culture 100,000 colonies *E. coli*

What would you recommend?
A. 3-day course of amoxicillin
B. 7-day course of ciprofloxacin
C. 3-day course of ciprofloxacin
D. 7-day course of nitrofurantoin
E. No treatment

Answer: _____

Asymptomatic Bacteriuria of Pregnancy

- 20–30x increased risk of progression to pyelonephritis compared to nonpregnant women
- Pyelonephritis is associated with prematurity, low birth weight, and increased perinatal mortality
- Appropriate length of treatment controversial (no 3-day course for beta-lactams)
- Preferred drugs: Amoxicillin (if sensitive), nitrofurantoin, amoxicillin/clavulanate, cephalosporin

AR 108

A 29-year-old asthmatic woman presents in January with sudden onset of fever, chills, sore throat, and myalgias. She is 28 weeks pregnant. The woman was feeling well until 12 hours ago.
Physical exam:
BP 90/60, P 120, RR 10, T 102.2° F (39.0° C)
Chest: Clear
Labs:
Rapid flu test and chest x-ray negative, WBC 10,000

What would you recommend?
A. Prednisone and azithromycin
B. Ceftriaxone
C. Zanamivir
D. Oseltamivir
E. Supportive/Symptomatic care

Answer: _____

Influenza in Pregnancy

- Treat all suspected or confirmed cases up to 2 weeks postpartum because of increased mortality/morbidity in pregnant patients
- Rapid flu test: Sensitivity as low as 10% (range 10–70%), so don't withhold treatment for negative result
- Treatment: Oseltamivir

AR 109

A 28-year-old woman with B2 HIV disease presents for prenatal care. She was diagnosed 4 years ago with HIV disease. At that time, she had oral and vaginal candidiasis, a CD4 count of 200, and a viral load of 30,000. She was treated with zidovudine/3TC and atazanavir and has had an increase in CD4 count to 370; she now has a nondetectable viral load.
She asks for your advice on what medications she can take during pregnancy.

What should you advise?
A. Stop 3TC and atazanavir; continue zidovudine.
B. Switch to DDI/D4T/amprenavir.
C. Stop antiretrovirals; restart zidovudine at 34 weeks.
D. Stop all antiretrovirals.
E. Continue with current regimen.

Answer: _____

HIV and Pregnancy

- Risk of vertical transmission is 25%, reduced to 8% with use of zidovudine in mother; Rate < 1% with 3-drug therapy
- Current recommendations are to treat mother with appropriate 3-drug therapy for HIV; Use zidovudine if at all possible; If mother does not need HAART, then it should be started by 28 weeks
- Do resistance testing in all patients with a positive viral load before starting therapy

- Concern for D4T + DDI-containing regimens — avoid them; Avoid efavirenz in the first trimester and nelfinavir
- Decreased risk of transmission with C-section, recommended for women with viral loads > 1,000 near the time of delivery
- Recommendations for Use of Antiretroviral Drugs in Pregnant HIV-Infected Women 2009 http://AIDSinfo.nih.gov

AR 110A

A pregnant 27-year-old female (late 1st trimester) presents with dyspnea and pleuritic chest pain. She reports she has had progressive left leg swelling over the past week.
ABG 7.48/22/80

The most appropriate initial diagnostic test would be:
A. V/Q scan
B. Bilateral venography
C. Pulmonary angiography
D. Duplex ultrasonography
E. CT angiogram

Answer: _____

AR 110B

She does have a confirmed DVT with likely PE.

What is the appropriate therapy?
A. Rivaroxaban
B. Warfarin
C. Enoxaparin
D. Heparin
E. Apixaban

Answer: _____

Treatment of Venous Thromboembolism in Pregnancy
- LMWH is preferred, considered safe and easier to administer than unfractionated heparin
- Warfarin contraindicated
- Do not use direct thrombin or Xa inhibitors

SLE and Pregnancy
- Normal fertility, but miscarriage rate 1.5–3x increased
- Neonatal lupus associated with anti-Ro (SSA) or anti-La antibodies in the mother
- Neonatal lupus includes congenital heart block

Medical Causes of Dysfunctional Uterine Bleeding

AR 111

A 26-year-old woman presents with a 4-month history of vaginal bleeding. She states she has had menstrual periods every 10–16 days, lasting 3–5 days at a time. She has had no pain and otherwise has felt well. The patient states she is not currently sexually active. Physical exam is normal, with normal speculum exam and normal uterine size. Pregnancy test is negative.

What would you recommend for this patient?
A. Endometrial biopsy.
B. Transvaginal ultrasound.
C. Dilation and curettage.
D. Begin on oral contraceptive.

Answer: _____

Abnormal Premenopausal Bleeding
- Heavy/Prolonged bleeding with normal intervals: Submucosal fibroids
- Irregular bleeding with intervals < 18 days: Luteal phase abnormality
- Spontaneous abortion/Ectopic pregnancy
- Postcoital bleeding

Medical Causes of Dysfunctional Uterine Bleeding
- Hypothyroidism
- Liver disease with coagulopathy
- Thrombocytopenia
- Chronic renal failure

AR 112

A 29-year-old woman presents for evaluation of postcoital bleeding. She has had a small amount of bleeding after intercourse 4 times over the past 2 weeks. She has had no pain and no other symptoms. She has had 2 normal Pap smears in the past 3 years.

What is the most likely finding on speculum exam?
A. Cervical HSV
B. Normal cervical exam
C. Endocervical polyp
D. Cervical cancer
E. Nabothian cyst

Answer: _____

Postcoital Bleeding
- Endocervical polyps
- Cervicitis (*Chlamydia*)
- Cervical erosions
- Cervical cancer

General Internal Medicine
Audience Response Answers

Audience Response 1
Answer: E. Calcium.

AR 2
Answer: D. TMP/SMX.

AR 3
Answer: A. Acetaminophen.

AR 4
Answer: C. Levofloxacin.

AR 5
Answer: D. Grapefruit juice.

AR 6
Answer: A. Doxycycline.

AR 7
Answer: C. TMP/SMX.

AR 8
Answer: F. Nifedipine.

AR 9
Answer: B. Stop tramadol.

AR 10
Answer: B. Topiramate.

AR 11
Answer: A. Fluoxetine.

AR 12
Answer: C. Alendronate.

AR 13
Answer: E. Paroxetine.

AR 14
Answer: C. In patients who have the disease, 25% have a negative test result.

AR 15
Answer: D. 25%.

AR 16
Answer: C. 15% of patients without bladder cancer test positive for this test.

AR 17
Answer: Point D.

AR 18
Answer: Point B.

AR 19
Answer: E. 99%.

AR 20
Answer: D. Sensitivity would increase; specificity would decrease.

AR 21
Answer: B. Increases the prevalence.

AR 22
Answer: B. Case-control trial.

AR 23
Answer: D. Cigarette smoking can cause lung cancer.

AR 24
Answer: B. 2.5%.

AR 25
Answer: D. Blood glucose monitoring is not associated with a statistically significant change in HbA1c.

AR 26
Answer: D. 1.2–4.0.

AR 27
Answer: B. 5.

AR 28
Answer: D. 1.33.

AR 29
Answer: D. 0.1.

AR 30
Answer: C. Stop nortriptyline.

AR 31
Answer: E. Check vitamin D level.

AR 32
Answer: D. Drug side effect of ciprofloxacin.

AR 33
Answer: C. Keep a sitter at the bedside.

AR 34
Answer: C. Chlordiazepoxide.

AR 35
Answer: C. Donepezil.

AR 36
Answer: B. Donepezil.

AR 37
Answer: A. Donepezil.

AR 38
Answer: B. Do not go to the bedroom until he is tired.

AR 39A
Answer: C. Ferritin level.

AR 39B
Answer: B. Pramipexole.

AR 40
Answer: E. Multiple sensory deficits.

AR 41
Answer: D. Epley maneuver.

AR 42
Answer: E. Brainstem ischemia.

AR 43
Answer: D. Amlodipine.

AR 44
Answer: D. Spironolactone.

AR 45
Answer: C. Fecal disimpaction.

AR 46
Answer: A. Depression.

AR 47
Answer: D. Mirtazapine.

AR 48
Answer: C. Detrusor overactivity.

AR 49
Answer: C. Recommend Kegel exercises.

AR 50
Answer: A. Terazosin.

AR 51
Answer: C. Finasteride.

AR 52
Answer: A. Intraurethral alprostadil (Muse).

AR 53
Answer: E. Do not give blood products.

AR 54
Answer: B. Treat with antibiotics because the patient has a life-threatening condition.

AR 55
Answer: A. Do not intubate patient; keep him comfortable.

AR 56
Answer: D. The nephew's request to discontinue IVF and antibiotics is within his capacity to act with the patient's durable power of attorney.

AR 57
Answer: A. Obtain an autopsy.

AR 58
Answer: A. Ask the patient if she would like to designate a family member to help make decisions about her care.

AR 59
Answer: D. Tell the patient you understand his feelings and that you will be available to talk to the family if he wants you to.

AR 60
Answer: A. The physician should terminate the professional relationship and wait a period of time before pursuing personal contacts with the patient.

AR 61
Answer: B. A dosage error was made, and he received 10x the insulin dose he was supposed to receive. He is receiving glucose to help prevent low blood sugar.

AR 62
Answer: D. 40 mg of IV morphine.

AR 63
Answer: C. Refill gabapentin/naproxen/taper oxycodone and start duloxetine.

AR 64
Answer: D. Check CMP, U/A, and TSH.

AR 65
Answer: B. Atorvastatin 80 mg.

AR 66
Answer: C. Pravastatin 40 mg.

AR 67
Answer: D. Stop atenolol and oral estrogen.

AR 68
Answer: D. Okay for immediate surgery.

AR 69
Answer: C. Risk-assess with dipyridamole thallium test.

AR 70
Answer: D. No further testing needed.

AR 71
Answer: E. None of the above.

AR 72
Answer: B. Stop warfarin 5 days before surgery, restart 1st post-op day.

AR 73
Answer: D. Delay surgery at least 4 months.

AR 74
Answer: D. Lipids.

AR 75
Answer: D. Mammogram, Pap smear, colonoscopy.

AR 76
Answer: A. Cholesterol.

AR 77
Answer: D. Lipid panel and chest CT.

AR 78
Answer: E. 66-year-old man with 60-pack-year Hx of smoking, quit 10 years ago.

AR 79
Answer: D. Ethylene glycol ingestion.

AR 80
Answer: C. Salicylate overdose.

AR 81
Answer: B. Methylene blue.

AR 82
Answer: C. Lisinopril-lithium interaction.

AR 83
Answer: D. Ecstasy.

AR 84
Answer: E. None of the above.

AR 85
Answer: C. Glaucoma.

AR 86
Answer: D. Carotid duplex.

AR 87
Answer: E. Ophthalmologic consultation.

AR 88
Answer: B. Immediate referral to ophthalmology for laser therapy of new vessel disease.

AR 89
Answer: C. Evaluation by ophthalmologist within 1–2 weeks.

AR 90
Answer: D. Chest x-ray and immediate referral to ophthalmology.

AR 91
Answer: D. Cerumen impaction.

AR 92
Answer: E. Prednisone.

AR 93
Answer: E. Sumatriptan.

AR 94
Answer: A. Bipolar disorder.

AR 95
Answer: D. Borderline personality disorder.

AR 96
Answer: A. Citalopram.

AR 97
Answer: D. Stop sertraline; begin bupropion.

AR 98
Answer: B. Avoid paroxetine; prefer fluoxetine.

AR 99
Answer: D. Paroxetine (Paxil).

AR 100
Answer: D. Bupropion.

AR 101
Answer: E. Discontinue citalopram and tramadol.

AR 102
Answer: D. Neuroleptic malignant syndrome.

AR 103
Answer: E. 1.25%.

AR 104
Answer: B. 1/9.

AR 105
Answer: E. No treatment.

AR 106
Answer: C. Labetalol.

AR 107
Answer: D. 7-day course of nitrofurantoin.

AR 108
Answer: D. Oseltamivir.

AR 109
Answer: E. Continue with current regimen.

AR 110A
Answer: D. Duplex ultrasonography.

AR 110B
Answer: C. Enoxaparin.

AR 111
Answer: D. Begin on oral contraceptive.

AR 112
Answer: C. Endocervical polyp.

MedStudy

Internal Medicine Video Board Review

Hematology

Presented by

Aric Parnes, MD
Instructor in Medicine — Harvard Medical School
Brigham & Women's Division of Hematology
Boston, Massachusetts

Table of Contents

© 2017 MedStudy Internal Medicine Video Board Review – Hematology • Aric Parnes, MD

Hematology Abbreviations

ABVD	Adriamycin, bleomycin, vinblastine, dacarbazine (chemotherapy regimen)
ACLA	Anti-cardiolipin antibody
ACD	Anemia of chronic disease
Ag	Antigen
AI	Anemia of inflammation
ALL	Acute lymphoblastic leukemia
AML	Acute myeloid leukemia
APC	Activated protein C
APL or aPML	Acute promyelocytic leukemia
ATG	Antithymocyte globulin
ATO	Arsenic trioxide
ATRA	All-trans retinoic acid
CALR	Calretinin
CHOP	Cyclophosphamide, Hydroxydaunomycin, Oncovin (Vincristine), and Prednisone
CLL	Chronic lymphocytic leukemia
CML	Chronic myelogenous leukemia
CVA	Cerebrovascular accident
DAT	Direct antiglobulin test
DFS	Disease free survival
DLBCL	Diffuse large B cell lymphoma
DIC	Disseminated intravascular coagulation
EDTA	Ethanol, dimethylsulfoxide, ethylenediaminetetraacetic acid
ESA	Erythropoiesis-stimulating agent
ET	Essential thrombocytosis
FDP	Fibrin degradation product
FFP	Fresh frozen plasma
FNA	Fine needle aspiration
GHS	Glycated human serum
GM-CSF	Granulocyte macrophage colony stimulating factor
HCL	Hairy cell leukemia
Hgb	Hemoglobin
HIT	Heparin-induced thrombocytopenia
HL	Hodgkin lymphoma
HUS	Hemolytic uremic syndrome
IBC	Iron binding capacity
IDA	Iron deficiency anemia
IFN beta	Beta-interferon
IL	Interleukin
INR	Insulin receptor
ISS	Insulin sliding scale
ITP	Immune thrombocytopenic purpura
IVIG	Intravenous immune globulin
LAP	Leukocyte alkaline phosphatase
LBL	Lymphoblastic lymphoma
LDH	Lactate dehydrogenase
LMWH	Low-molecular-weight heparin
mAb	Monoclonal antibodies
MCV	Mean corpuscular volume
MDS	Myelodysplastic syndromes
MF	Myelofibrosis
MGUS	Monoclonal gammopathy of undetermined significance
MM	Multiple myeloma
MMA	Methylmalonic acid
MPD	Myeloproliferative disorder
MPL	Myeloproliferative leukemia
MPV	Mean platelet volume
NHL	Non-Hodgkin lymphoma
NLPHL	Nodular lymphocyte predominant Hodgkin lymphoma
OCPs	Oral contraceptive pills
PAS	Periodic acid–Schiff
PC	Plasma cell
PFA	Platelet function assay
PNH	Paroxysmal nocturnal hemoglobinuria
PT	Prothrombin time
PTT	Partial thromboplastin time
PV	Polycythemia vera
PVSG	Polycythemia vera study group
RDW	Red cell distribution width
RIPA	Ristocetin-induced platelet aggregation
SOB	Shortness of breath
SPEP	Serum protein electrophoresis
TIBC	Total iron-binding capacity
TKI	Tyrosine kinase inhibitor
TNF	Tumor necrosis factor
TPN	Total parenteral nutrition
TRAP	Tartrate-resistant acid phosphatase stain
TTP	Thrombotic thrombocytopenic purpura
UPEP	Urine protein electrophoresis
URI	Upper respiratory infection
vWD	von Willebrand disease
vWF	von Willebrand factor
vWF:Ag	von Willebrand factor antigen
vWF:RCoF	von Willebrand ristocetin cofactor
WHO	World Health Organization
WM	Waldenström macroglobulinemia

Speaker Disclosure
Aric Parnes, MD, has documented that he has no commercial relationships to disclose.

Hematology

Anemia
Definition:
- Decrease in oxygen-carrying capacity
  - (Lower-than-normal hemoglobin and hematocrit)

Causes:
- Decreased production
  - Nutritional deficiencies
  - Marrow abnormality
- Increased destruction
- Blood loss

Workup tools include:
- Indices
- RDW (red cell distribution width)
- Reticulocyte count
- Review of peripheral smear

Audience Response 1A

A 62-year-old with diabetes and rheumatoid arthritis presents with fatigue and anemia. Her Hgb is 8 g/dL, and her Hct is 25% with an MCV of 79.

The best tests to evaluate this anemia would include:
A. Ferritin and RDW
B. Ferritin and total iron-binding capacity
C. Ferritin and percent iron saturation
D. Ferritin and soluble transferrin receptor

Answer: _____

AR 1B

The following labs return:
Iron 30 (30–150)
IBC 300 (250–450)
% Saturation 10% (15–50%)
Ferritin 30 (30–400)
Soluble transferrin receptor 2.6 (0.76–1.76)

The most likely cause of the anemia given these numbers would be:
A. Iron deficiency anemia
B. Beta thalassemia
C. Anemia of chronic disease
D. Folate deficiency

Answer: _____

Iron Deficiency Anemia (IDA)
- Most common cause of anemia
- Secondary to blood loss or insufficient dietary intake or malabsorption
- Pregnancy also associated with iron-deficient states
- Must <u>always</u> look for and identify a cause for iron deficiency

Hints for IDA diagnosis:
- Indices — microcytic and hypochromia
- RDW — elevated
- Reticulocyte count — inappropriately low
- Thrombocytosis

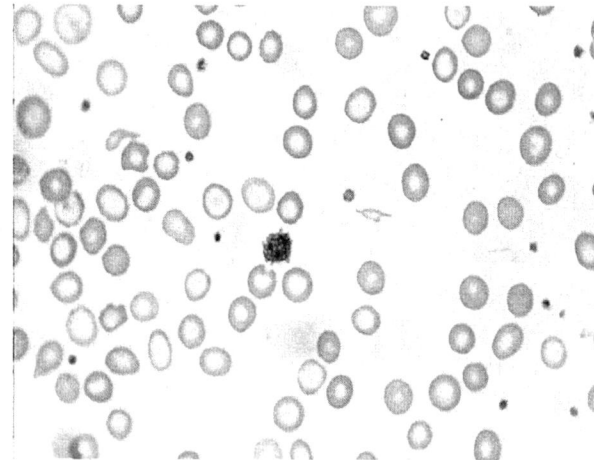

Laboratory tests:

Iron	low
Iron-binding capacity	high
Percent saturation	low
Ferritin	low

IDA (cont.)
Soluble transferrin receptor assay
- Can help differentiate between IDA and ACD
- Transferrin transports iron
- If iron low, then increase production of receptors to bind available iron + transferrin
- Should be increased with iron-deficient states

If unable to tell iron status after all blood tests completed, the final option is evaluation of iron stores in the bone marrow.

Treatment options:
- Should correct etiology if possible
- Oral iron replacement: Need 200–250 mg of elemental iron daily to replete stores ($FeSO_4$ 325 mg tid)

- Intravenous iron replacement
  - Iron dextran
  - Iron sucrose
  - Ferric gluconate
  - Ferumoxytol
  - Ferric carboxymaltose

AR 2
A 62-year-old with diabetes and rheumatoid arthritis presents with fatigue and anemia.
Lab studies are as follows:

Hgb 9.0	Fe 30
Retic 1.0	TIBC 150
MCV 85	Fe sat 20%
RDW 12	Ferritin 400

The cause for this anemia is most likely:
A. Iron deficiency
B. Anemia of inflammation
C. Beta thalassemia
D. Aplastic anemia

Answer: _____

Anemia of Inflammation (AI)
- Anemia of chronic disease (ACD)
- Inability to utilize available storage iron
- Mediated by inflammatory cytokines such as TNF, IL 1, IL 6, and IFN beta

- Mediated by hepcidin production — which is increased by inflammation
- Hepcidin impairs iron absorption
- Increased hepcidin results in anemia
- Usually associated with a decreased erythropoietin state

Clues for diagnosis:
- Usually normochromic normocytic RBCs
- Occasionally may be hypochromic microcytic
- Decreased reticulocyte count

Other laboratory tests include:

Iron levels	low
IBC	low
Ferritin	high
% Saturation	low/normal

AI (cont.)
Other lab tests include:

Soluble transferrin receptor	normal
Bone marrow assay	increased iron stores

Treatment options include:
- Exogenous erythropoietin
- Transfusion support
- Optimize associated medical illness

AR 3
A 60-year-old patient with hypothyroidism on replacement thyroid develops paresthesia, fatigue, and a macrocytic anemia.

He should be suspected to have which of the following?
A. Pernicious anemia
B. Anemia of inflammation
C. Folate deficiency
D. Iron deficiency anemia

Answer: _____

B_{12} Deficiency
- Poor diet or abnormality of small bowel
- Autoimmune in nature with associated antiparietal cell antibodies or intrinsic factor antibodies
- Seen in association with other autoimmune phenomena
- Neurological deficits associated

Folate Deficiency
- Secondary to dietary deficiency
  - Alcoholics
  - Drug addicts
- Malabsorption
- Chronic hemolytic states
- Pregnancy

B_{12} / Folate Deficiencies
Clues for diagnosis:
- Indices — macrocytic
- RDW — elevated
- Reticulocyte count — decreased
- Decreased WBC and platelet counts (pancytopenia)
- Hypersegmentation

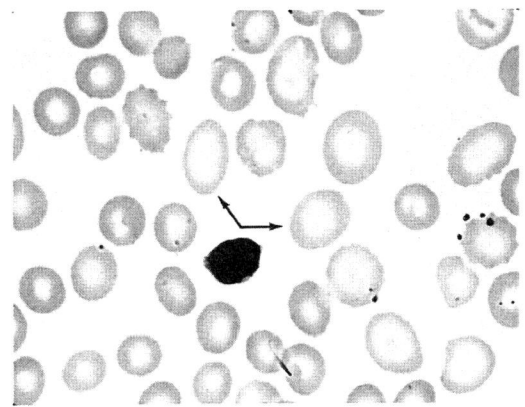

B_{12} / Folate Deficiencies (cont.)

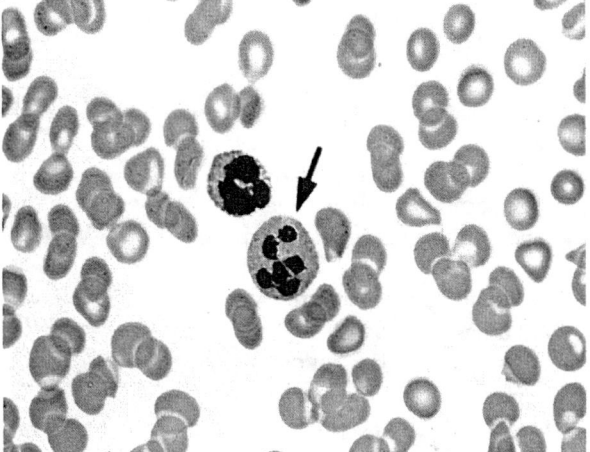

B_{12} / Folate Deficiencies (cont.)

Tests for Diagnosis:
- Vitamin B_{12} level $\longrightarrow$ low in B_{12} def
- Folate level check $\longrightarrow$ low in folate def
- MMA level $\longrightarrow$ high in B_{12} def
- Homocysteine level $\longrightarrow$ high in both

B_{12} Deficiency
Other tests include:
- Parietal cell antibodies
- Intrinsic factor antibodies

B_{12} / Folate Deficiencies (cont.)
Treatment options:
- B_{12} should be replaced by IM injection, and usually replacement is lifelong
  - Varying schedules
    - 1,000 mcg/day x 1 week
    - 1,000 mcg/week x 1 month
    - 1,000 mcg/month x life
- Folate is usually replaced PO 1 mg/day

Aplastic Anemia
- Pancytopenia
- Occurs secondary to a stem cell disorder
- The majority of cases are idiopathic; However, may be related to:
  - Drugs
  - PNH
  - Certain viral infections

Drug/toxin associated aplasia seen with:
- Benzene and radiation — dose-related
- Gold, sulfa drugs, chloramphenicol, and insecticides are usually idiosyncratic-type reactions

- Presentation is a result of cytopenias
  - Infections
  - Anemia symptoms
  - Bleeding symptoms
- All cell lines are diminished on peripheral smear but generally normal in appearance
- Bone marrow exam is hypocellular

Treatment options include:
- Immunosuppression with ATG/cyclosporine
  - Older patients
  - Younger patients with no marrow donor
- Bone marrow transplant
  - Younger patients with a donor

Paroxysmal Nocturnal Hemoglobinuria (PNH)
- Acquired stem cell defect
- Hemolytic picture
- Associated with risk for thrombosis
- RBCs more susceptible to complement degradation

Diagnostic tests:
- Older tests replaced by flow cytometry showing absence of:
  - **CD55**
  - **CD59**

Treatment options:
- RBC transfusions during episodes of hemolysis
- Steroids
- Androgens
- Anticoagulation
- Eculizumab
- Stem cell transplant

Eculizumab
- mAb against C5
- Blocks cleavage of C5, thus blocks formation of C5b-9 complex
- Reduces hemolysis, thus transfusion
- Reduces thrombosis
- Risks include encapsulated organism infections

Hemoglobinopathies
- Predominant types
  - Sickle cell disease
  - Alpha thalassemia
  - Beta thalassemia
- Inherited
- Shortened RBC survival

- Disruption of either α chain or β-chain production (normal $\alpha\alpha/\beta\beta$)
- Diagnosis is made by hemoglobin electrophoresis
- All should have an elevated reticulocyte count

AR 4

A 28-year-old man is admitted to the hospital for chest pain and SOB. He has a history of sickle cell disease and is on chronic folic acid. His evaluation includes a CXR with bilateral infiltrates, and his lab studies are as follows:

Hgb 8.2	87% segs
Hct 25%	13% lymphs
WBC 32,000	103 nRBCs
Platelets 450,000	
O_2 saturation on RA 85%	

The most appropriate next step would be:

A. CT chest.
B. Start hydroxyurea.
C. Begin antifungal coverage.
D. RBC exchange transfusion.

Answer: _____

Sickle Cell Trait
- Hemoglobin AS
  - One affected gene
  - No clinical significance
  - Unable to fully concentrate urine

Sickle Cell Disease
- Hemoglobin SS
  - Valine to glutamic acid substitution on the β-globin gene
  - RBC sickles under low oxygen tension, becoming unable to pass through small blood vessels
  - Associated with:
    - Pain crisis
    - Nonhealing leg ulcers
    - Avascular necrosis

Important points to remember:
- Aplastic crisis from parvovirus B19
- Functional asplenia
- Develop microinfarcts of organs, such as brain — CVA
- Also at risk for priapism and retinal detachment

Treatment options:
- Folate
- Symptomatic treatment
- Simple transfusion or RBC exchange
- Hydroxyurea

Alpha Thalassemia
- Decreased production of the α chain
- 4 α-chain alleles, thus 4 variations with increasing severity with increasing number of genes deleted

ααα-	α-α-	α---	----
		(Hgb H)	(Hgb Barts)

- Should be microcytic with increased RBC count
- Should have an elevated reticulocyte count if anemic

- Normal electrophoresis (cannot be distinguished from iron deficiency)
- Diagnosis can be made by α-chain gene analysis, although usually not necessary to do

Beta Thalassemia
- Decreased production of the β-globin chain
- 3 categories:
  1) β-thalassemia minor — mild anemia with marked microcytosis
  2) β-thalassemia intermedia — some β-globin production and usually does not require transfusional support
  3) β-thalassemia major (Cooley's) — minimal production of hemoglobin and transfusion dependent

- Should be microcytic
- Should have an elevated reticulocyte count
- Should see elevated levels of Hgb A_2 on hemoglobin electrophoresis

AR 5

A 26-year-old woman with a history of lupus presents with complaints of fatigue and SOB. She has been doing well while being treated with hydroxychloroquine (Plaquenil) and azathioprine (Imuran, Azasan). She goes to see her doctor and a CBC is performed. By physical exam, she is noted to be tachycardic with a soft flow murmur. She is mildly icteric.
Her CBC returns:

Hgb 4	WBC 6,000
Hct 16%	Platelets 130,000
MCV 102	Retic 14%

The most likely diagnosis is:

A. Drug-induced anemia
B. B_{12} deficiency anemia
C. Autoimmune hemolytic anemia
D. Refractory anemia with sideroblasts

Answer: _____

Autoimmune Hemolytic Anemia
- Expect macrocytosis secondary to an elevated reticulocyte count
- Should see spherocytes on peripheral smear
- Should have elevated levels of LDH and bilirubin (total and indirect)
- Low haptoglobin
- Diagnose with direct Coombs test (a.k.a. direct antiglobulin test [DAT])

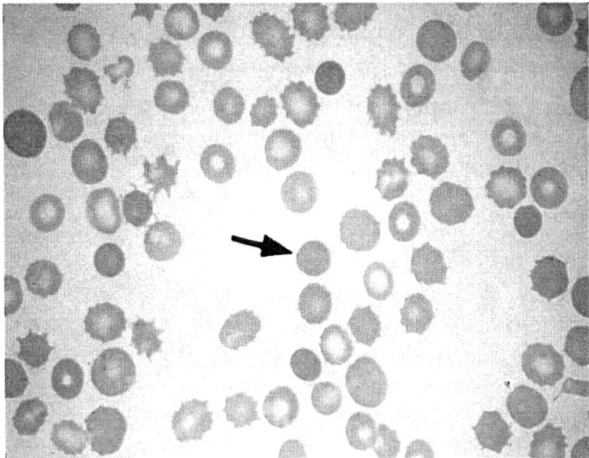

Direct Coombs Test
- Demonstrates antibody on the RBC surface
- Mix patient's blood with anti-IgG or C3 antibodies
- Agglutination indicates a positive test
- Positive test: Autoantibody

Indirect Coombs Test
- Demonstrates antibody in the serum
- Mix patient's serum with known panel of RBCs
- Agglutination indicates a positive test
- Positive: Alloantibody

Warm Autoantibodies
- IgG antibodies
- React at room temperature
- Associated with lymphoproliferative and collagen vascular diseases
- Usually respond to therapy with immunosuppression or splenectomy

Cold Autoantibodies
- IgM antibodies
- React at lower temperatures
- Hemolysis occurs through the complement pathway
- Associated with lymphoproliferative diseases or infection
- Not very responsive to therapy — stay warm!!

Hemochromatosis

AR 6
A 70-year-old diabetic man presents with c/o arthralgias in his knees.
You notice he is very tan despite his claim he is indoors most of the day. His exam is pertinent for bronzed skin and mild joint swelling in his knees. His liver edge is not palpable, and he has no splenomegaly.

Lab studies include:

WBC 8,400	Glu 210	AST 90
Plt 363,000	Creat 1.3	ALT 95
Hct 40		T Bili 1.6
MCV 82		
Normal Diff		

You suspect hemochromatosis.

Your initial screening test should be:
A. Serum Fe
B. Serum IBC
C. Transferrin saturation
D. Genetic test for *H63D*

Answer: _____

Hereditary Hemochromatosis
- Autosomal recessive inheritance
- Frequent in Caucasians
- Mutation in *C282Y* or *H63D* genes
- Modulates absorption of iron via HFE protein
- Affects hepcidin production

- Iron deposition
  - Liver   – Skin   – Joints
  - Heart   – Pancreas
- Best test(s) for diagnosis
  - Transferrin saturation
    - > 45% women
    - > 50% men
  - Ferritin
    - > 1,000
  - Gene studies

- Treatment
  - Phlebotomy to iron deficient state
- Slows progression of sequelae but does not reverse damage
- Test 1st degree family members

Myelodysplasia

AR 7

A 72-year-old man presents with fatigue and bruising. He has been noted to be mildly thrombocytopenic with a CBC as follows:

Hgb 11.4	WBC 4,300	Segs 25
Hct 34	Plt ct 65,000	Monos 15
MCV 102	Retic 0.4%	Lymphs 60

His peripheral smear shows basophilic stippling and a dimorphic population.

Which of the following is the most likely diagnosis?

A. Lymphoma with a leukemic phase
B. Evans syndrome
C. Myelodysplasia
D. Chronic lymphocytic leukemia

Answer: _____

Myelodysplastic Syndromes (MDS)

- Clonal stem cell disorders of the elderly
- Often present with pancytopenia although may have only 1 or 2 cell lines suppressed
- Prognosis depends on:
  - Percentage of blasts
  - Cytogenetics

- Peripheral smear and lab findings suggestive of an MDS state include:
  - Dimorphic RBC population
  - Macrocytic RBCs
  - Pseudo–Pelger-Huët anomaly
  - Large agranular platelets
  - Decreased reticulocyte count

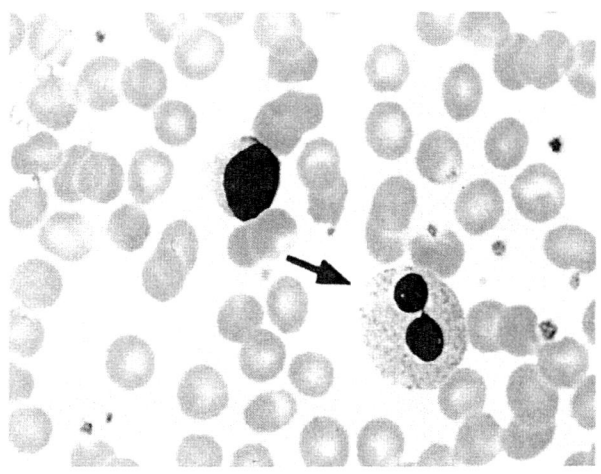

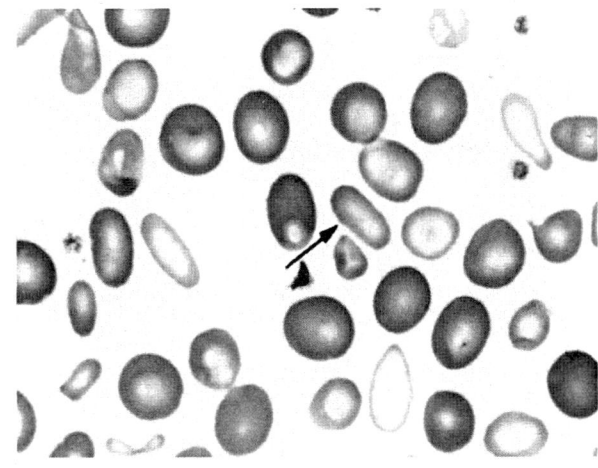

MDS (cont.)

- Diagnosis is made by bone marrow evaluation revealing dysplastic maturation of 1 to 3 cell lines
- Generally have a hypercellular bone marrow with evidence of dysplasia in 1 or all cell lines
- May also see ringed sideroblasts

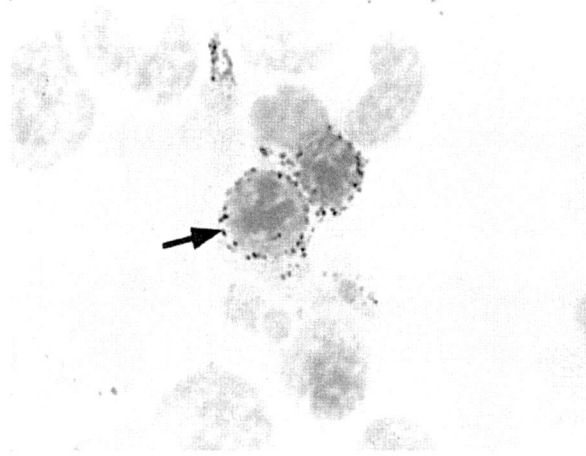

MDS (cont.)

- Differentiate subtypes by the percent of blasts and the percent of ringed sideroblasts
- Cytogenetic abnormalities also important
- WHO Classification scheme
  - 8 groups based on the above

- 5q deletion syndrome
  - Usually found in females
  - Thrombocytosis
  - Has a more favorable prognosis
  - High response rate to lenalidomide

General treatment options include:
- Supportive care
- Growth factors
- Chemotherapy
- Bone marrow transplant

AR 8A

A 45-year-old woman presents with fatigue, early satiety, and bruising. She has noted night sweats and a 10-lb weight loss over the last 6 weeks. Her PE is remarkable for splenomegaly and several large ecchymotic areas.

Her CBC is as follows:

Hgb 10   WBC 250,500
Hct 31   Plts 675,000
MCV 78

What would you like to do next?
A. Perform platelet aggregations.
B. PT, INR, PTT.
C. Fe, IBC, ferritin.
D. Review peripheral smear.

Answer: _____

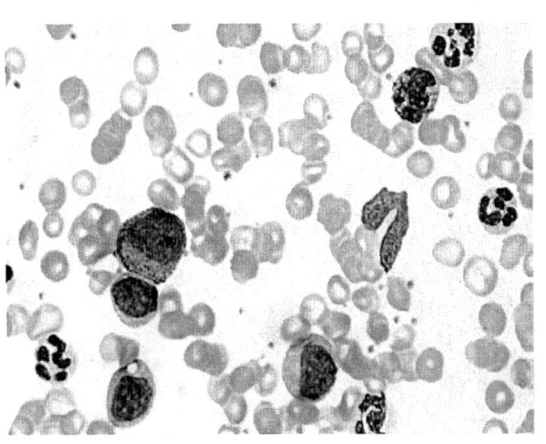

AR 8B
Which of the following is the most likely diagnosis?
A. Chronic myeloid leukemia
B. Polycythemia vera
C. Acute myeloid leukemia
D. Chronic lymphocytic leukemia

Answer: _____

Chronic Myeloid Leukemia (CML)

Myeloproliferative Disorders (MPD)
- Polycythemia vera
- Essential thrombocytosis
- Myelofibrosis
- Chronic myeloid leukemia

- Generally diseases of the elderly
- All clonal disorders classified by the cell line most affected
- Marrow will be hypercellular in all
- Splenomegaly is a common physical finding in all

Chronic Myeloid Leukemia (CML)
- Chronic course
- Presents with subjective symptoms, such as fatigue and early satiety, although often found on routine CBC
- Linked to radiation exposure, but not clearly to any other environmental or infectious etiologies

Typical laboratory presentation
- Markedly elevated WBC count
- Left shift to early precursors
- "Myelocyte spike"
- Eosinophilia and basophilia

- Diagnosis is made by finding:
  - Low LAP (leukocyte alkaline phosphatase)
  - Marrow that is hypercellular
  - Characteristic chromosomal abnormality
    - t(9;22) — Philadelphia chromosome
    - Additional chromosomal findings dependent upon the phase of the disease

Philadelphia Chromosome
- First chromosomal abnormality definitely linked to development of malignancy
- Found in over 95% of CML patients
- Moves the abl proto-oncogene on chr 9 to the bcr on chr 22
- Results in production of an abnormal tyrosine kinase

Natural Disease Progression

Chronic Phase
↓
Accelerated Phase
↓
Blast Crisis

Chronic phase:
- Usually relatively asymptomatic
- Easily controlled counts
- Disease duration
  - 2 years untreated
  - 3–4 years with hydroxyurea
  - 4–5 years with interferon
  - Unknown with TKI therapy

Accelerated phase:
- Increasingly difficult to control counts
- Increasing eosinophilia and basophilia
- Accumulation of additional cytogenetic abnormalities
- Treatment becomes more difficult

CML (cont.)
Blast crisis:
- Transformation to acute leukemia
  - 80% AML
  - 20% ALL
- Poor prognosis with survival measured in months despite therapy

Treatment options include:
- Oral drugs — hydroxyurea, busulfan
- Interferon
- Low-dose cytarabine
- Combinations of the above

Tyrosine Kinase Inhibitors:
- Drugs designed to take advantage of the t(9;22) abnormality
- Majority have a cytogenetic remission, but duration unknown
- Few side effects — primarily fluid retention/ GI toxicity/rash

| Imatinib | Nilotinib | Dasatinib |
| Bosutinib | | Ponatinib |

Bone marrow transplantation
- Still therapy of choice for young patients with a matched available donor
- Curative therapy
- Historically best when performed early in the disease
  - Chronic phase 50–70% (5-year DFS)
  - Accelerated phase 20–30%
  - Blast crisis 10–15%

Polycythemia Vera (PV)
- Expansion of the erythroid line but usually see mild degrees of leukocytosis and thrombocytosis as well
- Growth is independent of erythropoietin
- Typically affects an older patient population
- Symptoms may include aquagenic pruritus

Presentation is usually one of:
- Plethora
- Splenomegaly
- Thrombosis
- Hyperviscosity
- Gout

- Erythromelalgia
  - Erythema and pain of digits
- Headache, dizziness
- Small vessel thrombosis

Diagnostic criteria: (Modified from the PVSG)
- Increased RBC mass (difficult to do)
- Normal P_aO_2
- Splenomegaly
- JAK2 V617F or exon 12 mutations

JAK2
- JAK2 V617F genetic abnormality found to be associated with up to 95% of patients
- A tyrosine kinase activated in response to certain growth factors (GM-CSF and erythropoietin)
- If found, then diagnosis is PV, not secondary

PV (cont.)
- Other criteria include:
  - Elevated platelet count
  - Elevated WBC count
  - Low serum erythropoietin levels
  - Elevated LAP
  - Elevated B_{12}

- Diagnosis requires exclusion of secondary causes of erythrocytosis
  - Gaisböck syndrome
  - Hypoxic states
  - Renal disease
  - Malignancy

Natural history of this disorder is slow and indolent with:
- Progression occurs over many years to decades
- Progression to a fibrotic or spent phase (PPMM)
- Conversion to acute myeloid leukemia

Treatment options include:
- Phlebotomy — easy way to control red blood cell count
- Drugs — used primarily to help control platelet count or if phlebotomy not feasible: Hydroxyurea
- Low-dose ASA — if no contraindication

Ruxolitinib
- An inhibitor of both JAK1 and JAK2
- Now indicated in PV with an inadequate response to hydroxyurea
- Do not have to be JAK2+ to use
- Side effects primarily cytopenias

AR 9A
A 55-year-old woman presents for her routine physical exam. She is healthy and is on no medications.
She recently had a normal Pap smear and normal mammogram. She had a colonoscopy at age 50 that was normal.
Her physical exam was normal except for a BMI of 26.
Her CBC is:

| Hgb 12 | WBC 5,600 | Ferritin 40 |
| MCV 82 | Platelets 780,000 | |

Repeat CBC 2 months later: Hgb 12.3 and Plts 770,000

AR 9A (cont.)
The most likely diagnosis is:
A. Early iron deficiency anemia
B. Essential thrombocytosis
C. Occult malignancy
D. Polycythemia vera

Answer: _____

AR 9B
Appropriate intervention would be:
A. Oral iron replacement
B. Hydroxyurea
C. Imatinib
D. Observation

Answer: _____

**This is likely essential thrombocytosis,
and you should just observe.**

Essential Thrombocytosis (ET)
- By definition — unexplained thrombocytosis
  sustained for 6 months
- May be associated with splenomegaly
  but not usually massive
- $JAK2$ is abnormal in 50–60% of patients
- New mutation CALR found exclusive of $JAK2$ —
  associated with a different subset of ET
- MPL

Must rule out other causes for "reactive"
thrombocytosis:
- Iron deficiency anemia
- Malignancy
- Collagen vascular disease
- Infection
- Post-splenectomy state
- Other MPDs

- Complications may include either bleeding
  or thrombosis
- Platelet function tests are not indicative of tendency
  to bleed or clot
- May see erythromelalgia
- May see spurious hyperkalemia

- Treatment options include:
  – Observation
  – Hydroxyurea
  – Interferon-α
  – Anagrelide
- Little evolution to acute leukemia

Secondary Thrombocytosis
- Remember that secondary thrombocytosis **does not**
  put you at risk of bleeding or clotting
- There is **no** absolute number that denotes primary
  from secondary thrombocytosis

Idiopathic Myelofibrosis
- Agnogenic myeloid metaplasia or myelofibrosis
  with myeloid metaplasia
- Older patients
- Clonal disorder with cytopenias
- Marrow fibrosis
- Extramedullary hematopoiesis
- Massive splenomegaly

Myelofibrosis
- Characterized by a myelophthisic picture
  on peripheral smear
  – Teardrop-shaped RBCs
  – nRBCs
  – Left-shifted WBC series
- Anemia
- $JAK2$ positive in 50–60%
- CALR also found

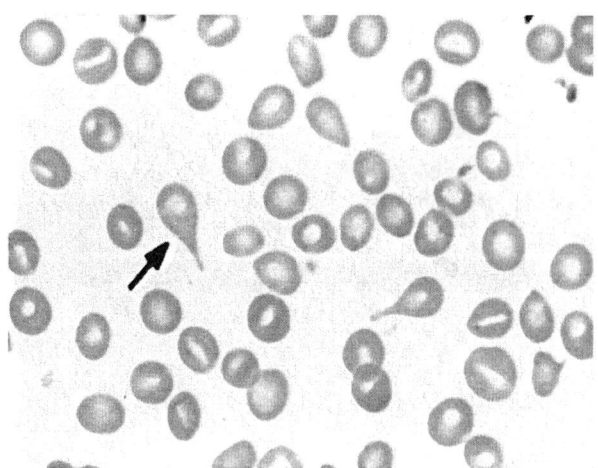

Myelofibrosis (cont.)
- Natural history is shorter than most MPDs
- Median survival is only 5 years
- Progressive marrow failure with increasing transfusion
  dependence and organomegaly
- Infectious complications
- May convert to acute leukemia

Treatment options include:
- Supportive care
- Growth factors
- Hydroxyurea
- Splenectomy
- Bone marrow transplant

Ruxolitinib
- An inhibitor of both *JAK1* and *JAK2*
- Also indicated in intermediate- or high-risk MF
- Do not have to be *JAK2*+ to use
- Side effects primarily cytopenias

Primary Hemostasis & Bleeding Disorders

AR 10
A healthy, 42-year-old female with complaints of epistaxis and easy bruising for 2 weeks is seen in the ED. She has the following CBC:

Hgb 10	WBC 6,200
Hct 30	Plts 38,000
MCV 72	Normal differential

Which of the following is the most likely diagnosis?
A. Acute leukemia
B. MDS
C. Chronic leukemia
D. ITP

Answer: _____

Hemostasis
Normal hemostasis involves 2 phases:
- **Primary — the platelet plug**
  and
- Secondary — the coagulation cascade

Bleeding Disorders
- Platelet abnormality vs. coagulopathy can be differentiated by the <u>type</u> of bleeding
- Primary platelet bleeding is mucosal with petechiae, epistaxis, gum bleeding, and GI tract bleeding
- Coagulation bleeds are generally joint and soft tissue bleeds

Tests to evaluate a bleeding patient include:
- Platelet count ➔ measures the number of platelets
- Platelet aggregation or PFA ➔ measures the function of platelets

Thrombocytopenia

Decreased platelets result from:

Decreased Production   Increased Destruction

Sequestration

*** Always Make Sure This is Real and Not Artifact ***
- Look at the peripheral smear
  - May see clumping (EDTA phenomena)
  - Look at platelet size (MPV)
  - Look at WBCs
  - Also get to look at RBCs

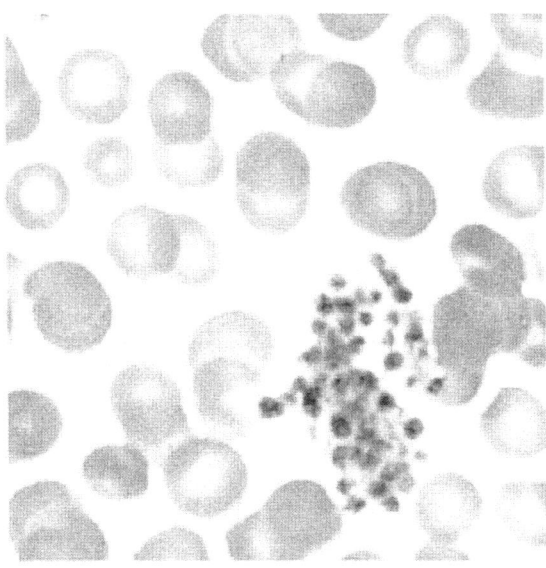

Thrombocytopenia (cont.)
As a general rule, if platelets are above 20,000, the risk of spontaneous bleeding is small. When the count goes below 10,000, the risk increases substantially and transfusions should be considered.

Decreased production
- Primary marrow failure (AA)
- Marrow replacement (leukemia, infiltration)
- Viral suppression
- Drug suppression

Sequestration
- Hypersplenism
- Generally mild and trilineage suppression
- Evidence of liver disease

Increased Destruction
- ITP
- TTP/HUS
- DIC
- HIT

Immune Thrombocytopenia (ITP)
- In childhood, this is usually post viral and a self-limited illness
- In adults, it is usually a chronic disease
- Antibody-mediated — IgG
- Significant bleeding rare

ITP (cont.)
- 30-30-30-10 rule
  - Idiopathic
  - Drugs
  - Disease states such as lymphoma, CLL, collagen vascular diseases
  - Viral illnesses such as HCV, HIV

- No diagnostic test
  - Primarily a diagnosis of exclusion
  - Rule out HIV and hepatitis C
  - Rule out SLE
  - Evaluate drug history

Treatment options:
- Platelets > 30,000 — observation
- Platelets < 30,000 — treatment
  - Steroids (dexamethasone, prednisone)
  - IVIG
  - Splenectomy
    - Up to 80% improved with these maneuvers

Optional therapies for patients failing steroids

- **Rituximab**   - **Danazol**
- **TPO receptor agonists:**   - **Vinca alkaloids**
  - Eltrombopag
  - Romiplostim

- **Splenectomy**   - **Anti-Rho (D)**

Thrombotic Thrombocytopenic Purpura (TTP)
Diagnostic Pentad:
1) Microangiopathic hemolytic anemia
2) Thrombocytopenia
3) Fever
4) Neurological signs
5) Renal dysfunction

- Associated with various disorders
  - Pregnancy
  - Metastatic cancer
  - Bone marrow transplant
  - Drugs
    - Mitomycin C
    - Ticlopidine
    - Cyclosporine
    - Tacrolimus

- The peripheral smear is helpful
  - Schistocytes
  - Retics
  - nRBCs
  - Thrombocytopenia
  - Normal WBC series

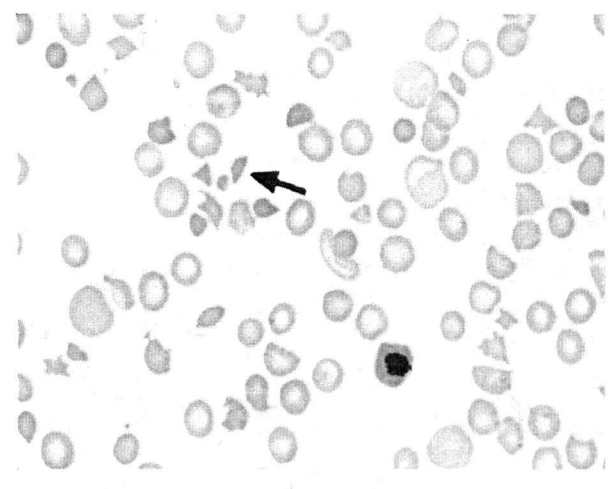

TTP (cont.)
- Other lab abnormalities confirm the hemolytic process
  - Elevated reticulocyte count
  - Elevated LDH
  - Elevated total and indirect bilirubin
  - Decreased haptoglobin
- DAT negative
- Normal coags

- ADAMTS13 (von Willebrand cleaving protease)
  - Cleaves unusually large vWF multimers
  - Congenital: *ADAMTS13* gene defect found in congenital disease
  - Acquired: Antibody against the protease (presence of an ADAMTS13 inhibitor)
  - Increased numbers of very large vW multimers that activate/clear platelets

This syndrome is considered a medical emergency, and treatment should be instituted immediately.
- Plasma exchange
- Steroids (for suspected autoantibody)
- Platelet transfusions are contraindicated unless there is a life-threatening bleed

Disseminated Intravascular Coagulation (DIC)
- Present with either bleeding or thrombosis
- Always secondary to an underlying illness, such as:
  - Obstetrical catastrophes
  - Malignancy
  - Trauma
  - Sepsis
  - APL

Laboratory findings include:
- Schistocytes
- Thrombocytopenia
- Elevated fibrin degradation products (D-dimer, fibrin split products)
- Prolonged PT and PTT
- Decreased fibrinogen

PT	Prolonged
PTT	Prolonged
PLT CT	Decreased
Fibrinogen	Decreased
FDP	Increased
D-dimer	Positive

DIC (cont.)
- Treatment of the underlying disorder
- Support with appropriate products
  - Cryoprecipitate
  - FFP
  - Platelets
  - pRBCs
- Heparin therapy — rarely needed

AR 11
A 56-year-old is admitted for revision of a recent total hip replacement and has a normal CBC at admission. He has an unremarkable surgery and requires no transfusions. He receives postoperative pain medications and is anticoagulated with LMWH. Two days postoperatively, he is noted to have the following CBC:

Hgb 12	WBC 5,600	INR 1.0
Hct 33%	Diff normal	PTT 33 secs
MCV 88	Platelets 25,000	

You should immediately:
A. Transfuse platelets.
B. Change anticoagulation to argatroban.
C. Investigate for source of bleeding.
D. Begin warfarin.

Answer: _____

You should stop LMWH and substitute a direct thrombin inhibitor, such as argatroban or bivalirudin.

Heparin-Induced Thrombocytopenia (HIT)
- Autoimmune phenomenon
- Antibody to heparin-PF4 complex
- Affects about 3% of patients treated with heparin
  - Less risk with LMWHs
  - Higher risk with surgical patients especially orthopedics

- Occurs 5–8 days after starting heparin therapy unless there has been prior exposure
- Amnestic response after prior exposure (generally within last 100 days) and can develop thrombocytopenia within 1–2 days
- If platelet count falls by 50% or falls below 100,000, immediately stop heparin
- 4 Ts — degree and likely cause of thrombocytopenia, timing, associated thrombosis

Two variants noted
- Type 1 (nonimmune-mediated)
  - Mild thrombocytopenia
  - No thrombosis associated
  - Usually resolves off heparin therapy and may resolve while still on heparin therapy

- Type 2 (immune-mediated)
  - More severe thrombocytopenia
  - Associated with both arterial and venous thrombosis
  - Remain hypercoagulable for weeks after heparin discontinued and thrombocytopenia resolved

Treatment includes:
- Discontinuation of heparin or LMWH
- Substitution with direct thrombin inhibitor: Bivalirudin (excreted in urine) or argatroban (metabolized by liver)
- Reversal with vitamin K if warfarin already started
- Initiate warfarin only after platelet count has recovered and anticoagulation with alternate agent is established

AR 12A
A 24-year-old with a history of epistaxis and heavy menses presents for a tonsillectomy. She gives a family history of excessive bleeding as well.
She has a preoperative workup with a normal PT and PTT.
Her CBC is normal.

A differential diagnosis for this patient should include:
A. DIC
B. May-Hegglin anomaly
C. ACLA syndrome
D. vWD

Answer: _____

AR 12B

The next step in the workup of this patient should include:

A. 1:1 mix of patient and normal plasma
B. von Willebrand factor Ag and activity
C. Antiplatelet antibodies
D. Factor VII level

Answer: _____

von Willebrand Disease (vWD)
- Most common inherited bleeding disorder
- Autosomal dominant inheritance
- Bleeding ranges from mild to severe and spontaneous

- von Willebrand factor is a multimeric protein with multiple functions
  - **Platelet adhesion**
  - **Carrier protein for Factor VIII**
- Exists as a series of proteins with varying molecular weights
- Defined as a quantitative or qualitative defect

- There are 3 main types of von Willebrand disease
- The diagnostic tests for vWD may vary from individual to individual and even from day to day in the same individual
- Plasma levels of vWF are influenced by blood type
  - Type O have lower levels

vWD Tests
- vWF:Ag — assay for the total vWF protein
- vWF:RCoF — assay for the ability of patient plasma to agglutinate normal platelets with the addition of ristocetin
- Factor VIII level
- RIPA — platelet aggregation in response to ristocetin
- Multimeric assay

- vWF:Ag — low
- vWF:RCoF — low
- Factor VIII level — normal to low
- RIPA — normal to low
- Multimeric assay — normal/abnormal to absent

vWD Types Include
- Quantitative — 1 (low levels)
- Qualitative — 2 (functional defect)
- Quantitative — 3 (absent)

vWD (cont.)
Treatment options:
- Desmopressin (DDAVP/Stimate) — raises plasma vWF and Factor VIII levels by release from the endothelium; Best used in mild Type 1 disease
- Should always test DDAVP response prior to surgery

- Develops tachyphylaxis after 48 hours
- Desmopressin may worsen the thrombocytopenia seen with Type 2b and will not work with Type 3
- Cryoprecipitate is rich in vWF and Factor VIII and may be used to treat emergent bleeding or for surgery

- vWF concentrates (typically also contain Factor VIII) may be used for all types of vWD
- Given twice daily for active bleeds or surgery and continued at least 48 hours

Rare conditions but favorite exam topics are: Bernard-Soulier syndrome and Glanzmann thrombasthenia

Bernard-Soulier Syndrome
- Also called the giant platelet syndrome
- Glycoprotein Ib platelet defect
- Unable to bind vWF, which is important for adhesion to the endothelium
- Have decreased ristocetin aggregation
- Have mild thrombocytopenia

Glanzmann Thrombasthenia
- Glycoprotein IIb–IIIa defect
- Unable to cross-link fibrinogen, which is important for aggregation
- Have abnormal platelet aggregation
- Platelet count is normal
- Platelet size (MPV) is normal

Hemostasis
Normal hemostasis involves 2 phases:
- Primary — the platelet plug
        and
- **Secondary — the coagulation cascade**

Clotting pathway may be activated by injury or intrinsic factors

Intrinsic	Common	Extrinsic
XII	X	
XI	V	VII
IX	II	
VIII	fibrinogen	

Bleeding Disorders
Appropriate tests for workup include:
PT ⟹ measures the extrinsic and common pathways
PTT ⟹ measures the intrinsic and common pathways

© 2017 MedStudy Internal Medicine Video Board Review – Hematology • Aric Parnes, MD

Evaluation of Prolonged PT or PTT
- 1:1 mix of patient and normal plasma
  - Will detect a factor deficiency — should see correction with mix
  - Will allow detection of an inhibitor — does not correct with mixing
  - May need to do a 2-hour incubation to reveal a slow inhibitor

Hemophilia

Hemophilia A   Hemophilia B
Factor VIII   Factor IX

- Both are X-linked recessive in inheritance
- Both are associated with soft tissue and joint bleeds
- Both result in prolongation of the PTT

Hemophilia A
- Factor VIII is synthesized in the liver
- Circulates bound to vWF
- Need 25% activity for normal hemostasis
  - Severe disease < 1% activity
  - Moderate disease 1–5% activity
  - Mild disease > 5% activity
- Risk of bleeding correlates with amount of Factor VIII

Hemophilia A treatment options include:
- Desmopressin (DDAVP) will increase the plasma level of Factor VIII two- to three-fold and is useful in mild hemophilia
- For more severe patients or bleeds, replacement with cryoprecipitate is feasible, but factor products are preferable

Factor VIII Inhibitors
- Develop in 10–20% of patients receiving factor infusions
- They are IgG antibodies
- Detected when the 1:1 mix does not correct
- Measured in Bethesda units
- Treat with activated PCC (prothrombin complex concentrate, activated Factors II+VII+IX+X, FEIBA), Factor VIIa (NovoSeven), porcine VIII, or immune tolerance

Hemophilia B
- Factor IX deficiency
- Synthesized in the liver
- Requires vitamin K as a cofactor for modification
- Also known as "Christmas disease"
- Clinically indistinguishable from hemophilia A

Hemophilia B treatment options:
- FFP
- Factor IX concentrates — plasma derived and recombinant are available
- Twice the volume of distribution to consider when calculating replacement doses

Other Factor Deficiencies

Factor X
- Deficiency is very rare
- Prolongs PT & PTT
- Acquired deficiency occurs with amyloidosis
- Treat with FFP or Factor X concentrate

Factor XI
- Third most common (hemophilia C)
- Autosomal recessive inheritance
- Correlation between factor level and bleeding tendency is poor
- Less spontaneous bleeding
- Treat with FFP

Factor XII
- Factor XII is also known as the Hageman factor
- Have prolonged PTT
- No clinical bleeding
- Normal hemostasis

Factor XIII
- Stabilizes fibrin clot after clot formation
- Normal screening coagulation tests
- Have late bleeding and poor wound healing
- Diagnosis with abnormal euglobulin clot lysis assay
- Treat with FFP or Factor XIII concentrate (long half-life)

Vitamin K Deficiency
- Vitamin K-dependent factors are:
  - II
  - VII
  - IX
  - X
- Vitamin K deficiency seen with:
  - **Liver disease**
  - **Poor absorption**
  - **TPN**
  - **Warfarin use**
  - **Antibiotic use**

- Factor VII with the shortest half-life, thus most sensitive
- Prolonged PT, normal PTT
- Treat with vitamin K (works within 8–12 hours)
- If bleeding, can use FFP, prothrombin concentrate complexes (Kcentra)

Thrombotic Disorders
- Hypercoagulable states result in unprovoked thrombosis
- Family history is important
- Most are undefined, but there are several deficiencies of the naturally occurring anticoagulants that are described

Antithrombin Deficiency
- Autosomal dominant inheritance
- Rare
- Inactivates activated II, IX, X, XI, XII
- Action is enhanced with heparin
- Usually have clots at a young age

- Should measure prior to the institution of heparin therapy but may be decreased secondary to thrombosis
- Can measure at the completion of AC therapy to confirm a low level
- Protein may be decreased or dysfunctional
- Should measure with both a functional assay and an antigenic assay

Treatment options include:
- Heparin — remember: These patients may be relatively "heparin resistant"
- Warfarin or direct anticoagulants for long-term anticoagulation
- Recombinant and plasma-derived AT is available for surgery

Protein C Deficiency
- Autosomal dominant inheritance
- Rare
- Cleaves activated Factors V and VIII
- Vitamin K dependent
- Should measure prior to the initiation of warfarin therapy or at the completion of warfarin

Protein S Deficiency
- Autosomal dominant inheritance
- Rare
- Functions as a cofactor with protein C
- Vitamin K dependent
- Should measure prior to the initiation of warfarin therapy or at the completion of warfarin

Protein C / S Deficiencies
Treatment:
- For an acute clot, patients should be anticoagulated with heparin
- Long-term therapy should be with warfarin

Warfarin-Associated Skin Necrosis
- Proteins C and S function as anticoagulants, and both are vitamin K dependent
- When warfarin is initiated, the levels of the anticoagulants may decrease more quickly than the procoagulant levels, resulting in a hypercoagulable state
- This is especially prominent in the patients who are protein C deficient, as protein C half-life is very short

APC Resistance / FVL
- Mutation in Factor V, resulting in resistance to activated protein C
- Most common inherited hypercoagulable defect
- Found in up to 25% of patients with recurrent thrombosis
- Additive to other risk factors (OCPs, pregnancy, other defects)

APC Resistance
- Treatment is with heparin/LMWH followed by warfarin
- Recommendations for duration of AC therapy are variable; Should take into account other risk factors — both temporary and inherited — as well as whether heterozygous or homozygous when deciding duration

Antiphospholipid Antibody Syndrome
- Prolonged PTT
- Clotting
  - May be venous or arterial
- Recurrent spontaneous fetal loss

Treatment options:
- Anticoagulation
  - Warfarin
  - Heparin/LMWH
- ASA

Direct Oral Anticoagulants
- Direct thrombin (II) inhibitor
  - Dabigatran
- Factor Xa inhibitors
  - Rivaroxaban
  - Apixaban
  - Edoxaban

Hematologic Malignancies

AR 13
An 80-year-old woman presents with pneumonia. She does not respond to antibiotics. Her exam is remarkable for crackles and small cervical nodes.

Her CBC is as follows:
Hgb 7.0   WBC 55,000
Hct 20   Plts 40,000
Many large blasts with granules are noted.

Which of the following is the most likely diagnosis?
A. Acute myeloid leukemia
B. Hairy cell leukemia
C. Myelodysplastic syndrome
D. Chronic lymphocytic leukemia
E. Chronic myelogenous leukemia

Answer: _____

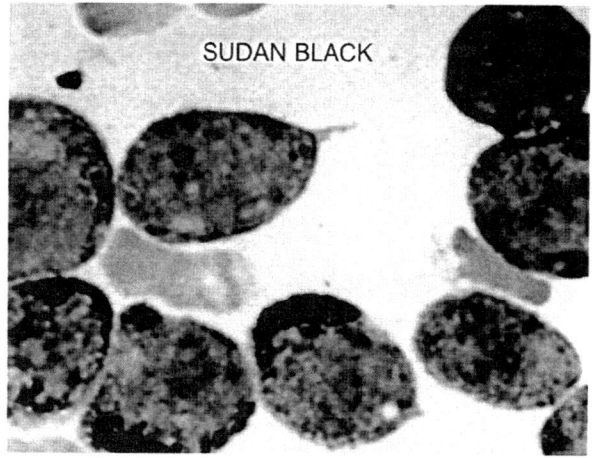

SUDAN BLACK

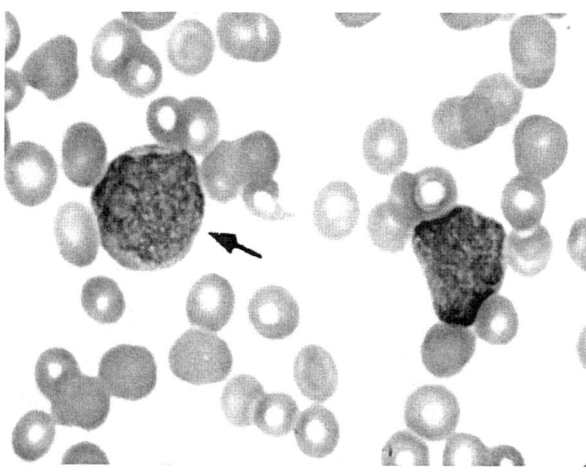

Acute Leukemia
- Accumulation of immature cells (blasts)
- Maybe myeloid or lymphoid
- Myeloid more common in adults

Myeloid	Lymphoid
Sudan black	PAS
Myeloperoxidase	Fewer nucleoli
Esterases	
Auer rods	
More nucleoli	

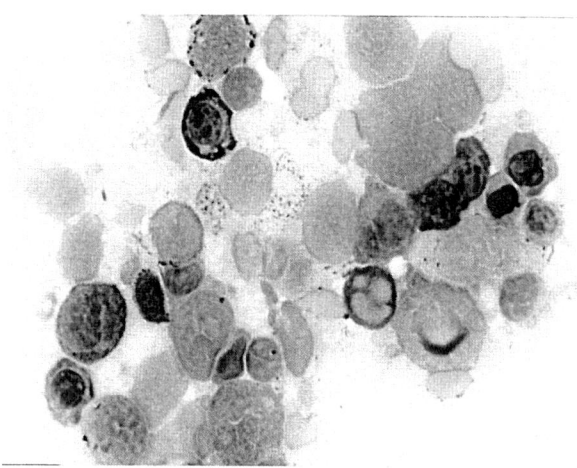

Acute Leukemia (cont.)
- Usually presents with an elevated WBC count but may be normal or low (aleukemic)
- Have accompanying anemia and thrombocytopenia
- May present with infectious complications

- Workup includes:
  - A bone marrow aspirate and biopsy
    - Blasts > 20%
  - Special stains on marrow or peripheral blood
  - Flow cytometry on marrow or peripheral blood
  - Cytogenetic and molecular studies on marrow

Acute Myeloid Leukemia (AML)
- Old FAB Classification is based on morphology (e.g., undifferentiated, promyelocytic, monocytic, megakaryocytic)
- WHO Classification is based on genetics
- Classification made using stains, flow cytometry results, and cytogenetics
- Classification only changes therapy for 1 class: APML

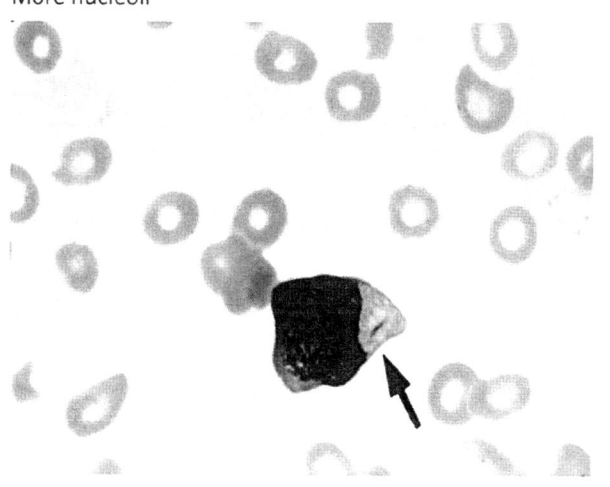

AML (cont.)

Best Prognostic Factor

Cytogenetics

Other prognostic factors include:
- Age — the older patient has an adverse prognosis
- Secondary AML — particularly resistant to therapy
- Performance status — a poor performance status is an adverse prognostic indicator

M3: aPML
- Associated with t(15;17)
- Translocation involving the retinoic acid receptor gene
- Good prognosis category
- Prominent Auer rods
- **Commonly associated with DIC**

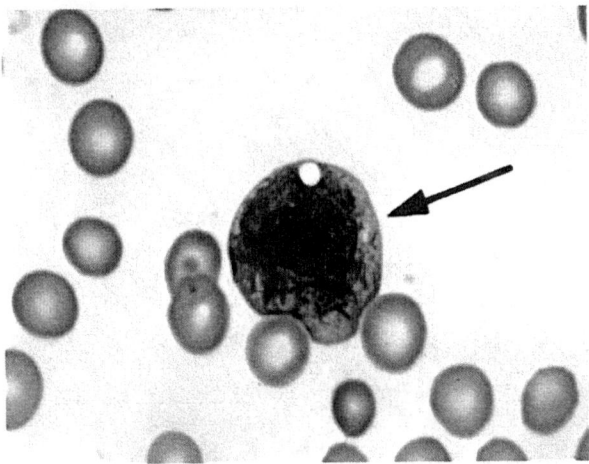

AML (cont.)

M5: Monocytic
- **Commonly associated with skin and soft tissue disease**
- **Gingival hyperplasia**
- CNS disease may occur

In general, treatment consists of:
- Supportive care with transfusions
- Leukapheresis, if blast count > 100,000, or for symptoms of hyperviscosity
- Combination chemotherapy
- Bone marrow transplant

Treatment scheme:
- Induction chemotherapy — designed to take a patient to aplasia with recovery of "normal" hematopoiesis and a remission state
- Consolidation chemotherapy — designed to reinforce the remission obtained; Usually multiple cycles given

Acute Promyelocytic Leukemia (APL)
- Treatment for this subtype is different
  - Based on the translocation of the retinoic acid receptor
  - Uses all-trans retinoic acid (ATRA) as a maturational agent
  - Avoids development or worsening of DIC
  - May also include chemotherapy with an anthracycline or arsenic trioxide (ATO)

- With standard chemotherapy
  - Remission rate is > 70%
  - Long-term, disease-free survival is 20–25%
- "Good" risk cytogenetic groups do better, with survivals up to 60%
- Bone marrow transplant is best curative option

Acute Lymphocytic Leukemia (ALL)
- Primarily occurs in children
- Lymphadenopathy and splenomegaly occur in 50%
- An anterior mediastinal mass is common with the T-cell subtypes
- CNS disease is common

- Classification made using stains, flow cytometry, and cytogenetics
- WHO Classification based solely on B- or T-cell lineage

Prognostic factors:
- Age — the young fare better (< 30)
- Blast count — > 30,000 do poorly
- Cytogenetics — hyperdiploidy is a good finding, whereas a Philadelphia chromosome t(9;22) is a poor prognostic finding

Treatment consists of:
- Supportive care with transfusions
- Leukapheresis is not usually necessary because the blasts are smaller and less likely to cause sludging
- Combination chemotherapy

Treatment scheme:
- Induction chemotherapy using multi-drug regimens
- Consolidation chemotherapy with multi-drug regimens for multiple cycles
- Maintenance
- CNS prophylaxis
- Total treatment time of 2–3 years

- The majority of children completing therapy will obtain a cure
- Adults have only a 30–40% long-term survival with standard therapy
- For relapsed and poor prognosis patients, bone marrow transplant offers long-term disease control

AR 14A

An 80-year-old woman is seen for her yearly checkup. She feels well. A screening CBC is done, and she has the following values:

Hgb 7   WBC 55,000   Lymphs 98%
Hct 20   Plts 40,000

Her physical exam is remarkable for 2-cm lymphadenopathy in the cervical chain and splenomegaly.

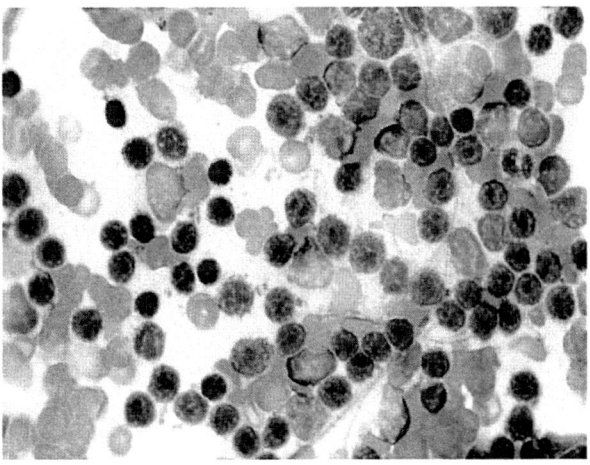

Which of the following is the most likely diagnosis?
A. Chronic myeloid leukemia
B. Chronic lymphocytic leukemia
C. Hairy cell leukemia
D. Prolymphocytic leukemia

Answer: _____

Chronic Lymphocytic Leukemia (CLL)

AR 14B
Which of the following statements is true?
A. She has Stage IV disease.
B. She should be observed rather than treated at this stage.
C. Her life expectancy from this leukemia is less than 6 months.
D. This is a leukemoid reaction.

Answer: _____

Chronic Leukemias
- Usually present with an elevated WBC count
- The cells here are **mature**
- Varying degrees of anemia and thrombocytopenia

- Workup initially involves review of the peripheral smear
- A bone marrow aspirate and biopsy
- Flow cytometry on peripheral blood
- Cytogenetics on bone marrow

Chronic Lymphocytic Leukemia (CLL)
- The most common leukemia in western countries
- Typically a disease of older individuals
- Commonly is asymptomatic at presentation with lymphocytosis found incidentally
- Lymphadenopathy and splenomegaly are common physical findings

- May present with infectious complications
  - Hypogammaglobulinemia
- May have autoimmune hemolytic anemia
- May have autoimmune thrombocytopenia

Workup includes:
- Flow cytometry, which is usually diagnostic
  - B-cell disorder with an abnormal pattern
  - CD19, CD20 (dim), CD23 positive
  - CD5 positive
  - Light chain restricted
  - Absolute clonal count > 5,000

Rai staging system		Survival
0	Lymphocytosis	> 10 yrs
I	Lymphadenopathy	9 yrs
II	Splenomegaly	6–7 yrs
III	Anemia	1–2 yrs
IV	Thrombocytopenia	1–2 yrs

Treatment options include:
- Observation — many patients have no indication for therapy at the time of presentation
- Indications for treatment include:
  - Symptomatic disease
  - Rapid doubling of the WBC count
  - Anemia
  - Thrombocytopenia

- Chlorambucil
- Fludarabine or combinations
- Rituximab/ofatumumab ± bendamustine
- Alemtuzumab
- Newer drugs: Ibrutinib, idelalisib, obinutuzumab

Commonly associated with second malignancies
- Lung cancer
- Head and neck cancer

Transformation of disease occurs and is known as Richter syndrome.
- Heralded by rapidly growing nodes or extranodal disease
- Upgrade to a more aggressive lymphoma such as diffuse large cell lymphoma

Hairy Cell Leukemia (HCL)

- Rare
- B-cell in phenotype
- Increased risk for infections
- Affects males over females 4:1
- Older patients affected

Usual presentation is:
- Pancytopenia
- Marked splenomegaly
- Inaspirable bone marrow

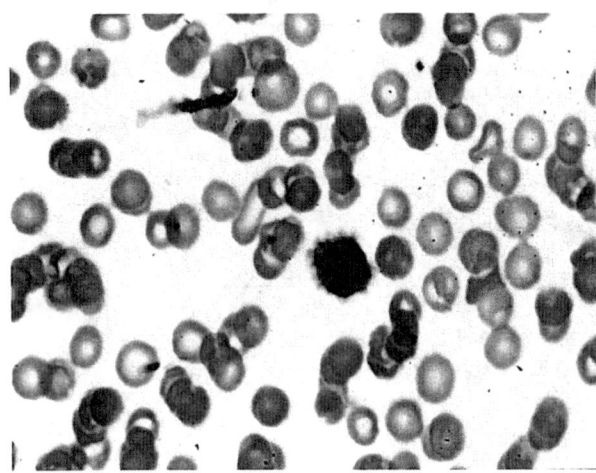

HCL (cont.)

Diagnosis hinges upon:
- Flow cytometry findings
  - CD19, CD20 positive
  - CD5 negative
  - CD11c, CD103 positive

Other diagnostic findings include:
- Bone marrow with hypercellularity and increased reticulin fibrosis "dry tap"
- TRAP stain positivity
  - Tartrate-resistant acid phosphatase stain

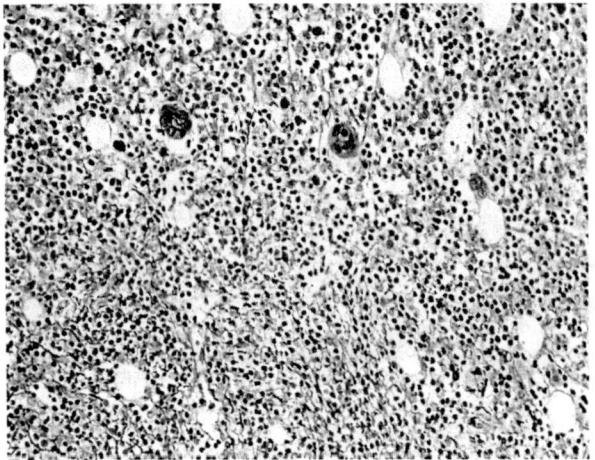

HCL (cont.)

- Usually follows an indolent course
- Indications for treatment include:
  - Symptomatic disease
  - Infectious complications
  - Anemia
  - Thrombocytopenia

- Treatment options include:
  - Splenectomy
  - 2-CDA (cladribine)
  - Other purine analogues (e.g., pentostatin)
- Results in prolonged disease-free survivals and possibly cures

AR 15A

A 24-year-old woman presents with painless lymphadenopathy that measures up to 3 cm in her cervical chain. She is asymptomatic and has not had any recent URI symptoms.
Physical exam is pertinent for the lymph nodes mentioned, as well as several small inguinal nodes measuring 2–3 cm.
She has an FNA of an inguinal node that is nondiagnostic.

The next step should be:

A. CT scan of chest, abdomen, and pelvis
B. Observation
C. Fine needle aspiration of the cervical nodes
D. Excisional biopsy of a cervical node

Answer: _____

Lymphoma

- Present with painless lymphadenopathy
- May have associated symptoms such as:
  - Fever
  - Night sweats
  - Weight loss
  - Pruritus

- Diagnosis is made by biopsy of an involved lymph node or mass
- Flow cytometry is helpful for diagnosis
  - Specific markers for subtypes of lymphoma
  - Clonality
  - Lineage (B vs. T)

AR 15B

Her pathology returns diffuse large cell lymphoma.
After discussion of the diagnosis with her, the next most appropriate step in her management would be:

The next most appropriate step in her management would be:
A. Referral to general surgery for debulking of all disease.
B. Check a GHS and begin chemotherapy with ABVD.
C. Check a B2MG, LDH, and ESR.
D. CT scans of chest, abdomen, and pelvis.

Answer: _____

Lymphoma (cont.)
- Staging involves CT chest, abdomen, and pelvis
- Bone marrow aspirate and biopsy
- PET scan
- LDH

AR 15C

Her CT scan returns with a mediastinal mass that measures 8 cm, as well as many nodes in her abdomen, the largest of which is 3 cm.
She has a bone marrow that is negative for disease.

What is the stage of her disease?
A. IIA
B. IB
C. IIBX
D. IIIA
E. IVAX

Answer: _____

Lymphoma (cont.)

Ann Arbor Staging System

Stage I	1 node or group
Stage II	2 or more lymph node groups, same side of the diaphragm
Stage III	Spans the diaphragm
Stage IV	Disseminated disease

- Subscripts with the staging system include
  - A: Means symptoms are absent
  - B: Means "B" symptoms present
  - X: Denotes bulky disease, defined as any mass that is > 10 cm or a mass > 1/3 the diameter of the chest
  - E: Extranodal disease

Hodgkin Lymphoma (HL)
- Bimodal age distribution
- Often see the "B" symptoms
  - Fever
  - Night sweats
  - Weight loss
- Pruritus is common
- Unusual complaint of pain with alcohol ingestion

- Diagnosis made by finding Reed-Sternberg cells
- WHO defines classical Hodgkin and nodular lymphocyte predominant Hodgkin lymphoma (NLPHL)

Treatment involves either:
- Combination chemotherapy
  - ABVD
- Radiation therapy
- Combined modality therapy with both

Prognosis is most closely linked to **stage** of disease
- Stage IA with survival rate of > 90%
- Stage IV with survival rate of > 60%

Long-term complications after treatment for Hodgkin lymphoma are common and include:
- Hypothyroidism
- Infertility
- Secondary malignancy, including
  - MDS/AML
  - Solid tumors such as breast and lung
  - Must screen early

Non-Hodgkin Lymphoma (NHL)
- Most are B-cell in origin
- Incidence is increasing in western countries
- Many associated with immunodeficiency states
- Currently classified by the WHO Classification scheme

Low-grade
- Indolent course
- Older patients
- Fewer "B" symptoms
- Higher stage at presentation

- Predominantly follicular lymphomas
- Sensitive to chemotherapy but not curable
- Long median survival: 7–10 years
- May transform to more aggressive disease

Intermediate/High-grade
- Aggressive histology
- Younger patients
- DLBCL predominates
- Includes lymphoblastic lymphoma (LBL) and Burkitt's

NHL (cont.)

Intermediate/High-grade
- Most are B-cell in origin
- Treat with curative intent
- Median survival is 1–2 years

NHL — Specific Types

Lymphoblastic Lymphoma = ALL
- Typically young adults and children
- Frequently a mediastinal mass at presentation
- Often Stage IV at presentation
- CNS involvement is common

Burkitt Lymphoma = L3 ALL

Endemic	Epidemic
African variety	U.S.
Jaw mass	Abdominal mass
EBV+++	EBV±

Burkitt Lymphoma
- Very rapid growth pattern/aggressive
- Looks like "starry sky" under low power
- Associated with a t(8;14)
  - Involves *C-MYC* proto-oncogene
  - Moves to immunoglobulin gene loci
- Involves CNS and marrow frequently

AR 16

Your patient has an intermediate-grade NHL, specifically DLBCL, that is Stage IIIA. She asks your advice concerning treatment options.

You should tell her:
A. She does not yet need treatment.
B. She should not agree to treatment because there is none with proven efficacy.
C. She should receive radiation therapy to her mediastinal mass followed by rituximab.
D. Multi-agent chemotherapy will offer her a chance for cure.

Answer: _____

NHL (cont.)

Treatment strategies:
- Low-grade lesions
  - "Watch and wait" with treatment reserved for symptomatic disease
  - Treat until symptoms resolve, then observation again
  - Treatment should be more aggressive if younger patient

Treatment strategies:
- Intermediate and high-grade lesions
  - Treat at time of diagnosis
  - Use combination chemotherapy ± radiation therapy
  - Standard of care is CHOP plus monoclonal antibody therapy with rituximab

AR 17

A 72-year-old man is seen for routine checkup. He has no complaints, and his physical exam is benign. Screening lab is as follows:

Hgb 12.0	T prot 10
Hct 37	Alb 2.0
WBC 3,300	AST 67
Plts 460,000	ALT 80

Initial workup should include which of the following?
A. Liver biopsy
B. Bone marrow aspirate and biopsy
C. SPEP/UPEP
D. β_2-microglobulin

Answer: _____

Serum Protein Electrophoresis and Urine Protein Electrophoresis

Multiple Myeloma (MM)
- Should be considered in older patients with unexplained anemia and CKD
- Should be considered in older patients with unexplained back pain
- May present with recurrent infections or hypercalcemia

Clues include:
- Rouleaux on peripheral smear
- An elevated globulin fraction (TP-Alb)
- A low anion gap

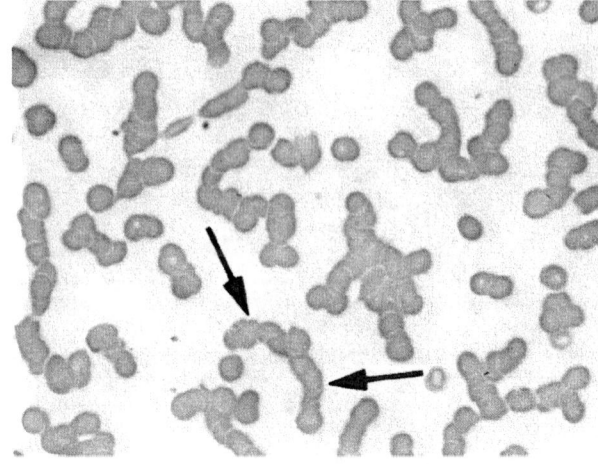

MM (cont.)
- 95% will have an abnormal protein on SPEP or UPEP
- The M spike is most commonly IgG followed by IgA, light chain disease, and IgD
- < 5% will be nonsecretory with no evidence of protein secretion

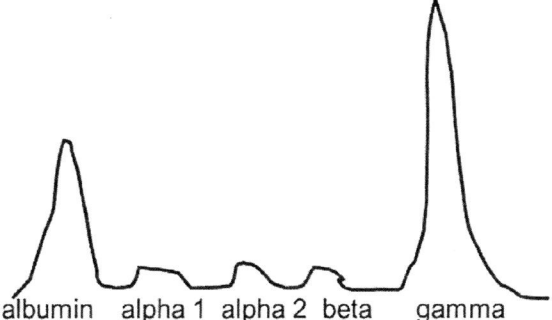

albumin   alpha 1   alpha 2   beta   gamma

Diagnosis
- MGUS
  - < 10% marrow PC and < 3-g M spike
  - No end-organ damage
- Smoldering MM
  - > 10% marrow PC or > 3-g M spike
  - No end-organ damage
- Active MM
  - > 10% marrow PC with an M spike and end-organ involvement
    - Calcium, anemia, renal dysfunction, bone disease

MM (cont.)
- Durie-Salmon staging system provides an assessment of tumor mass using:
  - Hgb
  - Calcium
  - # of lytic lesions
  - Protein levels
- ISS staging uses B2MG and albumin

- Remember that the bone lesions seen with myeloma are purely lytic lesions
- They should be assessed with metastatic bone survey, not bone scan

Treatment options include:
- Observation until clear progression of disease or the patient becomes symptomatic
- Melphalan and prednisone
- Combined chemotherapy regimens
- Thalidomide/lenalidomide/pomalidomide
- Bortezomib/carfilzomib
- Many others
- Bone marrow transplant

MGUS — Monoclonal Gammopathy of Undetermined Significance
No therapy is indicated, but these patients should be followed at least yearly for progression of their disease.

Waldenström Macroglobulinemia (WM)
- Increased IgM levels
- More common in older men
- More consistent with a lymphoma with lymphadenopathy and organomegaly

- Presentation is usually with:
  - Lymphadenopathy/Organomegaly
  - Purpura
  - Neuropathy
  - Hyperviscosity syndrome

Hematology "Pearls"

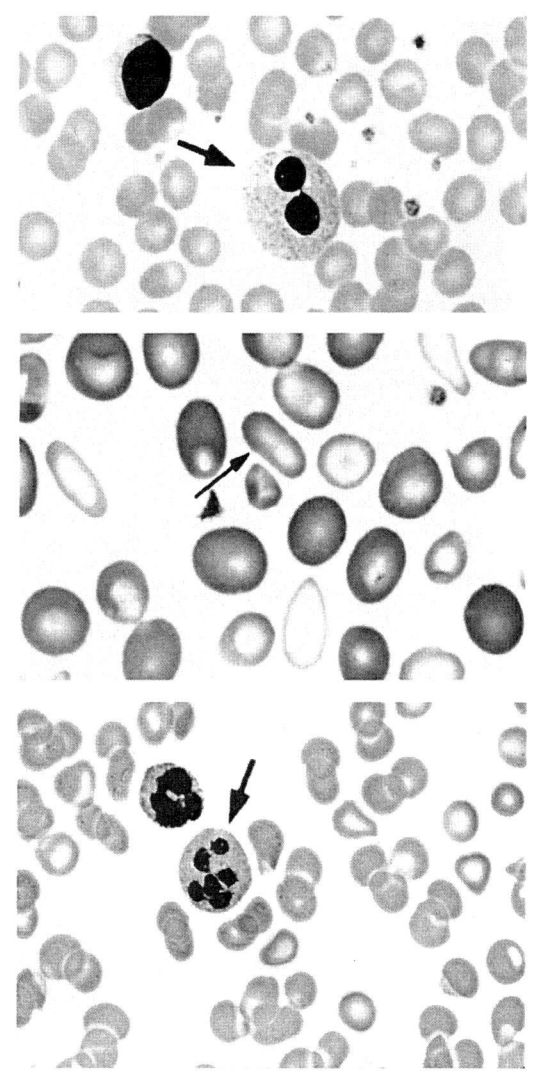

Hematology "Pearls" (cont.)

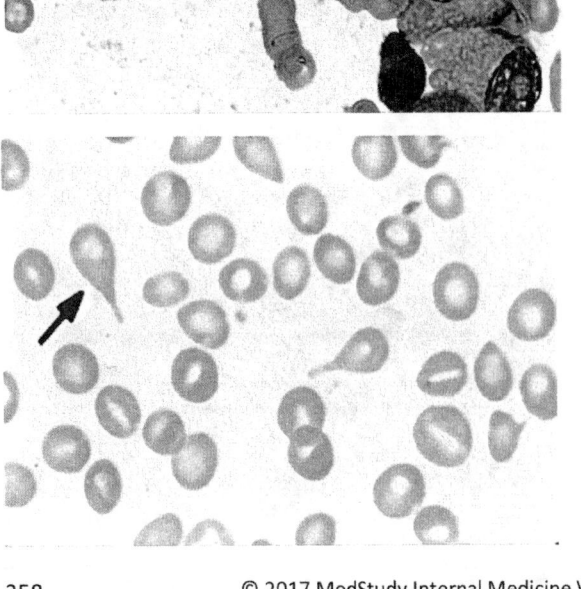

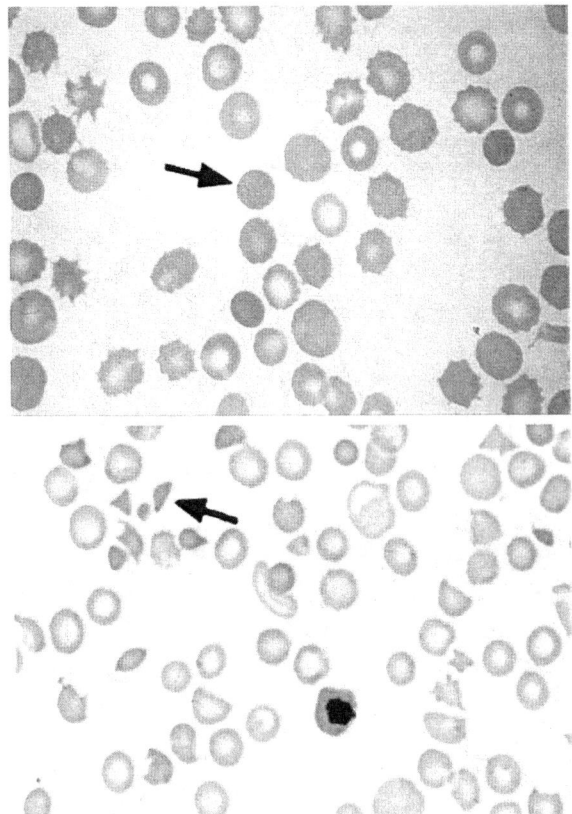

RBC "Clues"
- Cigar/Pencil shapes
- Macroovalocytes
- Spherocytes
- Schistocytes

- Bite cells
- Burr cells
- Target cells
- Teardrop cells

WBC "Clues"
- Smudge cells
- Basophilia/Eosinophilia
- Hairlike projections
- Hypersegmentation

- Döhle bodies
- Pelger-Huët cells
- Auer rods

Hematologic Malignancies
- Clues on peripheral smear:
  - Blasts = Acute leukemia
  - Auer rods = Myeloid blasts (AML)
  - Mature cells = Chronic leukemia
  - Mature lymphocytes = CLL
  - Maturing myeloid cells = CML

Hematology
Audience Response Answers

Audience Response 1A
Answer: D. Ferritin and soluble transferrin receptor.

AR 1B
Answer: A. Iron deficiency anemia.

AR 2
Answer: B. Anemia of inflammation.

AR 3
Answer: A. Pernicious anemia.

AR 4
Answer: D. RBC exchange transfusion.

AR 5
Answer: C. Autoimmune hemolytic anemia.

AR 6
Answer: C. Transferrin saturation.

AR 7
Answer: C. Myelodysplasia.

AR 8A
Answer: D. Review peripheral smear.

AR 8B
Answer: A. Chronic myeloid leukemia.

AR 9A
Answer: B. Essential thrombocytosis.

AR 9B
Answer: D. Observation.

AR 10
Answer: D. ITP.

AR 11
Answer: B. Change anticoagulation to argatroban.

You should stop LMWH and substitute a direct
thrombin inhibitor, such as argatroban or bivalirudin.

AR 12A
Answer: D. vWD.

AR 12B
Answer: B. von Willebrand factor Ag and activity.

AR 13
Answer: A. Acute myeloid leukemia.

AR 14A
Answer: B. Chronic lymphocytic leukemia.

AR 14B
Answer: A. She has Stage IV disease.

AR 15A
Answer: D. Excisional biopsy of a
cervical node.

AR 15B
Answer: D. CT scans of chest, abdomen, and pelvis.

AR 15C
Answer: D. IIIA.

AR 16
Answer: D. Multi-agent chemotherapy will offer her
a chance for cure.

AR 17
Answer: C. SPEP/UPEP.

MedStudy

Internal Medicine Video Board Review

Infectious Disease

Presented by

Fred A. Zar, MD
Professor of Clinical Medicine
Program Director, Internal Medicine Residency
University of Illinois at Chicago
Chicago, Illinois

Table of Contents

Infectious Disease Abbreviations

AACEK	*Aggregatibacter aphrophilus, Aggregatibacter actinomycetemcomitans, Cardiobacterium hominis, Eikenella* spp, and *Kingella kingae* (previously HACEK)
AFB	Acid-fast bacilli
AKI	Acute kidney injury
ASO	Antistreptolysin O
AVB	Atrioventricular block
BAL	Bronchoalveolar lavage
CDI	*Clostridium difficile* infection
CLABSI	Central line-associated blood stream infection
CMI	Cell-mediated immunity
CMV	Cytomegalovirus
CPK	Creatine phosphokinase
CRP	C-reactive protein
CSF	Cerebrospinal fluid
CSPN	Cephalosporin
DOE	Dyspnea on exertion
DTRs	Deep tendon reflexes
EBV	Epstein-Barr virus
ELISA	Enzyme-linked immunosorbent assay test
EM	Erythema multiforme
EOM	Extraocular movement
ESR	Erythrocyte sedimentation rate
FC	Flucytosine
FTA-ABS	Fluorescent treponemal antibody absorption test
GABHS	Group A beta-hemolytic streptococci
GC	Gonococcal
GNB	Gram-negative bacilli
GPC	Gram-positive cocci
HCAP	Health-care–associated pneumonia
HEENT	Head, eyes, ears, nose, throat
HIV	Human immunodeficiency virus
HSV	Herpes simplex virus
HUS	Hemolytic uremic syndrome
IBD	Inflammatory bowel disease
IFA	Immunofluorescence assay
IGRA	Interferon gamma release assay
IUD	Intrauterine device
IVDU	IV drug use
JC virus	John Cunningham polyomavirus
KOH	Potassium hydroxide
MAC	*Mycobacterium avium* complex
MRSA	Methicillin-resistant *Staphylococcus aureus*
MSM	Men who have sex with men
MSSA	Methicillin-sensitive *Staphylococcus aureus*

NAAT	Nucleic acid amplification testing
NHL	Non-Hodgkin lymphoma
NRTI	Nucleoside reverse transcriptase inhibitor
NNRTI	Nonnucleoside reverse transcriptase inhibitor
NSAID	Nonsteroidal antiinflammatory drug
NVD	Nausea, vomiting, diarrhea
OP	Opening pressure
PA	Polyarthritis
PJP	*Pneumocystis jiroveci* pneumonia (formerly PCP)
PCR	Polymerase chain reaction
PI	Protease inhibitor
PICC	Peripherally inserted central catheter
PID	Pelvic inflammatory disease
PMI	Point of maximal impulse
PPD	Purified protein derivative
PRBC	Packed red blood cell
RA	Rheumatoid arthritis
RMSF	Rocky Mountain spotted fever
RPR	Rapid plasma reagin
RSV	Respiratory syncytial virus
RUL	Right upper lobe
SEM	Systolic ejection murmur
SLE	Systemic lupus erythematosus
STI	Sexually transmitted infection
TB	Tuberculosis
TCAs	Tricyclic antidepressants
TEE	Transesophageal echocardiogram
TIG	Tetanus immunoglobulin
TMs	Tympanic membranes
TOA	Tubo-ovarian abscess
TPN	Total parenteral nutrition
TST	Tuberculin skin test
TTE	Transthoracic echocardiogram
UTI	Urinary tract infection
VDRL	Venereal disease research laboratory test
VRE	Vancomycin-resistant enterococci
VZV	Varicella-zoster virus

Speaker Disclosure
Fred A. Zar, MD, has documented that he has no commercial relationships to disclose.

**INFECTIOUS DISEASE
PART 1**

Audience Response 1 — History and Physical
Hx: A 17-year-old woman comes to ED with severe left biceps pain of 1-day duration. She is recovering from chickenpox and recalls a very itchy lesion in that area that she has been scratching for 2 days.
PE: T 101.8° F (38.7° C), BP 70/40, PR 110, RR 20
Many healing varicella lesions
L bicep tender, warm 6 cm x 8 cm swelling with woody induration

AR 1 — Labs, Imaging, Initial Rx
Hb 11.0 g/dL, WBC 21.0 x 10^3/mm^3 12% bands, Platelet 75,000/mm^3
Creat 2.0 mg/dL, AST 95 U/L, ALT 100 U/L
MRI: "Edema of soft tissues above the L biceps muscle belly with early fascial necrosis"
She receives a dose of vancomycin and piperacillin/tazobactam and goes to the OR for surgical debridement; Gram stain of surgical fluid reveals gram (+) cocci chains

Which of the following would you do now?
A. Continue vancomycin alone.
B. Continue piperacillin/tazobactam alone.
C. Continue vancomycin and piperacillin/tazobactam.
D. Switch to penicillin.
E. Switch to penicillin and clindamycin.

Answer: _____

Rapidly Progressive Cellulitis
- Group A strep
  - Lymphatic disease
    - Vein donor leg
    - Mastectomy
- Pasteurella multocida
  - Animal bites (dogs, cats)
- *Clostridium perfringens*
  - Contaminated trauma
- *Vibrio vulnificus*
  - Salt water and cirrhosis
- Necrotizing fasciitis

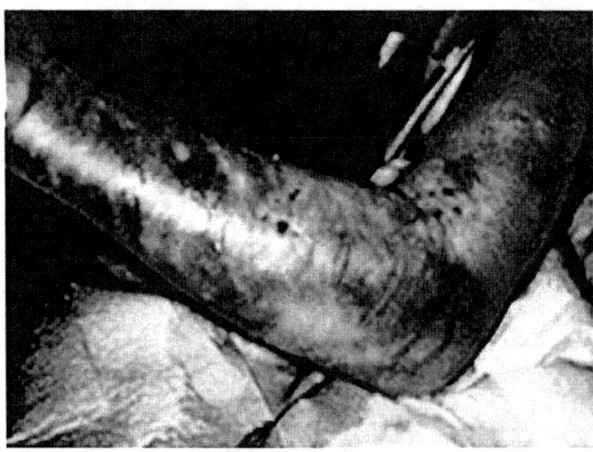

Group A strep necrotizing fasciitis

Necrotizing Fasciitis — Suggestive Findings
- Skin necrosis and blebs
- Disproportionate pain
- Late anesthesia
- Disproportionate systemic toxicity
- Crepitus or gas on x-ray
- Probe passing easily through fascia

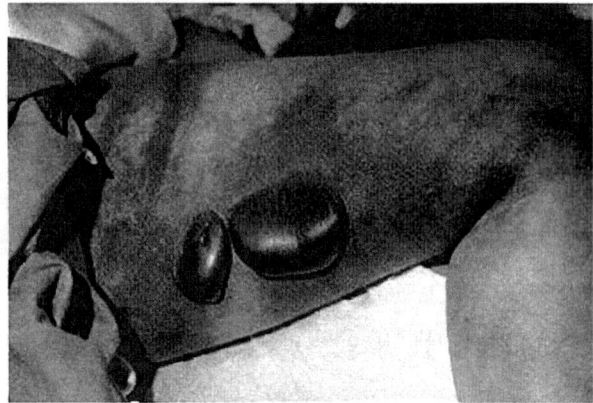

Necrotizing Fasciitis — Microbiology
- Type I (mixed aerobic/anaerobic)
  - At least 1 anaerobe
    - Usually *Bacteroides* or peptostreptococci
  - At least 1 aerobe (not group A strep)
    - Usually enteric GNB
- Type II (group A strep)
  - Group A strep ± *S. aureus*
- Type III (*Clostridium perfringens*)
- Other monomicrobial
  - *V. vulnificus*, group B strep, *S. aureus*, *Clostridia*
- Treatment
  - Surgery and antibiotics

Toxic Shock Syndrome
- <u>Presenting triad</u>
  - Fever, shock (or orthostatic hypotension), rash (late desquamation)
- <u>Involvement of > 3 organ systems</u>
  - GI (NVD), muscle (myalgia or CPK), AKI, transaminase/bili, thrombocytopenia, altered consciousness
- <u>Sources</u>
  - Strep: Soft tissue infection (BC usually positive)
  - Staph: Surgical wounds, foreign bodies, pneumonia
- <u>Treatment</u>
  - Site control + organism-specific antibiotics + clindamycin

AR 1 – Key Points
- Recognize rapidly progressive cellulitis
- Recognize necrotizing fasciitis
- Recognize toxic shock syndrome
- Know the treatment for toxic shock syndrome

AR 2 — History and Physical
Hx: A 68-year-old man with Type 2 diabetes presents with a draining foot ulcer at the base of his right big toe for 1 week. He denies fever. He takes his metformin regularly.
PE: T 100.2° F (37.9° C), BP, PR, RR are normal
Right foot circumferential distal redness and a purulent 4 x 5-cm ulcer that probes to bone

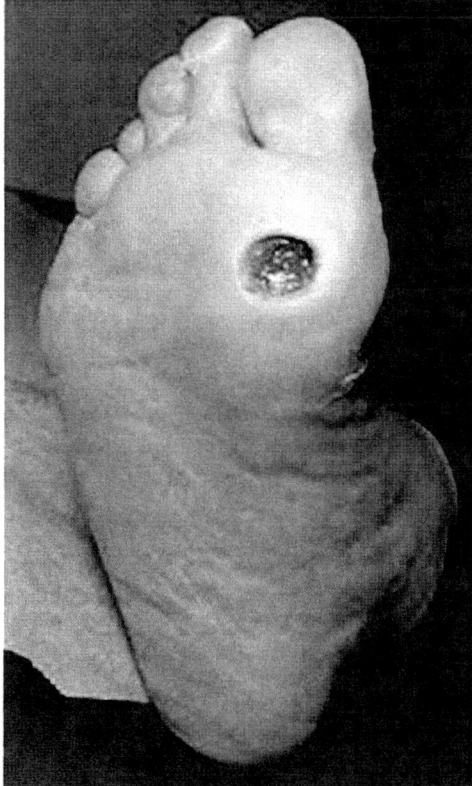

AR 2 — Labs and Imaging
Hb 12.5 g/dL, WBC 9,700/mm^3, Pl 245,000/mm^3
Plain radiograph: Ulceration of the plantar aspect of the head of the right 1st metatarsal with mild soft tissue swelling; No gas in tissue; Bony structures appear normal without evidence of osteomyelitis

Which of the following would you do now?
A. Radionuclide bone scan.
B. MRI of right foot.
C. Start vancomycin and piperacillin/tazobactam.
D. Culture the drainage prior to antibiotics.
E. Obtain a bone biopsy for culture prior to antibiotics.

Answer: _____

Concordance of Bone and Swab Cultures in DM Foot Osteo
- <u>The study</u>
  - 76 patients with 81 episodes
  - All had bone biopsy for culture
- <u>The results</u>

Organism	Concordance of both cultures
S. aureus	**21/49 (42.8%)**
GNB	12/42 (28.5%)
<u>Streptococci</u>	<u>8/31 (25.8%)</u>
Total	43/191 (22.5%)

Sonneville E. *Clin Infect Dis*. 2006;42:57–62.

Meta-Analysis of Dx Tests for DM Osteomyelitis — 9 Studies; 1,054 patients

Diagnostic Test	Sens (95% CI)	Spec (95% CI)
Probe-to-bone	0.60 (0.46–0.73)	**0.91 (0.86–0.94)**
MRI	**0.90 (0.82–0.95)**	0.79 (0.62–0.91)
Leukocyte scan	0.74 (0.67–0.80)	0.68 (0.57–0.78)
Radiography	**0.54 (0.44–0.63)**	0.68 (0.53–0.80)
Bone scan	0.81 (0.73–0.87)	**0.28 (0.17–0.42)**

Dinh MT. *Clin Infect Dis*. 2008;47:519–527.

AR 2 — Key Points
- Know the operating characteristics of various tests for diabetic foot osteomyelitis
- Recognize the nonspecific nature of drainage cultures
- Recognize the need for bone cultures for definitive treatment of diabetic foot osteomyelitis

AR 3 — History and Physical
Hx: A 53-year-old woman presents to the ED with a 2-day history of watery diarrhea 10–12 times a day. Three weeks ago, she had a UTI treated with a 7-day course of levofloxacin. She is able to take fluids and her hydrochlorothiazide for blood pressure control.

PE: T 101.5° F (38.6° C), BP 126/80, PR 100, RR 16
Abdomen has minimal bowel sounds and diffuse tenderness

AR 3 — Labs and Imaging
Hb 13.5 g/dL, WBC 19,700/mm^3, Pl 245,000/mm^3
Creatinine is 1.8 mg/dL (baseline 1.0)
Abdominal CT: No free air; Slight diffuse thickening of the colonic wall; No evidence of bowel obstruction

After obtaining a test for *C. difficile*, what would you do next?
A. Await result prior to treatment.
B. Start metronidazole PO.
C. Start vancomycin PO.
D. Start vancomycin PO and metronidazole PO.
E. Start vancomycin PO and metronidazole IV.

Answer: _____

Response to CDI Treatment When Stratified by Disease Severity

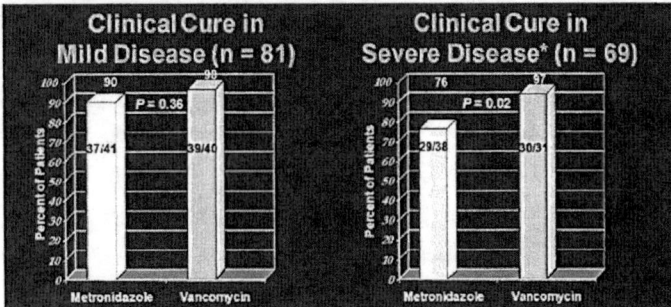

*Severe disease defined as intensive care unit admission;
Pseudomembranous colitis on endoscopy;
Or at least 2 of the following:
1) Age > 60 years,
2) Temperature > 101° F,
3) Albumin level < 2.5 mg/dL,
4) White blood cell count (WBC) > 15,000 cells/mm^3
Zar FA. *Clin Infect Dis*. 2007;45:302–307.

IDSA Severity of Disease Classification
- Mild-to-moderate
  - WBC < 15,000/mm^3 **and** creatinine increase < 50%
- **Severe**
  - **WBC > 15,000/mm^3 or creatinine increase > 50%**

- Severely complicated
  - Any of:
    - Ileus
    - Megacolon
    - Hypotension
    - Shock
Cohen SH. *Infect Control Hosp Epidemiol*. 2010;31:431–455.

Empiric Therapy of Initial Episode of CDI
- Mild or moderate disease
  - Metronidazole 500 mg PO q 8 h x 10–14 d
- **Severe disease**
  - **Vancomycin 125 mg PO q 6 h x 10–14 d**
- Severe complicated disease
  - Vancomycin 500 mg PO qid per NG tube, and/or metronidazole 750 mg IV q 8 h
  - If ileus, give vancomycin retention enema instead of PO (500 mg in 500 cc NS q 6 h)
European Society of Clinical Microbiology and Infectious Diseases Guidelines. *Clin Micro Infect*. 2009;15:1067–1079.
Infectious Diseases Society of America Guidelines. *Infect Control Hosp Epidemiol*. 2010;31:431–455.
Australasian Society for Infectious Diseases. *Med Jour Australia*. 2011;194:353–358.

AR 3 — Key Points
- Recognize the typical clinical setting in which *C. difficile* infection occurs
- Know how to assess the severity of *C. difficile* infection
- Know how to treat *C. difficile* diarrhea based on severity

AR 4 — History and Physical
Hx: A 29-year-old man is hospitalized with worsening neurologic symptoms over 8 weeks; symptoms include confusion, dysarthria, and left hemiparesis poor vision.
He was diagnosed with HIV infection 8 years ago and has been noncompliant with therapy.
Last CD4 count was 82, two years ago.
PE: VS are normal; 18/30 on Mini-Mental State Exam;
VA 20/200 OU, fundoscopy normal; left hemiparesis and hemianopia

AR 4 — Labs, Imaging, Initial Rx
Hb 9.2 g/dL, WBC 1.5/mm^3, 12% lymphs
Pl 130,000/mm^3

MRI

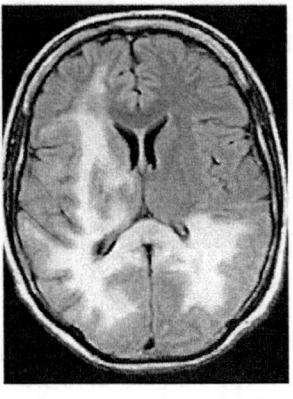

© 2017 MedStudy Internal Medicine Video Board Review – Infectious Disease • Fred A. Zar, MD

Which of the following is most likely?
A. Progressive multifocal leukoencephalopathy
B. Primary CNS lymphoma
C. Toxoplasmosis
D. Cytomegalovirus encephalitis
E. Herpes simplex encephalitis

Answer: _____

Progressive Multifocal Leukoencephalopathy
- Pathogenesis
  - JC polyomavirus, > 85% adults infected
  - Dormant in kidney and lymphoid tissue
  - Immunosuppression → lytic infection of oligodendroglia → demyelination
- Clinical manifestations
  - Subacute motor and visual changes
- Diagnosis
  - Images: Multifocal demyelination, not fitting a vascular territory, no mass effect or enhancement
  - CSF: JC virus PCR (+)
- Treatment
  - Decrease immunosuppression

AR 4 — Key Points
- Recognize the various CNS presentations of opportunistic infections and malignancies after HIV infection
- Know the treatments for CNS opportunistic infections after HIV infection

AR 5A — History and Physical
Hx: A 50-year-old man with acute myelogenous leukemia presents with fever and chills after completing his 3rd round of induction chemotherapy 7 days ago.
PE: T 104.0° F (40.0° C), PR 128, RR 24, BP 136/82
PICC line in left arm without redness, tenderness, or drainage
Rest of exam normal

AR 5A — Labs and Imaging
Hb 9.6 g/dL, WBC 1,200/mm^3 w/ 20% neutrophils, 5% bands
Platelets 115,000/mm^3
CXR normal

Blood and urine cultures are sent. Next step?
A. Await cultures to direct antibiotic therapy.
B. Start cefepime.
C. Start cefepime and vancomycin.
D. Start cefepime and piperacillin/tazobactam.
E. Start cefepime and gentamicin.

Answer: _____

Febrile Neutropenia
- Definitions
  - Fever: T > 101.0° F (38.3° C) x 1 or 100.4° F (38.0° C) > 1 h
  - Neutropenia: ANC at or expected to be < 500/mm^3
- Empiric treatment
  - Monotherapy
    - Piperacillin/tazobactam, imipenem/meropenem, cefepime
  - Add vancomycin only if:
    - Severe sepsis
    - Blood culture with gram (+) cocci
    - Pneumonia
    - Suspected line sepsis
    - MRSA colonization
    - Soft tissue infection
    - Mucositis

Freifeld, et al. Clinical practice guideline for the use of antimicrobial agents in neutropenic patients with cancer: 2010 update by the Infectious Diseases Society of America. *Clin Infect Dis.* 2011;52(4):e56–e93.

AR 5B
Antibiotics are started and his fever resolves over the next 48 hours. Blood and urine cultures are negative. Six days later, fever recurs along with shortness of breath.

AR 5B — Repeat Testing
Hb 8.9 g/dL, WBC 1,400/mm^3 w/ 25% neutrophils, no bands
Platelets 100,000/mm^3
Chest x-ray and CT are obtained (below)

AR 5B — Images

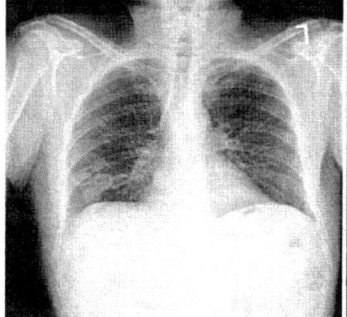
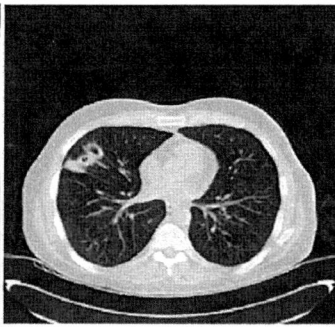

AR 5B — Bronchoalveolar Lavage

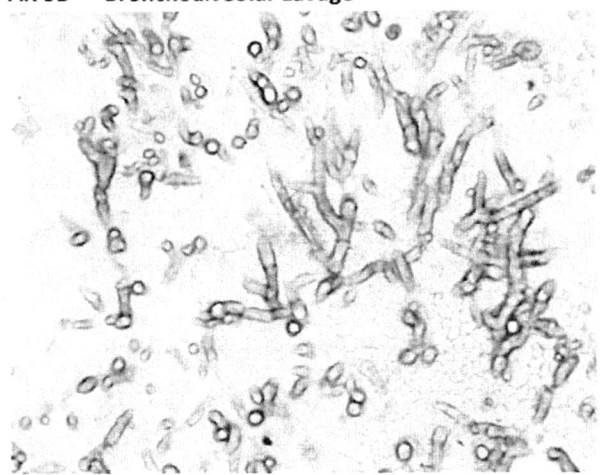

AR 5B

What would you do now?
A. Start IV fluconazole.
B. Start IV voriconazole.
C. Start IV lipid amphotericin B.
D. Start IV lipid amphotericin B and 5-flucytosine.

Answer: _____

Voriconazole vs. Ampho B for Invasive Aspergillosis

- <u>The study</u>
  - Randomized nonblinded trial, 277 pts
- <u>The results</u>

	Voriconazole $N = 144$	Ampho B $N = 133$	P
Response @ 12 wks	53%	32%	< 0.05
Complete	21%	16%	
Partial	32%	15%	
Survival @ 12 wks	71%	58%	< 0.05

Herbrecht R. *NEJM*. 2002;347:408–415.

Chronic Pulmonary Aspergillosis (> 3 months)

Disease	Description	Immune	Diagnosis	Treatment
Aspergilloma	Fungus ball	Competent	Culture, IgG Ab	Surgery if Sx; Vori if can't
Chronic cavitary	Multicavity	Competent	Culture, IgG Ab	Voriconazole
Chronic fibrosing	Fibrosis of above	Competent	Culture, IgG Ab	Voriconazole
Chronic necrotizing	Subacute invasive	Compromised	Culture, IgG Ab Galactomannan	Voriconazole

Chronic Pulmonary Aspergillosis

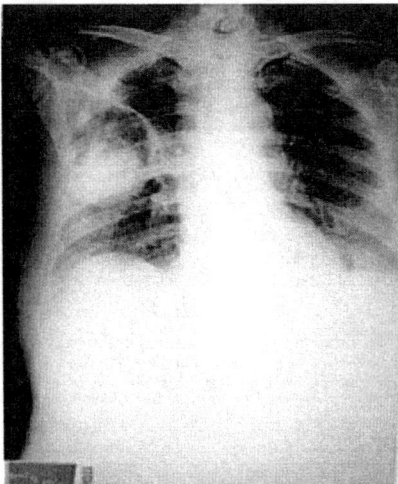

Aspergilloma

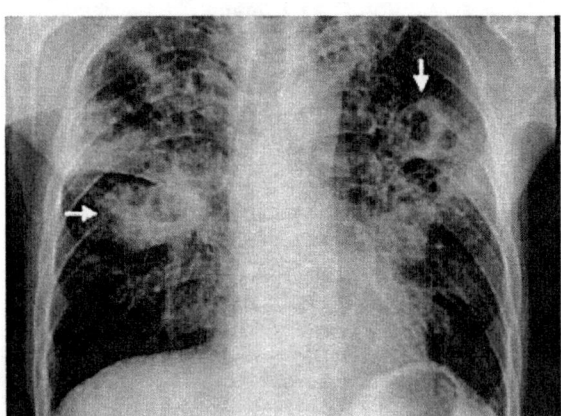

Cavitary

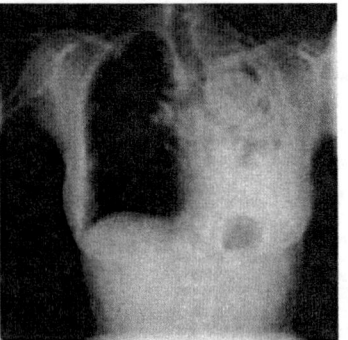

Fibrosing

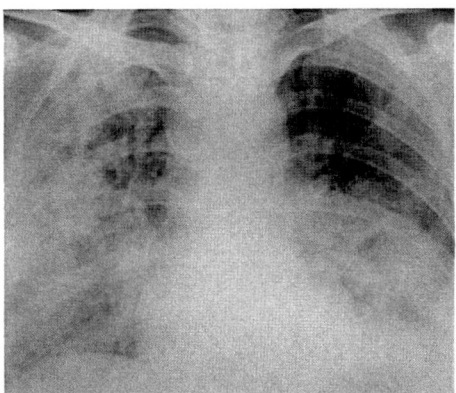

Necrotizing

AR 5 — Key Points
- Recognize febrile neutropenia
- Know which immediate antibacterial therapy is indicated
- Know the indications for empiric vancomycin
- Know how to recognize, diagnose, and treat invasive aspergillosis as a complication of prolonged neutropenia
- Know the forms of chronic pulmonary aspergillosis and how to treat them

AR 6 — History and Physical
Hx: A 25-year-old man is brought to the ED in July with acute onset of fever and hemoptysis. He is otherwise healthy. He works as an accountant and was at a pro basketball game last night with 12 coworkers. Eight of them have the same symptoms.
PE: T 102.4° F (39.5° C), BP 86/58, PR 128, RR 34
He is delirious and oriented only to person; Lungs have diffuse crackles without signs of consolidation

AR 6 — Labs
Hb 15.6 g/dL
WBC 31,000/mm^3 w/ 75% neutrophils, 10% bands, 3% metamyelocytes
Platelets 550,000/mm^3

AR 6 — Chest X-Ray

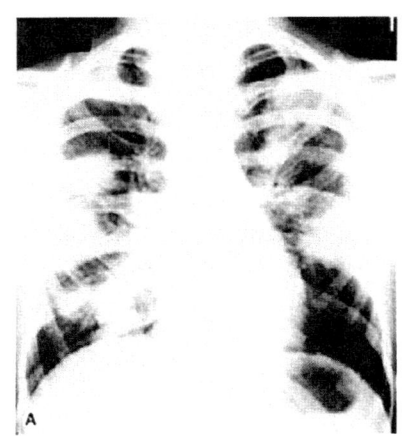

AR 6 — Peripheral Smear

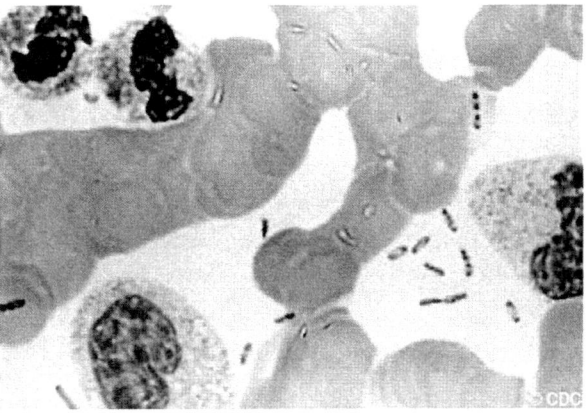

AR 6
What antibiotic(s) would you administer?
A. Ciprofloxacin
B. Penicillin
C. Ampicillin
D. Streptomycin
E. Piperacillin/tazobactam

Answer: _____

Differentiating Bioterrorist Bacteria

	Plague	Anthrax	Tularemia
Organism	Yersinia pestis	Bacillus anthracis	Francisella tularensis
Gram stain	GNCB	GPB	GNB
Incubation	Hours–2 d	1–7 d	3–5 d
Presentation	Hemoptysis	Flu → pneumonia	Fever + cough Nonproductive
Chest x-ray	Infiltrates	Hilar LN + Mediastinitis	Hilar LN + Infiltrates
Treatment	Streptomycin	Ciprofloxacin	Streptomycin
Contagious?	Yes	No	No

Anthrax
- Epidemiology
  - Spores in soil → animal acquisition
  - Human acquisition from animal contact
- Clinical types
  - Cutaneous (95%): Painless ulcer w/ eschar
  - GI/Pharyngeal: Ulcers with eschar
  - Inhalation: Wool sorters, bioterrorism
- Diagnosis
  - Culture
- Treatment
  - Fluoroquinolone

Anthrax (cont.)

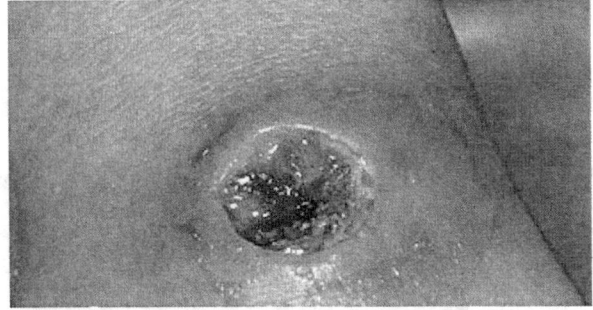

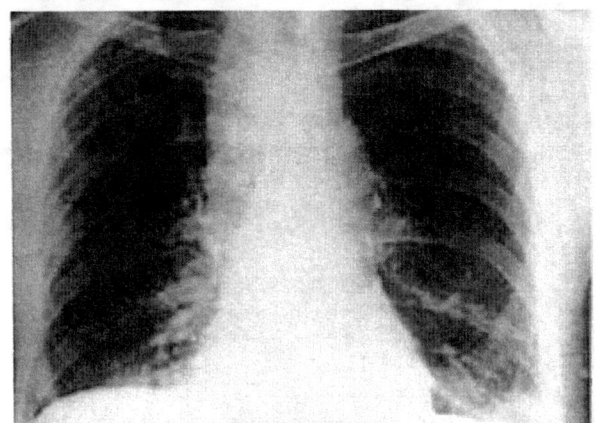

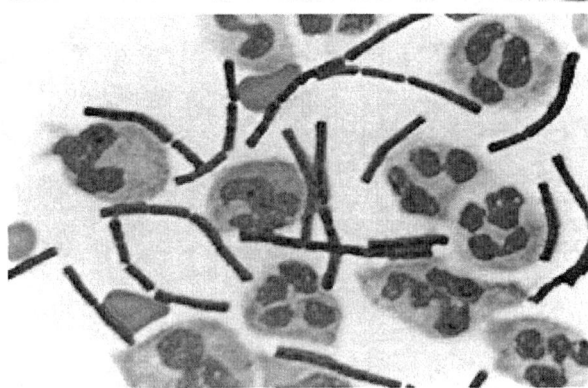

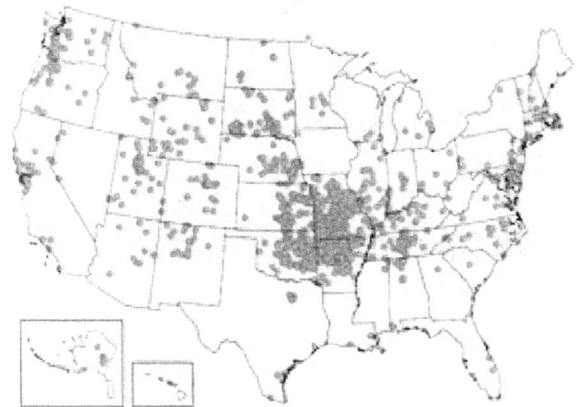

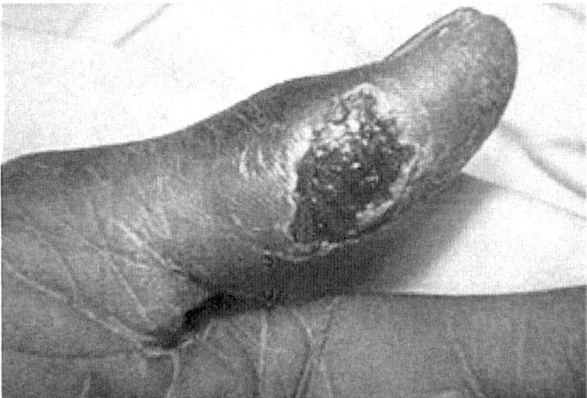

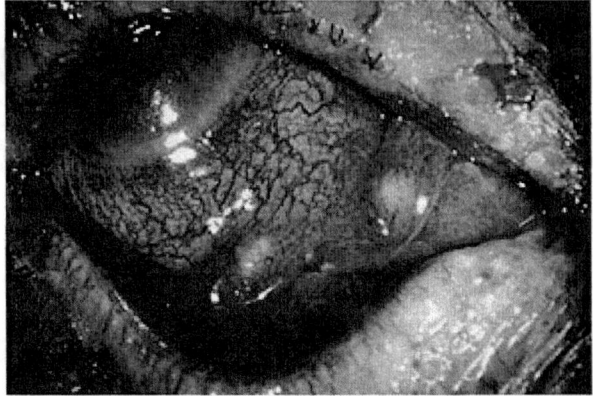

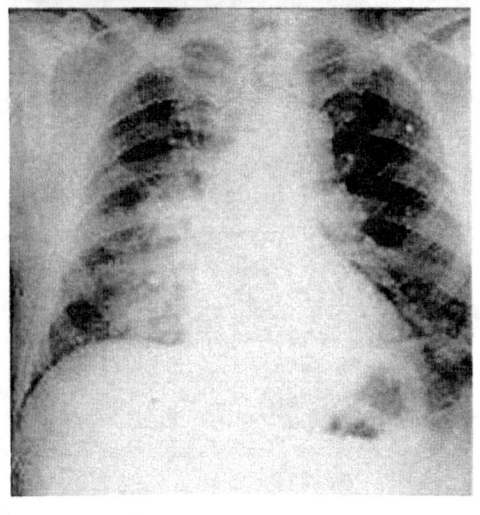

Tularemia
- <u>Epidemiology</u>
  - Large animal reservoir
  - Acquired by: Ticks, flies, direct contact
  - Inoculated, inhaled, ingestion
- <u>Clinical types</u>
  - Inoculation (most common)
    - Ulceroglandular, glandular, oculoglandular
  - Ingestion: Oropharyngeal
  - Inhalation: Pneumonic
  - No clear entry: Typhoidal
- <u>Diagnosis</u>
  - Culture (low yield), serology high titer/4-fold rise
- <u>Treatment</u>
  - Streptomycin (mild disease = Doxy, quin)

Indications for Streptomycin
- Drug of choice
  - Plague
  - Tularemia
- Second line
  - Tuberculosis
- Replaced by gentamicin
  - Endocarditis (viridans and GDE)
  - *Brucella*

AR 6 — Key Points
- Recognize a scenario suspicious for a bioterrorist attack
- Know 3 bioterrorism organisms that would present as clustered pneumonias
- Understand the different clinical manifestations of these agents
- Know the empiric treatment of these agents
- Know the few indications for streptomycin

AR 7A — History and Physical
Hx: A 58-year-old man presents to you in August with a 2-day history of fevers with myalgias and a mild headache. He is a New York City native and returned 6 days ago from a 2-week vacation in Cape Cod, MA. He has rheumatoid arthritis (RA) controlled by etanercept.
PE: T 101.8° F (38.8° C), PR 100, RR 20, BP 138/88
Jaundice
Heart and lungs are normal
Mild hepatosplenomegaly
Chronic changes of RA, no acute inflammation

AR 7A — Labs and Imaging
Hb 9.4 g/dL
WBC 9,200/mm^3 w/ 78% neutrophils, 2% bands, 11% lymphs
Platelets 85,000/mm^3
Haptoglobin < 20 mg/dL, LDH 800 U/L
Reticulocyte count 6.8%
AST 145 U/L, ALT 166 U/L
T bili 3.8 mg/dL, direct bili 0.8 mg/dL
CXR normal

AR 7A
What diagnostic test would you want next?
A. *Borrelia burgdorferi* serology
B. *Babesia microti* serology
C. *Anaplasma phagocytophilum* serology
D. *Ehrlichia chaffeensis* serology
E. Peripheral smear of blood

Answer: _____

AR 7B — Peripheral Smear

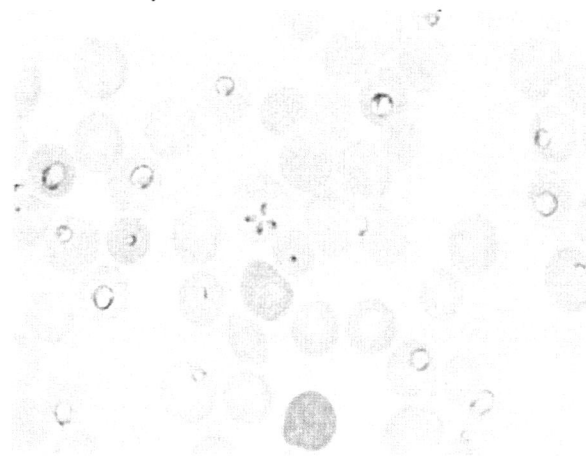

AR 7B
What antibiotics, if any, do you want to give?
A. Doxycycline
B. Amoxicillin/clavulanate
C. Chloroquine
D. Azithromycin and atovaquone
E. None

Answer: _____

Geography of Babesiosis

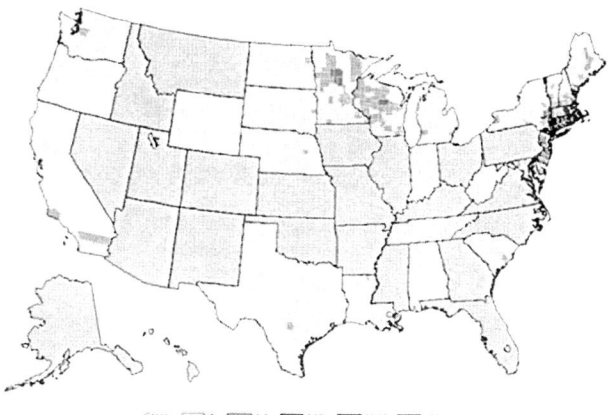

Source: Centers for Disease Control and Prevention. Number of reported cases of babesiosis, by county of residence* — 27 states,† 2013
N = 1,750; county of residence was unknown for 12 of the 1,762 patients. Cases are mapped to the patients' county of residence, which is not necessarily where they became infected.

AR 7C
He improves over the next 3 days, but then fevers — now with chills — recur, and he has a severe headache.
PE: T 104.0° F (40.0° C), PR 130, RR 20, BP 140/80
Jaundice is gone
Hepatosplenomegaly unchanged
Joint exam unchanged

AR 7C — Repeat Labs

Hb 10.4 g/dL
WBC 3,200/mm^3 w/ 40% neutrophils, 20% bands,
25% lymphocytes
Platelets 100,000/mm^3
Haptoglobin normal
Transaminases and bilirubin normal

What diagnostic test would you want next?

A. *Borrelia burgdorferi* serology
B. *Babesia microti* serology
C. *Anaplasma phagocytophilum* serology
D. *Ehrlichia chaffeensis* serology
E. Peripheral smear of blood

Answer: _____

AR 7D — Repeat Peripheral Smear

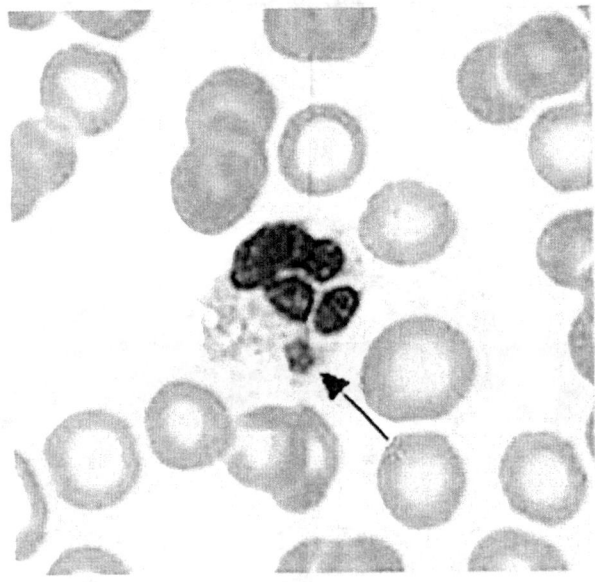

AR 7D

What antibiotics, if any, do you want to give?

A. Doxycycline
B. Amoxicillin/clavulanate
C. Chloroquine
D. Azithromycin and atovaquone
E. None

Answer: _____

Geography of Ehrlichiosis and Anaplasmosis

Ehrlichiosis Incidence, 2010

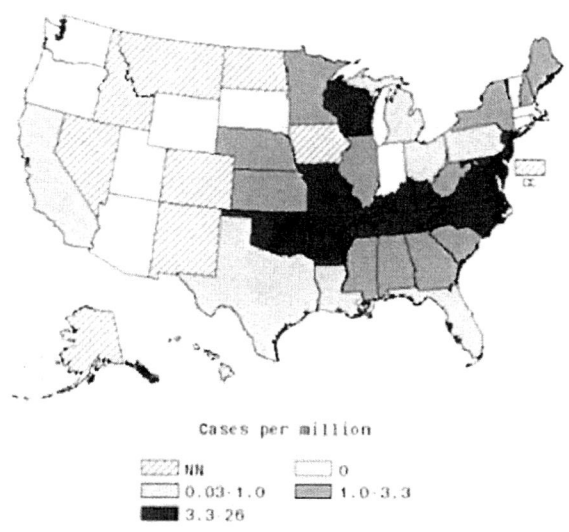

Cases per million

NN · 0 · 0.03-1.0 · 1.0-3.3 · 3.3-26

CDC 2011.

Anaplasmosis Incidence, 2010

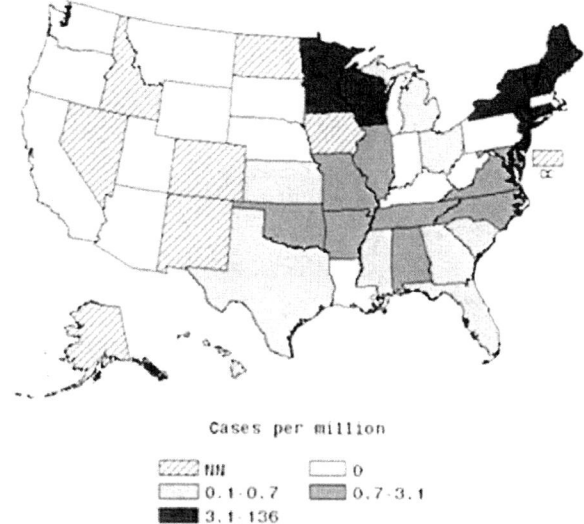

Cases per million

NN · 0 · 0.1-0.7 · 0.7-3.1 · 3.1-136

Tickborne Intracellular Organisms

	Babesiosis	Anaplasmosis	Ehrlichiosis
Tick	Ixodes scapularis	Ixodes scapularis	Amblyomma americanum
Organism	Babesia microti	Anaplasma phagocytophilum	Ehrlichia ewingii and chaffeensis
Incubation	1–6 weeks	1–2 weeks	1–2 weeks
Presentation	Fever, hemolysis	Flu-like with severe headache	Flu-like with severe headache
Rash	None	< 5%	~ 35%
CBC	Hemolytic anemia	Neutropenia	Lymphopenia ± pancytopenia
Diagnosis	Blood smear (PCR)	Blood smear PMN morulae	Blood smear Mono morulae
Treatment	Atovaquone + azithromycin	Doxycycline	Doxycycline

AR 7 — Key Points
- Diagnose and treat babesiosis in an immunocompromised host
- Recognize dual infection with tickborne illnesses
- Diagnose and treat anaplasmosis and ehrlichiosis

AR 8A — History and Physical
Hx: A 31-year-old man presents with a 4-day history of low-grade fever and nonproductive cough. He lives in Columbia, SC. He returned from a golf trip to Phoenix, AZ, 7 days ago.
He is otherwise healthy and continues to work as a bank teller.
PE: T 100.0° F (37.7° C), other VS normal
Lungs show bibasilar crackles

AR 8A — Labs and Imaging
Hb 14.6 g/dL
WBC 7,200/mm^3 with 54% neutrophils, 30% lymphocytes, no bands, 15% eosinophils

CXR:

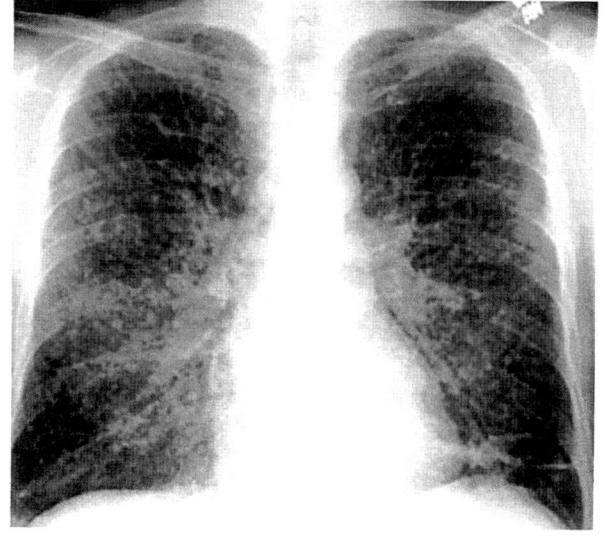

AR 8A
What causative organism do you suspect?
A. *Blastomyces dermatitidis*
B. *Histoplasma capsulatum*
C. *Coccidioides immitis*
D. *Cryptococcus neoformans*
E. *Aspergillus fumigatus*

Answer: _____

What antibiotic(s), if any, would you give?

A. Fluconazole

B. Itraconazole

C. Liposomal amphotericin B

D. None

Answer: _____

Areas Endemic for Coccidioidomycosis

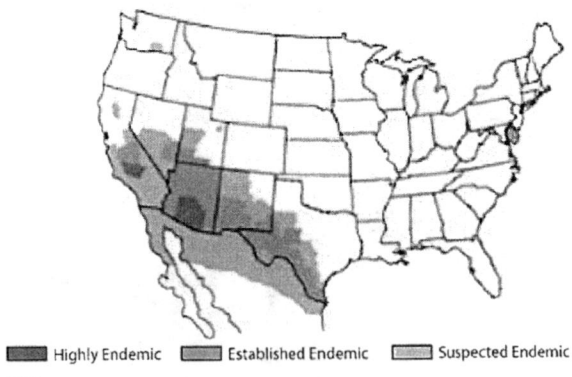

■ Highly Endemic   ■ Established Endemic   ■ Suspected Endemic

CDC

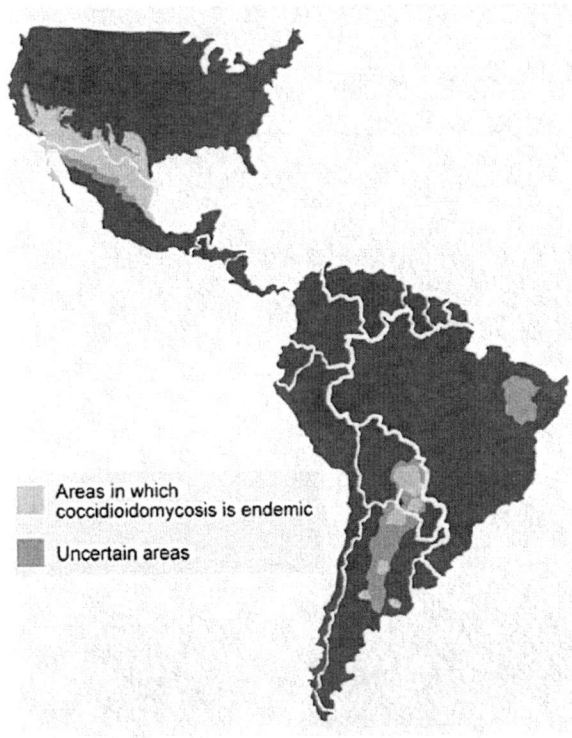

■ Areas in which coccidioidomycosis is endemic

■ Uncertain areas

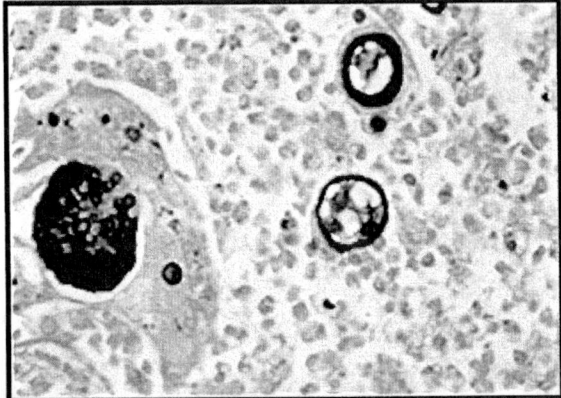

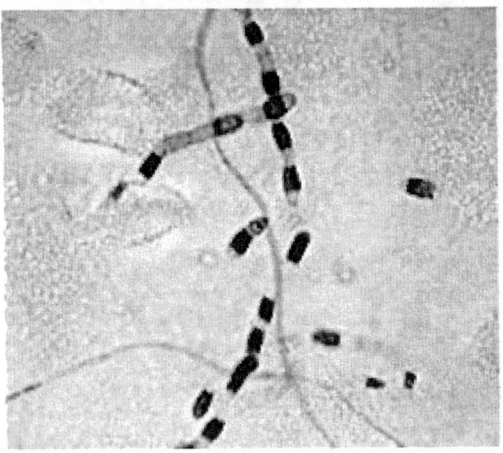

Coccidioidomycosis

- Epidemiology and pathogenesis
  - Southwestern U.S.
  - **Inhalation of arthroconidia (1)**
  - Worse in persons of color
  - Endospores → dissemination
- Microbiology
  - *Coccidioides immitis* and *C. posadasii*
- Clinical manifestations
  - Usually asymptomatic
  - **Valley fever** (fever, cough, flu-like, rash [EM], arthritis)
  - Acute/Chronic pneumonia ± cavitation
  - Skin, bone, joints, CNS
  - **Eosinophilia**

Blastomycosis

- Epidemiology and pathogenesis
  - **Ohio and Mississippi rivers**
  - Enters through lungs
- Microbiology
  - *Blastomyces dermatitidis*

- Clinical manifestations
  - **Acute, or chronic unresolving pneumonia**
  - **Fungating skin lesions**
  - Osteomyelitis
  - Brain abscess

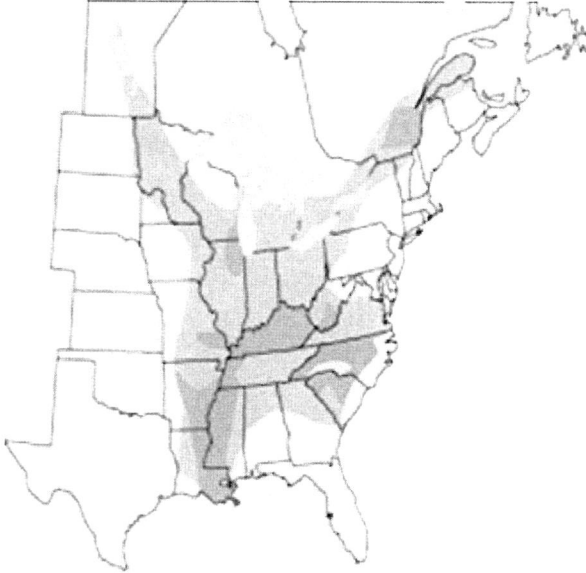

Gilchrist's 1st Case

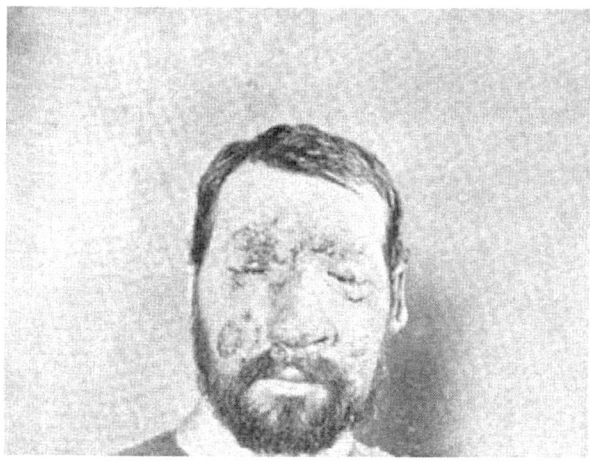

J. Hopkins Hosp Reports 1.269.1896.

Blastomycosis (cont.)
- Diagnosis
  - Tissue/Fluids: Broad-based bud
  - Culture
  - **Urinary antigen**
- Treatment[1]
  - Mild-to-moderate
    - **Itraconazole** x 6–12 mos
  - Severe
    - Ampho B x 1–2 wks or improvement, then itraconazole for total of 6–12 mos

[1]Chapman SW. *CID*. 2008;46:1801–1812.

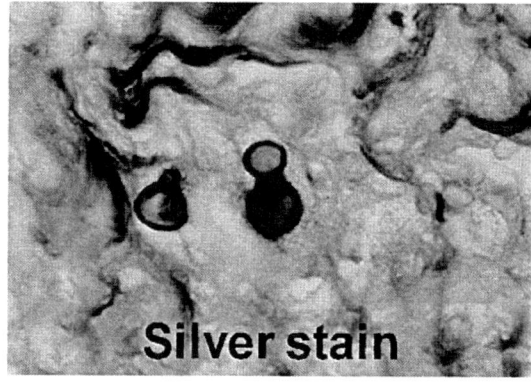
Silver stain

Histoplasmosis
- Epidemiology
  - **Ohio and Mississippi Rivers yet broader distribution**
- Microbiology
  - *Histoplasma capsulatum*
- Clinical manifestations
  - Usually none
  - **Acute/Chronic pneumonia ± cavitation**
  - **Mediastinitis**
  - Dissemination

Areas Endemic for Histoplasmosis

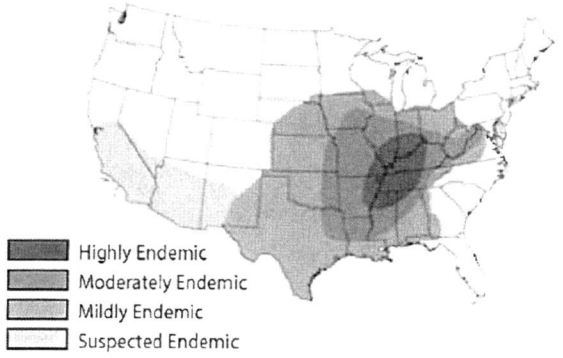

Highly Endemic
Moderately Endemic
Mildly Endemic
Suspected Endemic

Histoplasmosis (cont.)
- Diagnosis
  - Microscopic appearance
  - Culture
  - Serology
  - **Urinary Ag**

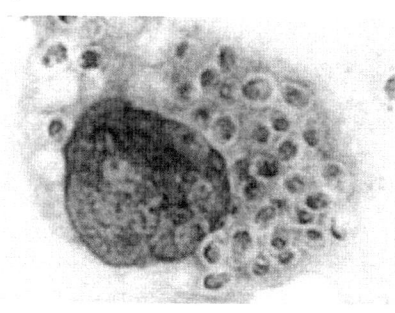

- Treatment
  - Chronic pneumonia of mild disseminated: **Itraconazole** x 12 mos
  - Severe pneumonia or disseminated: Ampho B x 1–2 wks → itracon to total 12 wks
  - CNS: Ampho B x 4–6 wks, then itracon x 12 mos

Antifungal Drugs of Choice
- Amphotericin B
  - Severe infection with endemic fungi, crypto, sporo, mucor
- Azoles
  - Fluconazole
    - Nonsevere *C. albicans*, *Cryptococcus*, *Coccidioides*
  - Itraconazole
    - Nonsevere endemic fungi, sporotrichosis
  - Posaconazole
    - Prophylaxis in high-risk pts (SCT, Prolonged Feb Neut)
  - Voriconazole
    - Invasive aspergillosis
  - Isavuconazole
    - Invasive aspergillosis, mucormycosis
- Echinocandins: Caspofungin (micafungin, anidulafungin)
  - Prolonged febrile neutropenia
  - Severe candidiasis
- 5-Flucytosine
  - Combo Rx of CNS crypto

Antifungal Therapy: 2017

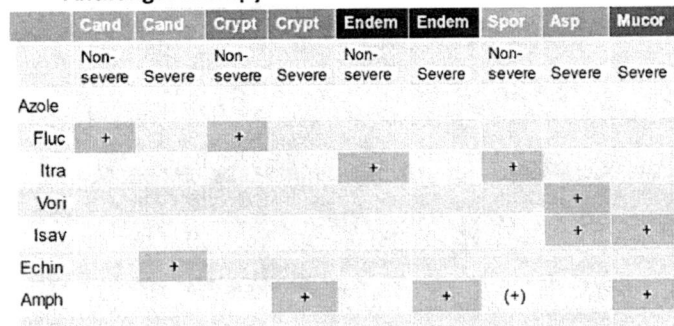

For CNS crypto, add 5-FC to amphotericin
For prolonged febrile neutropenia, add an echinocandin
For prophylaxis in stem cell transplant or anticipated
  prolonged feb neut, give posaconazole

AR 8 — Key Points
- Recognize the typical epidemiology and presentations of endemic fungi
- Know the methods of diagnosing these infections
- Understand the treatment of these infections based on severity and underlying host
- Know the antifungal drugs of choice

AR 9 — History and Physical
Hx: A 41-year-old woman presents to the ED after stepping on a nail that went through her work boot and 1 inch into her foot. She owns a farm in rural Indiana, and the nail was sticking out of a wooden board that had fallen off of her cow pasture fence.
She has had 4 prior tetanus toxoid immunizations, the last of which was 6 years ago.

AR 9
Which of the following should you give her?
A. Tetanus toxoid alone
B. Tetanus immunoglobulin
C. Tetanus toxoid and tetanus immunoglobulin
D. No tetanus prevention needed

Answer: _____

Tetanus — Wound Management

Past Toxoid	Clean and Minor	Tetanus Prone*
Unknown or < 3	Toxoid†	Toxoid† + TIG
≥ 3	Toxoid† if ≥ 10 yrs	Toxoid† if ≥ 5 yrs

*Crush, dirt/feces, puncture, missiles
† Toxoid + Pertussis (Tdap) once if ≥ 19 years old[1]
[1]CDC. *MMWR*. 2012;61(25):468.

AR 9 — Key Points
- Know how to characterize the risk of tetanus after a wound
- Know the indications for administering tetanus toxoid and tetanus immunoglobulin

---

AR 10A — History and Physical
An 18-year-old college freshman comes with her 2 roommates to campus health because of fever and a headache for 2 days. She is otherwise healthy.
PE: T 103.2° F (39.5° C), PR 128, RR 20, BP 96/66
Alert and oriented x 3
No papilledema
Presents with stiff neck
No rash
Neuro exam normal

Blood cultures are sent. In addition to a lumbar puncture what would you order next?
A. CT head
B. Procalcitonin level
C. Dexamethasone
D. Antibiotics

Answer: _____

Empiric Treatment of Bacterial Meningitis

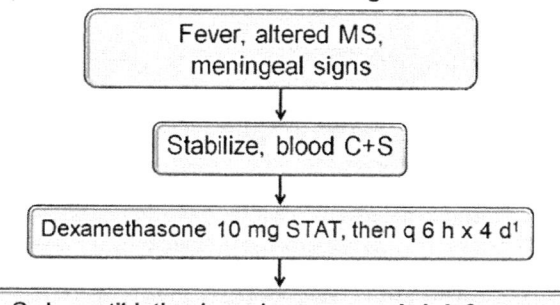

Fever, altered MS, meningeal signs

↓

Stabilize, blood C+S

↓

Dexamethasone 10 mg STAT, then q 6 h x 4 d[1]

↓

Order antibiotics based on **age and risk factors**

[1]de Gans J. *NEJM*. 2002;347:1549–1556.

AR 10B
What antibiotics would you give?
A. Ceftriaxone
B. Vancomycin and ceftriaxone
C. Vancomycin, ceftriaxone, and ampicillin
D. Vancomycin and ceftazidime

Answer: _____

Empiric Treatment of Bacterial Meningitis

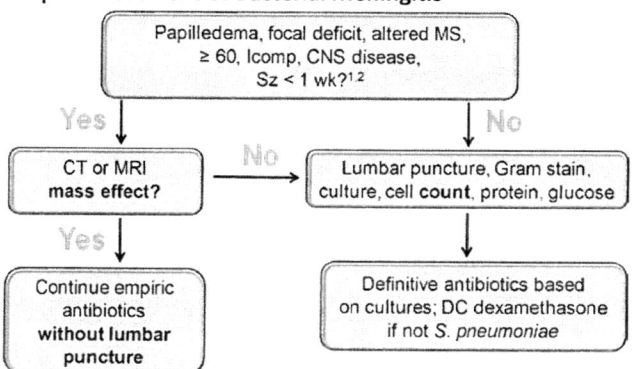

Papilledema, focal deficit, altered MS, ≥ 60, Icomp, CNS disease, Sz < 1 wk?[1,2]

Yes → CT or MRI **mass effect?** — No → Lumbar puncture, Gram stain, culture, cell **count**, protein, glucose

No → Lumbar puncture, Gram stain, culture, cell **count**, protein, glucose

Yes → Continue empiric antibiotics **without lumbar puncture**

Definitive antibiotics based on cultures; DC dexamethasone if not *S. pneumoniae*

[1]Gopal AJ. *Arch Intern Med*. 1999;159:2681–2685.
[2]Hasbun R. *NEJM*. 2001;345:1727.

Bacterial Meningitis, U.S. 2003–2007 (1,670 cases)

Age	S. pneumoniae	N. meningitidis	L. monocytogenes
18–34	50%	36%	2%
35–49	75%	8%	2%
50–64	78%	5%	6%
≥ 65	70%	5%	10%

Thigpen MC, et al. *NEJM*. 2011;364:2016–2025.

Empiric Therapy of Bacterial Meningitis — When the Gram Stain Doesn't Help

Patient	Likely Organisms	Antibiotics
18–50 yo	*S. pneumo, N. mening*	Ceftriaxone + vanc
> 50 yo	Above + *Listeria*	Above + ampicillin
Immunocompromised	*Listeria* + GNB	Amp + ceftazidime
Neurosurgery	*Staph* + GNB	Vanc + ceftazidime

Quigliarello VJ. *NEJM*. 336:708–16,1997.
Van de Beek D. *NEJM*. 354.44–53,2006.

AR 10C — CSF Findings
- Cloudy
- WBC 1,300/mm³: 94% neutrophils
- RBC 2/mm³
- Protein 145 mg/dL
- Glucose 44 mg/dL (serum 120)
- Gram stain (below)

AR 10C — CSF Gram Stain

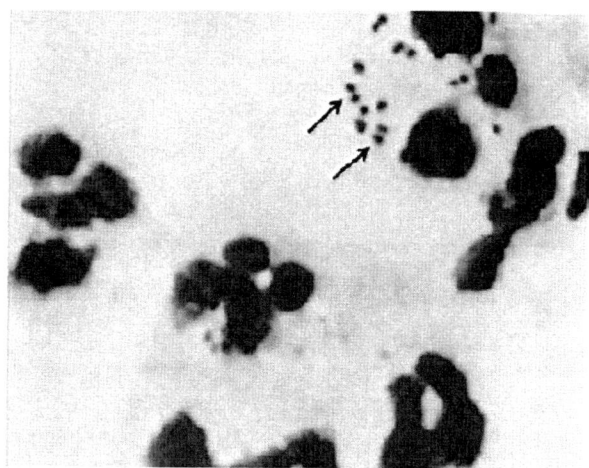

AR 10C
Which of the following is the best therapy pending susceptibilities?
A. Ceftriaxone alone
B. Ceftriaxone and dexamethasone
C. Vancomycin and ceftriaxone
D. Vancomycin, ceftriaxone, and dexamethasone

Answer: _____

AR 10D

Who should receive prophylaxis for exposure to her?

A. Her roommates

B. Her roommates and all health care workers

C. Her roommates, health care workers, and patients on her ward

D. No one

Answer: _____

Chemoprophylaxis for Meningococcal Meningitis
- Close contact definition
  - > 8 h within 3 feet, or
  - Direct contact with secretions
- Timing of significant exposure
  - 1 week prior to 1 day after presentation
- Drugs that are effective
  - Ciprofloxacin 500 mg PO x 1
  - Rifampin 600 mg PO bid x 2 days
  - Ceftriaxone 250 mg IM x 1
- Treat index case if not given ceftriaxone Rx

AR 10 — Key Points
- Recognize the importance of empiric dexamethasone in the treatment of bacterial meningitis
- Know when to do brain images prior to lumbar puncture in suspected bacterial meningitis
- Know the age-based empiric therapies for bacterial meningitis
- Know the definitive therapies for bacterial meningitis
- Know who should receive prophylaxis after exposure to meningococcal meningitis

AR 11 — History and Physical

Hx: A 67-year-old woman presents in July with a 2-day history of left lower extremity weakness and fever. She is retired and spends many of her days going for long walks around the pond behind her Dallas suburban home with many of her neighbors. None of them are ill.

PE: T 101.0° F (38.3° C), other VS normal

Alert and oriented x 3, lower extremity weakness

Decreased knee DTRs and absent ankle DTRs

Sensation intact

AR 11 — Labs and Imaging

CSF
- WBC 400/mm^3, 90% lymphocytes
- RBC 4/mm^3
- Glucose 89 mg/dL (serum 111)
- Protein 95 mg/dL

- MRI of lumbosacral spine normal

AR 11

Which of the following tests has the highest sensitivity in diagnosing her illness?

A. An IgM antibody assay

B. An IgG antibody assay

C. A viral PCR assay

D. A viral culture

Answer: _____

West Nile Virus — Neurologic Manifestations
- No symptoms in 80%
- Encephalitis
- Aseptic meningitis
- **Acute flaccid paralysis (~ polio)**
- Movement disorders
  - Tremors, myoclonus, parkinsonism
- Rhabdomyolysis
- Miscellaneous
  - Ataxia, cranial neuropathy, optic neuritis, polyradiculopathy

AR 11 — Key Points
- Know the epidemiology of West Nile Virus
- Recognize the neurologic manifestations of West Nile Virus
- Know the most sensitive test to diagnose symptomatic West Nile Virus infection

AR 12 — History and Physical

Hx: An 18-year-old woman is new to your practice, having just moved to town to attend college. She is complaining of left cheek and maxillary tooth pain for 3 days. She has a stuffed nose with purulent drainage. She says she gets "sinus infections" 2–3 times a year that always respond to antibiotics when given. She takes levothyroxine daily. She is allergic to trimethoprim/sulfamethoxazole and milk.

PE: T 99.5° F (37.5° C), other VS normal

Bilateral maxillary sinus tenderness and poor transillumination; Purulent nasal discharge seen

What further testing, if any, should you do?

A. CT or MRI of sinuses

B. CBC with differential

C. Immunoglobulin levels

D. Nitroblue tetrazolium reduction test

E. None

Answer: _____

 © 2017 MedStudy Internal Medicine Video Board Review – Infectious Disease • Fred A. Zar, MD

IgA Deficiency

- Presentations
  - **Recurrent sinusitis or pneumonia**
  - Recurrent giardiasis
  - **Food/respiratory allergies**
  - Autoimmune
    - Hashimoto's, celiac disease, PA, SLE, RA
  - False (+) **serum** pregnancy test
- Treatment
  - Usually none, except acute episodes
  - **Avoid** blood transfusions and IVIG
  - Acute episodes; IgA-poor IVIG

Common Variable Immunodeficiency

- Definition
  - New onset low IgG and IgA and/or IgM
  - Decreased response to immunizations
  - No known cause
- Manifestations (ages 1–5, 18–25)
  - **Sinopulmonary infection (encapsulated)**
  - Giardiasis
  - COPD and/or restrictive lung disease
  - IBD
  - NHL
  - Autoimmune
    - **Hashimoto's**, celiac disease, PA, SLE, RA
- Treatment
  - IVIG q 3–4 wks

Complement Deficiencies

- C2 > C4 > C1 (proximal pathway)
  - **Recurrent sinopulmonary, ear infections**
  - Encapsulated organisms
  - **SLE at early age**
- C5–C9 (terminal pathway)
  - Recurrent *Neisseria* infections
- Diagnosis
  - **CH50**, then specific components
- Treatment
  - Vaccinations (pneumococcal, meningococcal)
  - No other specific therapy

AR 12 — Key Points

- Recognize the need to pursue an etiology of recurrent sinopulmonary infections in young adults
- Know the common causes of recurrent sinopulmonary infections in young adults
- Know the diagnostic testing of each of these etiologies

AR 13 — History and Physical

Hx: A 58-year-old man with Type 2 diabetes comes to your office with tender swollen areas on the back of his neck that have been enlarging for the last 5 days.
He is allergic to trimethoprim/sulfamethoxazole.

PE: T 100.4° F (38.0° C), PR 98, RR 14
Labs: Blood glucose = 108

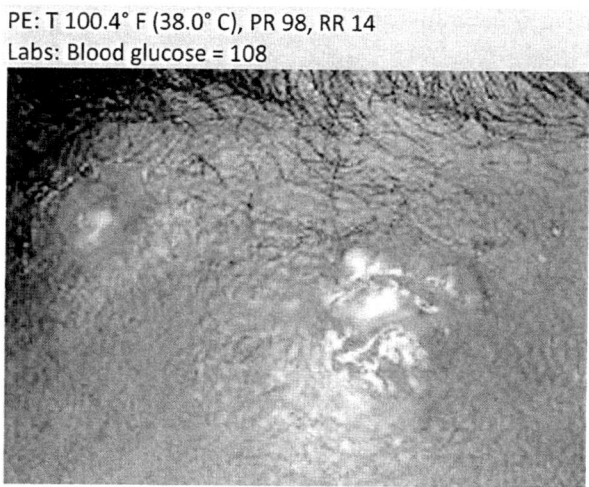

AR 13

After draining the lesions in your office, what would you prescribe next?
A. Cephalexin PO
B. Amoxicillin/clavulanate PO
C. Doxycycline PO
D. Vancomycin IV
E. Daptomycin IV

Answer: _____

The Anatomy of Soft Tissue Infections — "Cellulitis"

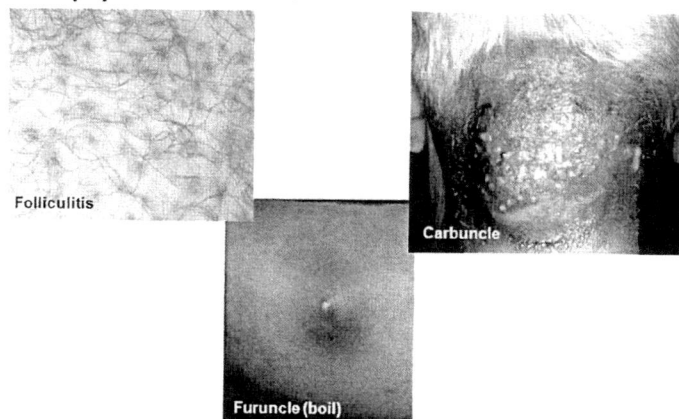

Staphylococcal Infections

Folliculitis

Carbuncle

Furuncle (boil)

Streptococcal Lymphangitis (Erysipelas)
- Face
- Arm, post-breast surgery
- Post-liposuction
- Leg, post-saphenous vein harvest

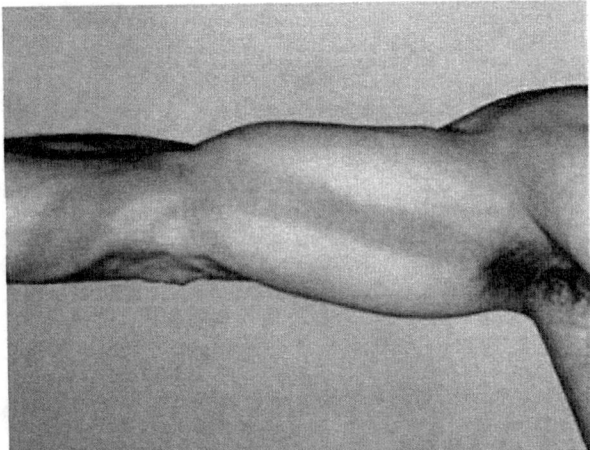

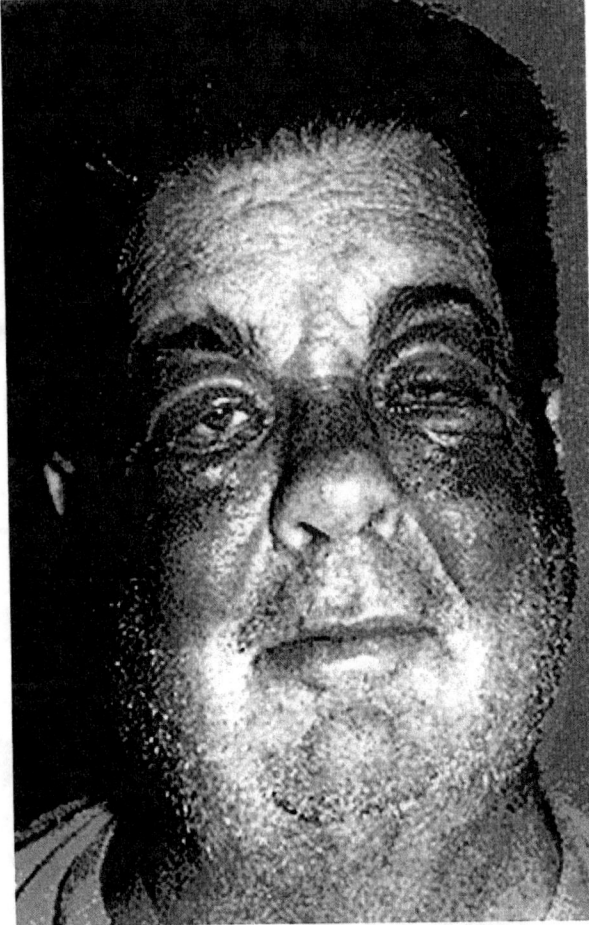

Classification of Skin and Soft Tissue Infections

Severity	Purulent	Nonpurulent
Mild	No systemic signs	No systemic signs
Moderate	Systemic signs	Systemic signs
Severe	Sepsis or failed Rx, immunocompromised	Sepsis or failed Rx, immunocompromised, bullae/slough, trauma

Stevens DL. *CID*. 59:147, 2014.

Treatment of Purulent Cellulitis
- <u>Mild disease</u>
  - Incision and drainage only
- <u>Moderate disease</u>
  - Incision and drainage
  - Culture
  - Empiric Rx
    - T/S or doxycycline
  - Definitive Rx
    - MRSA: PO T/S
    - MSSA: PO diclox or cephalexin
- <u>Severe disease</u>
  - Incision and drainage
  - Culture
  - Empiric Rx
    - Vanc, dapto, linezolid, telavancin, or ceftaroline
    - Clindamycin if resistance < 15%
  - Definitive Rx
    - MRSA: IV vancomycin
    - MSSA: IV nafcillin, cefazolin, clindamycin

Stevens DL. *CID*. 59:147, 2014.

T/S vs. Placebo for Skin Abscess
- <u>The study</u>
  - Uncomplicated abscess, I+D'd in ED
  - T/S vs. placebo for 7 d
  - Outcome assessed at 7–14 d
- <u>The results</u> (those who took ≥ 75% of doses)

	T/S	Placebo	P
N	524	533	
Cure	92.9%	85.7%	< 0.001
Repeat I+D	3.4%	8.6%	< 0.05
Infection in HHC	1.7%	4.1%	< 0.05

Talan DA. *N Engl J Med*. 2016;374:823-32.

Treatment of Nonpurulent Cellulitis
- <u>Mild disease</u>
  - PO: PCN, 1° CSPN, dicloxacillin, clindamycin
- <u>Moderate disease</u>
  - IV: Penicillin, cefazolin, ceftriaxone, clindamycin
- <u>Severe disease</u>
  - **Surgery** for C+S
  - Vancomycin + piperacillin/tazobactam

Stevens DL. *CID*. 59:147, 2014.

Newer Glycopeptides

Glycopeptide	T ½	Frequency	Indications
Telavancin (2013)	7–10 h	Daily	ABSSSI HCAP/VAP
Oritavancin (2014)	10 d	Weekly	ABSSSI
Dalbavancin (2014)	14 d	Biweekly	ABSSSI

ABSSSI = Acute bacterial skin and
  skin structure infection
HCAP = Health-care–associated pneumonia
VAP = Ventilator-associated pneumonia

AR 13 — Key Points
- Recognize a staphylococcal carbuncle by presentation and Gram stain
- Differentiate staphylococcal and streptococcal cellulitis
- Know that the majority of community-acquired *Staphylococcus aureus* are methicillin resistant
- Utilize inexpensive oral drugs to treat uncomplicated *S. aureus* skin infections regardless of methicillin sensitivity

---

AR 14A — History and Physical
Hx: A 32-year-old man comes to an urgent care center with a 2-day history of a sore throat. He denies cough, runny nose, or hoarseness. No one is sick at home. He works as a real estate agent.
PE: T 99.9° F (37.2° C)

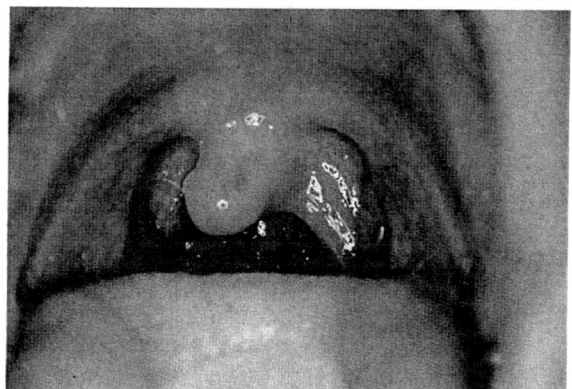

AR 14A
What would you do now?
A. Swab for rapid antigen testing for group A strep prior to treatment.
B. Swab for culture prior to treatment.
C. Swab for rapid antigen and start penicillin.
D. Swab for culture and start penicillin.
E. No testing, no penicillin.

Answer: _____

AR 14B
A rapid antigen test is performed and is negative. Now what would you do?
A. Swab for culture prior to treatment.
B. Swab for culture and start penicillin.
C. No further testing; treat with penicillin.
D. No further testing, no antibiotics.

Answer: _____

Approach to Strep Pharyngitis

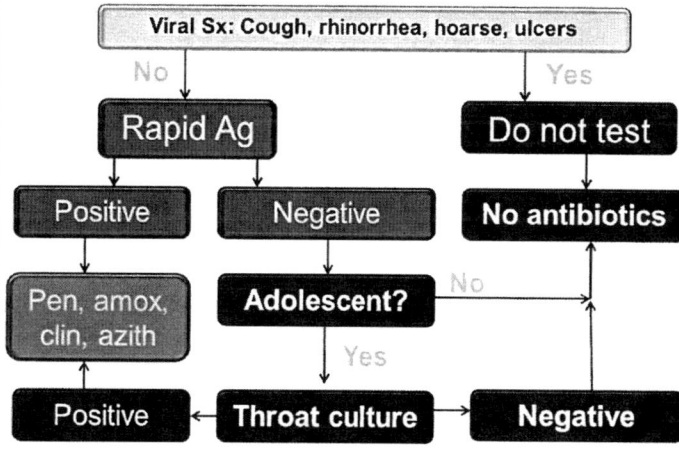

IDSA. *Clin Infect Dis.* 2012;55:1279–1282.

AR 14 — Key Points
- Know which adolescents and adults should be tested for group A strep pharyngitis
- Know the operating characteristics of rapid Ag testing for GABHS
- Know the treatment for group A strep pharyngitis

AR 15 — History and Physical
Hx: A 62-year-old man comes to a Montana ED in February complaining of 2 days of abdominal pain and vomiting and 1 day of blurred vision and trouble talking. His wife is with him and has similar symptoms. They live on a farm and have been eating stored food from their basement, riding out the recent heavy snow fall.
PE: VS are normal, no orthostasis
Alert but has dysarthria
Pupils and mouth exam (shown next)

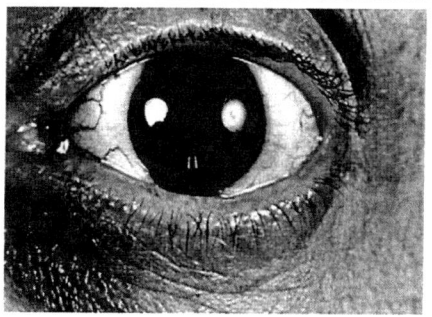

AR 15 (cont.)

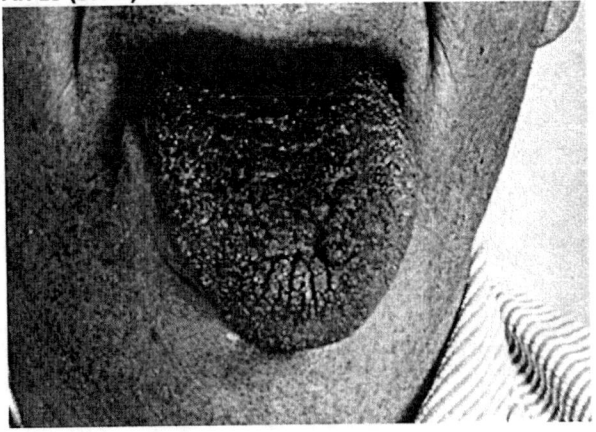

What should he be treated with?

A. Plasmapheresis
B. Intravenous immunoglobulin
C. A series of vaccines
D. High doses of an antibiotic
E. An equine antitoxin

Answer: _____

Clostridium botulinum — Botulism
- Toxin acquisition
  - **Foodborne: Direct ingestion of preformed toxin**
  - Wound: Spores → germinate → toxin production
  - Infantile and unknown: Ingestion of spores
- Toxin action
  - Prevents docking of ACh vesicles to presynaptic membrane in peripheral nerves
  - No sympathetic or CNS involvement

- Clinical features
  - Permanent prevention of ACh release
    - Descending motor paralysis
    - Parasympathetic cranial nerve paralysis
      - Dilated pupils, dry tongue, dysarthria, dysphagia, respiratory arrest
    - No fever
- Treatment
  - Equine antitoxin
  - Penicillin if wound source
  - Supportive

AR 15 — Key Points
- Recognize the epidemiologic setting of foodborne botulism
- Recognize the clinical manifestations of botulism
- Know the emergent treatment of foodborne botulism

AR 16 — History and Physical
Hx: A 19-year-old man comes to your office complaining of severe burning with urination for 2 days. He noted pus from his urethra today. He had vaginal intercourse without protection with a new female partner 4 days ago. She has no symptoms and denies any prior STIs.
PE: Exam normal except for easily expressible pus from the urethra

AR 16 — Labs
Nucleic acid amplification testing (NAAT) is not available in your office; a Gram stain of the urethral pus is performed and is also sent for culture (below).

AR 16 — Gram Stain

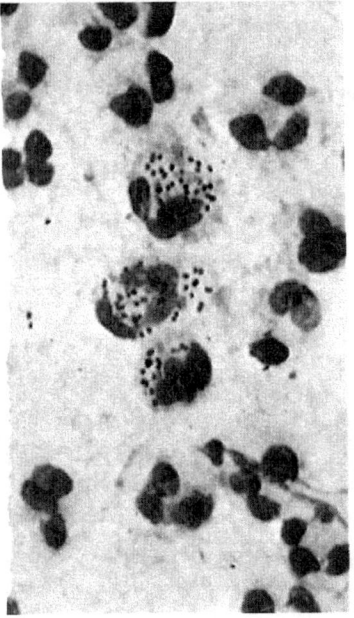

AR 16
What should be done next?

A. Send him to ED for NAAT prior to treatment.
B. Treat with ceftriaxone 250 mg IM x 1.
C. Treat with ceftriaxone 250 mg IM x 1 plus azithromycin 1 g PO x 1.
D. Treat with azithromycin 1 g PO x 1.

Answer: _____

Neisseria gonorrhoeae in Men
- Purulent, painful urethritis (rarely asymptomatic)
- **Incubation period 3–7 days**
- Complications
  - Epididymitis
  - Prostatitis
  - Periurethral abscess
- **Diagnosis**
  - **Gram stain or discharge: Useful and diagnostic**
    - **Sens = 90–95%, Spec = 95–100%**

© 2017 MedStudy Internal Medicine Video Board Review – Infectious Disease • Fred A. Zar, MD

- NAAT of urine
- Culture if above not (+)
- Treatment
  - Ceftriaxone 250 mg IM x 1 and
    azithromycin 1,000 mg PO x 1

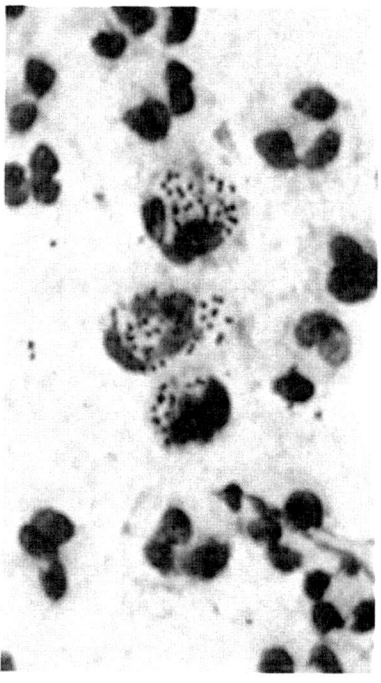

Neisseria gonorrhoeae in Women
- **Primary site = Endocervix (80% asymptomatic)**
  - Secondary spread to vagina, urethra, rectum
- Complications
  - Pelvic Inflammatory Disease
    - TOA, sterility, periurethral abscess
    - Rx: Foxy/Doxy vs. clinda/gent
  - Disseminated infection
    - Oligoarthritis and cutaneous pustules

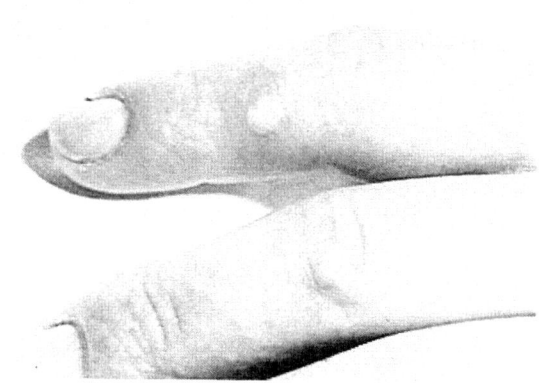

Neisseria gonorrhoeae in Women (cont.)
- Diagnosis
  - Gram stain of endocervix: **Not** useful
    - Sens = 50–70%, Spec = 80%
  - NAAT of urine/vaginal swabs or culture required
    (80–90% sensitive)
- Treatment (test for cure in 3 months)
  - Uncomplicated
    - **Ceftriaxone 250 mg IM x 1 and azithromycin
      1,000 mg PO x 1**
  - Disseminated
    - Ceftriaxone for 3 d, then total 7–10 d course
- Screening (annual)
  - H/O STI, new/mult partners, unsafe sex, sex for
    drugs/money

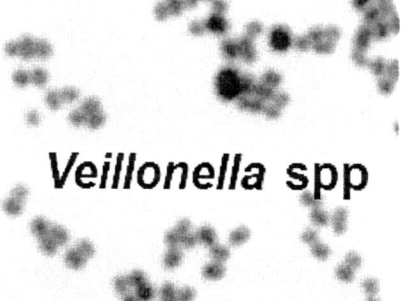

STD Treatment Guidelines *MMWR* 2015;64(RR-03):1.

Chlamydia trachomatis
- Epidemiology
  - The most common bacterial STI
  - Majority of women are asymptomatic →
    continuous reservoir
- Clinical manifestations **(7–14 d incubation)**
  - Women: Cervicitis > acute urethral syndrome > PID,
    perihepatitis
  - Men: Urethritis > epididymitis
- Diagnosis
  - **Nucleic acid amplification (e.g., PCR) of urine**
  - Immunoassays for *Chlamydia* antigens
- Treatment of uncomplicated infection
  - Azithromycin 1 g PO x 1 and ceftriaxone 250 mg IM
CDC 2010.

Differentiating Gonorrhea and *Chlamydia* Urethritis
	Gonococcus	*Chlamydia*
Incubation	< 7 days	> 7 days
Dysuria	Severe	Smarting
Amount of DC	Profuse	Slight
Color of DC	Yellow	Clear

Criteria for Diagnosis of PID

- Pelvic/Lower abd pain, no other cause and 1 of:
  - Uterine/Adnexal tenderness, **or**
  - Cervical motion tenderness
- Increased specificity if:
  - PO temperature > 101.0° F (38.3° C)
  - Cervical or vaginal discharge
  - WBCs on vaginal NaCl prep
  - Elevated ESR
  - Elevated CRP
  - Evidence of cervical GC or *Chlamydia*
- Definitive criteria
  - Endometritis on endometrial biopsy
  - US/MRI w/ tubo-ovarian abscess, fluid in tubes
  - Laparoscopic evidence of PID

CDC 2010.

Indications for Hospitalizing PID

- Surgical emergency cannot be excluded
- Pregnancy
- Failed to respond to outpatient therapy
- Nausea and vomiting
- HIV infection
- Tubo-ovarian abscess

CDC 2010.

Outpatient Regimens for PID

- Regimen A
  - Ceftriaxone 1 g IM
    + doxycycline 100 mg bid x 14 d
    ± metronidazole 500 mg bid x 14 d
- Regimen B
  - Cefoxitin 2 g IM + probenecid 1 g PO
    + doxycycline 100 mg PO bid x 14 d
    ± metronidazole 500 mg bid x 14 d
- Regimen C
  - Another 3rd generation CSPN
    + doxycycline 100 mg bid x 14 d
    ± metronidazole 500 mg bid x 14 d

CDC 2010.

Inpatient Regimens for PID

- Regimen A
  - Cefoxitin 2 g IV q 6 h or cefotetan 2 g IV q 12 h
    + doxycycline 100 mg PO/IV q 12 h
  - Continue 24 h after improvement then complete
    14 d course of doxycycline PO + clinda or metron
    if tubo-ovarian abscess (TOA)
- Regimen B
  - Clindamycin 900 mg IV q 8 h
    + gentamicin 2 mg/kg load, then 1.5 mg/kg q 8 h
  - Continue 24 h after improvement then complete
    14 d course of doxycycline or clindamycin PO if TOA

CDC 2010.

AR 16 — Key Points

- Know the differing presentations of *Chlamydia* and gonococcal urethritis
- Know the yields of diagnostic tests for *Chlamydia* and gonococcal urethritis
- Know the treatment of uncomplicated infection from each organism
- Understand the need to treat for *Chlamydia* in patients with gonorrhea
- Know how to diagnose PID
- Know the treatment regimens for PID depending on location of treatment

AR 17 — History, Physical, and Labs

Hx: A 33-year-old woman returns for follow-up after treatment of a syphilitic chancre on her labia 15 months ago. Her RPR at that time was (+) at a titer of 1:64 and her FTA-ABS was also (+). She was treated with 2.4 mU of benzathine penicillin IM x 1.
She has had 3 male sexual partners since then.
She has no other medical problems.
PE: Exam normal
Lab: RPR (+) at a titer of 1:32

What should be done next?

A. Retreat with benzathine penicillin 2.4 mU IM x 1.
B. Retreat with benzathine penicillin 2.4 mU IM q week x 3.
C. Perform a lumbar puncture prior to treatment.
D. Have her return in 6 months for repeat RPR.

Answer: _____

Syphilis — Stages

Stage	Time Post-infection	Pathogenesis
Incubation	Immediate	Silent multiplication/dissem.
Primary	3 weeks (3–90 d)	Tissue necrosis at inoculation
Secondary	6 weeks (2–12 w)	Huge organism load Immune complexes Remote multiplication
Latent, early	< 1 year	Asymptomatic, seropositive
Latent, late	> 1 year	Obliterative endarteritis of CNS/CV parenchyma
Tertiary (late) Neurosyphilis Cardiovascular Gummatous	2–30 years	

Syphilitic Chancre

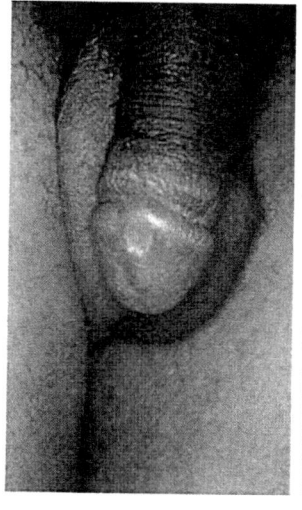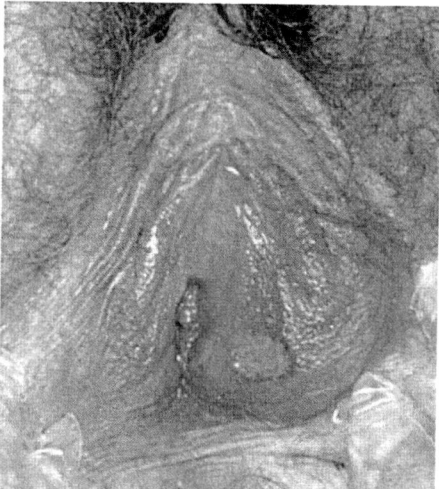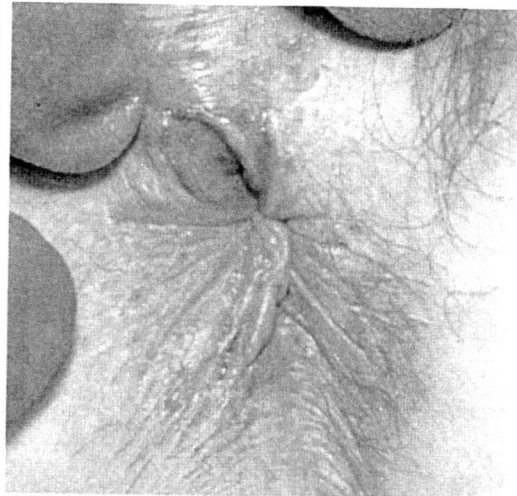

Secondary Syphilis

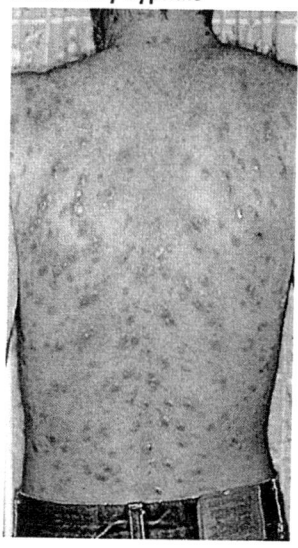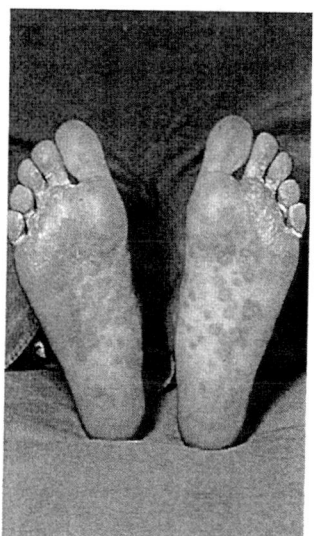

Syphilis — Mucous Patch (cont.)

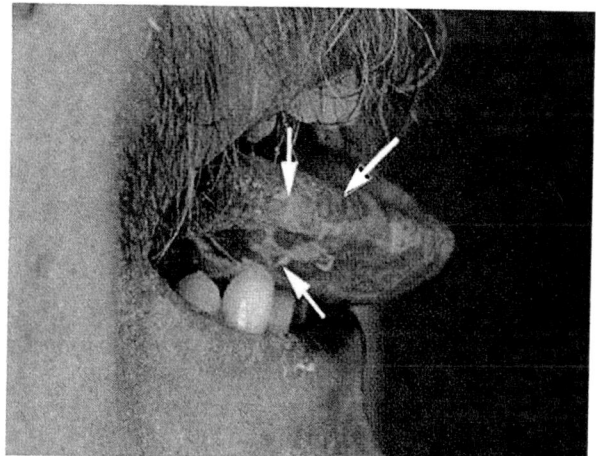

Oral hairy leukoplakia

Syphilis — Mucous Patch

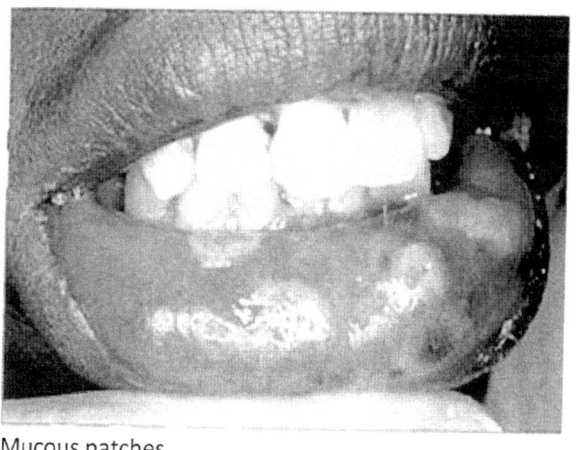

Mucous patches

Secondary Syphilis — Condyloma Lata

Secondary Syphilis — Condyloma Lata (cont.)

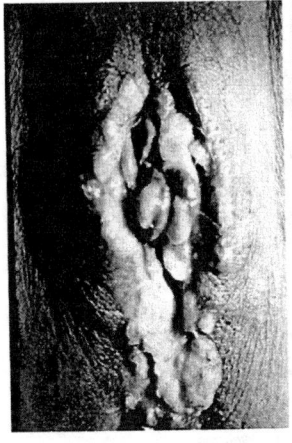
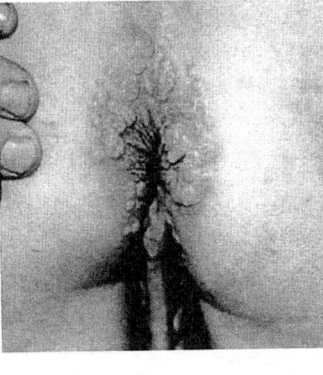

Cardiovascular Syphilis

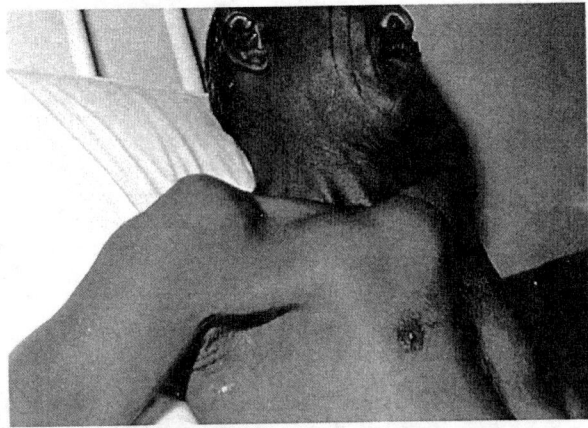

Neurosyphilis

- Only 2/3 are symptomatic
- Meningovascular syphilis (2–10 yrs post infection)
  - Endarteritis of meninges, brain, cord
- **Parenchymal neurosyphilis**
  - General paresis (15–20 yrs post infection)
    - **P**ersonality changes
    - **A**ffect changes
    - **R**eflexes increased
    - **E**ye (Argyll Robertson* pupils) →
    - **S**ensorium changes
    - **I**ntellectual deterioration
    - **S**peech defects
  - Tabes dorsalis (25–30 yrs post infection)
    - Demyelination of dorsal columns
    - Ataxia, lost vibration/position, incontinence
    - Lightning pains

*Douglas Moray Cooper Lamb Argyll Robertson, Scottish ophthalmologist, 1837–1909.

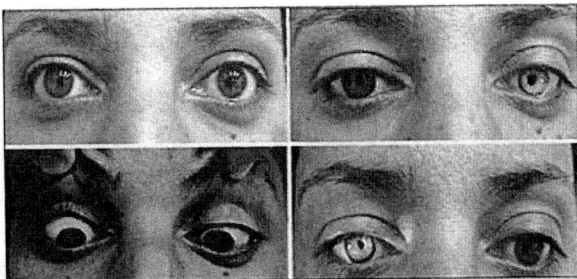

Figure. Argyll Robertson pupil.

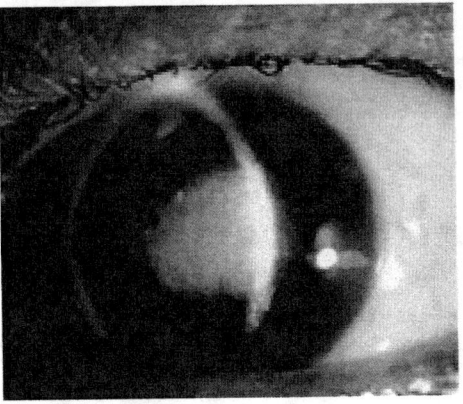

Syphilitic keratitis

Diagnosing Syphilis — Nontreponemal Reaginic Serology

- Lab aspects
  - IgG & IgM reacting with beef liver or heart
  - Current antigen is cardiolipin-cholesterol-lecithin
  - RPR = Card, VDRL = Slide flocculation
- Seroprevalence
  - Primary = 70%
  - Secondary = 99%
  - Tertiary = 70%
- Seroreversion with Rx
  - Primary = 1 year
  - Secondary = 2 years
  - Late latent = 5 years
- Failure to serorevert
  - Reinfection
  - Inappropriate therapy
  - Biological false (+)

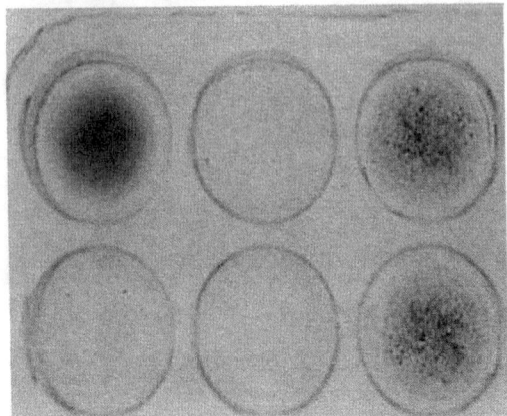

Syphilis Therapy

- Primary, Secondary, or Early Latent (< 1 yr)
  - **Benzathine penicillin G, 2.4 mU x 1**
  - **Ceftriaxone 1 g daily x 10 d**
  - Doxycycline 100 mg PO bid x 14 d
  - (Azithromycin 2 g PO x 1)
- Late Latent (or unknown duration) Late Nonneuro
  - **Benzathine penicillin G, 2.4 mU q wk x 3**
  - (Doxycycline 100 mg PO bid x 4 weeks)
- Neurosyphilis
  - Aqueous penicillin G 3–4 mU q4h x 10–14 d
    ± Benzathine penicillin G 2.4 mU x 1
  - Ceftriaxone 2 g IV x 10–14 d
  - (Procaine penicillin G 2.4 mU IM/d +
    probenecid 500 mg qid x 10–14 d)
  - Retap q 6 mo x 4, retreat if cells at 6 mo
    or CSF abnml at 24 mo
- Partners
  - Rx if contact w/ 1°, 2° or early latent w/in 90 d

CDC STD Guidelines. *MMWR.* 2010;59(RR–12):1–116.

Syphilis — CSF Exam in Syphilis

- Indications
  - Neurologic or ophthalmologic signs/Sx
  - Signs of active tertiary syphilis
    - Aortitis
    - Gumma
  - **Treatment failure**
- **Diagnostic of neurosyphilis (any of):**
  - VDRL (+)
  - Protein > 45 mg/dL
  - Lymphocytes > 5 cells//mm^3

CDC 2010.

AR 17 — Key Points

- Understand the time frame in which nontreponemal
  testing for syphilis should serorevert after
  appropriate Rx
- Know the reasons for failure to serorevert
- Understand the indications for performing a lumbar
  puncture in patients with syphilis
- Understand how to diagnose neurosyphilis

AR 18 — History and Physical

Hx: A 24-year-old woman presents with a 3-day history
of unpleasant smelling, continuous vaginal discharge.
She is sexually active with 1 partner for 3 years and is
currently 10 weeks pregnant.
PE: External genitalia normal; Opaque copious vaginal
discharge present with a fishy odor; Underlying vaginal
walls and cervix appear normal

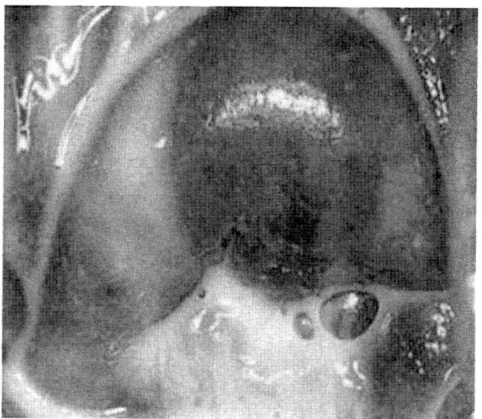

AR 18 — Labs

A sample of the discharge has a pH of 6.5.; addition
of KOH produces a fishy odor and reveals no fungal
elements on microscopy; a saline prep reveals:

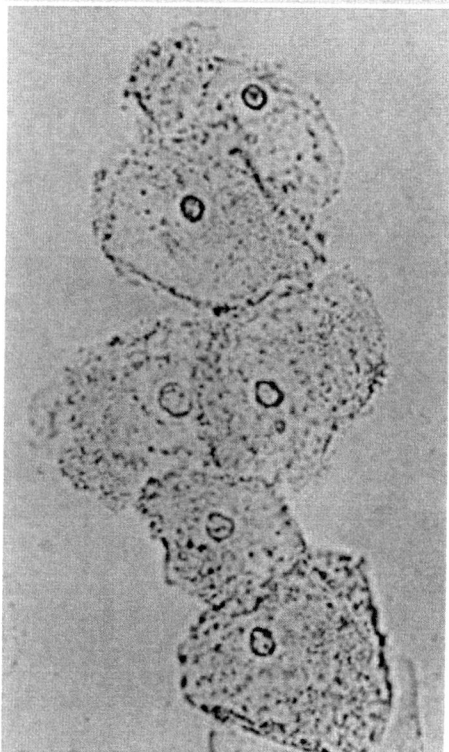

AR 18
What would you do next?

A. Metronidazole 500 mg bid x 7 d.

B. Metronidazole 2 g x 1.

C. Clindamycin 300 mg bid x 7 d.

D. No treatment, have her return in 2nd trimester and
treat if still symptomatic.

Answer: _____

Metronidazole in 1st Trimester
- The Study
  - Meta-analysis 1966–1996
    - 4 cohort (2 prospective), 1 case-control
  - N = 199,451
- The Results
  - Malformations
    - Exposed = 189/2,524 (7.5%)
    - Not exposed = 30,887/196,927 (15.7%)
    - p = 0.32

Caro-Paton T. *Br J Clin Pharmacol.* 44:179–82, 1997.

Vaginosis and Vaginitis
- Bacterial vaginosis
  - *Lactobacillus* replaced by anaerobes
    - *Mobiluncus, Gardnerella*
  - Clinical: Fishy odor, no irritation
- Vulvovaginal candidiasis
  - *C. albicans*
  - Clinical: Pruritus, white plaques on red base
  - If recurrent: Rule out DM and HIV
- *Trichomonas*
  - *Trichomonas vaginalis*
  - Clinical: Profuse discharge, ± foul

Vaginitis Diagnostic Tests

	Vaginal pH	Wet Prep	KOH Prep
Bacterial Vaginosis	> 5.0	Clue cells	Fishy odor
Candida	< 5.0	Fungal elements	Fungal elements
Trichomonas	> 5.0	Trichomonads	Not diagnostic

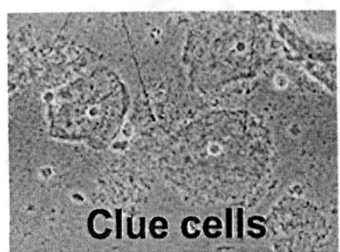
Clue cells

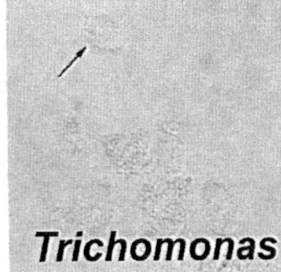
Trichomonas

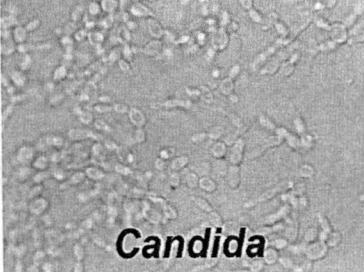
Candida

Vaginitis Treatment

	1st Line	Other Choices	Pregnancy
Bacterial Vaginosis	Metronidazole PO or gel x 7 d	Clindamycin PO or gel	Same
Candida	Fluconazole x 1	Topicals	Same?
Trichomonas	Metron 2 g x 1	Tinidazole	Same

Fluconazole During Pregnancy
- The Study
  - Denmark database 1997–2013
  - 1,405,663 pregnancies
    - 3,315 exposed during wks 7–22
  - 1:4 exposed:unexposed
- The Results

	Exposed	Not Exposed	P
Spont Ab	147/3,315 (4.4%)	563/13,246 (4.2%)	< 0.05
Stillbirth	21/5,382 (0.4%)	77/21,506 (0.4%)	NS

- Effect seen even if only topical use

Molgarrd-Nielsen D. *JAMA.* 315:58–57, 2016.

AR 18 — Key Points
- Differentiate the 3 common causes of vaginal discharge
- Know the treatment of infectious etiologies of vaginal discharge
- Know whether 1st trimester pregnancy affects these treatments

AR 19A — History, Physical, and Labs
Hx: A 38-year-old woman presents with a 2-day history of abdominal cramps and diarrhea 4–5 times per day. She is not vomiting.

She was at an office retreat at a resort 2 days prior to becoming ill. Eight of 21 other attendees are similarly ill. The Public Health Department requested stool specimens on all those who were ill, and she is here to follow up on the results.

PE: T 99.4° F (37.4° C), PR 90, RR 14, BP 118/80
No orthostasis
Abdominal exam normal
Lab: Stool culture growing *Shigella sonnei*

In addition to oral hydration, what would you do next?
A. Amoxicillin x 5 d
B. Trimethoprim/sulfamethoxazole x 5 d
C. Levofloxacin x 3 d
D. No antibiotic therapy

Answer: _____

AR 19B — History, Physical, and Labs

Hx: A 38-year-old woman presents with a 2-day history of abdominal cramps and diarrhea 4–5 times per day. She is not vomiting.

She was at an office retreat at a resort 2 days prior to becoming ill. Eight of 21 other attendees are similarly ill. The Public Health Department requested stool specimens on all those who were ill, and she is here to follow up on the results.

PE: T 99.4° F (37.4° C), PR 90, RR 14, BP 118/80

No orthostasis

Abdominal exam normal

Lab: Stool culture growing *Salmonella enterica*

In addition to oral hydration, what would you do next?

A. Amoxicillin x 5 d
B. Trimethoprim/sulfamethoxazole x 5 d
C. Levofloxacin x 3 d
D. No antibiotic therapy

Answer: _____

Meta-Analysis of Rx of Nontyphoidal *Salmonella* Enteritis

- <u>The study</u>
  - 12 trials of antibiotics vs. placebo, with 778 pts
- <u>The results</u>

	Effect of antibiotics	p value
Duration of illness	− 0.07 d	0.76
Duration of diarrhea	− 0.03 d	0.91
Duration of fever	− 0.45 d	0.09
Cure	81% vs. 75%	0.07
C+S (+) > 42 d	**11% vs. 3%**	**0.01**

Sirinavin S. *Cochrane Database Syst Rev.* 2000;CD001167.

AR 19C — History, Physical, and Labs

Hx: A 38-year-old woman presents with a 2-day history of abdominal cramps and diarrhea 4–5 times per day. She is not vomiting.

She was at an office retreat at a resort 2 days prior to becoming ill. Eight of 21 other attendees are similarly ill. The Public Health Department requested stool specimens on all those who were ill, and she is here to follow up on the results.

PE: T 99.4° F (37.4° C), PR 90, RR 14, BP 118/80

No orthostasis

Abdominal exam normal

Lab: Stool culture growing *Campylobacter jejuni*

In addition to oral hydration, what would you do next?

A. Amoxicillin x 5 d
B. Trimethoprim/sulfamethoxazole x 5 d
C. Levofloxacin x 3 d
D. No antibiotic therapy

Answer: _____

Meta-Analysis of *Campylobacter* Treatment

- <u>The study</u>
  - 11 randomized placebo controlled trials
  - 244 treated (5 quin, 6 EMN) vs. 235 placebo
- <u>The results</u>
  - Mean reduction in days of diarrhea = 1.32 d ($p < 0.001$)
  - All studies showed a decrease in carriage if treated
  - Mean duration of diarrhea
    - If treated in < 3 days = 2.4 d
    - If treated ≥ 3 days = 4.1 d
    - p = NS

Ternhag A. *CID. 2007*;44:696–700.

Antibiotics for *Salmonella* and *Campylobacter*

- <u>Severe disease</u>
  - Unremitting diarrhea (> 7 stools)
  - High-grade fever
  - Hospitalized
  - Extraintestinal
  - > 7 days
- <u>At risk for severe disease</u>
  - Immunocompromised
    - Immunosuppressed, extremes of age, pregnant
  - Inflammatory bowel disease

AR 19D — History, Physical, and Labs

Hx: A 38-year-old woman presents with a 2-day history of abdominal cramps and diarrhea 4–5 times per day. She is not vomiting.

She was at an office retreat at a resort 2 days prior to becoming ill. Eight of 21 other attendees are similarly ill. The Public Health Department requested stool specimens on all those who were ill, and she is here to follow up on the results.

PE: T 99.4° F (37.4° C), PR 90, RR 14, BP 118/80

No orthostasis

Abdominal exam normal

Lab: Stool culture growing *E. coli* O157:H7

In addition to oral hydration, what would you do next?

A. Amoxicillin x 5 d
B. Trimethoprim/sulfamethoxazole x 5 d
C. Levofloxacin x 3 d
D. No antibiotic therapy

Answer: _____

Risk Factors for HUS after _E. coli_ O157:H7 Infection
- The study
  - Prospective enrollment of 259 children
- Multivariable analysis

Risk factor	Odds ratio	_p_ value
WBC increase*	1.1	0.008
Vomiting	3.05	0.02
Antibiotic Rx	**3.62**	**0.02**

*Each 1.0 above 1.5

Wong CS. _Clin Infect Dis._ 2012;55:33–41.

Bacterial Diarrhea Rx Summary

Bacterial	Who to Treat	What to Use
Shigella	At risk	Quinolone
Salmonella	At risk	Quinolone
Campylobacter	At risk	Azithromycin, Quinolone
E. Coli O157	No one	N/A

AR 19 — Key Points
- Recognize the presentation of bacterial diarrhea
- Know which bacterial pathogens warrant therapy and what agents to use

AR 20 — History and Physical

Hx: A 66-year-old man presents to the ED with 4 days of left ear pain. It began mild; but for the last 36 hours, it has been 10/10 and radiates to the TMJ on that side. He required bilateral cerumen removal 2 years ago, and since then he irrigates his ears at least twice a week. He denies loss of hearing, fever, or cough. He has hypertension and diabetes, both controlled with oral medications.

PE: T 99.2° F (37.3° C), PR 100, RR 16, BP 138/88

Left ear (below)

AR 20 — Ear Exam and Labs
- WBC = 11.3
- Glucose = 211
- ESR = 110

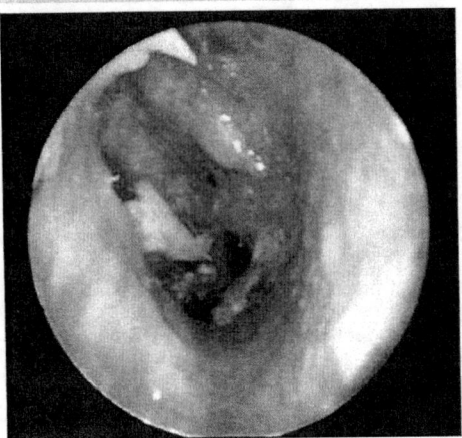

What would you do next?
A. Culture ear canal and treat based on results.
B. Send home on topical ciprofloxacin.
C. Send home on oral ciprofloxacin.
D. Admit and begin intravenous antibiotics.

Answer: _____

AR 20 — Key Points
- Differentiate between benign and malignant otitis externa
- Recognize the need for administration of intravenous therapy to prevent complications

AR 21A — History and Physical

Hx: A 37-year-old man presents to your office for the evaluation of fever, chills, severe headache, nausea, and myalgias. He was a participant in a Hawaiian triathlon 1 week ago. Several dozen others are similarly ill. Two other participants have been admitted to the hospital with acute kidney injury, meningitis, and hepatitis. He is penicillin allergic.

PE: T 102.4° F (39.1° C), PR 100, RR 20, BP 108/76

Alert, oriented x 3 and looks uncomfortable

Lungs and heart normal

Liver palpably enlarged

Eye exam (below):

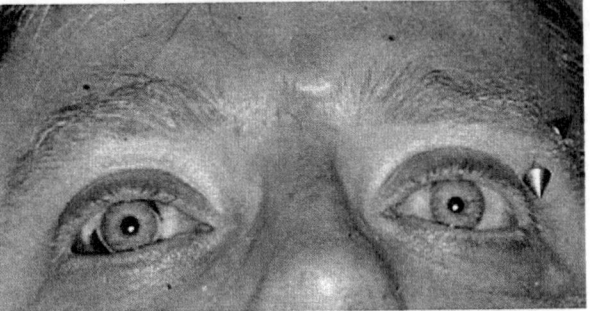

AR 21A — Labs

Hb 13.8 g/dL

WBC 9,300/mm^3 with normal differential

Platelets 150,000/mm^3

Total bili 6.6 mg/dL, direct bili 3.2 mg/dL

AST 82 U/L, ALT 88 U/L

Creatinine 2.1 mg/dL

U/A: Protein 100 mg/dL, RBC 8/hpf, WBC 12/hpf, trace (+) blood, LE (−), nitrite (−)

CSF: WBC 111/mm^3, RBC 2/mm^3, protein 97 mg/dL, glucose 89 mg/dL

Gram stain (−)

What test will give you the most timely diagnosis?
A. IgM serologies
B. IgG serologies
C. Blood culture
D. CSF culture
E. Stool culture

Answer: _____

AR 21B
He is admitted. How would you treat him pending results?
A. IV levofloxacin
B. IV doxycycline
C. IV streptomycin
D. IV aztreonam

Answer: _____

Leptospirosis
- <u>Epidemiology and pathogenesis</u>
  - Large animal reservoir
  - Acquired from contact with contaminated water or animals
  - Hawaii has most cases
  - **Triathlons, IRONMAN**
- <u>Microbiology</u>
  - *L. interrogans*
- <u>Clinical manifestations</u>
  - Abrupt fever, myalgia, headache
  - Rare multiorgan injury: AKI, liver, aseptic meningitis, coagulopathy, ARDS
  - **Conjunctival suffusion**
- <u>Diagnosis</u>
  - **IgM serology**, 4-fold IgG change
  - Microscopic agglutination test (CDC)
  - Culture takes 10 days, < 50% yield
- Treatment: Only if severe, doxycycline

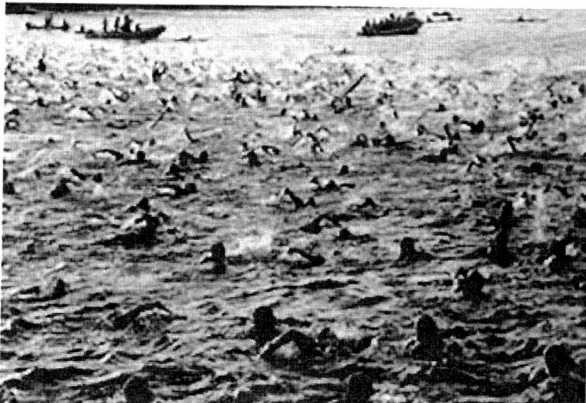

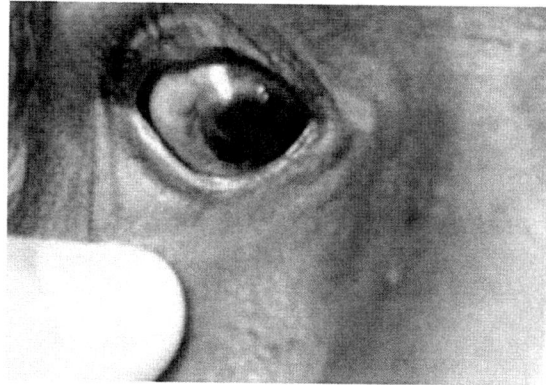

AR 21 — Key Points
- Recognize the epidemiologic setting of an outbreak of leptospirosis
- Recognize the clinical presentation of severe leptospirosis (Weil disease)
- Know the utility of various diagnostic tests for leptospirosis
- Know the treatment of leptospirosis

AR 22A— History and Physical
Hx: A 28-year-old man comes to the ED 1 hour after a dog bite. It occurred when he tried to break up a fight between his and a neighbor's dog.
He has had regular tetanus immunizations, the last of which was 4 years ago.
PE: VS are stable
           Hand photo (below)

AR 22A — Hand Photo

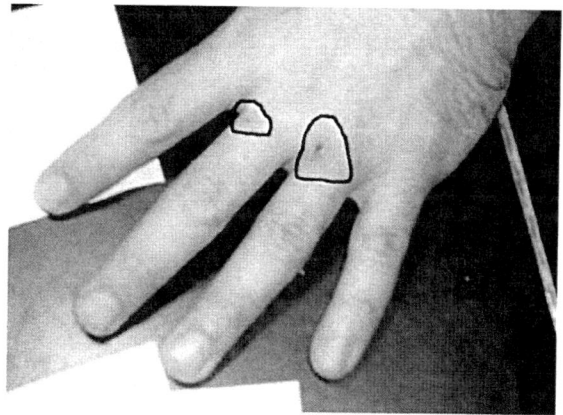

AR 22A
What tetanus treatment/prophylaxis is needed?
A. Tetanus toxoid alone
B. Tetanus immunoglobulin
C. Tetanus toxoid and tetanus immunoglobulin
D. No tetanus prevention needed

Answer: _____

Tetanus — Wound Management

Past Toxoid	Clean and Minor	Tetanus Prone*
Unknown or < 3	Toxoid	Toxoid + TIG
≥ 3	Toxoid if ≥ 10 yrs	Toxoid if ≥ 5 yrs

*Crush, dirt/feces, puncture, missiles

AR 22B

What oral antibiotics, if any, should be given?

A. Doxycycline
B. Clindamycin
C. Amoxicillin
D. Amoxicillin/clavulanate
E. None

Answer: _____

AR 22C

What should be done with respect to rabies?

A. Give rabies vaccine.
B. Give human rabies immunoglobulin (HRIG).
C. Give rabies vaccine and HRIG.
D. Observe dog for 10 days.
E. No prophylaxis needed.

Answer: _____

Animal Bites
- Risk of Infection
  - Humans > cats > dogs
- Approach
  - Debride
  - Image if needed
  - Tetanus prophylaxis
  - Rabies prophylaxis
  - Amoxicillin/clavulanate
    - All human bites
    - Immunocompromised, hand, near joint or bone, severe, crush, edema

Animal Bites — Rabies Prophylaxis
- Animal-specific approach
  - Bat, raccoon, fox, skunk
    - Begin prophylaxis
  - Dog, cat, ferret
    - Observe x 10 d
  - Small rodents
    - No prophylaxis needed
- Prophylaxis
  - Human rabies immunoglobulin
    - Infiltrate wound then rest IM
  - Human diploid cell vaccine
    - 1 mL on days 0, 3, 7, 14

AR 22 — Key Points
- Know the approach to tetanus prophylaxis in the setting of an animal bite
- Know the approach to rabies prophylaxis in the setting of an animal bite
- Know the indications for antibiotics after an animal bite
- Know the antibiotic of choice for animal bites when indicated

AR 23 — History and Physical

Hx: A 35-year-old Wisconsin man presents in August with low-grade fever, myalgias, and rash on his back for 1 week. He is otherwise healthy.
PE: T 100.4° F (38.0° C), other VS normal

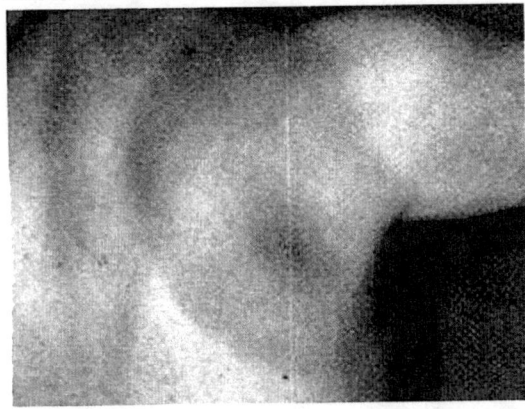

AR 23

What would you do next?

A. Test for Lyme IgM antibody and treat if (+).
B. Test for Lyme IgM antibody but begin treatment for Lyme disease.
C. Treat for Lyme disease without performing serology.
D. Do not test or treat for Lyme disease.

Answer: _____

Lyme Disease — CDC National Surveillance Definition
- Case definition
  - **Erythema migrans (> 5 cm), or**
  - **One late manifestation and lab confirmation of infection**
- Acceptable late manifestations
  - Musculoskeletal: Intermittent joint swelling, ± chronic pauciarticular
  - Nervous: Lymphocytic meningitis, cranial neuritis, radiculoneuropathy, encephalomyelitis
  - Cardiac: Acute 2nd/3rd AVB, resolves in wks, ± myocarditis
- Lab confirmation of infection
  - Culture (+), or IgM ± IgG Ab by ELISA confirmed with Western blot
  - CSF Ab > blood Ab

CDC 2011.

Lyme Disease Cases 2016

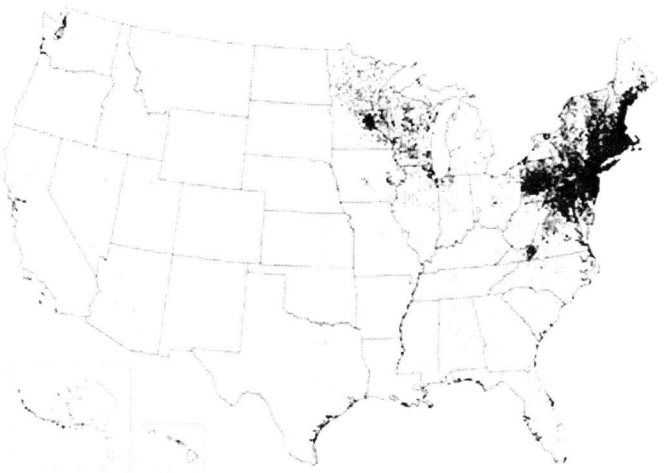

CDC 2016.

Lyme Disease — Treatment
- Antibiotics
  - PO: Doxycycline, amoxicillin, cefuroxime
  - IV: Ceftriaxone
- Manifestation   Route and Duration

Manifestation	Route and Duration
EM, Bell's palsy	PO x 14–21 d
1° AVB	PO x 14–21 d
Meningitis	**IV x 10–28 d**
2° to 3° AVB	**IV then** PO x 14–21 d
Arthritis	PO x 28 d
Recurrent	PO or IV 28 d

AR 23 — Key Points
- Recognize the primary stage of Lyme disease, in specific, erythema migrans
- Know that the presence of erythema migrans is diagnostic of Lyme disease
- Know that serology is not indicated, and may be misleading, in patients with erythema migrans

---

AR 24 — History and Physical
Hx: A 34-year-old man comes to your office with the lesions shown. They started as a solitary bump on the back of the hand and have progressed over the last 2 weeks. They are slightly painful and occasionally drain clear, odorless fluid. He is the owner of the Greenleaf Flower Shoppe in town.

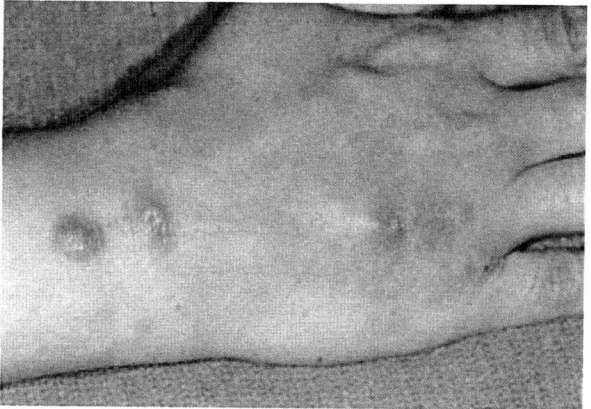

AR 24
Sending the drainage and/or biopsy for which of the following would be most likely to be diagnostic?
A. Viral culture
B. Bacterial culture
C. Mycobacterial culture
D. Fungal culture

Answer: _____

Sporotrichosis
- Epidemiology and microbiology
  - Inoculation of *Sporotrichum schenckii* in soil
- Clinical manifestations
  - Nodules/Ulcers along lymphatic drainage
- Diagnosis
  - Gram stain and culture
- Treatment
  - Itraconazole through 2–4 wks after resolution

AR 25 — History and Physical
Hx: A 34-year-old man comes to your office with the lesions shown. They started as a solitary bump on the back of the hand and have progressed over the last 2 weeks. They are slightly painful and occasionally drain clear, odorless fluid. He is the owner of the Aquarius Fancy Fish store in town.

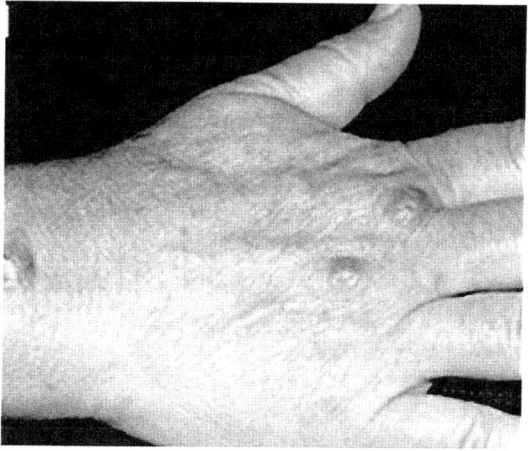

AR 25 (cont.)
Sending the drainage for which of the following would be most likely to be diagnostic?
A. Viral culture
B. Bacterial culture
C. Mycobacterial culture
D. Fungal culture

Answer: _____

Mycobacterium marinum
- Epidemiology
  - Fresh-water– and salt-water–free living
- Clinical manifestations
  - Indolent nodules without systemic symptoms
- Diagnosis
  - Culture of biopsy or drainage
- Treatment
  - Clarithromycin, doxycycline, or T/S

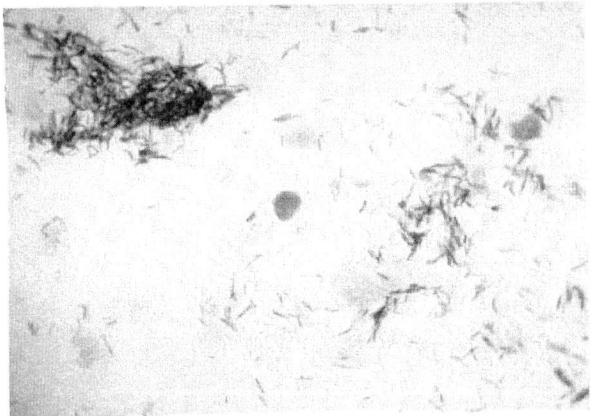

AR 24 and 25 — Key Points
- Recognize 2 common inoculation soft tissue infections of the hand
- Know the epidemiologic settings in which they occur
- Know what cultures should be taken in each setting
- Know what antibiotics should be administered to treat them

AR 26 — History and Physical
Hx: A 20-year-old woman is brought in by neighbors after being found confused in her home. She wears a medical alert bracelet that says "diabetes" on it.

PE: T 98.6° F (37.0° C), BP 100/68, PR 112, RR 30 Orthostatic, oriented only to name. Right eye proptosis with periorbital swelling and limited EOM on that side. Dusky area superior lateral nose as shown; Mucous membranes dry.

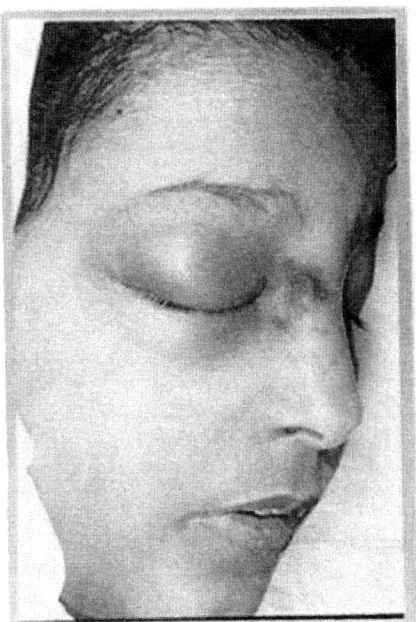

AR 26 — Labs and Initial Care
Labs:
Glucose 313 mg/dL, serum ketones (+)
Na^+ 132 mEq/L, K^+ 3.3 mEq/L,
Cl^- 95 mEq/L, HCO_3^- 13 mEq/L, AG 24
Phos 2.0 mEq/L, Creat 2.1 mg/dL
WBC 22,300/mm^3 with 11% bands
Hb 12.1 g/dL, Pl 456,000/mm^3
Initial care: Receives IVF, insulin infusion, K^+ and Phos with resolution of DKA and improved mental state; CT scan of orbits and sinuses is performed (below)

AR 26 — CT Orbits and Sinuses

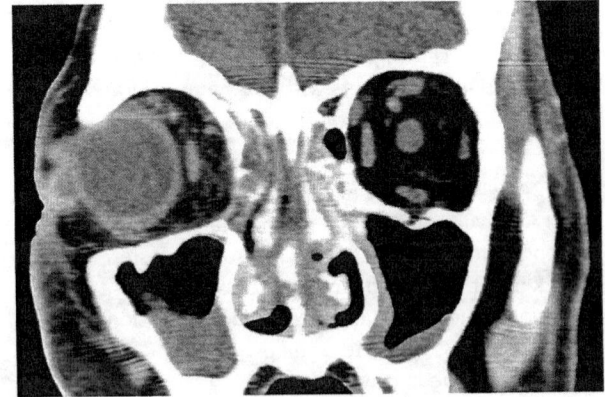

AR 26 (cont.)
Otolaryngology and ophthalmology are consulted.
In the meantime, what would you give her?
A. IV vancomycin and cefepime
B. IV vancomycin, cefepime, and metronidazole
C. PO posaconazole
D. IV itraconazole
E. Liposomal amphotericin B

Answer: _____

Mucormycosis
- Microbiology
  - Ubiquitous: *Rhizopus*, *Mucor*, and *Rhizomucor*
- Epidemiology
  - Prolonged neutropenia, immunosuppressed, DKA
  - Deferoxamine-iron chelation promotes growth
- Clinical manifestations
  - Rhinocerebral
  - Pulmonary
- Diagnosis
  - Broad nonseptate hyphae
  - Fragile, often culture negative

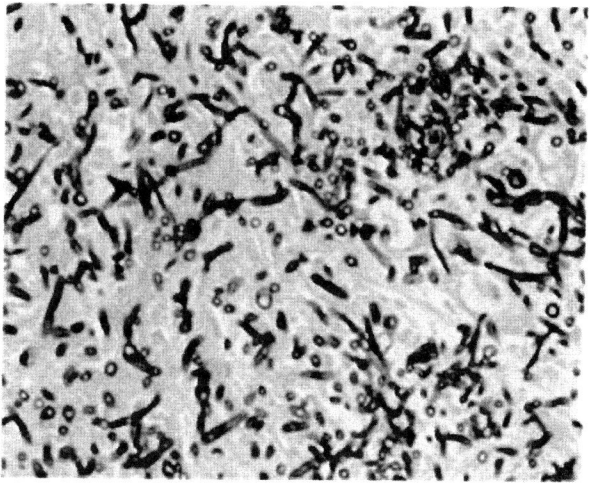

Rhinocerebral Mucormycosis
- Initial presentation
  - Unilateral headache, stuffiness, epistaxis
- Progression
  - Periorbital swelling, proptosis, ophthalmoplegia, blindness, stroke
- Images show bone destruction
- Treatment
  - Correct predispositions
  - Debridement
  - Amphotericin B
    - Posaconazole if not tolerated

AR 26 — Key Points
- Recognize the clinical settings in which mucormycosis occurs
- Recognize the need for emergent surgical intervention
- Know the initial and alternative therapy for mucormycosis

AR 27 — History and Physical
Hx: A 35-year-old man presents with a 10-day history of sudden onset of watery diarrhea. Five days ago, he noted RUQ pain worse with eating and a temperature of 100.9° F (38.3° C). Found to be HIV (+) 3 years ago but is not compliant with antiretrovirals. He has not been on any antibacterial drugs.
PE: T 101.3° F (38.5° C), BP 90/64, PR 120, RR 12
Orthostatic
Dry mucous membranes
Abd: RUQ tenderness and Murphy's sign (+)

AR 27 — Labs and Images
Labs:
Hb 10.3 g/dL
WBC: 4,300/mm³ 86% neutrophils, 6% lymphocytes
Platelets 129,000/mm³
Lytes, creatinine, lipase normal
AST 44 U/L, ALT 61 U/L, Alk phos 211 U/L (20–70)
RUQ U/S:
Thickening of gallbladder wall
No stones, pericholecystic fluid, bile duct dilation

Which of the following tests on his stool is most likely to reveal the causative agent of his symptoms?
A. Stool for bacterial culture
B. Stool for viral culture
C. Stool for ova and parasites
D. Stool for ova and parasites with acid-fast stain
E. Stool for *Clostridium difficile* toxin

Answer: _____

Opportunistic Parasites

	Cryptosporidiosis	Cystoisospora	Cyclospora	Microsporidiosis
Organism	C. parvum	C. belli	C. cayetanensis	Enterocytozooan sp.
Stain	Acid fast	Acid fast	Acid fast	Trichrome
Treatment	Nitazoxanide	T/S (quinolone)	T/S (quinolone)	Albendazole

1) All cause watery diarrhea and may cause acalculous cholecystitis
2) Stool yield enhanced by monoclonal antibody staining
3) *Cystoisospora* causes eosinophilia

AR 27 — Key Points
- Recognize the clinical presentation of opportunistic parasites that cause diarrhea and acalculous cholecystitis in HIV-infected patients
- Know the methods of diagnosing these infections
- Know the pathogen-specific treatment of these infections

INFECTIOUS DISEASE
PART 2

AR 28 — History and Physical
Hx: A 28-year-old female medical student presents to the campus health office with a 4-day history of fever. Fevers have occurred every other day, are as high as 104.9° F (40.5° C), and are followed by drenching sweats. The last episode was this morning.
She is a native of Honduras and just returned 1 week ago from visiting friends and relatives there for 2 weeks.
She thinks she has malaria.
PE: T 99.0° F (37.2° C), BP 98/70, PR 100, RR 12
Not orthostatic; Physical exam normal

AR 28 — Labs and Images
Labs:
Hb 12.3 g/dL, WBC: 6,300/mm^3,
Platelets 329,000/mm^3,
Malaria thin prep:

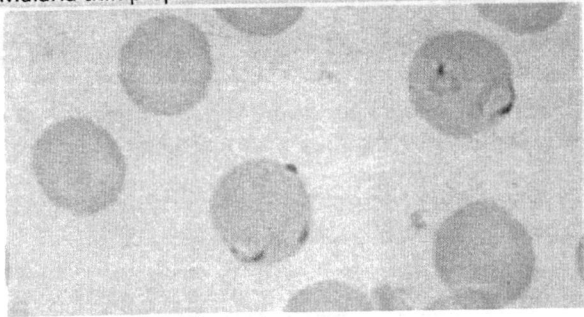

AR 28 (cont.)
What would you treat her with?
A. Chloroquine
B. Chloroquine then primaquine
C. Mefloquine then primaquine
D. Artesunate + mefloquine
E. Atovaquone + proguanil

Answer: _____

Global Distribution of Malaria

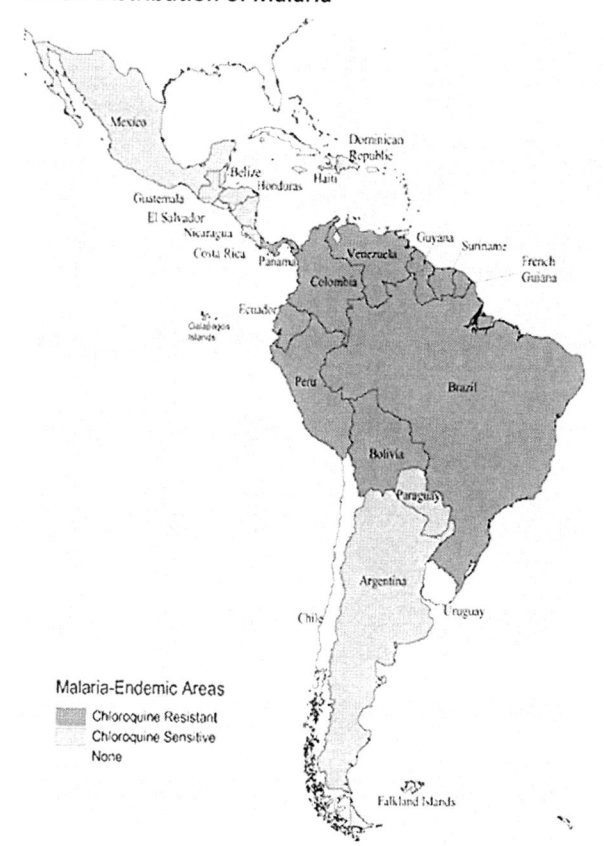

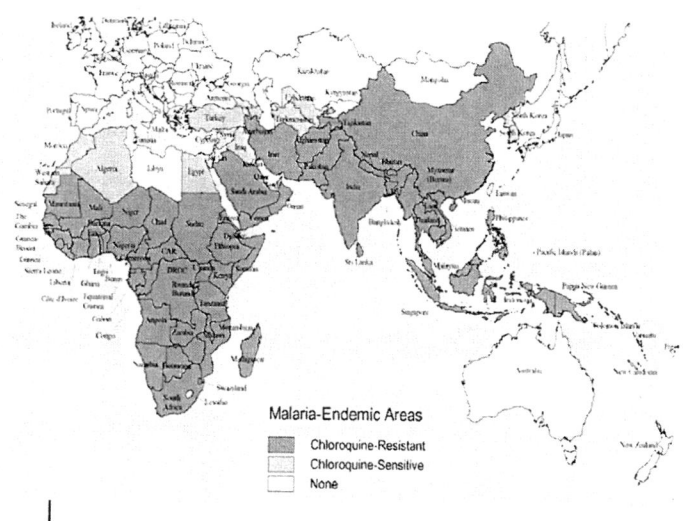

Malaria-Endemic Areas
- Chloroquine-Resistant
- Chloroquine-Sensitive
- None

Malaria-Endemic Areas
- Chloroquine Resistant
- Chloroquine Sensitive
- None

Importance of Recognizing *P. falciparum*
- Drug resistance
- High-level parasitemia
- End-organ damage
- Need for hospitalization

Diagnosis of *P. falciparum*
- Double chromatin knobs (headphones)
- Multiple parasitism
- High-level parasitism (> 5%)
- Banana gametocytes

Plasmodium falciparum

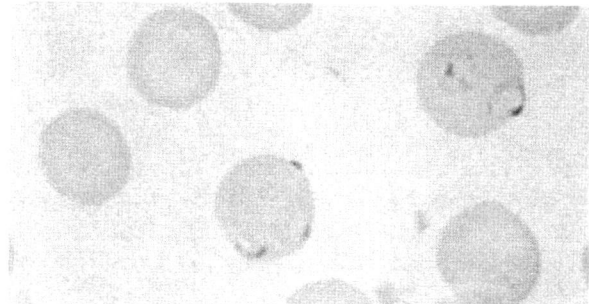

Multiple parasites per cell

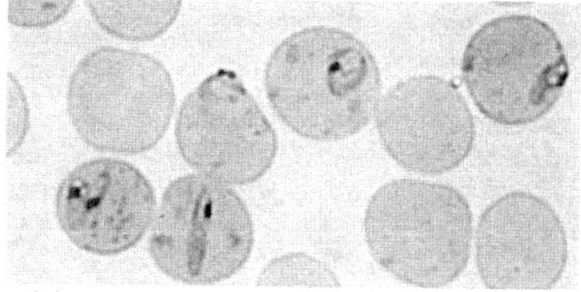

High-level parasitism

Plasmodium falciparum (cont.)

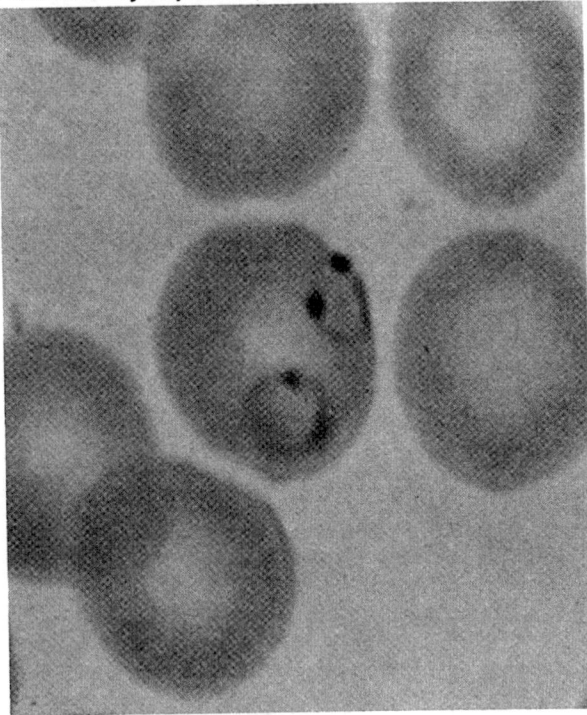

Double chromatin dots (headphones)

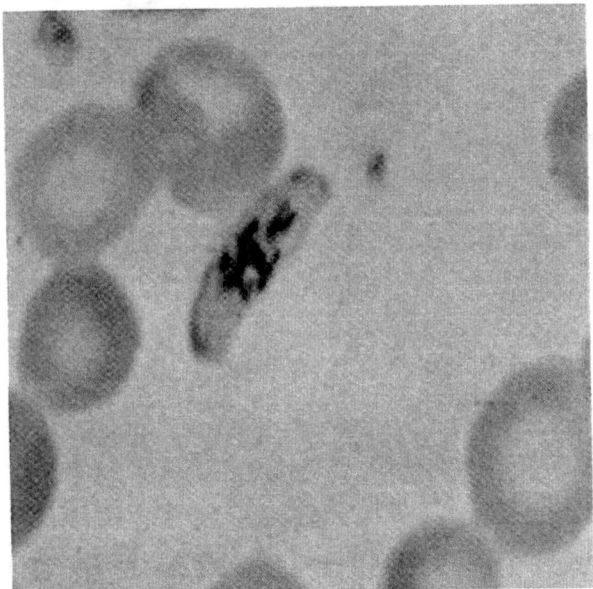

Banana gametocyte

Malaria Species Characteristics and Rx

Species	Fever Cycle	World Cases	Liver Stage?	RBCs Infected	Parasite Level	Chloroquine Resistance?
P. vivax	Tertian	51%	Yes	Retics	Low	Uncommon
P. ovale	Tertian	1%	Yes	Retics	Low	Rare
P. falciparum	Tertian	48%	No	All	High	Yes
P. malariae	Quartan	1%	No	Old	Low	No
P. knowlesi	Irregular	< 1%	No	All	May be high	No

1) Falciparum makes up > 75% of U.S. cases
2) Liver stage requires primaquine for cure
3) Chloroquine-resistance regimens
   - Mild: Atovaquone-proguanil
   - Severe: Quinidine, quinine
     - Artesunate (CDC)
     - Artemether and lumefantrine (IV not available in U.S.)

Malaria Chemoprophylaxis

Drug	Use	Dose	Start/End	Pros	Cons
Chloroquine	Chloroquine sensitive	500 mg (salt) q week	1–2 weeks/ 4 weeks	Cheap Easy dosing	Resistance prevalent
Mefloquine	Chloroquine resistant	250 mg (salt) q week	2 weeks/ 4 weeks	Easy dosing	Resistance in SE Asia
Atovaquone/ Proguanil	Choloruine resistant	250/100 mg q day	1–2 days/ 7 days	Short course Few side effects	Daily dosing ≠ pregnancy
Doxycycline	Cholorquine resistant	100 mg q day	1–2 days/ 4 weeks	Cheap	Daily dosing ≠ pregnancy Sun sens.
Primaquine	*P. vivax* *P. ovale*	52.6 mg salt q day	Upon return/ 14 days	Prevents late disease onset	G6PD ≠ pregnancy

Hill DR (IDSA). *Clin Infect Dis.* 2006; 43:1499.
Freedman DO. *NEJM.* 2008; 359:603.

AR 28 — Key Points
- Know the findings on a malarial smear that are specific for *P. falciparum*
- Know the general distribution of *P. falciparum* chloroquine resistance
- Know the WHO recommendations for the treatment of *P. falciparum* malaria
- Know when treatment with primaquine is indicated
- Know the regimens for prevention of malaria in travelers

AR 29A — History and Physical
Hx: A 34-year-old woman is brought in by her family after she suffered a generalized tonic-clonic seizure 2 hours ago at home. She has never had a prior seizure and is otherwise healthy. She emigrated from Mexico 9 years ago.
PE: VS normal
Slightly confused without focal neurologic deficit
Rest of the exam normal

AR 29A — CT Head

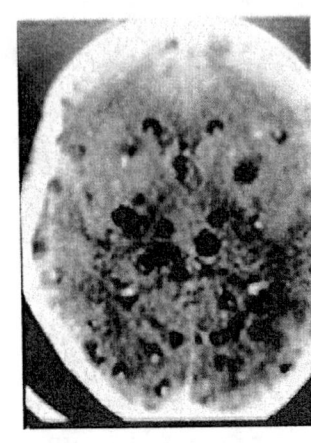

AR 29A (cont.)
What test would you do next?
A. Serum antibody assay
B. CSF antibody assay
C. Brain biopsy
D. Stool for ova and parasites
E. No test needed prior to treatment

Answer: _____

AR 29B
In addition to antiseizure medication, what additional treatment would you give her?
A. Praziquantel
B. Praziquantel and glucocorticoids
C. Albendazole
D. Albendazole and glucocorticoids
E. No antimicrobial treatment needed

Answer: _____

Global Distribution of *Taenia solium* Cysticercosis/Taeniosis

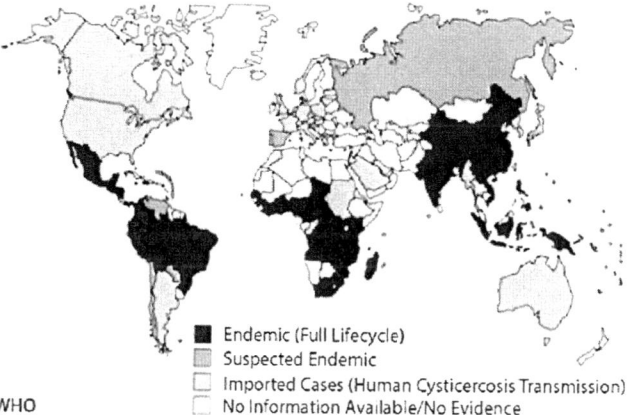

■ Endemic (Full Lifecycle)
▨ Suspected Endemic
▢ Imported Cases (Human Cysticercosis Transmission)
▢ No Information Available/No Evidence
WHO

T. solium — Tapeworm Cycle
- Tapeworm (human) → fecal eggs
- Eggs ingested by pigs
- Eggs release oncospheres in pig gut
- Oncospheres → muscle cysticerci
- Humans eat undercooked pork (oncospheres)
- Cysticerci develop into tapeworm
- Treatment: Praziquantel

T. solium — Cysticercus Cycle
- Human ingests eggs
- Eggs release oncospheres in human gut
- Oncospheres → cysticerci
  - Muscle
  - Brain
- Life cycle ends

Neurocysticercosis
- Clinical manifestations
  - Intraparenchymal: Seizures
  - Extraparenchymal: Hydrocephalus
- Diagnosis
  - Tapeworm: Ova and parasites
  - Neurocysticercosis
    - Imaging
    - Serology if needed
- Treatment
  - Albendazole x 3–14 d **and** steroids

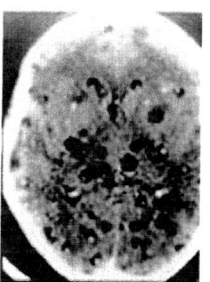

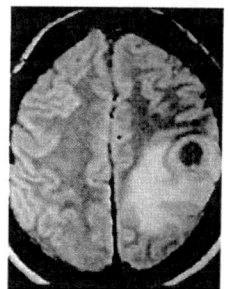

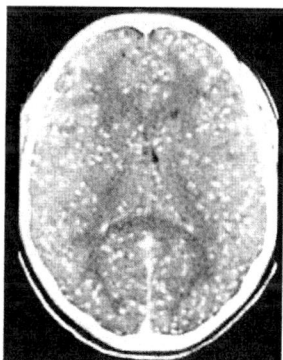

AR 29 — Key Points
- Understand the *Taenia* life cycle and the 2 outcomes of infection in humans
- Recognize the clinical presentation of neurocysticercosis in a patient from an endemic area
- Know that neuroimaging, when classic, is diagnostic of neurocysticercosis
- Know the indications for treatment and the drugs of choice for neurocysticercosis

AR 30 — History and Physical

Hx: A 22-year-old man presents to your clinic with a painful, itchy eruption on his penis for 2 days.
He has an unmeasured fever, body aches, headache, and burning with urination for 1 day. He has a new female sex partner who has a history of gonorrhea in the past.
He has no history of sexually transmitted diseases.
He has no trouble with medication compliance.

PE:

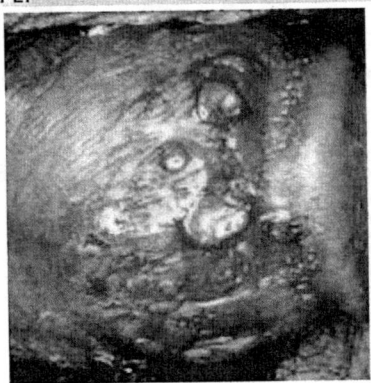

AR 30 (cont.)

You send vesicular fluid for HSV PCR. What next?

A. PO acyclovir
B. PO famciclovir
C. PO valacyclovir
D. No antiviral therapy needed

Answer: _____

Herpes Simplex Treatment

- Primary infection
  - Who to treat
    - Lesions < 72 hours
    - Immunocompromised
  - How long to treat
    - 7–10 days

Cost of Drugs to Treat HSV for 10 Days

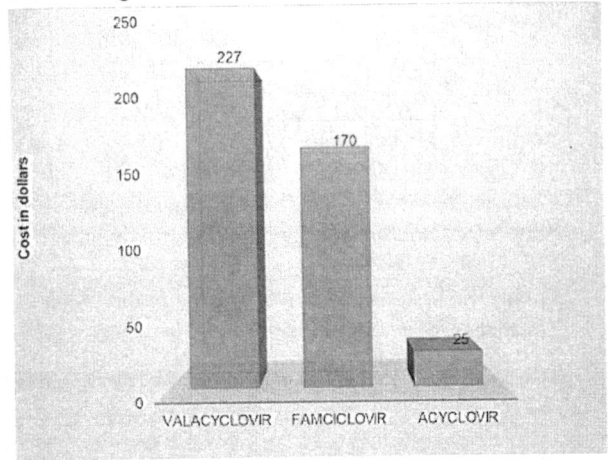

Herpes Simplex Treatment (cont.)

- Recurrences
  - Who to treat
    - Lesions < 48 hours
    - Severe symptoms
  - How long to treat
    - 5 days

- Suppressive Rx for recurrent
  - Who to treat
    - $\geq$ 6 x per year
    - EM, eczema herpeticum, aseptic meningitis
  - How to treat
    - Daily low dose

AR 30 — Key Points

- Recognize primary genital herpes simplex infection
- Recognize the utility of culture or PCR to identify which serotype is present
- Know the clinical scenarios in which treatment of genital herpes is of benefit
- Know the most cost-effective treatment of genital herpes

AR 31 — History and Physical

Hx: A 40-year-old woman is brought in by her husband because of 4 days of fever and 1 day of confusion and trouble talking. She is otherwise healthy and on no medications. He knows of no substance abuse.

PE: T 100.6° F (38.1° C), BP 120/82, PR 100, RR 16
Confused, oriented only to name
Expressive aphasia
Right homonymous hemianopia
No other abnormal neurologic findings

AR 31 — CSF and Image

CSF:
Slightly cloudy
WBC $112/mm^3$,
               40% neutrophils
               60% lymphocytes
RBC $1,200/mm^3$
Protein 80 mg/dL
Glucose 82 mg/dL

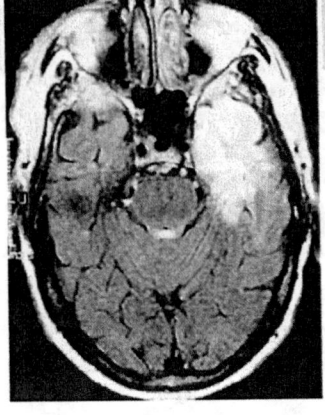

AR 31 (cont.)
IV acyclovir is started. What would you do next?
A. Send CSF for viral PCR.
B. Send CSF for viral antibody.
C. Send CSF for viral culture.
D. Obtain brain biopsy for viral culture.

Answer: _____

CSF HSV-1 PCR vs. Brain Biopsy Viral Culture

	Brain Biopsy Culture	
Author	HSV (+)	HSV (−)
Aurelius[1]	42/43 (98)	0/60
Lakeman[2]	53/54 (98)	3/47 (6)
Total	95/97 (98)	3/107 (3)

[1]*Lancet*. 1991;337:189.
[2]*JID*. 1995;171:857.

AR 31 — Key Points
- Recognize the clinical presentation of herpes simplex encephalitis
- Know the appropriate diagnostic tests for herpes simplex encephalitis
- Know how to treat herpes simplex encephalitis

AR 32 — History and Physical
Hx: A 30-year-old homeless woman presents to the ED with a 5-day history of rash and pain on her right side above her right hip. She intermittently comes to your student-run free clinic. She has a history of prostitution, which led to HIV antibody testing 2 months ago; it was negative. She denies any shortness of breath, chest pain, abdominal pain, nausea, or vomiting. She has no significant past medical history.
PE: VS normal
Neuro, lung, heart, abdominal exam normal
Skin exam (below)

AR 32 — Skin Exam

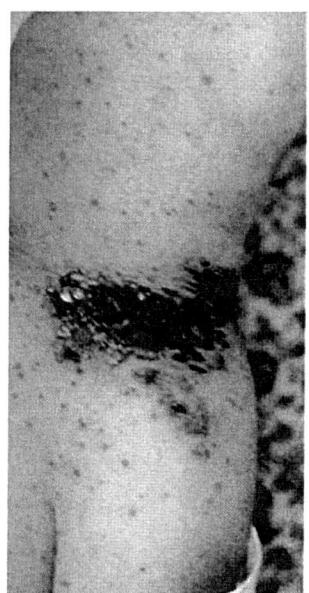

What would you do next?
A. Start high-dose acyclovir.
B. Start high-dose acyclovir and prednisone.
C. Start high-dose acyclovir, prednisone, and amitriptyline.
D. Observe without antiviral therapy.

Answer: _____

Varicella-Zoster Virus (VZV)
- Treatment
  - Immunocompetent
    - If > 50 yo and < 72 h
    - Disseminated
      - 3 dermatomes or
      - 30 lesions outside of primary dermatomes
  - Immunocompromised: All
  - Steroids and TCAs have no role
- Prevention
  - Zoster vaccine if > 50 (regardless of history)

Zoster Vaccine Trial
RDPCT of 38,546 adults ≥ 60, median f/u = 3.1 yrs

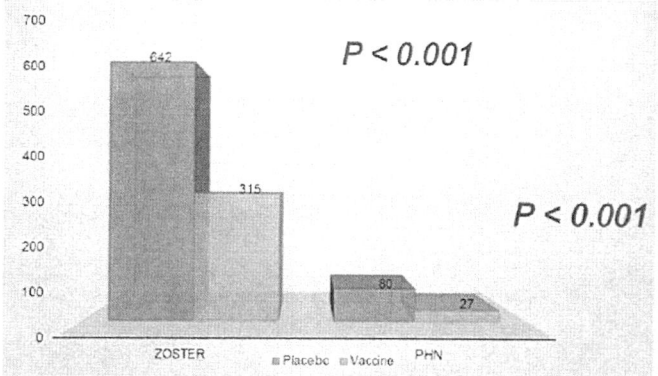

Oxman MN. *NEJM*. 2005;352:2271–2284.

Zoster Vaccine Trial
RDPCT of 22,439 adults 50–59, mean f/u = 1.1 yrs

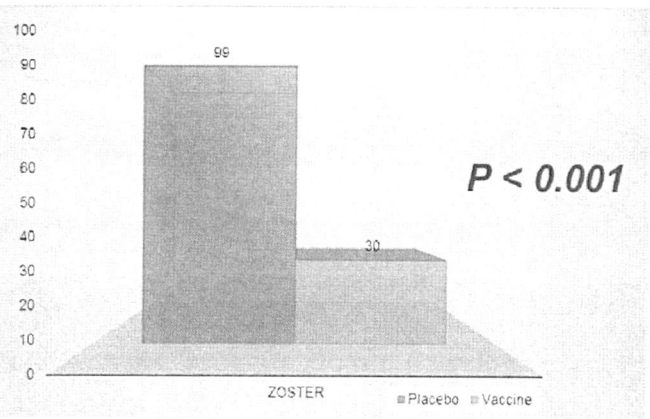

Schmader KE. *Clin Infect Dis. 2012*;54:922–928.

AR 32 — Key Points
- Make a clinical diagnosis of herpes zoster
- Recognize disseminated herpes zoster in an immunocompetent host
- Know when antiviral treatment for herpes zoster is beneficial
- Know that glucocorticoids and tricyclic antidepressants are not useful in acute zoster
- Know the indications for zoster vaccine

AR 33 — History and Physical
Hx: A 16-year-old high school student is seen in the student health center with 3 days of a sore throat, fever to 102.2° F (39.0° C), and fatigue. She is otherwise healthy and has had all required immunizations.
Her 2 older brothers and her parents are well at home. She has had 2 boyfriends in the last 18 months but denies sexual intercourse with either of them. Her only medication is an oral contraceptive.
PE: T 101.8° F (38.8° C), HR 110, RR 12, BP 110/75
Throat (below)
Posterior cervical adenopathy
Palpable spleen tip

AR 33 — Throat Exam

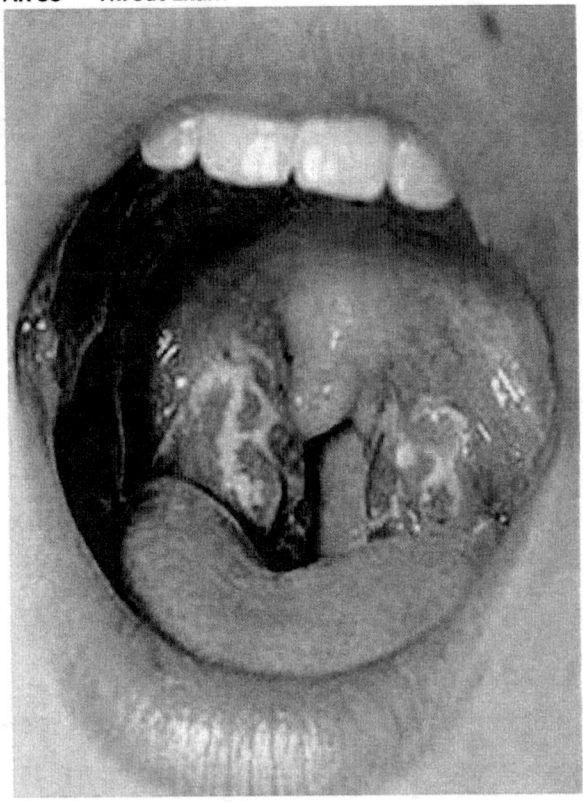

AR 33 — Labs
CBC:
  Hb = 15.1 g/dL
  WBC = 14,800/mm^3, 35% neutrophils, 50% lymphocytes (12% atypical), 10% monocytes
  Platelets = 150,000/mm^3
Group A strep rapid Ag (−)
Heterophile antibody (−)

Which of the following is likely to make an etiologic diagnosis?
A. EBV IgM capsid antibody
B. CMV IgM antibody
C. Toxoplasma IgM antibody
D. HIV antibody
E. HIV viral load

Answer: _____

Exudative Pharyngitis
- Bacterial
  - *Streptococcus* group A*, C, G
  - *Corynebacterium diphtheriae**
  - *Arcanobacterium haemolyticum*
  - Vincent's angina
  - (*Yersinia enterocolitica*)
  - (*Francisella tularensis*)
  - *Neisseria gonorrhoeae**
- Viral
  - Adenovirus (Types 3, 4, 7, 14, 21)
  - Epstein-Barr virus
  - (Herpes simplex virus*)

*Treatment is of proven benefit.

AR 33 — Key Points
- Recognize the clinical presentation of acute Epstein-Barr virus (EBV) infection (acute mononucleosis) in an adolescent
- Know the operating characteristics of heterophile antibody testing in the setting of acute mononucleosis
- Know what are the likely pathogens that cause heterophile antibody negative acute mononucleosis
- Know that EBV is the most common cause of heterophile antibody negative acute mononucleosis with exudative pharyngitis

AR 34A — History and Physical
Hx: A 24-year-old woman presents with progressive dyspnea on exertion over the last 3 days. She has HbSS sickle cell disease and has about 1 pain crisis per year. She has had a low-grade fever and bilateral small joint pains for about a week. She denies rash, cough, or chest pain.

PE: T 101.3° F (38.5° C), HR 120, RR 22, BP 100/68
Alert and slightly short of breath at rest
Conjunctiva pale
Lungs clear, heart with 2/6 SEM over pulmonic area
Abd benign, no hepatosplenomegaly
Fingers, wrists, and ankles with pain on ROM, no swelling

AR 34A — Labs and Image
CBC:
Hb = 4.2 g/dL, MCV 84 fL, Retic index = 0.3%
WBC = 4,800/mm^3 75% neutrophils, 12% lymphocytes, 5% monocytes
Platelets = 150,000/mm^3
Bone marrow aspiration:
    Normal white cell and platelet maturation;
    red cell arrest
Chest x-ray normal

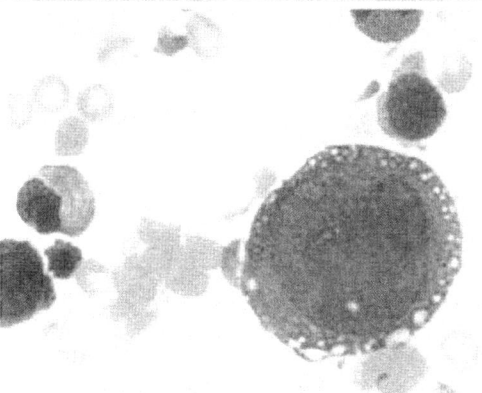

Marrow aspirate

AR 34A
What other testing would you do?
A.   Bone marrow culture
B.   Chest CT
C.   *Borrelia* serologies
D.   Fungal serologies
E.   Pregnancy test

Answer: _____

AR 34B
In addition to PRBC transfusions, what else would you administer?
A.   Intravenous immunoglobulin
B.   Acyclovir
C.   Ganciclovir
D.   Ribavirin
E.   Nothing

Answer: _____

Parvovirus — Lacy Rash on Trunk

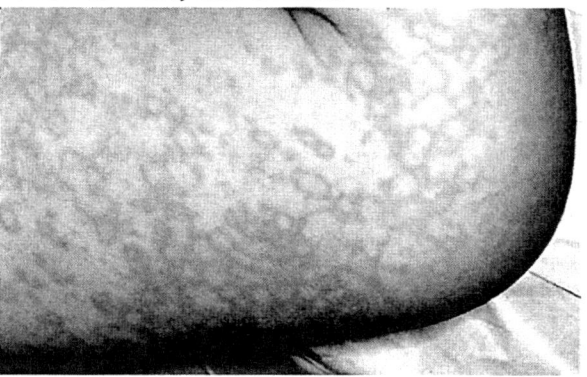

Parvovirus B19 — Troublesome Hosts
- Pregnant women
  - Fetal loss
  - Hydrops fetalis
- Hemoglobinopathies
  - Self-limited aplastic anemia
  - Support with transfusions
- Immunosuppressed (HIV, Txpl, CVI)
  - Prolonged aplastic anemia
  - Treat with intravenous immunoglobulin

AR 34 — Key Points
- Recognize the clinical manifestations of acute parvovirus infection
- Recognize the potential consequences of parvovirus infection in pregnancy
- Recognize hosts that are susceptible to aplastic anemia and how to treat them

AR 35 — History and Physical
Hx: A 27-year-old man presents with fever and severe headache and myalgias for 1 day. He is a medical student who returned 4 days ago from a trip to the Dominican Republic as part of the school's international medicine program. He took mefloquine for malaria prophylaxis.

PE: T 103.1° F (39.5° C), HR 90, RR 20, BP 90/68
Alert but in pain from his head and muscle aches
Neck supple
Lungs, heart, and abdomen benign
Fine petechial rash all over (below)

AR 35 — Leg Rash

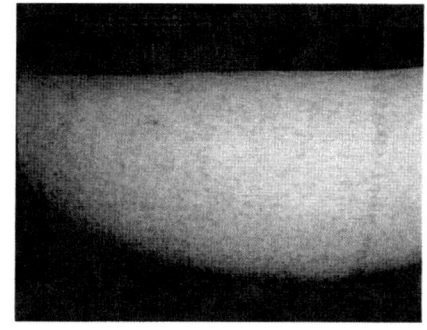

AR 35 — Labs
CBC:
  Hb 16.1 g/dL
  WBC 2,800/mm^3, neutrophils 82%, bands 8%,
  monocytes 5%
  Platelets 28,000/mm^3
Creat 2.4 mg/dL
AST 85 U/L, ALT 92 U/L
Alk phos normal, T bili 1.1 mg/dL
U/A: 2+ ptn, RBC 8/hpf
  WBC 2/hpf

What test is likely to confirm your diagnosis?
A. Skin biopsy for rickettsial fluorescent Ab
B. Blood malarial smear
C. Blood for bacterial culture
D. Blood for viral culture
E. Blood for viral serology

Answer: _____

Dengue Fever

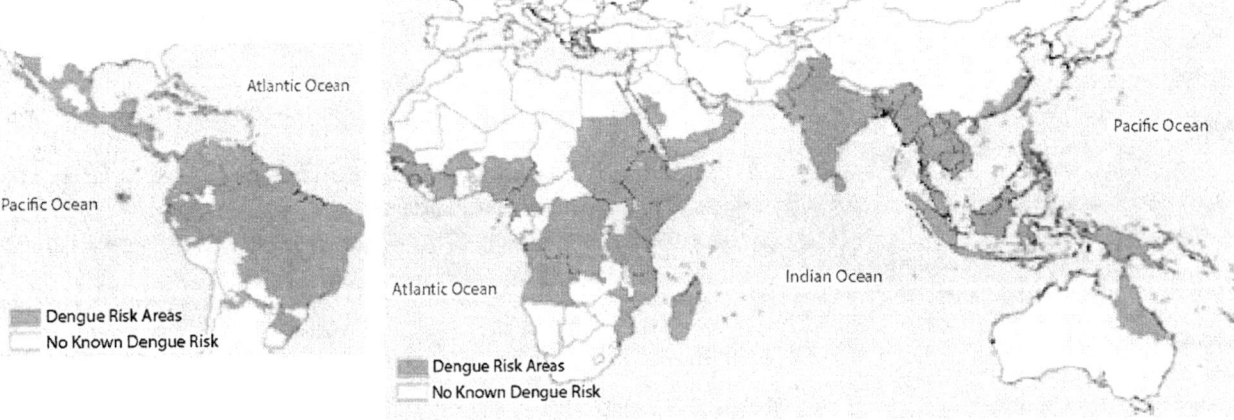

CDC

Dengue Fever (cont.)
- Epidemiology and pathogenesis
  - Most common mosquito-borne viral disease
    (*Aedes* mosquito)
- Classic Dengue fever (4- to 7-day incubation)
  - Severe HA, muscle and joint pains, fever
  - Hemorrhagic manifestations in 10–20%
    (epistaxis, petechiae, purpura, melena)
  - Self-limited ~ 7 days
- Dengue hemorrhagic fever
  - Capillary leak syndrome: Multiple hemorrhagic sites
    with shock
- Diagnosis
  - Serology
  - PCR (through CDC)

- Treatment
  - Support fluid status
  - Platelets only if < 10,000 and active bleed

AR 35 — Key Points
- Recognize the classic presentation of Dengue
  in a person recently visiting an endemic area
- Know the diagnostic test of choice for Dengue fever
- Know the treatment of Dengue

© 2017 MedStudy Internal Medicine Video Board Review – Infectious Disease • Fred A. Zar, MD

Ebola 2014

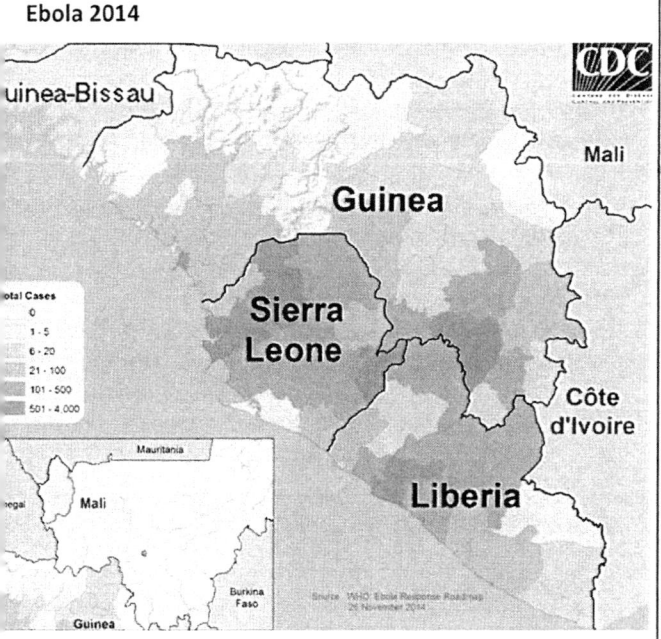

Zika 2017
- Microbiology
  - *Aedes*-mosquito–borne Flavivirus
    - ~ Dengue, Ebola, yellow fever
- Clinical manifestations
  - 80% of infections are asymptomatic
  - 2–12 days of incubation
  - Milder than Dengue, Ebola
    - Low fever, MP rash, mild distal arthralgias, nonpurulent conjunctivitis
    - Never hemorrhagic fever
    - Fetal: Microcephaly, CNS calcifications

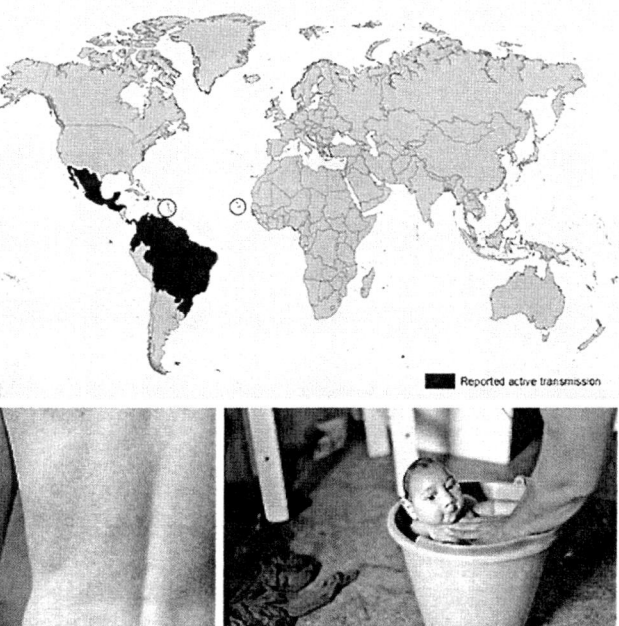

AR 36 — History and Physical

Hx: A 33-year-old man presents to your office in December with a 4-day history of acute onset of fever and cough. He denies shortness of breath or pleuritic chest pain. He is an otherwise healthy math teacher at a local high school. Influenza A has been diagnosed in 3 of his students.
PE: T 101.5° F (38.6° C), HR 106,
RR 20, BP 110/78
Alert and oriented
Lung and heart exams normal

AR 36 — Labs and Image
CBC:
  Hb 15.1 g/dL
  WBC 8,800/mm^3
      neutrophils 74%, lymphs 15%,
      monocytes 4%
  Platelets 328,000/mm^3
Chest x-ray normal

What would you do now?
A. Nasopharyngeal swab for rapid Ag testing for influenza.
B. Nasopharyngeal swab for PCR testing for influenza.
C. No testing, treat with oseltamivir.
D. Neither test nor treat with oseltamivir.

Answer: _____

Epidemic Influenza
- Epidemiology and pathogenesis
  - Highly contagious, winter months in North America
- Clinical manifestations
  - Acute fever and cough during seasonal disease (80% PPV)
- Testing
  - Immunoassays: (60% sens, 98% spec)
  - PCR: (> 90% sens and spec)
- Who to test
  - Immunocompetent at risk for severe disease
  - Immunocompromised
  - Inpatients with acute febrile resp. disease

Advisory Committee on Immunization Practices (ACIP). *MMWR*. 2012;61(32):613.

Influenza Treatment and Prevention
- Who to treat
  - Hospitalized
  - Lower respiratory tract disease
  - At risk for severe disease
    - LTCF residents
    - ≥ 65 years old
    - Pregnant
    - COPD, CHF, CA, CKD, CLD
    - DM
    - Sickle cell disease
    - Immunosuppressed
    - Trouble with secretions
    - Native American, Alaskan
    - BMI ≥ 40
- How to treat
  - Neuraminidase inhibitor
    - Oseltamivir PO
    - Zanamivir inhaler
  - **Give within 48 h**
- Influenza vaccine
  - Annually > 6 mo old[1]
  - Inactivated only
  - High-dose vaccine?
    - ≥ 65
    - Statin use

[1]Advisory Committee on Immunization Practices (ACIP). *MMWR.* 2012;61(32):613.

Neuraminidase Inhibitors in Hospitalized Patients with H1N1
- The study
  - Meta-analysis of 90 studies; 58,422 pts
  - Early Rx = Within 48 hours of 1st symptom
- The results

	Mortality OR (95% CI)
NAI vs. no NAI	0.72 (0.51–1.01)
Early NAI vs. late NAI	0.38 (0.27-0.53)
Early NAI vs. no NAI	0.35 (0.21–1.71)

Muthuri SG. *J Infect Dis.* 207:553–63, 2013.

Neuraminidase Inhibitors in Hospitalized Patients with H1N1
- The study
  - Meta-analysis of 78 studies; 59,234 pts
  - Early Rx = Within 48 hours of 1st symptom
- The results

	Mortality OR (95% CI)
NAI vs. no NAI	0.81 (0.70-0.93)
Early NAI vs. late NAI	0.48 (0.41–0.56)
Early NAI vs. no NAI	0.50 (0.37–0.67)

Muthuri SG. *Lancet Respir Med.* 2:395, 2014.

AR 36 — Key Points
- Recognize an influenza-like illness in the setting of an influenza epidemic
- Know the operating characteristics of clinical impression and various diagnostic tests for influenza
- Know in which clinical setting specific tests for influenza virus are useful
- Know who to treat for influenza

AR 37A — History and Physical
Hx: A 28-year-old woman comes to you because she has been found to be HIV antibody (+) last week. She has been a sex worker for 8 years and has never been tested before. She has unintentionally lost 15 pounds over the last 2 years and currently weighs 100 pounds.
PE: VS normal
Exam completely normal

AR 37A — Labs
CBC:
　Hb 9.1 mg/dL, MCV 88 fL
　WBC 3,800/mm³,
　　　neutrophils 87%, lymphocytes 5%
　　　monocytes 4%
　Platelets 178,000/mm³
CD4 count 38/mm³
Interferon gamma release assay (−)
Chest x-ray normal

If genotypic sensitivity testing permits, which antiretroviral therapy would you start?
A. 3 nucleoside reverse transcriptase inhibitors (NRTIs)
B. 2 NRTIs and an integrase inhibitor
C. An NRTI, an rPI, and a nonnucleoside reverse transcriptase inhibitor (NNRTI)
D. An NRTI, an rPI, and an integrase inhibitor

Answer: _____

Treatment of HIV Infection[1,2]
- Who to treat
  - Everyone
- Initial genotypic resistance testing
  - Everyone
- What to start
  - 2 NRTIs + integrase inhibitor
    - Emtricitabine + tenofovir + any integrase inhibitor
    - Abacavir + lamivudine + dolutegravir **(test for HLA B*5701)**
  - 2 NRTIs plus a boosted protease inhibitor
    - Emtricitabine + tenofovir + darunavir/ritonavir

[1] Panel on Antiretroviral Guidelines for Adults and Adolescents. Guidelines for the use of antiretroviral agents in HIV-1-infected Adults http://www.aidsinfo.nih.gov/ContentFiles/AdultandAdolescentGL.pdf .

[2] International Antiviral Society–USA Panel. *JAMA.* 2016;316(2):191-210.

Antiretroviral Drugs 2017

- NRTIs
  - Abacavir
  - Didanosine
  - Emtricitabine
  - Lamivudine
  - Stavudine
  - Tenofovir
  - Zidovudine
- NNRTIs
  - Delavirdine
  - Efavirenz
  - Etravirine
  - Nevirapine
  - Rilpivirine

NRTIs = Nucleoside reverse transcriptase inhibitors
NNRTIs = Nonnucleoside reverse transcriptase inhibitors

- PIs
  - Atazanavir
  - Darunavir
  - Fosamprenavir
  - Indinavir
  - Lopinavir
  - Nelfinavir
  - Ritonavir
  - Saquinavir
  - Tipranavir
- P450 Inhibitor
  - Cobicistat
- Fusion Inhibitors/CCR5 antag
  - Enfuvirtide
  - Maraviroc
- Integrase Inhibitors
  - Elvitegravir
  - Dolutegravir
  - Raltegravir

PIs = Protease inhibitors

Antiretroviral Fixed-Dose Combinations 2017

- Abacavir-lamivudine
- Abacavir-lamivudine-zidovudine
- Efavirenz-tenofovir-emtricitabine
- Elvitegravir-cobicistat-tenofovir-emtricitabine
- Tenofovir-emtricitabine
- Rilpivirine-emtricitabine-tenofovir
- Zidovudine-lamivudine
- Dolutegravir-abacavir-lamivudine

AR 37B

What antimicrobials should be given to prevent opportunistic infections?
A. Trim/sulfa and azithromycin
B. Trim/sulfa, azithromycin, and fluconazole
C. Trim/sulfa, azithromycin, and valganciclovir
D. Trim/sulfa, azithromycin, fluconazole, and valganciclovir

Answer: _____

HIV — 1° Prophylaxis of Opportunistic Infections

Infection	Trigger	Regimen
Pneumocystis	CD4 < 200	T/S DS daily or tiw
Toxoplasmosis	CD4 < 100 + serology	T/S DS daily
MAC	CD4 < 50	Azithromycin q wk
Tuberculosis	TST > 5 mm or IGRA (+)	INH x 9 mos

HIV Preexposure Prophylaxis

- The studies
  - Used tenofovir-emtricitabine daily for 1 month vs. placebo
- The results
  - Decreased rates of transmission
    - 45% in MSM[1]
    - 62% in heterosexual high risk (Botswana)[2]
    - 67% in discordant heterosexual couples[3]
- The consequences
  - FDA approves tenofovir-emtricitabine for preexposure prophylaxis in HIV (–) persons at risk[4]:
    - Infected partner, recent STI, multiple partners, no condoms, sex worker
    - ≤ 90-day supply, check HIV status before renewal

[1]*NEJM.* 2010;363:2587. [2]*NEJM.* 2012;367:423.
[3]*NEJM.* 2012;367:399. [4]USPHS Clinical Practice Guideline 2014.

Preexposure Prophylaxis

- Who to offer to:
  - Background incidence > 2%
  - Recent STI Dx
  - Postexposure prophylaxis given > 1 in last year
  - IVDU and sharing needles
- What to offer:
  - Emtricitabine and tenofovir
  - Counseling!

International Antiviral Society-USA Panel. *JAMA.* 2014;312:390-409.

HCW Postexposure Prophylaxis

- If the answer is <u>yes</u> to these 2 questions, then give postexposure prophylaxis
  1) Is the fluid bloody?
  2) Is the skin integrity compromised?
- Insignificant exposures
  - Urine, skin intact

HCW Postexposure Prophylaxis (cont.)
- What to give?
  - If known HIV (+) source, base on resistance if known
  - Three drugs for 4 weeks
    - Emtricitabine + tenofovir + raltegravir
- Test for HIV at 0, 6, and 16 wks
Kuhar DT. *ICHE.* 34:875–92, 2013.

Other Postexposure Prophylaxis
- Who to give it to:
  - Exposure of: Mucosa, nonintact skin, percutaneous
  - From: Blood/Bloody fluid, semen, vaginal/anal secretions, breast milk
  - Occurred in < 72 hours
  - Known or suspected HIV in source patient
- What to give:
  - Emtricitabine and tenofovir and raltegravir or dolutegravir
  - Give for 28 days
- How to follow:
  - Test for HIV Ag/Ab
    - Baseline, 4–6 wks, 3 mo, 6 mo
  - Test for syphilis, gonorrhea, *Chlamydia*
  - Test for pregnancy
CDC: *Updated Guidelines for Antiretroviral Postexposure Prophylaxis After Sexual, Injection Drug Use, or Other Nonoccupational Exposure to HIV—United States.* 2016.

AR 37C
Her brother has accompanied her and asks if he should be tested. He is 18 and has been sexually active with 3 women. He denies STIs (or known STIs in his partners) and IVDU.

What HIV screening, if any, should you do?
A. No testing indicated.
B. Test him once now.
C. Test him once now and repeat if new partner.
D. Test him once now and repeat every year.

Answer: _____

HIV — Screening
- Risk stratification
  - High risk
    - IVDU, MSM, STI diagnosis, STI testing
  - Risk
    - Unprotected intercourse, partners at risk, sex for drugs/money
  - No risk
    - Not sexually active, monogamous (−) partner
- Screening recommendation
  - High risk: ≤ 12 mo[1] or 3–6 mo[2]
  - Risk: At least once as adults (15–65[1])
  - No risk: No screening unless pregnant[1]
[1]USPSTF *Annals Intern Med.* 2013;159:51–60.
[2]International Antiviral Society-USA Panel.
  JAMA. 2014;312:390–409.

AR 37 — Key Points
- Know when to treat antiretroviral naïve HIV-infected persons
- Know how to select an initial antiretroviral regimen
- Know the groups that may benefit from preexposure prophylaxis
- Know the approach to a needlestick sustained by a health care worker
- Know who should be screened for HIV

AR 38 — History and Physical
Hx: A 34-year-old man presents to the ED with 2 weeks of slowly worsening shortness of breath, low-grade fever, and cough. He has had HIV infection for 12 years and has intermittently been on antiretrovirals. He had Stevens-Johnson syndrome after receiving trim/sulfa 10 years ago for a prior pneumonia.
PE: T 100.2° F (37.9° C), PR 94, RR 20, BP 128/78
Alert, oriented, and in moderate respiratory distress
Lungs with bilateral diffuse crackles, no signs of consolidation
Rest of the exam normal

AR 38 — Labs and Image
CBC:
  HB 9.8 g/dL
  WBC 7,600/mm^3
      88% neutrophils
      6% lymphocytes
  Platelets 178,000/mm^3
ABG on room air
  pO$_2$ 59 mmHg, pCO$_2$ 20 mmHg
  pH 7.56
Chest x-ray

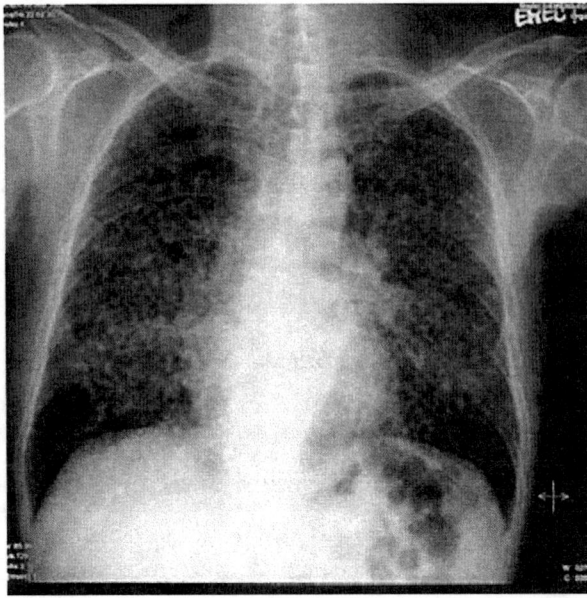

© 2017 MedStudy Internal Medicine Video Board Review – Infectious Disease • Fred A. Zar, MD

AR 38 — Induced Sputum

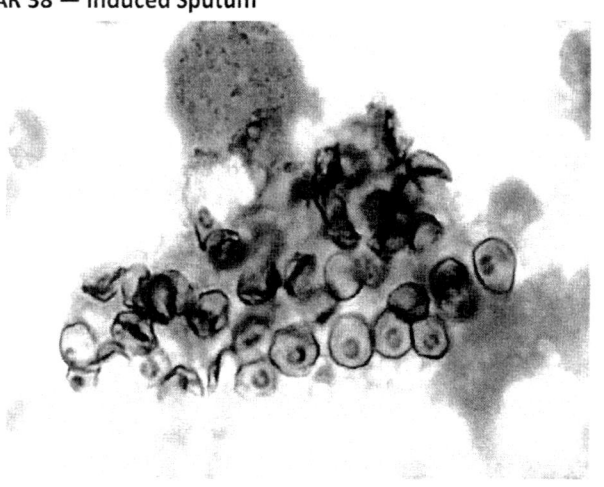

AR 38

In addition to oxygen, what else would you give?
A. Atovaquone
B. Atovaquone and prednisone
C. Pentamidine
D. Pentamidine and prednisone

Answer: _____

Pneumocystis jiroveci — An Odd Bug
- Looks like a protozoon
- Genetically a fungus
- Killed by antibacterials and antiprotozoal agents, but not antifungals

Severity of *Pneumocystis* Pneumonia
(Determines antibiotic and need for steroids)

Severity	pO_2	A-a Gradient
Mild	> 70	< 35
Moderate	60–70	35–45
Severe	< 60	> 45

Guidelines for the Prevention and Treatment of Opportunistic Infections in HIV-Infected Adults and Adolescents. *MMWR.* 58 (RR-4):1–216, 2009.

Treatment of *Pneumocystis* Pneumonia
- <u>Mild-to-moderate</u>
  - T/S 2 DS bid x 21 d
  - 2nd line
    - Atovaquone
    - Clindamycin + primaquine
- <u>Severe</u>
  - T/S IV 5 mg/kg q 8 h
  - 2nd line
    - Pentamidine
- <u>Steroids</u>
  - If P_aO_2 is less than 70 mmHg or A-a gradient > 35

AR 38 — Key Points
- Know the clinical presentation of *Pneumocystis jiroveci* pneumonia (PJP; formerly PCP)
- Know the appropriate treatment for PJP based on severity and drug allergies
- Know the indications for adjunctive glucocorticoids in PJP

AR 39A — History and Physical
Hx: A 26-year-old presents with fever, rash, and joint aches. Fever began 4 days ago, followed by bilateral knee pain. This got a little better, but then her ankles, followed by her elbows, became achy. Her husband noticed a rash on her back today. She teaches first grade, and 5 of her students were out over the last month with strep throat. She currently denies a sore throat.
PE: T 100.6° F (38.1° C), PR 90, RR 12, BP 124/74
Alert and oriented
Pharynx normal, no lymphadenopathy
Lungs, heart, abdomen normal
Pain on ROM of knees, ankles, elbows; No effusions
Neuro exam normal
Skin exam (below)

AR 39A — Rash

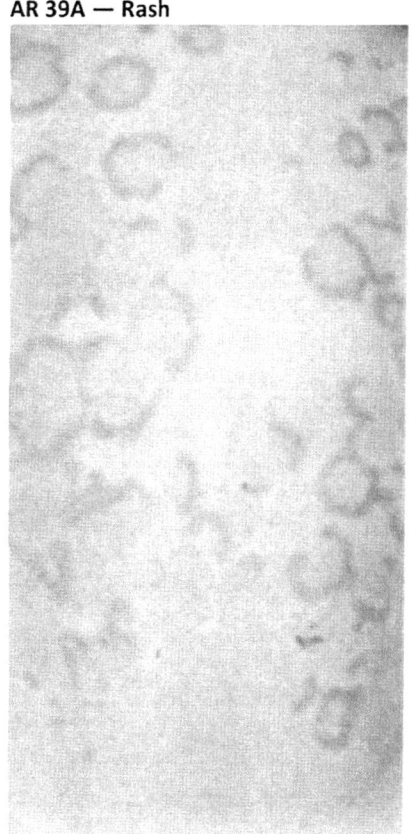

AR 39A (cont.)
What should you diagnostically do next?
A. Echocardiogram
B. Skin biopsy
C. Knee joint aspiration
D. Antistreptolysin O (ASO) antibody titer

Answer: _____

Re-Modified Jones Criteria for Acute Rheumatic Fever
- Diagnostic guidelines
  - Evidence of antecedent group A strep infection
    - (+) Throat culture or rapid Ag, **or**
    - Elevated or rising strep Ab titer, **and**
  - 2 major, ~~+ 1 minor~~, or 1 major and 2 minor criteria
- Major criteria
  - Carditis: Valvulitis, myocarditis **(can be echo only)**
  - Polyarthritis: Migratory, large joints **(mono or arthralgias only, if high risk)**
  - Chorea: (Sydenham's)
  - Erythema marginatum
  - Subcutaneous nodules: Firm, painless, extensor surfaces
- Minor criteria
  - Polyarthralgia **(mono if high risk)**
  - Fever ($\geq$ 38.5° C) **(38.0° C if high risk)**
  - Elevated ESR or CRP
  - Prolonged PR interval

Dajani AS. *JAMA* 1993;268:2069–2073
Gewitz MH. *Circ* 2015;131:1806–1818

AR 39B
- ASO titer is markedly elevated
- An echocardiogram reveals no myocardial or valvular abnormalities
- She receives amoxicillin and aspirin for 10 days, and her symptoms resolve over the next 2 weeks

What duration of antibiotic prophylaxis should be given to prevent recurrences?
A. 5 years
B. 10 years
C. 20 years
D. For life
E. No prophylaxis needed

Answer: _____

Duration of 2° Rheumatic Fever Prophylaxis
- Carditis and residual heart disease
  - 10 years or until 40 (whichever longer)
- Carditis with no residual heart disease
  - 10 years or until 21 (whichever longer)
- No carditis
  - 5 years or until 21 (whichever longer)

Gerber MA. *Circulation.* 2009;119:1541–1551.

AR 39 — Key Points
- Recognize the clinical presentation of rheumatic fever
- Use the modified Jones criteria to confirm the diagnosis
- Know the treatment of an initial episode of rheumatic fever
- Know the appropriate drugs and duration of treatment to prevent recurrences of rheumatic fever

AR 40A — History and Physical
Hx: A 68-year-old comes to the ED with fever for 5 days and no other symptoms. He has a past history HTN, Type 2 DM, and asymptomatic aortic stenosis.
PE: T 101.2° F (38.4° C), PR 98, RR 16, BP 158/98
Alert and oriented
HEENT normal
Heart PMI sustained, 3/6 SEM radiating to carotids
Lungs clear
Abd benign
Extremities show an open ulcer of right heel, nonfoul exudate, does not probe to bone
Skin otherwise normal

AR 40A — Labs, Images, and Course
Labs
 CBC:
  Hb 10.2 g/dL, MCV 86 fL
  WBC 8.8, 84% neutrophils, no bands
  Platelets 298,000/mm^3
Images
 X-ray right foot: No osteomyelitis or gas in tissues
 Chest x-ray: Cardiomegaly, no pulmonary infiltrates
Course
 Started on vancomycin and piperacillin/tazobactam
 Day 2: T 100.8° F (38.2° C)
  3 of 3 blood cultures with gram-positive cocci in clusters

What would you do next?
A. MRI of right heel
B. CT head
C. Lumbar puncture
D. Transthoracic echo
E. Transesophageal echo

Answer: _____

© 2017 MedStudy Internal Medicine Video Board Review – Infectious Disease • Fred A. Zar, MD

Major Criteria for Infectious Endocarditis (IE)
(Need 2 major, 1 major + 3 minor, 5 minor)
- Positive Blood Culture for Endocarditis
  - Typical organism in 2 or more BCs, **or**
    - Viridans strep, *S. bovis*, AACEK, *S. aureus*, **or**
    - Enterococcus, community-acquired, no 1° focus
  - Persistent bacteremia, **or**
    - ≥ 2 BCs, > 12° apart, **or** 3/3 **or** > 50% of > 3, > 1° apart
  - One BC for *Coxiella burnetii* or antiphase IgG Ab > 1:800

Durack DT. *Am J Med*. 1994;96:200–209.
Li JS. *CID*. 2000;30:633–638.

Major Criteria for IE (cont.)
(Need 2 major, 1 major + 3 minor, 5 minor)
- Evidence of Endocardial Involvement
  - Positive echocardiogram, **or**
    - Oscillating mass (unexplained) on valve, or supporting structure or in path of regurgitant jet, or implanted device, **or**
    - Abscess, **or**
    - New prosthetic dehiscence
  - New valvular regurgitation

Durack DT. *Am J Med*. 1994;96:200–209.
Li JS. *CID*. 2000;30:633–638.

Proposed Minor Criteria for IE
(Need 2 major, 1 major + 3 minor, 5 minor)
- Predisposition
  - Endocardial disease or IVDU
- Temperature > 38° C (100.4° F)
- Vascular Phenomena (1 of):
  - Major arterial embolus, septic pulmonary emboli, mycotic aneurysms, intracranial bleed, conjunctival hemorrhages, Janeway lesions (not petechiae/splinters)

Durack DT. *Am J Med*. 1994;96:200–209.
Li JS. *CID*. 2000;30:633–638.

Proposed Minor Criteria for IE (cont.)
(Need 2 major, 1 major + 3 minor, 5 minor)
- Immunologic Phenomena (1 of):
  - Glomerulonephritis, Osler's, Roth's, (+) RhF
- Microbiologic Evidence
  - BC (+) yet not meeting major criteria
  - Seropositive: *Brucella, Chlamydia, Coxiella, Legionella, Bartonella*

Durack DT. *Am J Med*. 1994;96:200–209.
Li JS. *CID*. 2000;30:633–638.

AHA / ACC Algorithm for Echo in Infective Endocarditis

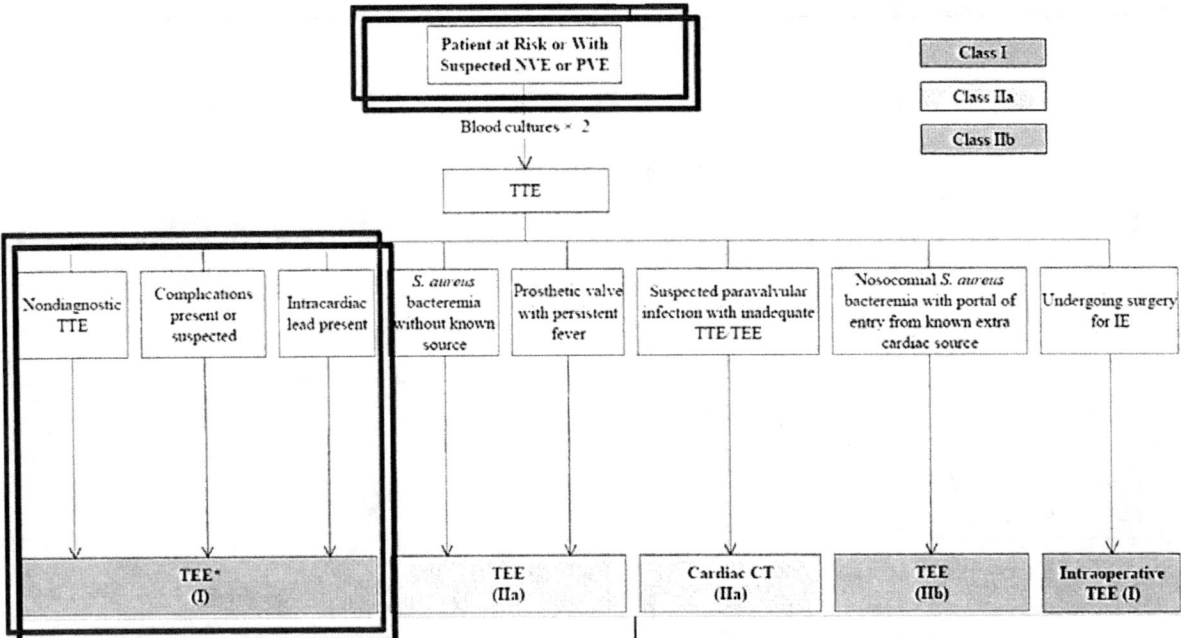

AHA/ACC ePub 3/4/2014 *Circulation*.

Indications for TEE in Infective Endocarditis
- Suspected or known IE and TTE (–)
- Suspected or known complications of IE
  - Abscess
  - Perforation
  - Papillary muscle rupture
- Intravascular device leads

AHA/ACC ePub 3/4/2014 *Circulation*.

AR 40B
- Blood cultures grow methicillin-sensitive *S. aureus*
- Echocardiogram shows a 5-mm vegetation on the left aortic valve cusp

What antibiotic(s) would you give IV for 6 wks?
A. Vancomycin alone
B. Nafcillin alone
C. Nafcillin with gentamicin for the first 3–5 days
D. Nafcillin with gentamicin for the first 2 weeks

Answer: _____

Low-Dose Gentamicin is Nephrotoxic[1]
- The study
  - Review of nephrotoxicity in prior trial of daptomycin vs. standard Rx for staph endocarditis with gent x 4 d[2]
- The results

	Nephrotoxicity
ASPen + gent	16/63 (25)
Vanc + gent	10/46 (22)
Daptomycin	9/120 (8)

[1]Cosgrove SE. *Clin Infect Dis*. 2009;48:713.
[2]Fowler VG. *NEJM*. 2006;355:653.

Cardiac Conditions Requiring Endocarditis Prophylaxis
- **Prosthetic valve**
- **Prior infective endocarditis**
- Congenital heart disease
  - Unrepaired cyanotic disease
  - Repaired cyanotic disease with prosthesis < 6 months
  - Repaired cyanotic disease with residual defects
- **Cardiac valvulopathy S/P cardiac transplantation**

Wilson W. *Circulation*. 2007;115:1736–1754.
Nishimura RA. *Circulation*. 2008;118:887–896.

Procedures Requiring Endocarditis Prophylaxis
- Prophylaxis indicated
  - Dental procedures if:
    - Manipulation of gingiva or periapical
    - Perforation of oral mucosa
  - Respiratory procedures
    - Cutting mucosa
    - Tonsillectomy, bronch and incision
- Prophylaxis **not** indicated
  - All others

Wilson W. *Circulation*. 2007;115:1736–1754.
Nishimura RA. *Circulation*. 2008;118:887–896.

Antibiotic Regimens for Prophylaxis of Endocarditis

Route/Situation	Agent	Regimen*
Oral	Amoxicillin	2 g
NPO	Ampicillin	2 g IM/IV
	Cefazolin	1 g IM/IV
	Ceftriaxone	1 g IM/IV
Pen Allergy		
Oral	Cephalexin	2 g PO
	Clindamycin	600 mg
	Azith/Clarith	500 mg
NPO	Cefazolin/Ceftriaxone	1 g IM/IV
	Clindamycin	600 mg

*1 dose 30–60 minutes before
Nishimura RA. *Circulation*. 2008;118:887–896.

AR 40 — Key Points
- Recognize the potential for endocarditis when there is high-grade bacteremia with a typical endocarditis pathogen
- Know that *S. aureus* usually has large vegetations detectable via TTE
- Know the definitive therapy for *S. aureus* native valve endocarditis
- Know the current recommendations for prophylaxis of endocarditis

AR 41 — History and Physical
Hx: You are consulted from the psychiatry service to evaluate a patient with a urinary tract infection.
She is a 44-year-old woman admitted with suicidal ideation. She admits to recent use of crack cocaine. A urinalysis and drug screen were sent as part of her admission labs. She denies dysuria, frequency, or urgency.
She has no other medical problems.
VS normal
Physical exam normal

AR 41 — Labs
Urine toxicology
   (+) for cocaine and cannabinoids
Urinalysis
   pH 5.5
   Protein negative
   Glucose negative
   Leukocyte esterase 2+
   Nitrites 3+
   WBC 25/hpf
   RBC 3/hpf
   Bacteria moderate
Urine culture
   > 10^5 *E. coli*
Pregnancy test negative

What would you recommend to the psych service?
A. Trimethoprim/sulfamethoxazole x 3 days
B. Levofloxacin x 3 days
C. Nitrofurantoin x 5 days
D. Fosfomycin x 1
E. No treatment at this time

Answer: _____

Treatment of Asymptomatic (+) Urine Cultures

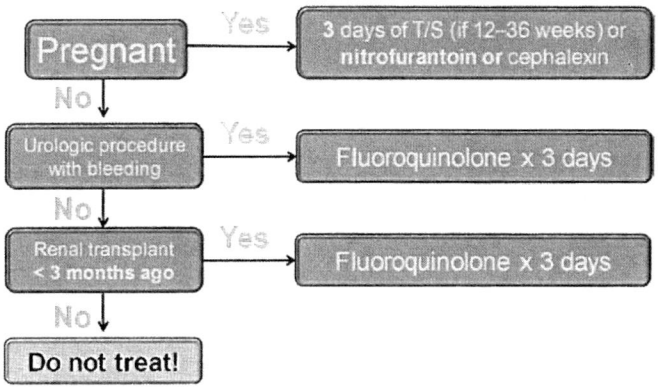

Nicolle L, et al. *CID*. 2005;40(5):643–654.
Lee JR. *Transplantation*. 96:732–738, 2013.

Asymptomatic Bacteruria in Renal Transplant Recipients
- The study
  - 1,166 txpl recipients over 5 years at Cornell
  - Incidence and risk factors for UTI in 1st 3 months
- The results
  - 247 (21%) had a UTI
    - 168 (68%) were asymptomatic

Rx status	HR for rejection	P
Treated (147)	0.92	0.88
Untreated (100)	**2.80**	**0.01**

Lee JR. *Transplantation*. 96:732–738, 2013.

AR 41 — Key Points
- Recognize asymptomatic urinary tract infections
- Know the few indications to treat asymptomatic urinary tract infections
- Know what regimens to use when treatment is indicated

AR 42 — History and Physical
Hx: A 28-year-old woman calls your office with dysuria and frequency x 2 days. She denies fever, abdominal pain, or flank pain. She is an established patient of yours being treated with fluoxetine for depression.
She has never had a urinary tract infection before.
She is sexually active only with her husband of 7 years.
According to the microbiology lab of the hospital in your community, 25% of *E. coli* are resistant to trimethoprim/sulfamethoxazole.

AR 42 (cont.)
What do you recommend to her?
A. Trimethoprim/sulfamethoxazole x 3 days.
B. Levofloxacin x 3 days.
C. Nitrofurantoin x 5 days.
D. Fosfomycin x 1.
E. Come in for a culture prior to treatment.

Answer: _____

Complicated vs. Uncomplicated UTIs
- Definition of complicated UTI
  - Diabetes mellitus
  - Immunocompromised
  - Structural anomaly
  - Foreign body
  - Resistant organism
  - Male
- All others are uncomplicated

Treatment of Symptomatic UTIs

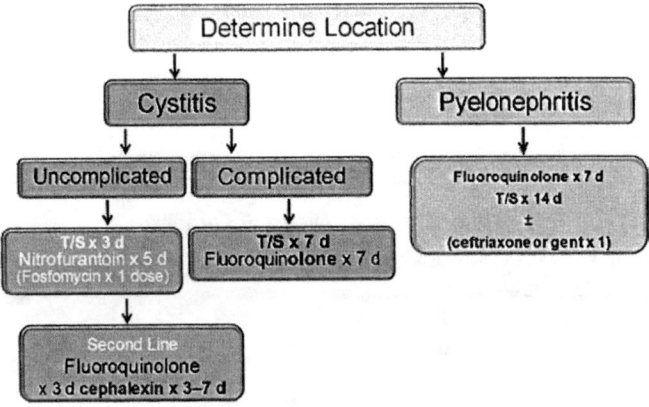

Gupta K. *CID*. 2011;52:561–564.

Caveats about Antibiotics for UTIs
- Trimethoprim/sulfamethoxazole
  - No allergy, no antibiotics or inpatient x 90 d,
    T/S if resistance ≤ 20%
- Nitrofurantoin
  - No suspicion of pyelonephritis
- Fosfomycin use
  - No suspicion of pyelonephritis, less efficacy
- Ceftriaxone or AG use
  - If quinolone resistance ≥ 10%
- β-lactams
  - Routinely less effective than other agents

FDA Warning: Fluoroquinolones
- Side effects
  - Tendinopathy, tendon rupture
  - Myopathy
  - Neuropathy
  - Arthropathy
  - CNS: Insomnia, mood alteration, dizzy

- Only use if no alternative for:
  - Acute sinusitis
  - Exacerbation of COPD
  - Uncomplicated UTI
FDA: Posted July 26, 2016.

AR 42 — Key Points
- Know what constitutes a complicated urinary tract infection
- Know the antibiotics recommended to treat uncomplicated and complicated cystitis
- Know how to use local antibiotic susceptibilities to determine empiric treatment

---

AR 43 — History and Physical
Hx: A 16-year-old boy is brought to the ED complaining of an unmeasured fever and severe headache for 2 days. Yesterday, a rash began on his wrists and ankles that is spreading to his trunk today.
P/E: T 103.0° F (39.4° C), PR 90, RR 20, BP 100/68
In distress from headache
Neck supple and lungs, heart, and abdomen normal
Petechial rash distal extremities (below)

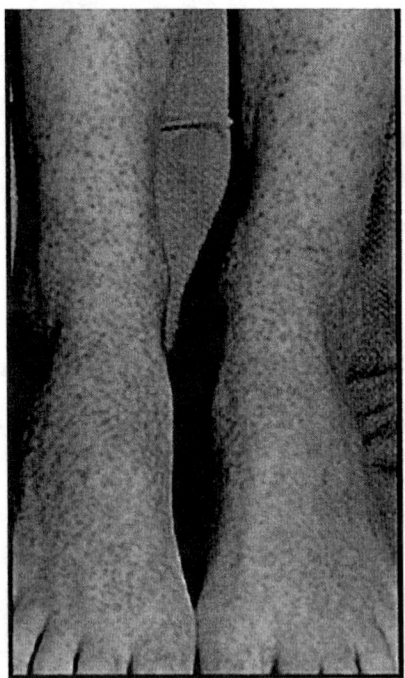

AR 43 — Labs
CBC: Hb 14.8 g/dL, WBC 4,900/mm³
       platelets 96,000/mm³
Lytes: Na⁺ 126 mEq/L, K⁺ 4.9mEq/L,
       Cl⁻ 101mEq/L, HCO₃⁻ 27mEq/L
Glucose 78 mg/dL
U/A: WBC 7/hpf, RBC 44/hpf

What antibiotic(s) would you give?
A. Doxycycline
B. Levofloxacin
C. Vancomycin and piperacillin/tazobactam
D. Vancomycin and ceftriaxone
E. Streptomycin

Answer: _____

Rocky Mountain Spotted Fever — *Rickettsia rickettsii*
- Pathogenesis
  - Transmitted by *Dermacentor variabilis* (dog tick)
  - Infects capillary endothelial cells
- Clinical manifestations
  - Fever and **severe** headache
  - Rash day 3: Maculopapular → petechiae
  - Wrists and ankles → palms, soles → trunk
  - Hyponatremia, thrombocytopenia

Relative Bradycardia
- Definition
  - Temp   Pulse
    - 102°   < 110
    - 103°   < 120
    - 104°   < 130
    - 105°   < 140
    - 106°   < 150
  - Adult
  - Simultaneous
  - Sinus rhythm
  - No beta-blockers
- Etiologies
  - Infectious diseases
    - Viral
      - Dengue, yellow fever
    - Bacterial
      - Brucellosis, legionella*, tularemia mycoplasma, typhoid, leptospira psittacosis, RMSF, typhus, Q fever
    - Malaria
  - Noninfectious diseases
    - Central fever*
    - Drug fever*
    - Tumor fever*
    - Factitious fever*
*Nosocomial causes

RMSF Cases, U.S. 2010, CDC

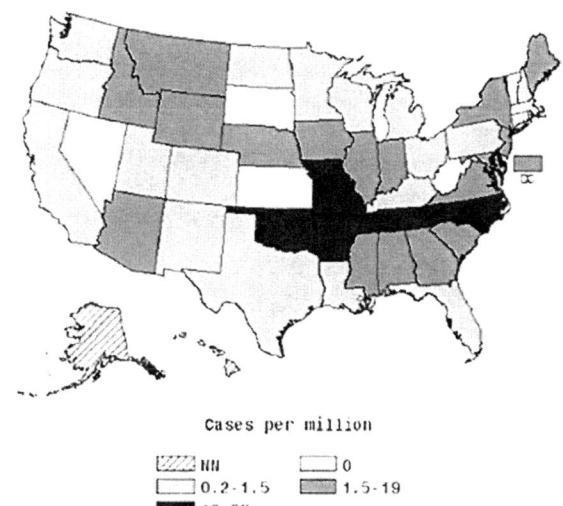

Cases per million

- NN
- 0.2-1.5
- 19-63
- 0
- 1.5-19

RMSF — Diagnosis and Treatment
- Diagnosis
  - Cultures (tissue, blood)
    - Biohazard
    - Too hard, too long
  - Immunohistochemistry
    - Skin Bx (70–90%)
  - Serology
    - IFA: IgM (+) at ~ 7 d, IgG in ≥ 10 d
- Treatment
  - Empiric doxycycline

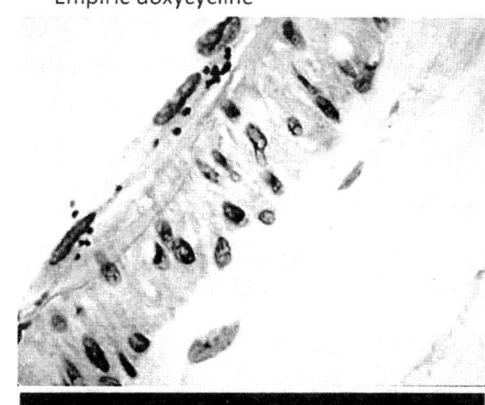

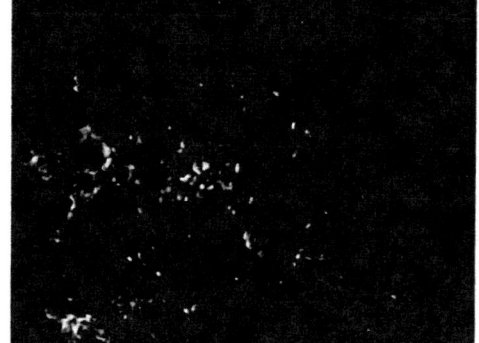

AR 43 — Key Points
- Recognize the clinical presentation of Rocky Mountain spotted fever
- Recognize the importance of empiric antibiotics prior to the microbiologic diagnosis of Rocky Mountain spotted fever
- Be aware of the clinical utility of relative bradycardia

AR 44A — History and Physical
Hx: A 78-year-old woman admitted with an L middle cerebral thrombotic stroke develops fever on day 4.
PE: T 101.0° F (38.3° C), RR 16, PR 100, BP 128/84
Exam normal other than aphasia and R hemiparesis
PICC line in her R arm

AR 44A — Labs and Images
CBC: Hb 11.4 g/dL, WBC 14,800/mm³
      Platelets 300,000/mm³
Glucose 98 mg/dL
U/A normal
Chest x-ray normal
Two peripheral and 1 PICC hub culture drawn

Which of the following would you give?
A. Vancomycin
B. Vancomycin + cefepime
C. Vancomycin + fluconazole
D. Vancomycin + cefepime + fluconazole

Answer: _____

Dx of Central Line-Associated Blood Stream Infection (CLABSI)
- If line removed:
  - Catheter tip and BC with same organism
- If line retained:

Hub	Peripheral	Diagnosis
+	+	CLABSI if: Hub quant ≥ 3 x blood quant Hub growth ≥ 2 hours prior to blood
+	−	Catheter colonization
−	+	Bacteremia unrelated to line

IDSA. *Clin Infect Dis*. 2009;49:1–45.

CLABSI — Empiric Treatment
- Vancomycin alone, but add:
  - Antipseudomonal GNB coverage if
    - Severe sepsis
    - Neutropenia
    - Colonized with resistant GNB
    - Femoral line

- Antifungal therapy (echinocandin)
  - (Fluconazole if no azole x 3 mos, resistance low)
  - Prior broad-spectrum antibacterials
  - ≥ 1 site colonized with *Candida*
  - Heme malignancy
  - Femoral line
  - TPN

IDSA. *Clin Infect Dis*. 2009;49:1–45.

AR 44B
In 24 hours, the cultures from the periphery and PICC hub growth shows GPCs in clusters, which is identified 24 hours later as MRSA with an MIC of 0.5 µg/mL vancomycin.
She has defervesced and her exam is unchanged.

When should the PICC be pulled?
A. Now
B. If BCs stay (+) 3 days after vancomycin
C. If BCs stay (+) 1 week after vancomycin
D. If TEE shows vegetations 3 days after vancomycin
E. If TEE shows vegetations 1 week after vancomycin

Answer: _____

CLABSI — Line Removal Criteria
- Clinical indications
  - Severe sepsis, hemodynamic instability
  - Metastatic (meningitis, osteo, endocarditis)
  - Suppurative thrombophlebitis
  - BC (+) > 72 h into appropriate therapy

Organism Indications	ST (< 14 d)	LT (≥ 14 d)
S. aureus	Remove	Remove
P. aeruginosa	Remove	Remove
Fungi	Remove	Remove
Mycobacteria	Remove	Remove
Other GNB	Remove	Can retain
Enterococci	Remove	Can retain

IDSA. *Clin Infect Dis*. 2009;49:1–45.

AR 44C
The line is pulled as scheduled.
BCs on days 3 and 7 of vancomycin are (−). On day 7, her vital signs are normal and the exam is unchanged.
WBC and blood glucose are normal.
A TEE on day 8 is without vegetations.

How long would you continue antibiotics?
A. Discontinue now.
B. Total of 2 weeks.
C. Total of 4–6 weeks.
D. Total of 8 weeks.

Answer: _____

© 2017 MedStudy Internal Medicine Video Board Review – Infectious Disease • Fred A. Zar, MD

CLABSI — Duration of Treatment (After First Negative BC)

- 7–14 days
  - Unless listed below
- 2 weeks
  - Fungal
  - *S. aureus* only if:
    - No DM, Isupp, prostheses, metastatic, **and**
    - TEE (−), BC (−) w/in 72 h, catheter out
- 4–6 weeks
  - *S. aureus*
  - BC (+) > 72 hours on Rx
  - Metastatic (endocarditis, meningitis)
- 6–8 weeks
  - *S. aureus* osteomyelitis

IDSA. *Clin Infect Dis.* 2009;49: 1–45.

AR 44 — Key Points

- Know the diagnostic criteria for central line associated blood stream infection (CLABSI)
- Choose the appropriate empiric therapy for CLABSI depending on patient characteristics
- Choose the appropriate duration of treatment for CLABSI depending on clinical and microbiologic data

AR 45 — History and Physical

Hx: A 71-year-old man is admitted with fever and chills off and on for 2 weeks. He denies other symptoms. He has not seen a physician for over 20 years. He has smoked for 55 years and drinks at least 6 beers a day.
PE: T 100.6° F (38.1° C), PR 98, RR 16, BP 160/95
Conjunctival hemorrhages
Osler node on left little finger
CVS: Gr 3/6 systolic crescendo-decrescendo murmur aortic area, radiating to carotids

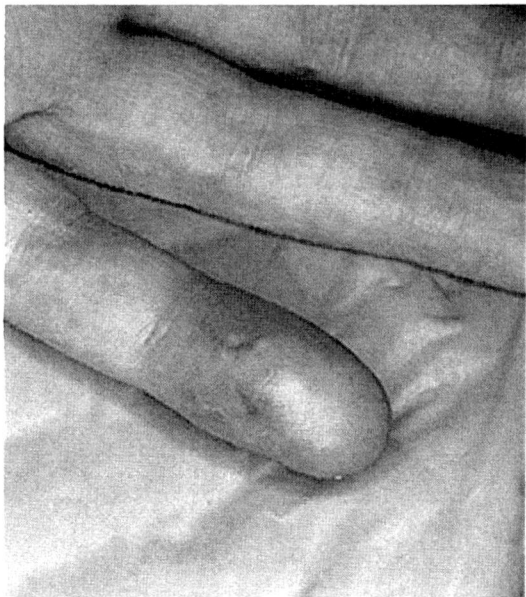

AR 45 — Labs and Course

Labs:
CBC: Hb 9.8 g/dL WBC 11,000/mm^3
   platelets 285,000/mm^3
U/A: WBC 10/hpf, RBC 110/hpf, LE trace
Lytes: Normal
Course:
Blood cultures: 3/3 *Streptococcus bovis* biotype I (*S. gallolyticus*)
Transthoracic echo: 0.8-cm vegetation on aortic valve

What exam would best reveal why he developed endocarditis?

A. Chest x-ray
B. Transesophageal echo
C. CT abdomen
D. CT pelvis
E. Colonoscopy

Answer: _____

S. bovis Bacteremia Association with Colon CA and Endocarditis

- The study
  - Meta-analysis of 11 case series
- The results
  - Colon Ca in 128/340 (38%)
    - *S. bovis* I vs. II = 7.26
  - Endocarditis in 150/344 (44%)
    - *S. bovis* I vs. II = 16.61

Boleij A. *Clin Infect Dis.* 2011;53:870–878.

S. bovis New Names

Old names	New names	Synonyms
S. bovis biotype I	*S. gallolyticus*	*S. gallolyticus* subsp. *gallolyticus*
S. bovis biotype II.1	*S. lutetiensis*	*S. infantarius* subsp. *coli*
	S. infantarius	*S. infantarius* subsp. *infantarius*
S. bovis biotype II.2	*S. pasteurianus*	*S. gallolyticus* subsp. *pasteurianus*

Schlegel L. *Int J Syst Evol Microbiol.* 2003;53:631.

Malignancy in *C. septicum* Bacteremia

Cancer/Total (%)	Heme	GI	Other	Occult	Mortality
65/86 (76)[1]	35	19	11	12	62%
7/7 (100)[2]	2	4	1	2	71%
31/51 (61)[3]	12	18	1	12	67%
7/8 (88)[4]	1	6	0	4	62%
42/59 (71)[5]	16	14	12	NS	68%
131/162 (81)[6]	65	55	11	41	65%
283/373 (76)	46%	41%	13%	29%	65%

[1]*JAMA.* 1969;209:385–388.
[2]*Ann Surg.* 1981;193:361–364.
[3]Multiple Case Reports reported in next ref.
[4]*Arch Surg.* 1984;119:546–550.
[5]*Am J Med.* 1979;66:63–66.
[6]*Medicine.* 1989;68:30–37.

AR 45 — Key Points
- Learn the latest nomenclature for species previously known as *Streptococcus bovis*
- Recognize the strong association between *Streptococcus bovis* and colon cancer
- Recognize the strong association between *Clostridium septicum* and colon cancer
- Recognize the need for diagnostic colonoscopy in patients with bacteremia from these 2 organisms

AR 46A — History and Physical
Hx: A 27-year-old man presents to your student-run free clinic with a 2-week history of low-grade fever and fatigue. He has a 3/10 new headache. He is homeless. HIV infection was diagnosed 7 years ago, but he has never been able to maintain antiretroviral therapy due to the cost. He is on no medications.
PE: T 100.0° F (37.7° C), PR 76, RR 12, BP 90/60
Ht 5'10", Wt 125
Mental status normal and fundi benign
Neck supple, no nodes
Heart, lungs, abdomen normal

AR 46A — Labs and Images
CBC:
Hb 9.8 g/dL, MCV 90 fL
WBC 3,400/mm^3
   80% neutrophils, 0 bands, 9% lymphs
Platelets 112,000/mm^3
Lytes and creatinine normal

What next?
A. CD4, HIV viral load/genotype, RTC 1 wk for antiretrovirals
B. Head CT
C. Lumbar puncture
D. Chest x-ray
E. Three blood cultures

Answer: _____

Cryptococcal Meningitis Presentation

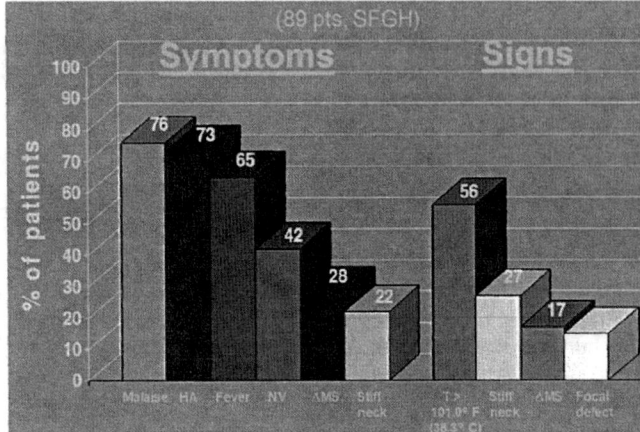

Chuck SL. *NEJM.* 1989;321:794–9.

Cryptococcal Meningitis Laboratory Data

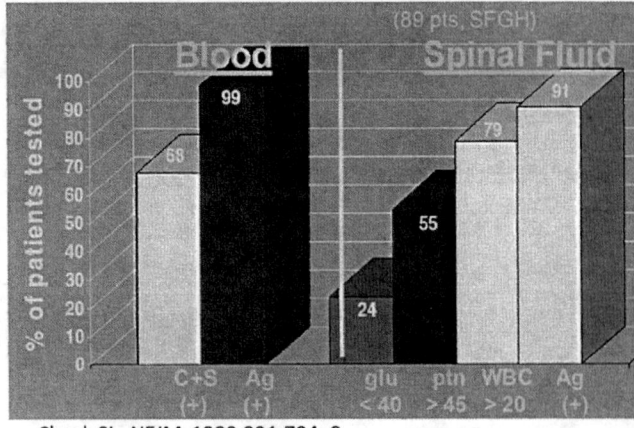

Chuck SL. *NEJM.* 1989;321:794–9.

Cryptococcal Meningitis: Dx
- CSF
  - India Ink: Sens: ~ 75% (immediate)
  - Crypto Ag: Sens = 91–100%, Spec = 93–98%
  - Culture: Sens = 95%, Spec = 100%
- Blood
  - Crypto Ag: Sens = 91%, Spec = 83%
  - Culture: Sens ~ 50%, Spec = 100%

AR 46B — Course
CT head normal
$CD4 = 5/mm^3$
HIV viral load 100,000 copies/mL
Blood cultures are sent (eventually negative)
Chest x-ray normal
Lumbar puncture
    Opening pressure is 27 cm
    $WBC = 8/mm^3$, $RBC = 0/mm^3$
    Glucose = 78 mg/dL, Protein = 64 mg/dL
    Cryptococcal Ag (+) 1:1024

What antifungal would you start?
A. Fluconazole
B. Itraconazole
C. Amphotericin B deoxycholate
D. Liposomal Amphotericin B
E. Liposomal Amphotericin B +5-flucytosine

Answer: _____

Cryptococcal Meningitis — Rx
- Induction (2 weeks)
  - Liposomal amphotericin B + 5 FC
  - Repeat LPs to keep OP normal
- Consolidation (8 weeks)
  - Fluconazole 400 mg/d
- Maintenance (≥ 1 year)
  - Fluconazole 200 mg/d
    - DC once CD4 > 100

IDSA. *Clin Infect Dis*. 50:291–322, 2010.
Hamill RJ. *Clin Infect Dis*. 51:225-232, 2010.

AR 46 — Key Points
- Recognize the clinical presentation of cryptococcal meningitis in an HIV-infected person
- Know the operating characteristics of tests used to diagnose cryptococcal meningitis
- Implement the 3 phases of treatment of cryptococcal meningitis in an HIV-infected person
- Recognize the need to control CSF opening pressures in cryptococcal meningitis

AR 47 — History and Physical
Hx: A 47-year-old man presents to the ED with fever and SOB x 2 days. He was a recipient of a living donor renal transplant 5 months ago. The donor was CMV IgG Ab (+), and had (−) Ab for HIV, toxo, HSV, and VZV. His RPR and PPD were nonreactive, and he had not traveled outside of the U.S. The patient had (−) Ab for CMV, HSV, VZV, HIV, and his RPR and IGRA were (−).

Current medications include trimethoprim/sulfamethoxazole, mycophenolate, tacrolimus, and valganciclovir.
PE: T 101.0° F (38.3° C), PR 102, RR 20,
  BP 100/68, SpO_2 = 88%
Lungs have diffuse scattered rales without bronchial BS
Heart, abdomen, neuro exams normal

AR 47 — Labs and Images
CBC: Hb 9.8 g/dL, MCV 88 fL
$WBC\ 6,400/mm^3$
88% neutrophils, 0 bands, 7% lymphs
Platelets $285,000/mm^3$
Lytes normal
Creatinine 1.8 mg/dL (which is his baseline)
U/A normal

Chest x-ray as shown

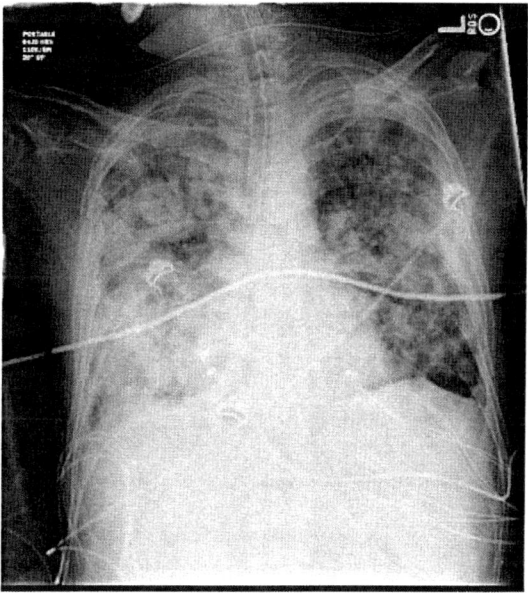

AR 47
He receives oxygen. What is the next diagnostic step?
A. Blood for bacterial, mycobacterial, viral, and fungal culture.
B. Sputum for bacterial, mycobacterial, viral, and fungal culture.
C. Blood for viral and fungal serologies.
D. Obtain lung tissue for histology and culture.

Answer: _____

Post-Transplant Infections
General principles:
- Timing is predictive
- Symptoms and signs muted
- Altered anatomy alters exam reliability
- Antibiotic resistance more common
- Multiple pathogens may be present

Post-Transplant Infections (cont.)
- Diagnosis
  - Cultures, Ag detection, biopsy
  - Serologies usually not helpful

Transplant Infections < 1 mo
- Recipient derived
  - Surgical site, lines, HCAP, UTI
  - Hep B and C reactivation
  - *Clostridium difficile*
  - *Strongyloides stercoralis*
- Donor-derived infections
  - Screened for: HSV, CMV, HIV, syphilis
  - Resistant bacteria: VRE, MRSA
  - Fungi: Resistant *Candida* species
  - Toxoplasmosis

Transplant Infections 1–6 mos
- Opportunists
  - Fungi: PJP, endemic
  - Viral: HSV, VZV, CMV, BK, JC
  - Bacterial: Mycobacteria
  - Parasitic: Toxo, Cryptosporidium, Microsporidium
  - Prophylaxis:
    - Pneumocystis (T/S)
    - Herpes viruses (valganciclovir)

Transplant Infections > 6 mos
- Community-acquired infections
- Late viral infections
  - CMV, HSV
  - Post-transplant lymphoproliferative disease (EBV)
  - BK
  - Progressive multifocal leukoencephalopathy (JC)
- Fungi:
  - *Aspergillus, Mucor, Cryptococcus*
- Bacteria
  - *Nocardia*
  - *Rhodococcus*

Post-Transplant Pneumonia
Rapidly Progressive Causes
- Bacterial
  - Usual pathogens
  - *Nocardia, Legionella, Rhodococcus*
- Fungal
  - PJP, *Aspergillus, Cryptococcus*, endemics
- Viral
  - CMV, VZV, HSV, influenza, RSV

Risk of CMV Disease by Donor Serostatus

	Donor	Serostatus
Recipient Serostatus	+	−
+	50%	20%
−	75%	< 5%

CMV Disease in the Immunosuppressed Host
- Pulmonary
  - Pneumonia
- Ocular
  - Retinitis
- Gastrointestinal
  - Esophagitis, enteritis, colitis
- Neurologic
  - Encephalitis, meningitis, myelitis, polyradiculopathy

Diagnosis of CMV Disease
- Blood DNA and Ag assays
  - Indicate infection, not necessarily disease
- Cultures
  - Blood indicates infection, not disease
  - Tissue may be false (+) from viremia
  - Take time
- Serology
  - Not helpful due to immunosuppression
- **Tissue biopsy**
  - **Inclusions and/or histochemical stains diagnostic**

AR 47 — Key Points
- Know the timeline of infections that occur after solid organ transplant
- Recognize that post-transplant pneumonia is a medical emergency and the various agents that cause it
- Determine the relative risk of CMV disease based on serostatus of donor and recipient
- Know the best way to diagnose CMV infection in an immunocompromised host

AR 48 — History and Physical
Hx: A 30-year-old man presents with a fever for 4 days and rash for 2 days. He has had malaise for a week. The rash began on his face, progressed to his neck and upper trunk yesterday, and now involves most of his body. His only other symptoms are burning of his eyes and a runny nose. He works as a ride attendant at Disneyland. He is on no medications and is otherwise healthy, which he attributes to his parents refusing to vaccinate him as a child.

PE: T 103.6° F (39.7° C), PR 126, RR 20, BP 120/80
Mild bulbar conjunctivitis bilaterally
Swollen nasal mucosa, throat normal
Tiny axillary and supraclavicular adenopathy
Rash (next page)

AR 48 — Rash

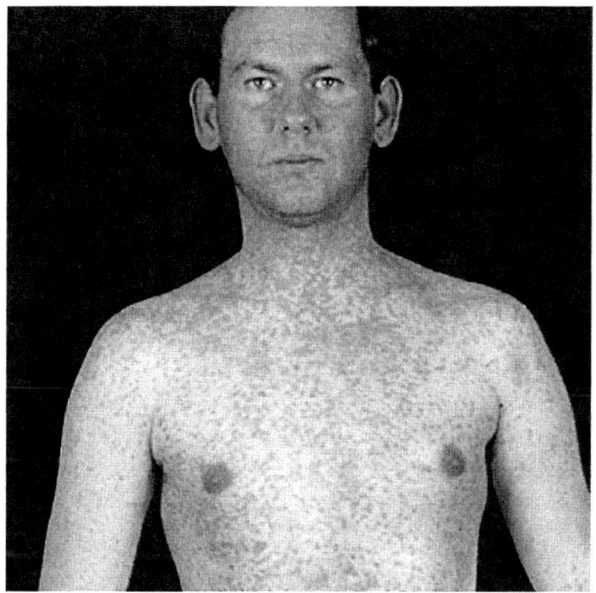

AR 48
What is your presumptive diagnosis?
A. Rubeola (measles)
B. Rubella (German measles)
C. Acute HIV
D. Varicella (chicken pox)

Answer: _____

Rubeola (Measles) — Epidemiology
- Reservoir only in humans
- Airborne spread (airborne for hours)
- Pre-vaccine
  - 90% by age 15
  - 75% contact attack rate
  - 4 million cases/year in U.S.
- Post-vaccine (1968)
  - 1990: 27,000 cases (epidemic)
  - 21st C: Median 63 cases/year

December 28, 2014 - February 6, 2015

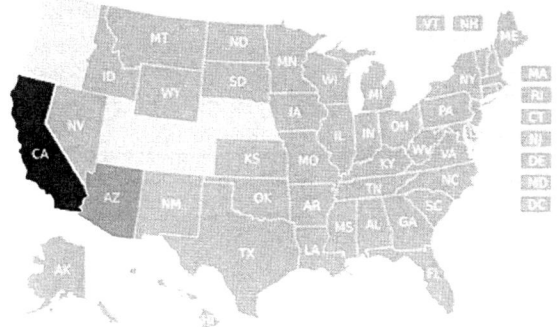

Cases*:
- 0
- 1-4
- 5-9
- 10-19
- 20+

From December 28 to February 6, 2015, 114 people from 7 states [AZ (7), CA (99), CO (1), NE (1), OR (1), UT (3), WA (2)] were reported to have measles and are considered to be part of a large, ongoing outbreak linked to an amusement park in California*.

Rubeola (Measles) — Clinical Phases
- Incubation (7–21 d)
- Prodrome (2–3 d)
  - Fever, coryza, cough, ± conjunctivitis
- Exanthem (develops over 2–3 d)
  - Contagious 4 days on either side of rash onset
  - Maculopapular blanching rash
  - Face → neck → trunk → extremities
  - Lymphadenopathy
  - Koplik spots (diagnostic)
- Recovery (~ 2 weeks)
  - Rash darkens, fades, desquamates
  - Cough wanes

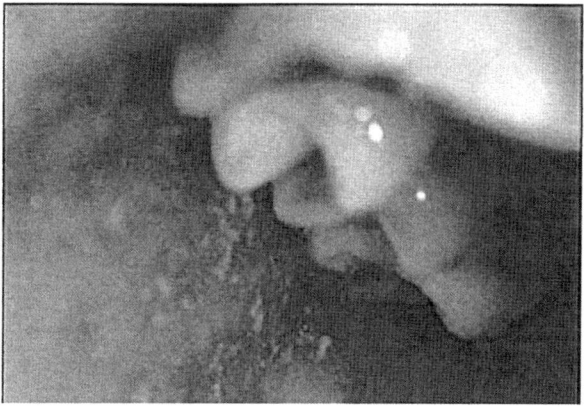

Rubeola (Measles) — Complications (25%)
- Diarrhea (10%)
- Pneumonia (5–10%)
- Otitis media (5–10%)
- Neurologic
  - Encephalitis (0.1%)
  - Acute disseminated encephalomyelitis (ADEM)
    - Autoimmune, ~ 2 weeks after rash
    - Common residual, 10–20% mortality
  - Subacute sclerosing panencephalitis (SSPE)
    - 1:100,000
    - 7–10 years after measles, ? variant virus
    - 100% mortality

Rubeola (Measles) — Diagnosis, Prevention, and Treatment
- Diagnosis
  - Clinical
  - PCR assays available
  - Serology retrospective
- Prevention
  - Live attenuated vaccine (1968)
  - Initial dose 10–15 months
  - 2nd dose (1990) ≥ 28 days later (before age 4)
  - > 95% effective
  - Lifelong immunity (~ to disease)
- Treatment
  - No specific treatment

AR 48 — Key Points
- Be aware of the risk of measles in the unvaccinated adult
- Recognize the clinical presentation of measles
- Know the clinical sequelae of measles

AR 49 — History and Physical
Hx: A 74-year-old woman presents to the ED in January with 36 hours of fever, productive cough, and SOB. She has hypertension. She sees her internist regularly. She has no known lung or heart disease. She received her influenza vaccination last November and both pneumococcal vaccines (PCV13 and PPV23). Five days ago, she visited her 4-month-old great-grandson who had the flu.

PE: T 102.6° F (39.2° C), PR 115, RR 22, BP 144/90, SpO_2 94% on room air
Alert and in mild respiratory distress
HEENT and neck normal
Heart and abdomen normal
Lungs with bilateral diffuse rales and wheezing

AR 49 — Labs and Image
CBC: Hb 13.8 g/dL
WBC 11,000/mm³
    74% neutrophils, 4% bands, 10% lymphs
Platelets 300,000/mm³
Rapid Ag detection for influenza (–)

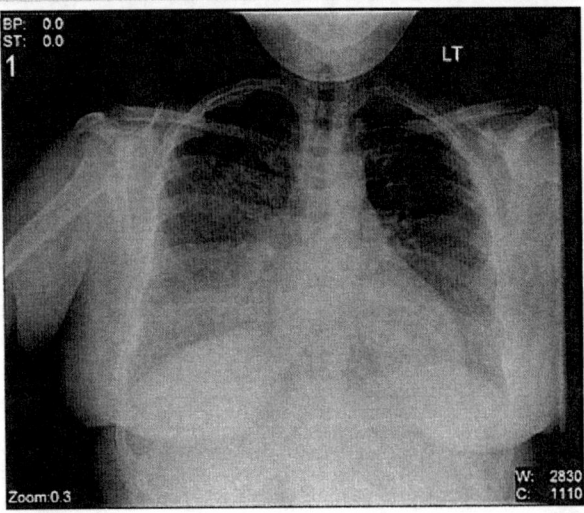

AR 49 (cont.)
What diagnostic test would you do next?
A. Secretions for adenovirus Ag
B. Secretions for respiratory syncytial virus PCR
C. Sputum for viral culture
D. Serology for mycoplasma
E. Blood for CMV PCR

Answer: _____

Respiratory Syncytial Virus (RSV)
- Epidemiology
  - Peak in January and February
  - Transmitted via secretions and fomites
  - Children < 1, adults > 65
  - Universal by age 3, yet immunity wanes
- Clinical
  - Incubation 4–6 days
  - Bronchitis, bronchospasm, pneumonia
- Diagnosis
  - Rapid Ag detection
- Treatment
  - Ribavirin if immunocompromised

How common is RSV in adults?
- The study
  - Prospective, 4 winters
  - 3 cohorts
    - Elderly (> 65)
    - Younger with cardiopulmonary disease ("at risk")
    - Hospitalized for acute cardiopulmonary disease
  - Influenza and RSV diagnosed by:
    - PCR
    - Culture
    - Serology

Falsey AR. *NEJM. 2005*;352:1749–1759.

How common is RSV in adults?

Cohort	Influenza	RSV
Elderly	2–5%	3–7%
At risk	2–7%	4–10%
Hospitalized	2–20%	8–13%

Mortality: Influenza 8%, RSV 7%
Falsey AR. *NEJM.* 2005;352:1749–1759.

AR 49 — Key Points
- Understand the epidemiology of RSV infection in adults
- Recognize the clinical presentation of RSV pneumonia in adults
- Know to test for RSV in those with influenza-like presentations but negative rapid Ag detection for influenza

AR 50 — History and Physical

Hx: A 28-year-old man comes to the neighborhood free clinic complaining of fever for 5 days, sore throat for 3 days, and 2 days of a rash. He feels tired and his muscles ache. He is a heroin user and has had episodic bisexual unprotected sex. His last partner was 3 weeks ago. He says he tested negative for HIV and syphilis 2 months ago.

PE: T 102.2° F (39.0° C), PR 112, RR 16, BP 90/60

HEENT: Pharyngeal erythema without exudate

Neck: Several tiny supraclavicular nodes; also bilateral axillary nodes

Heart, lungs, abdomen normal

AR 50 — Rash

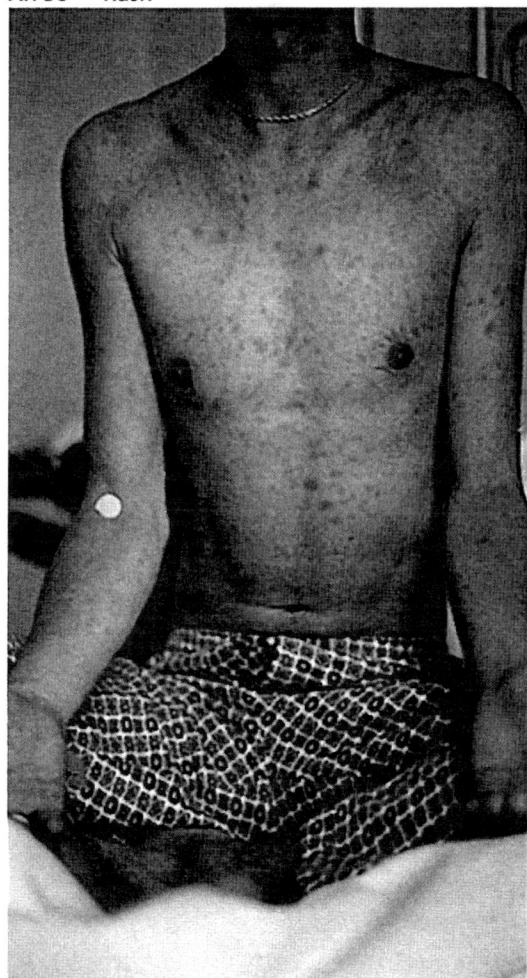

AR 50 — Labs

CBC: Hb 13.8 g/dL, MCV 94 fL

WBC 4,400/mm³

    78% neutrophils, 0 bands

    11% lymphs, 3% eosinophils

Platelets 165,000/mm³

Lytes, LFTs, and creat normal

Which test is most likely to be diagnostic?

A. RPR

B. EBV capsid IgM Ab

C. CMV IgM Ab

D. Parvovirus B19 PCR

E. HIV viral load

Answer: _____

Acute Retroviral Syndrome

- Epidemiology
  - Occurs in ~ 90% of new HIV infections
  - Incubation = 2–4 wks, lasts 2–4 wks
- Clinical manifestations (> 50% occurrence)
  - Fever, LNs, pharyngitis, rash, myalgia/arthralgia
- Diagnosis
  - HIV antibody is **negative**
  - Viral detection via p24 assay or PCR
- Treatment
  - Initiate antiretroviral therapy

HIV Infection Assays

Assay	Days to positivity
HIV IgG Ab	25–35
HIV IgM Ab	20–30
HIV p24 Ag	15–20
HIV PCR (50 copy cutoff)	10–15
HIV PCR (1–5 copy cutoff)	5

Diagnosing HIV Infection

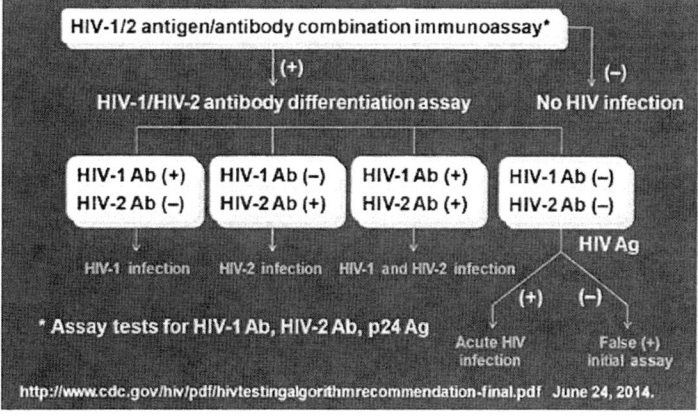

Sore Throat, Rash, and Fever
- <u>Noninfectious diseases</u>
  - Pemphigus/pemphigoid
  - SLE
  - Kawasaki disease
  - Erythema multiforme major
  - Toxic epidermal necrolysis
- <u>Infectious diseases</u>
  - *Streptococcus pyogenes*
  - HIV
  - *Arcanobacterium hemolyticum*
  - *Mycoplasma pneumoniae*
  - Epstein-Barr virus
  - Coxsackievirus
  - Toxic shock syndrome

Scarlet Fever

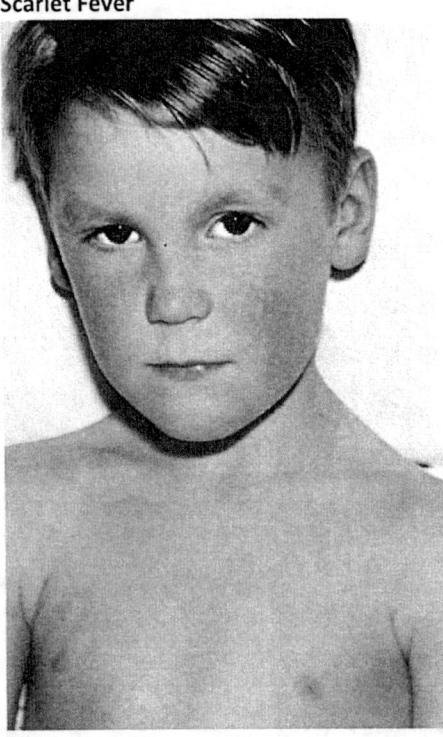

Scarlet Fever — Sandpaper Rash

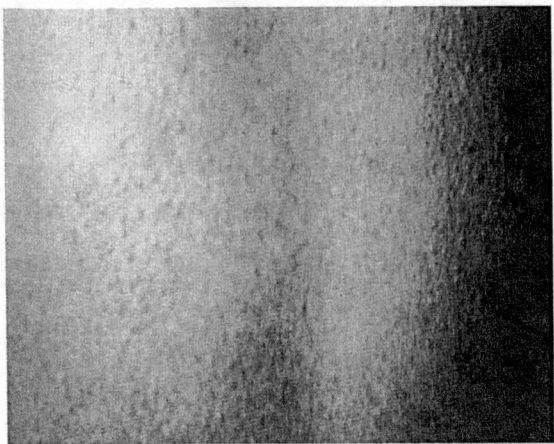

Scarlet Fever — Pastia's Sign

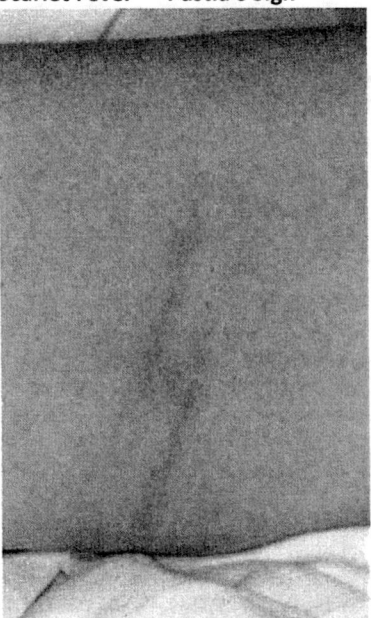

Strawberry Tongue
- Kawasaki disease
- Toxic shock syndrome
- Scarlet fever

Scarlet Fever — White Strawberry Tongue

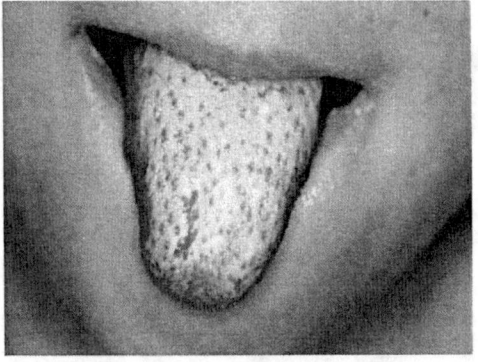

Scarlet Fever — Red Strawberry Tongue

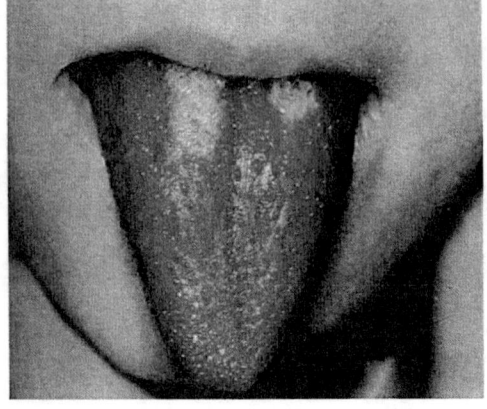

Mycoplasma pneumoniae — EM

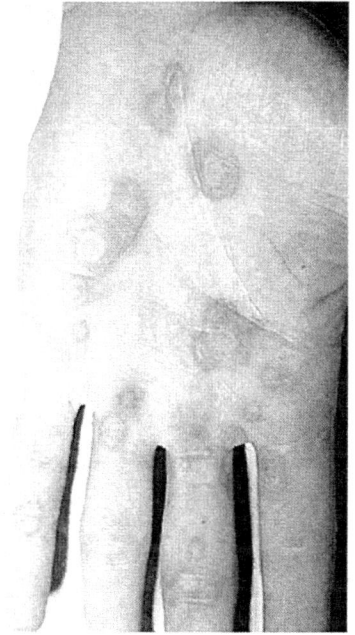

Infectious Mononucleosis Rash

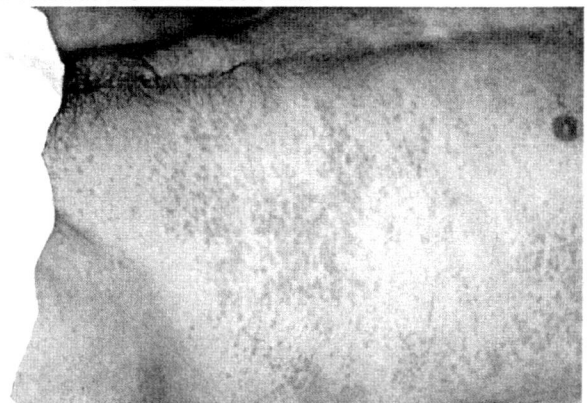

Infectious Mononucleosis — Ampicillin Rash

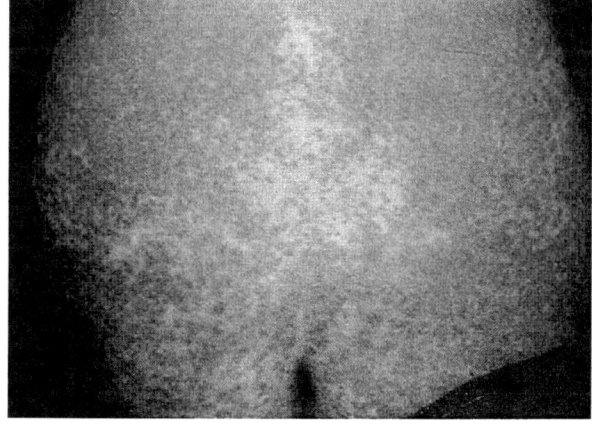

AR 50 — Key Points
- Recognize the short differential diagnostic possibilities for fever, sore throat, and rash
- Recognize the clinical presentation of the acute retroviral syndrome in a person at risk
- Know the appropriate testing to diagnose the acute retroviral syndrome

AR 51 — History and Physical

Hx: A 57-year-old man is referred to you from the ENT clinic after undergoing a biopsy for suspected head and neck cancer.

He presented with a 2-month history of progressive, painless swelling of his right jaw. He has poor dental hygiene, DM, and has smoked for 40 years.

AR 51 — Right Jaw Mass

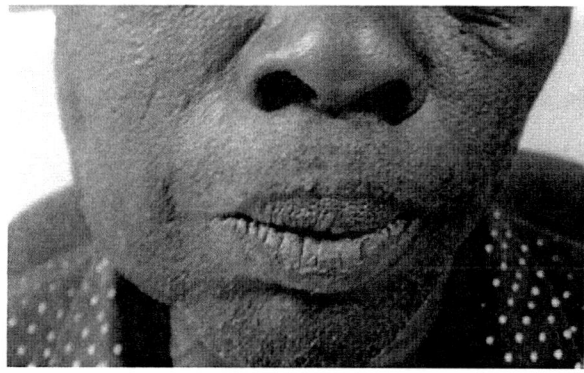

AR 51 — Biopsy Results

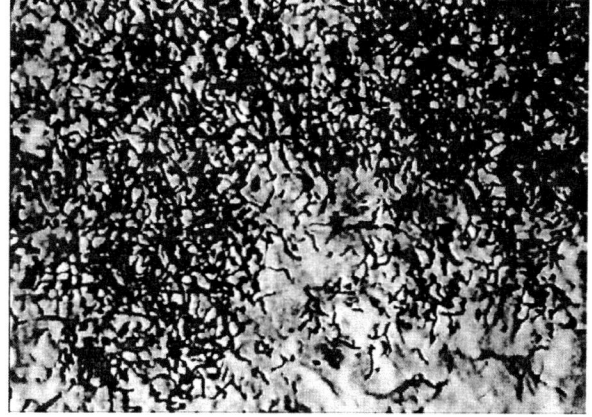

AR 51

What antibiotic would you recommend?
A. Penicillin
B. Trimethoprim/sulfamethoxazole
C. Levofloxacin
D. Metronidazole
E. Fluconazole

Answer: _____

Actinomyces israelii
- Epidemiology
  - Anaerobic normal flora of mouth, gut, vagina
- Clinical manifestations
  - Cervicofacial
  - Abdominal abscess
  - IUD intrapelvic
- Diagnosis
  - Gram stain and culture
- Treatment
  - Penicillin
  - (Doxycycline, clindamycin)

AR 51 — Key Points
- Recognize the clinical presentation of cervicofacial actinomycosis
- Know the Gram stain appearance of *Actinomyces israelii*
- Prescribe the appropriate presumptive therapy for actinomyces infection

AR 52 — History and Physical

Hx: A 37-year-old man presents to the clinic with a 10-day history of a new right-sided headache, weakness of his left arm > left leg, and sleepiness. He has noted a mild cough and DOE, which he ascribes to his severe persistent asthma for which he takes inhaled albuterol + salmeterol, and prednisone 40 mg/d. He has never been tested for HIV or TB.

PE: T 99.8° F (37.6° C), PR 88, RR 20, BP 128/84, P_aO_2 95%
Lethargic
Strength L arm 3/5, L leg 4/5
Lungs: Decreased breath sounds RUL
Heart and abdomen normal

AR 52 — Images

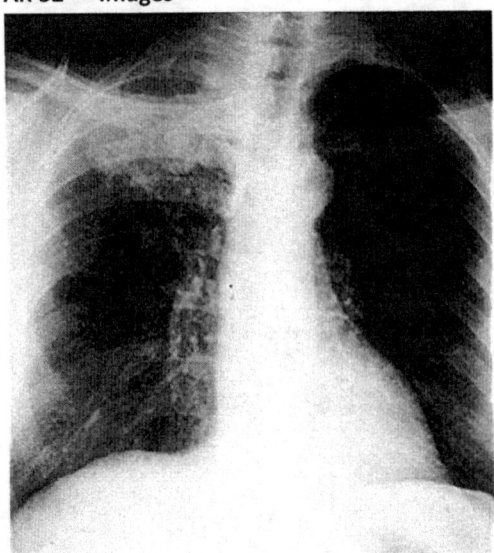

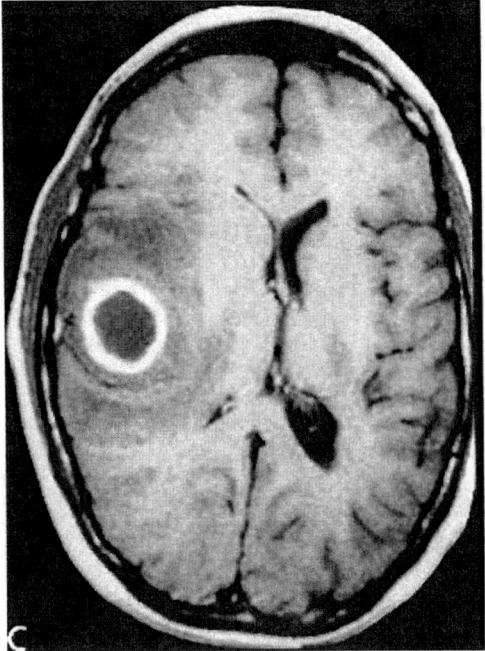

AR 52 — Course and Labs
- Started on INH, rifampin, pyrazinamide, and ethambutol
- IGRA (–) for TB
- HIV antibody (–)
- Sputum AFB (–) x 3
- BAL reveals image below

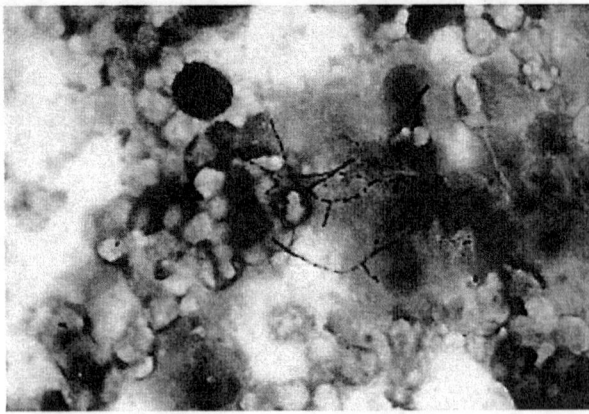

AR 52
What antibiotic would you recommend?
A. Penicillin
B. Vancomycin and metronidazole
C. Trimethoprim/sulfamethoxazole and imipenem
D. Fluconazole
E. Liposomal amphotericin B

Answer: _____

Nocardia asteroides
- Epidemiology
  - Aerobic, never normal flora
  - 70% of pts have compromised CMI
- Clinical manifestations
  - CNS
  - Pulmonary
  - Cutaneous
- Diagnosis
  - Gram stain and culture
- Treatment
  - T/S ± imipenem (if severe)

Actinomyces vs. *Nocardia*

Organism	Growth	Sites	Treatment
Actinomyces	Anaerobe	Jaw Abdomen Pelvis	Penicillin (clindamycin) (doxycycline)
Nocardia	Aerobe	CNS Lung Skin	Trim/sulfa ± imipenem

AR 52 — Key Points
- Recognize the clinical presentation of *Nocardia* in an immunocompromised host
- Know the Gram stain appearance of *Actinomyces israelii*
- Prescribe the appropriate presumptive therapy for *Nocardia* infection

AR 53 — History and Physical
Hx: A 38-year-old man presents with 5 days of nasal congestion, temp to 100.5° F (38.3° C), and nonpurulent nasal drainage. He is otherwise healthy and on no medications.
PE: T 100.9° F (38.3° C), PR 98, RR 12, BP 110/76
No conjunctivitis, TMs normal
Nasal mucosa inflamed, no purulence noted
Throat and neck normal
Heart, lungs, abdomen normal

What would you do next?
A. Nasal saline, RTC 5 days if worse/no better.
B. Prescribe trimethoprim/sulfamethoxazole.
C. Prescribe amoxicillin/clavulanate.
D. Prescribe levofloxacin.
E. Order CT sinuses.

Answer: _____

Rhinosinusitis — Indications for Antibacterial Therapy
- Persistent and not improving ≥ 10 d
  - 60% will have bacterial infection*
- Severe for ≥ 3 days
  - T > 102.0° F (38.9° C) and purulent drainage, **or**
  - Facial pain
- Double-sickening, new onset ≥ 3 days
  - Headache
  - Discharge
IDSA. *CID.* 2012;54(8):1041–1045.
*Gwantney J. *Allergy Clin Immunol.* 1992;90:457–461.

Microbiology of Acute Bacterial Sinusitis
Pathogen	% of Cases
Streptococcus pneumoniae	41%
Haemophilus influenzae	35%
Anaerobes	7%
Streptococcal species	7%
Moraxella catarrhalis	4%
Staphylococcus aureus	3%
Other	4%

Meltzer EO. *J Allergy Clin Immunol.* 114:S115–S212, 2004.

Rhinosinusitis — Assessing Risk for Resistant Organisms
- At risk for antibiotic resistance
  - Age < 2 or > 65
  - Daycare
  - Antibiotics in last month
  - Hospitalized in last 5 days
  - Comorbidities (heart, lung)
  - Immunocompromised
IDSA. *CID.* 2012;54(8):1041–1045.

Rhinosinusitis — Antibiotics
- 1st line (not at risk of resistance)
  - Amoxicillin/clavulanate
- 2nd line (at risk of resistance)
  - Doxycycline
  - Fluoroquinolone
- **Do Not Use**
  - Macrolides
  - Trimethoprim/sulfamethoxazole
  - Cephalosporins
IDSA. *CID.* 2012;54(8):1041–1045.

Rhinosinusitis — Adjunctive Rx
- Intranasal saline
- Intranasal steroids
  - If suspected allergic etiology
- No benefit
  - Decongestants
  - Antihistamines
IDSA. *CID.* 2012;54(8):1041–1045.

Rhinosinusitis — Duration of Rx

- Improvement after 3–5 days
  - 1st line drugs: Complete 5- to 7-day course
  - 2nd line drugs: Complete 7- to 10-day course
- Worsening or no improvement 3–5 days
  - Broaden or switch coverage
  - If no improvement after 3–5 more days
    - Consider noninfectious etiology
    - Image (CT) to look for suppurative complications
    - Meatal cultures for pathogen-specific therapy

IDSA. *CID*. 2012;54(8):1041–1045.

CT Scan of Rhinovirus Rhinosinusitis

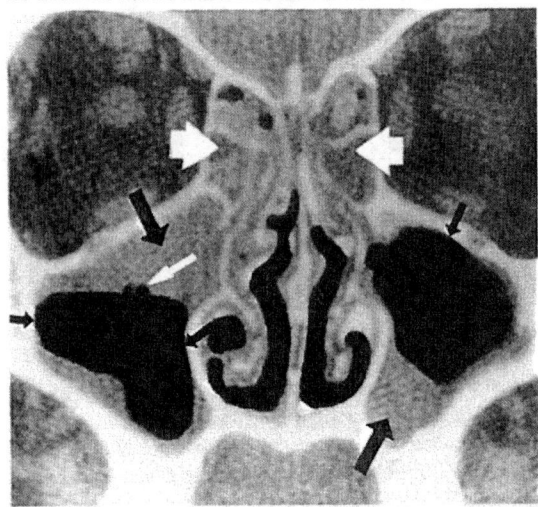

| Large black arrows = Thick exudates in maxillary sinuses |
| Small black arrows = Normal air, bone interfaces |
| Large white arrows = Opacification of ethmoid sinuses |
| Small white arrows = Gas bubbles in exudate |

Gwaltney JM. *CID*. 1996;23:1209-25.

Incidental Sinus CT Abnormalities
Head CTs for Nonsinus Reasons, 666 Cases

Result	Ethmoid	Maxillary	Sphenoid	Frontal
Normal	72%	76%	91%	95%
Mucosal thickening	25%	15%	7%	3%
Mucosal polyp	0.4%	6%	1%	0.2%
Opacification	1%	2%	1%	0.8%
Bone destruction	1%	2%	1%	0.3%

Havas TE. *Arch Otol Head Neck Surg*. 1988;114:856–859.

AR 53 — Key Points

- Know the clinical findings indicative of bacterial rhinosinusitis
- Know the 1st and 2nd line treatments for rhinosinusitis and when to choose between them
- Understand the indications for imaging in patients with rhinosinusitis
- Know the indications for sinus cultures in rhinosinusitis

AR 54 — History and Physical

Hx: A 23-year-old medical student presents to University Health Services with 14-day history of fever up to 104.0° F (40.0° C) the last 2 days. The fever began 10 days after returning from a 3-week stay in India. She developed nonbloody diarrhea the last 5 days associated with moderate abdominal cramping. She is otherwise healthy and on no medications other than OTC NSAIDs which temporarily relieve her fever. She has received hepatitis A and B vaccines in the past.
PE: Looks exhausted on exam
T 103.0° F (39.4° C), PR 94, RR 16, O_2 sat 98%
Mucous membranes dry, no jaundice
Rash on abd (image below)
Abd: Mild diffuse abdominal tenderness, (+) spleen tip
Heart, lungs, and neurologic normal

AR 54 — Rash

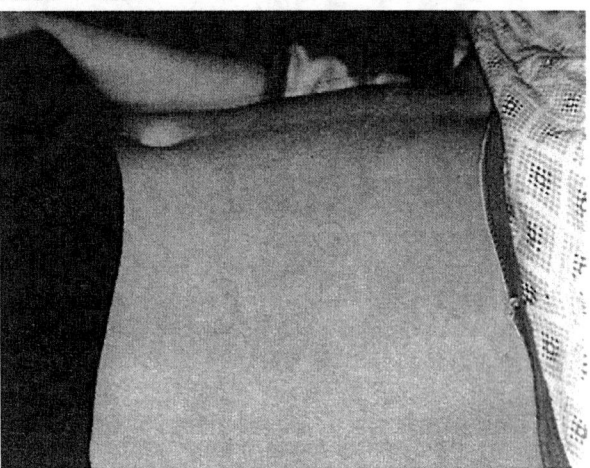

AR 54 — Labs

CBC: Hb 11.8 g/dL, MCV 90 fL
WBC 3,400/mm^3
    68% neutrophils, 8% bands
    12% lymphs, 8% monocytes
Platelets 140,000/mm^3
Lytes, creat, and glucose normal
AST 97 U/L, ALT 113 U/L
T bili = 1.2 mg/dL
U/A: Normal

AR 54 — Course

Blood and stool cultures are sent.
She is given ciprofloxacin 500 mg bid.
Three days later, she is still febrile.
Blood and stool cultures are negative.

What would you do next?
A. Repeat stool culture.
B. Repeat blood culture.
C. Culture the urine.
D. Culture a punch biopsy of the rash.
E. Culture her bone marrow.

Answer: _____

Typhoid Risk

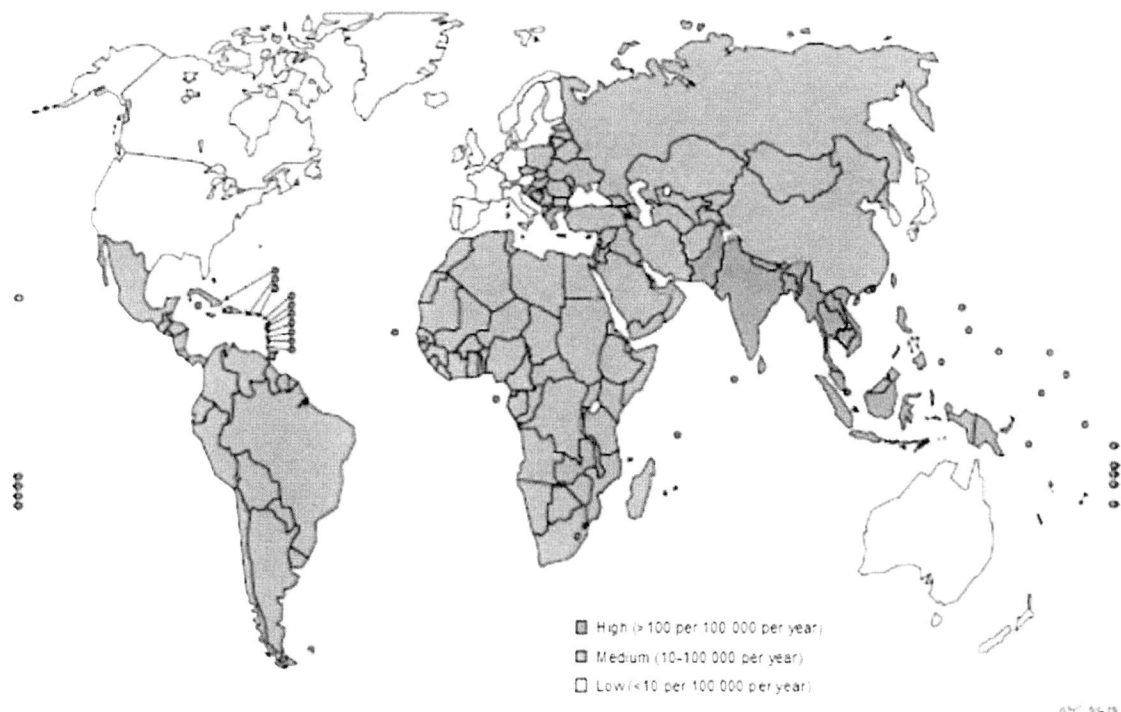

- High (> 100 per 100 000 per year)
- Medium (10-100 000 per year)
- Low (<10 per 100 000 per year)

Typhoid
- Epidemiology
  - *S. enterica* serotype typhi
  - Human reservoir
  - See map
- Clinical manifestations
  - Incubation 5–21 days
  - Week 1: Stepwise fever, relative bradycardia
  - Week 2: Abdominal pain, rose spots
  - Week 3: HSmegaly, GI bleed

Typhoid — Lab and Cultures
- Laboratory findings
  - Pancytopenias, often w/ L shift
  - Transaminase elevations
- Culture yields
  - Urine   10–25%
  - Stool   10–25%
  - Rose spots   40–50%
  - Blood   40–80%
  - Marrow   80–95%

Typhoid Antibiotic Resistance

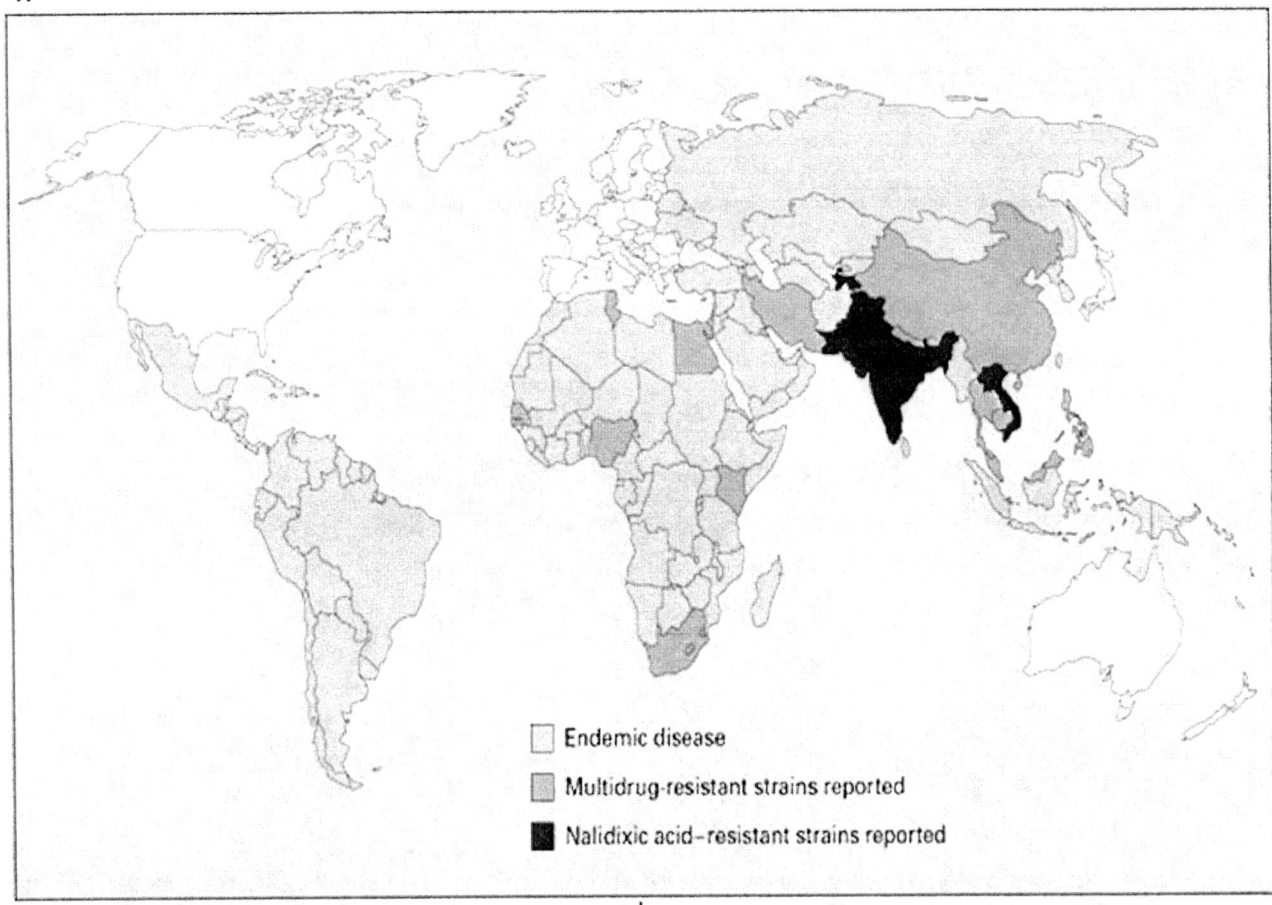

Endemic disease

Multidrug-resistant strains reported

Nalidixic acid–resistant strains reported

Typhoid — Treatment and Prevention
- Treatment
  - 1st line
    - Fluoroquinolone
    - Also for carriers [stool/urine (+) > 12 mos]
  - Alternate regimens
    - Azithromycin, ceftriaxone, chloramphenicol
- Prevention (efficacy at 1 year)*
  - Inactivated parenteral vaccine: 69%
  - Oral live vaccine: 35%

*Cochrane Database Syst Rev. 2014;1:CD001261.

AR 54 — Key Points
- Recognize the clinical presentation of typhoid in a traveler from an endemic area
- Know the diagnostic yields of various culture sites for typhoid
- Realize the risk of resistance to fluoroquinolones and know alternative treatment choices
- Know the limitations of current preventative vaccines

Infectious Disease
Audience Response Answers

Audience Response 1
Answer: E. Switch to penicillin and clindamycin.

AR 2
Answer: E. Obtain a bone biopsy for culture
prior to antibiotics.

AR 3
Answer: C. Start vancomycin PO.

AR 4
Answer: A. Progressive multifocal
leukoencephalopathy.

AR 5A
Answer: B. Start cefepime.

AR 5B
Answer: B. Start IV voriconazole.

AR 6
Answer: D. Streptomycin.

AR 7A
Answer: E. Peripheral smear of blood.

AR 7B
Answer: D. Azithromycin and atovaquone.

AR 7C
Answer: E. Peripheral smear of blood.

AR 7D
Answer: A. Doxycycline.

AR 8A
Answer: C. *Coccidioides immitis*.

AR 8B
Answer: D. None.

AR 9
Answer: A. Tetanus toxoid alone.

AR 10A
Answer: C. Dexamethasone.

AR 10B
Answer: B. Vancomycin and ceftriaxone.

AR 10C
Answer: A. Ceftriaxone alone.

AR 10D
Answer: A. Her roommates.

AR 11
Answer: A. An IgM antibody assay.

AR 12
Answer: C. Immunoglobulin levels.

AR 13
Answer: C. Doxycycline PO.

AR 14A
Answer: A. Swab for rapid antigen testing
for group A strep prior to treatment.

AR 14B
Answer: D. No further testing, no antibiotics.

AR 15
Answer: E. An equine antitoxin.

AR 16
Answer: C. Treat with ceftriaxone 250 mg IM x 1
plus azithromycin 1 g PO x 1.

AR 17
Answer: C. Perform a lumbar puncture prior
to treatment.

AR 18
Answer: A. Metronidazole 500 mg bid x 7 d.

AR 19A
Answer: C. Levofloxacin x 3 d.

AR 19B
Answer: D. No antibiotic therapy.

AR 19C
Answer: D. No antibiotic therapy.

AR 19D
Answer: D. No antibiotic therapy.

AR 20
Answer: D. Admit and begin intravenous antibiotics.

AR 21A
Answer: A. IgM serologies.

AR 21B
Answer: B. IV doxycycline.

AR 22A
Answer: D. No tetanus prevention needed.

AR 22B
Answer: D. Amoxicillin/clavulanate.

AR 22C
Answer: D. Observe dog for 10 days.

AR 23
Answer: C. Treat for Lyme disease
without performing serology.

AR 24
Answer: D. Fungal culture.

AR 25
Answer: C. Mycobacterial culture.

AR 26
Answer: E. Liposomal amphotericin B.

AR 27
Answer: D. Stool for ova and parasites
with acid-fast stain.

AR 28
Answer: A. Chloroquine.

AR 29A
Answer: E. No test needed prior to treatment.

AR 29B
Answer: D. Albendazole and glucocorticoids.

AR 30
Answer: A. PO acyclovir.

AR 31
Answer: A. Send CSF for viral PCR.

AR 32
Answer: A. Start high-dose acyclovir.

AR 33
Answer: A. EBV IgM capsid antibody.

AR 34A
Answer: E. Pregnancy test.

AR 34B
Answer: E. Nothing.

AR 35
Answer: E. Blood for viral serology.

AR 36
Answer: D. Neither test nor treat with oseltamivir.

AR 37A
Answer: B. 2 NRTIs and an integrase inhibitor.

AR 37B
Answer: A. Trim/sulfa and azithromycin.

AR 37C
Answer: B. Test him once now.

AR 38
Answer: D. Pentamidine and prednisone.

AR 39A
Answer: D. Antistreptolysin O (ASO)
antibody titer.

AR 39B
Answer: A. 5 years.

AR 40A
Answer: D. Transthoracic echo.

AR 40B
Answer: B. Nafcillin alone.

AR 41
Answer: E. No treatment at this time.

AR 42
Answer: C. Nitrofurantoin x 5 days.

AR 43
Answer: A. Doxycycline.

AR 44A
Answer: A. Vancomycin.

AR 44B
Answer: A. Now.

AR 44C
Answer: B. Total of 2 weeks.

AR 45
Answer: E. Colonoscopy.

AR 46A
Answer: C. Lumbar puncture.

AR 46B
Answer: E. Liposomal Amphotericin B +
5-flucytosine.

AR 47
Answer: D. Obtain lung tissue for histology
and culture.

AR 48
Answer: A. Rubeola (measles).

AR 49
Answer: B. Secretions for respiratory syncytial
virus PCR.

AR 50
Answer: E. HIV viral load.

AR 51
Answer: A. Penicillin.

AR 52
Answer: C. Trimethoprim/sulfamethoxazole
and imipenem.

AR 53
Answer: A. Nasal saline, RTC 5 days
if worse/no better.

AR 54
Answer: E. Culture her bone marrow.

MedStudy

Internal Medicine Video Board Review

Nephrology

Presented by

Manish Suneja, MD
Director, Internal Medicine Residency Program
Co-Strand Director, Clinical and Professional Skills
Professor of Internal Medicine
Dr. William and Sondra Myers Professor
University of Iowa Hospitals and Clinics
& Carver College of Medicine
Iowa City, Iowa

Table of Contents

Nephrology Abbreviations

ABG	Arterial blood gas
ACEI	Angiotensin-converting enzyme inhibitor
ADH	Antidiuretic hormone
ADPCKD	Autosomal dominant polycystic kidney disease
AG	Anion gap
AIN	Acute interstitial nephritis
AKI	Acute kidney injury
AMI	Acute myocardial infarction
ANCA	Antineutrophil cytoplasmic antibody
ARB	Angiotensin receptor blocker
ASO	Antistreptolysin O
ATN	Acute tubular necrosis
BUN	Blood urea nitrogen
CAD	Coronary artery disease
CCB	Calcium channel blocker
CKD	Chronic kidney disease
CVA	Cerebrovascular accident
DAH	Diastolic arterial hypertension
DBP	Diastolic blood pressure
DD	Differential diagnosis
DM	Diabetes mellitus
EABV	Effective arterial blood volume
ECF	Extracellular fluid
EGPA	Eosinophilic granulomatosis with polyangiitis
ESRD	End-stage renal disease
FE_{Na}	Fractional excretion of sodium
FHH	Familial hypocalciuric hypercalcemia
FMD	Fibromuscular dysplasia
FSGS	Focal segmental glomerulosclerosis
GBM	Glioblastoma multiforme
GFR	Glomerular filtration rate
GN	Glomerulonephritis
HAGMA	High anion gap metabolic acidosis
HPF	High power field
HPT	Hyperparathyroidism
IgA	Immunoglobulin A
IUAN	Idiopathic uric acid nephrolithiasis
JVD	Jugular venous distention
LRTI	Lower respiratory tract infection
MPGN	Membranoproliferative glomerulonephritis
MPO	Mast cell peroxidase
NAGMA	Nonanion gap metabolic acidosis; Normal anion gap metabolic acidosis
PAC	Plasma (aldosterone)
PCKD	Polycystic kidney disease
P_{Osm}	Plasma osmolality
PRA	Plasma renin activity

PTH	Parathyroid hormone (phosphate-trashing hormone)
RF	Risk factor
RPGN	Rapidly progressive glomerulonephritis
RTA	Renal tubular acidosis
SBP	Systolic blood pressure
SIADH	Syndrome of inappropriate antidiuretic hormone secretion
SLE	Systemic lupus erythematosus
TSH	Thyroid-stimulating hormone
UA	Uric acid
U/A	Urinary analysis
UAG	Urine anion gap
URTI	Upper respiratory tract infection

Speaker Disclosure
Manish Suneja, MD, has documented that he has no
commercial relationships to disclose.

Nephrology

Topics
- Acute Kidney Injury
- Glomerular Diseases (Nephritic Syndrome)
- Glomerular Diseases (Nephrotic Syndrome)
- Nephrolithiasis
- Metabolic Acid-Base Disorders with Special Attention
  to Renal Tubular Acidosis (RTA)
- Hypertension (Including Secondary Hypertension)
- Hyponatremia and Hypernatremia
  (Disorders of Water Balance)
- Other Electrolyte and Mineral Disorders
- Pregnancy and Kidney
- Chronic Kidney Disease
- Polycystic Kidney Disease

Acute Kidney Injury

Acute Kidney Injury
- Sudden loss of renal function over hours to days
- Commonly **reflected by rise in creatinine and/or
  decrease in urine output**

**Classification of the Etiologies of Acute Kidney Injury
(AKI)**

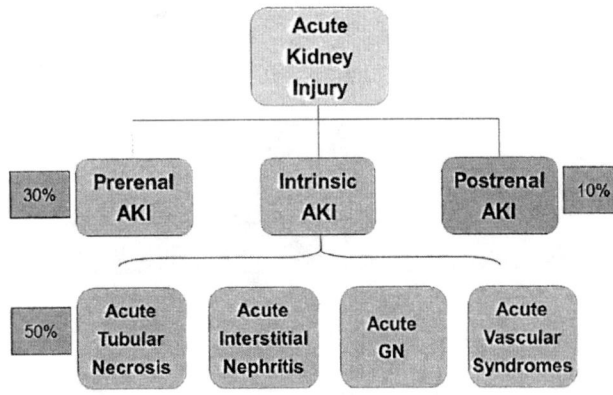

Prerenal Acute Kidney Injury

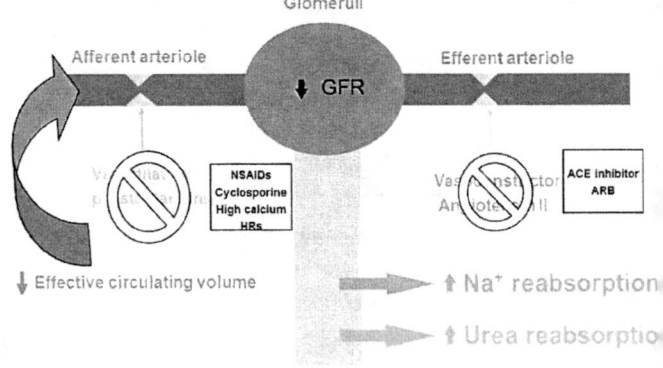

Urine Indices in AKI

	Prerenal	Intrinsic ATN
U_{Osm}	> 500	< 350
Na^+ (mEq/L)	< 20	> 40
Bun/Cr (mg/dL)	> 20:1	< 10:1
FE_{Na}	< 1%	> 2%
FE_{Urea}	< 35%	> 55%
U/P Creat	> 40	< 20
Sediment	Bland	Muddy brown, Granular casts

Useful marke[r]
when someo[ne]
is on
diuretics

Trumps all t[he]
urine indice[s]
** ATN

Acute Tubular Necrosis

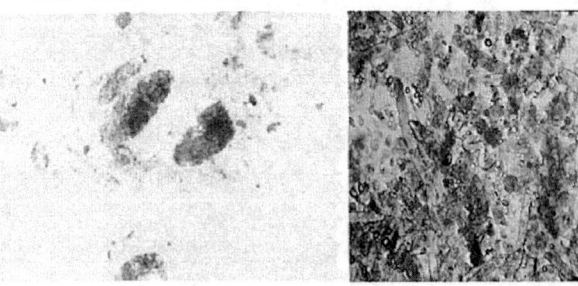

Pigmented granular ("muddy brown") casts
Marker of acute tubular necrosis

- **Ischemic:** Prerenal → ATN
- **Nephrotoxic**
  - **Endogenous**
    - Free myoglobin (**rhabdomyolysis:** Cocaine, statins,
      trauma, and electrolytes → **low phos and low K^+**)
    - Free hemoglobin (intravascular hemolysis)
  - **Exogenous**
    - Contrast
    - Drugs (**gentamicin**, amphotericin, cisplatin)
    - **Osmotic nephropathy:** Sucrose/mannitol/dextran,
      especially in patients with underlying chronic kidney
      disease

ATN Rhabdo vs. Hemolysis
Heme+ on dipstick but no RBC on micro:
Differential Diagnosis
$\downarrow$

1) **Myoglobinuria (rhabdo)** → check CPK/aldolase
2) **Hemoglobinuria (hemolytic anemia)** → peripheral blood smear/LDH/hapto/indirect bilirubin
- Treatment
  - <u>Early aggressive hydration with isotonic saline</u>
    - May need > 10 L IVF to achieve euvolemia*
  - Urine alkalinization — pH > 6.5
  - Keep UO 250–300 mL/hr

*Ron D, et al. Prevention of acute renal failure in traumatic rhabdomyolysis. *Arch Intern Med.* 1984 Feb;144(2):277–280.

Acute Interstitial Nephritis
(Drugs vs. Inflammatory Condition)
- Acute renal failure due to lymphocytic infiltration of the interstitium
- #1 Cause: <u>Drugs</u>; #1 drug = <u>NSAIDs/PPIs</u>
- Nondrug causes —

(pearl → exams like Sjögren's and sarcoidosis)
U/A → WBC or WBC cast in urine with no evidence of infection
(<u>Eosinophils in the urine on Wright or Hansel stain</u>)
- Classic triad of:
  - Fever
  - Rash
  - Eosinophilia
- Rx: Discontinue medication, PO steroids (early within 2 weeks)

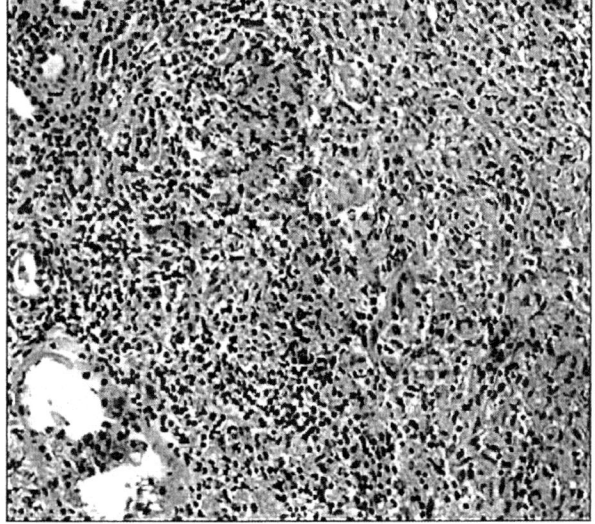

Clinical Features of PPI-Associated AIN

Finding	Frequency
Pyuria	72%
Fatigue and nausea	39%
Eosinophilia	33%
Weakness	22%
Fever	10%
Rash	< 10%

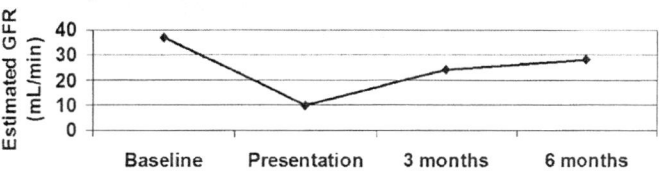

Geevasinga N, et al. Proton pump inhibitors and acute interstitial nephritis. *Clin Gastroenterol Hepatol.* 2006;4:597–604.

AKI after Arterial Catheterization
- **Post contrast**
  - AKI within 24–48 hours
  - Prevention with hydration pre- and postprocedure
  - Possible benefit from *N*-acetylcysteine (1,200 mg bid dose)

*154 mEq/L NaHCO₃ bolus 3 mL/kg/hr 1 hr before;
1 mL/kg/hr infusion for 6 hours after
Recently a negative study!!
*Merten GJ, et al. Prevention of contrast-induced nephropathy with sodium bicarbonate: A randomized controlled trial. *JAMA.* 2004 May 19;291(19):2328–2334.

Bottom line → Hydration with NS

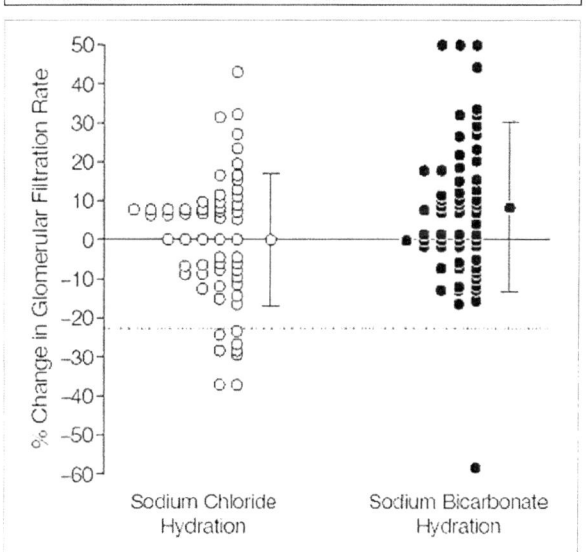

AKI after Arterial Catheterization (cont.)

- **Atheroembolic disease:** If not recovering by day 5 post contrast, must consider atheroembolic disease **(Pearl)**
  - Can occur spontaneously or after other vascular trauma
  - Hollenhorst plaque, livedo reticularis, and peripheral emboli
  - Eosinophiluria/Eosinophilia, low complement, high amylase
  - RX
    - Consider stopping anticoagulation (if not a strong indication)
    - **Statins?** Otherwise supportive care

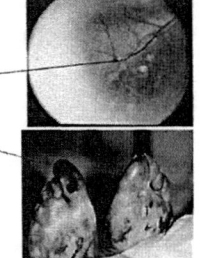

Some Other Important Stuff!!
Phosphate Nephropathy

- Develops within days after exposure (to an oral sodium phosphate bowel preparation)
- Generally recognized only when lab studies are performed at some later time
- **Clue: Hyperphosphatemia is out of proportion** to the degree of kidney injury and urinalysis has minimal findings
- **Risk factor → underlying CKD & diabetes (older age)**

Abdominal Compartment Syndrome

Intravesical Pressure Monitoring

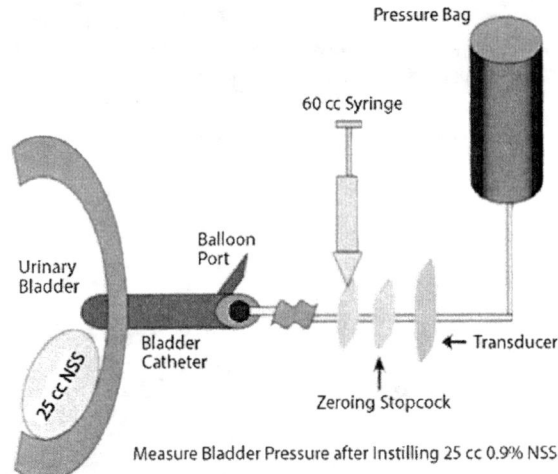

Measure Bladder Pressure after Instilling 25 cc 0.9% NSS

Diagnosis → Sustained IAP > 20 with AKI (often looks prerenal)

Pathophysiology → Decreased renal perfusion from increased renal vein pressure

Treatment → Decompressive laparotomy

Abnormal Urinalysis

- Cells
  - RBCs
    - **Dipstick blood+, no RBCs: Rhabdo or hemolysis
    - RBC casts = Glomerulonephritis
  - WBCs
    - **Sterile pyuria:** *Interstitial nephritis vs. tuberculosis, prostatitis, **analgesic abuse nephropathy (chronic, sterile pyuria, acetaminophen may contribute, imaging: ± Papillary necrosis)
    - **Nonsterile:** Urinary tract infection (upper vs. lower)
  - Eosinophils
    - *Drug-induced interstitial nephritis, atheroembolic disease
- Casts
- Crystals

Audience Response 1

A 77-year-old man with nausea, vomiting, and general malaise: 10 cc urine output in the last 2 days
PMH: Hyperlipidemia, HTN, T2DM, cigarettes x 40 years
Exam: Pale and stuporous, BP 170/70, HR 88
   Loud carotid bruits; Faint systolic ejection murmur
   Clear lungs
   Obese abdomen that is soft and without peritoneal signs
Labs: Glu 142, K^+ 5.4, Creat 6.4, BUN 165
Urinalysis: Bland

Which of the following is the most appropriate next step in management?

A. Order ANCA and anti-GBM antibodies.
B. Insert a temporary pacemaker in case hyperkalemia worsens.
C. Obtain a CT of the abdomen and pelvis with contrast.
D. Place a Foley catheter in the bladder.
E. Place a temporary dual lumen dialysis catheter.

Answer: _____

Glomerular Diseases (Nephritic Syndrome)

Proteinuria

- **Normal**
  - 24-hour urine = < 150 mg/d
  - "Spot" urine protein:creatinine ratio < 200 mg/g (0.2) roughly equivalent to 24-hour sample
- **Glomerular disease:**
  - If spot protein:creatinine ratio > 1.5–2.0 or 24-hour urine > 1.5–2.0 g/24 hr
- **Tubulointerstitial disease:** > Normal but < glomerular
  - If spot protein:creatinine ratio < 1.0 or 24-hour urine < 1.0 g/24 hr

Clinical "Syndromes"

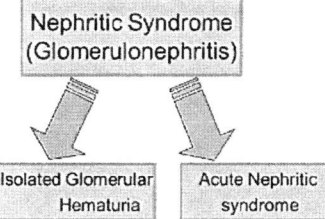

Chronic Glomerulonephritis / Chronic Kidney Disease

Nephrotic vs. Nephritic

	Nephrotic	Nephritic	Chronic GN
Proteinuria	> 3.5 g	< 1 g	Variable
RBCs	Minor, if any	Significant	Variable
Casts	Fatty casts, lipid droplets	RBC casts	Broad waxy casts

Nephritic Syndrome — Features
- Hematuria (main feature RBC cast/dysmorphic RBC)
- Proteinuria (1–3 g/24 hours)
- Hypertension and edema
- Azotemia (elevated BUN/creatinine)

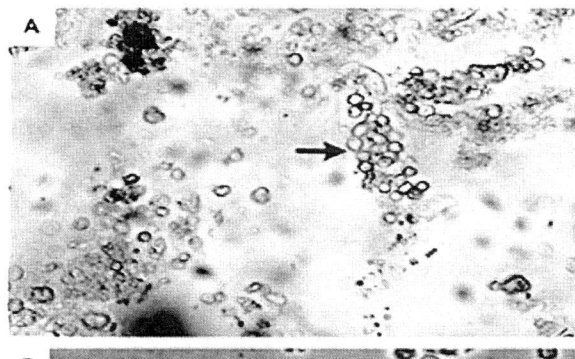

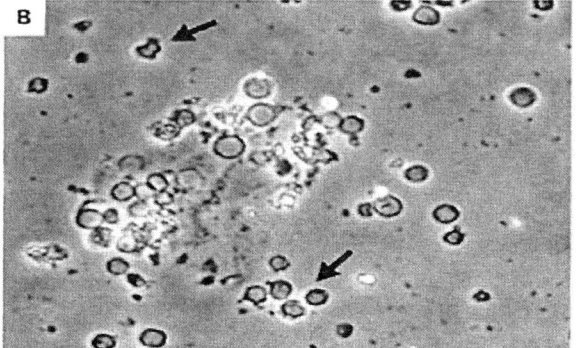

Nephritic Syndrome — Isolated Glomerular Hematuria
- **IgA Nephropathy**
  - Mesangial immune deposits staining for IgA
  - Recurrent frank hematuria after an upper respiratory tract infection
- **Alport Syndrome**
  - X-linked — defect in type IV collagen α5 chain in 85%
  - Most often has associated hematuria (positive family history)
  - Associate proteinuria, renal dysfunction as well as sensorineural deafness

Urine Sediment in Nephritic Syndromes

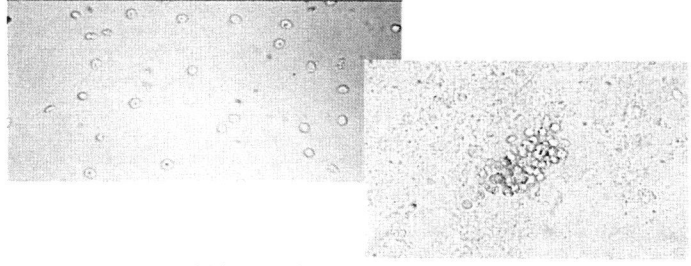

Proteinuria: Mild (< 1–2 g)
Hematuria: 1–3$^+$

Nephritic Syndrome

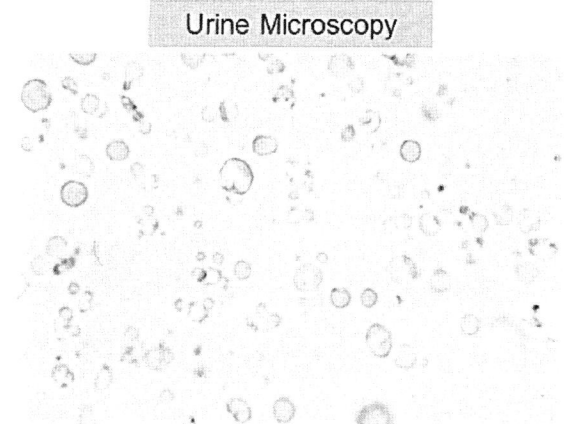

Nephritic Syndrome (cont.)

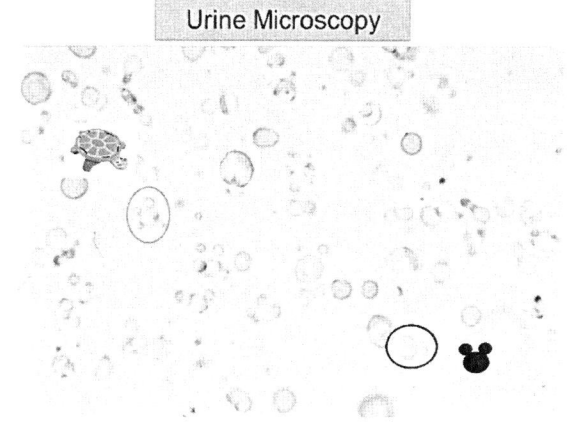

Glomerulonephritis / RPGN

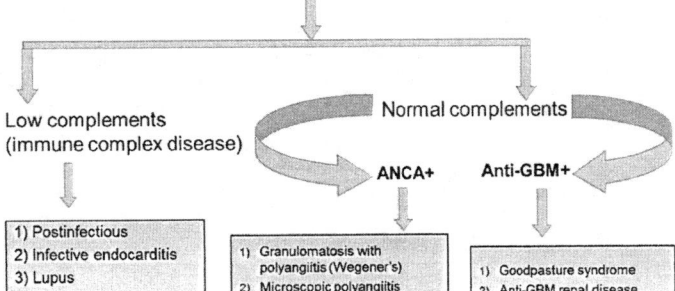

1) IgA nephropathy (most common GN)	1) Hematuria/RBC casts
2) Henoch-Schönlein	2) Proteinuria (1–3 g/day)
	3) HTN
	4) Renal failure

Low complements (immune complex disease)

Normal complements — ANCA+ — Anti-GBM+

Low complements:
1) Postinfectious
2) Infective endocarditis
3) Lupus
4) Cryoglobulinemia
5) Membranoproliferative

ANCA+:
1) Granulomatosis with polyangiitis (Wegener's)
2) Microscopic polyangiitis
3) Eosinophilic granulomatosis with polyangiitis (EGPA; formerly Churg-Strauss)
4) Renal limited ANCA

Anti-GBM+:
1) Goodpasture syndrome
2) Anti-GBM renal disease

IgA Nephropathy
(**Immune complex disease with normal serum complements)

- IgA nephropathy is the **most common primary GN** worldwide; IgA reacts to unidentified antigens
- **Recurrent hematuria** (can have sub-nephrotic range proteinuria)
- Episodes of **gross/microscopic hematuria are precipitated by flu-like illness**
- Diagnosis is made clinically or on **percutaneous renal biopsy**

IgA Nephropathy — Berger's
(**Immune complex disease with normal serum complements)

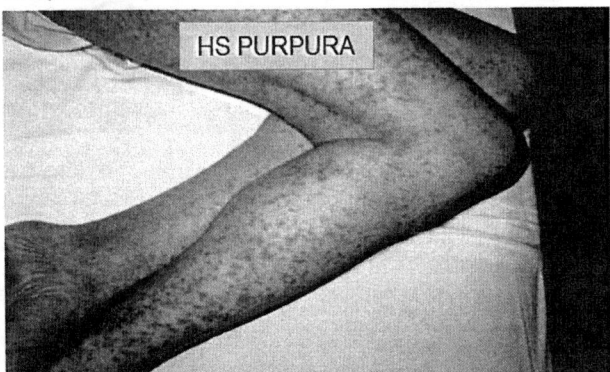

HS PURPURA

Kids or young adults
1) Palpable purpura
2) Arthritis/Arthralgia
3) Abdominal pain
4) Renal involvement

Acute Postinfectious GN

- Usually occurs in children — poststreptococcal GN is the most common cause of postinfectious GN
- Occurs after a streptococcal <u>pharyngitis or impetigo</u>
- Latent period: Acute onset of gross hematuria (<u>cola-colored</u>) or microscopic hematuria occurs 7–10 days after pharyngitis and up to 30 days after skin infection
- Caused by group A beta-hemolytic streptococci, particularly nephritogenic strains

Pearl

Nephritic syndrome after (skin Infx. or URI)
Decreased complement level (especially C3)
Increased ASO titer

Cryoglobulinemic GN

- Cryoglobulin is a generic term given to immunoglobulins that precipitate on cooling and resolubilize on warming
- 3 types:
  - Type 1 — monoclonal Ig (usually IgM)
  - **Type 2** — monoclonal Ig directed against Fc portion of polyclonal Ig (**hepatitis C**)
  - Type 3 — polyclonal Ig directed against Fc portion of polyclonal Ig

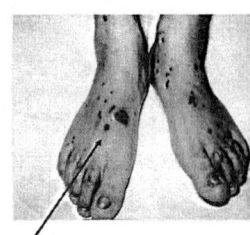

Pearl
Purpuric rash
Pseudo-Raynaud phenomenon
C4 depressed whereas C3 levels are low normal
Renal disease may improve with Rx of hepatitis C

Lupus Nephritis

- SLE is a multisystem, autoimmune disease with antibodies directed against a wide variety of cellular components
- Predominantly affects young women
- Various organ systems like skin, joints, serous membranes, heart, neurologic, blood, and the kidneys are involved
- **Type 4 lupus nephritis (diffuse proliferative)** most common; most worrisome
- **ANA, anti-dsDNA, depressed complement level (both C3 and C4)**

Rx
Induction → Cyclophosphamide/MMF + steroids
Maintenance → MMF/azathioprine

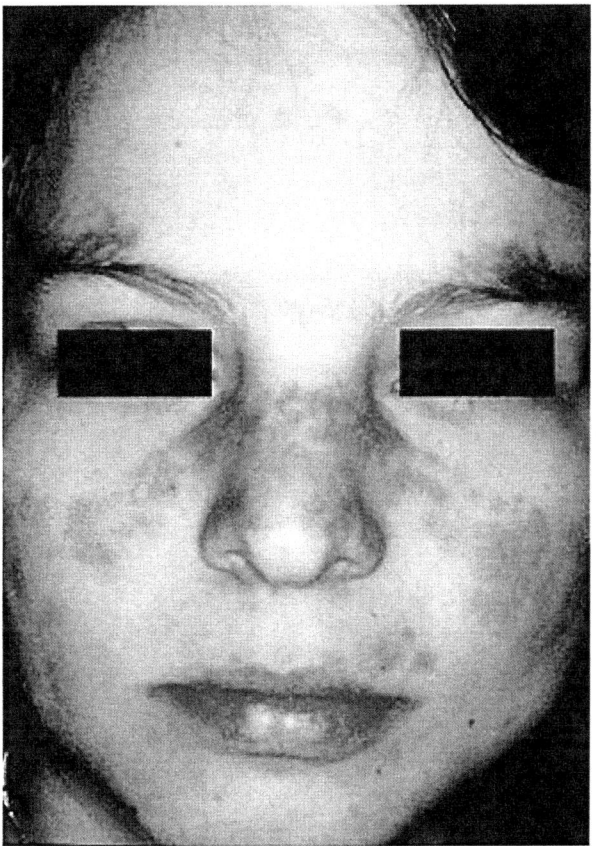

Membranoproliferative GN (MPGN)
- Group of disorders generally presenting with proteinuria, hematuria, and hypertension
- Gen associated with *hepatitis C and hepatitis B (clue risk factors or elevated liver enzymes)
- Can present as both nephrotic and nephritic syndromes
- **Low C3 level is seen in up to 70% of patients**
- Biopsy diagnosis

!!! New: Problems with alternate complement pathway: C3 glomerulopathy

Glomerular Diseases Associated with Low Complement Levels
- Postinfectious GN
- Lupus nephritis
- Infective endocarditis
- Membranoproliferative GN (MPGN)
  - Hepatitis B
  - Hepatitis C
- Cryoglobulinemia-associated GN

Nephritis with Normal Complements (ANCA Vasculitis & Anti-GBM)
- Granulomatosis with polyangiitis (formerly Wegener's)
  - **URTI** (sinusitis, epistaxis)
  - LRTI (infiltrates, cavitary lesions, DAH)
  - c-ANCA → anti-PR3
- Microscopic polyangiitis
  - Pulmonary hemorrhage
  - **Mononeuritis multiplex**
  - Cutaneous small vessel vasculitis (palpable purpura)
  - p-ANCA → anti-MPO
- Eosinophilic granulomatosis with polyangiitis (EGPA; formerly Churg-Strauss)
  - Asthma/Atopy
  - **Eosinophilia**

How to Remember All of This?
- Look for clues in history and lab results
- Place the case in a broad category like nephrotic syndrome, **nephritic syndrome**
- **Narrow differential based on complement level**
- **Renal-pulmonary syndrome** — Look at the nephritic syndrome table
- Look for key features

AR 2
A 19-year-old: Tea-colored urine x 1 day
H/O rhinorrhea and a cough x 2 days
PE: BP 138/92
Normal exam
U/A: TNTC RBCs, 2+ protein
ASO titer positive, C3/C4 normal,
Creat normal

Which of the following is the most likely diagnosis?
A. Postinfectious glomerulonephritis
B. Endocarditis
C. Poststreptococcal glomerulonephritis
D. Lupus nephritis
E. IgA nephropathy

Answer: _____

Glomerular Disease (Nephrotic Syndrome)

Nephrotic Syndrome — Features
- Proteinuria > 3.5 g/day
- Edema
- Hypoalbuminemia
- Hyperlipidemia
- Lipiduria

Hypercoagulable
Urinary loss of antithrombin III and plasminogen
Hemoconcentration

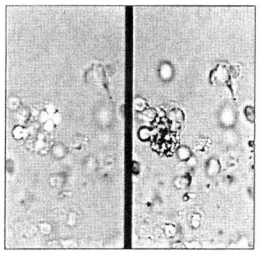

Nephrotic Syndrome — Histologic Classification
- Minimal change disease
- Membranous glomerulopathy
- Focal segmental glomerulosclerosis
- Membranoproliferative GN

Minimal Change Disease — Clinical Clues and Features
- **Most common in children/young adults (sudden onset of severe nephrosis)**
- Patient usually normotensive, nephrotic sediment, normal renal function
- Secondary etiologies:
  - Idiopathic
  - Drugs — **NSAIDs**
  - Toxins — mercury, lead
  - Tumors — **Hodgkin disease**
- **Rx: Steroids; Adults may require cytotoxics**

Focal Segmental Glomerulosclerosis — Clinical Clues and Features
- Most common primary renal disease in **African Americans**
- Patient usually hypertensive; Usually progresses to ESRD over 5–20 years
- **Primary (idiopathic)**
- **Secondary etiologies**
  - Familial — **gene mutations**
  - Drugs — intravenous heroin, pamidronate
  - Infections — **HIV (collapsing FSGS)**, parvovirus
  - Adaptive — reflux nephropathy, **obesity**
- **Rx: ACEIs/ARBs, steroids**

Membranous Nephropathy — Clinical Clues and Features
- Most common cause of idiopathic nephrotic syndrome in **Caucasian adults**
- Heavy proteinuria is common; Hypertension and azotemia develops as disease progresses
- **Increased incidence of renal vein thrombosis (Flank pain/hematuria/high LDH)*****
- **Secondary etiologies**
  - Drugs — NSAIDs, gold, penicillamine
  - Infections — hepatitis B/C, syphilis
  - **Tumors — carcinoma*****
  - Immunologic — SLE, RA
- **Rx: ACEI ± immunomodulation**

Nephrotic Syndrome — Systemic Disease Diabetic Nephropathy
- Most common cause of nephrotic syndrome in adults
- Leading cause of ESRD in U.S.
- 30% of patients with Type 1 and 20% of patients with Type 2 DM develop diabetic nephropathy
  - **Initially microalbuminuria** followed by heavy proteinuria and decline in renal function

- Diagnosis usually made on clinical grounds (unless no retinopathy present)
  - Up to 30% without retinopathy might have another etiology for their nephrotic syndrome

Drug of choice → ARB/ACEI

Nephrotic Syndrome — Systemic Disease Amyloidosis/Multiple Myeloma***
- **Amyloid:** Biochemical forms
  - Amyloid AL — immunoglobulin origin → MM
  - Amyloid AA — inflammatory states
- **Multiple myeloma (very important to recognize these clues)**
  - Renal failure with hypercalcemia
  - Discrepancy in urine dipstick and urine prot/creat ratio
  - Low anion gap
  - Total protein to albumin ratio > 2:1
  - Back pain in elderly

Nephrotic Syndrome

	Primary*	Secondary
Minimal Change Disease (Clue: Young adults/kids)		**NSAIDs** Lymphoma
Focal Segmental Glomerulosclerosis (Clue: African American)		**Genetic** (*APOL 1* & *MYH9* in AA) HIV Heroin Obesity
Membranous Glomerulopathy (Clue: Adults — cancer?)		**Solid tumors** SLE (lupus nephritis)
Membranoproliferative GN (Clue: Low complements)		**Hepatitis C**

*Primary = *de novo* renal disease = idiopathic

How to Remember All of This? Summary Principles
- Look for clues in history and lab results
- Place the case in a broad category like nephrotic syndrome, nephritic syndrome, etc.
- Just remember key features

AR 3

An 84-year-old man with T2DM and HTN:
Severe low back pain and increasing confusion
3-month history of 20-lb weight loss
Exam: Frail and generally decompensated with normal vital signs and point tenderness over L3
Labs: Na⁺ 139, K⁺ 5.9, Cl⁻ 115, HCO₃⁻ 18, Albumin 2.5, Total protein 8 BUN 68, Creat 3.6, Ca²⁺ 11.1, Glu 145 U/A 1.020, pH 6.0, 2 RBCs/HPF, trace protein
24-hour urine: Clearance 18 cc/m;
24-hour urine protein 5.5 g

Which of the following is the most appropriate next step in patient care?
A. Prostate-specific antigen (PSA)
B. Colonoscopy
C. Complement levels
D. Urine and serum electrophoresis
E. Urine for Hansel stain for eosinophils

Answer: _____

AR 4
A 64-year-old male with PMH of HTN, hyperlipidemia, OA:
New onset lower extremity edema
Recent history: Fatigue/tiredness; Weight loss 5 lbs
Meds: Acetaminophen, metoprolol, simvastatin
Exam: BP 122/74, HR 82
Fundi not visible, abdomen is slightly obese; 3+ pitting edema of the lower extremities to mid-calf
Fasting BMP: Creat 1.1 mg/dL, Albumin 2.1, total Cholesterol is 314, fasting glucose is 98 mg/dL
U/A: 4+ protein, micro shows fat droplets
Urine protein to creatinine ratio is 7.5
Hemoglobin is 9.8 and stool occult is positive

What is the most likely diagnosis?
A. FSGS (focal segmental glomerulosclerosis)
B. Minimal change disease
C. Amyloidosis
D. Membranous nephropathy
E. Membranoproliferative glomerulonephritis

Answer: _____

Nephrolithiasis

Renal Stones

Nephrolithiasis → The Afflicted
• Prevalence
  – Estimated **12% of men** and **6% of women** will develop a stone during lifetime
• Recurrence
  – 30–50% will have recurrence within 5 years
  – However, treatment can reduce this risk by up to 50%

~ 80% contain calcium with calcium oxalate — the most common

Types of Stones
• Basically 2 types
  1) **Calcium-based**
     • **Calcium oxalate — 70% (most common)**
     • Calcium phosphate — 10% → think distal RTA
  2) **Everything else**
     • **Uric acid — ~ 10%**
     • *Struvite — ~ 10% → Urease-splitting organisms
     • Cysteine — 1%
     • Drug-induced

Drugs Associated with Stones
• **Triamterene**
• **Indinavir**
• Sulfonamides
• Acetazolamide
• Ascorbic acid
• Chemotherapy (increased urate load)

Urinary Risk Factors
• **High (promoters)**
  – High urine calcium (hypercalciuria)
  – High urine oxalate (hyperoxaluria)
  – High urine uric acid (hyperuricosuria)
• **Low (inhibitors)**
  – Low urine citrate (hypocitraturia)
  – Low urine volume (very important in all stone formers)
Increase in promoters or decrease in inhibitors!

Risk Factors for Calcium Oxalate Stone
• **Hypercalciuria → most important**
• **Hyperoxaluria**
• Hyperuricosuria
• Hypocitraturia
• Low urine volume (common to all stones)

Risk Factor — Idiopathic Hypercalciuria

R/O ↑ Ca²⁺, Vit D, TSH, or cancer, sarcoidosis, etc.
↓
Idiopathic Hypercalciuria
Men > 300 mg/day
Women > 250 mg/day

• Treatment:
  – Anticalciuric diuretics (thiazides)
    • HCTZ
    • Chlorthalidone
    • Indapamide
• Diet:
  – Reduce animal protein
  – Reduce Na⁺

Risk Factor — Hyperoxaluria

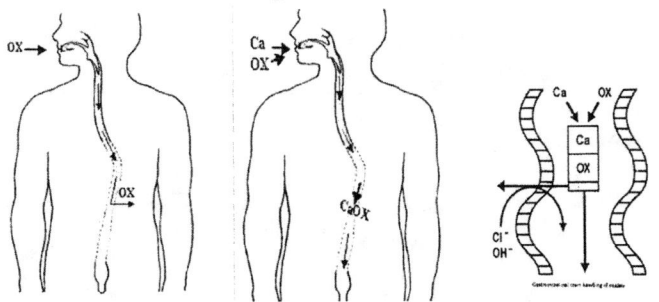

Current Understanding → Oxalate

Treatment of Idiopathic Hyperoxaluria
- Diet
  - Reduce oxalate-containing food (spinach, rhubarb, beetroots, nuts)
  - Avoid low-calcium diet

Calcium and the Risk of Symptomatic Kidney Stones in Males

	Group 1	Group 2	Group 3	Group 4	Group 5
Calcium intake (mg)	< 605	605–722	723–848	849–1,049	> 1,050
Incidence/100,000 person/yr	435	310	279	266	243
Multivariate RR (95% CI-)	1.0	0.74 (0.57–0.97)	0.68 (0.52–0.90)	0.68 (0.51–0.90)	0.66 (0.49–0.90)

$p = 0.018$ for trend

Curhan GC, et al. A prospective study of dietary calcium and other nutrients and the risk of symptomatic kidney stone. *NEJM*. 1993;328:833–838.

Risk Factors for Uric Acid Stone!!
(Becoming more common with diabetes and obesity)
- Acidic urine pH**
- Hyperuricosuria
- Low urine volume

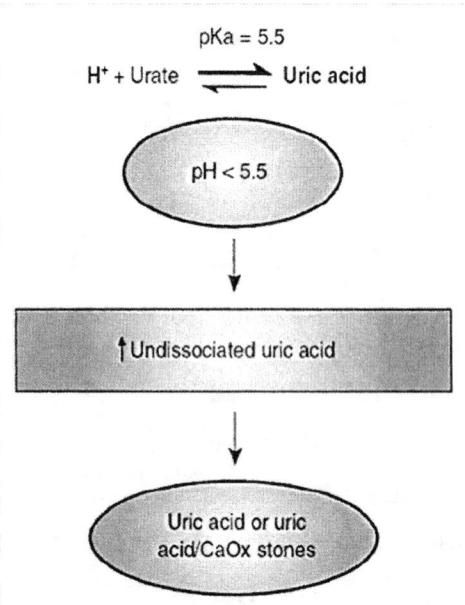

pKa = 5.5

$H^+ + Urate \rightleftharpoons$ Uric acid

pH < 5.5

↑Undissociated uric acid

Uric acid or uric acid/CaOx stones

Prevention and Rx of IUAN
- Increase urine pH > 6
  - Potassium citrate 20–30 mEq 2–3 times daily
- Allopurinol
  - If urine UA level is increased
- Improve the metabolic risk factors

Medical Treatment of Nephrolithiasis
- Thiazides: ↑ Renal tubular calcium absorption Rx for hypercalciuria
- Potassium citrate: Rx for hypocitraturia

Dietary Prescription

- Urinary Volume → Increase fluid intake to maintain a urine volume > 2 L (fluids: 2.5–3 L/d)
- High U. Calcium →
  1) Reduce nondairy animal protein intake (5 servings of meat/week)
  2) Reduce sodium intake (< 2.4 g/day)
  3) Reduce sucrose intake
- High U. Oxalate →
  1) Avoid high oxalate foods
  2) **Adequate dietary calcium (> 700 mg at least)**
  3) Avoid vitamin C supplements
- High U. Uric acid → Reduce purine intake
- Low U. Citrate →
  1) Increase fruit and vegetable intake (phytates)
  2) Reduce nondairy animal protein intake

Stones → Key Points
- Calcium oxalate (**1° HPT**, idiopathic hypercalciuria, low urine citrate, hyperoxaluria) **most common**
- Calcium phosphate (**distal renal tubular acidosis**)
- Uric acid 10% (**low urine pH** & hyperuricosuria — assoc. with gout, chronic diarrhea, ileostomy) → **Radiolucent → Rx: Increase the urine pH**

- Struvite — magnesium ammonium phosphate (**infection with bacteria** that expresses urease) → Staghorn calculi
- Cystine (cystinuria) — **hexagonal**

Metabolic Acid-Base Disorders with Special Attention to Renal Tubular Acidosis (RTA)

Metabolic Acid-Base Disorders
- **Metabolic acidosis**
  - High anion gap (HAGMA)
  - Normal anion gap (NAGMA)
- **Metabolic alkalosis**

The Henderson-Hasselbalch Formula is the Mantra of Acid-Base Physiology

The Mantra

$$pH = pKa + \log \frac{[HCO_3^-]}{[CO_2]}$$

$$pH \propto \frac{[HCO_3^-]}{[CO_2]}$$

$$Acidity = \frac{Bicarbonate}{Carbon\ Dioxide}$$

$$A = {}^B/_{CD}$$

There Are 4 Primary Ways That pH Can Change

1) Increase in **HCO₃⁻** increases **pH:** **Metabolic alkalosis**

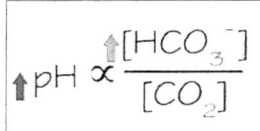

2) Increase in HCO₃⁻ increases pH: Metabolic alkalosis

   Decrease in **HCO₃⁻** decreases **pH:** **Metabolic acidosis**

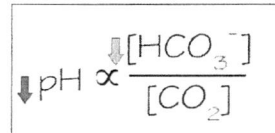

3) Increase in HCO₃⁻ increases pH: Metabolic alkalosis

   Decrease in HCO₃⁻ decreases pH: Metabolic acidosis

   Increase in **pCO₂** decreases **pH:** **Respiratory acidosis**

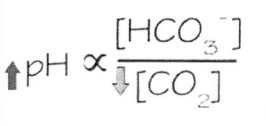

4) Increase in HCO₃⁻ increases pH: Metabolic alkalosis

   Decrease in HCO₃⁻ decreases pH: Metabolic acidosis

   Increase in pCO₂ decreases pH: Respiratory acidosis

   Decrease in **pCO₂** increases **pH:** **Respiratory alkalosis**

Approach to the Data …

Think about the history …
what do their symptoms/signs suggest?

Six-Step Approach to Acid-Base Analysis
1) Is the patient acidemic or alkalemic?
2) Is the overriding disturbance metabolic or respiratory?
3) If respiratory … is it acute or chronic based on compensation?
4) If metabolic … is the respiratory system compensating appropriately?
5) Is there a high anion gap?
   (*****Always check an anion gap!!**)
6) In cases of increased anion gap —
   Is there a second metabolic disturbance?
   (check corrected bicarbonate)

Step 1 — Acidemia or Alkalemia?
- Remember compensation is never 100%
- pH < 7.4 — acidemia
- pH > 7.4 — alkalemia
- pH = 7.4 — you're fine (or … mixed)

Step 2 — Is it Metabolic or Respiratory?
- If it's **acidosis** (or alkalosis) look for the source of acid (or base)
- **HCO₃⁻ < 24**   **Metabolic acidosis**
- HCO₃⁻ > 24   Metabolic alkalosis
- **CO₂ > 40**   **Respiratory acidosis**
- CO₂ < 40   Respiratory alkalosis

Determine the Primary Disorder

pH / pCO$_2$ / pO$_2$ / HCO$_3^-$

1) Acidosis or alkalosis
   – If the pH is < 7.4, it is acidemia
   – If the pH is > 7.4, it is alkalemia
2) Determine if it is metabolic or respiratory
   – If the pH, bicarbonate, and pCO$_2$ all move in the same direction (up **or** down), it is metabolic
   – If the pH, bicarbonate, and pCO$_2$ move in discordant directions (up **and** down), it is respiratory

What are the Acid-Base Disorders?

Case	pH	pCO$_2$ mmHg	[HCO$_3^-$] mEq/L
A	7.32	28	14

Metabolic acidosis

What are the Acid-Base Disorders?

Case	pH	pCO$_2$ mmHg	[HCO$_3^-$] mEq/L
A	7.47	20	14

Respiratory alkalosis

What are the Acid-Base Disorders?

Case	pH	pCO$_2$ mmHg	[HCO$_3^-$] mEq/L
A	7.08	49	14

Respiratory acidosis and metabolic acidosis

Step 3 — Compensations
After you come up with "primary disturbance," your next question should ALWAYS BE =
"Is there compensation?"

Simple Acid-Base Disorders

	Primary process	Compensation
Metabolic acidosis	⇩[HCO$_3^-$]	⇩ pCO$_2$
Metabolic alkalosis	⇧[HCO$_3^-$]	⇧ pCO$_2$
Respiratory acidosis	⇧ pCO$_2$	⇧[HCO$_3^-$]
Respiratory alkalosis	⇩ pCO$_2$	⇩[HCO$_3^-$]

***Compensation is always in the same direction as the primary disorder

Compensation if the Primary Disorder is Respiratory

Δ PCO$_2$:   Δ HCO$_3^-$

	Respiratory acidosis	Respiratory alkalosis
Acute	**10:1**	**10:2**
Chronic	**10:3**	**10:5**
	For every rise of 10 in the pCO$_2$ the HCO$_3^-$ will rise by 1 or 3	For every fall of 10 in pCO$_2$ the HCO$_3^-$ will fall by 2 or 4

Step 4 — Compensation if the Primary Disorder is Metabolic
Metabolic acidosis: Winter's formula
$$1.5 \times HCO_3^- + 8 \pm 2$$
Metabolic alkalosis:
   pCO$_2$ rises 0.7 per mEq rise in HCO$_3^-$

Step 5 — Is There a High Anion Gap?
- [Cl$^-$] + [HCO$_3^-$] + U Anions = [Na$^+$] + U Cations
- U Anions – U Cations = [Na$^+$] – [Cl$^-$] – [HCO$_3^-$]
- **Anion Gap = [Na$^+$] – [Cl$^-$] – [HCO$_3^-$]**
- Major unmeasured cations
  Ca^{2+}, K$^+$, Mg^{2+}, paraproteins (and lithium)
- Major unmeasured anions
  – **Albumin**
  – **Phosphates**
  – **Sulfates**
  – **Organic anions**

Calculating the Anion Gap
- Anion gap = Na$^+$ – (HCO$_3^-$ + Cl$^-$)
- Normal is 10–12
  – Varies by hospital
  – Average anion gap in healthy controls is 6 ± 3

Causes of HAGMA
- **MUDPILES**
  – **Methanol** (increased osmolal gap)
  – **Uremia**
  – **Diabetic ketoacidosis**
  – **Paraldehyde** → replaced with Propylene glycol
  – **Isoniazid, iron** (very uncommon)
  – **Lactate**
  – **Ethylene glycol** (increased osmolal gap)
  – **Salicylates** (resp. alkalosis → mixed resp. alkalosis + HAGMA)

**Mnemonic for the 21st century —
GOLDMARK: This acronym represents **G**lycols (ethylene and propylene), **O**xoproline, **L**-lactate, **D**-lactate, **M**ethanol, **A**spirin, **R**enal failure, and **K**etoacidosis

Causes of HAGMA (cont.)
If you do not like mnemonics!!!

Type	Increased Anions
Diabetic **ketoacidosis** Alcoholic **ketoacidosis** Starvation **ketoacidosis**	β-hydroxybutyrate, acetoacetate β -hydroxybutyrate, acetoacetate, lactate
Lactic acidosis	Lactate
Renal failure	Phosphate, sulfate, organic anions
Toxins: Methanol Ethylene glycol Salicylates	Formate, lactate Oxalate, glycolate Salicylates

Step 6 — If You Have an Anion Gap, Determine What the Bicarbonate was Before the Anion Gap
Corrected bicarbonate: Δ Anion gap + HCO_3^-
　　　Where Δ Anion gap = Anion gap − 12

The Acid-Base Time Machine
- Assume that the loss of bicarbonate due to addition of an anion is roughly 1:1
- So for every increase in the anion gap of one, the bicarbonate should drop by one
　　　Δ HCO_3^- = Δ Anion Gap

　　HCO_3^- before − HCO_3^- now = $AG_{current}$ − AG_{normal}

　　　　Corrected bicarbonate
　HCO_3^- before = HCO_3^- now + ($AG_{current}$ − AG_{normal})

**Osmolal gap
- In the presence of a large anion gap (> 20–25) of undetermined etiology, you must rule out a toxic alcohol
  − Methanol (retinal edema)
  − Ethylene glycol (oxalate crystals)
- Osmolal Gap:
  − Measured osmolality − calculated osmolality
  − > 10 consider methanol or ethylene glycol***
- Molecular weights
  − Methanol: 32
  − Ethylene glycol: 62

Examples: What is the Acid-Base Diagnosis?
　　　　Blood gas: 7.50 / 20
　　　Na^+ = 140, Cl^- = 103, HCO_3^- = 15
Respiratory alkalosis and anion gap metabolic acidosis
　　　　　　Ex 1

Case
- Anion gap metabolic acidosis
- Normal gap metabolic acidosis
- Respiratory acidosis

136	105	38
1.5	10	1.8

pH = 7.1
pCO_2 35
Anion gap = 21

Evaluate:
- **Acidosis** or alkalosis
- **Metabolic** or respiratory
- Isolated metabolic acidosis?
  ✓ Yes.
- **Anion gap** or nonanion gap
- Additional metabolic disorder?
  ✓ Yes
  ✓ Nonanion gap metabolic acidosis

7.14 / 18 / 212 / 6
pH / pCO$_2$ / pO$_2$ / HCO$_3^-$

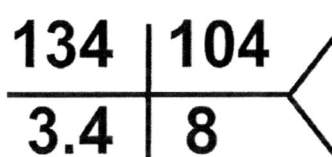

- Predicted pCO_2
  ✓ (8 x 1.5) + 8 ± 2 =
  ✓ 18–22
- Anion gap
  ✓ 134 − (104 + 8) =
  ✓ 22
- Bicarbonate prior to anion gap
  ✓ HCO_3^- + (AG − 12) = HCO_3^- before
  ✓ 8 + (22 − 12) =
  ✓ 18

Possible RTA??
　　　　RTA should be suspected
　　　　　　⇩
　　　　Metabolic **acidosis** +
　　　　Hyperchloremia +
　　　Normal plasma anion gap

(In a patient without evidence of gastrointestinal HCO_3^- losses)

Urine Anion Gap
- UAG = Urine ($Na^+ + K^+ - Cl^-$)
- The UAG is **negative** in patients with a normal AG metabolic acidosis

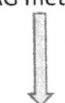

This is secondary to an appropriate **increase in urinary ammonium** (unmeasured cation) in order to excrete the excess acid

Urinary Anion Gap
Nonanion Gap Metabolic Acidosis (NAGMA)
- UAG = Urine ($Na^+ + K^+ - Cl^-$)
- Type 1 (distal) RTA: **Urine AG is positive** (unable to excrete ammonium normally; It is also positive in Type 4)
- Diarrhea: **Urine AG is negative**

Urinary Anion Gap NAGMA (cont.)
- In diarrhea, UAG becomes "negative"
- If renal tubular function is impaired Type 1 (distal) RTA, UAG is "positive"

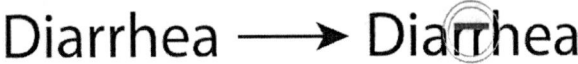

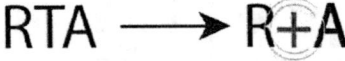

Types of RTA
Pearl: Exams like Sjögren syndrome + Distal RTA
Proximal RTA (Type 2) — Hypokalemia
- Isolated bicarbonate defect
- Fanconi syndrome (**multiple myeloma**), drugs
Distal RTA (Type 1) — Hypokalemia
- Classic type (**Sjögren syndrome**) or **SLE**
- Urine anion gap → positive
- **Associated with stones and nephrocalcinosis (hypercalciuria → calcium phosphate)**
RTA Type 4 (low renin/low aldo) — Hyperkalemia
(**diabetes**, HIV, obstruction)
- Urine anion gap → positive

AR 5
A 26-year-old Caucasian female referred for further evaluation of hypokalemia and acidosis:
She was in her usual state of excellent health until 4 months back when she developed dry mouth and muscle weakness. She was found to have a serum potassium of 2.8 mEq/L and a bicarbonate level of 15 mEq/L during her lab check. She was treated with oral potassium and bicarbonate supplements, and then she

stopped taking these medications. Six weeks later, she developed myalgias and collapsed due to profound weakness. She was found to have a serum bicarbonate level of 14 mEq/L with a serum potassium of 2.0 mEq/L.

140 | 114 | 13 Calcium 9.1
2.0 | 14 | 1   Phosphorus 3.5

ABG: pH 7.29, pCO₂ 30, pO₂ 100
Urine K⁺ 46, Urine Na⁺ 36, Urine Cl⁻ 42,
Urine_osm 580
U/A: pH 6.8, no casts

Which of the following is the correct diagnosis?
A. Type 4 RTA
B. Diarrhea
C. Type 1 RTA (distal RTA)
D. Renal tubular alkalosis
E. Type 2 RTA (proximal RTA)

Answer: _____

**Metabolic Alkalosis —
(Exams like metabolic alkalosis and urine chloride)

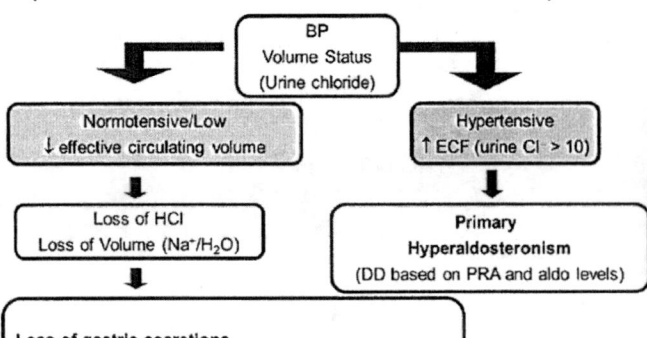

Clues to Acid-Base Disorders*
- Normal ABGs & ↑ AG = Mixed metabolic acidosis/alkalosis
- Low AG (< 8) = **Hypoalbuminemia, paraproteinemia,** hypercalcemia/magnesemia, lithium intoxication
- Osmolal gap > 10 = **Methanol (blindness), ethanol, ethylene glycol (oxalate crystals)**
- Isopropyl alcohol **osmolal gap without acidosis**

Hypertension
(Including Secondary Hypertension)

Hypertension — JNC 8
- Classification of BP (JNC 7): Definition **not addressed** in JNC 8
  - Normal = < 120/ < 80
  - Pre-hypertension: 120–130/80–89
  - HTN, Stage 1: 140–159/90–99
  - HTN, Stage 2: > 160/ > 100
- **Goals of treatment:** Threshold for pharmacologic treatment was defined in JNC 8 based on **age, diabetes, and chronic kidney disease**
  - General population < 60 years → < 140/90
  - General population **> 60 years** → **< 150/90**
  - All ages, no CKD, **diabetes +** → **< 140/90**
  - All ages **CKD+**, with/without diabetes → **< 140/90**

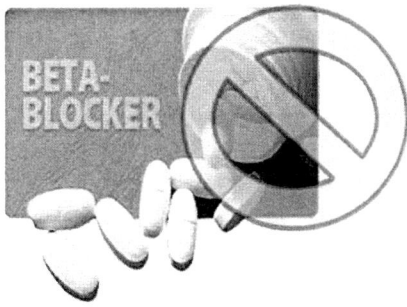

JNC 8 — Treatment of HTN
- **Lifestyle interventions for all**
- **Drug Therapy**
  - Recommended based on **race and CKD**
    - **Race** (general population < 60 years or > 60 years, diabetics without CKD)
      - **Black** (including those with diabetes): Thiazide or CCB
      - **Nonblack** (including those with diabetes): ACEI or ARB, CCB or thiazide diuretics
    - **CKD** (regardless of race or diabetes, population > 18 years): Treatment should include **ACEI or ARB**

Can begin with 2 drugs:
- SBP > 160 or DBP > 100
- SBP > 20 mmHg above goal
- DBP > 10 mmHg above goal

Hypertension in the Elderly
- **Rx of patients older than 60 years of age**
  - Threshold for pharmacologic treatment (> 150/90): Strong recommendation — Grade A **(JNC 8)** ... **Questions raised by SPRINT trial** (among patients at **high risk for cardiovascular events but without diabetes**, targeting a systolic blood pressure of < 120 mmHg, as compared with < 140 mmHg, resulted in lower rates of fatal and nonfatal major cardiovascular events and death from any cause)
  - If Rx results in lower achieved SBP (e.g., < 140 mmHg) and is well tolerated, without adverse effects on health or quality of life, treatment does not need to be adjusted
- Evaluate for secondary cause, if new diagnosis after age 55 years

Antihypertensive Diuretic
- Chlorthalidone recommended over hydrochlorothiazide (HCTZ)
  - HCTZ less potent & shorter acting
  - Problems: Lack of fixed-dose combinations & no 12.5 mg tablet, more likely to induce hypokalemia
- Loop diuretics for **CHF & CKD**

ARB + ACEI (Do Not Use Together)
- > 2x risk
  - Acute kidney injury
  - Hyperkalemia
  - ONTARGET (Negative study: Rx to prevent vascular events in patients with CAD/DM)
- Previous indication for combination was persistence of proteinuria > 1 g following trial on ARB or ACEI:
  - **Lancet retracted the COOPERATE trial in 2009**
  - Would recommend adding nondihydropyridine CCB (diltiazem) or spironolactone

Indicators of Secondary HTN
- Abrupt or accelerated
- Malignant/Refractory HTN
- Systolic-diastolic epigastric or renal bruits
- Hypokalemia with metabolic alkalosis

Common Causes of 2° HTN
- **Structural**
  - Coarctation of aorta (UE BP > LE BP)
- **Renal**
  - Chronic kidney disease
- **Renovascular**
  - Renal artery stenosis (atherosclerosis vs. FMD → young females)

Common Causes of 2° HTN (cont.)
- **Endocrine**
  - Adrenal
    - **Primary aldosteronism (very important — know the workup)**
    - **Cushing syndrome (cortisol acts like aldosterone)**
    - Pheochromocytoma
  - Thyroid disorders/parathyroid disorders
- **Medication (important cause of resistant HTN)**
  - Pseudoephedrine
  - NSAIDs
  - Herbals
  - Excessive salt intake
- **Sleep apnea (important cause of resistant HTN)**

Hypokalemic Hypertensive

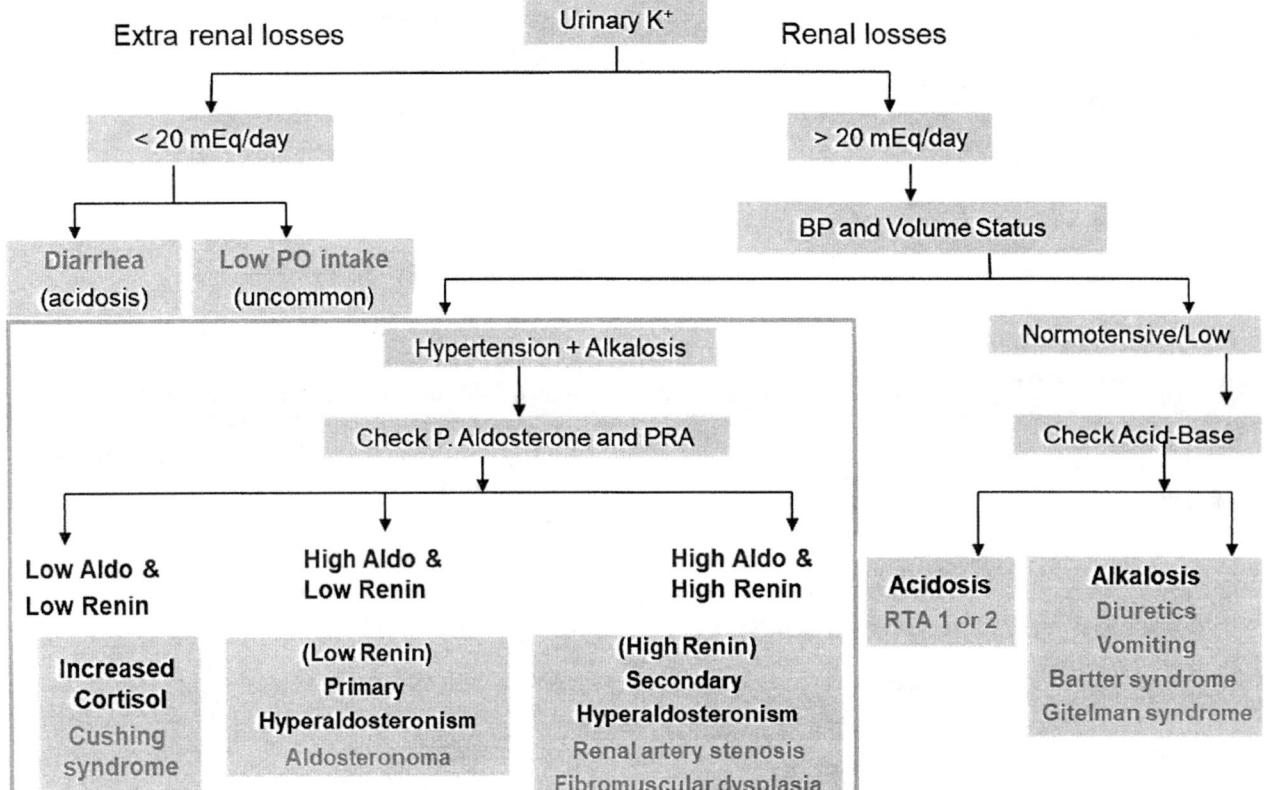

Source: Manish Suneja, MD

The Hypokalemic Hypertensive
- If you have no idea what I'm talking about …
- If "hyperreninemic" and "hyperaldo" sound like gibberish to you …
- When you see a **hypertensive patient** with **hypokalemia**, think:

  PAC:PRA!

Primary Aldosteronism

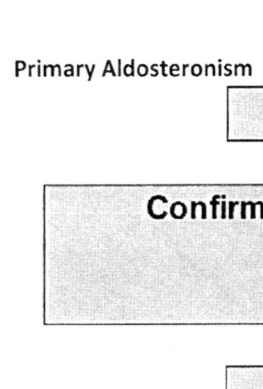
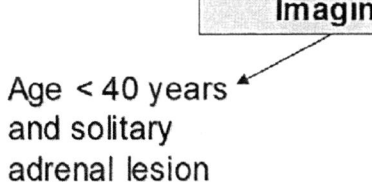

Screening → Ratio of PAC to PRA > 20

Confirmation → 24-hour urine for aldo and creatinine on a high-salt diet (aldo > 12 μg/24 hrs)

Imaging → CT with adrenal cuts

Age < 40 years and solitary adrenal lesion

→ Surgery

Age > 40 years or B/I lesions or negative imaging

→ Adrenal vein sampling

Lateralization → Consider surgery

No lateralization → Medical Rx: Spironolactone vs. eplerenone

---

AR 6

A 22-year-old woman referred from GYN for BP eval:
Previous BPs 149/92 and 154/95
Review of systems negative
No family history of HTN
PE: 155/94, HR 86, Afebrile, RR 14
Examination normal
Na^+ 142, K^+ 2.9, Cl^- 104, HCO_3^- 32,
BUN 10, Creat 0.6, Glu 102
CBC normal

Which of the following is the most appropriate next step in her management?
A. CT scan of the adrenals
B. Ratio of plasma aldosterone concentration to plasma renin activity
C. Helical CT of the renal vasculature
D. A.M. cortisol level
E. Captopril renal scintigraphy

Answer: _____

AR 7

Based on the last question, which of the following is the most likely diagnosis, if both PRA and plasma aldosterone levels returned high?
A. Renal artery stenosis
B. Fibromuscular dysplasia
C. Conn syndrome (adrenal adenoma)
D. Bilateral adrenal hyperplasia
E. Cushing syndrome

Answer: _____

**Hyponatremia and Hypernatremia
(Disorders of Water Balance)**

Hypernatremia → $[Na^+]$ > 145 mEq/L

and

Hyponatremia → $[Na^+]$ < 135 mEq/L

**Represent
disorders of water homeostasis
(or the concentration of serum Na^+)**

$$P_{Osm} = 2[Na^+] + Glu/18 + BUN/2.8$$

ADH Regulates Water Balance

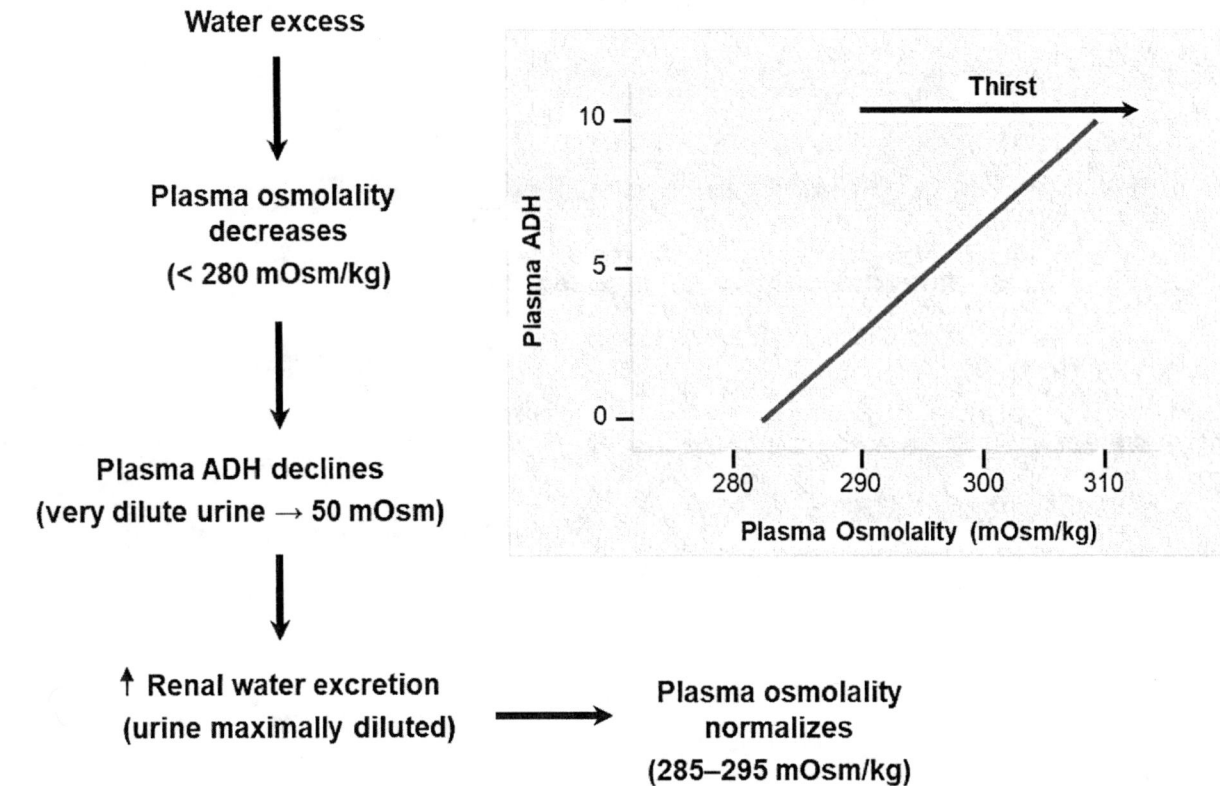

Water excess

↓

Plasma osmolality decreases
(< 280 mOsm/kg)

↓

Plasma ADH declines
(very dilute urine → 50 mOsm)

↓

↑ **Renal water excretion**
(urine maximally diluted) → **Plasma osmolality normalizes (285–295 mOsm/kg)**

ADH Regulates Water Balance (cont.)

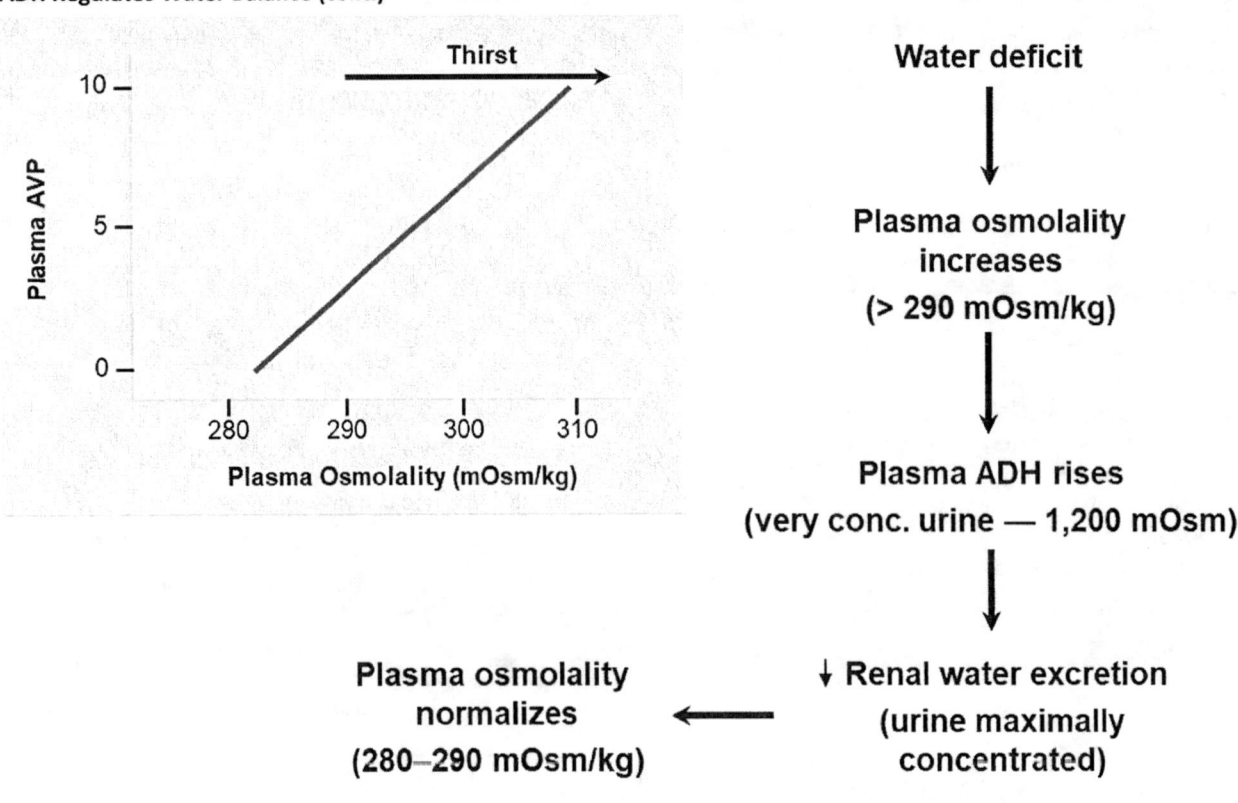

Water deficit

↓

Plasma osmolality increases
(> 290 mOsm/kg)

↓

Plasma ADH rises
(very conc. urine — 1,200 mOsm)

↓

↓ **Renal water excretion**
(urine maximally concentrated)

← **Plasma osmolality normalizes (280–290 mOsm/kg)**

Physiological Stimuli for ADH Release
- **Elevated plasma osmolality**
- **Decreased effective arterial blood volume**
  - Hypotension
  - Hypovolemia
- **Endogenous stimuli**
  - Nausea
  - Pain

How Does Hyponatremia Develop?
- **Physiology:**
  - **Huge water intake** with normal water excretion (i.e., psychogenic polydipsia)

    <u>Or</u>

    Normal water intake with **impaired water excretion** (common)

    Factors causing impaired water excretion
    1) **High ADH** — promotes water reabsorption in collecting duct
    2) **Low EABV**
       - Enhances ADH secretion → Promotes proximal fluid reabsorption resulting in decreased distal delivery

---

Water intake > Water excretion
<u>Must</u> have water intake!

Approach to Hyponatremia
- **Measure plasma osmolality** → **need to know P_{Osm}**
  - **When low, defines true hypo-osmolal state or clinical hyponatremia**
  - If high → plasma glucose; If normal → protein and lipids
- **Assess volume status** → **need to know volume status**
  - Clinical parameters — **orthostatics, JVD, S_3 gallop, lung exam/pedal edema, skin turgor**
  - Objective assessment of volume status — $U_{Na} < 20$, FE_{Na} and $FE_{Urea} < 35$ **consistent with hypovolemic state**
- **Urine osmolarity and Urine sodium → Need U_{Osm}, U_{Na}**
  - Urine osmolarity → Presence of ADH
  - Urine Na^+ → If low, suggests volume depletion

Approach to Differential Diagnosis — Hyponatremia

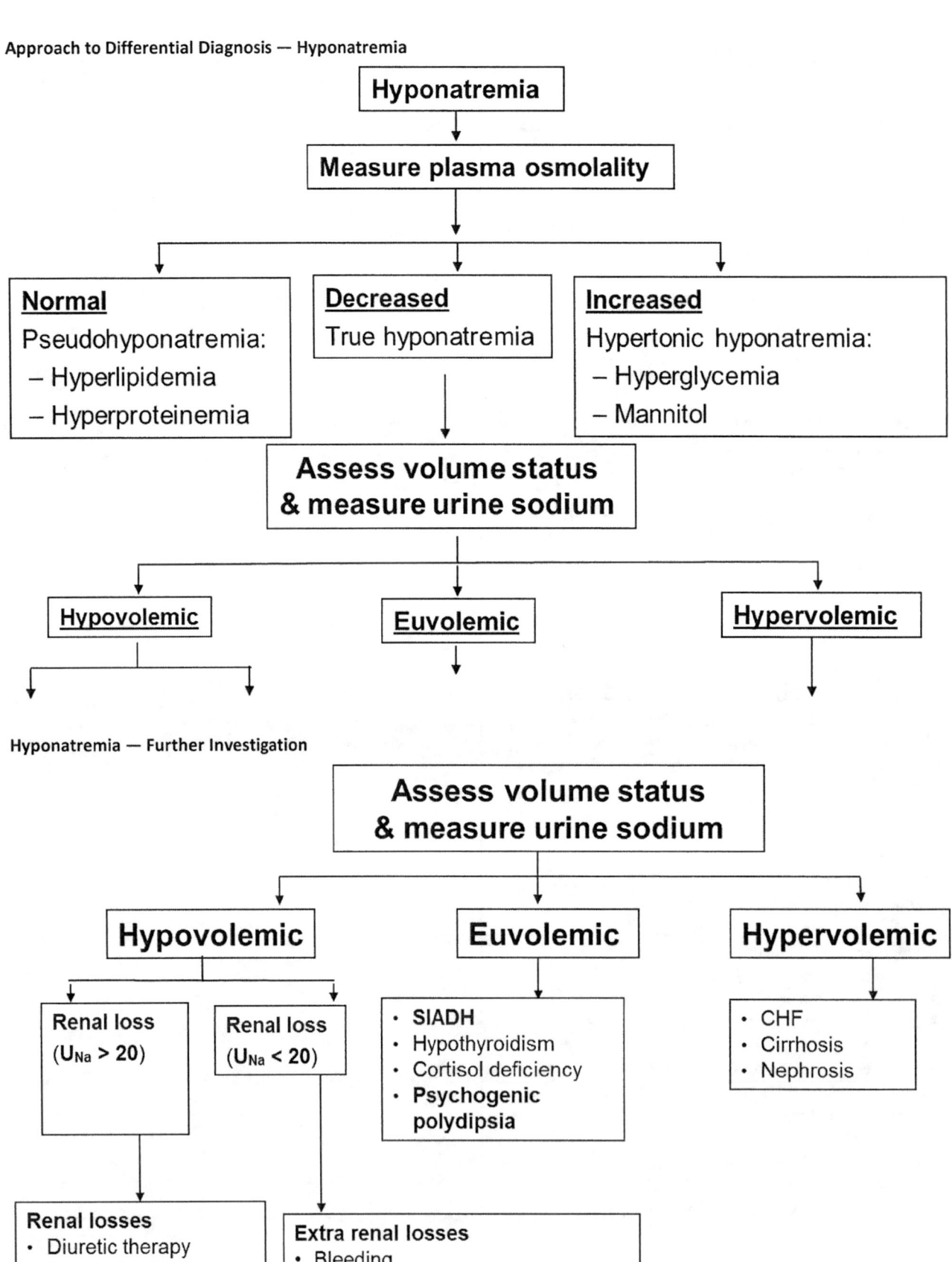

Hyponatremia

Measure plasma osmolality

Normal
Pseudohyponatremia:
– Hyperlipidemia
– Hyperproteinemia

Decreased
True hyponatremia

Increased
Hypertonic hyponatremia:
– Hyperglycemia
– Mannitol

Assess volume status & measure urine sodium

Hypovolemic   **Euvolemic**   **Hypervolemic**

Hyponatremia — Further Investigation

Assess volume status & measure urine sodium

Hypovolemic   **Euvolemic**   **Hypervolemic**

Renal loss
($U_{Na} > 20$)

Renal loss
($U_{Na} < 20$)

- SIADH
- Hypothyroidism
- Cortisol deficiency
- **Psychogenic polydipsia**

- CHF
- Cirrhosis
- Nephrosis

Renal losses
- Diuretic therapy & osmotic diuresis

Extra renal losses
- Bleeding
  – GI (N/V, diarrhea)

SIADH
- **Diagnosis:**
  - Low serum osmolality/Na$^+$ conc. associated with:
    1) In a euvolemic patient (***No suggestion of volume depletion and urine Na$^+$ > 20**)
    2) An inappropriately concentrated urine (**High urine osmolarity suggesting presence of ADH**)
    3) Always rule out <u>cortisol deficiency and thyroid disease</u>

Inappropriate Stimuli for ADH Release

SIADH

- **Drugs (SSRI, phenothiazines, cyclophosphamide ...)**

- **Pulmonary diseases**

- **CNS disease**

- **Malignancies (small cell cancer)**

A Prudent Approach to the Treatment of Hyponatremia
Symptomatic Hyponatremia
(Acute — duration < 48 hours)
1) Risk for complication of **cerebral edema greater than risk of treatment of complication**
2) Treat with hypertonic NaCl: **3% NaCl (1 mL/kg/hr) until convulsions subside**

Symptomatic Hyponatremia
(Chronic or Unknown Duration)
1) Do not increase serum sodium by **more than 8 mEq/day**
   **(If the serum sodium increases too rapidly, interrupt the increase by starting hypotonic fluids and/or desmopressin [DDAVP] 4 µg s.c.)
2) Long term
   - H$_2$O restriction
   - Demeclocycline 300–600 mg bid
   - V$_2$ receptor antagonist → aquaretics (tolvaptan)

Points to Remember!!!
- In evaluating patients with <u>hyponatremia</u>
  - First determine the <u>osmolarity</u>
  - If patient is hypoosmolar, then assess the <u>volume status</u>
  - Differential would depend on the volume status

How Does Hypernatremia Develop?
Physiology
- Increase in plasma osmolality should stimulate ADH secretion and thirst with decreased water excretion and increased water intake → **persistent hypernatremia does not occur in normal subjects**
- Must have **defect in thirst mechanism** (e.g., hypothalamic lesion)
                    Or
- **Limited access to free water** (e.g., infants or adults with impaired mental status)

Points to Remember!!!***
- In evaluating patients with **hypernatremia**
  - Remember both ADH secretion and thirst are necessary physiologic responses to defend against the development of hypernatremia
  - **If urine osmolality is high → water deprivation** (access to water) or thirst problems (hypodipsic)
  - **If urine osmolality is low → central or nephrogenic diabetes insipidus**

Central Diabetes Insipidus
- Etiologies
  - Idiopathic
  - Tumor or infiltration (sarcoid, histiocytosis, TB)
  - Surgery or trauma
  - CVA
- With water restriction
  - <u>Will respond to ADH administration</u>
- Treatment
  - <u>Desmopressin</u> is primary therapy

Nephrogenic Diabetes Insipidus
- Collecting tubule does not respond to ADH → polydipsia
- Etiologies
  - Hereditary: X-linked defect in V2 receptor gene
  - Drugs: <u>Lithium</u>, demeclocycline, ampho B
  - <u>Hypercalcemia</u>, hypokalemia, <u>Sjögren's</u>
- Rx: <u>Thiazide diuretics</u>
  - Cause volume depletion and increase proximal water absorption, so little is delivered to distal tubules

Evaluation of Polyuria
(Urine output exceeding 3 L per day)

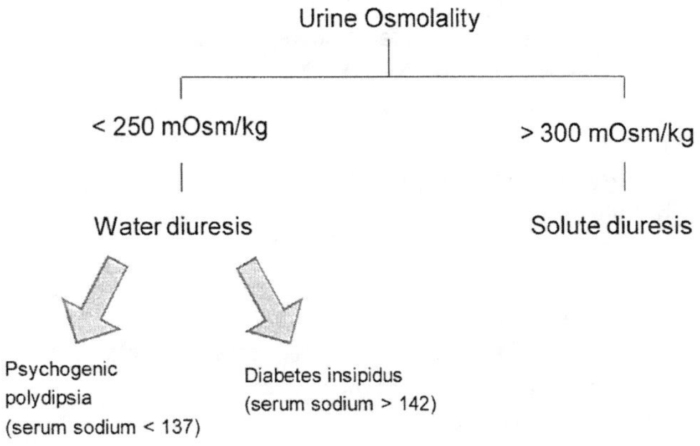

Urine Osmolality

< 250 mOsm/kg   > 300 mOsm/kg

Water diuresis   Solute diuresis

Psychogenic polydipsia (serum sodium < 137)

Diabetes insipidus (serum sodium > 142)

AR 8

A 76-year-old male smoker:
Admitted with 3 weeks of falling and dizziness
Lost 20 lbs in the past 6 months
Exam: BP 120/80, HR 85 (lying and standing)
Chest: End-expiratory wheezes
Na^+ 116, S_{Osm} 241,
Urine Na^+ 25, U_{Osm} 673
TSH normal, cortisol is normal

Which of the following is the most likely diagnosis?
A. Central diabetes insipidus
B. Nephrogenic diabetes insipidus
C. Beer potomania
D. SIADH
E. Volume depletion

Answer: _____

AR 9

In SIADH, what would you expect?
A. High urine osmolarity and high urine Na^+
B. Low serum osmolarity and low urine Na^+
C. High urine osmolarity and low urine Na^+
D. Low urine osmolarity and high urine Na^+

Answer: _____

Other Electrolyte and Mineral Disorders
• **Hypokalemia and hyperkalemia**
• **Calcium homeostasis**
• **Hypomagnesemia**

Hypokalemic — the Hypokalemic Hypertensive

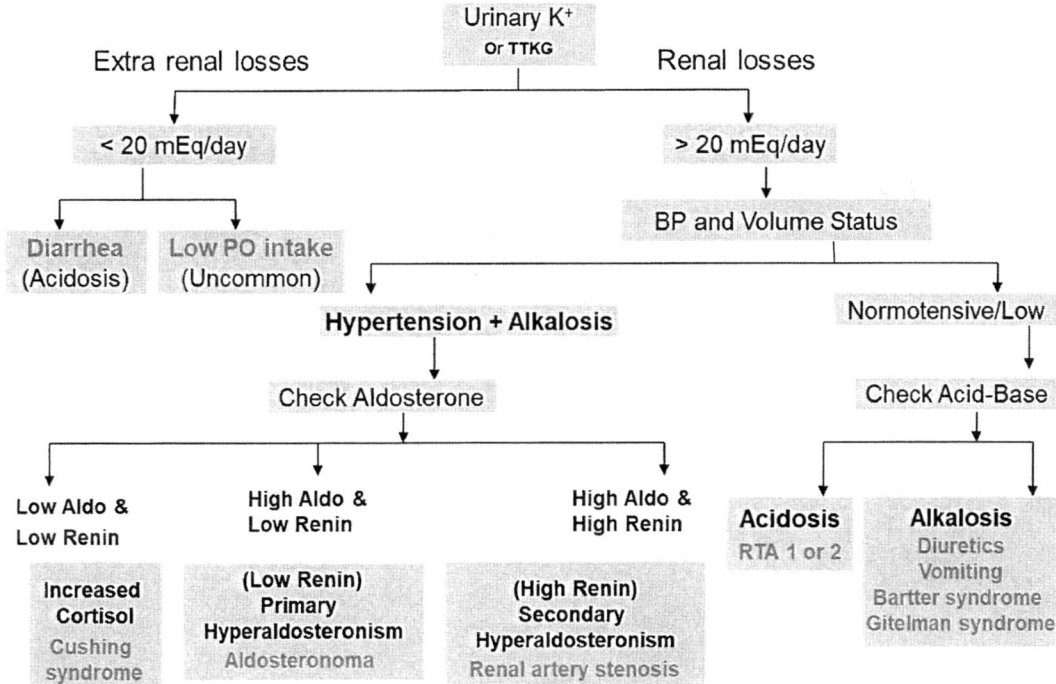

Source: Manish Suneja, MD

Hypokalemia

- Management issue: <u>AMI</u>
  - GISSI-2 Study, 1998
    - 2x increased risk of <u>ventricular fibrillation</u> when $K^+ < 3.6$
    - Recommendation: Keep <u>$K^+ > 4.0$</u> and <u>$Mg^{2+} > 2.0$</u> in patients post-MI

Hyperkalemia — Inhibitors of the Renin-Angiotensin-Aldosterone System

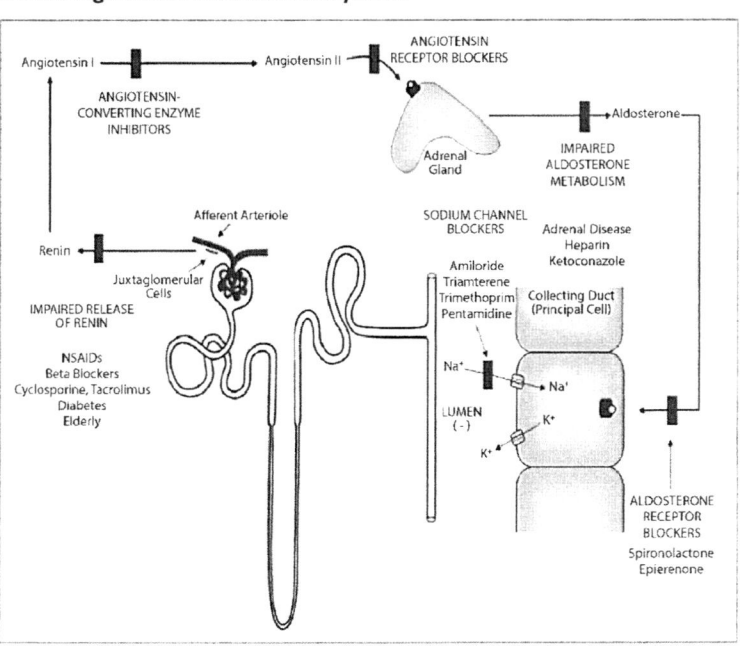

Acute Hyperkalemia

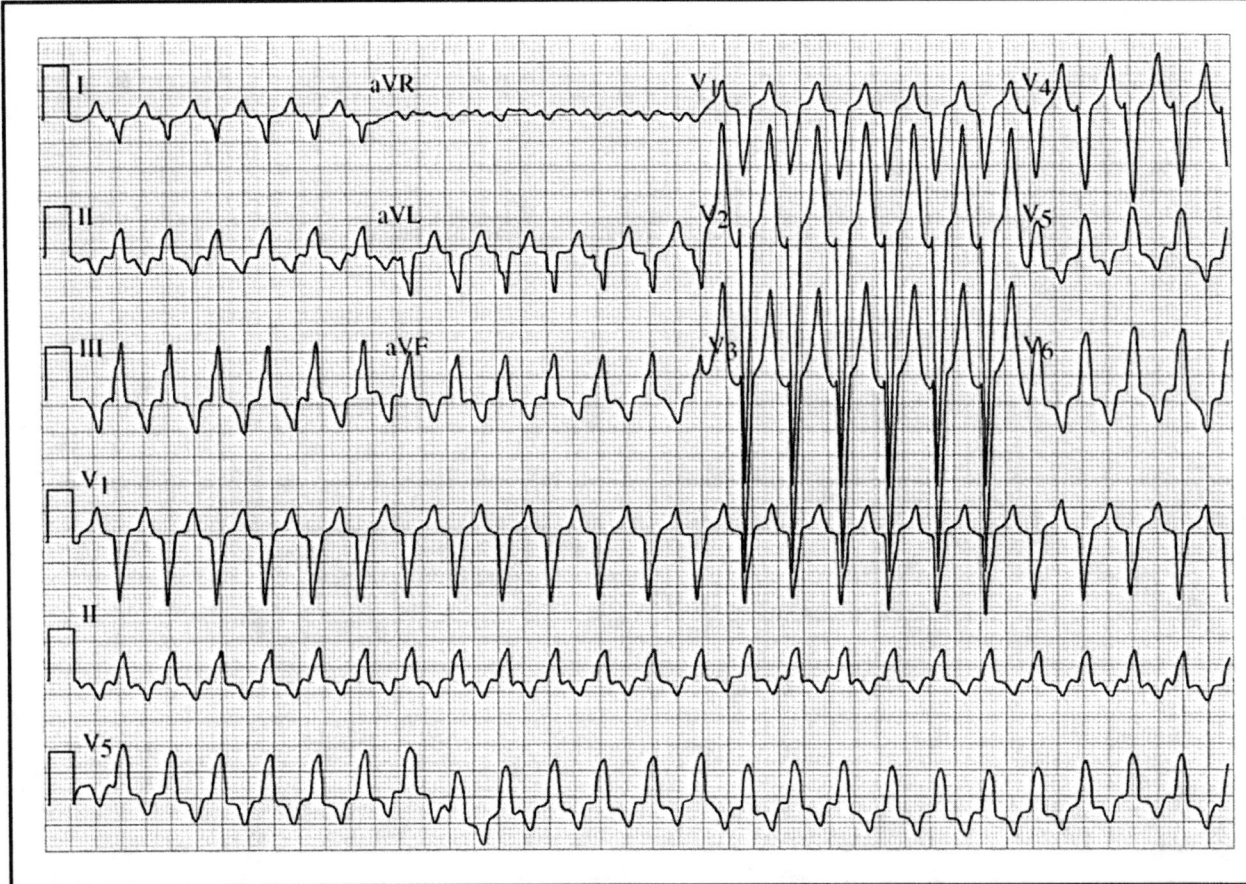

ECG Changes

Peaked T waves

Widened QRS

Loss of P waves

Bradyarrhythmias

Hyperkalemia — Treatment

Treatment is urgent if K^+ > 7 mEq/L

1) **Cardioprotection (first thing to do if ECG changes present)**
   - Calcium gluconate for membrane stabilization
   - ECG monitor

2) **Redistribution**
   - Glucose + insulin
   - Bicarbonate
   - β-adrenergic agonist (albuterol inhaled)

3) **Loss**
   - Ion-exchange resins/sodium polystyrene sulfonate (Kayexalate)
   - Diuretics (furosemide)
   - Dialysis

Causes of Hypercalcemia

(First test → PTH)**

- Malignancy → **low PTH**
  - Multiple myeloma: IL6
  - Lymphomas: Increased production of 1,25 hydroxy vitamin D
  - Solid tumors (squamous cell cancer or lung, etc.): PTH-related peptide
- Granulomatous disease, including fungal infections → **low PTH**
- Milk alkali syndrome or excessive calcium and vitamin D intake → **low PTH**

Causes of Hypercalcemia (cont.)

(First test → PTH)**

- Primary hyperparathyroidism → **high PTH**
  - Asymptomatic
  - **Bones** (osteoporosis/osteopenia)
  - **Stones** (calcium oxalate)
  - **Moans** (constipation)
  - **Groans** (weakness & fatigue)
  - Osteitis fibrosa cystica: Subperiosteal bone resorption radial middle phalanges
- Familial hypocalciuric hypercalcemia (FHH) → **high PTH**

Primary Hyperparathyroidism
- Diagnosis is simple
  - ↑ Ca^{2+} and low phos
  - Normal or ↑ PTH
    - This is clearly inappropriate if the Ca^{2+} is high
    - Be aware: Even normal PTH is inappropriate!**
  - **High urine calcium increases the risk of stones **(Pearl: Distinguishes it from FHH)**

Familial Hypocalciuric Hypercalcemia (FHH)
- Common distractor on exams when primary hyperparathyroidism is the correct answer
- Autosomal dominant (defect in **calcium-sensing receptor**)
- No clinical features of hypercalcemia
  - Ca^{2+} with normal or ↑ PTH
  - > 99% urine calcium absorption (these patients are **hypocalciuric**)** in contrast to **hypercalciuria** with primary hyperparathyroidism
- No treatment

Primary vs. Secondary Hyperparathyroidism
- Both have **increased PTH (phosphate-trashing hormone) levels**
- Primary occurs when PTH is **inappropriately** released → HIGH calcium and LOW phosphorus
- Secondary occurs when calcium is **LOW/NML** in CKD and **phosphorus is HIGH**
- **Look at the clinical case; Is CKD present or not? **Pearl: Hyperphosphatemia → secondary due to CKD****

Calcium Management Issues
- Hypercalcemia
  - **Saline: 1st (loop diuretics are out)
  - Calcitonin (1st 48°)
  - *Bisphosphonates
    - Pamidronate
    - Etidronate
    - Zoledronic acid
    - Don't forget about jaw osteonecrosis
  - Steroids
- Hypocalcemia
  - Always check Mg^{2+}
  - Long QT

AR 10
A 55-year-old female:
PMH: Squamous cell lung cancer 2 years ago
Doing fine

Exam normal

Calcium 11.4 (9–10.5)
Calcium over previous 3 years 9.0–10.0
PO_4 2.1
Alk phos 180 (36–92)
Creatinine 1.2
PTH 108 (10–60)
25-$(OH)_2$-D 15 (30–80)

Which of the following is the most likely cause of her hypercalcemia?
A. Hypercalcemia of malignancy
B. Vitamin D deficiency
C. Primary hyperparathyroidism
D. Osteoporosis
E. Familial hypocalciuric hypercalcemia

Answer: _____

Hypomagnesemia
- Etiologies
  - Diarrhea
  - Drugs: Thiazides, aminoglycosides, penicillins
  - Alcohol abuse
  - New: Chronic use of proton pump inhibitors!
    - Sometimes refractory to supplementation unless PPI is discontinued!
- Treatment
  - Magnesium sulfate PO or IV

Pregnancy and Kidney

Physiology of Pregnancy

GLOMERULAR HEMODYNAMICS
- Vasodilatation
- Increase in RPF and GFR

ANATOMICAL
- Increase in kidney size (1 cm)
- Dilation of the collecting system (R>L)

TUBULAR FUNCTION
- Altered tubular reabsorption of protein, glucose, amino acids and uric acid

ELECTROLYTE BALANCE
- Increased total body sodium up to 900–1,000 meq
- Increased total body potassium up to 320 meq
- Decrease in set point for thirst and ADH release
- Expansion of plasma volume

Hypertension in Pregnancy
- BP falls in normal pregnancy; BP > 120/80 is abnormal, though level at which to treat depends on many factors
- Safest for Rx: Methyldopa and hydralazine
  - Also safe: Labetalol, β-blockers
  - Less data: Calcium channel blockers
  - Avoid if possible: Diuretics
  - Do not use: ACEI/ARB*

- Chronic HTN
  Hypertension present before 20 weeks
- Preeclampsia:
  HTN and proteinuria after 20 wks, no prior history of HTN
- Gestational HTN: After 20 wks with no prior history, no proteinuria
- Chronic HTN with superimposed preeclampsia:
  Worse HTN, new onset or worsening proteinuria after 20 wks

Chronic Kidney Disease

Chronic Kidney Disease
- Structural/Functional kidney abnormalities x 3 months

  or
- Decreased GFR, with or without evidence of kidney damage

Staging and Action Plan for CKD

Stage	Description	GFR (mL/min/1.73 m²)	Action
1	Kidney damage with NI GFR	> 90	Dx and Rx co-morbid conditions, slow progression, CVD risk reduction
2	Kidney damage with mild ↓ GFR	60–89	Estimate progression
3	Moderate ↓ GFR	30–59	Evaluate and Rx complications
4	Severe ↓ GFR	15–29	Prepare for kidney replacement therapy
5	Kidney failure	< 15 (or dialysis)	Replacement (if uremia present)

Slowing the Progression of Chronic Kidney Disease
- Aggressive treatment of BP
- Blockade of the renin-angiotensin system: ACEI, ARB ± spironolactone
- Tight control of glucose if diabetic
- Treat hypercholesterolemia

CKD and CHD
- Substantial increase in CHD risk
  - RFs: HTN, DM, metabolic risk
  - Increase in CHD even without these RFs
- Know that the risk of death from CHD is higher than progression to dialysis in patients with CKD
- ? Coronary artery calcification related to increased calcium phosphate product

Miscellaneous Management CKD
- **ACEI/ARBs:** OK if creatinine ↑ up to 30% over baseline if stabilizes within 4 months; Do not discontinue! Reduce proteinuria — don't use ACEI and ARB together; Blood pressure goal < 140/90
- **NaHCO₃:** Treat acidosis to maintain **HCO₃⁻ > 22** (slows progression & improves nutrition in Stage 4)
- Secondary hyperparathyroidism & CKD-associated bone and mineral disease
  - **Inability to excrete PO₄ → ↑ PO₄ → ↑ PTH ← ↓ 1,25 vitamin D**
    - **First →** Control phosphorus levels
    - **Second →** Start active 1,25 hydroxy vitamin D (calcitriol)

Control of Hyperphosphatemia and Secondary Hyperparathyroidism in CKD
1) **Diet:** Reduce dietary P intake (< 800 mg)
2) **Binders (1ˢᵗ):** Prevent gut absorption of P with binders
   - **Calcium-based, if ↓ Ca²⁺**
     1) Calcium acetate
     2) Calcium carbonate

   With meals

   - **Noncalcium-, nonaluminum-based if normal or high serum Ca²⁺**
     1) Sevelamer (Renagel, Renvela)
     2) Lanthanum carbonate (Fosrenol)
3) **Vitamin D (2ⁿᵈ):** Prevent severe secondary hyperparathyroidism and attendant effluxes of P and Ca²⁺ from bone
   - Rx elevated PTH with vitamin D/vitamin D analogues → calcitriol

Miscellaneous Management CKD (cont.)
- Do not forget **anemia recommendations:**
  - Replace iron first
  - Erythropoietin-stimulating agents to target Hgb 10–12 mg/dL (Hct 33–36%)
- Gadolinium and CKD (****Nephrogenic systemic fibrosis**)
  - Fibrosing disorder (thickening and hardening of skin and fibrosis in organs); Related exposure to gadolinium-containing agents in patients with reduced kidney function
  - **FDA recommends avoidance in CKD with GFR < 30, ESRD, and acute kidney injury**
  - American College of Radiology states to avoid it for patients with GFR of < 44

Indications for Renal Replacement Therapy CKD
- Fluid and electrolyte disturbances refractory to medical therapy
- Pericarditis
- Encephalopathy, seizure, neuropathy
- Uremic symptoms: Nausea, vomiting, anorexia, altered food taste, disturbance in sleep-wake cycle
- Evidence of malnutrition: Decreased BUN/Cr, hypoalbuminemia

Polycystic Kidney Disease
- Autosomal dominant inheritance
- Affects 1 in 400 to 1 in 1,000 live births (4–6% of ESRD)
- Affects all ethnic groups worldwide
- No family history in 40%

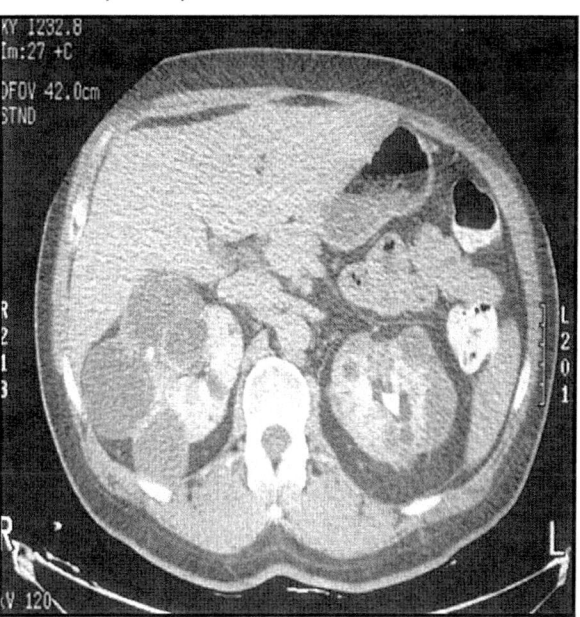

ADPCKD
- Two genes identified
  - *PKD1* (chromosome 16) 85% of cases, encodes polycystin 1
  - *PKD2* (chromosome 4) 15% of cases, encodes polycystin 2
- Identical manifestations, but *PKD2* patients present later in life and have longer renal survival (ESRD mean age 69 in *PKD2* vs. 57 in *PKD1*)

Complications of PCKD
- Progressive renal insufficiency and hypertension (80%)
- Hemorrhage into cysts
- Infected cysts → **use ciprofloxacin**
- Stones

Systemic Manifestations of ADPCKD
- Cysts in kidney (100%), liver (75%), pancreas
- Cardiac valvular abnormalities
  - Mitral valve prolapse
  - Tricuspid and aortic regurgitation
- Intracranial aneurysms (5% overall and 20% with family history)

**Don't screen unless h/o aneurysms in first-degree relative or high-risk occupation

Nephrology
Audience Response Answers

Audience Response 1
Answer: D. Place a Foley Catheter in the bladder.

AR 2
Answer: E. IgA Nephropathy.

AR 3
Answer: D. Urine and serum electrophoresis.

AR 4
Answer: D. Membranous nephropathy.

AR 5
Answer: C. Type 1 RTA (distal RTA).

AR 6
Answer: B. Ratio of plasma aldosterone concentration to plasma renin activity.

AR 7
Answer: B. Fibromuscular dysplasia.

AR 8
Answer: D. SIADH.

AR 9
Answer: A. High urine osmolarity and high urine Na^+.

AR 10
Answer: C. Primary hyperparathyroidism.

MedStudy

Internal Medicine Video Board Review

Neurology

Presented by

Jitesh Kar, MD, MPH
Clinical Assistant Professor
Department of Neurology
University of Alabama at Birmingham,
Huntsville Regional Medical Campus
Huntsville, Alabama

Neurology

Table of Contents

© 2017 MedStudy Internal Medicine Video Board Review – Neurology • Jitesh Kar, MD

Neurology Abbreviations

ABG	Arterial blood gas
ACA	Anterior cerebral artery
AD	Alzheimer disease
ADC	Apparent diffusion coefficient
ADHD	Attention-deficit/hyperactivity disorder
AEDs	Antiepileptic drugs
AHC	Alternating hemiplegia of childhood
ALS	Amyotrophic lateral sclerosis
AMS	Altered mental status
APCKD	Adult-type polycystic kidney disease
ART	Antiretroviral treatment
AVM	Arteriovenous malformation
AZT	Azidothymidine
BPPV	Benign paroxysmal positional vertigo
CA	Cancer
CAD	Coronary artery disease
CAG	Cytosine-adenine-guanine
CCB	Calcium channel blocker
CIDP	Chronic inflammatory demyelinating polyneuropathy
CJD	Creutzfeldt-Jakob disease
CK	Creatine kinase
CMP	Comprehensive metabolic panel
CMT	Charcot-Marie-Tooth disease
CN	Cranial nerve
CNS	Central nervous system
COMT	Catechol-O-methyltransferase
CPA	Cerebellopontine angle
CRP	C-reactive protein
CSF	Cerebrospinal fluid
CTA	Computed tomographic angiogram
CTD	Connective tissue disease
CTMR	Choriocarcinoma carcinoid thyroid melanoma renal cell
CTS	Carpal tunnel syndrome
CUS	Carotid ultrasound
DBP	Diastolic blood pressure
DBS	Deep brain stimulation
DM	Diabetes mellitus
DTR	Deep tendon reflexes
DWI	Diffusion weighted (magnetic resonance) imaging
EEG	Electroencephalogram
EMG	Electromyography
EOM	Extraocular muscle
ESR	Erythrocyte sedimentation rate
FB	Forebrain
FFP	Fresh frozen plasma
FLAIR	Fluid attenuation inversion recovery
FND	Focal neurologic deficits
FTD	Frontotemporal dementia

FVC	Forced vital capacity
GBS	Guillain-Barré syndrome
GRE	Gradient recalled echo
GTC	Generalized tonic-clonic
HA	Headache
HAART	Highly active antiretroviral treatment
HC	Homocysteine
HH	Homonymous hemianopsia
HIV	Human immunodeficiency virus
HLD	Hyperlipidemia
HSV	Herpes simplex virus
ICA	Internal carotid artery
ICH	Intracerebral hemorrhage
ICP	Intracranial pressure
IIH	Idiopathic intracranial hypertension
INO	Internuclear ophthalmoplegia
INR	International normalized ratio
IVIG	Intravenous immune globulin
JC	John Cunningham (virus)
LBD	Lewy body dementia
LE	Lower extremity
LMN	Lower motor neuron
LOC	Loss of consciousness
LP	Lumbar puncture
MAO-B	Monoamine-oxidase-B
MAP	Mean arterial pressure
MCA	Middle cerebral artery
MEP	Maximal expiratory pressure
MFV	Miller Fischer variant
MG	Myasthenia gravis
MHA-TP	Microhemagglutination assay for *Treponema pallidum* antibodies
MI	Myocardial infarction
MIP	Maximal inspiratory pressure
MMA	Methylmalonic acid
MMSE	Mini-mental state examination
MOCA	Montreal Cognitive Assessment
MRA	Magnetic resonance angiogram
MRI	Magnetic resonance imaging
MS	Multiple sclerosis
NCS	Nerve conduction studies
NMO	Neuromyelitis optica
NMS	Neuroleptic malignant syndrome
NPH	Normal pressure hydrocephalus
NSAIDs	Nonsteroidal antiinflammatory drugs
NTD	Neural tube defect
OCD	Obsessive compulsive disorder
OCP	Oral contraceptive pill
OMD	Oromandibular dystonia
OP	Opening pressure
OPCA	Olivopontocerebellar atrophy
OSA	Obstructive sleep apnea

PCA	Posterior cerebral artery
PCR	Polymerase chain reaction
PD	Parkinson disease
PDD	Parkinson disease dementia
PET	Positron emission tomography
PLEDs	Periodic lateralized epileptiform discharges
PLEX	Plasma exchange
PML	Progressive multifocal leukoencephalopathy
PMR	Polymyalgia rheumatism
PNA	Pneumonia
PSG	Polysomnogram
PSM	Primary sensorimotor (cortex)
PSP	Progressive supranuclear palsy
RA	Rheumatoid arthritis
RAPD	Relative afferent pupillary defect
RAS	Reticular activating system
RCC	Renal cell carcinoma
RPR	Rapid plasma reagent
SACD	Subacute combined degeneration
SAH	Subarachnoid hemorrhage
SBP	Systolic blood pressure
SC	Spinal cord
SND	Striatonigral degeneration
SPECT	Single photon emission computed tomography
SPEP	Serum protein electrophoresis
SSPE	Subacute sclerosing panencephalitis
SSRI	Selective serotonin reuptake inhibitor
TCA	Tetracyclic antidepressant
TCD	Transcranial Doppler
TCP	Thrombocytopenia
TEE	Transesophageal echocardiogram
TIA	Transient ischemic attack
tPA	Tissue plasminogen activator
TSH	Thyroid stimulating hormone
TTE	Transthoracic echocardiogram
UDS	Urine drug screen
UE	Upper extremity
UMN	Upper motor neuron
UPEP	Urinary protein electrophoresis
UTI	Urinary tract infection
VDRL	Venereal disease research laboratory test
VFC	Vascular flow capacity
VZV	Varicella zoster virus

Speaker Disclosure
Jitesh Kar, MD, MPH, has documented that he has no commercial interests to report.

Neurology

Overview of Neurology
- Coma
- Seizures
- Dementia
- Demyelinating Diseases
- Movement Disorders
- CNS Infections
- Headache
- Stroke & TIA
- Myelopathies
- Motor Neuron Disease
- Neuropathies
- Myopathies
- Dizziness
- CNS Metastasis
- Metabolic & Toxic Disorders

Objective
Question: Why did I decide to do this project?
A. Because no one else was ready to do it.
B. As a Neurologist, I have ample free time.
C. I am a big nerd and don't have a life.
D. I like Neurology and I love to teach.

Answer: _____

Things to Keep in Mind
- This is a **review** course
- This lecture/presentation is **for you**!
- Updates/Disputable topics will not be discussed
- Key words
- Questions are very specific

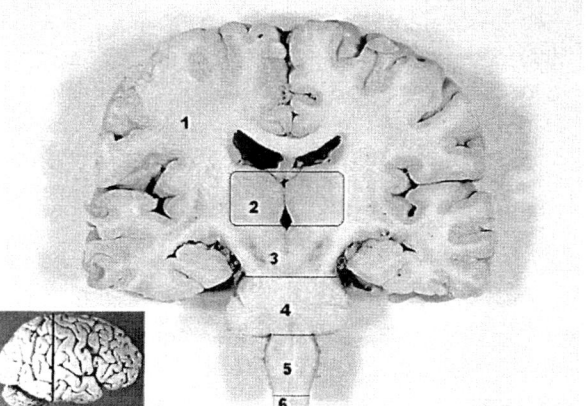

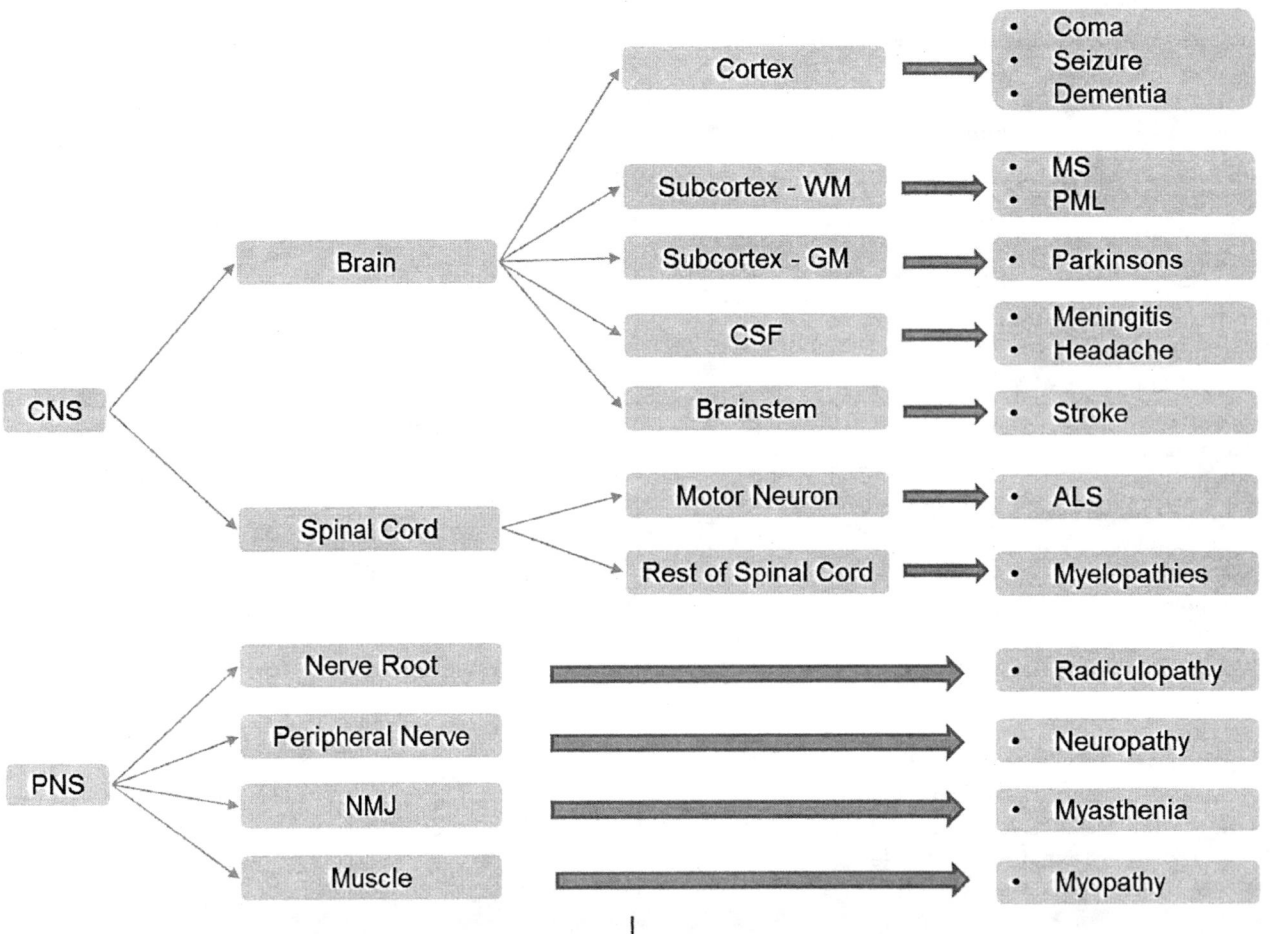

The following is a diagram of the nervous system:

- **CNS**
  - **Brain**
    - **Cortex** → Coma, Seizure, Dementia
    - **Subcortex - WM** → MS, PML
    - **Subcortex - GM** → Parkinsons
    - **CSF** → Meningitis, Headache
    - **Brainstem** → Stroke
  - **Spinal Cord**
    - **Motor Neuron** → ALS
    - **Rest of Spinal Cord** → Myelopathies
- **PNS**
  - **Nerve Root** → Radiculopathy
  - **Peripheral Nerve** → Neuropathy
  - **NMJ** → Myasthenia
  - **Muscle** → Myopathy

Coma

Overview — Coma
- Definitions
- Causes
- Examination:
  - Herniation syndrome
  - Reflexes
  - Breathing pattern
  - Posturing
- Workup
- Differential diagnosis

Definitions
- Awake, alert — normal
- Confusion — cannot maintain a coherent thought
- Delirium — confusion plus autonomic symptoms
- Stupor — can arouse to painful stimuli
- Coma — no response even to most painful stimuli
- **Awareness:**
  - "High" level of function
  - Requires a functioning cerebral cortex
  - Allows us to understand our environment

- **Arousal:**
  - More primitive
  - Requires a working brainstem
  - Mediated through RAS (sleep-wake cycles)

Coma
- Bilateral cortical damage
- Bilateral RAS — brainstem
- Medications/Intoxication
- Metabolic
  - Causes:
    - Supratentorial
    - Infratentorial
    - Metabolic
    - Diffuse
    - Multifactorial

Examination is the Key!
- **No** response to commands or pain
- Make sure patient is **not** sedated
- Where is the lesion?
  - Cortical vs. brainstem
  - Motor response — posturing
  - Breathing pattern
  - Pupillary reflex

© 2017 MedStudy Internal Medicine Video Board Review – Neurology • Jitesh Kar, MD

Neurological Exam in Coma
- **Decorticate posturing (C):** <u>Motor response: Posturing</u>
  - Arms towards cords
  - Lesion is cortical
  - Flexion and adduction of arms and extension of legs
  - Lesion is above red nucleus (midbrain)
- **Decerebrate posturing (E):**
  - Extension of arms
  - Lesion is below red nucleus (midbrain)
  - Posterior fossa lesions, herniation

Coma — Motor Responses

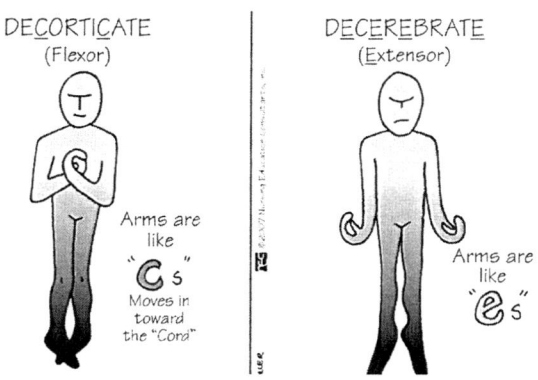

Breathing Pattern

Type of Breathing	Description	Localization
Cheyne-Stokes	Hyperventilation alternating with apnea	Bilateral cortical damage — Supratentorial
Central neurogenic hyperventilation	Increase in rate and depth of respiration	Lower midbrain-upper pontine
Apneustic	Slow deep inspiration f/b apneic pause, rate — 1.5 bpm	Pontine lesion
Ataxic	Irregular	Medulla

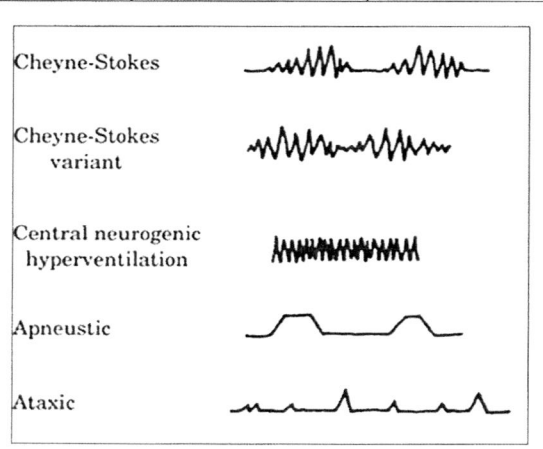

Coma — Pupils

Size	Description	Dysfunction	Example
● ●	One dilated and fixed	Parasympathetics	• Uncal herniation on the dilated side
● ●	Both Midpoint and fixed	Sympathetics, Parasympathetics	• Midbrain injury • Barbiturates • Anoxia • Atropine • Hypothermia
· ·	Both Pinpoint	Sympathetics	• Pontine injury • Opiates
● ●	Both fixed and dilated	Sympathetics, Parasympathetics	• Medullary lesion • Anoxia • Barbiturates • Hypothermia • Anticholinergics
· ●	One pinpoint	Sympathetics	• Lateral medulla • Horner syndrome

What are you talking about?
How am I going to remember all these?
- **Midpoint B**oth: Midbrain and Barbiturates
- **Pin P**oint: Pontine and Opiates
- Both **L**arge: Medu**LL**A
- Unilateral dilated fixed pupil: Uncal herniation on the side of dilated pupil
- One pupil small, one normal: Miosis on smaller pupil side; ? Horner syndrome

Workup
- Metabolic:
  - CBC
  - Electrolytes
  - Renal function
  - Hepatic function
  - Glucose
- Toxic: Urine drug screen
- Septic: U/A, CXR, BC, UC, sputum, LP, ABG
- Structural: CT head, MRI brain
- Postictal: EEG

Causes of Coma

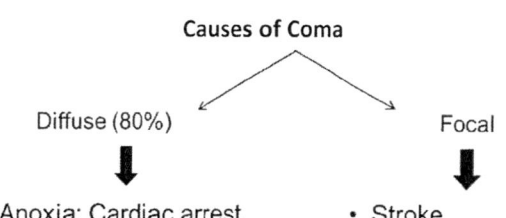

Diffuse (80%)	Focal

• Anoxia: Cardiac arrest
• Metabolic:
  – Hyper/Hypoglycemia
  – Hypercalcemia
  – Acidosis/Alkalosis
  – Hypothyroidism
  – Hypothermia
  – Renal failure — uremia
  – Hepatic failure
• Sepsis
• Poisoning: CO, cyanide
• Drugs: Alcohol, barbiturates
	• Stroke
	• ICH
	• Tumor

Herniation Syndromes

Supratentorial

3 — Subfalcine

2 — Central

1 — Uncal

Tentorium

4

Infratentorial

Upward — 5

Tonsillar — 6

Uncal Herniation

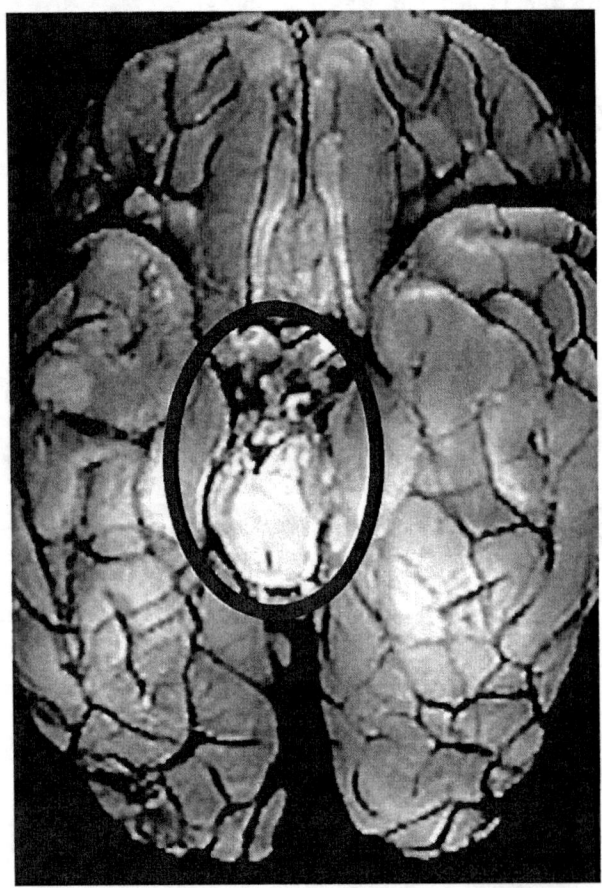

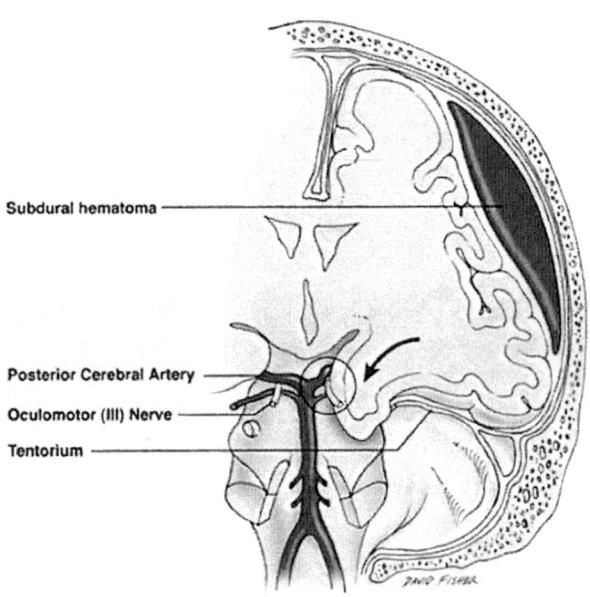

Subdural hematoma

Posterior Cerebral Artery

Oculomotor (III) Nerve

Tentorium

Ipsilateral dilated fixed pupil in a comatose patient: **Think of uncal herniation**

Coma — "Mimics"
- **Locked-in syndrome**
  - Lesion of a specific region of the **pons (basis pontis)**
  - Spares the RAS (reticular activating system)
  - Disrupts corticospinal/bulbar pathways
    - Patient is alert
    - Cannot talk (corticobulbar paths)
    - Cannot move (corticospinal paths)
    - Can communicate only with blinking
  - Normal EEG — Remember, the cortex is normal

Coma — "Mimics" (cont.)
- **Vegetative state:**
  - Severe, diffuse injury of the cerebral cortex (B/L)
    - Most common cause is anoxia
    - Other causes — terminal Alzheimer's or CJD
  - After > 4 weeks of coma, the patient will show some arousal, but no awareness
  - No purposeful behavior
  - Normal sleep-wake cycle
- **Persistent vegetative state:**
  - > 3 months of vegetative state

- **Akinetic mutism** — B/L anterior frontal lobe lesions
- **Catatonia**
  - Typically seen in psychiatric illnesses
  - Keep the limb in same position/maintain posture for long time
- **Brain death**
  - Absence of cerebral function
  - Absence of brainstem function
  - No reversible cause (e.g., no barbiturates, not hypothermic)
  - Apnea test ($pCO_2 > 60$)
  - Supportive tests **not** required, but they may be helpful
    - EEG — no cerebral activity
    - Cerebral blood flow test — no blood flow

Audience Response 1
A 30-year-old man is brought to the ED after being found by his landlord. No medical history is available. The patient's general physical exam is remarkable for bradypnea and hypothermia. Neurologic exam reveals a comatose, unresponsive man with bilateral, small, reactive pupils.

What is the most likely diagnosis for the person in this case?
A. Pontine stroke or hemorrhage
B. Opiate intoxication
C. Seizure
D. Left middle cerebral artery stroke

Answer: _____

Seizures

Seizures
- Abnormal excessive electrical discharges
- Motor manifestation: Convulsion
- Epilepsy: Recurrent seizures
- Aura: May occur before focal seizure

- Partial seizures:
  - Simple partial: No LOC
  - Complex partial: LOC +
  - Partial seizure with secondary generalization
- Generalized seizures:
  - Nonconvulsive: Absence seizure
  - Convulsive:
    - Tonic
    - Myoclonic
    - Clonic
    - Tonic-clonic
- Pseudo seizure: No electrographic correlation

Seizures — Causes
- Primary (idiopathic)
- Secondary (due to something)
  - **V**ascular: AVM, aneurysm, HTN urgency
  - **I**nfection: Meningitis, encephalitis, UTI, PNA
  - **T**rauma, toxin
  - **A**lcohol withdrawal
  - **M**etabolic (glucose, Na^+, Mg^{2+}, phos), medications
  - **I**diopathic
  - **N**eoplasms
  - **S**troke

Workup
- Vitals: Fever, HTN
- CBC: Infection
- CMP, Mg^{2+}, phos: Metabolic
- UDS, alcohol level: Toxic
- U/A, CXR, LP, B/C, sputum: Infection
- CT: To rule out ICH
- MRI Brain: Stroke, tumor
- MRA/CTA: Vascular malformation
- EEG: Normal EEG does **not** exclude

Fosphenytoin vs. Phenytoin

	fosphenytoin	phenytoin
IV infusion rate	150 mg/min	50 mg/min
pH	8.5	12
Route of admin	IM & IV	IV & po
ECG/BP monitor	yes	yes
Serum level	10–20 mcg/mL	10–20 mcg/mL

Treatment — Algorithm

Time (min)	Action
0–5	Diagnose, serum tests, etc.
6–10	D50 + thiamine; lorazepam
10–20	fosphenytoin 20 mg PE/kg
20–30	fosphenytoin 5–10 mg PE/kg
30–60	phenobarbital 20 mg/kg; intubation
> 60	Addt'l phenobarb or iatrogenic coma

Chronic Treatment
- Partial sz: Carbamazepine, oxcarbazepine
- GTC: Rest all
- When to stop the medication?
  Individualized
  – 2–4 years without seizure, normal EEG
  – 40% risk of recurrence in 2 years
- Surgery
- Vagus nerve stimulator
- Ketogenic diet

Women & AEDs
- AEDs which reduce the efficacy of OCP
  – Phenytoin
  – Phenobarbital
  – Carbamazepine
  – Oxcarbazepine
  – Topiramate
- **Lamotrigine and contraceptive pills:**
  – Estrogen-containing OCP: Reduces lamotrigine level
  – Lamotrigine reduces progesterone level, so women on progestin-only pill will have higher risk of becoming pregnant

Seizures in Pregnancy
- Birth defect is 2–3%
- Uncontrolled seizure: Abruptio, premature labor
- No one-to-one trial for epilepsy in pregnancy
- Valproate is associated with NTD, reduced risk with folic acid
- AEDs are associated with increased risk of hemorrhage, no data for vitamin K
- Teratogenicity
  – Pregnancy "D": Phenytoin, phenobarbital, carbamazepine, valproate
  – Pregnancy "C": All others
- Recommend: One med, lowest dose
- **Folate, folate, folate!**

Dementia

Dementia
- Remember, dementia is **not** a diagnosis
- **Must** find the **cause** of the dementia

Dementia — Definition
- Cognitive and behavioral impairments
  – Progressive
  – Not due to delirium
  – No psychiatric illness
- Impairment in 2 or more of 5 domains
  – Memory
  – Executive function
  – Perception
  – Language
  – Behavior

Dementia — Treatable Causes
- Normal pressure hydrocephalus
- Chronic subdural hematoma
- Hypothyroidism
- B_{12} deficiency
- Heavy metal poisoning (mercury, lead, arsenic)
- Syphilis
- **Depression** (a.k.a. pseudodementia)
- Multiple infarcts
- Chronic medical conditions (renal or hepatic failure)
- Infection (HIV-AIDS, Creutzfeldt-Jakob disease)
- Post-irradiation
- Tumors
- Vasculitis

Dementia — Differential Dx
- Alzheimer's (80% of dementias)
- Depression/Pseudodementia
- Multi-infarct dementia
- Dementia with Lewy bodies
- Fronto-temporal dementia

Normal Pressure Hydrocephalus (NPH)
- **Clinical triad (3 Ws)**
  1) Apraxic gait (magnetic) (wobbly)
  2) Incontinence (wet)
  3) Dementia ("weird")
- Often occurs after trauma, meningitis, or SAH
- Few findings on examination
- **No** papilledema
- Possibly due to poor reabsorption of CSF
- Neuroimaging (NPH vs. *ex vacuo*)
  – **LP — diagnostic and "therapeutic"**
  – Radionuclide cysternography
- Rx: Medical — acetazolamide (decrease CSF prod.)
- Sx: Surgical — V-P shunt (ventriculoperitoneal)

Normal Pressure Hydrocephalus (NPH) (cont.)

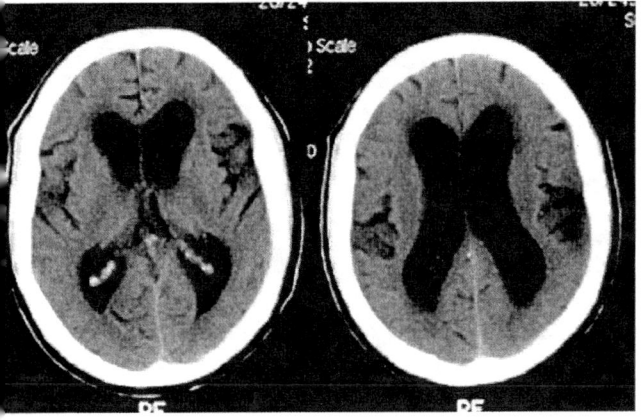

Dementia — Multi-Infarct
- Second most common cause
- Abrupt onset
- Stepwise deterioration
- Mild confusion; impairment in memory, perception, and executive function, followed by difficulties in judgment and orientation; Neuropsychiatric symptoms are late
- Treatment: Prevent further injury
  - **ASA, statin**
  - Risk factors management

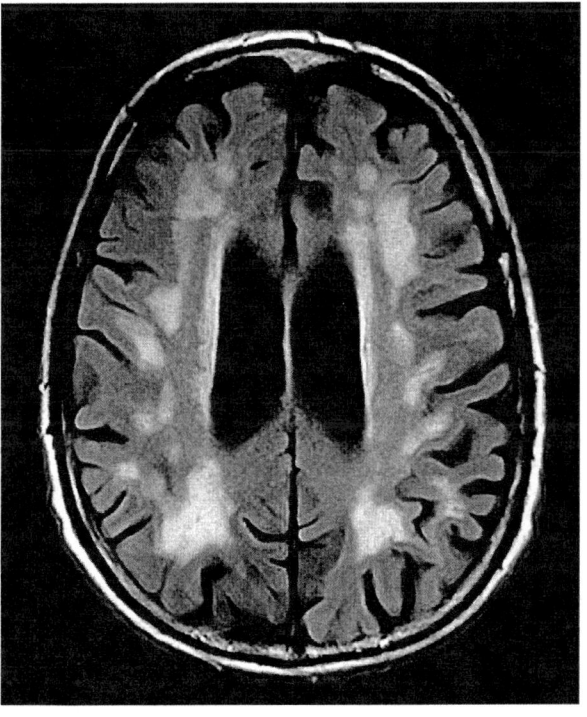

> # Exam topics:
> - Multiple vascular risk factors
> - WM disease on MRI

Alzheimer's Dementia
- Most common cause of dementia after age 60
- Diagnosis
  - Insidious onset, usually over years
  - Remember: More common in Down syndrome
- *ApoE4* gene
- Temporal/Parietal lobes are affected first
  - Poor memory (short term), anomia, aphasia
  - Decreased spatial orientation
- Frontal lobes are affected later
  - Decreased social inhibitions
  - Incontinence
  - Apraxia

Dementia — Treatment of Alzheimer's
- First line: Cholinesterase inhibitors
  - Donepezil (Aricept)
  - Rivastigmine (Exelon)
  - Galantamine (Razadyne)
  - Best results in mild-to-moderate AD
- Additive treatment
  - *N*-methyl-*D*-aspartate receptor antagonist — memantine (Namenda)

Frontotemporal Dementia
- Younger patients (5th and 6th decades)
- Onset and progression similar to Alzheimer's (really, you cannot tell them apart clinically)
- More rapid change in **personality and behavior**
- CT/MRI: Frontal/Temporal atrophy
- Diagnosis is made at autopsy
  - Pick bodies — argentophilic intranuclear inclusions (argentophilic = Silver staining)

Frontotemporal Dementia

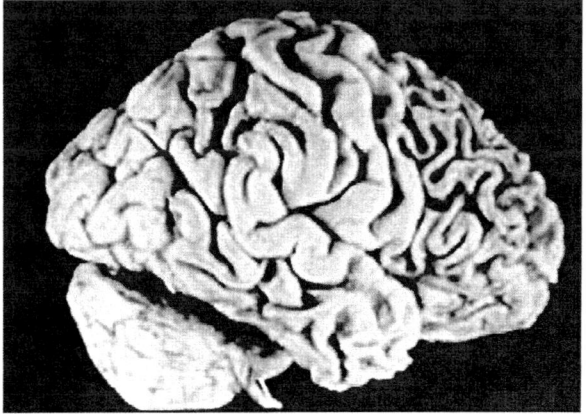

Dementia — Creutzfeldt-Jakob Disease (CJD)
- Rapidly progressive (acute or subacute)
- Infected prion (proteins)
- 4 variants:
  1) Sporadic: 95%, we do **not** know why
  2) Familial: Rare
  3) Iatrogenic: Infected instrument, transplant, human tissue/hormone
  4) Variant: Bovine spongiform encephalopathy

- Associated signs
  - **Myoclonus (startle)**
  - Cerebellar signs
  - Rigidity
  - Psychiatric symptoms
- Dx test: Brain biopsy
- CSF 14-3-3 protein, MRI shows cortical ribbon sign
- EEG: Generalized periodic epileptiform discharges
- Fatal

Creutzfeldt-Jakob Disease (CJD)

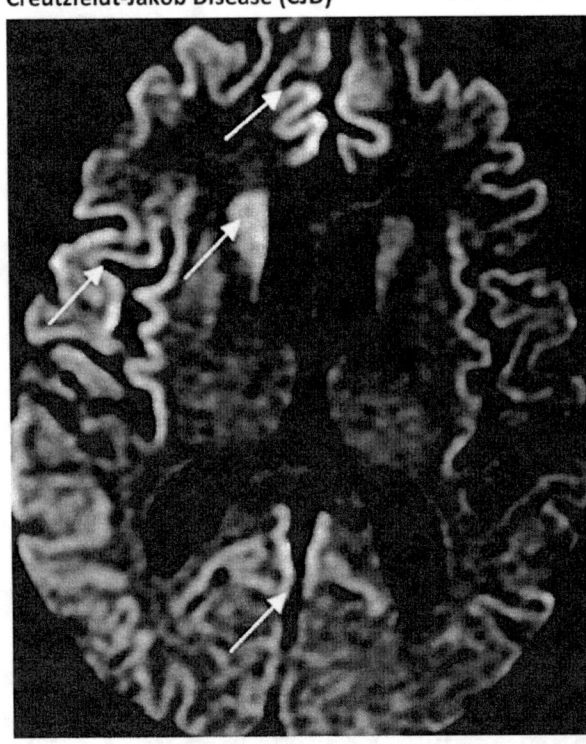

Parkinson Disease Dementia
- PD symptoms first, eventually dementia
- If dementia develops **within 1 year** of motor dysfunction → Lewy body dementia

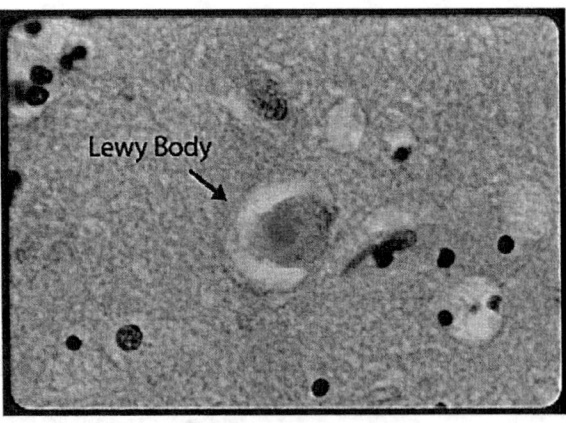

Parkinson Disease Dementia vs. Lewy Body Dementia
- PDD vs. LBD
- In PDD, dementia develops after at least 1 year of Parkinson features
- If patient with Parkinson features developed dementia in the 1st year, it is LBD

Progressive Supranuclear Palsy
- Supranuclear ophthalmoplegia — vertical gaze palsy
- Frequent falls
- **Vertical gaze palsy, dementia, fall: PSP**
- Pseudobulbar palsy
- Axial dystonia
- 6th decade
- Extension of neck

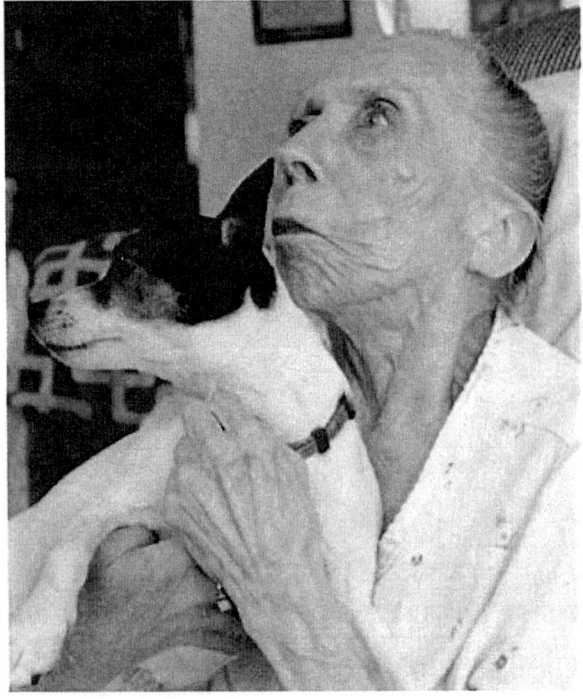

Huntington Dementia

- AD, starts between 35 and 40 years of age:
  Young patient
- Genetic: Chrom. 4 – **hunting 4 food**, trinucleotide repeat **CAG**
- C/F: Chorea, personality changes, psychiatric symptoms
- Positive family history
- Patho: Affects the basal ganglia — caudate, putamen
- CT or MRI: **Atrophy of caudate**
- PET decreased metabolism — caudate, putamen
- Treatment is palliative
- Treat chorea:
  - Tetrabenazine
  - Dopamine-depleting drugs
    - Haloperidol
    - Chlorpromazine

Wait a second — Something is missing!

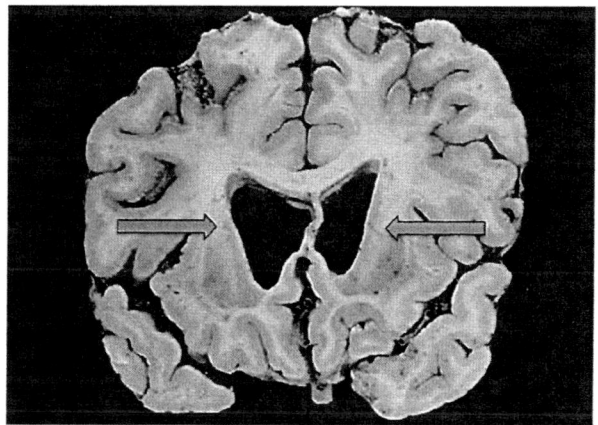

Dementia in AIDS

- MC cause of dementia in a young patient with HIV
- Low CD4 count
- Not on HAART
- Usually irreversible
- Antidepressant
- HAART

Depression — Pseudodementia

- Symptoms of depression
- SIGECAPS
- Good insight
- Poor concentration/attention
- MMSE/MOCA score: Good
- No aphasia or apraxia
- Frontal lobe release signs are usually absent
- Rx: Antidepressant

Chronic Traumatic Encephalopathy

- Chronic trauma/concussion
- NFL Players
- Dementia
- Depression

Dementia

Type	Lobe	Particular Feature
AD	Parietal Temporal Later on frontal	Global delay Daily activities are impaired Family history
FTD	Frontal Temporal	Change in personality Behavioral problem
LBD	Occipital	Hallucination
PDD	Parietal Occipital	PD features for > 1 year Dementia — late
Pseudodementia	None	Attention/concentration Depression symptoms
NPH	Normal Enlarged ventricles	Triad

Dementia — Cases

AR 2

A 66-year-old Portuguese man is brought in by his family for memory problems and "trouble walking right." His exam reveals a quiet, reserved man who has a slow, halting gait. During the interview, he urinates and seems unaware of what has happened.

What is the most likely diagnosis?

A. Alzheimer's disease
B. Parkinson disease
C. Normal pressure hydrocephalus
D. Progressive supranuclear palsy
E. Creutzfeldt-Jakob disease

Answer: _____

AR 3

A 69-year-old man is brought to your office by his wife. He has gradually worsening forgetfulness for the last 2–3 years. During the interview, you discover that he used to organize all of the finances but is no longer able to do so. At times, he has uncharacteristically angry outbursts. His exam reveals a disheveled man with grasp and snout reflexes.

What is the 1ˢᵗ line treatment for his condition?

A. Tacrine
B. Donepezil
C. Levodopa
D. Sertraline

Answer: _____

AR 4

A 72-year-old woman complains of memory problems. She has mild HTN, history of a "mild" MI 5 years ago, and recent loss of her husband of 45 years.
General physical exam is normal. Neurologic exam is remarkable for 1/3 recall on MMSE (mini-mental status examination) — her total score was 29/30.
Neuro exam was otherwise normal.

What treatment would you recommend?

A. "Watch and wait."
B. Donepezil.
C. Sertraline.
D. Levodopa.
E. Memantine.

Answer: _____

Demyelinating Diseases
- Multiple sclerosis
- Optic neuritis
- Neuromyelitis optica
- Progressive multifocal leukoencephalopathy
- Central pontine myelinolysis

Multiple Sclerosis (MS)
- Young women 20–40s
- Male to female = 1:2
- ? Initial infection → autoimmune response
- Demyelination of white matter in CNS
- Incidence is higher in northern latitudes
- Vitamin D: Environmental risk factor
  - Eye: Optic neuritis
  - Spinal cord: Transverse myelitis
  - Brain: Periventricular WM lesions

Types of Multiple Sclerosis
1) Primary progressive
2) Secondary progressive
3) Relapsing-remitting: Most common

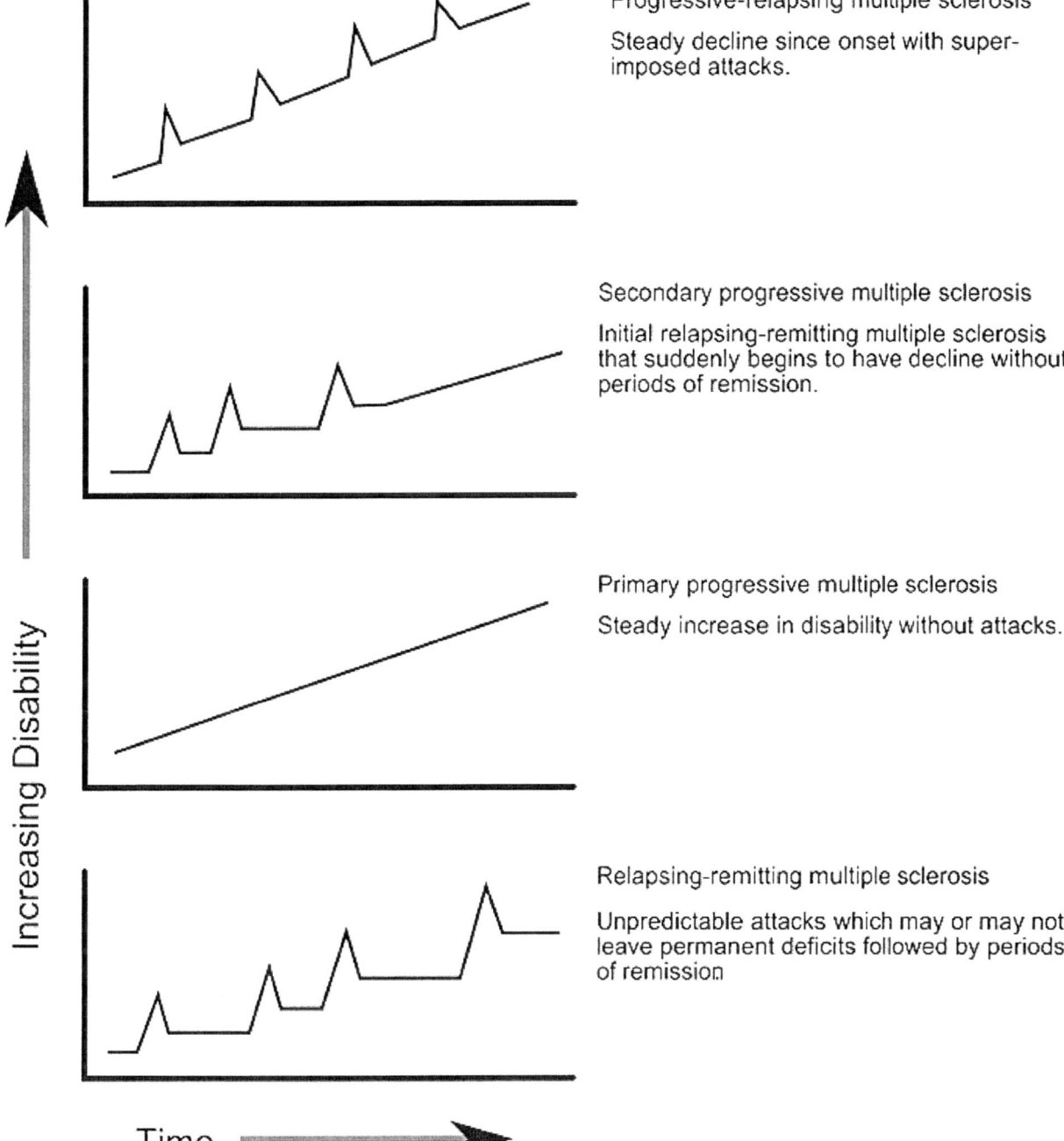

Progressive-relapsing multiple sclerosis

Steady decline since onset with super-imposed attacks.

Secondary progressive multiple sclerosis

Initial relapsing-remitting multiple sclerosis that suddenly begins to have decline without periods of remission.

Primary progressive multiple sclerosis

Steady increase in disability without attacks.

Relapsing-remitting multiple sclerosis

Unpredictable attacks which may or may not leave permanent deficits followed by periods of remission

Clinical Features of MS
- Painful vision loss
- Eye findings: RAPD, INO
- Relapsing-remitting symptoms
- UMN signs on exam
- Spasticity, sensory deficits, ataxia, bladder problem
- Fatigue, cognitive deficits

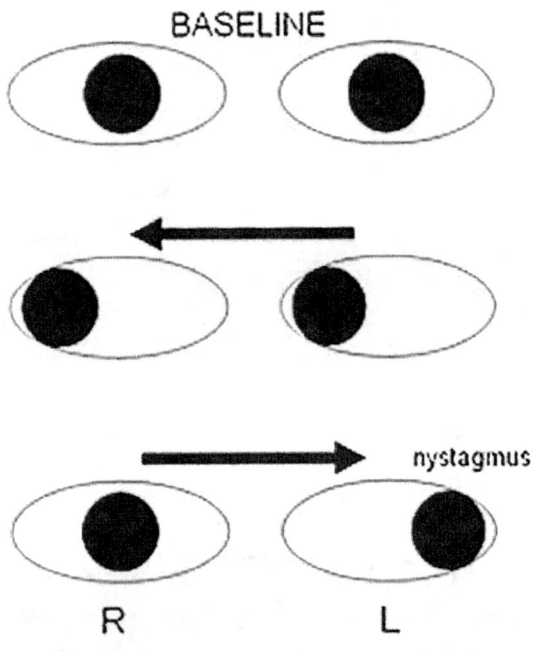

BASELINE

nystagmus

R   L

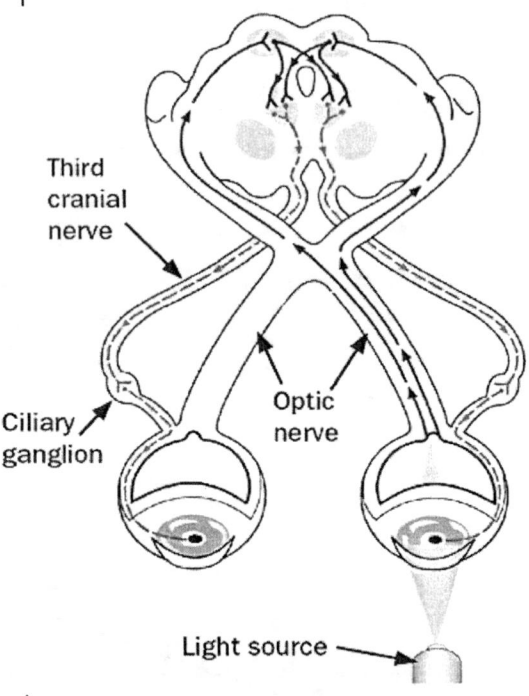

Third cranial nerve

Ciliary ganglion

Optic nerve

Light source

Diagnosis of MS
- Revised McDonald's
- MRI brain w, w/out
- MRI spine w, w/out
- Visual evoked potential
- Lumbar puncture:
  - Oligoclonal bands
  - IgG index

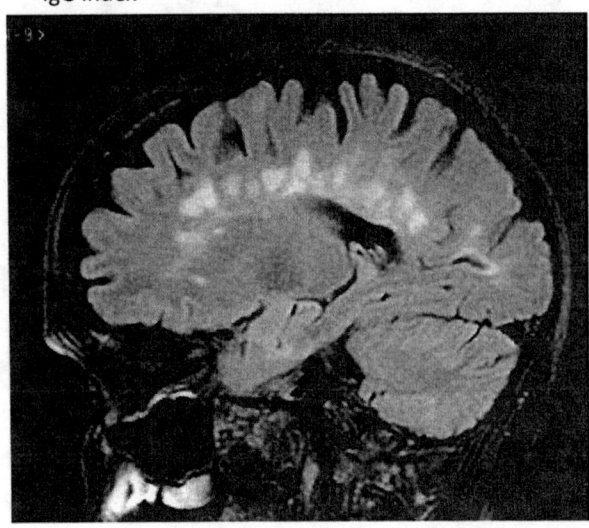

Treatment of MS
- Acute exacerbations: Steroids IV vs. PO
- Optic neuritis: IV steroids
- Outpatient:
  - Interferon beta-1a: Avonex, Rebif
  - Interferon beta-1b: Betaseron
  - Glatiramer acetate SC injection (Copaxone)
  - Fingolimod
  - Natalizumab: Side effect — PML

Vitamin D supplement is an adjunctive treatment

Progressive Multifocal Leukoencephalopathy
- Severe white matter demyelination
- T-cell immunodeficiency
- Associated with JC virus
- HIV-positive patient with CD4 < 200
- Chronic steroid therapy
- Patient on MS medication — which one?
- Acute to subacute onset
- Progressive
- Mortality is high, around 3–6 months
- CSF PCR for JC virus
- Diagnostic test: Brain biopsy
- Rx: ? HAART in HIV-positive patients

Progressive Multifocal Leukoencephalopathy (cont.)

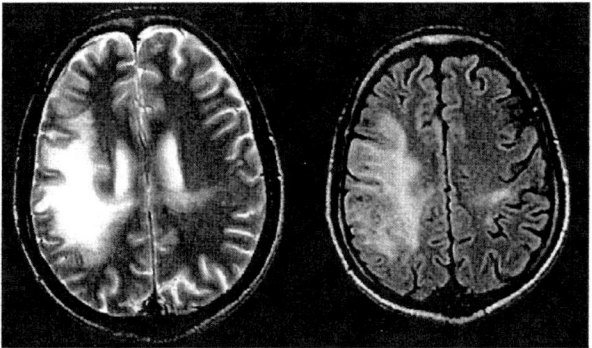

Central Pontine Myelinolysis
- Rapid correction of hyponatremia
- Pontine demyelination due to osmotic damage
- Can be seen in extra-pontine area
- Locked-in syndrome: Quadriparesis
- Swallowing difficulty
- Flaccid paralysis, may progress to spastic

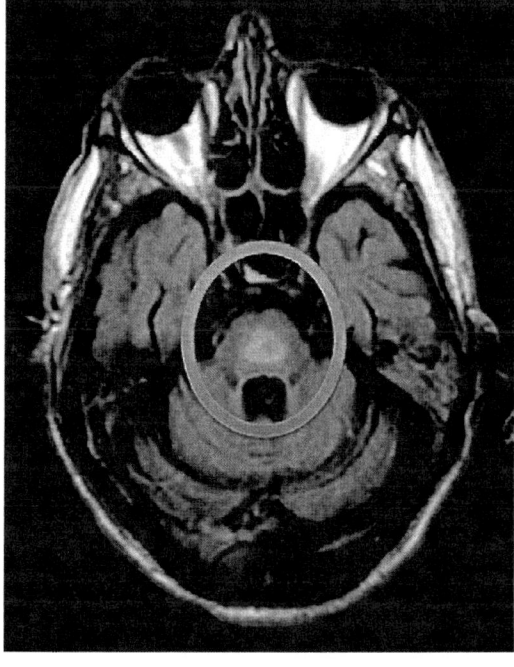

Movement Disorders

Overview — Movement Disorders
- Parkinson disease
- Progressive supranuclear palsy
- Tremor
- Tardive dyskinesia
- NMS
- Hemifacial spasms
- Tourette syndrome
- Focal dystonias

Movement Disorders

Movement Disorders → Hypokinetic / Hyperkinetic

Hypokinetic → Low dopamine → PD

Hyperkinetic → High dopamine →
- Akathisia
- Dyskinesia

Parkinson's Disease / Normal — Substantia nigra

- Bradykinesia
- Rigidity
- Resting tremor
- Postural instability

→ Parkinsonism

→ Need to identify the cause

- Idiopathic Parkinson disease → Dementia: 20–30% / Depression: 50%
- Secondary parkinsonism → MC: Drug-induced parkinsonism

Drug-Induced Parkinsonism

Anything which reduces dopamine

- Neuroleptics (dopa. blockade)
  - Phenothiazines, butyrophenones
- Antiemetics (weak dopa. blockade)
  - Prochlorperazine, metoclopramide
- Catecholamine analogs/depleting drugs
  - Reserpine, tetrabenazine

If medication is causing it, what is the treatment?

Neurology is easy — stop the medication!

Parkinson Disease (PD) — Pathology
- Loss of dopaminergic neurons in SN
- Nigrostriatal pathway
- Intracytoplasmic eosinophilic inclusion — faint halo

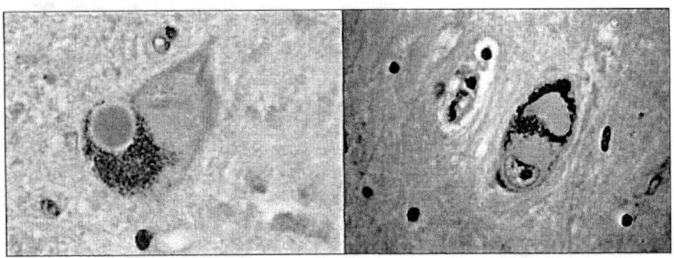

Non-Motor Symptoms of PD*
- Constipation
- Olfactory deficits
- Periodic REM sleep behavioral disorder
- Depression
- Possible:
  - RLS
  - Apathy
  - Fatigue
  - Erectile dysfunction
  - Urinary incontinence

Treatment — Overview

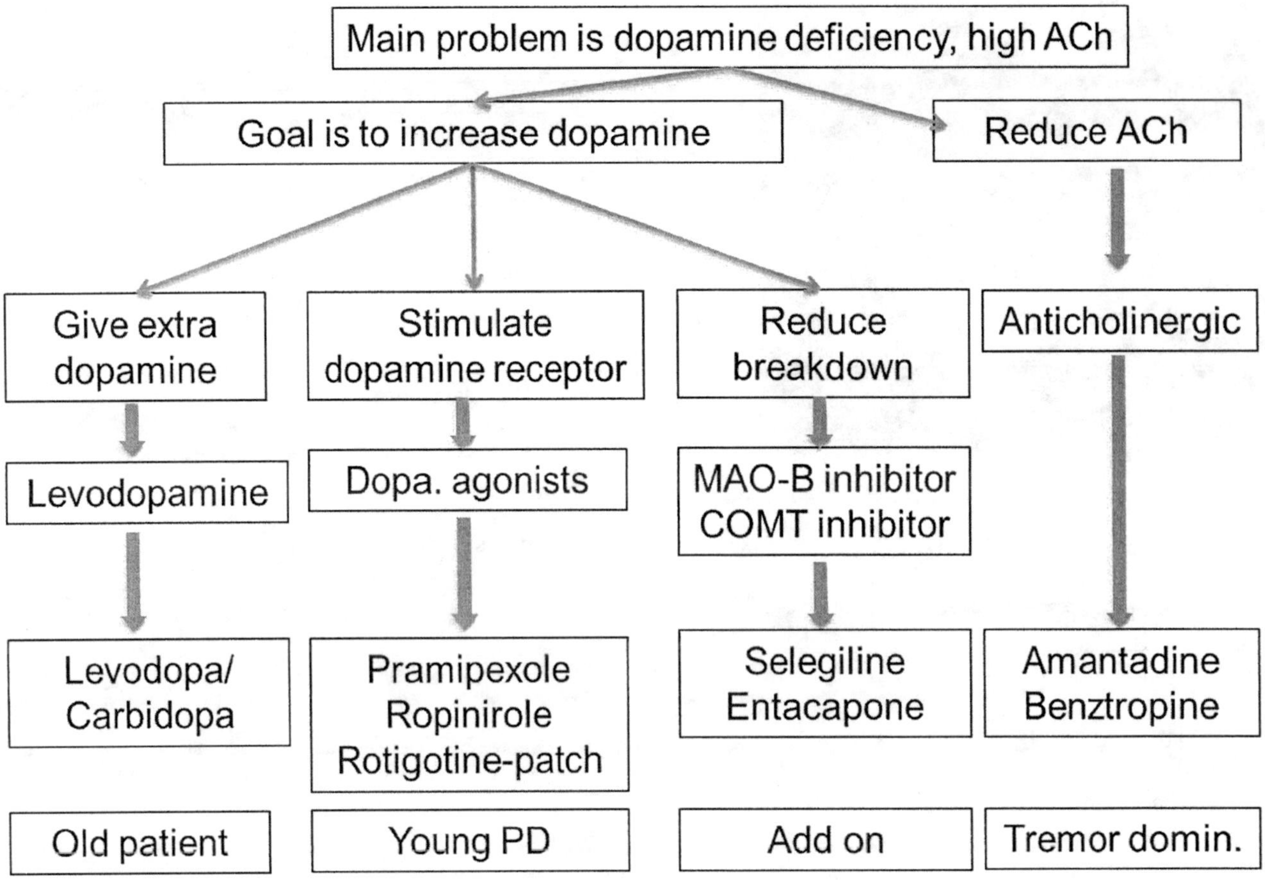

```
            ┌─────────────────────────────────────────────┐
            │  Main problem is dopamine deficiency, high ACh │
            └─────────────────────────────────────────────┘
              │                                      │
  ┌──────────────────────────────┐      ┌──────────────────┐
  │  Goal is to increase dopamine │      │    Reduce ACh    │
  └──────────────────────────────┘      └──────────────────┘
```

Give extra dopamine	Stimulate dopamine receptor	Reduce breakdown	Anticholinergic
Levodopamine	Dopa. agonists	MAO-B inhibitor COMT inhibitor	
Levodopa/ Carbidopa	Pramipexole Ropinirole Rotigotine-patch	Selegiline Entacapone	Amantadine Benztropine
Old patient	Young PD	Add on	Tremor domin.

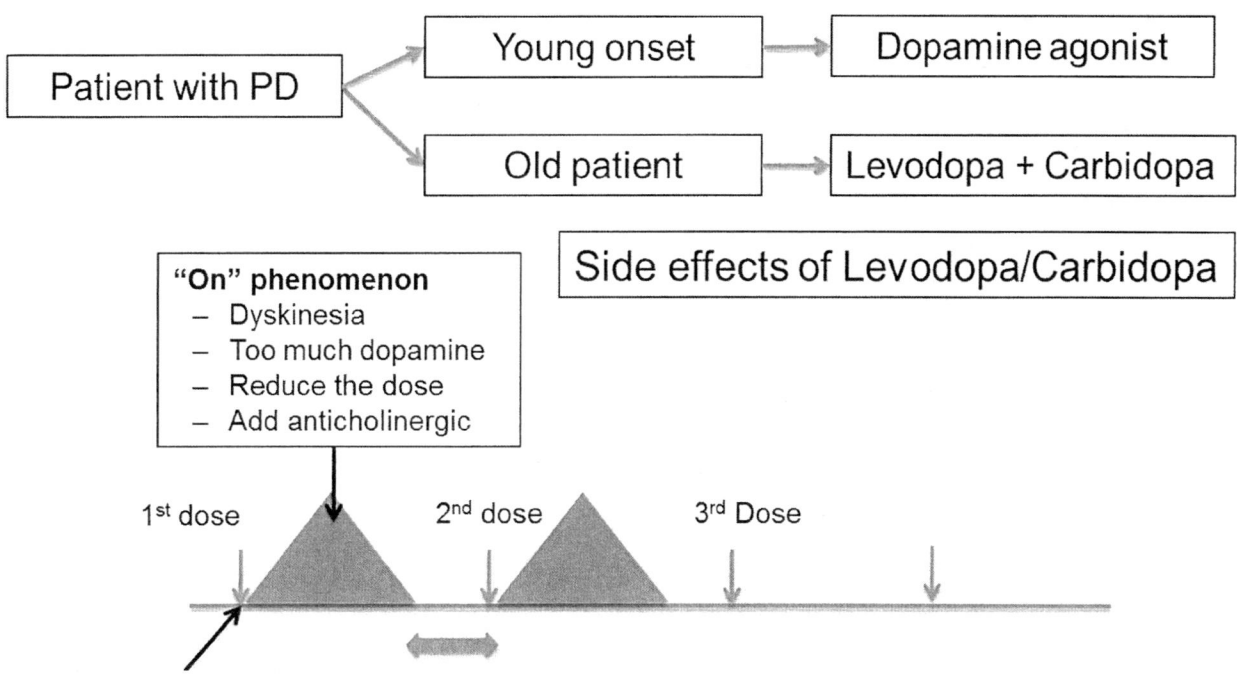

Patient with PD
→ **Young onset** → **Dopamine agonist**
→ **Old patient** → **Levodopa + Carbidopa**

Side effects of Levodopa/Carbidopa

"On" phenomenon
- Dyskinesia
- Too much dopamine
- Reduce the dose
- Add anticholinergic

1st dose   2nd dose   3rd Dose

Nausea
- 30 mins before food
- Reduce levodopa
- Increase carbidopa

"Off" phenomenon
- Worsening of symptoms
- Medication wear off
- Use COMT inhib.
- Increase the frequency

Things to Remember about PD Meds
- Dopa. agonists: Compulsive shopping, pathological gambling, hypersexuality
- Anticholinergics in elderly: **Careful**
- Neuroprotective therapy for PD: None
- Selegiline + TCA/SSRI: Serotonin syndrome
- Levo + carbidopa in young: Dyskinesia
- Sudden stopping of PD meds: Parkinson hyperpyrexia syndrome

Surgical Treatment — PD
- Thalamotomy (ventrolateral nucleus)
- Pallidotomy
- Deep brain stimulation (high-frequency stimulation of ventralis intermedius)

Intestinal Gel / Infusion
- Infusion of levodopa/carbidopa — GI
- PEG

Parkinson Plus Syndrome
- PSP: Vertical gaze palsy, bulbar symptoms
- Shy-Drager syndrome: Autonomic insufficiency
- OPCA: Cerebellar signs, pseudobulbar signs
- SND: Dementia (?)

Progressive Supranuclear Palsy
- Supranuclear ophthalmoplegia — can't look down
- Pseudobulbar palsy
- Axial dystonia
- 6th decade
- Extension of neck

PSP = Progressive supranuclear palsy
OPCA = Olivopontocerebellar atrophy
SND = Striatonigral degeneration

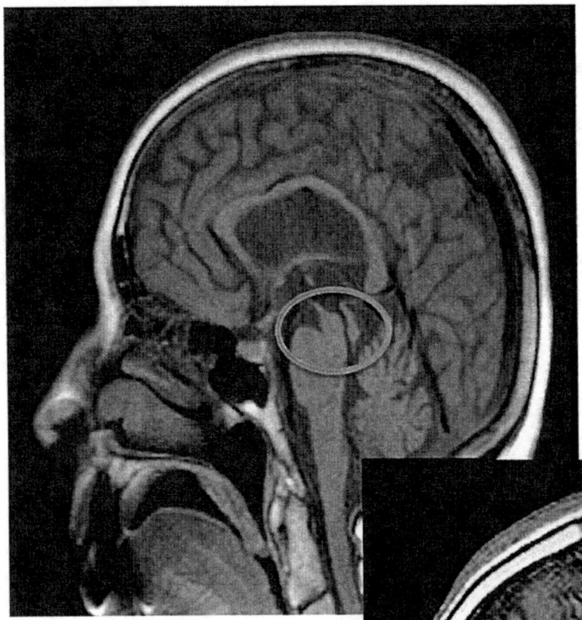

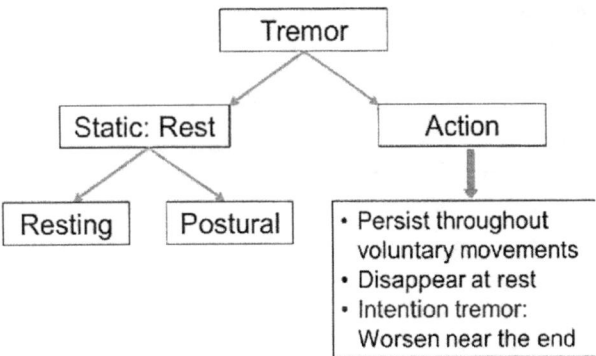

PSP

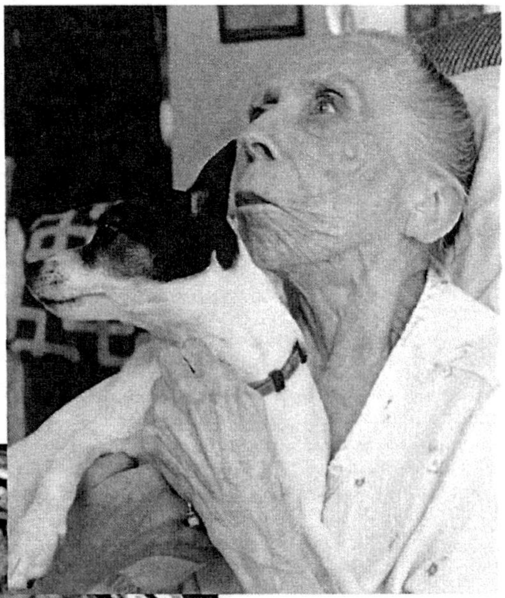

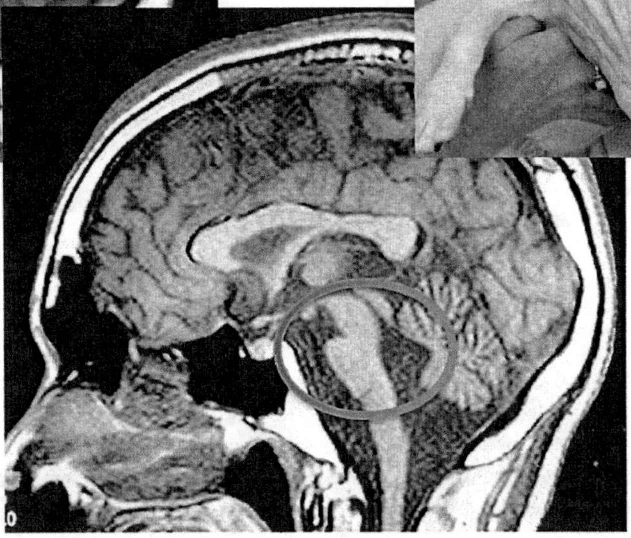

OPCA

```
              ┌──────────┐
              │  Tremor  │
              └────┬─────┘
         ┌─────────┴─────────┐
    ┌─────────┐         ┌──────────┐
    │Static: Rest│        │  Action  │
    └────┬─────┘         └────┬─────┘
    ┌────┴────┐               ▼
 ┌───────┐ ┌────────┐   ┌──────────────────────┐
 │Resting│ │Postural│   │• Persist throughout  │
 └───────┘ └────────┘   │  voluntary movements │
                        │• Disappear at rest   │
                        │• Intention tremor:   │
                        │  Worsen near the end │
                        └──────────────────────┘
```

Essential Tremor
- Postural tremor
- Autosomal dominant: Family history
- Improves with alcohol
- Head tremor
- Voice tremor
- PD tremor involves jaw and mouth
- Rx: Propranolol, primidone, gabapentin, topiramate, botulinum toxin, DBS

Tardive Dyskinesia
- Many involuntary movements
- Dystonia, chorea, tremor, athetosis
- Face, mouth, tongue, eyelid, arching of back
- Long history of antipsychotic medication
- Use 2nd generation of antipsychotics
- Clozapine (BM suppression), quetiapine
- Rx: Clonazepam (mild), ginkgo, reserpine (dopamine depletion), botulinum toxin, DBS

Neuroleptic Malignant Syndrome
- Unusual response to typical and atypical antipsychotics (depletes dopa. — severe PD)
- Rigidity, hyperthermia, autonomic instability, rhabdomyolysis
- Mortality rate is very high if untreated
- Rx:
  - Dopa. agonist: Bromocriptine, dantrolene
  - Supportive therapy
  - Stiff muscle — ventilation → paralyzed, intubation

Hemifacial Spasms
- Half of face is having spasms
- Facial nerve is getting compressed
- Causes:
  - Basilar dolichoectasia (80%)
  - MS
  - Acoustic neuroma
- Treatment:
  - Rx: Carbamazepine, gabapentin
  - Ix: Botulinum toxin
  - Sx: Decompression surgery

Tourette Syndrome
- Developmental neuropsychiatric problem
- Duration > 1 year
- Onset: 2–15 years
- Tics: Motor, vocal tics
- OCD, ADHD, conduct disorder
- Rx:
  - Mild: Clonidine
  - Moderate-to-severe: Haloperidol, risperidone

Focal Dystonia

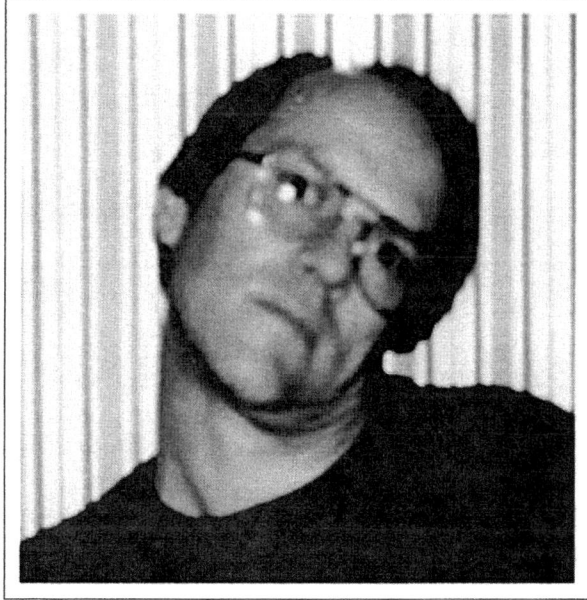

Spasmodic torticollis

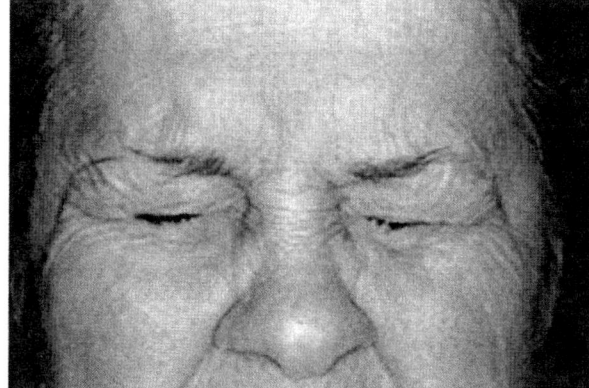

Blepharospasms

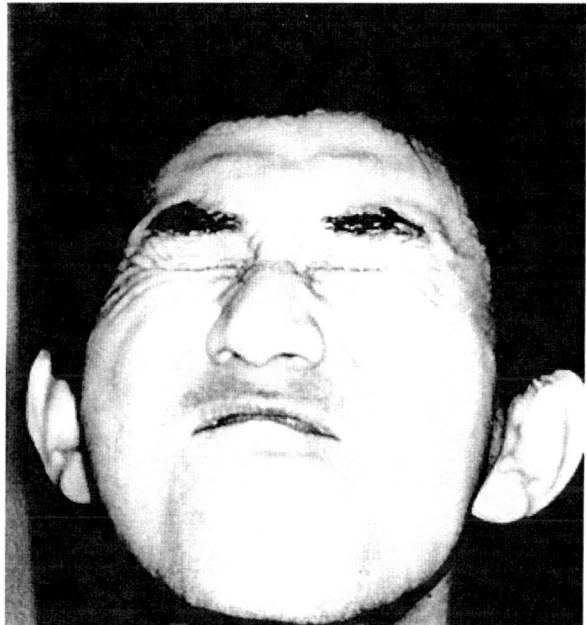

Meige syndrome: Eye + OMD

Movement Disorders — Cases

AR 5

A 65-year-old man complains of "stiffness" and difficulty walking. Exam reveals hypophonia, masked facies, bradykinesia, and shuffling gait. There is no resting tremor.

What is the most likely diagnosis?
A. Parkinson disease
B. Progressive supranuclear palsy
C. Huntington disease
D. Shy-Drager syndrome
E. Wilson disease

Answer: _____

AR 6

A 66-year-old woman presents with right arm tremor and side-to-side head tremor that has gradually worsened over 2 years. The arm tremor is worse when she brings a spoon or teacup to her lips. She has noticed that a glass of wine improves the tremor transiently. Exam shows a positional tremor.

What is the 1st line treatment?
A. Drink alcohol — it helps!
B. Levodopa.
C. Propranolol.
D. Primidone.
E. Thiamine.

Answer: _____

AR 7

A 78-year-old woman has gradual onset of very bothersome tongue-thrusting movements. She has a history of diabetes and gastroparesis that has been treated for 4 years with metoclopramide.

What is the most likely diagnosis?
A. Parkinson disease.
B. Huntington disease.
C. Tardive dystonia.
D. Tardive dyskinesia.
E. This is why I don't like Neurology — too many terms!

Answer: _____

CNS Infections

Acute Bacterial Meningitis
- Sick patient
- Meningeal signs ±
- LP, blood culture and antibiotics
- CT before LP
  - Focal neurological deficits
  - Raised ICP signs
- Broad coverage of antibiotics
- Steroids ±
- Streptococcal pneumonia, *H. influenza*, *N. meningitidis*

Brain Abscess
- Headache, fever, focal neurological deficits
- Extension of local infection: Sinus
- Hematogenous spread
- Base of the skull fracture
- Cribriform plate fracture
- Smooth margin on imaging
- Neurosurgical procedure
- Staph, strep, *Nocardia*

Viral Infections
- Lymphocyte predominant CSF
- Herpes encephalitis: HSV-1 (MC) and HSV-2
  - Young or old patient
  - New onset seizure
  - Change in personality/Hallucinations
  - High mortality if untreated
  - Temporal lobe: Hemorrhage & necrosis
- Dx: HSV PCR CSF
- Rx: Acyclovir
- Do **not** forget about **V**ZV: **V**esicle, **v**ascular complication (**stroke & ICH**)
- Encephalitis with flaccid paralysis: West Nile
- EEG: PLEDs, think of SSPE — measles

Progressive Multifocal Leukoencephalopathy
- AMS, hemiparesis, quadriparesis, speech
- JC virus — polyomavirus
- HIV patient with WM disease
- Newer medications, **not** only HIV
- Natalizumab for MS
- Rituximab
- CSF: JC virus PCR
- Dx test: Biopsy
- Rx: ART

© 2017 MedStudy Internal Medicine Video Board Review – Neurology • Jitesh Kar, MD

Progressive Multifocal Leukoencephalopathy

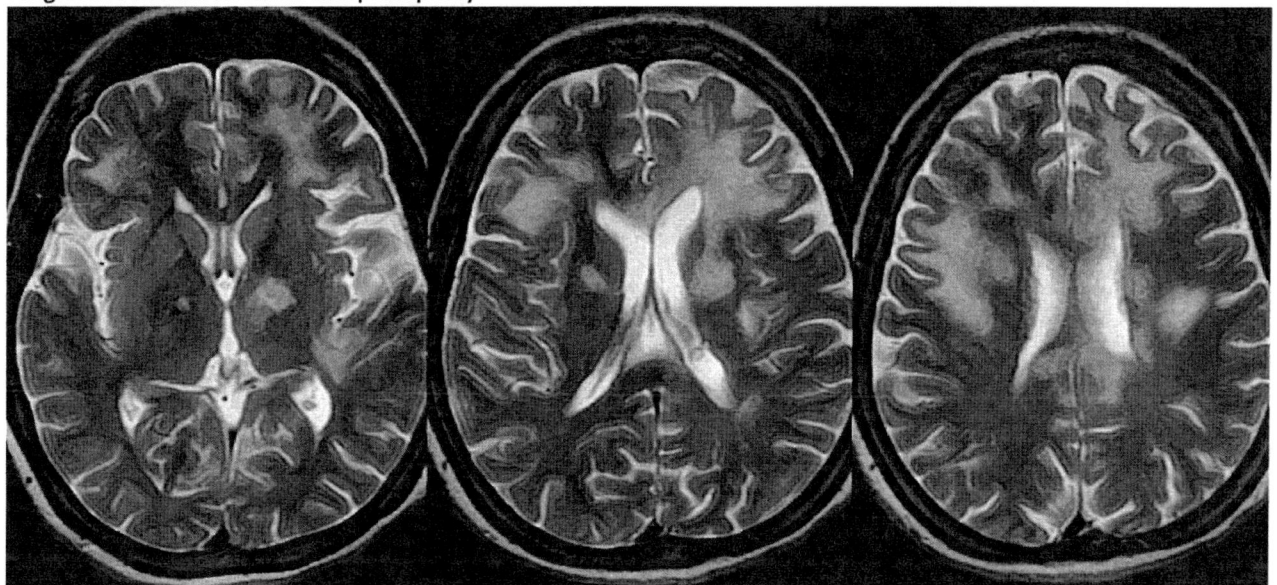

HSV Encephalitis

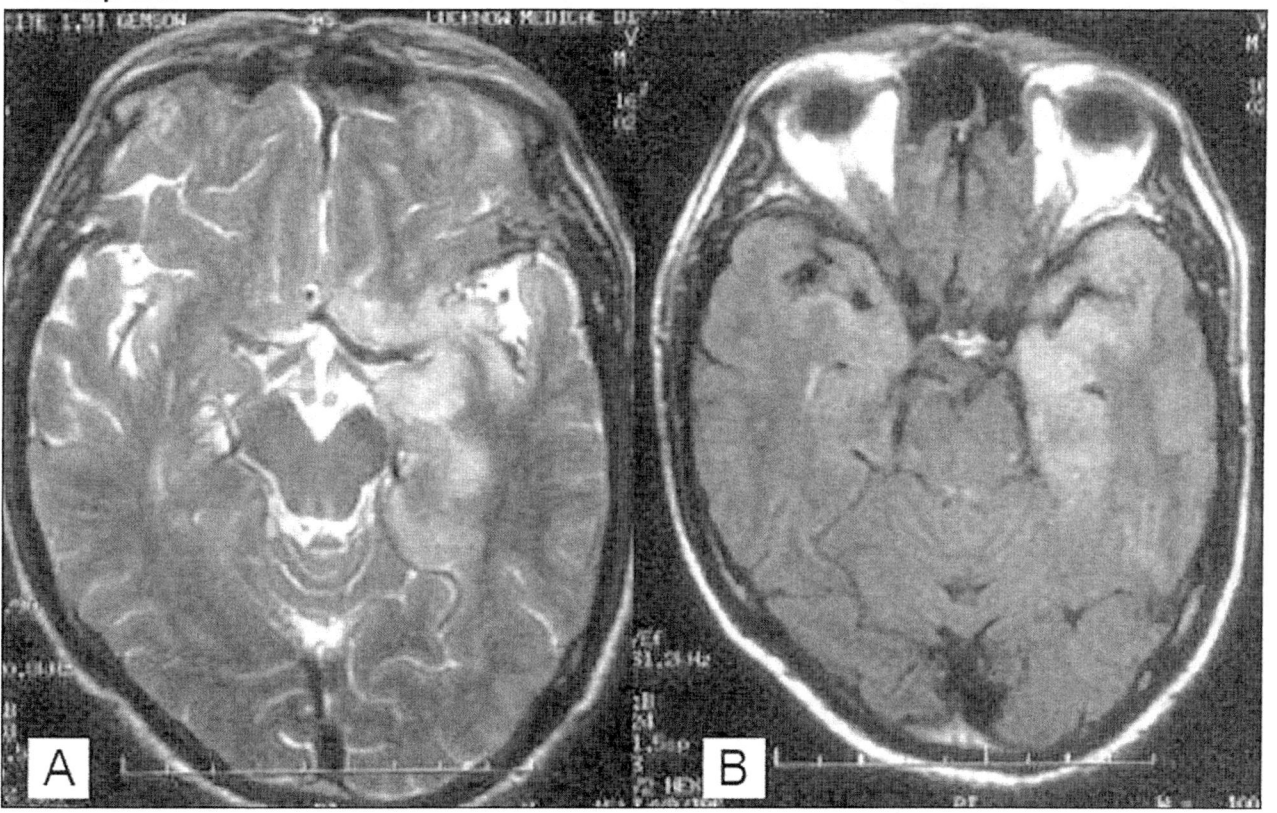

Parasitic Infection — Toxoplasmosis
- HIV patient
- **Multiple ring enhancing lesion**
- IgG antibody: **Not** diagnostic
- Rx: Pyrimethamine, sulfadiazine
- Recurrence is common

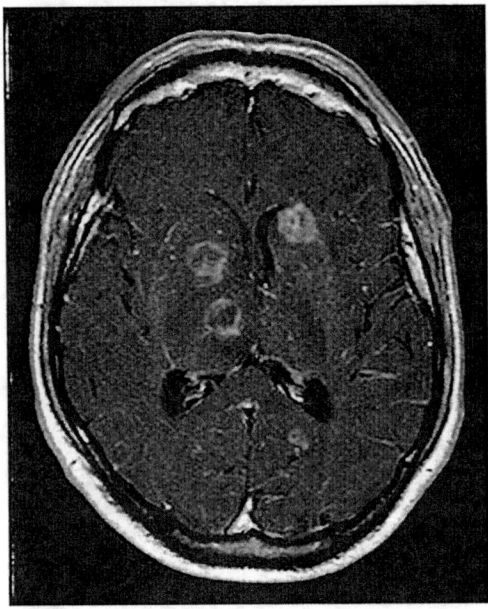

Parasitic Infection — Neurocysticercosis
- Contaminated food/water
- Taenia solium
- Cyst in brain
- Ruptured cyst → edema
- Calcification
- Seizure
- Rx: Albendazole ± steroids
- AEDs if seizure +

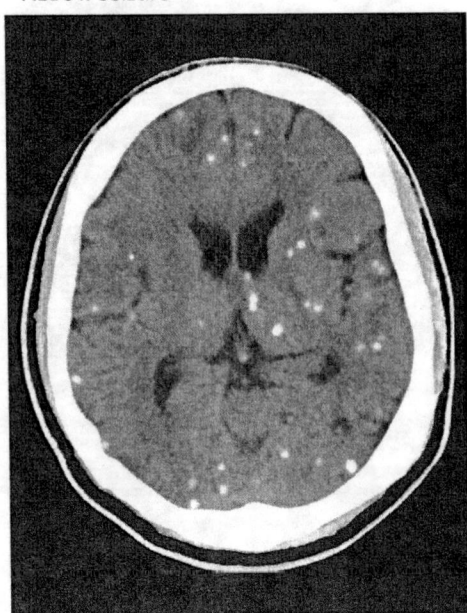

Fungal CNS Infections
- Cryptococcal meningitis
- Immunocompromised patient: HIV/steroids
- Elevated OP
- Cryptococcal antigen titer in serum, CSF
- Rx: Amphotericin B, flucytosine for 2 weeks, f/b oral fluconazole for 8 weeks
- Raised ICP management

Headache

Headache Syndromes
- Primary
  - Migraine
  - Tension
  - Cluster
  - Autonomic cephalgia
- Secondary
  - Hemorrhage
  - Increased intracranial pressure
  - Trauma
  - Giant cell arteritis
  - Sinus/Dental diseases
  - Infection

Red Flag signs of HA — SNOOP
- **S**: Systemic features — fever, weight loss, sz
- **N**: Neurological deficits
- **O**: Old age, > 50 years
- **O**: Onset — sudden
- **P**: Progression of HA, pattern of HA changed

Headache — Migraine
- Character: Unilateral, throbbing, pulsatile
- Associated with nausea (90%), vomiting (30%), photophobia, phonophobia, positive family history
- Onset: Gradual, over 30–60 minutes
- Duration: 2–72 hours
- Triggers: Certain foods, smells, physical exercise, stress, alcohol, premenstrual
- 17% women, 6% men

- Without aura (common)
- With aura (classic — about 35% have this)
  - Aura precedes headache by up to 1 hour
  - Aura consists of neurologic symptoms (scintillating scotomata, numbness, weakness)
- Other types
  - Complicated
  - Basilar
  - Acephalic migraine
  - Status migrainosus: 72 hours

Migraine — Acute / Abortive Rx
- Abortive (< 2 headaches/month)
  - Over-the-counter analgesics
  - NSAIDs
  - Ergotamines (Cafergot Ergomar)
  - 5-HT agonists ("triptans"): Chest tightness and flushing
- Do not use ergotamines and triptans together or in patients with uncontrolled hypertension, h/o stroke, or heart disease!
- **Avoid triptans in (look for these conditions):**
  - Complicated migraine
  - Coronary heart disease or angina
  - History of stroke
  - Uncontrolled BP
  - Pregnancy

Migraine — Prophylaxis
- Preventive (> 4 headaches/month)
  - Antidepressants (TCAs > SSRIs)
  - Anticonvulsants: Topiramate, valproate, gabapentin
  - **Beta-blockers (propranolol, timolol): Asthma!**
  - Botulinum toxin (Botox)
  - CCB (verapamil): Bradycardia and constipation
  - **Topiramate (Topamax):**
    - Topa will make you dopa. — confusion
    - Renal stones

Headache — Cluster
- Men > women, ages of 20–40 years
- **Night – alarm clock** HA
- **Cluster**, restless
- Associated with rhinorrhea or nasal congestion, lacrimation, red conjunctiva, miosis
- Abortive Rx: High-flow O_2, triptans
- Prophylactic Rx: Verapamil, lithium, steroids, topiramate

Tension HA
- HA that starts during or after Neuro lecture
- Bilateral, squeezing
- Worse at the end of the day
- Stress makes it worse
- Relaxation technique and sleep help
- Abortive Rx: ASA, NSAIDs, acetaminophen
- Prophylactic Rx: TCAs

Sexual Headache / Coital Headache
- Tension/Throbbing type
- Increases with sexual excitement
- Benign
- Rx: NSAIDs before sexual activity

Post-Traumatic Headache
- After trauma/concussion
- Benign, reassurance

Giant Cell Arteritis
- Vasculitis of temporal artery
- Temporal HA and blurry vision
- Jaw claudication
- Temporal artery pulsation/tenderness
- Order — CRP, ESR: High
- Pathology: Giant cell arteritis
- Patchy lesion: ? Normal biopsy
- Do **not** wait for biopsy
- Start prednisone
- Complications: Blindness
- Associated with PMR

Pseudotumor Cerebri or IIH
- Idiopathic intracranial hypertension (IIH)
- HA, blurry vision, papilledema
- Raised ICP
- Obese woman, OCP, steroids
- Recent acne treatment — vitamin A overuse

Headache — Pseudotumor Cerebri
- Hallmark is morning headache **and** papilledema
- Headache worsened by coughing, straining
- Visual disturbance
  - Enlarged blind spot
  - Decreased peripheral vision
- Horizontal diplopia: Ophthalmoplegia (CN 6)
- Diagnosis is clinical; Headache and papilledema are most common features
- CT brain and MRI brain will be **normal**
- **Lumbar puncture**
  - LP: Opening pressure (OP) is > 25 cm H_2O

Pseudotumor Cerebri — Treatment
- Goal is to preserve vision
  - Weight loss, low-sodium diet
  - Diuretics:
    - Acetazolamide 250–500 mg daily up to tid
    - Furosemide 40–80 mg/day
  - Steroids — only used acutely as it can also **cause** pseudotumor
    - Prednisone 40–60 mg/day
    - Dexamethasone 6–12 mg/day
- Surgery
  - Lumboperitoneal shunt (50% benefit)
  - Optic nerve sheath fenestration
- Most cases resolve in 6–12 months

Intracranial Hypotension Headache*
- Positional headache
- Worse on standing/sitting
- Improves on lying down
- Post LP headache
- CSF leak headache
- Find a leak

Intracranial Hypotension Headache (cont.)
- Treatment:
  - Blood patch
  - IV fluids
  - Caffeine

Headache — Trigeminal Neuralgia
- Sharp shooting-like pain over trigeminal nerve area
- Pain is **lancinating**
  - Affects the $V_2 > V_3$ distribution of the trigeminal
  - Often, the person has trigger points:
    Pain is brought on by touching the face, toothbrushing, chewing, yawning
- If < 40 years of age, think multiple sclerosis
  - Demyelination of the trigeminal entry zone can cause this

Trigeminal Neuralgia — Treatment
- Anticonvulsants
  - Carbamazepine, oxcarbazepine, phenytoin, and gabapentin (also probably pregabalin)
- Baclofen (Lioresal, Gablofen)
- Glycerol injection — in the trigeminal cistern
- Surgery
  - Radiofrequency rhizotomy = Destroy the pain fibers
  - Microsurgery to reposition a blood vessel that crosses the 5th cranial nerve

Thalamic Pain Syndrome
- Post stroke in thalamic area
- Days, weeks, months, or years later
- Hemibody sensory loss or pain

Headache
- Tension HA:
  - At the end of the day
- Migraine HA:
  - Debilitating
  - Sensitive to light, sound
  - Aura ±
- Cluster HA:
  - Autonomic features
  - **Night**
  - In **cluster**

In headache questions look for:
- Secondary causes of headache
- Contraindications for medications!

Types of headaches by pain distribution:

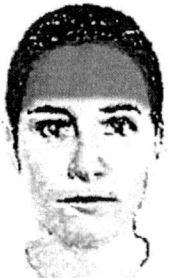 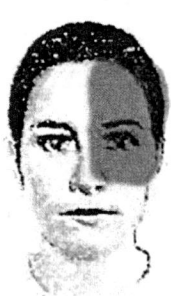 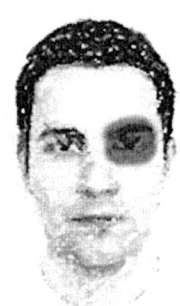

Tension   Migraine   Cluster

Source: Zanjabee Integrative Medicine & Primary Care

Headache — Cases

AR 8

An 18-year-old woman complains of a left unilateral, throbbing headache that was preceded by "flashing lights in the right eye." The headache worsened over 30 minutes and has persisted for 3 hours. The patient now complains of right hand and foot weakness. Exam shows a mild right hemiparesis and word-finding difficulty.

What is the diagnosis?
A. Right middle cerebral artery stroke
B. Left middle cerebral artery stroke
C. (Complex) migraine
D. Cluster headache
E. Transient ischemic attack

Answer: _____

AR 9

A 26-year-old male attorney has a severe retro-orbital stabbing headache for 20 minutes. It wakes him from sleep each morning at 2 a.m. and has done so for the past 5 days. He has no history of headache. Neurologic exam is normal.

What is the most likely diagnosis?
A. Coital headache
B. Migraine
C. Cluster headache
D. Subarachnoid hemorrhage
E. Pseudotumor cerebri

Answer: _____

AR 10

A 38-year-old woman complains of a global headache and occasional double vision.
She is obese, and her exam is only remarkable for mild possible papilledema bilaterally.

What is the greatest concern that you have for this woman, if untreated?
A. Potential for intracranial hemorrhage.
B. Intracranial tumor.
C. Possible loss of vision.
D. Pituitary apoplexy.
E. Yikes, I don't know!

Answer: _____

AR 11

A 75-year-old woman with diabetes, HTN, and a history of "mild" myocardial infarction complains of a unilateral, severe, constant headache. She also has a low-grade fever and malaise. Exam reveals no nuchal signs, but the patient has left temporal artery tenderness. ESR is 125.

What is the next step in management?
A. Indomethacin.
B. Prednisone.
C. Sumatriptan.
D. Propranolol.
E. Oxygen by nasal cannula.
F. Temporal artery biopsy.
G. No need for any medication; just wait and watch!

Answer: _____

AR 12

A 23-year-old man complains of an excruciating headache that began abruptly during intercourse and has persisted for 2 hours. General physical exam is normal. Neurologic exam is normal.

What is the most likely diagnosis?
A. Coital headache
B. Subarachnoid hemorrhage
C. Migraine
D. Cluster headache
E. Temporal arteritis

Answer: _____

Stroke & TIA

Transient Ischemic Attack
- Ischemia without infarction
- Duration — **no more than** 24 hours
- $ABCD^2$ score
- Hospitalization within 72 hours of event if:
  - $ABCD^2$ score ≥ 3
  - Cannot complete workup in less than 48 hours
- TIA workup: Will discuss in next session with stroke

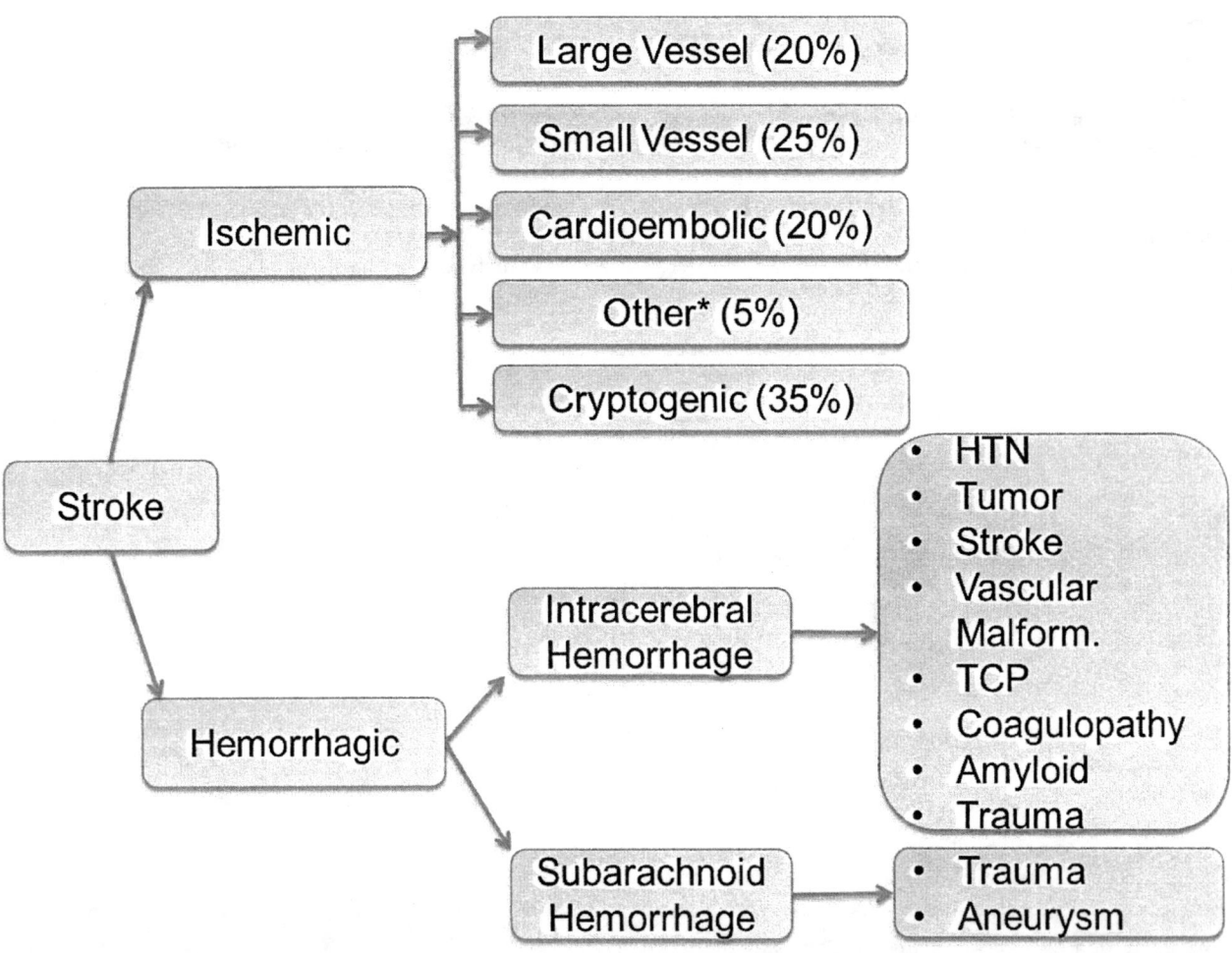

Stroke
- Ischemic
  - Large Vessel (20%)
  - Small Vessel (25%)
  - Cardioembolic (20%)
  - Other* (5%)
  - Cryptogenic (35%)
- Hemorrhagic
  - Intracerebral Hemorrhage
    - HTN
    - Tumor
    - Stroke
    - Vascular Malform.
    - TCP
    - Coagulopathy
    - Amyloid
    - Trauma
  - Subarachnoid Hemorrhage
    - Trauma
    - Aneurysm

Prevention of Stroke
- BP, lipid control
- Smoking cessation, diet and exercise
- Treatment of A-fib
  - ASA
  - Warfarin
  - ASA + clopidogrel
  - Dabigatran: Direct thrombin inhibitor
    - 110 mg dose — non-inferior to warfarin
    - 150 mg bid — superior to warfarin
    - Trend of more frequent MI — careful in CAD
- Carotid endarterectomy or stent: > 70% stenosis
- Treatment of OSA
- Screening for aneurysm in patients with:
  - Family history of SAH
  - ADPKD

Neuroimaging 101
- CT head:
  - To rule out bleed
  - Hyperdense (bright), hypodense (dark)
- CTA: For blood vessel abnormality
- MRI brain:
  - Hyperintense (bright), hypointense (dark)
  - Bright on DWI, dark on ADC: Acute stroke
  - Dark on GRE: Hemosiderin – blood

Stroke — Evaluation
- CT (usually done first to r/o hemorrhage)
- MRI: DWI, ADC (acute stroke)
- ECG
- Echocardiogram: TTE, TEE
- CTA > MRA > CUS and TCD
- A1c
- Lipid panel
- Urine drug screen
- Hypercoag. panel if young patient
- Cerebral angiogram: Case by case

Stroke Localization 101
- X & Y axis model
- First think of X axis: Right vs. left
- Y axis levels:
  - Cortex:
    - Cortical signs: Aphasia; Neglect; Visual field cut
    - For lobe localization: Think of Homunculus
  - Subcortex
  - Midbrain: 3, 4 cranial nerves
  - Pons: 5–8 cranial nerves
  - Medulla: 9–12 cranial nerves
- **Crossed findings (Keep in mind)!**

Stroke — Aphasia
- Broca aphasia (dominant frontal): **Nonfluent**
  - Repetition is impaired
  - Inarticulate, short phrases, simple grammar
  - Comprehension is preserved
- Wernicke's (dominant posterior temporal): **Fluent**
  - Repetition is impaired
  - Good articulation, but meaningless ("word salad")
  - Poor comprehension (speech and writing)

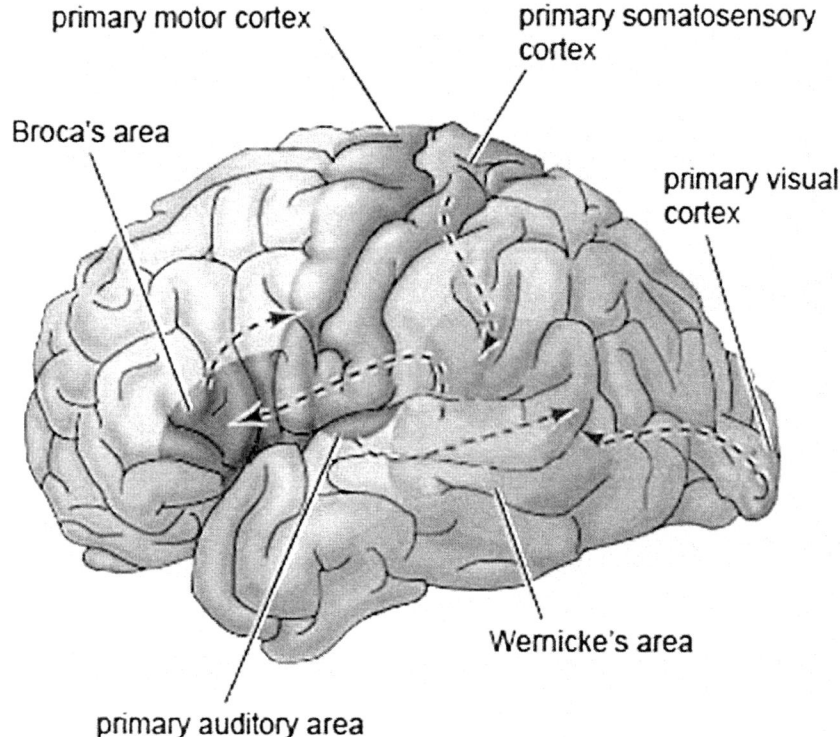

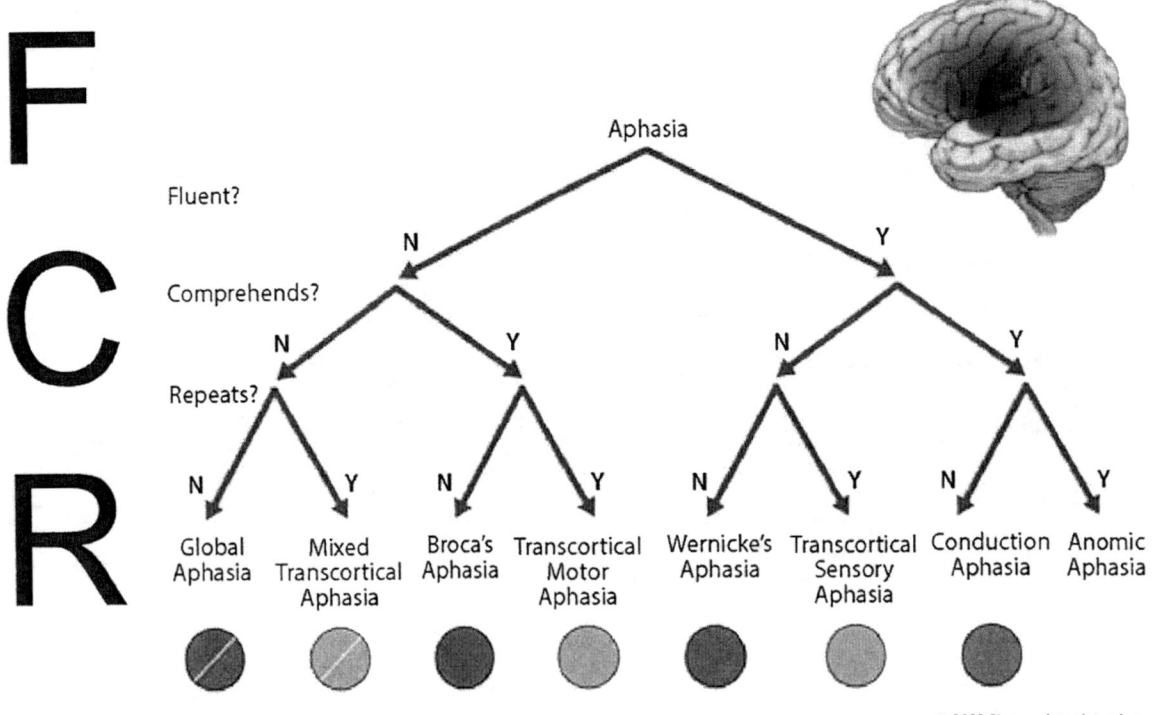

F C R

Aphasia

Fluent?

N   Y

Comprehends?

N   Y   N   Y

Repeats?

N   Y   N   Y   N   Y   N   Y

Global Aphasia — Mixed Transcortical Aphasia — Broca's Aphasia — Transcortical Motor Aphasia — Wernicke's Aphasia — Transcortical Sensory Aphasia — Conduction Aphasia — Anomic Aphasia

© 2002 Sinauer Associates, Inc.

Stroke — Neglect
- Lack of attention to 1/2 of self or environment
- Due to lesions of the nondominant parietal lobe
- Can also occur in lesions of dominant parietal and dominant frontal lobes (these are less common)

Vessel	Clinical Features
MCA	• Contralateral hemiplegia • Contralateral hemianesthesia • Contralateral homonymous hemianopsia • Aphasia (dominant) • Neglect (nondominant)
ACA	• Contralateral monoparesis (foot and leg) • Contralateral grasp • Abulia (lack of spontaneity) • Urinary incontinence
PCA	• Contralateral homonymous hemianopsia • Color anomia (can't name colors, dominant hemisphere) • Mild contralateral hemiparesis • Mild contralateral hemianesthesia

Cortical Vascular Territories

Anterior Cerebral Artery
Middle Cerebral Artery
Posterior Cerebral Artery

Cranial Nerves
- Arise from midbrain: 3, 4
- Arise from pons: 5, 6, 7, 8
- Arise from medulla: 9, 10, 11, 12
- **Do not** come from brainstem: 1, 2
- **All** are ipsilateral, **except** 4, which crosses posterior to the midbrain

Cranial Nerve Dysfunction — Symptoms

Cranial Nerve	Symptom
3, 4, 6	Double vision
5	Numbness of face
7	Weak face
8	Hearing loss
9, 10, 12	Dysarthria and dysphagia
11	Weak shoulder and neck

Cerebellar Stroke
- Special case
  - Edema causes brainstem compression
  - Always admit and observe
  - Surgical decompression if edema is severe (to prevent herniation syndrome)

Ischemic Stroke — Vertebrobasilar
- Lateral medullary syndrome (Wallenberg)
- Clinical features
  - Dysphagia/Dysarthria (CN 9, 10, which innervate muscle of palate and throat)
  - Ipsilateral Horner syndrome (autonomic tracts)
  - Ipsilateral facial numbness (damage to nucleus 5)
  - Ipsilateral ataxia (damage to inferior cerebellar peduncle)
  - Contralateral decreased pain and temperature (damage to spinothalamic tract)

Ischemic Stroke — Lacunar Type
- 90–95% are due to lipohyalinosis
  - Most commonly associated with HTN and DM
- 5–10% are due to emboli
- Clinical features
  - Pure motor or sensory symptoms (face = arm = leg)
  - Clumsy hand — dysarthria syndrome
  - Ataxic hemiparesis (clumsiness >> weakness)
  - Internuclear ophthalmoplegia

Internuclear Ophthalmoplegia (INO)
- Adduction weakness
- Ipsilateral
- Lesion in **medial longitudinal fasciculus**
- If young, think multiple sclerosis; If old, think lacunar stroke

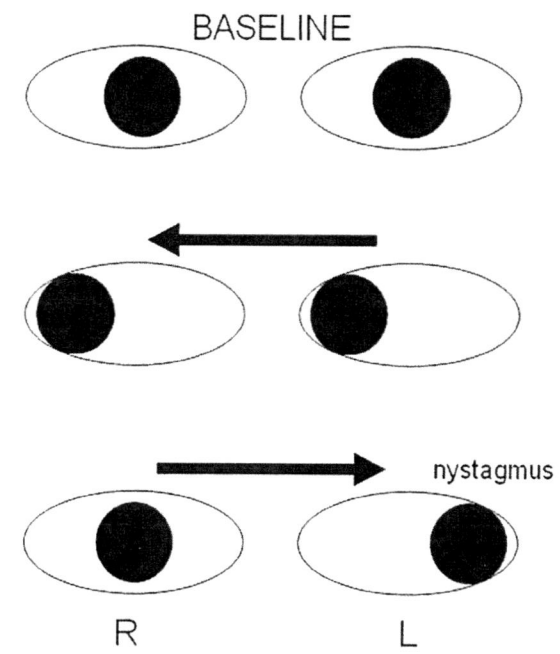

Ischemic Stroke — Treatment
- Supportive measures (ABCs)
- Hypertension (MAP > 130 or SBP > 220)
  - Rarely require IV antihypertensives
  - **No** sublingual nifedipine
- Possibly use thrombolytics (tPA)

Ischemic Stroke — tPA
- Tissue plasminogen activator (tPA)
- Given within 4.5 hours after onset of deficits
- Contraindications
  - Intracranial hemorrhage on CT
  - Hypodensity on CT (tPA could convert an ischemic to a hemorrhagic stroke)
  - Surgery in past 2 weeks (tPA may restart bleeding)
  - Severe uncontrolled hypertension (SBP > 185; DBP > 110)

Ischemic Stroke — Intra-arterial tPA
- Must be infused via arterial access
- Up to 6 hours after onset of stroke
- Lower dose of tPA is needed
- Improved rate of opening vessel
- Highly trained team
- Must have rapid access to these resources

Ischemic Stroke — Prevention
- Reduce risk factors (smoking, EtOH)
- Control blood pressure, diabetes, lipids
- Antiplatelet agents
  - Aspirin (81–325 mg) and clopidogrel (75 mg)
- Carotid endarterectomy
  - Good benefit if > 70% stenosis
  - Small benefit if 50–70% stenosis

Intracerebral Hemorrhage
- Intraparenchymal hemorrhage — ICH
- SAH
- Epidural hematoma
- Subdural hematoma

Hemorrhagic Stroke — Causes
- Hypertension: MC
  - Putamen
  - Thalamus
  - Pons
  - Cerebellum
- Amyloid: Second MC, lobar
- Coagulopathy: INR > 3
- Trauma
- Tumor (or arteriovenous malformation)
  - Cocaine associated with AVM formation

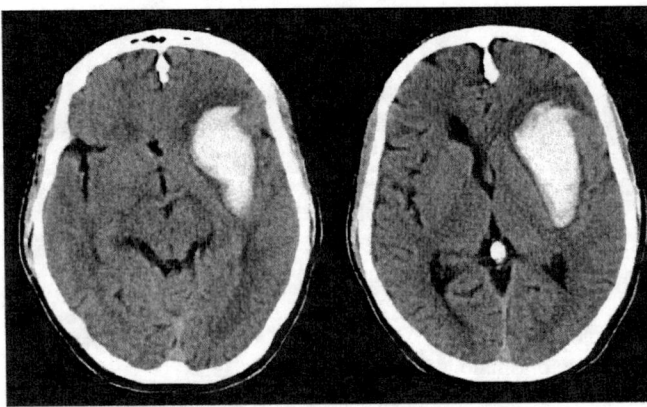

Hemorrhagic Stroke — Treatment
- Supportive measures
- HTN — aggressively treat, nicardipine
- Coagulopathy: Vitamin K, FFP
- **Surgical management:**
  - Cerebellar hemorrhage
  - Lobar hemorrhage > 30 cc
  - Around 1 cm of surface
  - Life-threatening

Subarachnoid Hemorrhage (SAH)
- Blood in subarachnoid space
- Causes: Traumatic vs. nontraumatic
  - Aneurysm
  - AVM
  - Cocaine abuse
- **"Worst headache"**
- CT + in 85–90%
- LP + in > 95%
- Angiogram is gold standard
- Watch for:
  - Cardiac arrhythmias
  - **Vasospasm**

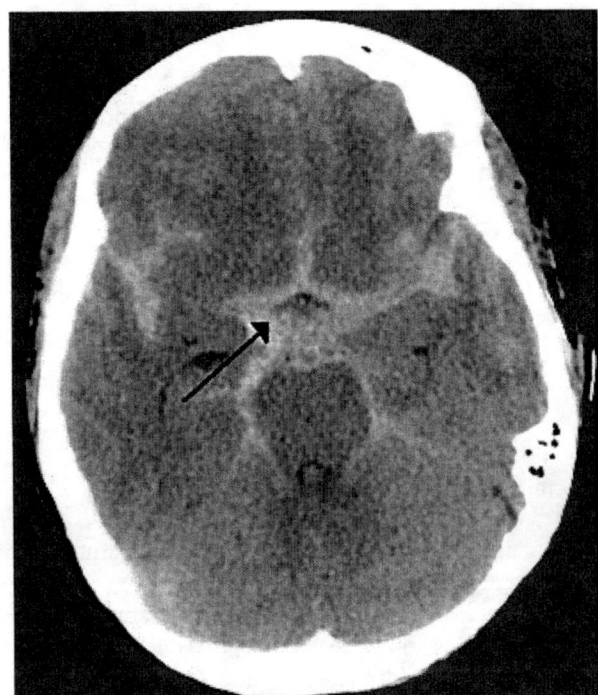

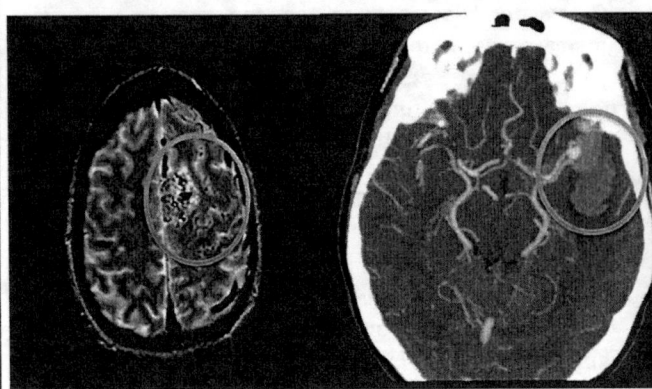

SAH (cont.)
- 80% anterior circulation
  - 40% in ICA
  - 30% anterior communicating artery
- 20% posterior circulation
- 25% of aneurysms are **multiple: APCKD**

Treatment of SAH and its Complications
- AVM/Aneurysm repair: Clip/Coil
- HTN: Aggressively treat
- Vasospasm: 3–5 days after SAH, peak 7 days
  - Focal neurologic deficits
  - Several days (up to 2 weeks) after bleed
  - Treat with nimodipine (usually for about 3 weeks)
- Hydrocephalus: Shunt

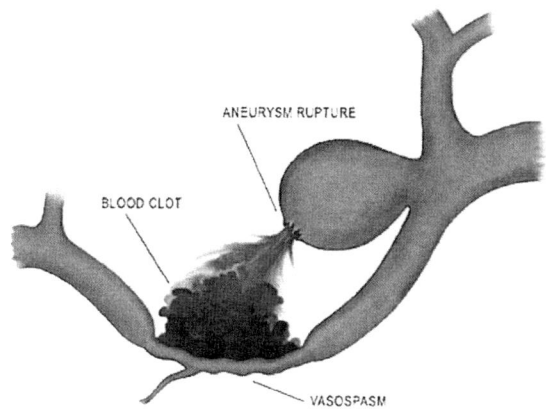

SAH (cont.)
- 1st degree relatives have higher risk
- Screen for aneurysm
- **Mycotic aneurysm**
  - Secondary to septic emboli
  - Blood culture
  - Antibiotics

Subdural Hematoma
- Under dura
- Crescent shape
- Lucid interval
- Acute or chronic
- Elderly patient with fall
- Bridging vein rupture
- MRI (FLAIR): Most sens.
- Rx: Surgical

Epidural Hematoma
- Above dura
- Biconvex
- Lucid interval: ±
- Acute
- Temporal trauma
- Middle meningeal artery
- MRI (FLAIR): Most sens.
- Rx: Evacuation of hematoma — craniotomy

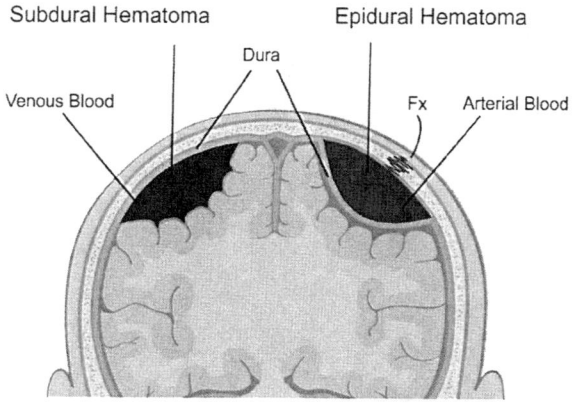

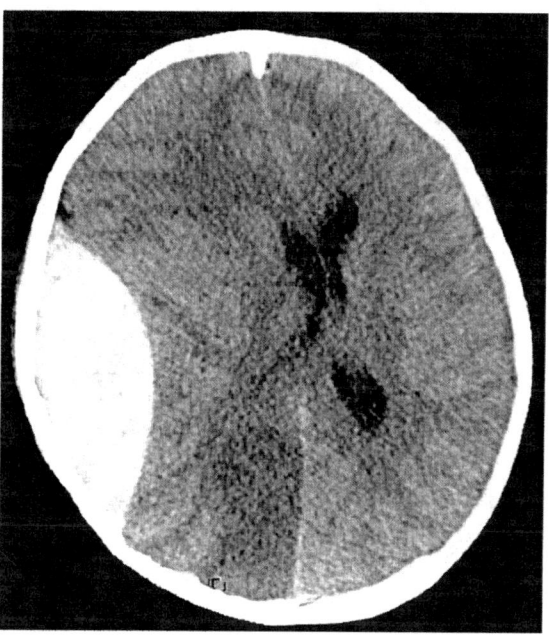

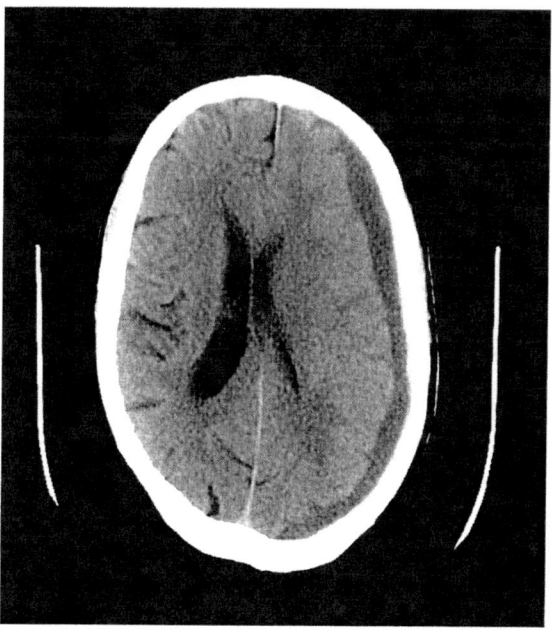

Epidural Hematoma (cont.)

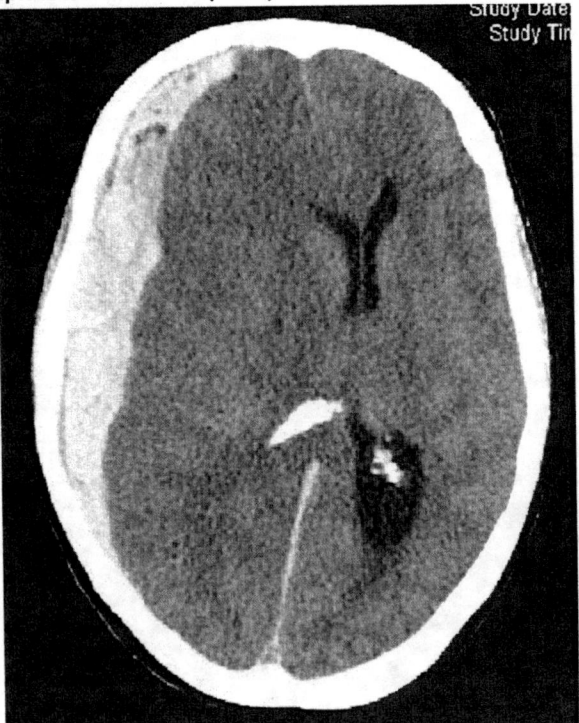

Transient Global Amnesia
- Abrupt onset
- Anterograde amnesia and retrograde ±
- Almost recover completely in 24 hours
- Precipitating event in the question
- Intense emotion, stress
- MRI normal
- PET, SPECT: Hypometabolism in hippocampus and mesial temporal lobe during event, and normal after the event
- Self-resolve
- No treatment

Stroke Localization Questions
- Side of weakness/numbness: R/L
- Distribution: UE, LE, LE > UE
- Side of cranial nerve deficits: R/L
- Cortex:
  - Cortical signs — aphasia, neglect, VFC
  - LE > UE: ACA — think of Homunculus
- Subcortex: Exclusion – dense hemiplegia
- Brainstem:
  - Midbrain: CN 3, 4
  - Pons: CN 5–8
  - Medulla: CN 9–12
- Crossed findings:
  - Right-sided weakness with left-sided CN
  - Brainstem lesion

Stroke — Cases

AR 13
A 60-year-old with DM, HTN, and hypercholesterolemia has sudden onset of right-leg weakness. Exam shows right LE > UE weakness and incontinence.

Where is the lesion?
A. Left middle cerebral artery (MCA) stroke
B. Left anterior cerebral artery (ACA) stroke
C. Right MCA stroke
D. Right ACA stroke
E. Left posterior cerebral artery (PCA) stroke

Answer: _____

AR 14
A 60-year-old man with DM, HTN, and hypercholesterolemia has sudden onset of mild right hemiparesis and hemianesthesia. Exam shows right upper homonymous quadrantanopsia.

Where is the lesion?
A. Left middle cerebral artery (MCA) stroke
B. Left anterior cerebral artery (ACA) stroke
C. Right MCA stroke
D. Right ACA stroke
E. Left posterior cerebral artery (PCA) stroke

Answer: _____

AR 15
A 60-year-old with DM, HTN, and hypercholesterolemia has sudden onset of right hemianesthesia and hemiplegia. Exam shows left-sided past-pointing and dysmetria.

Where is the lesion?
A. Left middle cerebral artery (MCA) stroke
B. Left anterior cerebral artery (ACA) stroke
C. Right MCA stroke
D. Left posterior cerebral artery (PCA) stroke
E. Vertebrobasilar stroke

Answer: _____

© 2017 MedStudy Internal Medicine Video Board Review – Neurology • Jitesh Kar, MD

AR 16

A 60-year-old with DM, HTN, and HLD has sudden onset of confusion and agitation. Exam shows left hemiplegia and hemianesthesia. Patient has right gaze preference.

Where is the lesion?
A. Left middle cerebral artery (MCA) stroke
B. Left anterior cerebral artery (ACA) stroke
C. Right MCA stroke
D. Right ACA stroke
E. Vertebrobasilar stroke

Answer: _____

AR 17

A 60-year-old man with long-standing HTN and poor medical compliance is brought to the ED with acute onset of right hemiplegia, right hemianesthesia, and aphasia.

Where is the lesion?
A. Left middle cerebral artery (MCA) stroke
B. Left anterior cerebral artery (ACA) stroke
C. Left posterior cerebral artery (PCA) stroke
D. Right MCA stroke
E. Right ACA stroke

Answer: _____

Myelopathies

Myelopathies
- Diseases of spinal cord
- Spasticity, **sensory level**
- Bladder and bowel involvement

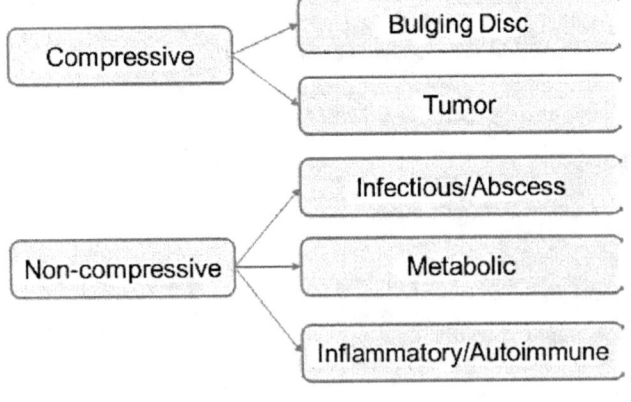

Metabolic Myelopathy — SACD
- B_{12} deficiency causes myelin loss
- Dorsal and lateral column
- Slow onset — frequent falls or dizziness
- B/L LE weakness, spasticity, position, vibration sense loss, ataxia with eyes closed!
- Brisk knee jerk with absent ankle jerk
- Neurological deficits can occur without anemia
- Lab: B_{12} level, MMA, homocysteine level
- Normal or low B_{12}, with elevated MMA, HC
- **Gastric bypass: Now neuropathy – Cu, Zn**

Metabolic Myelopathy — SACD
- **HIV vacuolar myelopathy:**
  – Posterior column tract symptoms in a pt. with HIV
- **Epidural abscess:**
  – Back pain, fever, chills, tenderness
  – LE weakness
  – *S. aureus*
  – Rx: Drainage & antibiotics
  – If TB is the cause, anti-TB medications
- **Tuberculous osteomyelitis:**
  – Pott disease
  – Clinical scenario
  – TB test
  – Extension → SC compression

Neurosyphilis
- Potential complications of untreated syphilis
- Eye, SC, and brain
- Argyll Robertson pupil: Accommodate +; Do **not** react
- Tabes dorsalis: Post. column tract damage
  – Position and vibration gone, ataxia
  – Dx: Screening — RPR or VDRL
  – Specific: MHA-TP
  – Do LP and MRI brain and SC depending on exam

Inflammatory Myelopathy
- Transverse myelitis
- One or 2 segments of SC
- Acute onset of progressive weakness
- Thoracic level
- Autoimmune: Lupus, Sjögren's, NMO
- Dx: MRI spine with contrast, NMO Ab
- Steroids
- No response, PLEX

Compressive Myelopathy
- **Cervical myelopathy:**
  – Compression of N. root: Radiculopathy
  – Compression of SC: Myelopathy
  – **Radiculopathy: Pain, absent reflexes**
  – **Myelopathy: Brisk reflexes**
- Elderly pt, leg weakness, brisk ankle jerk, do not forget to look at C spine!

Compressive Myelopathy (cont.)
- RA patient, post-op FND: C1–C2 injury
- **Thoracic myelopathy:** (Nipple: T4, umbilicus: T10)
  - Transverse myelitis, tumor

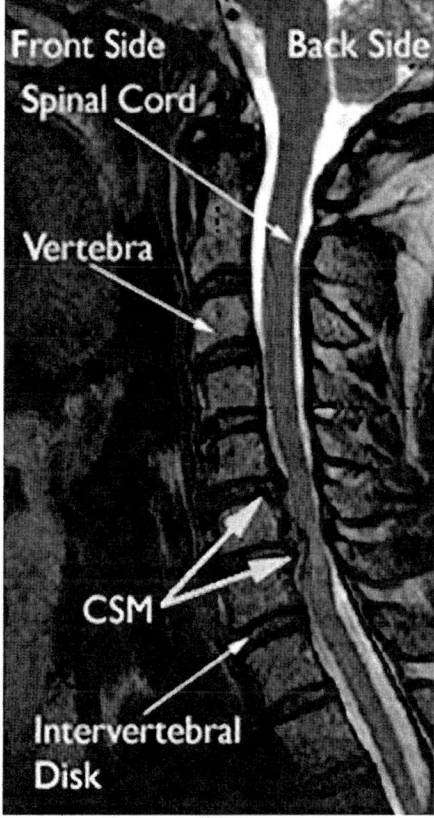

Lumbosacral Myelopathy
- L4 dermatome: Medial aspect of leg
- L5 dermatome: Anterolateral aspect of leg and dorsum of foot, large toe
- S1 dermatome: Lateral side of foot and small toe
- L5 myotome: Toe and ankle extensor weakness: **Foot drop**
- S1 myotome: Weakness of ankle plantar flexion
- **Key points for exam:**
  - **Patient cannot walk on his toes: S1**
  - **Patient cannot walk on his heels: L5**
  - **Back pain improves with leaning forward — lumbar spinal stenosis**

Syringomyelia
- Syrinx = Cavity
- Cavity inside the central canal
- Associated with Chiari 1 malformation
- Painless weakness of hands and arms
- Pain and temp. loss in both UE
- Position and vibration sense intact
- MRI of C spine

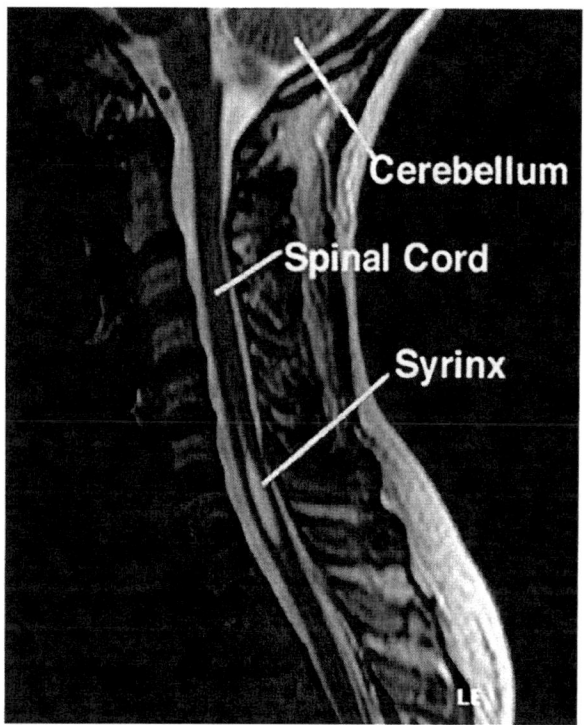

Motor Neuron Disease

Amyotrophic Lateral Sclerosis (ALS)
- UMN signs: Spasticity, brisk reflexes
- LMN signs: Atrophy, fasciculations, weakness
- Progressive disease
- Bulbar involvement
- Terminal stage in 3–5 years
- Riluzole to reduce the progression of the disease

Polio, Post-Polio Syndrome
- Polio was the MC cause of AHC disorder
- Post-polio: Areflexia with progressive weakness
- Consider: West Nile encephalitis

Conditions with UMN, LMN findings
- ALS
- B_{12} deficiency with SACD
- Cervical myelopathy
- Syringomyelia
- Friedreich ataxia
- Syphilis
- Hyperthyroidism

Neuropathies
- Mononeuropathies
- Mononeuropathy multiplex
- Diabetic mononeuropathies
- Polyneuropathy: Demyelinating vs. axonal
- GBS
- CIDP
- CMT
- Diabetic neuropathy
- Alcohol-related neuropathy

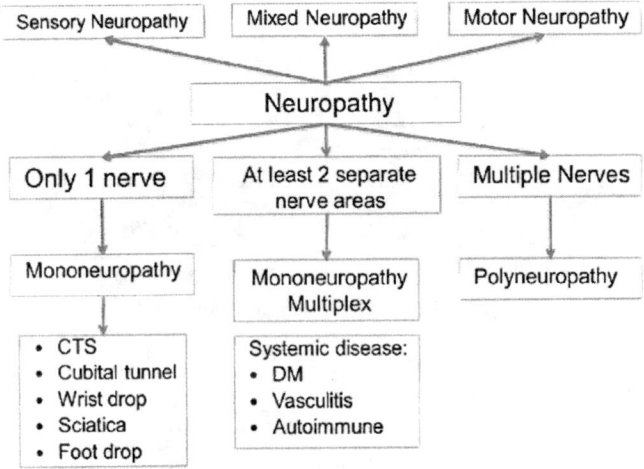

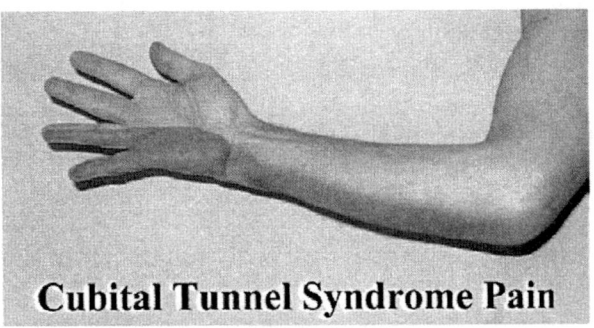

Cubital Tunnel Syndrome Pain

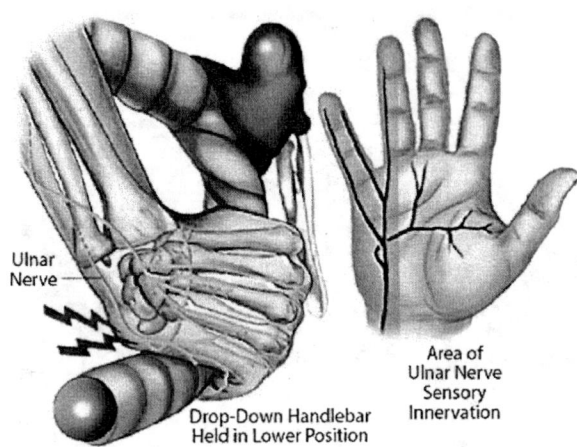

Ulnar Nerve

Drop-Down Handlebar
Held in Lower Position

Area of
Ulnar Nerve
Sensory
Innervation

Workup for Neuropathy
- Glucose tolerance test, HbA1c
- Free T_4, TSH
- Vitamin B_{12}
- ESR
- CBC, creatinine
- Chest x-ray
- SPEP, UPEP
- Urine heavy metals, urine drug screen
- EMG/NCS

Mononeuropathies in Upper Extremity
- Wrist drop: Radial nerve (radial groove humerus)
  - Saturday night palsy
  - Cannot extend the wrist!
- Carpal tunnel syndrome: Medial nerve (wrist)
  - Medial nerve at wrist, Tinel sign, Phalen sign
  - Tingling & numbness: First 3–4 fingers, hand, shoulder
  - B/L CTS: Thyroid, acromegaly, pregnancy
  - Wrist splint, refractory or EMG showed muscle loss: Surgery
- Ulnar neuropathy:
  Ulnar nerve (cubital tunnel)
  - Sensory symptoms: 3rd and little finger
  - Weakness of finger abductors and adductors
  - Elbow pads, splint, surgery

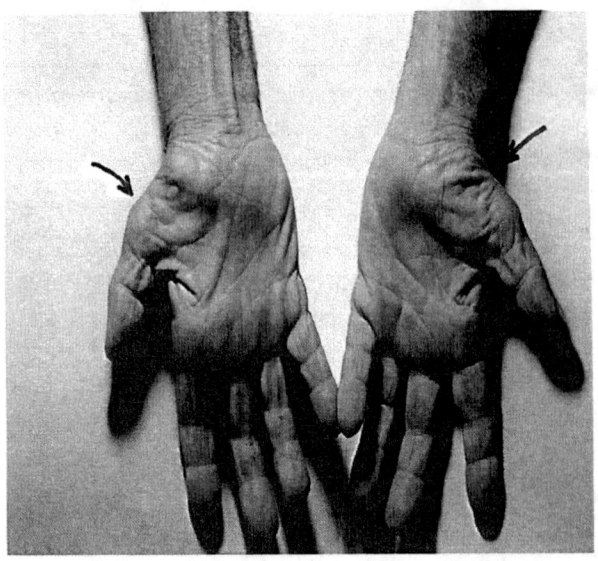

Mononeuropathies in Upper Extremity (cont.)

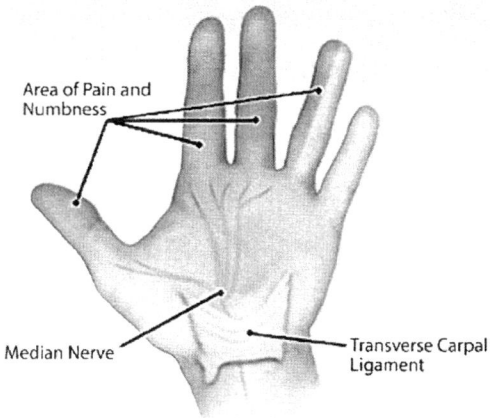

Area of Pain and Numbness

Median Nerve

Transverse Carpal Ligament

Carpal Tunnel Syndrome

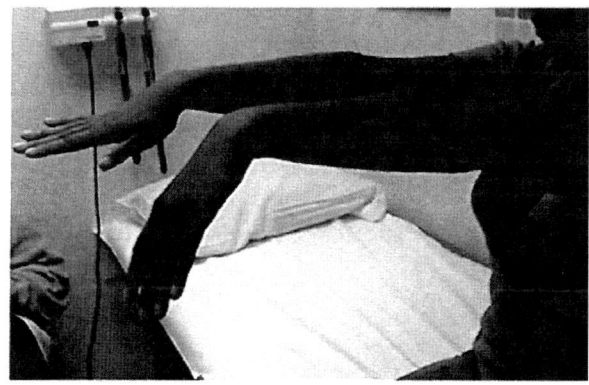

Mononeuropathies in Lower Extremity
- **Sciatic nerve compression:**
  - Posterior compartment
  - Difficulty standing on toes
  - **Ankle reflex preserved (absent in S1 radiculopathy)**
- **Peroneal nerve compression:**
  - Foot drop (UE equivalent?)
  - Prox. end of fibula
  - Eversion and dorsiflexion weak
  - **Inversion normal (L5 radiculopathy: Inversion weakness, L5 innervated muscles in thigh are weak)**

Mononeuritis Multiplex
- 2 or more segments of nerves
- Consider systemic diseases
- RA
- DM
- CTD
- Vasculitis
- Polyarteritis
- Lyme disease

Bell's Palsy

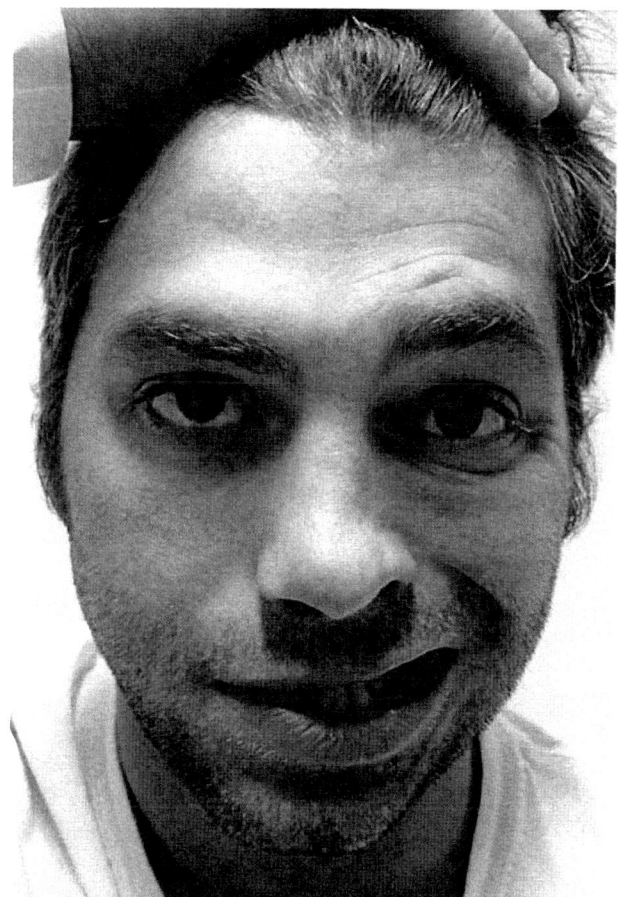

Source: James Heilman, MD

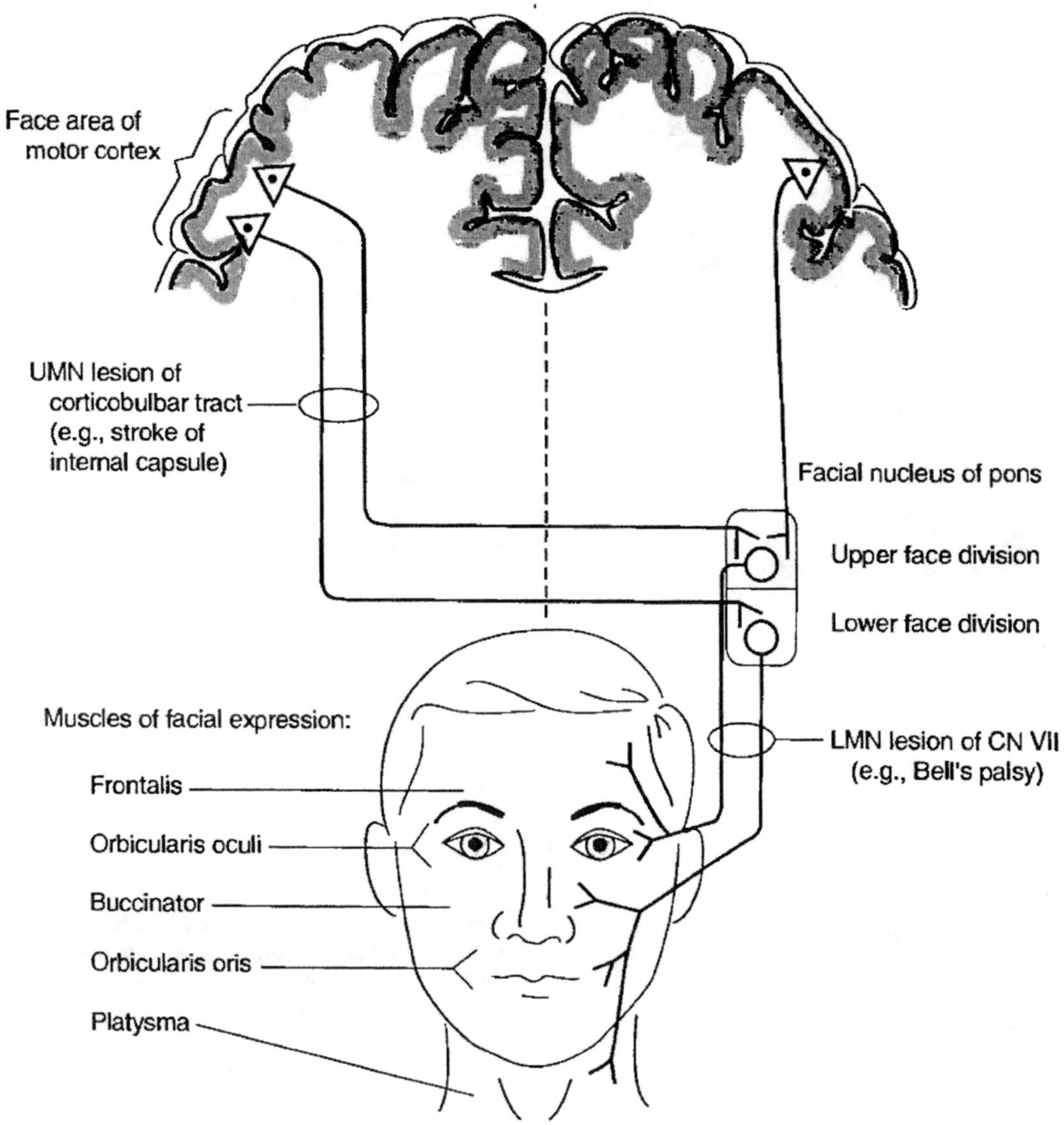

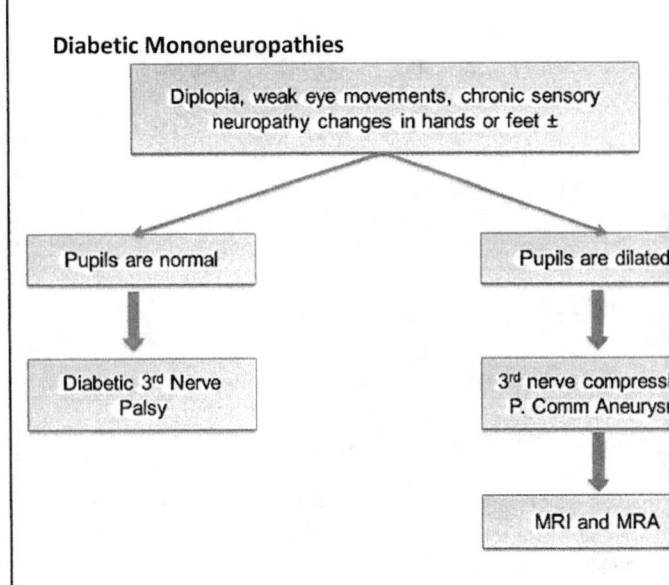

Face area of motor cortex

UMN lesion of corticobulbar tract (e.g., stroke of internal capsule)

Facial nucleus of pons

Upper face division

Lower face division

Muscles of facial expression:

Frontalis

Orbicularis oculi

Buccinator

Orbicularis oris

Platysma

LMN lesion of CN VII (e.g., Bell's palsy)

Bell's Palsy (LMN Facial Nerve Palsy)
- Causes:
  - Idiopathic
  - HSV
  - VZV: Vesicles around tympanic membrane
  - Lyme disease
  - Acute HIV
  - Parotid tumor
  - Cerebropontine angle tumor
  - **B/L facial palsy: MS, neurosarcoidosis**
- **When do you need imaging for Bell's palsy?**
  - Progressive worsening
  - Associated other cranial nerve deficits
  - Twitching/Seizure before the palsy
- Treatment:
  - Protect eye
  - Prednisone 60 mg ± antiviral
  - House-Brackmann grading system

Diabetic Mononeuropathies

Diplopia, weak eye movements, chronic sensory neuropathy changes in hands or feet ±

Pupils are normal

Pupils are dilated

Diabetic 3rd Nerve Palsy

3rd nerve compressi P. Comm Aneurysr

MRI and MRA

Diabetic Mononeuropathies (cont.)

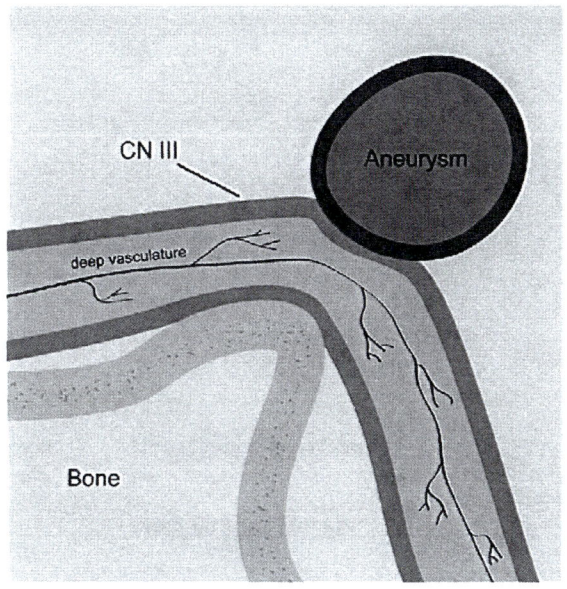

Unilateral Dilated Fixed Pupil
- If patient is comatose — uncal herniation
- Walk in to your clinic — to rule aneurysm/SAH
  - CT head without contrast
  - LP
  - CTA head

Diabetic Lumbosacral Plexopathy
- Also known as amyotrophy
- Leg pain followed by weakness
- Proximal muscles
- Autonomic symptoms, weight loss
- Sensory symptoms +
- Chronic history
- Partial recovery
- No specific treatment, trial of steroids

Polyneuropathies
- Peripheral nerve = Electrical wiring
- Insulation/Sheath: Myelin
- Copper wire: Axonal
- Demyelinating: **M**otor = Speed
  - Conduction velocity slow
  - Latency will be prolonged
  - Motor fibers are affected: Weakness
- **A**xonal: Low **a**mplitude
  - Sensorimotor features, sensory 1st

Guillain-Barré Syndrome (GBS)
- Acute inflammatory demyelinating polyneuropathy
- Postinfectious: GI or respiratory
- Autoimmune pathology: Antibody attacks myelin
- C/F: Ascending paralysis with areflexia, mainly motor
- Miller Fischer variant: Ophthalmoplegia, areflexia, ataxia

- LP: Albuminocytological dissociation
- MFV: Anti-GQ1b antibody
- Axonal variant: EMG, Anti-GQ1b antibody, *C. jejuni*
- Treatment: IVIG vs. plasma exchange
- Monitor: 20-30-40
  - FVC: < 20 mL/kg
  - MIP: < −30 cm H_2O
  - MEP: < 40 cm H_2O

Chronic Inflammatory Demyelinating Polyneuropathy (CIDP)
- GBS which did not resolve for **8 weeks**
- Begins insidiously and progresses slowly
- Chronic symmetric sensorimotor symptoms
- LP, EMG same as GBS
- Rule out systemic diseases: HIV, hepatitis, Lyme, thyroid, DM, sarcoid, autoimmune
- Rx: **Glucocorticoids**, IVIG, plasma exchange

Charcot-Marie-Tooth Disease (CMT)
- Hereditary neuropathy
- Myelin is not properly formed, genetic defect
- Family history present
- Symptoms are progressive, since childhood
- Sensorimotor symptoms
- EMG: **D**emyelinating

Diabetic Polyneuropathy
- Most common
- Sensory symptoms more — **Pain**, T, N
- Starts distally, symmetrical, length depen.
- Vibration and position sense: Absent
- Rx: Duloxetine (Cymbalta), pregabalin (Lyrica), TCA, gabapentin
- Treat the underlying problem
- Metformin side effect: B_{12} deficiency, which causes peripheral neuropathy

Alcoholic Polyneuropathy
- Axonal mainly, can be demyelinating
- Pain, tingling, numbness, symmetric, ascending
- Loss of reflexes and position, vibration sense
- Rx: DC alcohol, MV
- Acute thiamine deficiency: Wernicke encephalopathy, polyneuropathy, EOM involvement, ataxia

Neuromuscular Junction Pathology
- Myasthenia gravis
- Lambert-Eaton syndrome

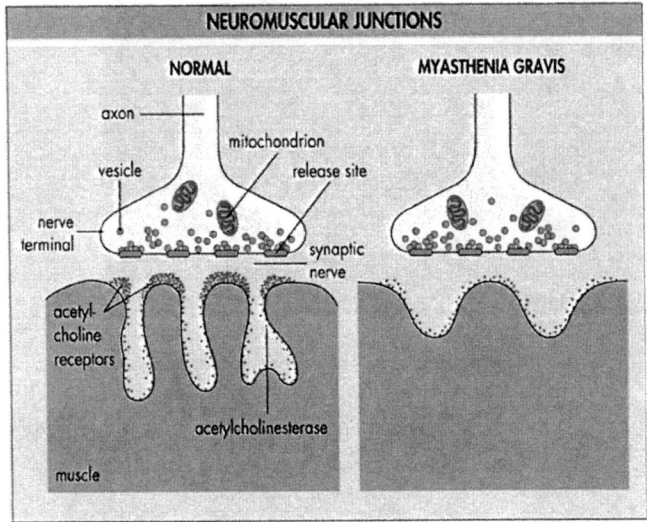

Myasthenia Gravis (MG)
- Autoimmune
- Seropositive: Antibody positive
  - **ACh receptor antibody (Post-synaptic)**
  - **MuSK Antibody**
- Seronegative: Neither
- Thymoma (15%)
- Thymic hyperplasia (60%)
- CT chest with contrast

MG — Clinical Features
- Generalized MG
  - Episodic weakness with repetitive movements
  - Worse in the evening, improves with rest
  - Prox. muscles, ptosis, muscles of face
  - DTRs are usually normal
- Ocular MG:
  - Weakness localized to eyes

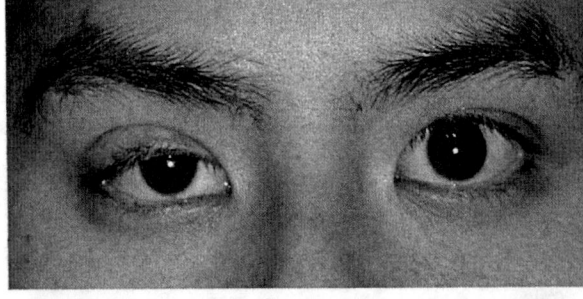

Diagnostic Tests
- Lid lag test: Look up for 30 seconds — ptosis
- Ice pack test: Ptosis improves
- Tensilon/Edrophonium tests: Rarely used
- Thyroid tests: 30% of patients have autoimmune thyroiditis

- Look for autoimmune disorders like lupus, RA
- CT chest for thymoma
- Repetitive Stimulation test: Electrodecremental response
- Single fiber EMG: Increase jitter — **most** sensitive test

	ACh. Recept. Ab	MuSK Ab
Generalized MG	85–90% +	50% in patients with negative ACh. Receptor Ab.
Ocular MG	60% +	

Treatment of MG
- Symptomatic: Pyridostigmine
- Immunomodulator:
  - Steroids
  - Steroid-sparing agent: Cyclosporine
- Treatment of myasthenia crisis: IVIG vs. PLE
- Thymectomy
  Watch for medications that can worsen myasthenia crisis:
  - Beta-blocker
  - Penicillin
  - Aminoglycosides

Lambert-Eaton Syndrome
- **Presynaptic Ca recep. Ab: Reduces ACh release**
- **Paraneoplastic: Small cell lung cancer**
- C/F: Same as MG except:
  - Rarely involves eyes
  - Symptoms improve with exercise
  - DTRs are hypoactive
- Diagnosis:
  - Anti-VGCC
  - EMG: Electro incremental response
- Rx:
  - Treat the cancer
  - Pyridostigmine
  - IVIG or steroid

Myopathies
- Inflammatory:
  - Polymyositis: Prox. muscle
  - Dermatomyositis: Prox. muscle + skin
  - Inclusion body myositis: Distal muscle
- Endocrine: Thyroid
- Medication: Statin
- Metabolic: Ragged red fiber myopathy
- Duchenne: 2 years of age, X-linked, prox. muscle weakness with elevated CK
- Myotonic: Adult onset, myotonia +, cataract, hypogonadism, cardiac defect, insulin resistance
- HIV-related myopathies:
  - Secondary to HIV vs. AZT
  - Discontinue ART

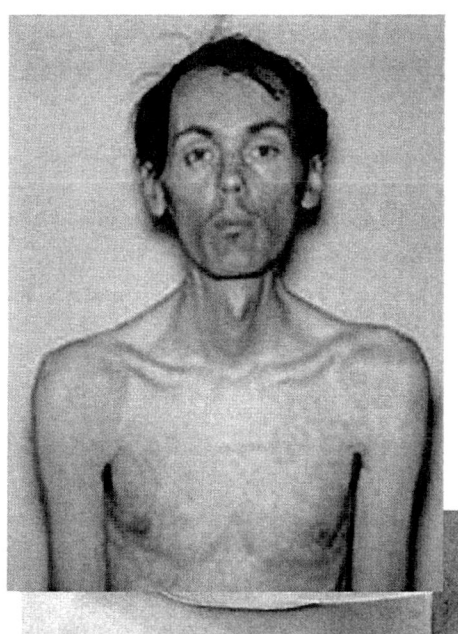
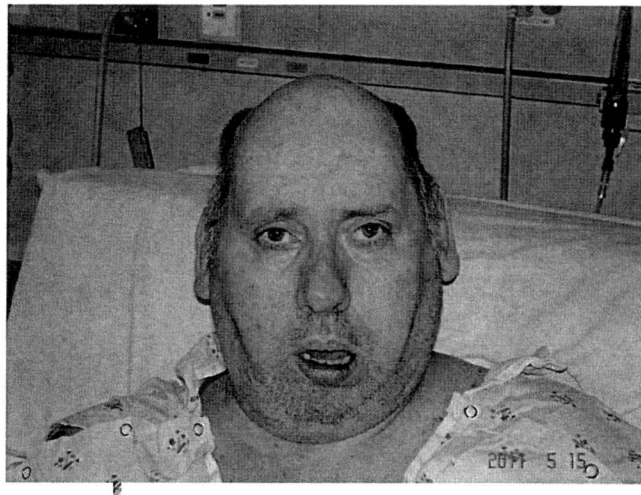
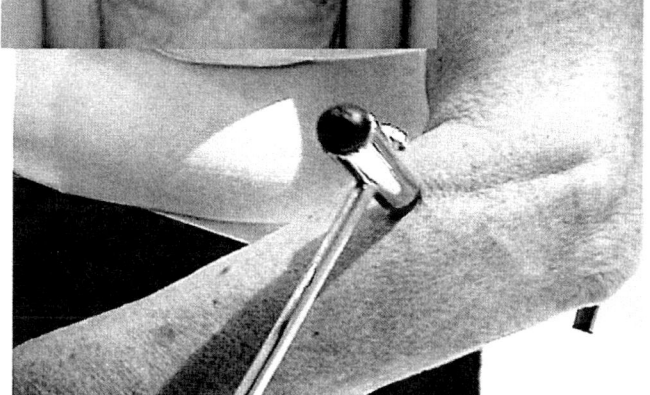
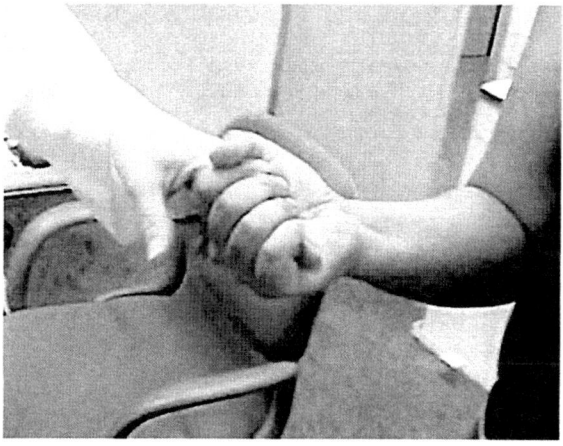

Dizziness

Dizziness — Definitions
- Dizziness
  - Vertigo — illusion of movement
  - Presyncope — lightheadedness
  - Dysequilibrium — sense of imbalance
  - Vaguely defined — emotional?

Dizziness — Vertigo (Exam)
- Nystagmus
  - Peripheral — unilateral with the fast component away from the affected ear
  - Central
    - Multidirectional = Drugs
    - Vertical = Brainstem or midline cerebellum
- Calorics
  - Slow component to cold ear
- Hearing loss

Dizziness — Vertigo

Features	Peripheral	Central
Onset	Sudden	Sudden/slow
Severity of vertigo	Intense	Less intense
Pattern	Intermittent	Constant
Associated nausea	Frequent	Variable
Nystagmus	Horizontal, Vertical	Vertical
Hearing loss	+/−	−
Tinnitus	+/−	−
CNS features	−	+

Causes of Vertigo
- Peripheral
  - Vestibular neuronitis
  - BPPV
  - Post-traumatic
  - Ménière's
  - Labyrinthitis
  - Ototoxic drugs
  - Motion sickness

- Central
  - Brainstem TIA/stroke
  - Cerebellar infarct or ICH
  - CPA tumors
  - Basilar migraine

Vestibular Neuritis
- Inflammation of vestibular nerve
- Sudden onset of **nonpositional vertigo**
- Sudden **prolonged** vertigo
  - Lasts hours to weeks (usually a few days)
  - Associated with nausea/vomiting, dysequilibrium
- Typically occurs in young adults
- Nystagmus — horizontal
- Usually **without tinnitus or hearing loss**
- If hearing loss + → vestibular labyrinthitis
- **Persistent symptoms and no hearing loss: Helps to differentiate from Ménière disease**
- Treatment is symptomatic vs. steroids

Benign Paroxysmal Positional Vertigo
- Vertigo is precipitated by movements of the head
- Few seconds
- Due to dislocation of an otolith
- Nystagmus is usually horizontal
  - Transitory and fatigable
- **No** tinnitus or hearing loss
- Treatment is symptomatic, sometimes self-resolving
- (Epley maneuver can restore otolith to normal)
- Meclizine does **not** cure the condition

Ménière Disease
- Onset in 20s and 30s
- **Triad: Vertigo, hearing loss, tinnitus**
- Relapsing and remitting course
- Increased endolymph in scala media (endolymphatic hydrops)
- Decreased salt (sodium) intake, alcohol, nicotine
- Diuretics
  - Thiazide diuretics (furosemide)
  - Acetazolamide (? decrease endolymph formation)
- Surgery:
  - Endolymphatic sac surgery
  - Labyrinthectomy
  - Vestibular nerve sections

Causes of Vertigo
- Vertebrobasilar TIA:
  - Posterior circulation
  - N, V, N, V: Nausea, Vomiting, Nystagmus, Vertigo
  - Ataxia
- Aminoglycoside toxicity:
  - Sensorineural hearing loss

Tinnitus
- Ringing sensation in ear
- Without any auditory stimuli
- Multiple causes: ASA overdose, MS, FB
- For exam: If you see tinnitus, it is **not** a case of vestibular neuritis

Dizziness — Cases

AR 18
A 64-year-old woman has noticed a sudden sense of spinning whenever she turns her head to the left and extends the neck. The sensation will last minutes to hours. Her exam is negative. Nylen-Barany produces lateral nystagmus to the left only.

What treatment would most likely help?
A. Meclizine.
B. Epley maneuver.
C. No treatment needed; this will resolve spontaneously.
D. Furosemide.
E. Refer to Psychiatry.

Answer: _____

AR 19
A 36-year-old man complains of vertigo, hearing loss, and ringing in the left ear.
He has had 8 severe episodes in 10 years. During each episode, he experienced severe nausea and vomiting. His physical exam is normal. His neurologic exam reveals marked hearing loss in the left ear.

What is the most likely diagnosis?
A. Shy-Drager syndrome
B. Orthostatic hypotension
C. Ménière disease
D. Benign positional vertigo
E. Vestibular neuronitis

Answer: _____

CNS Metastasis
- Parenchymal:
  - Nonhemorrhagic metastasis:
    - Lung
    - Renal
    - Breast
    - Lymphoma
  - Hemorrhagic metastasis: **(CTMR)**
    - Choriocarcinoma
    - Thyroid CA
    - Melanoma
    - RCC
- Dural: Breast, prostate
  - Prostate, breast, lung

- **Epidural:** Elderly patient with cancer history, now back pain, new onset of bladder and bowel dysfunction
- Meningeal: Lymphoma, breast, melanoma
- Rx: Depends on no. of lesions and functional status of patient
  - Single: Surgery + radiation
  - Inaccessible lesion: Stereotactic radiosurgery
  - Multiple metastases: Whole brain radiation and chemotherapy

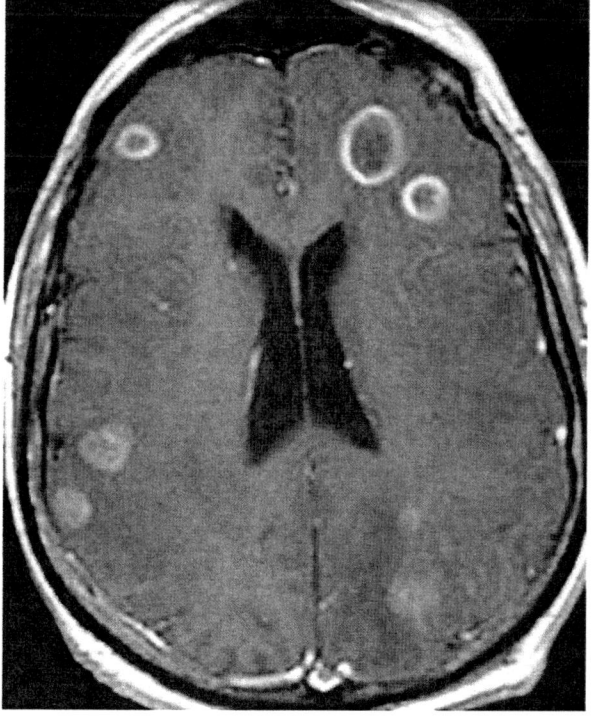

Overview
- Wernicke's
- Korsakoff syndrome
- Lithium toxicity
- Anticholinergic toxicity

Wernicke's / Korsakoff's
- Thiamine (B_1) deficiency
- Alcoholism, PEM, malabsorption, dialysis
- Confused, walks drunk, trouble moving eyes
- Severe: Amnesia — anterograde + retrograde
- Confabulate
- Hemorrhage or necrosis in mammillary bodies
- Rx:
  - IV thiamine before IV glucose
  - Prevents Korsakoff's

Lithium Toxicity
- Confusion, ataxia
- Asterixis
- Nystagmus
- Opsoclonus
- Seizure, myoclonus
- Low Na^+ increases Li resorption
- Rx: Dialysis

Anticholinergic Toxicity
- Cut. vasodilation
- Anhidrosis
- Hallucinations
- Mydriasis
- Urinary retention
- Hyperthermia

Narcolepsy
- Clinical (4 criteria: Only 50% will have all 4)
  1) Sleep attacks (irresistible)
  2) Cataplexy (sudden loss of muscle tone, no LOC, few seconds)
  3) Daytime sleepiness
  4) Hypnagogic & hypnopompic hallucinations
- Pathology: Loss of hypocretin — neurotransmitter
- Evaluation
  - PSG (polysomnogram): Reduce sleep latency

Think about Dr. Kar's boring Neurology board review lecture!

Oh no, not again! You're kidding me?!!!?!!

Immediately, you go to sleep! = Reduced latency on PSM

Reduced latency on PSM — Narcolepsy

Narcolepsy — Treatment

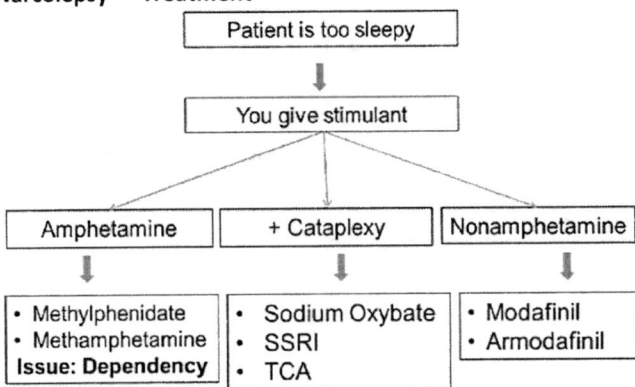

Optic Pathways
- U/L blindness: Optic N. lesion
- Bitemporal hemianopia: Optic chiasm lesion
- Homonymous hemianopia: C/L lesion of the optic tract
- Superior quadrantanopia: Temporal loop radiations
- Inferior quadrantanopia: Parietal lobe radiations — superior
- HH with macular sparing: Cortical lesion

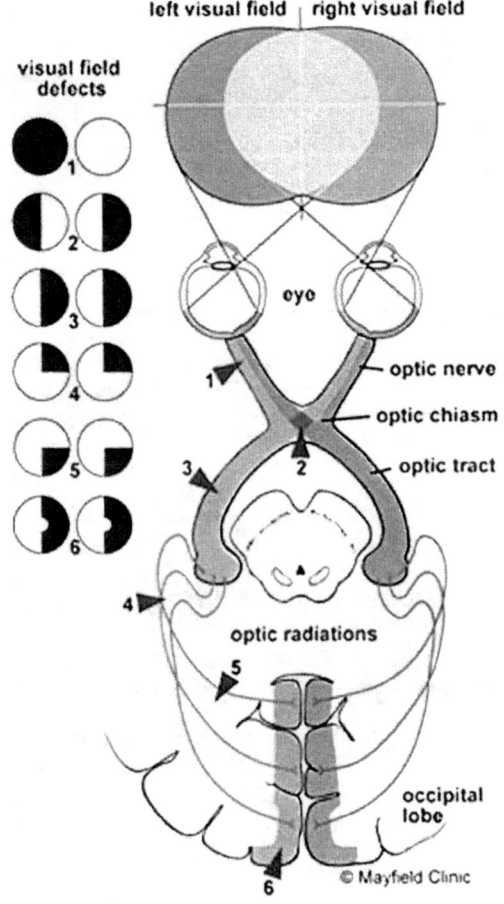

Neurology
Audience Response Answers

Audience Response 1
Answer: B. Opiate intoxication.

AR 2
Answer: C. Normal pressure hydrocephalus.

AR 3
Answer: B. Donepezil.

AR 4
Answer: C. Sertraline.

AR 5
Answer: A. Parkinson disease.

AR 6
Answer: C. Propranolol.

AR 7
Answer: D. Tardive dyskinesia.

AR 8
Answer: C. (Complex) migraine.

AR 9
Answer: C. Cluster headache.

AR 10
Answer: C. Possible loss of vision.

AR 11
Answer: B. Prednisone.

AR 12
Answer: A. Coital headache.

AR 13
Answer: B. Left anterior cerebral artery (ACA) stroke.

AR 14
Answer: A. Left middle cerebral artery (MCA) stroke.

AR 15
Answer: E. Vertebrobasilar stroke.

AR 16
Answer: C. Right MCA stroke.

AR 17
Answer: A. Left middle cerebral artery (MCA) stroke.

AR 18
Answer: B. Epley maneuver.

AR 19
Answer: C. Ménière disease.

MedStudy

Internal Medicine Video Board Review

Oncology

Presented by

Rishi Sawhney, MD
Medical Director, Bayhealth Cancer Institute
Hematology/Medical Oncology
Dover, Delaware

Table of Contents

Oncology Abbreviations

ACBE	Air-contrast barium enema
ACTH	Adrenocorticotropic hormone
ADH	Antidiuretic hormone
ALL	Acute lymphoblastic leukemia
AML	Acute myeloid leukemia
ASCUS	Atypical squamous cells of undetermined significance
ASGUS	Atypical glandular cells of undetermined significance
BEP	Bleomycin, etoposide, and cisplatin
BPH	Benign prostatic hyperplasia/hypertrophy
BRCA	Breast cancer gene
BSE	Breast self-exam
BSO	Bilateral salpingo-oophorectomy
CBE	Clinical breast exam
CF	Cystic fibrosis
CIN	Cervical intraepithelial neoplasia
CLL	Chronic lymphocytic leukemia
CML	Chronic myelogenous leukemia
CPK	Creatine phosphokinase
CR	Complete remission
DCBE	Double contrast barium enema
DCIS	Ductal carcinoma *in situ*
DRE	Digital rectal exam
DVT	Deep vein thrombosis
EBV	Epstein-Barr virus
EGFR	Epidermal growth factor receptor
EMG	Electromyogram
EP	Etoposide and cisplatin
ER/PR	Estrogen receptor/progesterone receptor
ESR	Erythrocyte sedimentation rate
ET	Epithelial tumor
FAP	Familial adenomatous polyposis
FNA	Fine needle aspiration
FOBT	Fecal occult blood test
GCT	Germ cell tumor
GVHD	Graft-versus-host disease
HD	Hodgkin disease
HER2	Human epidermal growth factor receptor 2
HGSIL	High-grade squamous intraepithelial lesion
HNPCC	Hereditary nonpolyposis colorectal cancer
HPSCT	Hematopoietic stem cell transplantation
HPV	Human papillomavirus
HR	Hormone receptor
HRT	Hormone replacement therapy
IBD	Inflammatory bowel disease
IP	Intraperitoneal
IVP	Intravenous pyelogram
LCIS	Lobular carcinoma *in situ*
LDH	Lactate dehydrogenase
LGSIL	Low-grade squamous intraepithelial lesion
LHRH	Luteinizing-hormone releasing hormone
MDS	Myelodysplastic syndrome
MEN1	Multiple endocrine neoplasia
MMG	Mammogram
MOPP	Mechlorethamine, oncovin, procarbazine, prednisone
NHL	Non-Hodgkin lymphoma
NSC	Non–small cell (cancer)
ONJ	Osteonecrosis of jaw
PBSC	Peripheral blood stem cells
PDGF	Platelet-derived growth factor
PGE_2	Prostaglandin E2
PSA	Prostate-specific antigen
PTH	Parathyroid hormone
PTHrP	Parathyroid hormone related peptide
RANKL	Receptor activator of nuclear factor kappa-B ligand
RFA	Radio frequency ablation therapy
RPLND	Retroperitoneal lymph node dissection
SC	Small cell (cancer)
SIADH	Syndrome of inappropriate antidiuretic hormone secretion
SOB	Short of breath
SVC	Superior vena cava syndrome
TAH	Total abdominal hysterectomy
TKI	Tyrosine-kinase inhibitor
TNM	Tumor size, nodal involvement, metastases
TRUS	Transrectal ultrasound
VEGF	Vascular endothelial growth factor
VIC	Variable intensity conditioning
VTE	Venous thromboembolism
WNL	Within normal limits
XRT	Radiation therapy
αFP	Alpha fetoprotein
β-hCG	Beta human chorionic gonadotropin

Speaker Disclosure

Rishi Sawhney, MD, has documented that he has no commercial relationships to disclose.

Oncology

Paraneoplastic Syndromes

Audience Response 1

A 65-year-old woman with breast cancer comes to your office for a checkup. She complains of abdominal pain and fatigue.
You request a chemistry panel while evaluating her complaints. The lab calls you with a panic value.
Her calcium is 13.5 mg/dL.

Which of the following statements is correct?

A. Since patient is asymptomatic, nothing needs to be done at present — observation only.
B. A corrected calcium should be calculated using the total protein.
C. She should receive treatment with IV D5W at 50 cc/hr.
D. Treatment should be initiated with a bisphosphonate.

Answer: _____

Paraneoplastic Syndromes
- A distant effect of malignancy mediated by factors secreted or triggered by the malignancy
- May develop before or during the malignancy
- May parallel the course of the disease
- Endo, neuro, renal, heme, rheum, derm, pulm, cardiac

- Paraneoplastic syndromes include:
  - Hypercalcemia
  - SIADH
  - Cushing syndrome
  - Dermatomyositis
  - Hypertrophic pulmonary osteoarthropathy
  - Lambert-Eaton syndrome

Hypercalcemia
- The most common paraneoplastic syndrome
- Malignancy is the most common cause in inpatients
- Occurs frequently with squamous cell carcinomas, breast cancer, and renal cell carcinoma
- Also commonly seen with multiple myeloma

- Symptoms resulting from hypercalcemia include:
  - Fatigue
  - Anorexia, abdominal pain, constipation
  - Polyuria, polydipsia $\rightarrow$ profound hypovolemia
  - Mental status changes
  - Sudden death
  - Stones, bones, and abdominal groans
  - Psychiatric moans

- Objective findings will usually include:
  - Renal dysfunction
  - Shortened QT interval, PR prolongation, bradycardia
  - Hyporeflexia

- Occasionally may herald an occult cancer
- Usually in someone with advanced malignancies
- For most malignancies, indicates a poor prognosis with life expectancy < 6 months

- Most affected patients will have bony metastasis
  - But extent of bone disease may not correlate with degree of hypercalcemia
- Mediated by multiple mechanisms
  - Direct bone invasion
  - Humoral mechanisms
    - Can occur without bone involvement
    - PTH-like factor: PTHrP
- Workup – PTH; PTHrP; 1,25-$(OH)_2$-vitamin D
  - Correct calcium for albumin level

- Treatment options:
  - Vigorous hydration with normal saline
  - Diuresis after patient rehydrated
  - Effective tumor therapy when possible

- Several medications available for use:
  - Steroids (selected cases)
  - Calcitonin
  - Bisphosphonates

- Steroids
  - Used primarily in multiple myeloma, where the tumor is responsive
  - Also useful in lymphoma and occasionally in breast cancer
  - Blocks production of the "activating factors"
  - May also increase calcium excretion in the urine

- Calcitonin
  - Inhibits bone reabsorption by binding to osteoclasts
  - Works very quickly, within hours, to decrease calcium with peak action at 48 hours
  - May develop tachyphylaxis
  - More effective with the addition of steroids

- Bisphosphonates
  - Mainstay of therapy for hypercalcemia
  - Concentrated in areas of high bony turnover
  - Taken up by the osteoclasts and inhibit their action
  - May also have effects on the osteoblasts

Hypercalcemia (cont.)
- Bisphosphonates (cont.)
  - Pamidronate has proven efficacy in all types of hypercalcemia and also associated with decreased skeletal events in both breast cancer and multiple myeloma
  - Zoledronic acid now preferred agent for malignant hypercalcemia
  - Toxicity is primarily renal insufficiency and osteonecrosis of jaw (ONJ)

- Denosumab
  - Monoclonal antibody to RANKL
  - Important in pathway of osteoclasts
  - Approved to prevent skeletal events in solid tumors
  - Approved to clear bone mass in high-risk cancer groups

AR 2

A 59-year-old heavy smoker presents to the emergency department with a 4-week history of cough with scant hemoptysis, a 15-lb weight loss, and intermittent bouts of confusion. Physical exam is notable for coarse breath sounds at the right lung base and mild temporal wasting. Neurologic exam is nonfocal. Laboratory studies include a serum K^+ of 3.3, Cr of 0.6, BUN of 10, Na^+ of 125, with a normal CBC. Chest x-ray suggests a 4-cm mass in the right lower lung lobe. Brain MRI with contrast returns negative.

Which of the following represents the most appropriate measure to address the cause of this patient's altered mental status?
A. Start chemotherapy and radiation for management of lung cancer.
B. IV hypotonic saline.
C. IV potassium supplementation.
D. Conivaptan.
E. Consult radiation oncology for possible brain metastasis.

Answer: _____

SIADH
- Primarily caused by small cell lung cancer
- Associated with medications such as cyclophosphamide
- Arises secondary to production of ectopic ADH, which acts in the kidneys to cause retention of free water
- Results in hyponatremia in the setting of less-than-maximally dilute urine and a normal volume status

- May be mild and asymptomatic
- May be more severe, with symptoms of mental status changes, nausea, anorexia, and weakness
- When extreme, may result in coma, seizures, and death
- The rate of development may dictate symptoms

- Treatment options include:
  - Fluid restriction — works best in mild cases with restriction of 500 mL to 1 L per day
  - IV saline (0.9–3%) plus furosemide
  - Conivaptan for acute treatment
  - Demeclocycline for chronic treatment
  - Treat the underlying malignancy

Cushing Syndrome
- Occurs frequently in small cell carcinoma, carcinoid tumors, and in association with MEN I syndrome
- Ectopic ACTH production
- Excessive production of glucocorticoids and mineralocorticoids by the adrenal glands

- Also see weakness, hypertension, and hyperglycemia
- Presentation is commonly seen with hypokalemic alkalosis
- If develops slowly, will see the syndrome with a buffalo hump, moon facies, hyperpigmentation, and hirsutism

- Diagnosis is made by finding:
  - Elevated ACTH levels
  - Elevated cortisol levels that typically do not suppress with dexamethasone
- Treatment options include:
  - Treatment of the primary tumor
  - Inhibitors of steroid synthesis such as ketoconazole or aminoglutethimide

Dermatomyositis
- Commonly associated with visceral adenocarcinomas such as stomach, breast, lung, and ovary
- Should consider malignancy in the older patient with dermatomyositis

- Polymyositis associated with skin changes
  - Proximal painless muscle weakness
  - Violaceous rash on exposed parts, especially the eyelids
  - Dysphagia is common
  - May develop weakness of the respiratory muscles

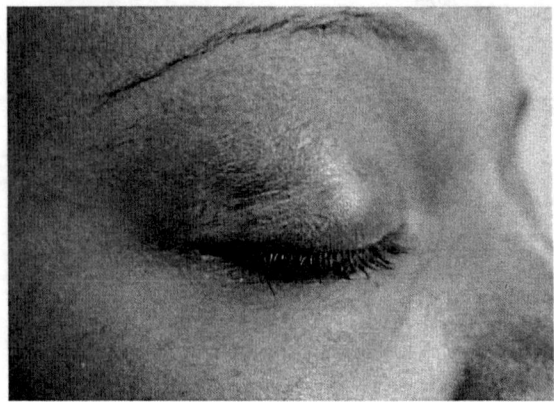

Dermatomyositis (cont.)
- Diagnosis is made by finding:
  - Elevated CPK, aldolase, LDH, and ESR
  - Abnormal EMG
  - Muscle biopsy with necrosis of muscle fibers and an inflammatory reaction
- Treatments include:
  - Steroids
  - Immunosuppressive agents
  - Treatment of the underlying malignancy

Hypertrophic Osteoarthropathy
- Commonly associated with lung cancers, although may be seen with CF, chronic pulmonary infections, or IBD
- May range from clubbing to severe periostitis and arthritis
- Cause is related to PGE_2, cytokines

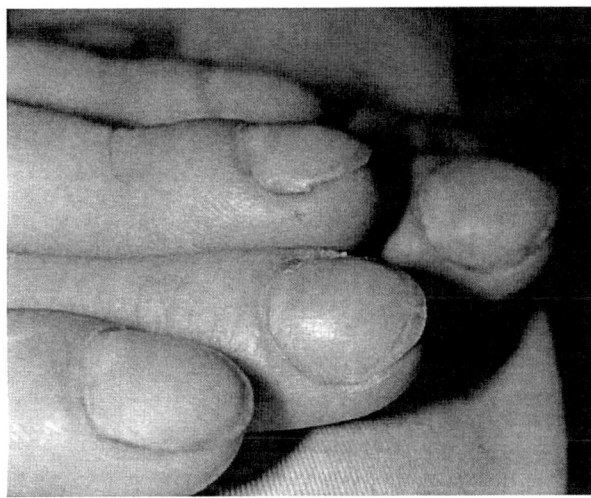

Hypertrophic Osteoarthropathy (cont.)
- Full syndrome
  - Clubbing
  - Periosteal proliferation
- Diagnose with x-rays or bone scan
  - Primarily see involvement of the tibia and femur

- Treatment
  - Salicylates/NSAIDs
  - Steroids
  - Effective tumor therapy
- In general, treatment is not very satisfying

Lambert-Eaton Syndrome
- Occurs primarily in small cell lung cancer
- Variant of myasthenia gravis
- Initial symptom: Weakness of the proximal muscles
- Autoimmune in nature, secondary to autoantibodies that result in impaired release of acetylcholine

- Diagnosis is made by finding an abnormal EMG with improvement in strength upon repetitive stimulation
- EMG is usually unaffected by addition of edrophonium chloride

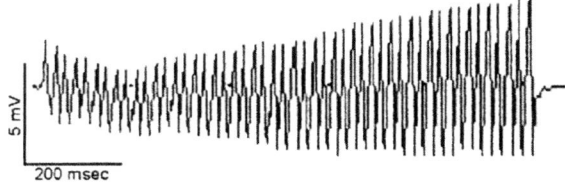

Lambert-Eaton Syndrome: 50 hz; Train of 50 stimulations

- Treatment includes:
  - Guanidine
  - Plasma exchange
  - IVIG
  - Immunosuppression
  - Treatment of malignancy

Direct Tumor Effects
- Superior vena cava (SVC) syndrome
- Bone metastases
- Spinal cord compression
- Brain metastases
- Malignant pleural effusions
- Malignant pericardial effusions

Superior Vena Cava (SVC) Syndrome
- Results from occlusion of the superior vena cava either by external compression or internal thrombus
- Most cases of external compression are secondary to malignancy
  - Lung cancer
  - Lymphoma
  - Metastatic disease

- Symptoms depend on the rate of obstruction, with more severe symptoms if occluded rapidly
- With slow compression, develop collateral drainage, which decreases the symptoms

- Symptoms include:
  - Facial and neck swelling
  - Dyspnea
  - Headaches
  - Hoarseness
  - Mental status changes

- Physical findings include:
  - Facial plethora
  - Edema of the neck, upper extremities, and face
  - Neck vein distention
  - Collateral veins on the anterior chest
  - Mental obtundation

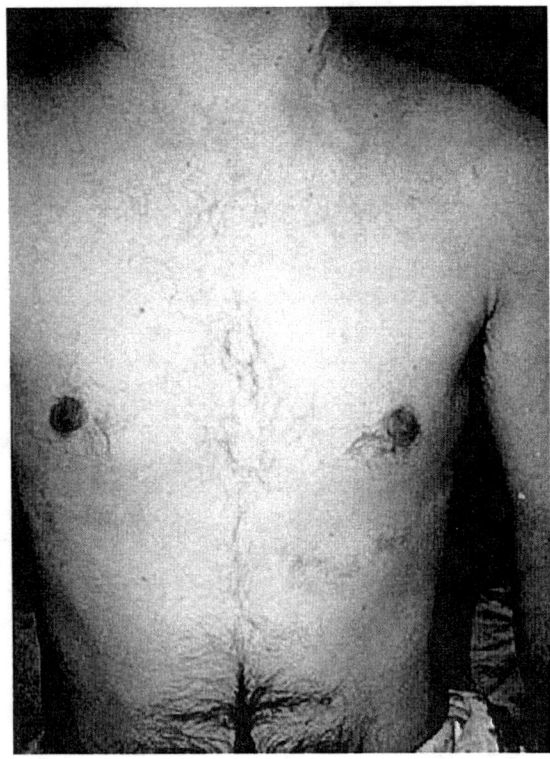

SVC Syndrome (cont.)
- Diagnosis is clinical and radiological
  - CXR
  - CT scan of the chest
- Need tissue diagnosis prior to instituting definitive therapy
  - Can safely perform bronchoscopy, mediastinoscopy, or thoracotomy

- While diagnosis being established, treatment should be initiated
  - Symptomatic relief with O_2 and diuresis
  - Steroids are used to decrease edema
  - For chemotherapy-sensitive tumors (small cell, germ cell, and lymphoma), choose primary chemotherapy
  - Radiation therapy for those tumors that do not respond rapidly to chemotherapy

- Other treatment options
  - Anticoagulation
  - Thrombolysis
  - Endovascular stenting

Bone Metastases
- Any malignancy may metastasize to the bone
- Most common would include:
  - Prostate
  - Breast
  - Lung
  - Renal cell
  - Myeloma

- Presenting symptoms include:
  - Pain
  - Pathologic fracture
- Common sites for bony involvement:
  - Vertebral bodies
  - Femur
  - Ribs
  - Pelvis

- Diagnosis should be made with:
  - Bone scan
  - PET scan
  - Metastatic bone survey
    - Remember that purely lytic lesions will not appear on a bone scan
    - Should always confirm a "hot" bone scan with plain films

- Treatment should include:
  - Radiation therapy for pain control
  - Evaluation for need for prophylactic rod placement
  - Developing therapies: RFA, vertebroplasty
  - Bisphosphonates
    - Solid tumors and multiple myeloma
  - Osteoclast inhibitors
    - Solid tumors only

AR 3

You see a 57-year-old woman in your office for fatigue and back pain. She has a history of hypertension, peptic ulcer disease, and breast cancer — for which she had a modified radical mastectomy and subsequent chemotherapy 2 years ago. She has been disease free since then.
Six months ago, she was in a motor vehicle accident and states she has had lower back pain since the accident. She usually performs back stretches twice per week. Several recent episodes of urinary incontinence prompted her to seek an evaluation.

She describes the pain as dull but worsening over the past 5 weeks. The pain is worse when she lies in bed. Her legs feel weak, and she is fatigued. There has been no weight loss. There is no other medical history.
She takes HCTZ and omeprazole. She has no allergies. Neurologic exam is significant for 4/5 power in the legs bilaterally, 3+ patellar and ankle reflexes, and uncoordinated gait. Straight leg raises cause bilateral back pain with some radiation down the legs. Pulses are 2+ and equal bilaterally.

AR 3 (cont.)
Which of the following is the most appropriate next step in the management of this patient?
A. Dexamethasone intravenously, emergent spine MRI
B. X-rays of the spine
C. Physical therapy for lumbar spinal stenosis
D. Referral to orthopedics for elective surgical evaluation
E. STAT neurology consultation; EMG

Answer: _____

Spinal Cord Compression
- An oncologic emergency
- Should **always** be suspected in a patient with a diagnosis of malignancy and a complaint of back pain
- Most common tumors are:
  - Lung
  - Breast
  - Prostate
  - Myeloma

- Symptoms include:
  - Back pain that is worsened by sneezing, coughing, or lying supine
  - Radicular pain
  - Loss of bowel and bladder control
  - Sensory changes typically precede motor loss

- Involvement of the spine is:
  - Thoracic in 70%
  - Lumbosacral in 20%
  - Cervical in 10%
- Area may be predicted by a sensory level with the upper limit of the level usually 1–2 vertebral bodies below the compression

- Diagnosis involves:
  - Plain spine films
  - CT scan
  - Myelogram
  - MRI
- MRI is the gold standard for diagnosis
  - Screen all levels of cord
- If presenting sign of malignancy, need tissue diagnosis to decide best treatment

- Treatment best if done early
- If the patient is ambulatory at the initiation of therapy, then they are likely to remain so
- If they are already paraplegic, then only 10% recover the ability to walk

- Treatment options:
  - Administer IV steroids at first suspicion to reduce edema
  - Radiation therapy is often the mainstay of therapy
  - Surgical decompression in selected patients
    - Unstable spine
    - Need tissue diagnosis
    - Radioresistant tumors
  - Chemotherapy can be combined with radiation for those with sensitive tumors

Brain Metastases
- Occur in about 1/4 of patients with cancer
- Associated with major morbidity and are associated with early death
- Usually occur in the setting of known neoplasm with systemic disease

- Most common tumors associated are:
  - Lung
  - Breast
  - Melanoma
  - Renal cell carcinoma

- Symptoms include those of increased intracranial pressure
  - Headache
  - Nausea
  - Seizures
  - Progressive neurological changes

- Diagnosis is usually made with:
  - CT or MRI of the head (contrast)
  - MRI is the more sensitive for small lesions and frequently reveals multiple lesions not seen with CT
  - Should look for surrounding edema or associated hemorrhage

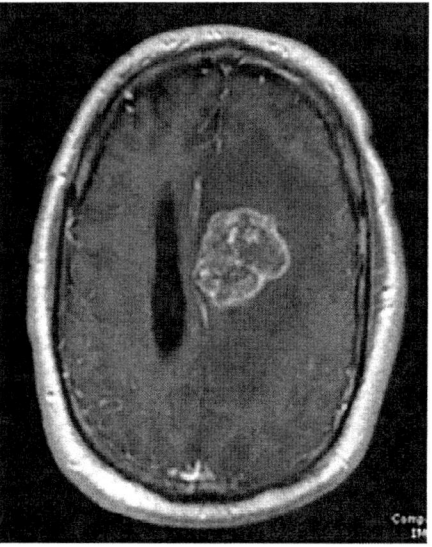

© 2017 MedStudy Internal Medicine Video Board Review – Oncology • Rishi Sawhney, MD

Brain Metastases (cont.)

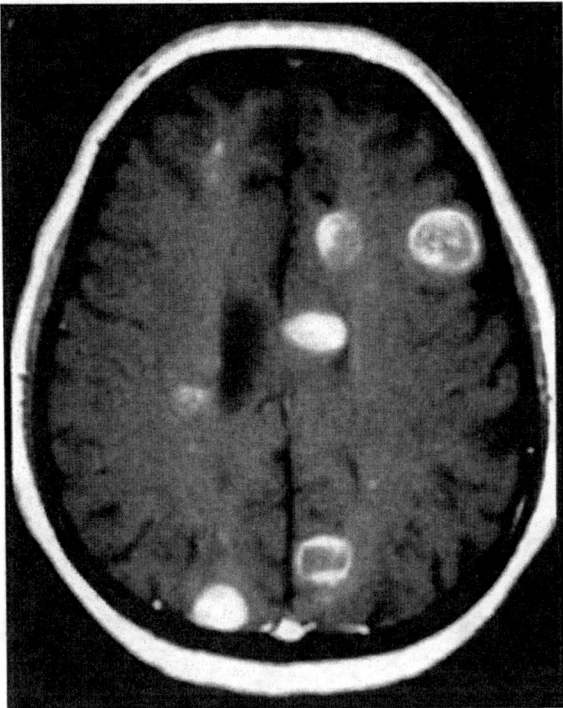

Brain Metastases (cont.)
- Treatment includes:
  - Immediate large doses of steroids (usually IV dexamethasone)
  - If the lesion is single, resection or stereotactic treatment may be tried
  - Consider stereotactic radiosurgery for those with ≤ 3 brain mets that are all ≤ 3 cm in size
  - For more extensive lesions, and after any resection, whole brain radiation therapy should be given

Malignant Pleural Effusions
- Occur either as an exudative reaction to a tumor or from lymphatic obstruction by the tumor
- Common tumors are those that metastasize to mediastinal nodes
  - Lung
  - Breast
  - Lymphoma

- Diagnosis is by pleural fluid cytology
  - Exudative
- May require multiple samples and large volume for diagnosis
- Occasionally may need pleural biopsy or thoracoscopy for diagnosis

- Treatment involves:
  - Symptomatic management with thoracentesis
  - Definitive management for recurrent effusions
    - Pleurodesis — talc, tetracycline, bleomycin
    - PleurX catheter
  - Therapy directed to the primary tumor

Malignant Pericardial Effusions
- Commonly occur in those tumors in the vicinity (direct extension)
  - Lung
  - Breast
- However, may occur via hematogenous spread
  - Leukemia
  - Lymphoma

- May cause tamponade
- Symptoms depend upon the rate of accumulation of the fluid
- Other restrictions, such as radiation fibrosis or large local tumor burden, may enhance the symptoms from a small effusion

- Symptoms include:
  - Dyspnea
  - Cough
  - Chest pain typically relieved by leaning forward
- Objective findings include:
  - Distended neck veins
  - Hepatomegaly
  - Edema

Malignant Pericardial Effusions (cont.)
- Diagnosis involves:
  - CXR with an enlarged cardiac silhouette
  - ECG with low voltage and electrical alternans

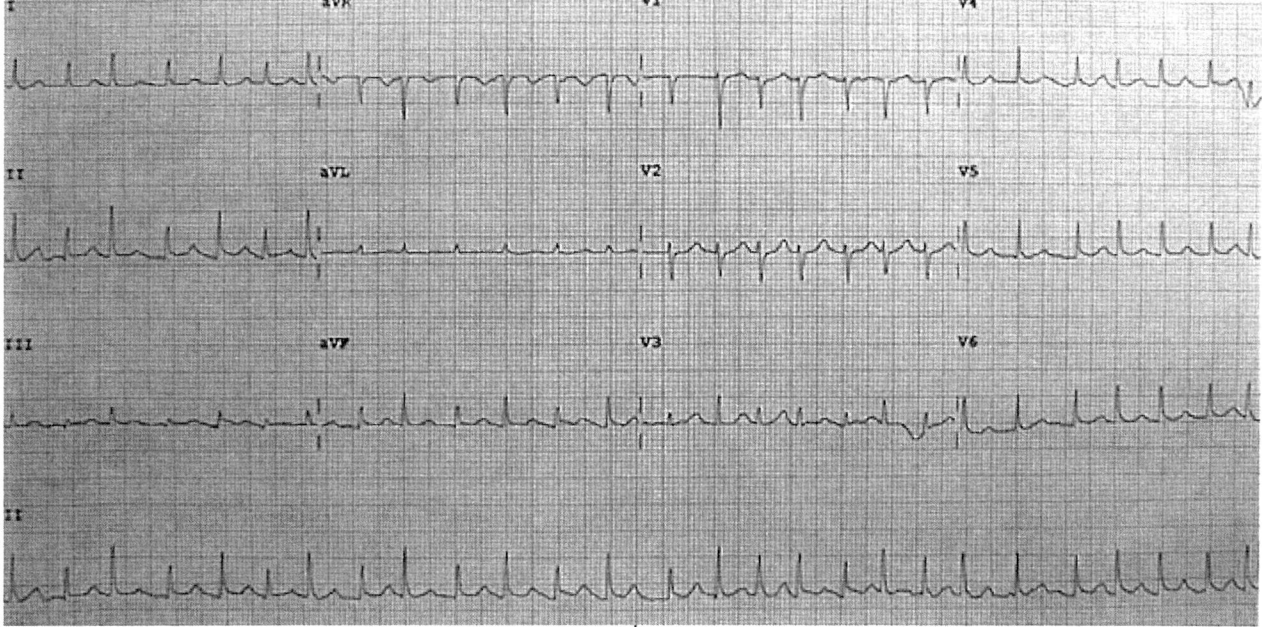

Source: James Heilman, MD

Malignant Pericardial Effusions (cont.)
- Echocardiography is the most sensitive test
  - May show right ventricular collapse
  - Demonstrates the size of the effusion

- Need pericardiocentesis for acute relief of symptoms
- Must institute definitive tumor therapy to prevent recurrence
- Long-term management may require a pericardial window, catheter drainage, and sclerosis or pericardiectomy

Cancer Incidence
- Males
  - Prostate > Lung > Colorectal
- Females
  - Breast > Lung > Colorectal

Cancer Death
- Males
  - Lung > Prostate > Colorectal
- Females
  - Lung > Breast > Colorectal

Breast Cancer

AR 4
A 65-year-old woman presents to your office after finding a mass in her breast. She discovered the mass during her monthly self-exam. She has observed it for 3 months and feels that it has enlarged slightly. It is not tender, and she does not have any other symptoms such as fatigue or weight loss. She has a 2-cm mass on exam and had a normal MMG.

Appropriate management would be:
A. Repeat mammogram in 6 months.
B. Observation for 6 months with a biopsy if it persists.
C. Tamoxifen therapy for prevention.
D. Referral to a surgeon for biopsy.
E. Reassurance, since it is not visible on MMG.

Answer: _____

AR 4 (cont.)
If a mass is solid, it should be biopsied; if it is cystic, it should be aspirated. If the fluid is bloody, recurs, or fails to resolve, then the mass should be biopsied.

Breast Cancer
- The most common malignancy in women
- The second leading cause of cancer death in women (lung is first)
- Occurs as a malignant proliferation of the cells lining the ducts of the breast

- Screening options include:
  - BSE — breast self-exam
  - CBE — clinical breast exam
  - **Mammography**
    - **Screening**
    - **Diagnostic**
  - **MRI for those at high risk**

ACS Recommendation 2015 (Average-Risk Women)
- Age 40–44 years: Give women option to start annual screening
- Age 45–54 years: Annual mammography
- Age > 55 years: Mammography every 1–2 years
- Regular clinical breast exam and breast self-exam not recommended

USPSTF 2016
- Age 40–49 years: Option to choose mammogram every 2 years
- Age 50–74 years: Mammogram every 2 years
- Age ≥ 75 years: Insufficient evidence to assess role of mammography

MMG — Where Guidelines Agree
- Current evidence recommends screening for 50–74 years of age (biennial vs. annual)
  - Most benefit in this age range
- Before age 50, and after age 74, mammography screening has less utility
- Breast self-exams and clinical breast exams are probably not useful in preventing breast cancer

Breast Cancer Risk
- Risk is difficult to define
  - Age is the most significant risk factor
    - Risk rises to 1 in 8 by 85 years of age
  - Family history is important
    - Involvement of 1st degree relatives with early or bilateral breast cancer increases the risk substantially

AR 5

A 33-year-old woman presents to discuss options for breast cancer prevention. Her family history is positive for breast cancer, as shown in this diagram.

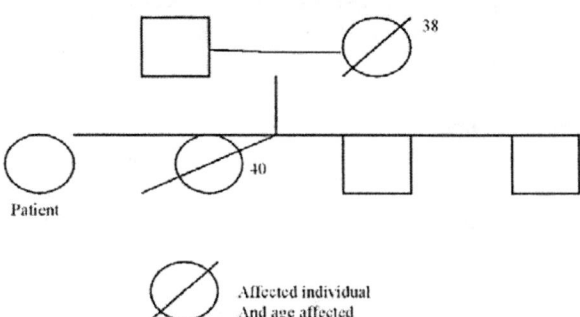

Which of the following would be appropriate to tell her?
A. Tell her not to worry; her risk of breast cancer is the same as that for any other woman.
B. Tell her bilateral mastectomy will prevent any possibility for malignancy.
C. Tell her the risk is increased at least 3-fold that of normal, and she should have testing for *BRCA1* and *BRCA2* genes.
D. Tell her to start mammograms at 50 years of age and have one done every other year.

Answer: _____

Breast Cancer Risk (cont.)
- Genetic syndromes
  - Tend to occur at young age
  - More likely to be bilateral
  - Multiple family members usually affected
- Only 10% of breast cancer is genetically linked
- Several genes identified

- Breast cancer — ovarian cancer syndrome
  - Led to the description of the *BRCA1* and *BRCA2* genes
  - Together, these account for 30–50% of all inherited breast cancer

- *BRCA1*
  - Chromosome 17: AD
  - Lifetime risk of developing breast cancer is 50–85%
  - Also increases the lifetime risk of developing ovarian cancer to 40%
  - Associated with an increase in the risk of breast and prostate cancer in men

Breast Cancer Risk (cont.)
- *BRCA2*
  - Chromosome 13: AD
  - Similar risk for breast cancer
  - Somewhat smaller risk for ovarian cancer (10–20%)
  - Associated with increased incidence of breast cancer in men

- Hormone-dependent disease; Thus, anything that increases your exposure to estrogen increases your risk of:
  - Early menarche
  - Late menopause
  - Fewer pregnancies
  - Late first pregnancy or no pregnancy
  - Exogenous estrogen

- Benign breast disease increases risk of subsequent breast cancer
  - Atypical ductal hyperplasia
  - DCIS
  - LCIS
- Previous breast cancer also increases the risk of a second breast cancer

Breast Cancer — Genetics
- Breast cancer screening should be individualized for patients at high risk
  - Earlier testing
  - More frequent testing
  - More intense testing
- *BRCA1*- or *BRCA2*-positive
  - Prophylactic mastectomy?
  - Prophylactic BSO?
  - MRI screen if no surgery
  - Chemoprevention

Breast Cancer — Clinical
- Presentation can vary:
  - Asymptomatic routine mammogram abnormality
  - A painless breast mass detected by the patient
  - Asymmetric eczema — think Paget's disease
  - Nipple discharge — nonmilky, unilateral
  - May develop nipple retraction or dimpling of the skin
  - Inflammatory cancer — warmth, erythema, peau d'orange

Breast Cancer — Workup
1) Mammogram/Ultrasound ± MRI
2) Aspiration (FNA) or biopsy
3) If cancer, then check hormone receptors and *HER2/neu*
4) Treat as indicated
- Palpable mass without abnormality on mammogram
  - Should biopsy

Breast Cancer — Staging
- The staging system has been developed by the AJCC and involves assessment of:
  - Tumor size
  - Involvement of axillary nodes
  - Occurrence of distant metastatic disease

TNM System

Breast Cancer — T, N
- Prognosis is best described by assessment of:
  - Tumor size
    - Greater than 2 cm denotes a worse prognosis
  - Number of involved axillary nodes
    - This is the most important prognostic factor
    - Prognosis worsens with each positive node
    - Can use sentinel node evaluation to assess

Breast Cancer — Prognosis
- Stage I: < 2 cm, 0 nodes, 10-yr surv: 75%
- Stage II: 2–5 cm or + nodes, 10-yr surv: 50%
- Stage III: > 5 cm or fixed nodes, chest wall/skin involvement, 10-yr surv: 27%
- Stage IV: Metastatic, 10-yr surv: < 10%

Breast Cancer — Pathology
- Other prognostic features include:
  - Hormone receptor status
    - If ER/PR receptor-negative, then expect a higher incidence of recurrence
  - *HER2/neu* status
    - Overexpression of *HER2/neu* denotes a more aggressive tumor

AR 6
A 58-year-old postmenopausal female is diagnosed with breast cancer. She has a 5-cm primary left breast tumor, that is estrogen receptor(+), with negative axillary lymph nodes.

Which of the following represents the most appropriate management plan?
A. Modified radical mastectomy alone
B. Modified radical mastectomy followed by endocrine therapy (aromatase inhibitor)
C. Modified radical mastectomy followed by chemotherapy and then endocrine therapy (aromatase inhibitor)
D. Lumpectomy followed by radiation
E. Lumpectomy followed by ovarian ablation and chemotherapy

Answer: _____

Breast Cancer — Management
Management of the patient with infiltrating ductal carcinoma of the breast is based on the previously mentioned factors, including staging, receptor status, and *HER2/neu* status.

Breast Cancer — Local Rx
- First decision should concern appropriate surgical management
  - Modified radical mastectomy **or**
  - Breast conserving surgery
    - Lumpectomy with axillary node evaluation
    - Should always be paired with local radiation therapy to decrease the local recurrence rate
    - Gives equivalent results to mastectomy

- Axillary lymph node evaluation
  - Provide prognostic information
  - Prevent recurrence
  - Sentinel node biopsy

Systemic Rx — Endocrine
- Tamoxifen
- In patients with ER+ tumors, 5 years of therapy reduces recurrence risk by approximately 50%
- Benefit for pre- & postmenopausal women
- Benefit in invasive & noninvasive tumors
- Other adjuvant Tx
  - Ovarian suppression
  - Aromatase inhibitors

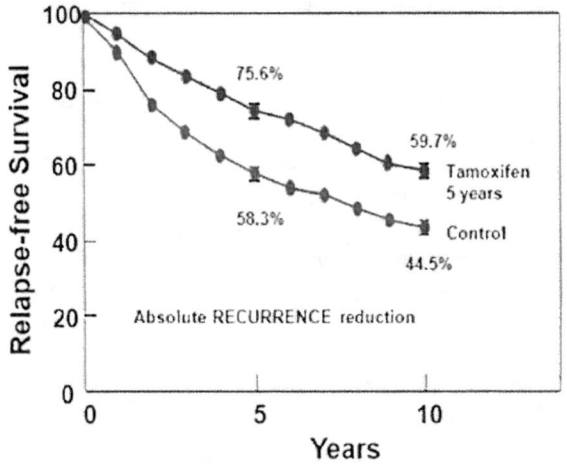

Systemic Rx — Endocrine (cont.)
- Aromatase Inhibitors
  - Prevent conversion of adrenally produced androgens into estrogens but do not prevent ovarian estrogen production

- Modest advantage over tamoxifen alone in postmenopausal women
  - As initial Tx instead of tamoxifen
  - Following tamoxifen
- Different side-effect profile
  - Less risk of endometrial cancer & VTE
  - Higher risk of osteoporosis, fractures, musculoskeletal symptoms

Systemic Rx — Chemotherapy
- Various regimens: TC, AC-T, TAC, CMF
- For operable invasive cancer, reduces recurrence risk by approximately 1/3
- Benefit decreases with increasing age
- Benefit greatest in node positive, HR negative, and premenopausal women
- Incorporation of trastuzumab for *HER2/neu*+ tumors further reduces recurrence risk

Breast Cancer — Adjuvant
- Basic rules for therapy:
  - All patients with hormone receptor positive tumors should receive endocrine therapy for at least 5 years
  - Patients with higher risk of relapse may also benefit from chemotherapy
    - Lymph node positive
    - Larger tumor size (> 1 cm)
    - High-risk gene expression profile (Oncotype)
  - If *HER2/neu* positive tumor, add trastuzumab to chemo

AR 7
A 50-year-old postmenopausal woman finds a breast lump. Ultrasound and mammography confirm a suspicious 3-cm mass. A core biopsy is positive for infiltrating ductal carcinoma.
A lumpectomy and axillary node dissection are done. The cancer is 3 cm with 2 positive axillary nodes. ER and PR receptors are negative. *HER2/neu* staining is negative.

Which of the following should you recommend?
A. Close follow-up with an exam every month.
B. Chemotherapy plus radiation.
C. Repeat surgery with conversion to a modified radical mastectomy followed by chemotherapy.
D. Local radiation therapy plus tamoxifen for 5 years.
E. Local radiation therapy alone.

Answer: _____

Breast Cancer — Summary
- Recap:
  - If hormone receptor (+) → endocrine therapy
    - **Premenopausal — tamoxifen ± ovarian suppression**
    - **Postmenopausal — aromatase inhibitor**
  - If higher risk tumor (node+, larger size, high-risk Oncotype) → give chemotherapy
  - If *HER2/neu+*, give trastuzumab plus chemo
  - Neoadjuvant: For locally advanced/inflammatory disease **or** for breast conservation
  - Emerging use of gene expression profiles for prognosis and predictive benefit of chemotherapy

AR 8

A 65-year-old female undergoes a lumpectomy and axillary sentinel lymph node evaluation for a 1-cm invasive ductal right breast cancer. Sentinel nodes return negative. The tumor is estrogen receptor positive and *HER2/neu* negative. She denies known personal or family history of cancer. She receives adjuvant radiation therapy and is then placed on letrozole once daily.

Which of the following would be the most appropriate diagnostic test as part of her follow-up?
A. Genetic testing for *BRCA1* & *BRCA2* mutations
B. Annual pelvic ultrasound and Pap smear
C. Bone density monitoring every 1–2 years
D. Annual CT scan of chest/abdomen/pelvis with contrast
E. Tumor markers studies every 6 months (CA 27.29, CA 15-3)

Answer: _____

Breast Cancer — Metastatic
- Not curable
- Most common sites:
  - Bone
  - Lung
  - Liver
  - CNS
- Treatment options:
  - Endocrine therapy
  - Chemotherapy
  - Radiation
  - Trastuzumab

- Choosing appropriate therapy
  - Low intensity therapy — endocrine
    - Hormone receptor positive disease
    - Bone/soft tissue/lymph node predominant
  - High-intensity therapy — chemotherapy
    - Hormone receptor negative disease
    - Visceral organ involvement
- Bisphosphonate therapy for osseous metastasis

Carcinoma *In Situ*
- Ductal (DCIS)
  - Benign
  - More common than lobular
  - See microcalcifications on mammogram
  - High-grade has higher risk of evolving into invasive disease
- Treatment is mastectomy vs. breast conservation surgery ± XRT followed by endocrine therapy

- Lobular (LCIS)
  - Nonpalpable with no reliable mammographic changes
  - Marker for cancer development in either breast
  - Frequently is multifocal and bilateral
- Treatment varies from observation only to tamoxifen to bilateral mastectomy

Breast Cancer — Prevention
- Prevention
  - The use of endocrine therapy has been demonstrated to reduce the risk of developing breast cancer in patients with increased risk
  - Choice of agents
    - Tamoxifen
    - Raloxifene
    - Aromatase inhibitors
  - Should be used in those women felt to be at high risk for breast cancer development
    - Previous cancer
    - Strong family history
    - *BRCA1*- or *BRCA2*-positive

- Risks to prolonged tamoxifen use include:
  - Increased risk of endometrial cancer
  - Risk of thrombosis
    - DVT
    - Pulmonary embolism
  - Cataracts
- Risks with aromatase inhibitors include:
  - Osteoporosis
  - Arthralgias
  - No thrombosis or malignancy risk

AR 9

A 25-year-old woman who received the HPV vaccine in the past has a routine Pap smear. All of her previous Pap smears have been negative. The results of this Pap smear show LGSIL (low-grade squamous intraepithelial lesion).

What do you recommend?
A. Repeat Pap in 6 months.
B. Repeat Pap in 1 year.
C. Administer booster dose of HPV vaccine.
D. Refer for colposcopy.
E. HPV testing.

Answer: _____

AR 9 (cont.)
The best answer would be further evaluation with colposcopy and biopsies of any abnormal areas that are visualized.

Cervical Cancer
- The 3rd most common female genital tract cancer after uterine and ovarian
- Mortality has dropped significantly with the introduction of effective screening
- Peak age is 20–30 years with a later peak in the 60s
- Usually, slowly progressive disease

- Risk factors:
  - A sexually transmitted disease
  - Associated with:
    - Early age at first intercourse
    - Multiple sexual partners
    - Low socioeconomic status
  - HIV

- The primary risk factor is HPV (human papillomavirus) infection
  - Viral isolates found in > 90% of lesions
  - Primarily see HPV types 16, 18
  - Testing for HPV not a good screening tool because up to 30% of women with normal Pap smears have infection

- Newly approved vaccination for HPV types 6, 11, 16, and 18
  - 6 and 11 estimated to cause 90% of genital warts
  - 16 and 18 cause 70% of cervical cancer
- Recombinant vaccine
- Recommended for ages 9–26 years
  - Best if given before sexually active
  - Give to males and females

Cervical Cancer — Screening
- ACOG recommendations (2016):
  - Pap smear screening for all women over 21 years of age
  - Every 3 years until 30 years of age
  - After 30 years of age, if 3 negatives obtained, may screen every 5 years (co-test HPV and cytology) or every 3 years (cytology alone) unless risk factors present
  - May stop at 65–70 years of age or if have a TAH

- USPSTF recommendations (2012):
  - 21–65 years of age every 3 years with Pap smear, or
  - 30–65 years of age every 5 years with Pap smear and HPV
  - Cessation of screening at 65 years of age if recent screens negative and no risk factors
  - Stop after total hysterectomy for benign disease

- These all share:
  - Begin at 21 years of age
  - 21–30 years of age do every 3 years
  - After 30 years of age do every 3 years (cytology alone) or every 5 years (cytology and HPV co-testing)
  - Stop after hysterectomy for benign disease or 65 years of age

- Pap smear technique is important
  - Must include cells from the transition zone
  - Usually sample the endocervix followed by the exocervix
  - Newer techniques to limit collection of poor samples and increase sensitivity
  - New computer-assisted screening systems to limit errors in interpretation

- Pap smear classified using the Bethesda system
  - WNL
  - Benign cellular changes
  - Atypical squamous cells/glandular cells of undetermined significance (ASCUS)/(ASGUS)
  - LGSIL (low-grade squamous intraepithelial lesion)
  - HGSIL (high-grade squamous intraepithelial lesion)
  - Cancer

- Abnormal Pap smear requires biopsy to further define the diagnosis

- ASCUS diagnosis ⟷ repeat in 3 mos*
                    check HPV
                    colposcopy
  *Abnormal repeat Pap needs colposcopy
- ASGUS diagnosis ⟶ colposcopy
- LGSIL or HGSIL ⟶ colposcopy

Cervical Cancer (cont.)
- Typically, LGSIL and HGSIL will require further evaluation with colposcopy and biopsy
  - LGSIL occasionally (15%) progresses to invasive cancer
  - HGSIL is more likely to be higher-grade dysplasia with increased risk of malignancy

- Biopsy results are reported as:
  - CIN I ⟶ mild dysplasia
  - CIN II ⟶ moderate dysplasia
  - CIN III ⟶ severe dysplasia, carcinoma *in situ*

  - LGSIL = CIN I
  - HGSIL = CIN II or CIN III

- Treatment
  - CIN I: Observation vs. cryotherapy
  - CIN II: Ablation or excision
  - CIN III: Ablation or excision
- After definitive therapy, must follow with frequent Pap smears (3–4 mos, then every 6 mos)

- Invasive cancer presents with:
  - Abnormal vaginal bleeding
  - Pelvic pain
  - Hematuria
  - Fistulas

- Most common tumor types:
  - Squamous cell (80%)
    - Develops from CIN
    - Arises at transition zone or ectocervix
    - Forms exophytic masses
  - Adenocarcinoma (20%)
    - Arises at transition zone or deeper in cervix
    - Barrel-shaped cervix

- Staging is by the FIGO guidelines
- Spreads primarily by direct extension
- Clinically staged with:
  - Physical exam
  - CXR
  - IVP if CT scan not done
  - CT scan/MRI

- Treatment options:
  - Influenced by tumor size, nodal involvement, and depth of tumor invasion
  - Early-stage disease may be treated with surgical resection (hysterectomy or cone biopsy) only
  - More advanced local disease is treated with radical surgery or radiotherapy
  - Bulky disease or disease that has invaded the parametria or nodes is treated with combination chemoradiotherapy
- Close follow-up is necessary because most recurrences occur within the first 2 years
- Pelvic recurrence may be treated with exenteration

AR 10

A 65-year-old is found to have an ovarian mass at the time of her annual Pap and pelvic exam.
She is asymptomatic.
Her gynecologist recommends that she have an ultrasound, which reveals a large, complex mass in her ovary.

The next step in the workup of this mass should include:
A. Measure β-hCG and αFP.
B. Repeat exam and U/S in 4–6 months.
C. Evaluation for *BRCA1* and *BRCA2* gene mutations.
D. CA-125 testing.
E. A CT-directed needle biopsy of the mass.

Answer: _____

Ovarian Cancer
- 5th most common cancer in women in the U.S.
- Accounts for the majority of deaths from gynecologic cancers in women
- More common with advancing age
- Rare before 40 years of age
- Peaks in the 8th decade

Ovarian Cancer — Risk
- Risk factors for ovarian carcinoma include:
  - "Incessant ovulation"
    - Nulliparity
    - Low parity
    - Infertility
    - Obesity

- Genetic risk factors (family history):
  - Most significant risk factor
  - Up to 10% may be genetically based
  - Breast/Ovarian syndrome
    - *BRCA1* — 40% risk
    - *BRCA2* — 10–20% risk
  - Lynch syndrome
    - 12% risk

© 2017 MedStudy Internal Medicine Video Board Review – Oncology • Rishi Sawhney, MD

Ovarian Cancer — Protective
- Protective factors include:
  - Oral contraceptive use
  - Breastfeeding
  - Early menopause
  - Multiple pregnancies (10% decrease in risk with each)

Ovarian Cancer — Screening
- Possible screening tests
  - Pelvic exam
    - Insensitive
  - Transvaginal ultrasound
    - High false-positive rate
  - CA-125
    - Not sensitive

CA-125
- Not a sensitive tool, but elevated in at least 80% of patients with ovarian cancer
- May be positive in multiple tumor types, including:
  - Cervix
  - Endometrial
  - Pancreas
  - Breast
  - Lung
  - Colon
- Better as disease monitoring tool

- Also elevated in nonmalignant states such as:
  - Pelvic inflammatory disease
  - Endometriosis
  - Pregnancy
  - Fibroids
  - Pancreatitis
  - Cirrhosis

- Recommended screening at this time is restricted to those with an increased risk (such as known *BRCA1* or *BRCA2*) and combines:
  - Pelvic exam
  - Transvaginal ultrasound
  - CA-125
- This strategy has not been shown to reduce mortality

Ovarian Cancer — Clinical
- Presentation
  - Usually advanced-stage disease at diagnosis because localized disease is asymptomatic
  - Abdominal pain
  - Bloating
  - Urinary symptoms
  - Occasionally torsion with an acute abdomen

Ovarian Cancer (cont.)
- 50% may present with ascites or with a palpable abdominal mass
- May see anorexia, weight loss, nausea, vomiting, or constipation
- Pelvic exam may reveal a mass
- Rectovaginal exam may detect a "Blumer shelf" with "wall-to-wall" tumor

Ovarian Cancer — Pathology
- Pathology
  - Epithelial tumors comprise the majority of tumors
    - May be benign
    - May be "borderline" or of low malignant potential
    - May be malignant
  - Rarely germ cell tumors in young patients

- Tumors of low malignancy potential
  - Typically in younger patients
  - Have malignant features but are not invasive
  - Diagnosed at early stage
  - Long-term survival of > 90%
  - Managed primarily with surgery

Ovarian Cancer — Staging
- Staging includes:
  - CA-125 level
  - CT scan chest/abdomen/pelvis
  - Surgical exploration, which should be performed by a surgeon skilled in gynecologic surgery

Ovarian Cancer — Surgery
- Surgery should include:
  - Full examination of the pelvis and peritoneal surfaces with biopsies
  - Aspiration of ascites or peritoneal lavage
  - Maximal cytoreduction of all visible tumor
  - TAH-BSO with omentectomy and lymph node sampling

Ovarian Cancer (cont.)
- Staging is done using the FIGO system
  - Stage I is confined to the ovary
  - Stage II has extension to the adjacent structures in the pelvis
  - Stage III has peritoneal spread
  - Stage IV has metastasis outside the abdomen or with parenchymal liver metastasis

Ovarian Cancer — Prognosis
- Prognostic factors include:
  - Stage
  - Age
  - Extent of disease at the completion of surgery
  - Performance status
  - Tumor grade

Ovarian Cancer — Rx

- Treatment options
  - Primary surgical resection
    - The amount of remaining disease has a direct correlation to long-term survival
  - Chemotherapy
    - Combinations of paclitaxel and cisplatin are standard of care
  - Radiation therapy
    - Not used often

Ovarian Cancer — Staging (cont.)

- Early-stage disease
  - Only 25% of patients at diagnosis
  - Stage I with no residual tumor is treated with surgical resection only
  - Chemotherapy is added if poorly differentiated tumor
- Later-stage disease with or without residual disease after laparotomy
  - Primarily treated with chemotherapy, either systemic or IP

Ovarian Cancer (cont.)

- Other cell types include:
  - Germ cell
    - Fewer than 5%
    - Usually large tumors
    - May secrete αFP or β-hCG
    - Presents with early-stage disease
- Treated with surgery, followed by chemotherapy with agents that include BEP (bleomycin, etoposide, and cisplatin)

AR 11

A 19-year-old man presents with a 2-month history of having a testicular mass. An ultrasound is done and reveals a solid mass. Testicular cancer is suspected.

Which of the following are the most appropriate next steps in the diagnostic workup?

A. Serum tumor markers and transscrotal orchiectomy.
B. Serum tumor markers and magnetic resonance imaging of scrotum.
C. Serum tumor markers and radical inguinal orchiectomy.
D. Serum tumor markers and transscrotal biopsy.
E. Obtain serum tumor markers.

Answer: _____

Testicular Cancer

- Uncommon tumor but most common in men 15–35 years of age
- Incidence is slowly rising, with seminoma increasing in the HIV population
- Occurs most often in Caucasian men
- In men > 50 years of age, consider a testicular mass to be a lymphoma until proven otherwise

- Risk factors for testicular cancer include:
  - Cryptorchidism
    - Abdominal >> inguinal
  - Prior testicular cancer
  - Family history of testicular cancer
  - Testicular feminization syndromes
  - HIV
  - Klinefelter syndrome with mediastinal germ cell

- 90% present in the testicles, 10% are extragonadal
- Presentation is most commonly described as a painless mass
- May have pain or swelling suggestive of orchitis
- Back pain may occur with spine metastasis
- Cough, SOB, and dyspnea with pulmonary metastasis

- Diagnosis
  - Often an initial trial of antibiotics is given if epididymitis or orchitis is suspected
  - Testicular ultrasound is indicated for a painless mass or painful one that does not resolve after antibiotics
  - Ultrasound can distinguish between a solid mass and inflammatory changes
  - Markers, including β-hCG, αFP, and LDH, are common

- If a mass is identified, then an inguinal orchiectomy is indicated for diagnosis
- Remember: The blood supply and lymphatics all originate in the abdomen
- A transscrotal approach is contraindicated because it may introduce tumor cells to different drainage pathways

Almost all testicular cancers are germ cell in origin

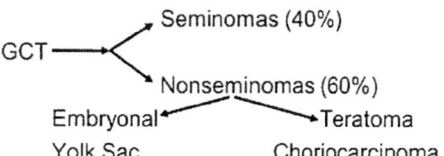

GCT → Seminomas (40%)
Nonseminomas (60%)
Embryonal
Yolk Sac
Teratoma
Choriocarcinoma

Testicular Cancer (cont.)
- Seminomas
  - Usually present in the 4th decade
  - Absence of any other cell type
  - If any other elements are present, it is classified as a nonseminoma
  - May have some cells of trophoblastic origin and produce β-hCG

Seminomas
never
produce αFP

- Seminomas usually present as localized disease
- Only 5–10% will present with metastatic disease
- Very radiosensitive
- Even metastatic disease is considered curable

- Nonseminomas
  - Typically present in the 3rd decade
  - May be composed of any one of the 4 histological cell types — or more than one (mixed germ cell tumors)
  - Can see elevated β-hCG **and** αFP tumor markers
  - Higher likelihood of metastatic disease at presentation
  - 1/3 confined to the testis; 1/3 metastatic

- Genetics
  - > 80% of germ cell tumors have an isochromosome 12p (an extra copy of the short arm of 12)
  - Most are hyperdiploid

- Tumor markers include:
  - αFP
    - Has half-life of 5–7 days
  - hCG
    - Has half-life of 24–36 hours
  - LDH
- These markers should be checked before and after surgery and are valuable to predict response to therapy and relapse

- Staging follows the TNM system or the system devised by the IGCCCG
- Staging requires:
  - The surgical removal of the tumor
  - Evaluation of the tumor markers
  - CT scan of the abdomen

- TNM system
  - Stage I ⟶ confined to the scrotum
  - Stage II ⟶ retroperitoneal disease
  - Stage III ⟶ distant metastases

- Treatment options
  - Orchiectomy
  - RPLND
  - Radiation therapy — primarily in seniors and in masses ≤ 5 cm

- Treatment options (cont.)
  - Combination chemotherapy
    - Most common combination is BEP (bleomycin, etoposide, and cisplatin)
    - Also use EP (etoposide and cisplatin)
  - High-dose chemotherapy with stem cell transplant support

- Any remaining mass after completion of chemotherapy may require resection
  - In nonseminomas, find:
    - Necrosis/Fibrosis
    - Viable tumor
    - Teratoma
- If you find viable tumor, should proceed with 2 additional cycles of chemotherapy

AR 12

A 24-year-old male presents to the primary care clinic for a routine physical. He has a history of a nonseminomatous testicular germ cell cancer treated 3 years ago with inguinal orchiectomy and adjuvant chemotherapy with bleomycin, etoposide, and cisplatin, achieving complete response. He feels well with no complaints. Exam demonstrates clear lungs, benign abdomen, and postoperative changes in the right inguinal region, with no contralateral testicular masses. Laboratory studies, including beta-HCG and AFP levels, return to normal.

In counseling this patient and devising a follow-up plan, you discuss the potential late sequelae of therapy for him.

Which of the following best represents a potential late complication of this patient's treatment program?
A. Bladder cancer
B. Chemotherapy-related cardiomyopathy
C. Secondary malignancies, including germ cell tumors, leukemia, and gastrointestinal malignancies
D. Hypothyroidism
E. Hemorrhagic cystitis

Answer: _____

Testicular Cancer (cont.)
- Late sequelae of therapy include:
  - Infertility
  - Second primary germ cell tumor
  - Secondary AML
  - Secondary gastrointestinal malignancies

Extragonadal Germ Cell Tumors
- May be primary retroperitoneal or mediastinal
- Should look for testicular primary
- Seminomas respond well to therapy and should be treated with BEP or EP

- Nonseminoma of the retroperitoneum is similar to those of testicular origin
- Primary mediastinal has a poor prognosis
- Mediastinal disease is associated with the i(12p)
- Mediastinal disease is associated with increased risk of heme malignancies such as AML (M7), MDS, or ET

AR 13

A 68-year-old man is seen for nocturia and hesitancy upon urinating. These symptoms have been present for years but have recently worsened. He has had serial prostate exams and measurements of his PSA. His last exam was 1 year ago and was consistent with BPH. His PSA was 3.5. Today, his PSA has risen to 10, and his exam is unchanged.

Evaluation that should be performed at this time includes:
A. Observation only.
B. Transrectal ultrasound with multiple biopsies.
C. Repeat rectal exam and PSA.
D. Bone scan.

Answer: _____

He should have a biopsy because his PSA is in the abnormal range. He also has an elevated PSA velocity, which is correlated with the likelihood of detecting malignancy and a poorer outcome from his malignancy.

Prostate Cancer
- A disease of aging men, cancer of the prostate increases after 50 years of age
- More than 70% of men over 80 years of age will have malignant cells in their prostate
- 8:1 incidence to death ratio
- Now, men are more typically diagnosed with early-stage disease

- Risk factors for prostate cancer:
  - Age — the most important risk factor
  - Family history of prostate cancer
  - Environmental — increased intake of animal fats is associated with increased risk
  - Race — African Americans more commonly affected

- Risk factors for prostate cancer (cont.)
  - Prostatic hypertrophy is not associated with an increased risk of developing invasive cancer
  - Cigarette smoking is not linked
  - Previous vasectomy is controversial

AR 14

A 50-year-old African American male is seen in your office for his routine health maintenance exam. He asks what you recommend for prostate screening.

Which of the following should you tell him?
A. Screening is not recommended by the American Cancer Society.
B. The U.S. Preventive Services Task Force recommends PSA and digital rectal exam for all men between the ages of 50 and 75.
C. A bone scan and PSA should be done yearly.
D. The American Cancer Society recommends that physicians discuss the benefits and risks of prostate cancer screening for men who have at least a 10-year life expectancy.
E. Screening should include a transrectal U/S yearly.

Answer: _____

Prostate Cancer — Screening
- Remains controversial
- Screening tests that are available include:
  - Digital rectal exam (DRE)
  - Prostate-specific antigen (PSA)
- No definitive clinical trial evidence that screening results in a decreased mortality from prostate cancer
- Does result in earlier diagnosis: "Stage shift"

PSA
- A marker relatively specific to prostate tissue
- Normal levels increase with age
- May be elevated in other settings
  - Prostatitis
  - Prostate hypertrophy
  - After prostate biopsy

© 2017 MedStudy Internal Medicine Video Board Review – Oncology • Rishi Sawhney, MD

- Not a very sensitive or specific marker
- Elevated in 65% of patients with prostate cancer
- Combination with DRE increases the utility of the marker
- May be more sensitive with use of the age-specific PSA or the percentage of free PSA

Prostate Cancer (cont.)
- Screening recommendation from the ACS (2010):
  - Discuss with physician to make informed decision after 50 years of age or after 45 years of age for high-risk individuals
- 2012 USPSTF: Recommends against PSA-based screening or prostate cancer

Prostate Cancer — Clinical
- Now diagnosed primarily in asymptomatic individuals after routine screening
- Before the use of screening, the common presentation was:
  - Urinary obstructive symptoms
  - Back pain

- Diagnosis involves the same tools as screening:
  - DRE
    - Usually detect a firm, hard nodule, but may just find diffuse enlargement or a normal gland
  - PSA
    - Levels over 4 ng/mL are considered abnormal

Diagnostic algorithm
Normal DRE
Normal PSA ⟶ annual exam
 (< 2.5 can do every 2 years)

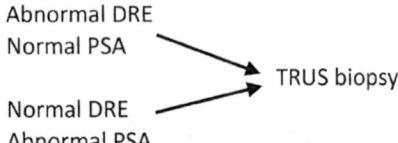

Abnormal DRE
Normal PSA
 ⟶ TRUS biopsy
Normal DRE
Abnormal PSA

Prostate Cancer — Diagnosis
- The diagnostic procedure of choice is a TRUS (transrectal ultrasound)-guided biopsy of the prostate gland
- Typically, 12 biopsies are done encompassing the peripheral zones of the gland
- Remember that BPH usually involves the transition zone, whereas cancer involves the periphery
- Pathology is almost always adenocarcinoma

Prostate Cancer — Path
- Gleason's histological grade is the most important prognostic feature for prostate cancer
- Gives a grade to both the predominant and secondary growth pattern, and adds the scores
- Total will be 2–10, with higher grade correlated with higher incidence of spread and mortality
- Gleason score of ≥ 7 is high-risk disease

Prostate Cancer — Staging
- Staging is done using the TNM system
  - Tumor size
  - Nodal involvement
  - Metastases
  - Most important predictors of pathologic stage and recurrence risk:
    - Gleason grade
    - Tumor stage
    - PSA level

- Staging includes:
  - Bone scan
    - Correlated with plain films
  - CT abdomen or MRI to assess pelvic nodes
    - Both are suboptimal in sensitivity
  - Many times, staging is surgical at the time of prostatectomy

- Multiple options for treatment exist:
  - Surveillance
  - Surgery
  - Radiation
  - Hormonal manipulation
  - Chemotherapy

Prostate Cancer — Local
- Localized disease (Stage I and II)
  - Goal is curative therapy
  - Radical prostatectomy vs. radiotherapy are both reasonable options if life expectancy > 10 years
  - Different side-effect profiles
  - Selection is patient dependent: If patient is elderly, then observation is a viable option

Prostate Cancer — Locoregional
Stage III disease, which penetrates the capsule into surrounding structures, is best treated with radiation therapy ± androgen deprivation therapy.

Prostate Cancer — Metastasis
- Stage IV disease with spread to nodes or distant sites is not a curable illness
- Common sites of spread include:
  - Skeletal system
  - Lung
  - Liver

- Pattern of bony spread is typically:
  - Spine
  - Pelvis
  - Femur
  - Skull
  - Ribs

Prostate Cancer — Hormonal
- Treatment at this stage is designed to palliate symptoms and preserve quality of life
  - Frontline therapy is generally hormonal manipulation
    - Remember that the prostate is androgen-dependent, and most cancers maintain some degree of sensitivity to androgens

- Hormonal manipulation may be accomplished using:
  - Antiandrogens
  - LHRH agonists
  - Orchiectomy
- Progression treated with antiandrogen withdrawal or second-line hormonal therapy
- All therapy is palliative

Drugs in Prostate CA
- Hormonal: Abiraterone acetate, bicalutamide, enzalutamide, leuprolide
- Chemo: Docetaxel, cabazitaxel
- Immunotherapy: Sipuleucel-T
- Steroids: Prednisone
- Antifungal: Ketoconazole

Prostate Cancer Prevention
- Finasteride associated with decreased risk of cancer after 7 years
- **But** ... increased percentage of diagnosed cancers were high grade

AR 15
A 60-year-old man with a history of chronic alcoholism and chronic tobacco use (2–3 packs a day for 40 years) presents as a referral from the emergency department with a new neck mass. He states that the mass is nontender and he just noticed it last week.

Exam: 3.4-cm left midcervical neck mass
Mass is firm and nontender to palpation.
Liver span 10 cm, slightly tender.
An excisional biopsy is done of the neck mass and shows squamous cell carcinoma.

Which of the following is the most appropriate workup at this time?
A. Neck dissection followed by radiation therapy.
B. Endoscopic visualization of the nasopharynx and larynx, and integrated PET-CT scan.
C. CT of the brain alone.
D. Proceed directly to chemotherapy.
E. CT of the neck alone.

Answer: _____

Head and Neck Cancer
- Many are older individuals in the 5th and 6th decades of life
- Men are affected more often than women
- Majority of patients are abusers of alcohol and tobacco
- Related to certain occupations such as woodworkers and textile workers

- Previous H and N cancer increases risk
- A viral association is also noted
  - EBV is strongly associated with nasopharyngeal cancer
  - HPV 16 and 18 have also been linked to cancers of the nasopharynx and oropharynx
  - HPV positivity is associated with improved disease survival

- The areas involved with head and neck cancer include:
  - Oral cavity
  - Oropharynx
  - Nasopharynx
  - Hypopharynx
  - Larynx

- Clinical presentation
  - The majority of patients present with advanced-stage disease
  - Symptoms depend upon the site of involvement and may include:
    - Hoarseness
    - Dysphagia
    - Odynophagia
    - Ulcerations
    - Weight loss

© 2017 MedStudy Internal Medicine Video Board Review – Oncology • Rishi Sawhney, MD

- The majority of head and neck tumors are squamous cell in origin
- There is an increased risk of secondary malignancy, including:
  - Lung cancer
  - Esophageal cancer

- Evaluation
  - Complete exam of the entire area, including fiberoptic evaluation
  - CT scans of the areas
- Diagnosis is generally made by FNA of a mass

- Prognosis is defined primarily by the stage of the tumor
- Also important is the differentiation of the tumor and involvement of lymphatics
- Staging utilizes the TNM system, with a worsening prognosis with advanced-stage disease

- Treatment modalities:
  - Surgical resection
  - Radiation therapy
  - Chemotherapy
- Goal of therapy is preservation of function, if possible, in addition to eradication of disease

- In general, early-stage disease is treated either with surgical resection or radiation therapy
- More advanced disease is treated with combination therapy, with surgery followed by radiation therapy
- Neoadjuvant chemoradiotherapy may be of benefit for preservation of function, particularly in laryngeal cancer

---

AR 16

A 55-year-old female presents to her primary care physician with a 2-month history of episodic diarrhea. Her medical history is notable only for hyperlipidemia that is diet controlled.

Her physical exam is notable for mild abdominal tenderness in the right upper quadrant, without peritoneal signs. Lungs are clear bilaterally, and heart sounds are normal with no murmurs on auscultation. A CT scan of the abdomen with contrast demonstrates the presence of 3 distinct enhancing liver lesions ranging from 2–3 cm, suspicious for metastasis.

A subsequent colonoscopy reveals a sessile polyp in the appendix. Biopsy of the rectal polyp reveals a well-differentiated neuroendocrine neoplasm consistent with carcinoid tumor.

Which of the following is the best initial step in the workup?

A. Serum calcitonin and ACTH levels
B. Pulmonary function tests including spirometry
C. 24-hour urine for 5-HIAA and serum chromogranin A level
D. CEA and CA 19-9 levels
E. 2-dimensional echocardiogram

Answer: _____

Carcinoid
- Very uncommon tumors usually found in appendix or small bowel
- Usually asymptomatic until spread to the liver or occasionally to the lung
- Indolent disease with long survival even with metastatic disease
- Seen in the MEN1 syndrome

- Neuroendocrine tumor type with secretion of multiple substances, including:
  - Serotonin
  - Kinin
  - Histamine
  - Prostaglandins

- The clinical syndrome is usually described as episodic
  - Flushing
  - Abdominal cramping
  - Diarrhea
  - Palpitations
  - Wheezing

- Valvular heart disease may occur with carcinoid syndrome
- Associated findings include:
  - Endocardial fibrosis
  - Often affects the pulmonary and tricuspid valves

- Diagnosis
  - 24-hour urine for 5-HIAA (5-hydroxyindoleacetic acid)
    - End product of serotonin metabolism
  - Serum chromogranin level
    - Protein stored and released with peptides and amines in neuroendocrine tissues

- If diagnosis is made when the tumor is localized, then long-term prognosis is good
- Surgical resection is often curative
- Small lesions (< 1–2 cm) have a low potential for metastatic spread

Carcinoid (cont.)
- With metastatic spread to the liver or the lung, carcinoid syndrome is seen
- Curative treatment is not available at this stage
- Must treat the symptoms
  - Antidiarrheal medications
  - Cyproheptadine

- Most effectively treated with the somatostatin analogue, octreotide
  - Can give as a monthly injection
  - Can reduce symptoms related to hormonal secretion, and slow progression of tumors
- Use of chemotherapy is limited but has involved the drug streptozocin

---

AR 17

A 67-year-old man with a 100-pack-year history of smoking (2 ppd for 50 years) is essentially dragged in by his wife, who says that he has withered away to nothing and has been acting very confused lately. He says he is fine but keeps calling you his grandchild. You do not get much more information out of him.

PMH: HTN controlled on lisinopril; Prostatectomy 5 years ago
ROS: 30-lb weight loss/6 mos.
Exam: Oriented only to person. Chest: Coarse, scattered crackles; No focal findings
Abd: Soft, benign
Laboratory:
  CXR: Central/Hilar mass with area of cavitation
  Calcium = 11.5 mg/dL

Based on your findings, which of the following types of lung cancer does this man most likely have?
A. Small cell
B. Adenocarcinoma
C. Squamous cell carcinoma
D. Bronchoalveolar carcinoma
E. Large cell

Answer: _____

Lung Cancer
- Major cause is smoking
- Most common cause of cancer-related deaths in the U.S. for men and women
- Most patients diagnosed with lung cancer will die of their disease
- Nonsmokers more commonly women than men

Lung Cancer — Risk
- Risk factors:
  - Smoking
    - Length of time
    - Number of cigarettes/day
    - Secondhand
  - Radon
  - Asbestos
  - Radiation exposure

Lung Cancer — Screening
- The USPSTF recommends yearly lung cancer screening with low-dose CT scan for people who:
  - Have a history of heavy smoking ($\geq$ 30 pack years) **and**
  - Smoke now or have quit within the past 15 years **and**
  - Between 55 and 80 years of age
- Radiation dose exposure is < 1/3 of a standard-dose diagnostic chest CT
- When should screening stop?
  - $\geq$ 81 years of age **or**
  - Has not smoked in 15 years **or**
  - Develops a health problem that makes him or her unwilling or unable to have surgery if lung cancer is found

Lung Cancer — Pathology
- Pathology
  - Non–small cell
    - Adenocarcinoma — most common
    - Squamous cell carcinoma
    - Large cell carcinoma
  - Small cell

- Major differences in the NSC and the SC types:
  - Sensitivity to treatment
  - Rapid growth
  - Association with paraneoplastic syndromes

Lung Cancer — Staging
- Staging
  - CT scans, including chest and abdomen/pelvis
  - Bone scan
  - PET scan
  - MRI brain
  - $\pm$ Mediastinoscopy
  - Obtain tissue biopsy for diagnosis

Lung Cancer — Prognosis
- Prognostic factors:
  - Stage (TNM)
  - Performance status
  - Absence of weight loss
  - Female
    - Not age
    - Not cell type

Lung Cancer — Treatment
- Treatment:
  - Resection of disease, if possible
    - Consider adjuvant treatment
  - If unresectable (locally advanced)
    - Chemotherapy + radiation
  - Metastatic disease
    - Chemotherapy

Lung Cancer — Special
- Pancoast tumor
  - Horner syndrome
  - Shoulder pain and arm pain
  - Attempt diagnosis prior to treatment to help with planning
  - Treat with chemotherapy and radiation, followed by resection, if possible

- Pearls
  - Remember that squamous and small cell are usually central
  - Adenocarcinoma and large cell are peripheral
  - Bronchoalveolar is the one **not** associated with cigarette smoking and may have better prognosis
  - Large cell is the "scar carcinoma"

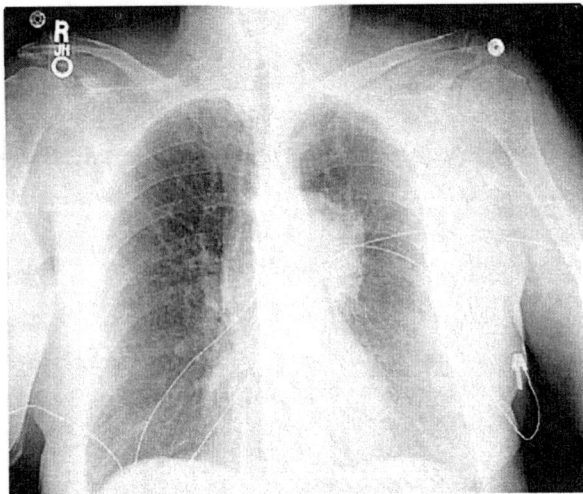

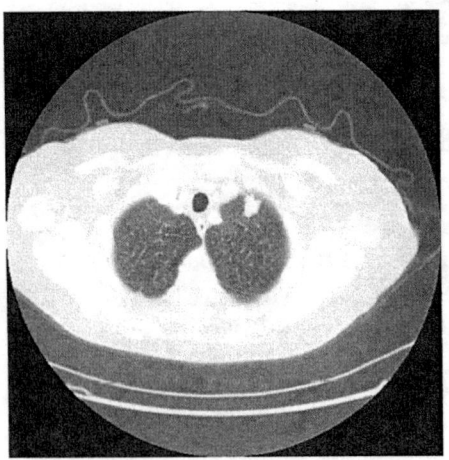

- Pearls (cont.)
  - Adenocarcinoma is the most common
  - Squamous cell cavitates
  - Mesothelioma is associated with asbestos exposure

  - Squamous cell is associated with hypercalcemia
  - Small cell is associated with SIADH, Cushing syndrome, and Lambert-Eaton syndrome
  - All may be associated with clubbing
  - All may be associated with hypertrophic pulmonary osteoarthropathy

Renal Cell Carcinoma
- Unusual cancer
- Affects men more often
- Linked to smoking
- More common in patients with acquired renal cystic disease
- Common in patients with von Hippel-Lindau disease

- Classic triad
  - Flank pain
  - Hematuria
  - Abdominal mass
- Now commonly found incidentally on CT abdomen exams and asymptomatic

- Paraneoplastic syndromes are common
  - Erythrocytosis
  - Hypertension
  - Hypercalcemia
  - Amyloidosis

- Diagnosis is usually by an imaging technique
  - CT scan
  - MRI
  - Ultrasound
- Pathology is typically clear cell carcinoma
- Medullary in sickle cell

- Therapy is most successful if the tumor is confined to the kidney and is capable of being resected
- Radical nephrectomy vs. partial nephrectomy
- Solitary metastases may be resected
- May resect venous involvement

- For metastatic disease, treatment historically disappointing, but now evolving with many new targeted drugs
- Chemotherapy is not very effective

Renal Cell Carcinoma (cont.)
- Immunotherapy can produce durable responses in minority of patients, with α-interferon and interleukin-2 used — but very toxic
- New targeted drugs — VEGF and PDGF tyrosine kinase inhibitors

- Other treatment options:
  - Sunitinib
  - Temsirolimus
  - Sorafenib
  - Pazopanib

Colon Cancer
- Second leading killer in the U.S.
- Increasing incidence in developed countries
- Decreasing incidence over last decade in U.S.
- Shift in location for disease to more proximal

- Risk factors:
  - Diet high in red meat (Western society)
  - Obesity
  - HRT is protective
  - NSAID is protective
- Increased in inflammatory bowel disease patients
  - Primarily ulcerative colitis
  - Occasionally Crohn's
- Familial

Colon Cancer — Screening
- Screening:
  - Digital rectal exam
  - FOBT
  - Sigmoidoscopy
  - Colonoscopy
  - ACBE
- Despite availability, there is relatively poor compliance with any screening test

ACS Screening Recommendations
- Men and women over 50 years of age
  - Flexible sigmoidoscopy every 5 years **or**
  - Colonoscopy every 10 years **or**
  - DCBE every 5 years **or**
  - Virtual colonoscopy every 5 years **or**
  - FOBT yearly
- Prefer test to screen for polyps and cancer

USPSTF Recommendations (2008)
- Yearly FOBT **or**
- Sigmoidoscopy every 5 years **or**
- Colonoscopy every 10 years from 50 to 75 years of age

Colon Cancer Screening Consensus
Screen after 50 years of age with a wide choice of available screening options.

Colon Cancer (cont.)
- Screening is routinely offered after 50 years of age, but there is no proven standard
- FOBT only test shown to decrease mortality
- Screen those with a genetic syndrome (FAP or HNPCC) early and often
- Prophylactic colectomy is used in inflammatory bowel disease and the genetic syndromes

AR 18
A 67-year-old female who presented with rectal bleeding underwent diagnostic colonoscopy. A 2.5-cm tumor was noted in the mid-descending colon, and biopsy results revealed the diagnosis of adenocarcinoma. Computed tomography of the abdomen and pelvis revealed evidence of localized disease only.

Of the following, which intervention is most likely to result in cure?
A. Immunotherapy
B. Radiation therapy
C. Surgical excision
D. Chemotherapy
E. NSAID therapy

Answer: _____

Colon Cancer (cont.)
- Treatment
  - Early stage — surgery is curative
  - Later-stage disease — need adjuvant treatment after surgery
  - Metastatic disease — consider resection; Primary treatment is with combination chemotherapy, such as FOLFOX or FOLFIRI

- Other treatment options
  - Bevacizumab
  - Cetuximab
  - Panitumumab
  - Regorafenib
  - Aflibercept

Melanoma
- Increasing in the U.S. and worldwide
- Interaction between susceptibility and environmental factors
- Increased risk if there is history of nonmelanoma skin cancer
- Prevention occurs by reducing sun exposure

- Remember: Depth of invasion is important in staging and planning the surgical resection margins
- Metastatic disease is poorly responsive to chemotherapy and may respond best to immune modulation with α-interferon or interleukin-2

- Other treatment options
  - Chemo
    - Temozolomide, dacarbazine
  - Immuno
    - Ipilimumab, nivolumab, interferon
  - Targeted BRAF inhibitors, MEK inhibitors
    - Vemurafenib, dabrafenib

Chemotherapy Complications
- Common complications
  - Nausea and vomiting
  - Tumor lysis syndrome
  - Neutropenic fever
  - Neutropenic colitis
  - Mucositis

Nausea and Vomiting
- Coordinated through both the CNS and the gastrointestinal system
- The vomiting center is in the medulla, and the chemoreceptor trigger zone is also involved in the pathway
- Neurochemicals like serotonin and dopamine are involved in the signaling

Antiemetic Therapy
- Many drugs useful to prevent nausea in conjunction with chemotherapy
- May have acute emesis, delayed emesis, or even anticipatory emesis
- Should tailor the regimen to the individual patient; Dependent on the drugs used and the pattern of nausea and emesis

- Drugs that are effective in combating nausea include:
  - Serotonin antagonists
  - Antihistamines
  - Phenothiazines
  - Steroids
  - Antianxiety agents such as benzodiazepines
  - Substance P/NK-1 receptor antagonist
    - Aprepitant

AR 19

A 24-year-old male with a known history of HIV presents with scattered peripheral lymphadenopathy. He is referred for biopsy, and the pathologist reports Burkitt lymphoma. In consultation with oncology, the patient is admitted for staging and initiation of therapy. On the second day of treatment, you are called by nursing, who report a marked decrease in urine output. Laboratory results:

Serum creatinine: 2.2   LDH: 1,100
Potassium: 6.1   Phosphorus: 5.2
Calcium: 7.2   Uric acid: 14.2
Hemoglobin: 10.3

Early treatment with which of the following would have likely prevented this patient's condition?
A. Intravenous steroids
B. Intravenous rasburicase
C. Intravenous furosemide
D. IV calcium infusion
E. IV sodium bicarbonate

Answer: _____

Tumor Lysis Syndrome
- Another side effect of chemotherapy
- Occurs when tumor breakdown occurs rapidly
- Should be anticipated in rapidly growing tumors or those tumors that are sensitive to chemotherapy, such as Burkitt lymphoma or other non-Hodgkin lymphomas

- Release of intracellular contents results in the development of:
  - Hyperuricemia
    - Uric acid nephropathy
  - Hyperkalemia
    - Cardiac arrhythmias
  - Hyperphosphatemia
    - Potentiate uric acid nephropathy and renal failure
  - Hypocalcemia
    - Tetany or arrhythmias

- Prevention is the key
- Should use adequate hydration plus pretreatment with allopurinol or rasburicase
- Urinary alkalinization has been used, but now falling out of favor
- Should follow electrolyte values closely after treatment

Neutropenic Fever
- An oncologic emergency
- The most common cause of chemotherapy-related death
- Fever may result from infection but may also be a manifestation of:
  - The tumor itself
  - Medication reactions
  - Blood products

Neutropenic Fever (cont.)
- By definition, a host becomes more susceptible to infection when the absolute neutrophil count is below 1,000 cells/mm^3
- The risk increases as the value decreases
- The duration of neutropenia is important also
- The longer the neutropenic state persists, the higher the risk of infection

- The usual manifestations may be absent because there is a lack of neutrophils to mount an inflammatory response
- Remember: You cannot make pus without white cells
- May not see infiltrates on CXR or see erythema at an IV site

- In all patients suspected of neutropenic fever, do a thorough exam
- Should always look for perirectal abscess, IV site infection
- Cultures of blood and any suspected site should be obtained as well as a CXR
- Empiric antibiotics should then be initiated

- Antibiotic therapy should be initiated immediately (no delays for transfer of patients, etc.)
- Should always empirically cover for a bacterial source
- Gram-negative infections, especially *Pseudomonas*, are the most deadly and should always be covered initially

- Gram-positive organisms are becoming more common in patients with neutropenia
- Should always include coverage for any obvious sites (lines, cellulitis, etc.)
- Should adjust coverage for any identified organism from culture

- If fever persists for prolonged period, consider a fungal etiology such as candidiasis
- These patients should receive an empiric trial of an antifungal agent
- Treatment should continue until the neutropenia is resolved or adequate therapy is delivered

Neutropenic Colitis / Typhlitis
- Occurs in patients after prolonged neutropenia and treatment with broad-spectrum antibiotics
  - Abdominal pain
  - Diarrhea that may be bloody
- Gram-negative bacteria
- May be fatal
- Seen most commonly in patients with leukemia
- Reserve surgical intervention for perforation

Mucositis
- One of the most difficult complications to manage
- Very painful ulceration of the oral and esophageal mucosa
- May lead to dehydration and may be source for fever and sepsis
- Usually self-limiting

AR 20
A 43-year-old female is diagnosed with oropharyngeal cancer. She will be receiving cisplatin with concurrent irradiation.

In discussing with the patient, which of the following represents a well-documented, and potentially irreversible toxicity of cisplatin to be aware of?
A. Cardiomyopathy
B. Tinnitus/Ototoxicity
C. Pulmonary fibrosis
D. Skin rash
E. Hypersensitivity reactions

Answer: _____

Chemotherapy
- General caveats:
  - Drugs fall into general categories
    - Alkylating agents
    - Platinum compounds
    - Antimetabolites
    - Topoisomerase I inhibitors
    - Antibiotics
    - Alkaloids

AR 21
Your patient is a 33-year-old female with a history of Hodgkin lymphoma, which was diagnosed 3 months ago. During her treatment for this disease, she has been receiving chemotherapy, including doxorubicin, bleomycin, vincristine, and dacarbazine. With each cycle of chemotherapy, she requires frequent doses of ondansetron for control of nausea and vomiting. She presents to clinic at this time with complaints of a burning sensation in both feet. Vascular examination of the lower extremities is normal.

Which of the following medications is most likely to be related to her current symptoms?
A. Ondansetron
B. Doxorubicin
C. Bleomycin
D. Vincristine
E. Dacarbazine

Answer: _____

Alkylating Agents
- DNA becomes alkylated and disrupted
- Able to affect slowly cycling cells (stem cells)
- Infertility is a common side effect
- Secondary malignancy (MDS/AML) common

- Nitrogen mustard
  - Oldest
  - MOPP
- Melphalan
  - Myeloma
- Chlorambucil
  - CLL

Cyclophosphamide
- Unique alkylating agent because it must be activated in the liver
- Breakdown product is acrolein
- Acrolein causes hemorrhagic cystitis
- Prevent with hydration or mesna
- Marrow toxicity and leukemia less likely

Platinum Compounds
- Inorganic compound with 2 amine groups and 2 chlorines attached
- Binds to DNA, much as the alkylators do
- Can actually cross-link DNA
- Most active in cells in G1, but can act across all cell phases (phase nonspecific)

Cisplatin
- Cleared by the kidneys; Thus, primary toxicity is renal damage
- May experience magnesium wasting
- Prevent with hydration
- Also causes peripheral neuropathy and ototoxicity
- Many uses — testicular, ovarian, lung

Carboplatin
- Causes more myelosuppression (especially thrombocytopenia)
- Causes less renal toxicity
- Not always interchangeable with cisplatin
  - Inferior results in testicular cancer
  - Probably equivalent in ovarian cancer

Antimetabolites
- Drugs that are similar to metabolites in the DNA and RNA synthesis pathways
- Usually compete for a critical enzyme or substitute into the backbone of DNA or RNA, causing disruption
- Maximally effective in cycling cells

- Not associated with profound or prolonged myelosuppression
- Not associated with risk of secondary leukemia
- Examples of commonly used drugs include:
  - 5-fluorouracil
  - Methotrexate
  - Cytarabine

5-Fluorouracil
- Resembles the pyrimidines, uracil, and thymidine
- Incorporates into RNA and disrupts the transcription
- Toxic to the GI epithelium, resulting in significant mucositis and diarrhea
- Enhanced by the addition of leucovorin

Methotrexate
- A folic acid analog
- Blocks the enzyme dihydrofolate reductase
- Blocks DNA synthesis due to the lack of thymidine
- Leucovorin is the "antidote" providing the necessary reduced folate to overcome methotrexate
- Works best in cells actively cycling

- Must be careful in patients with effusions because the drug will accumulate in the effusion and slowly leak out, causing prolonged exposure and increased toxicity
- Side effects generally include mucositis and diarrhea
- Used in many tumors, such as ALL, head and neck tumors, bladder, and breast cancer

Cytarabine
- Inhibits the binding of deoxycytidine to the DNA polymerase; Thus, effectively blocking the production of DNA
- Most active in S-phase cells
- In high doses, enters the CNS and may cause cerebellar toxicity
- Used in AML and lymphoma treatment

Topoisomerase I Inhibitors
- Parent compound is camptothecin
  - Topotecan, Irinotecan
- Unique action, with damage occurring by the interruption of the normal nick and repair mechanism performed by the topoisomerase I enzyme
- Again, cell–cycle-specific drug for S phase

Topotecan
- Dose-limiting toxicity is neutropenia
- May see nausea, fever, and skin rash
- Used for the treatment of ovarian cancer and lung cancer

Antibiotics
- Primarily
  - Anthracyclines
  - Actinomycin D
  - Bleomycin
  - Mitomycin C
- A very diverse group, all derived from microbial fermentation

Anthracyclines
- Daunorubicin and doxorubicin
- Intercalates DNA and disrupts replication
- May generate DNA breaks by the creation of free radicals
- Active throughout the cell cycle
- Must reduce dosage for hepatic toxicity

- Toxicity profile is unique
  - Cardiac toxicity occurs with increasing cumulative dosage of the drugs
  - Chronic congestive heart failure that is difficult to treat
  - Monitor by serial ejection fraction assessments and by endomyocardial biopsy
  - Reduced by dexrazoxane, which inhibits free radical formation

AR 22

Your patient is a 23-year-old female with a history of Hodgkin lymphoma diagnosed at 21 years of age. During her treatment for this disease, she received chemotherapy, including doxorubicin, bleomycin, vincristine, and dacarbazine, and involved field radiation therapy to cervical and supraclavicular region. She presents to clinic at this time with complaints of shortness of breath and a persistent, dry, hacking cough.

Which of the following treatments is most likely to be related to her current complaints?
A. Dacarbazine
B. Doxorubicin
C. Bleomycin
D. Radiation therapy
E. Vincristine

Answer: _____

Bleomycin
- Can be given IV, IM, or intracavitary
- Toxicity profile is unusual
  - Fever is common, and occasionally anaphylaxis may be seen
  - Skin reactions include erythema and hyperpigmentation
  - Pulmonary fibrosis is seen with increasing doses or in those having had chest radiation

Alkaloids
- Plant derivatives
- Includes:
  - Vincristine
  - Vinblastine
  - Etoposide
  - Taxanes

Vincristine
- From the periwinkle plant
- Binds to tubulin to interrupt the microtubule formation
- Metaphase-specific
- Primary toxicity is neurotoxicity
- Used in ALL, lymphomas

Vinblastine
- Almost exactly the same drug
- Mechanism is identical
- Side-effect profile is different
  - Primarily myelotoxicity
  - Little neuropathy

Taxanes
- Found in the bark of the Pacific yew tree
- Now can be manufactured from other parts of the tree and other species of the yew
- Bind to microtubules, preventing their breakdown into tubulin dimers
- Primarily disrupts mitosis
- Paclitaxel and docetaxel

Paclitaxel
- Associated with hypersensitivity reactions, which can be prevented by premedication with steroids and histamine blockers
- Causes bradyarrhythmias
- Causes neuropathy, mucositis, and almost universal alopecia that is total body

Monoclonal Antibodies
- Take advantage of tumor-specific properties such as cell surface markers or protein products of the tumor
- Has benefit of little toxicity to normal tissues, unless they express the marker
- May see infusion-related toxicity

Trastuzumab
- Anti-*HER2/neu*
- Effective in breast cancer that overexpresses *HER2/neu*
- Binds to a transmembrane receptor in the family of EGFR to block the cascade that drives cell growth and division
- Most effective when combined with chemotherapy
- **Cardiomyopathy, reversible**

Rituximab
- Anti-CD20
- Effective in CD20-positive lymphomas (B-cell)
- Has been modified by the addition of radioactive isotopes to add tumor toxicity
- Watch for hypersensitivity reactions and opportunistic infections!

Many New Targeted Therapies
- Proteasome inhibitors
- TKIs
- Antiangiogenesis drugs
- EGFR blockers

Hematopoietic Stem Cell Transplantation

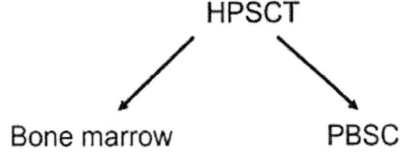

Stem Cells
- Pluripotent cells found in the bone marrow
- Rare (less than 1 in 100,000 cells)
- No identifiable morphological characteristics
- CD34+ (stem cell antigen)
- Thy 1–, HLA–, DR–

- Can be induced to circulate in the peripheral blood
- Need $2–5 \times 10^6$ CD34+ cells/kg of recipient body weight

HPSCT
Types of transplants:
- Syngeneic
- **Autologous**
- **Allogeneic**
  - Related
  - Unrelated

Autologous Transplant
- Use patient's own cells
- Has less acute mortality
- Higher relapse rate

Mobilization
- Goal is to collect sufficient cells for use as chemotherapy rescue
- Must manipulate the release of stem cells into the peripheral blood for collection or perform a bone marrow harvest
- Marrow harvest product has higher "contamination" rate than PBSC collection if disease involved the marrow

- May use high-dose chemotherapy with growth factors to mobilize stem cells from the marrow
- Also may use growth factors alone for mobilization
- Data for G-CSF

Collection
- PBSC collection is achieved by using a cell separator
- Target cell dose is $> 2 \times 10^6$ CD34+ cells/kg
- May take several collections to achieve an adequate cell dose

Autologous Transplant
- After adequate cells are cryopreserved
- Patient receives high-dose chemotherapy and/or radiation therapy for treatment of malignancy
- Stem cells given as rescue from high-dose chemotherapy

Toxicity
- Mucositis
- Neutropenic fever
- Pancytopenia requiring blood product support
- Mortality is 5–7% during the first 100 days of autologous transplant

Indications
- Some accepted indications for autologous transplant include:
  - Lymphoma, including NHL and HD
  - Leukemia, including AML and ALL in CR
  - Multiple myeloma
  - Testicular cancer for relapsed disease
  - No benefit in breast cancer

Allogeneic Transplant
- Related donor or unrelated donor (from NMDP or other registry)
- Has a higher acute mortality rate
- Long-term risk of GVHD
- Less relapse risk

- Identify a donor
  - Relative
  - NMDP or other registry
- Patient receives high-dose chemotherapy
  - For immunosuppression
  - For tumor treatment
  - To "make room" ??

Allogeneic Transplant (cont.)
- Donor cells given as rescue and as therapeutic maneuver
- Toxicity is similar to that of the autologous transplant, **plus**:
  - Veno-occlusive disease of the liver — can see with either but more common with allo-BMT — damage to hepatic venules from the chemotherapy; May be fatal

Toxicity (cont.)
- GVHD — a unique toxicity to allogeneic transplant — higher risk with unrelated donor source; May be fatal; Acute looks like fever, skin rash, GI tract involvement; Chronic looks like scleroderma
- GV"T" — a benefit of GVHD is graft vs. tumor effect, which may decrease relapse rate — mediated by T lymphocytes

Variable Intensity Conditioning
- VIC transplant attempts to take advantage of the GV"T" effect without all the toxicity of high-dose chemotherapy
- Uses immunosuppressant chemotherapy to allow chimerism and eventual total engraftment of the donor cells
- Still experience risk of GVHD

Indications
- Some accepted indications for allogeneic transplant:
  - Chronic leukemia, including CML and CLL
  - Relapsed acute leukemia, including AML and ALL
  - Myelodysplasia
  - Multiple myeloma (VIC)

© 2017 MedStudy Internal Medicine Video Board Review – Oncology • Rishi Sawhney, MD

Oncology
Audience Response Answers

Audience Response 1
Answer: D. Treatment should be initiated
with a bisphosphonate.

AR 2
Answer: D. Conivaptan.

AR 3
Answer: A. Dexamethasone intravenously, emergent
spine MRI.

AR 4
Answer: D. Referral to a surgeon for biopsy.

AR 5
Answer: C. Tell her the risk is increased at least 3-fold
that of normal, and she should have testing for *BRCA1*
and *BRCA2* genes.

AR 6
Answer: C. Modified radical mastectomy followed
by chemotherapy and then endocrine therapy
(aromatase inhibitor).

AR 7
Answer: B. Chemotherapy plus radiation.

AR 8
Answer: C. Bone density monitoring every
1–2 years.

AR 9
Answer: D. Refer for colposcopy.

The best answer would be further evaluation
with colposcopy and biopsies of any abnormal
areas that are visualized.

AR 10
Answer: D. CA-125 testing.

AR 11
Answer: C. Serum tumor markers and radical
inguinal orchiectomy.

AR 12
Answer: C. Secondary malignancies, including germ cell
tumors, leukemia, and gastrointestinal malignancies.

AR 13
Answer: B. Transrectal ultrasound with multiple
biopsies.

He should have a biopsy because his PSA
is in the abnormal range. He also has an elevated
PSA velocity, which is correlated with the likelihood
of detecting malignancy and a poorer outcome from
his malignancy.

AR 14
Answer: D. The American Cancer Society recommends
that physicians discuss the benefits and risks of prostate
cancer screening for men who have at least a
10-year life expectancy.

AR 15
Answer: B. Endoscopic visualization of the nasopharynx
and larynx, and integrated PET-CT scan.

AR 16
Answer: C. 24-hour urine for 5-HIAA and serum
chromogranin A level.

AR 17
Answer: C. Squamous cell carcinoma.

AR 18
Answer: C. Surgical excision.

AR 19
Answer: B. Intravenous rasburicase.

AR 20
Answer: B. Tinnitus/Ototoxicity.

AR 21
Answer: D. Vincristine.

AR 22
Answer: C. Bleomycin.

MedStudy

Internal Medicine Video Board Review

Pulmonary Medicine

Presented by

Raj Dasgupta, MD
Professor of Clinical Medicine
Keck School of Medicine of USC
Department of Medicine
Division of Pulmonary, Critical Care, and Sleep Medicine
Assistant Program Director of Internal Medicine Residency
Associate Program Director of the Sleep Medicine Fellowship
Los Angeles, California

Table of Contents

Pulmonary Abbreviations

ABG	Arterial blood gas
ABPA	Allergic bronchopulmonary aspergillosis
ACE	Angiotensin-converting enzyme
ACOS	Asthma-COPD overlap syndrome
ACTH	Adrenocorticotropic hormone
AFB	Acid fast bacilli
AIP	Acute interstitial pneumonia
ANA	Antinuclear antibody
APRV	Airway pressure release ventilation
aPTT	Activated partial thromboplastin time
ARDS	Acute respiratory distress syndrome
ASD	Atrial septal defect
ASV	Adaptive servo ventilation
AVAPS	Average volume assured pressure support
BAL	Bronchoalveolar lavage
BCG	Bacillus Calmette-Guerin
BD	Bronchodilator
BHR	Bronchial hyperresponsiveness
BiPAP	Bilevel positive airway pressure
BT	Bronchial thermoplasty
CA-MRSA	Community-acquired methicillin-resistant *Staphylococcus aureus*
CAP	Community-acquired pneumonia
CAT	COPD assessment test
CBT	Cognitive behavioral treatment
CF	Cystic fibrosis
CFTR	Cystic fibrosis transmembrane conductance regulator
COP	Cryptogenic organizing pneumonitis
COPD	Chronic obstructive pulmonary disease
CPAP	Continuous positive airway pressure
CSA	Central sleep apnea
CTEPH	Chronic thromboembolic pulmonary hypertension
DIP	Desquamative interstitial pneumonia
DLCO	Linear diffusion of carbon monoxide
DOA	Direct oral anticoagulant
DPLP	Diffuse parenchymal lung disease
DVT	Deep vein thrombosis
EBUS	Endobronchial ultrasound
EMG	Electromyogram
FEV_1	Forced expiratory volume in 1 second
FPP	Free portal pressure
FVC	Forced vital capacity
GERD	Gastroesophageal reflux disease
GFR	Glomerular filtration rate
GPA	Granulomatosis with polyangiitis (Wegener's)
HA-MRSA	Hospital-acquired methicillin-resistant *Staphylococcus aureus*

HF	Heart failure
HIT	Heparin-induced thrombocytopenia
HRCT	High resolution contrast tomography scan
IDU	Injection drug user
IGRAs	Interferon-gamma release assays
ILD	Interstitial lung disease
INH	Isoniazid
INR	International normalized ratio
IPF	Idiopathic pulmonary fibrosis
IVC	Inferior vena cava
JVD	Jugular venous distention
JVP	Jugular venous pressure
LABA	Long-acting beta-agonist
LAM	Lymphangioleiomyomatosis
LAMA	Long-acting muscarinic antagonist
LIP	Lymphocytic interstitial pneumonia
LMWH	Low-molecular-weight heparin
LTBI	Latent TB infection
LV	Left ventricle
LVRS	Lung volume reduction surgery
MAC	*Mycobacterium avium* complex
MAT	Multifocal atrial tachycardia
MDI	Metered-dose inhaler
MDR	Multidrug-resistant
MICU	Medical intensive care unit
MTX	Methotrexate
MV	Mitral valve
MVA	Motor vehicle accident
NSIP	Nonspecific interstitial pneumonia
NTM	Nontuberculous mycobacteria
OHS	Obesity hypoventilation syndrome
OSA	Obstructive sleep apnea
P_AO_2	Alveolar PO_2
P_aO_2	Arterial PO_2
PAH	Pulmonary arterial hypertension
PAP	Pulmonary artery pressure
PASP	Pulmonary artery systolic pressure
PCI	Percutaneous coronary intervention
PCR	Polymerase chain reaction
PCWP	Pulmonary capillary wedge pressure
PDA	Patent ductus arteriosus
PE	Pulmonary embolism
PEEP	Positive end-expiratory pressure
PEF	Peak expiratory flow
PFO	Patent foramen ovale
PFT	Pulmonary function test
PH	Pulmonary hypertension
PIOPED	The prospective investigation of pulmonary embolism diagnosis
PNA	Pneumonia
PNX	Pneumothorax
PPD	Purified protein derivative

PT	Prothrombin time
PVL	Panton-Valentine leukocidin
PVR	Pulmonary vascular resistance
RA	Rheumatoid arthritis
RAP	Right atrial pressure
RBILD	Respiratory bronchiolitis interstitial disease
RERAs	Respiratory effort-related arousals
RR	Respiratory rate
RV	Residual volume; right ventricle
S_aO_2	Arterial oxygen saturation of hemoglobin
SBP	Systolic blood pressure
SLE	Systemic lupus erythematosus
SVC	Slow vital capacity
SVR	Systemic vascular resistance
TBB	Transbronchial biopsy
TDR	Totally drug-resistant
TEE	Transesophageal echocardiogram
TLC	Total lung capacity
TPMT	Thiopurine-S-methyltransferase enzyme
TR	Tricuspid regurgitation
TRALI	Transfusion related acute lung injury
TRV	Tricuspid regurgitation peak velocity
TTE	Transthoracic echocardiogram
TV	Tidal volume
UFH	Unfractionated heparin
UIP	Usual interstitial pneumonia
UPPP	Uvulopalatopharyngoplasty
V/Q	Ventilation/Perfusion ratio
V/Q scan	Ventilation/Perfusion lung scan
VATS	Video-assisted thoracoscopic lung surgery
VSD	Ventricular septal defect
VTE	Venous thromboembolism
XDR	Extensively drug-resistant

Speaker Disclosure
Raj Dasgupta, MD, has documented that he has
no commercial relationships to disclose.

Pulmonary Medicine

Course Outline
- **Pulmonary Medicine**
  - Respiratory Physiology
    - O_2 Content
    - A-a Gradient
    - Etiology of hypoxemia
  - PFT
  - Asthma
  - COPD
  - Bronchiectasis
    - Cystic Fibrosis
  - Interstitial Lung Disease
  - Pulmonary Hypertension
  - PE and DVT
  - Pleural Effusions
  - Pneumothorax
  - Pneumonias
  - Tuberculosis
- **Critical Care Medicine**
  - ARDS and Ventilator Management
  - Early Goal-Directed Therapy in the MICU
- **Sleep Medicine**
  - OSA and CSA
- **Lung Cancer and Nodules**

Pulmonary Medicine

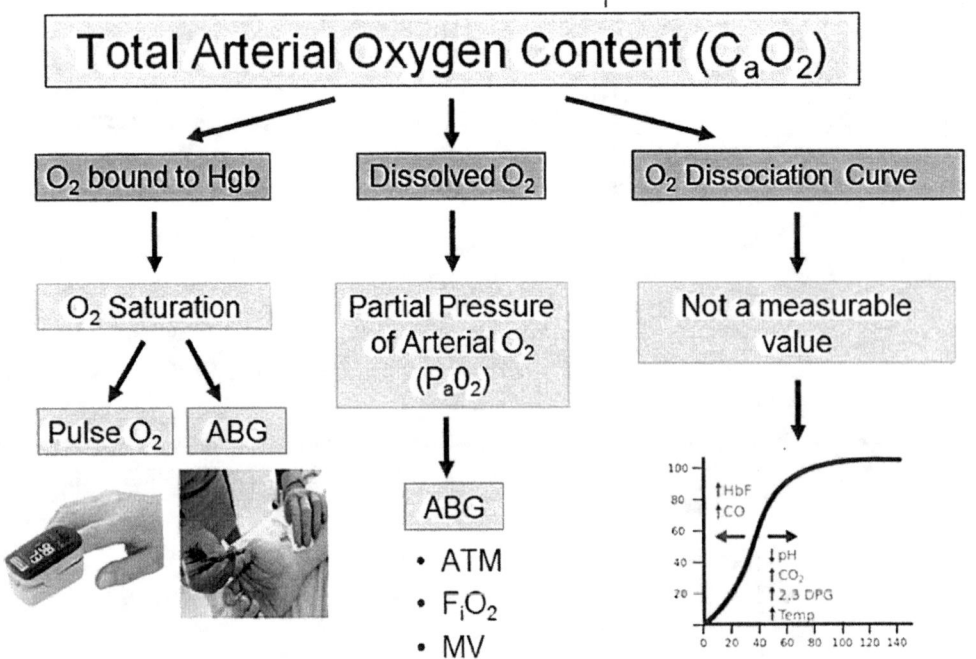

Systemic Arterial Blood and Total Oxygen Content

Summary of the effects of anemia, polycythemia, and carbon monoxide poisoning

	PO_2	Hb Concentration	O_2 per g Hb	O_2 Content
Anemia	N	↓	N	↓
Polycythemia	N	↑	N	↑
CO poisoning (acute)	N	N	↓	↓

Audience Response 1

A 42-year-old female has severe **smoke inhalation** from a house fire. In the emergency room, the patient complains of a severe headache and has a cherry-red discoloration of her skin and mucous membranes.

Which of the following laboratory findings is most likely present?

A. Decreased arterial O_2 saturation (S_aO_2)
B. Decreased arterial PO_2 (P_aO_2)
C. Increased alveolar arterial gradient
D. Increased serum bicarbonate
E. Normal O_2 content

Answer: _____

Audience Response 1 (cont.)

- CO poisoning commonly occurs in house fires
- Produced by incomplete combustion of carbon-containing materials and has a 240x greater binding affinity for heme groups than O_2
- S_aO_2 (average % of O_2 bound to heme groups in hemoglobin) is decreased in CO poisoning
- If co-oximetry is not used in measuring the arterial blood gas, the S_aO_2 will be normal, because it is calculated from the P_aO_2, which is normal in CO poisoning

AR 2

A 60-year-old male has just undergone a bronchoscopy with transbronchial biopsies of the RLL, and is noted to be tachypneic and cyanotic soon after the procedure was finished. His **O₂ sat** is noted to **be 87%**. His cyanosis does **not** improve with the addition of supplemental oxygen. B/L breath sounds and chest rise are noted.

Which of the following interventions is most likely to improve his condition?

A. Administer hyperbaric oxygen.
B. Administer methylene blue.
C. Obtain an ABG and CXR.
D. Intubate.
E. Place bilateral chest tubes.

Answer: _____

AR 2 (cont.)

- **Methemoglobinemia:** The ferrous (Fe^{2+}) irons of heme are oxidized to the ferric (Fe^{3+}) state, can't bind O_2
- **Etiology:**
  1) Congenital
  2) Topical anesthetics, nitrates, dapsone
- **Diagnosis:** ABG by co-oximetry
- **Presentation:**
  1) < 20%: Asymptomatic
  2) 20–40%: Headache, fatigue, dyspnea, and lethargy
  3) > 40%: Respiratory depression, altered consciousness, shock, seizures, death
- **Treatment:** Discontinue medication, methylene blue 1–2 mg/kg

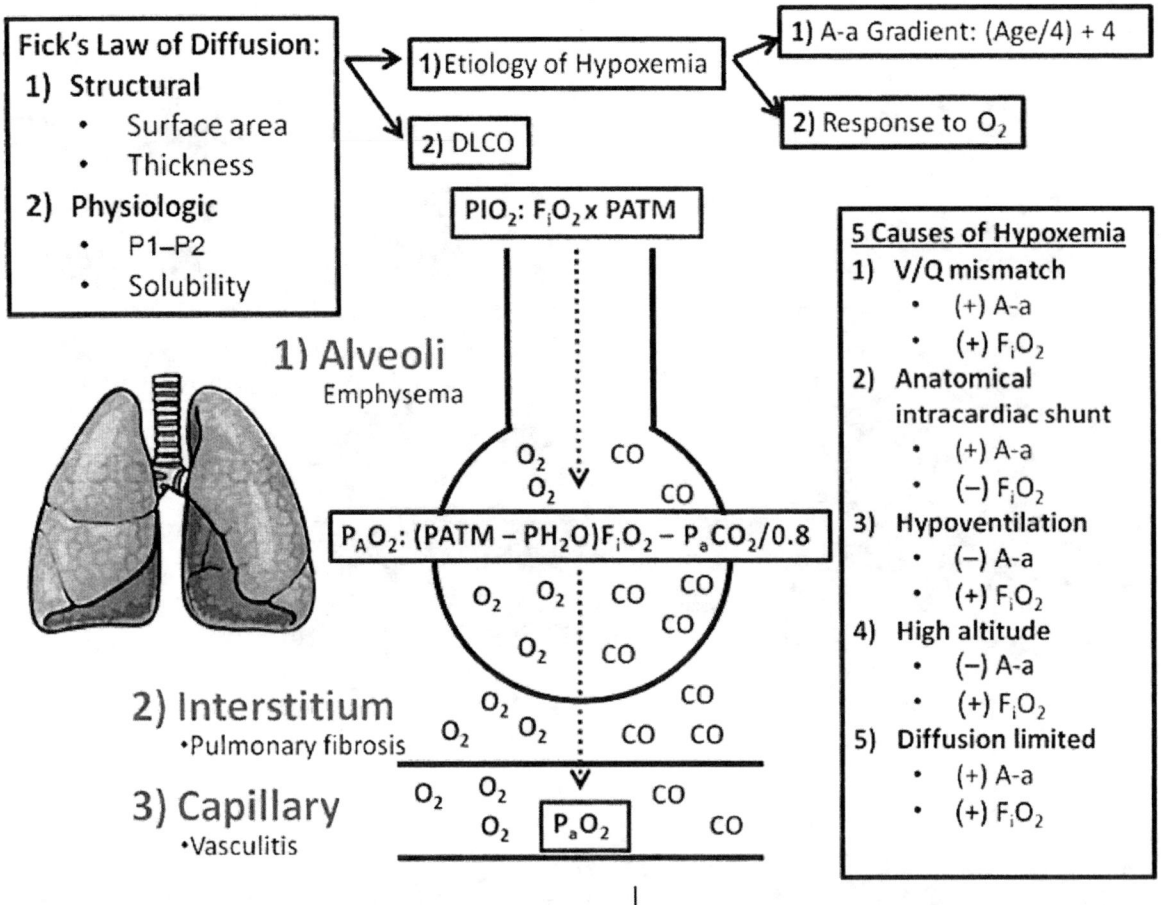

Fick's Law of Diffusion:
1) **Structural**
   - Surface area
   - Thickness
2) **Physiologic**
   - P1–P2
   - Solubility

1) Etiology of Hypoxemia

2) DLCO

1) A-a Gradient: (Age/4) + 4

2) Response to O_2

PIO_2: F_iO_2 x PATM

1) Alveoli
Emphysema

2) Interstitium
- Pulmonary fibrosis

3) Capillary
- Vasculitis

P_AO_2: $(PATM - PH_2O)F_iO_2 - P_aCO_2/0.8$

P_aO_2

5 Causes of Hypoxemia
1) **V/Q mismatch**
   - (+) A-a
   - (+) F_iO_2
2) **Anatomical intracardiac shunt**
   - (+) A-a
   - (−) F_iO_2
3) **Hypoventilation**
   - (−) A-a
   - (+) F_iO_2
4) **High altitude**
   - (−) A-a
   - (+) F_iO_2
5) **Diffusion limited**
   - (+) A-a
   - (+) F_iO_2

5 Causes of Hypoxemia
1) **V/Q mismatch**
   - The main cause of hypoxemia in lung diseases
     - Examples: PE, COPD, ARDS
   - Responds to oxygen
   - Widening of the A-a gradient
   - It may be due to:
     1) Airspace not being perfused (**dead space**)
     2) Perfused areas not being ventilated (**shunt**)

5 Causes of Hypoxemia (cont.)
2) **Anatomical shunting (2 types)**
   I. **Intracardiac shunting**
      - **Left to right**
        - ASD, VSD, PDA, PFO
      - **Right to left**
        - Terrible T's
        - Eisenmenger's complex
   II. **Intrapulmonary**
      - Hepatopulmonary syndrome
      - Pulmonary AV malformation

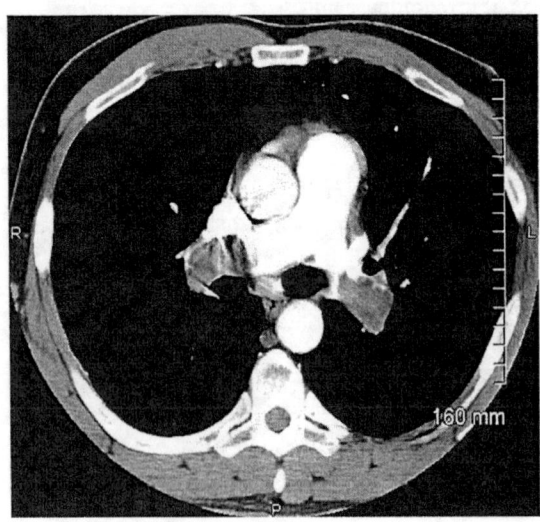

Eisenmenger's Complex

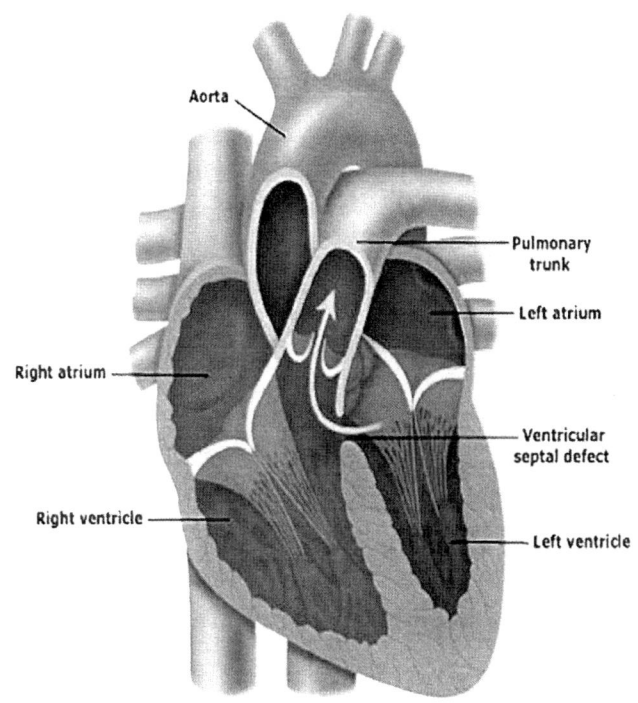

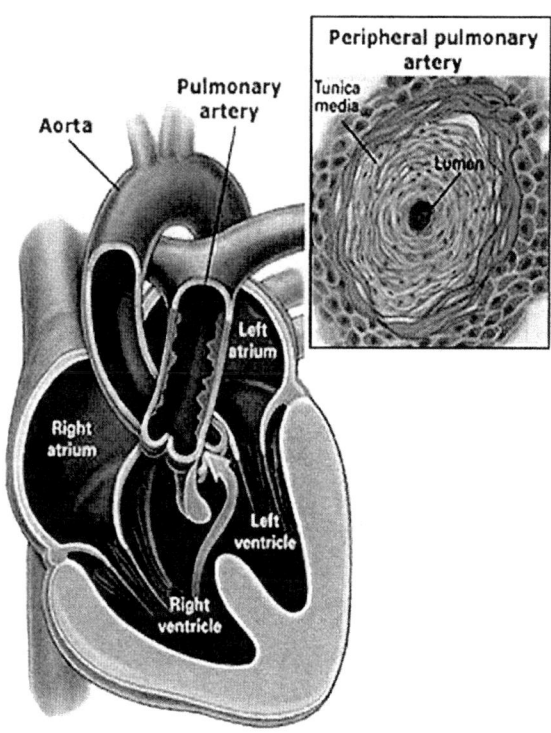

5 Causes of Hypoxemia (cont.)

3) **Hypoventilation**
   - A-a gradient is normal and responds to supplemental O_2
   - Think drug overdose and neuromuscular disorders
4) **High Altitude**
   - A-a gradient is normal and responds to supplemental O_2
5) **Decreased Diffusion**
   - Thickening of the alveolar-capillary interface to decrease diffusion of oxygen
   - Widening of A-a gradient and responds to supplemental O_2
   - Example: Interstitial lung disease

AR 3

A 48-year-old patient is evaluated for dyspnea during sleep.

The patient undergoes PFT with the following ABG: $P_aCO_2 = 65$; $P_aO_2 = 55$

Which of the following is most consistent with the clinical picture?

A. COPD
B. Neuromuscular disease
C. CHF
D. Idiopathic pulmonary fibrosis

Answer: _____

AR 3 (cont.)

- $P_AO_2 = 150 - P_aCO_2/0.8$
- A-a gradient = $P_AO_2 - P_aO_2$
- $P_AO_2 = 150 - 65 / 0.8 = 150 - 81 = 68$
- A-a gradient = $68 - 55 = 13$
- Normal A-a gradient = (age/4 + 4)
- $48/4 + 4 = 16$ (age appropriate A-a)

Pulmonary Function Test and Flow-Volume Loop

Pulmonary Function Tests
- **Consist of 3 tests:**
  1) **Static lung compartments**
     - Measured by lung volumes
       - TLC, RV
  2) **Airflow**
     - Dynamic compliance
       - FEV_1/FVC, FEF 25–50%
  3) **Alveolar membrane permeability**
     - **DLCO**

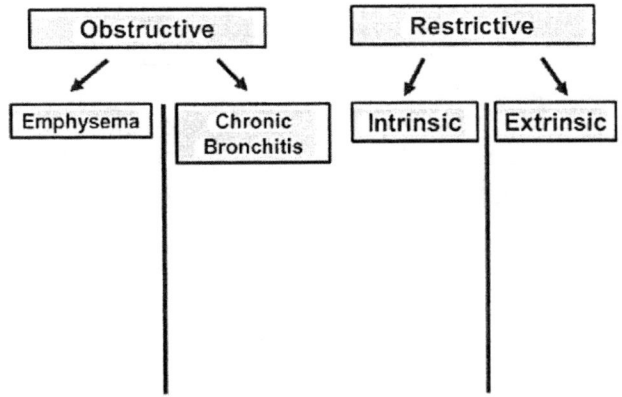

Pulmonary Function Tests (cont.)
- **In Your Office:**
  - With spirometry you can determine most of the:
    - Lung volumes & capacities
    - Flow-volume loops
    - Bronchodilator response
- **Pulmonary Function Lab:**
  - Total lung capacity
    - Helium dilution
    - Nitrogen wash-out
      - Good for PNX
    - Plethysmography
  - DLCO
    - Corrected for VA & Hgb
  - Methacholine challenge

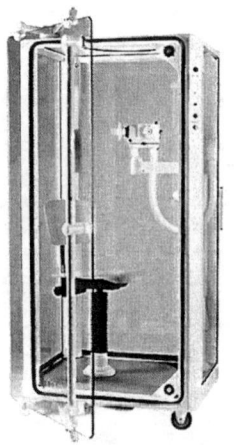

- **In general:**
  - **TLC** to assess restrictive lung disease
  - **FEV_1/FVC** to assess obstructive lung disease
    - < 70% of predictive is abnormal

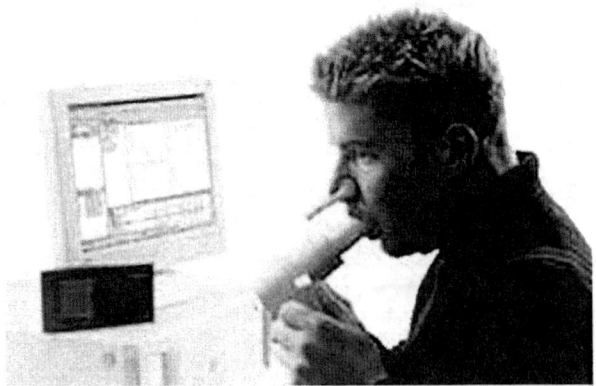

Pulmonary Function Tests (cont.)

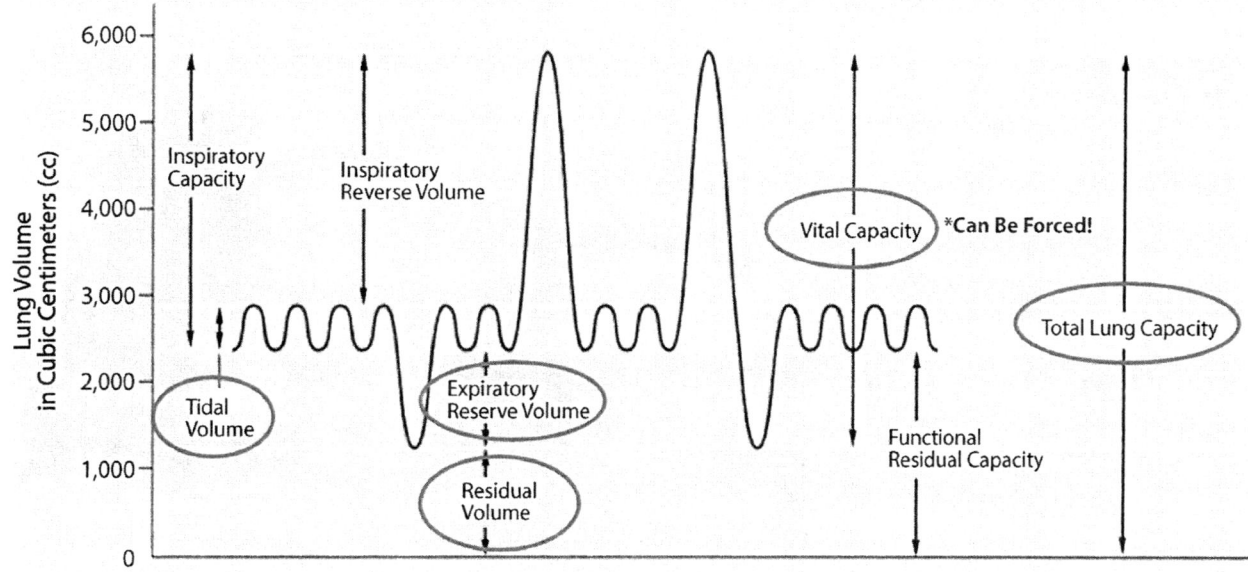

Forced Expiratory Volumes

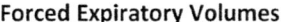

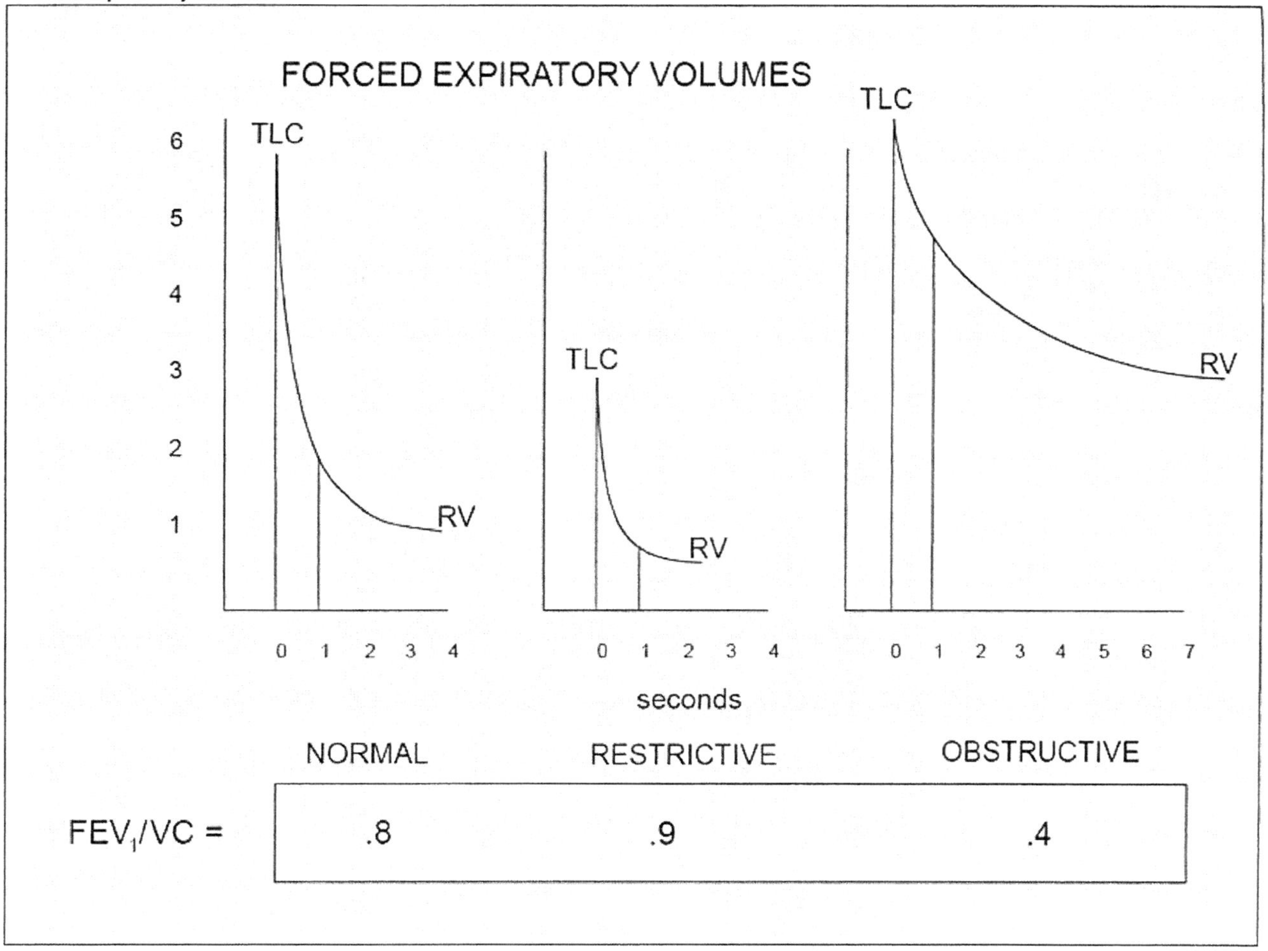

FORCED EXPIRATORY VOLUMES

	NORMAL	RESTRICTIVE	OBSTRUCTIVE
$FEV_1/VC =$	.8	.9	.4

Carbon Monoxide Diffusing Capacity (DLCO)
- Decreased by anything that interrupts **gas-blood** oxygen exchange:
  1) Alveoli
  2) Interstitium
  3) Capillary
- Decreased DLCO is seen in anemia
  - Correct for hemoglobin
- Usually normal to high DLCO in chronic asthma

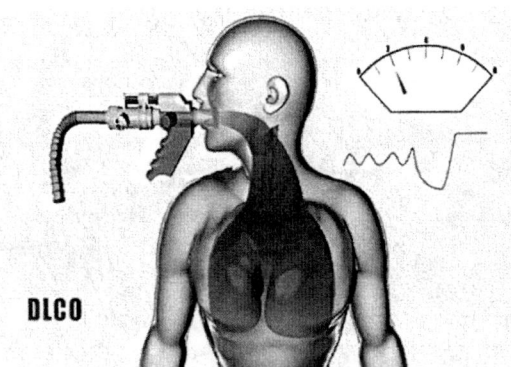

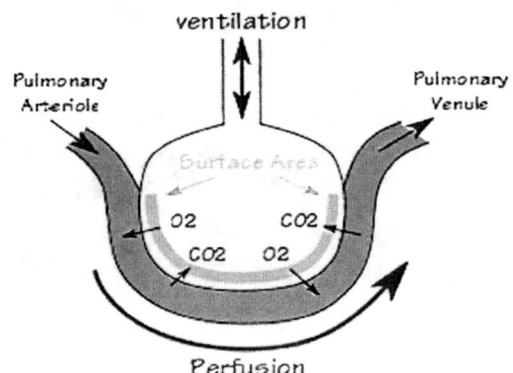

What Happens to the DLCO?
- Pulmonary embolism
- ASD or VSD
- Valsalva maneuver
- Supine position

Flow Volume Loops
- Common way of expressing **airflow** in the different lung diseases
- Derived from spirometry data, are plotted on a:
  - y axis (flow rate)
  - x axis (volume in liters)
- We get most of our information by the **shape** of the loop

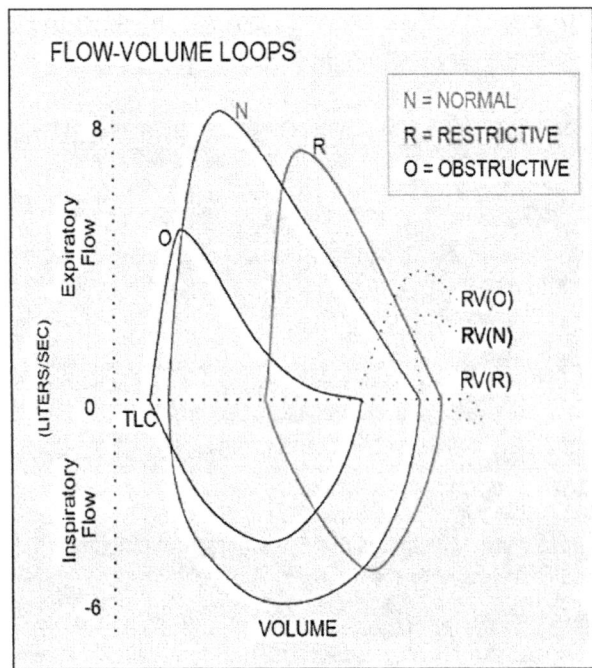

Diagnose Pulmonary Disease

	Asthma	COPD: Chronic Bronchitis	COPD: Emphysema	Pulmonary Fibrosis	PAH
FEV₁/FVC	nl or ↓	↓	↓	↑	nl
TLC	nl	nl	↑	↓	nl
DLCO	nl	nl	↓	↓	↓

Flow Volume Loops for Upper Airway Obstruction
1) **Fixed**
   - Tracheal stenosis
   - Compressive tumor
2) **Dynamic**
   - Extrathoracic
     - Flattening of the **inspiratory loop**: Vocal cord dysfunction
     - Flattening of the **expiratory loop**: Tracheomalacia
       - Flaccidity of the tracheal **support cartilage**, which leads to tracheal collapse
       - Trachea normally dilates slightly during inspiration and narrows slightly during expiration
       - These processes are exaggerated in tracheomalacia, leading to airway collapse on expiration

Flow Volume Loops for Upper Airway Obstruction (cont.)

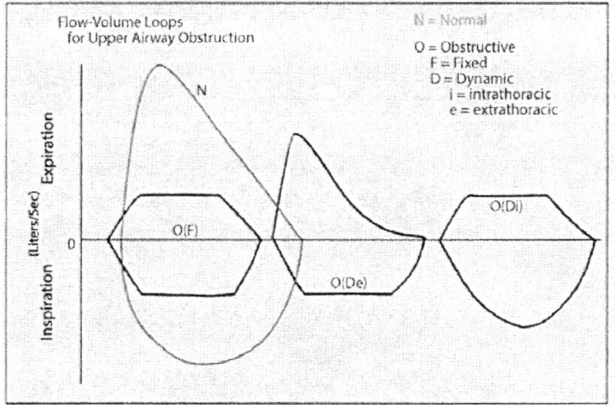

AR 4

A 50-something-year-old male presents with cough and breathlessness.

Test	Pre-BD			Post-BD	
	Actual	Pred	% Pred	Actual	% Chg
FVC (L)	3.17	4.22	75	3.98	25
FEV_1 (L)	2.16	3.39	63	2.86	30
FEV_1/FVC (%)	68	80		72	

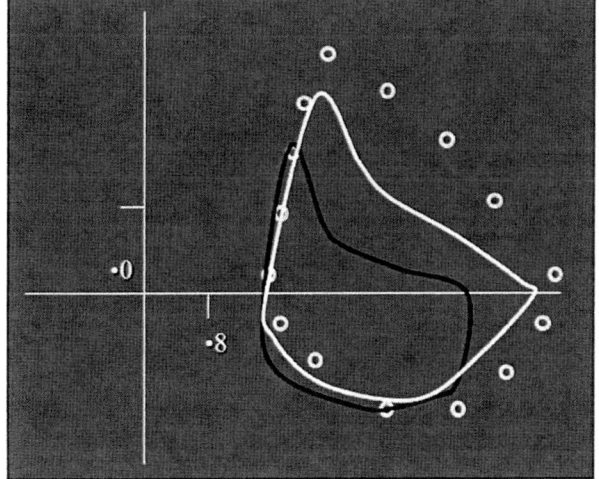

AR 4 (cont.)

Which of the following is the patient's most likely diagnosis?

A. Variable extrathoracic obstruction
B. Mild lower airway obstruction with reversibility
C. Severe lower airway obstruction without reversibility
D. Variable intrathoracic obstruction
E. Fixed obstruction

Answer: _____

AR 5

A 40-something-year-old female smoker and IDU presents with exertional breathlessness.

Test	Pre-BD			Post-BD	
	Actual	Pred	% Pred	Actual	% Chg
FVC (L)	0.92	3.10	30	0.72	– 17
FEV_1 (L)	0.47	2.53	19	0.42	– 10
FEV_1/FVC (%)	51	82		58	8
RV (L)	3.80	1.47	258		
TLC (L)	4.72	4.41	107		
DLCO	0.73	25	2.92		

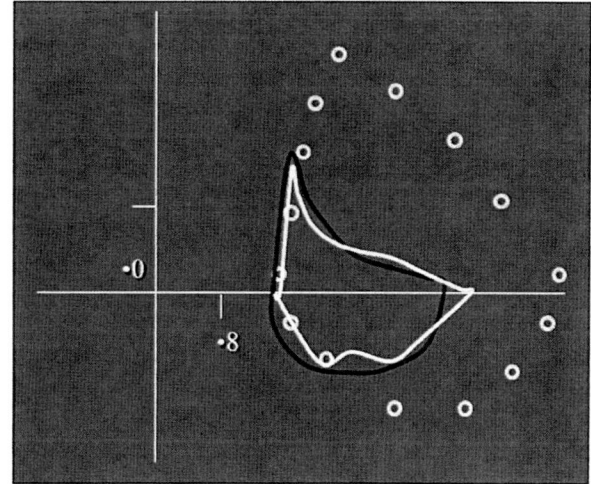

AR 5 (cont.)

Which of the following is the patient's most likely diagnosis?

A. Asthma
B. Hypersensitivity pneumonitis
C. Pulmonary arterial hypertension
D. COPD
E. Vocal cord dysfunction

Answer: _____

AR 6

A 20-something-year-old male with history of prolonged tracheal intubation, after Guillain-Barré 2 years ago, presents with breathlessness and wheezing.

Test	Pre-BD			Post-BD	
	Actual	Pred	% Pred	Actual	% Chg
FVC (L)	4.70	4.33	108	–	–
FEV_1 (L)	2.52	3.70	68	–	–
FEV_1/FVC (%)	54	85			

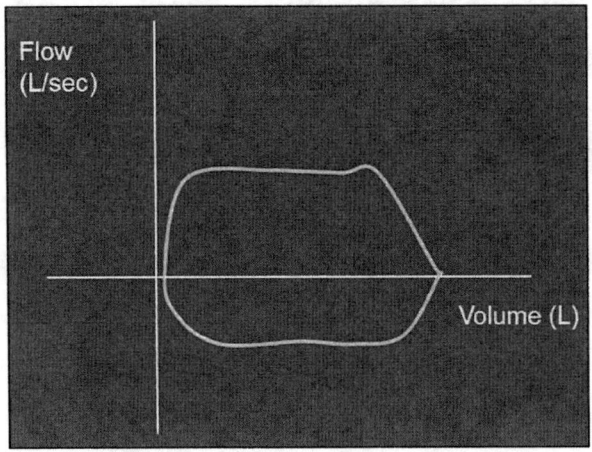

Flow (L/sec)

Volume (L)

AR 6 (cont.)

Which of the following best describes the patient's abnormality?

A. Restrictive defect
B. Variable intrathoracic obstruction
C. Variable extrathoracic obstruction
D. Fixed obstruction
E. Lower airway obstruction

Answer: _____

AR 7

A 30-something-year-old female tax accountant with a German shepherd and a cockatiel develops dyspnea.

Test	Pre-BD			Post-BD	
	Actual	Pred	% Pred	Actual	% Chg
FVC (L)	1.70	4.38	39	1.76	4
FEV_1 (L)	1.55	3.62	43	1.54	0
FEV_1/FVC (%)	91	83		88	−3
RV (L)	1.03	1.98	52		
TLC (L)	2.66	6.10	44		
DLCO	5.00	31.98	16		

AR 7 (cont.)

Which of the following flow-volume loops would be expected for this patient?

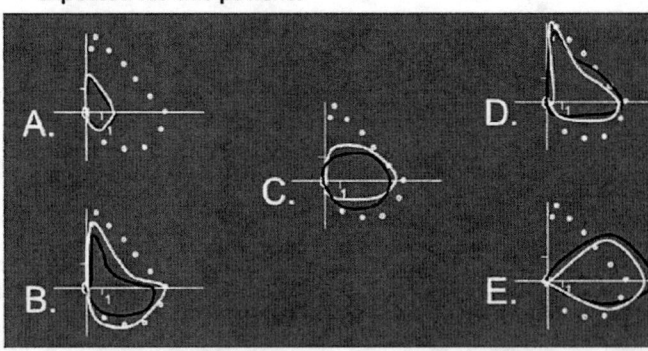

Answer: _____

AR 8

A 40-year-old female presents complaining of progressive dyspnea on exertion without chest pain.

Test	Pre-BD			Post-BD	
	Actual	Pred	% Pred	Actual	% Chg
FVC (L)	2.35	2.85	82	2.20	−6
FEV_1 (L)	1.97	2.29	86	1.98	0
FEV_1/FVC (%)	84	80		90	
RV (L)	1.67	1.58	105		
TLC (L)	4.23	4.37	97		
DLCO	9.90	22.85	43		

Which of the following is the best <u>next</u> step in this patient's management?

A. Direct laryngoscopy
B. Prescription of continuous positive pressure ventilation during sleep
C. Inhaled albuterol as needed
D. Echocardiogram
E. CT pulmonary angiography

Answer: _____

Bonus Question

A 58-year-old female with recurrent otitis media presents with cough.

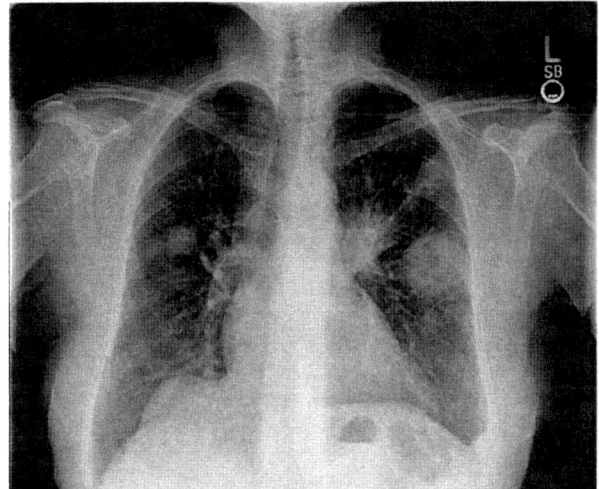

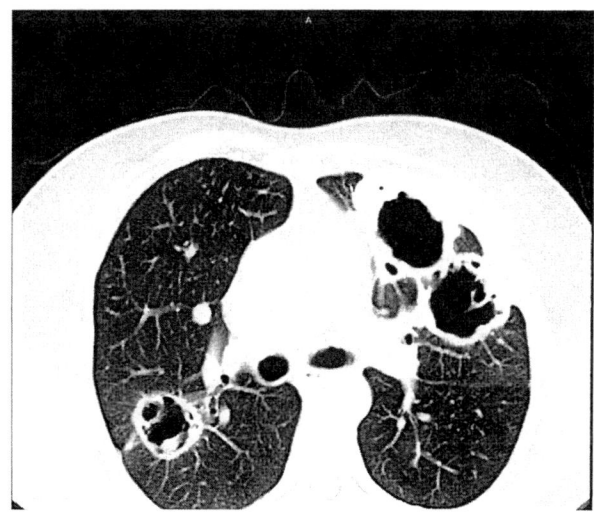

Diagnosis
Granulomatosis with polyangiitis (Wegener's)

6 Months Later …
- Patient is having increased SOB and wheezing
- Treated with:
  - Bronchodilators
  - Inhaled corticosteroids
- No improvement
  - Pulmonary consulted
  - CT Chest
  - PFTs

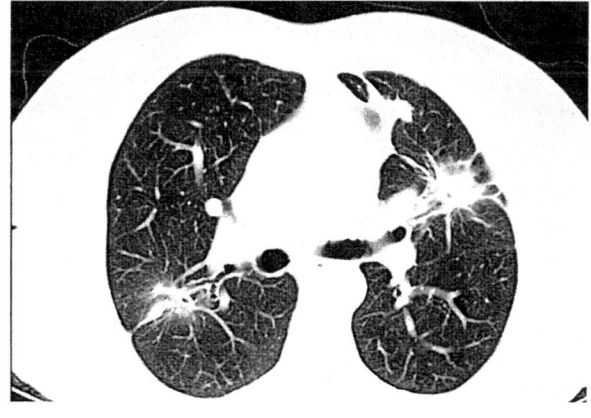

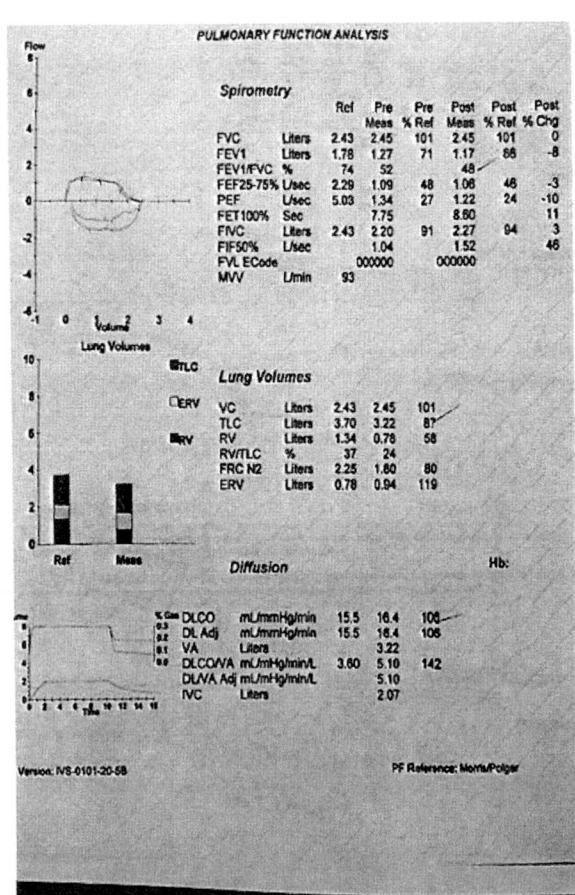

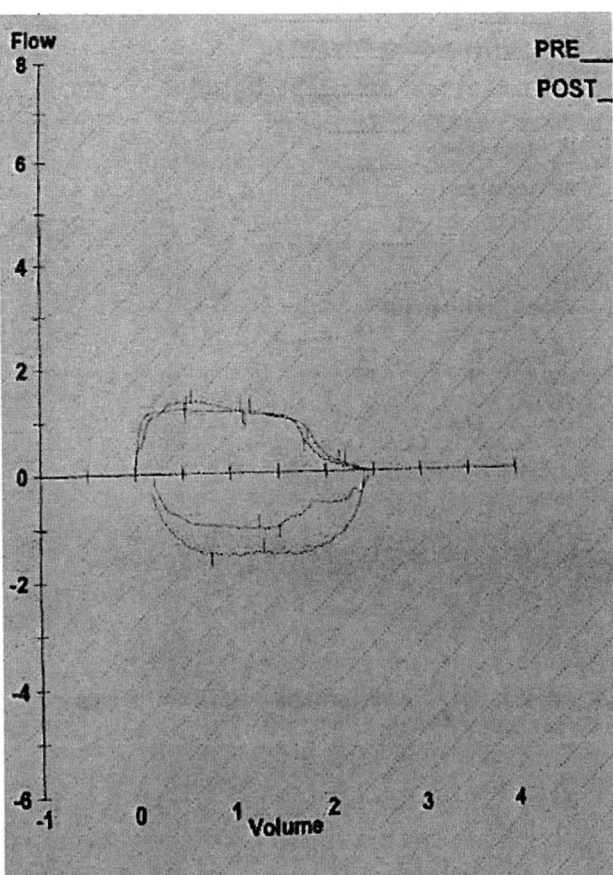

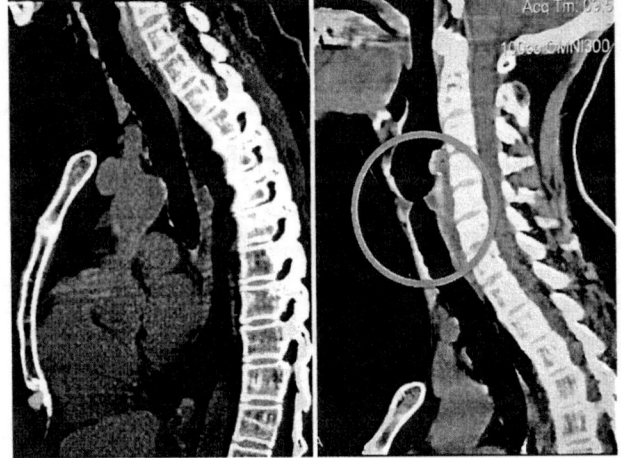

Subglottic stenosis secondary to GPA

Asthma

Asthma Definition & Diagnosis
- **Definition:**
  - **Chronic** inflammatory disease of the respiratory tree to various **sensitizing** stimuli, resulting in **reversible** airway obstruction
  - Characterized by:
    1) **Bronchial hyperresponsiveness** (BHR)
       - Challenge testing
    2) Abnormalities in airway **smooth muscle** function
       - Bronchial thermoplasty

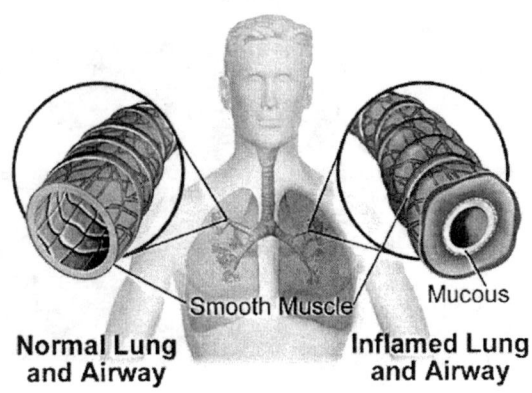

Asthma Diagnosis
Traditional:
- Pattern of symptoms and response to therapy
- Spirometry and/or PFTs + BD response
  - FEV_1/FVC, FEV_1, PEF
  - TLC, DLCO
- Challenge testing
  - Exercise-induced bronchoconstriction
    & chronic cough
    - Exercise, cold air, methacholine

Other considerations:
- Fraction of exhaled NO (FE_{NO})
  - Eosinophilic inflammation in the airways stimulates airway epithelial cells to produce NO
- Sputum "eosinophils"
  - Charcot-Leyden crystals
    - They are indicative of a disease involving eosinophilic inflammation
  - Curschmann's spirals
    - Spiral-shaped mucous plugs in the sputum

Asthma Signs & Classification
- The **classic** signs and symptoms of asthma are:
  - Intermittent dyspnea
  - Cough
  - Wheezing
- Clinically classified according to:
  - Frequency of symptoms
  - Forced expiratory volume in 1 second (FEV_1)
  - Peak expiratory flow rate
- Asthma may also be classified as:
  1) Atopic (extrinsic)
     - IgE (omalizumab [Xolair])
  2) Nonatopic (intrinsic)

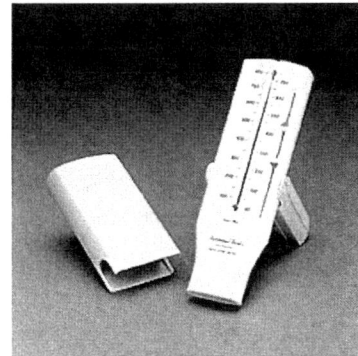

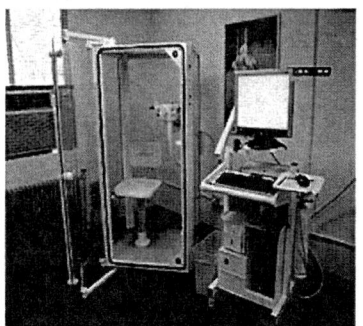

AR 9
What is the main antigen-presenting cell in the lung for asthmatics?
A. Mast cell
B. Eosinophil
C. Dendritic cell and macrophage
D. Neutrophil

Answer: _____

Dendritic Cell & Macrophage
1) **Dendritic cells**
   - Langerhans cells are dendritic cells (antigen-presenting immune cells) and contain large granules called Birbeck granules
2) **Macrophages**

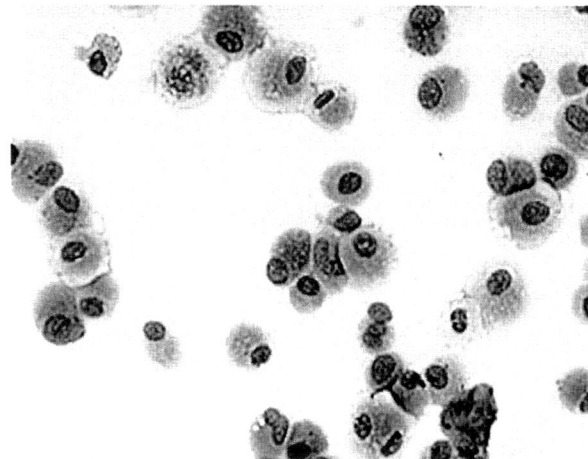

BAL showing an abundant amount of macrophages

AR 10
What is the main inflammatory cell in the airways of asthmatics?
A. Mast cell
B. Eosinophil
C. Neutrophil
D. Basophil

Answer: _____

Eosinophil

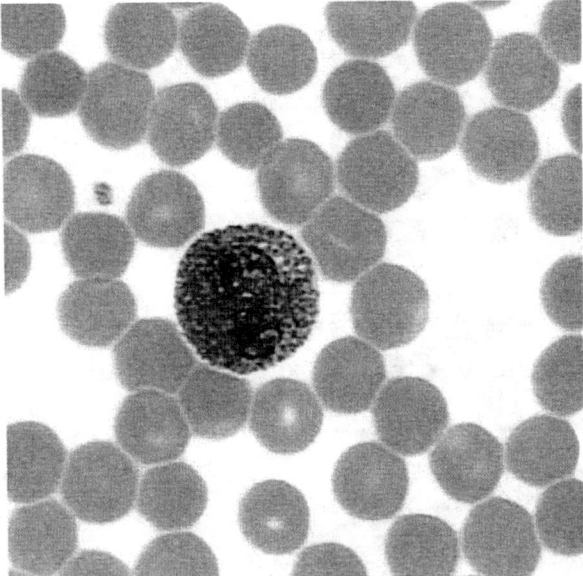

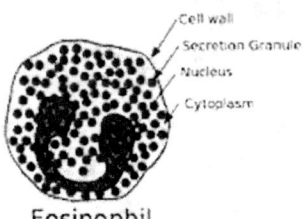

Eosinophil

Pharmacologic Asthma Treatment
- **Antiinflammatory medicines**
  - **Corticosteroids**
    - Route: Oral, inhaled, IV, and intramuscular
- **Direct bronchodilators** (short- and long-acting)
  - **β_2-agonists** (increases cAMP)
    - Salbutamol, albuterol, levalbuterol
  - **Anticholinergics** (M3 receptor in smooth muscle)
    - Helpful & recommended in the acute setting
    - Ipratropium bromide
  - **Methylxanthines** (relaxes bronchial smooth muscle)
    - Theophylline
    - Aminophylline (short-acting)
  - **Adrenergic agonists** (inhaled epinephrine)
    - Primatene Mist
      - OTC MDI
      - Removed 12/31/2011
    - Racemic epinephrine (Asthmanefrin)
      - OTC hand-held atomizer

- **Mast-cell stabilizers**
  - Cromolyn sodium and nedocromil
    - Not for asthma attack
    - 2 puffs qid
    - 4 weeks to get optimal effect
- **Leukotriene inhibitors**
  - Zileuton
    - Leukotriene synthesis inhibitor
  - Montelukast
    - Leukotriene receptor antagonist

The Dangers of Inhalers

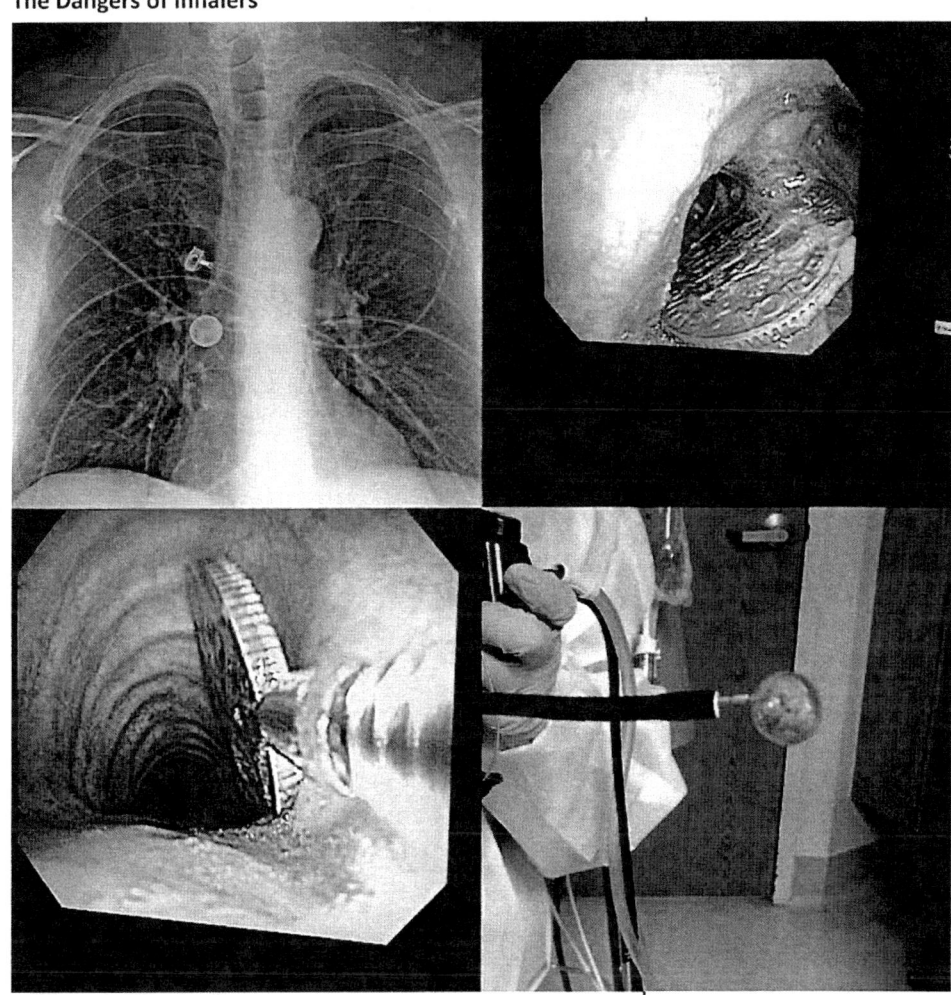

AR 11

Which of the following treatments for adult patients who have severe allergic asthma has been demonstrated to significantly reduce the requirement for oral steroid therapy in multiple trials?

	Mepolizumab	Omalizumab	Bronchial thermoplasty
A.	Yes	Yes	No
B.	Yes	No	No
C.	No	No	Yes
D.	Yes	Yes	Yes

Answer: _____

Answer: D

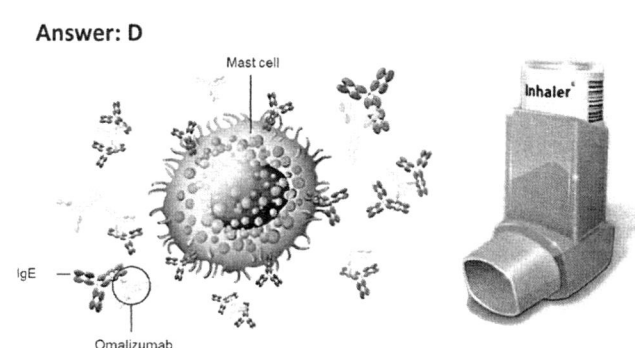

© 2017 MedStudy Internal Medicine Video Board Review – Pulmonary Medicine • Raj Dasgupta, MD

Asthma Immunologic Therapy
- **Omalizumab**
  - Subcutaneous injection for people who are 12 years of age and older
  - Moderate-to-severe persistent asthma that is triggered by year-round allergens in the air
  - Dosed on **IgE levels** and weight
  - Epinephrine auto-injector

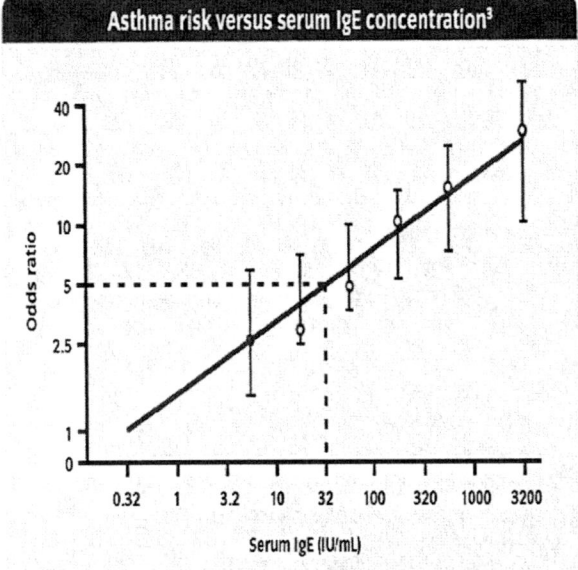

Asthma risk versus serum IgE concentration³

Burrows B, et al. Association of asthma with serum IgE levels and skin-test reactivity to allergens. *N Engl J Med.* 1989;320:272–277.

AR 12
Should you follow IgE levels after starting omalizumab?
A. Yes.
B. No.
C. Please tell me.

Answer: _____

AR 12 (cont.)
- Total IgE levels are elevated during treatment above the patient's baseline and remain elevated for up to 1 year after the discontinuation of treatment
- Retesting of IgE levels during omalizumab treatment is unnecessary and cannot be used as a guide for dose determination

AR 13

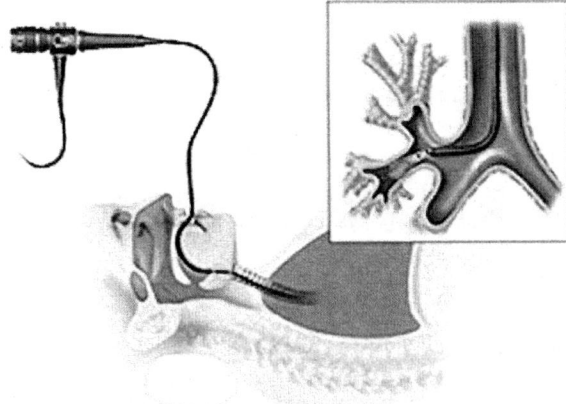

Is bronchial thermoplasty (BT) FDA approved for severe persistent asthma?
A. Yes.
B. No.
C. Only when it is sunny outside.

Answer: _____

AR 13 (cont.)
- FDA approved on April 27, 2010
- Nonpharmacologic therapy for severe asthma in patients 18 years of age and older not well controlled with currently available medical therapies
- Targets airway remodeling by reducing airway smooth muscle mass that is responsible for:
  - Bronchoconstriction
  - Mucus production
  - Airway hyperresponsiveness

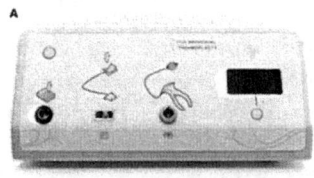

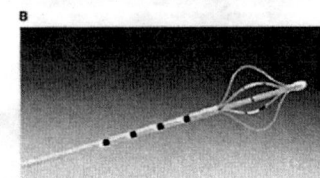

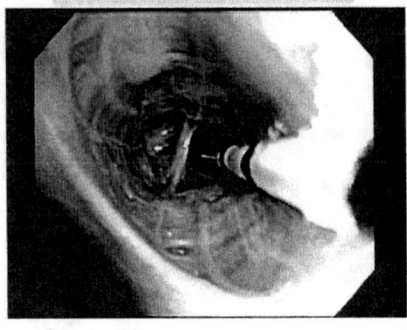

Bronchial Thermoplasty
- **3 separate procedures**:
  - 1 for each lower lobe
  - 1 for both upper lobes
  - Performed approximately 3 weeks apart
- **Benefits (5-year data)**:
  - 32% reduction in asthma attacks
  - 84% reduction in ED visits
  - 66% reduction in days lost from work, school, or other daily activities
  - 73% reduction in hospitalizations
- **Risks**
  - Immediately following the procedure, there is an expected transient increase in the frequency and worsening of respiratory-related symptoms
    - Patients are premedicated with steroids

The catheter delivers a series of 10-second temperature-controlled bursts of radio frequency energy that heat the lining of the lungs to 149.0° F (65.0° C).

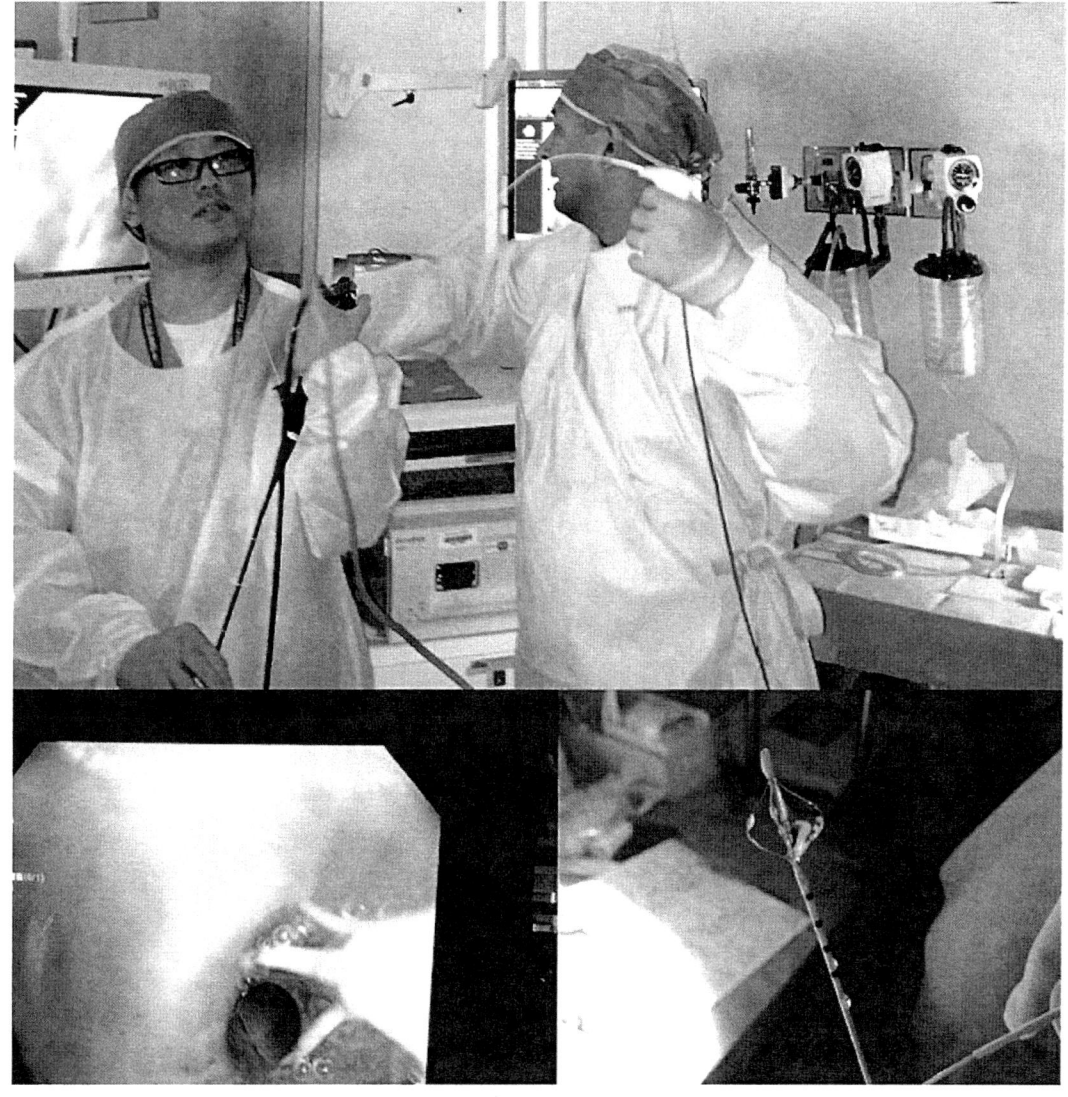

© 2017 MedStudy Internal Medicine Video Board Review – Pulmonary Medicine • Raj Dasgupta, MD

"What's New"
- FDA has recommended **mepolizumab** for add-on maintenance treatment in patients age 18 years or older with severe eosinophilic (peripheral) asthma
- Monoclonal antibody that binds to and inactivates interleukin-5

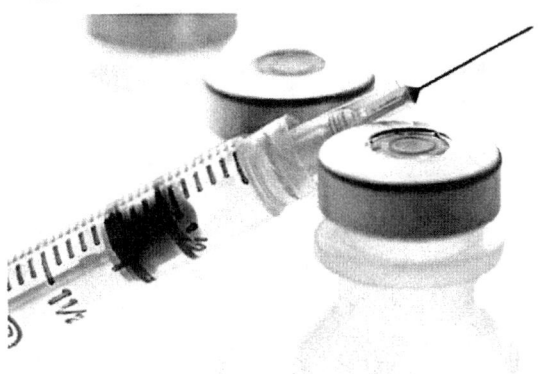

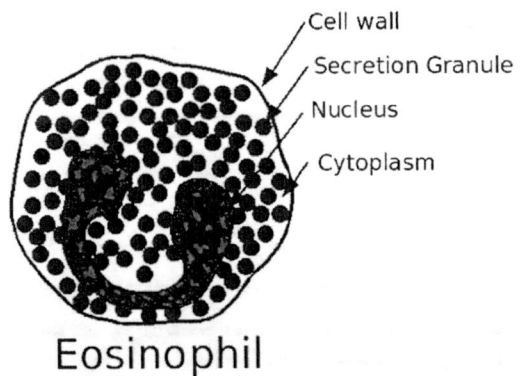

Cell wall
Secretion Granule
Nucleus
Cytoplasm

Eosinophil

Drugs to Be Careful of in Asthma
- Aspirin & NSAIDs
  - Samter's triad:
    1) Nasal polyps
    2) Asthma
    3) Aspirin intolerance
- Nonselective beta-blockers
- ACE inhibitors

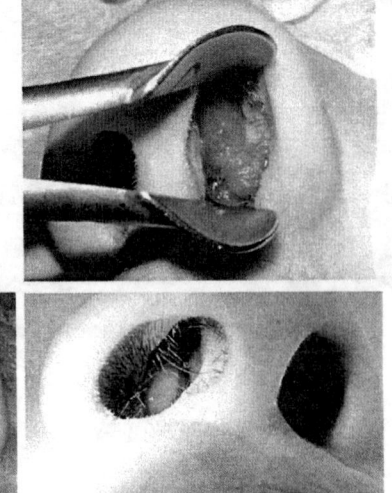

Asthma-Related Diseases
ABPA
- The major diagnostic features of classic ABPA include:
  - History of asthma
  - Immediate skin test reactivity to *Aspergillus* antigens
  - Precipitating serum antibodies to *A. fumigatus*
  - Elevated serum total IgE
  - Peripheral blood eosinophilia
  - Central bronchiectasis on chest CT
  - Elevated specific serum IgE and IgG to *A. fumigatus*

Churg-Strauss
- "Eosinophilic granulomatosis with polyangiitis"
- The ACR has established 6 criteria:
  1) Asthma
  2) Greater than 10% peripheral eosinophils on the differential
  3) Mononeuropathy or polyneuropathy
  4) Migratory or transient pulmonary opacities detected radiographically
  5) Paranasal sinus abnormality
  6) Biopsy containing a blood vessel showing the accumulation of eosinophils in extravascular areas

SEVERITY COMPONENTS	INTERMITTENT	PERSISTENT ASTHMA: daily medication		
		MILD	MODERATE	SEVERE
Symptoms	Less than once a week	More than twice per week but not daily	Daily	Throughout the day
Nocturnal Symptoms	Less than twice a day per month	Three-four times per month	More than once a week but not every night	Often every night per week
Interference with activity	Brief exacerbations	Exacerbations may cause minor limitation of activity and sleep	Exacerbations more than twice a week and may cause some limitation of activity and sleep	Frequent exacerbations with marked limitation of physical activity
SABA use	≤ 2 days per week	>2 days per week, but not daily and not more than once on any day	Daily	Several times per day
Pulmonary Function Test	• Normal FEV_1 between exacerbations • FEV_1 >80% predicted • FEV_1/FVC normal	• FEV_1 >80% predicted • FEV_1/FVC normal	• FEV_1 >60% but <80% predicted • FEV_1/FVC reduced 5%	• FEV_1 <60% predicted • FEV_1/FVC reduced 5%
Recommended Treatment Strategy	STEP-1 *Preferred:* SABA PRN	STEP-2 *Preferred:* Low-dose ICS *Alternative:* Cromolyn, LTRA, Nedocromil, or Theophylline	STEP-3 *Preferred:* Low-dose ICS + LABA *OR* Medium-dose ICS *Alternative:* Low-dose ICS + either LTRA, Theophylline, or Zileuton	STEP-4 or 5 STEP-4: Preferred: Medium-dose ICS + LABA Alternative: Medium-dose ICS + either LTRA, Theophylline, or Zileuton STEP-5: Preferred: High-dose ICS + LABA AND Consider Omalizumab for patients who have allergies
			Consider Oral Steroids	Consider Oral Steroids

Step-up if needed (First, check adherence, environmental control, and comorbid conditions)

ASSESS CONTROL

Step down if possible (and asthma is well controlled at least 3 months)

Each Step: patient education, environmental control, and management of comorbidities.
Steps 2-4: Consider subcutaneous allergen immunotherapy for patients who have allergic asthma.

Quick-relief medication for all patients:
- SABA as needed for symptoms. Intensity of treatment depends on severity of symptoms: up to 3 treatments at 20-minute intervals as needed. Short course of oral systemic corticosteroids may be needed.
- Use of SABA >2 days a week for symptom relief (not prevention of EIA) generally indicates inadequate control and the need to step up therapy.

Adapted from National Heart, Blood, and Lung Institute Expert Panel Report 3 (EPR 3). Guidelines for the Diagnosis and Management of Asthma. NIH Publication no. 08-4051,2007.

COPD

COPD Definition
- The Global Initiative for Chronic Obstructive Lung Disease (**GOLD**):
  - Is a **preventable** and treatable disease
  - Its pulmonary component is characterized by airflow limitation that is **not fully reversible**
  - Associated with an abnormal inflammatory response of the lungs to **noxious** particles or gases

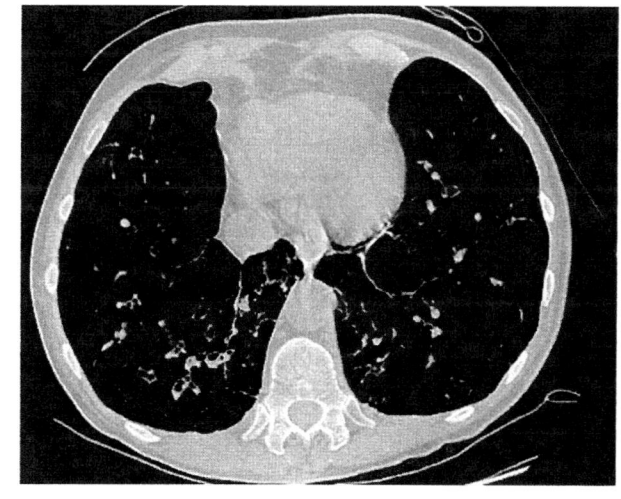

© 2017 MedStudy Internal Medicine Video Board Review – Pulmonary Medicine • Raj Dasgupta, MD

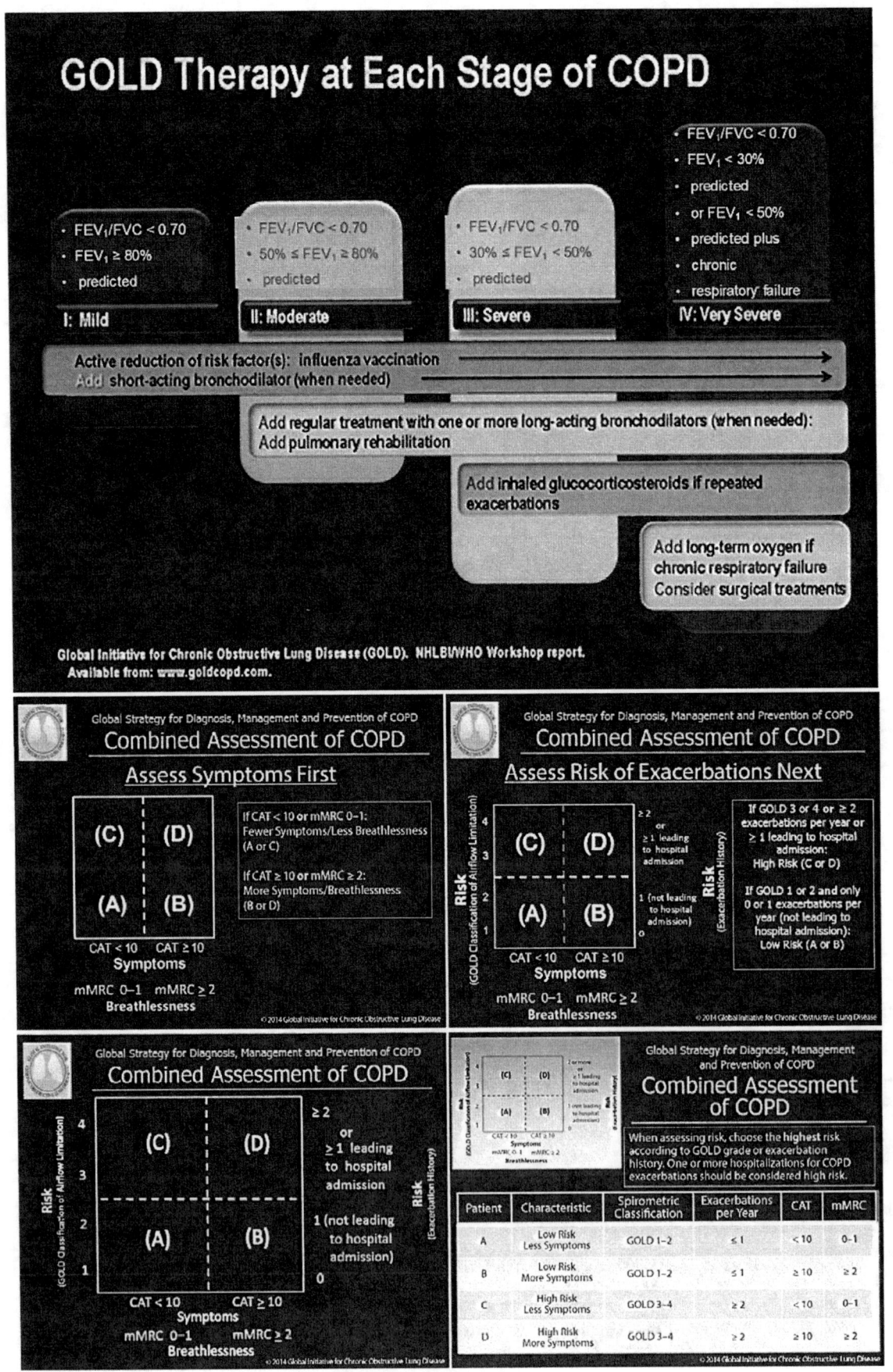

GOLD Therapy at Each Stage of COPD

- $FEV_1/FVC < 0.70$
- $FEV_1 \geq 80\%$
- predicted

I: Mild

- $FEV_1/FVC < 0.70$
- $50\% \leq FEV_1 \geq 80\%$
- predicted

II: Moderate

- $FEV_1/FVC < 0.70$
- $30\% \leq FEV_1 < 50\%$
- predicted

III: Severe

- $FEV_1/FVC < 0.70$
- $FEV_1 < 30\%$
- predicted
- or $FEV_1 < 50\%$
- predicted plus
- chronic
- respiratory failure

IV: Very Severe

Active reduction of risk factor(s): influenza vaccination
Add short-acting bronchodilator (when needed)

Add regular treatment with one or more long-acting bronchodilators (when needed):
Add pulmonary rehabilitation

Add inhaled glucocorticosteroids if repeated exacerbations

Add long-term oxygen if chronic respiratory failure
Consider surgical treatments

Global Initiative for Chronic Obstructive Lung Disease (GOLD). NHLBI/WHO Workshop report.
Available from: www.goldcopd.com.

Global Strategy for Diagnosis, Management and Prevention of COPD
Combined Assessment of COPD

Assess Symptoms First

| (C) | (D) |
| (A) | (B) |

CAT < 10   CAT ≥ 10
Symptoms
mMRC 0–1   mMRC ≥ 2
Breathlessness

If CAT < 10 or mMRC 0–1:
Fewer Symptoms/Less Breathlessness (A or C)

If CAT ≥ 10 or mMRC ≥ 2:
More Symptoms/Breathlessness (B or D)

© 2014 Global Initiative for Chronic Obstructive Lung Disease

---

Global Strategy for Diagnosis, Management and Prevention of COPD
Combined Assessment of COPD

Assess Risk of Exacerbations Next

Risk (GOLD Classification of Airflow Limitation) — 4, 3, 2, 1

| (C) | (D) |
| (A) | (B) |

CAT < 10   CAT ≥ 10
Symptoms
mMRC 0–1   mMRC ≥ 2
Breathlessness

Risk (Exacerbation History):
≥ 2 or ≥ 1 leading to hospital admission
1 (not leading to hospital admission)

If GOLD 3 or 4 or ≥ 2 exacerbations per year or ≥ 1 leading to hospital admission:
High Risk (C or D)

If GOLD 1 or 2 and only 0 or 1 exacerbations per year (not leading to hospital admission):
Low Risk (A or B)

© 2014 Global Initiative for Chronic Obstructive Lung Disease

---

Global Strategy for Diagnosis, Management and Prevention of COPD
Combined Assessment of COPD

Risk (GOLD Classification of Airflow Limitation) — 4, 3, 2, 1

| (C) | (D) |
| (A) | (B) |

CAT < 10   CAT ≥ 10
Symptoms
mMRC 0–1   mMRC ≥ 2
Breathlessness

Risk (Exacerbation History):
≥ 2 or ≥ 1 leading to hospital admission
1 (not leading to hospital admission)
0

© 2014 Global Initiative for Chronic Obstructive Lung Disease

---

Global Strategy for Diagnosis, Management and Prevention of COPD
Combined Assessment of COPD

When assessing risk, choose the highest risk according to GOLD grade or exacerbation history. One or more hospitalizations for COPD exacerbations should be considered high risk.

Patient	Characteristic	Spirometric Classification	Exacerbations per Year	CAT	mMRC
A	Low Risk Less Symptoms	GOLD 1–2	≤ 1	< 10	0–1
B	Low Risk More Symptoms	GOLD 1–2	≤ 1	≥ 10	≥ 2
C	High Risk Less Symptoms	GOLD 3–4	≥ 2	< 10	0–1
D	High Risk More Symptoms	GOLD 3–4	≥ 2	≥ 10	≥ 2

© 2014 Global Initiative for Chronic Obstructive Lung Disease

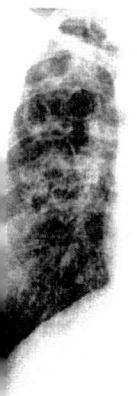
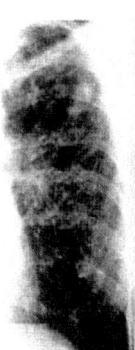
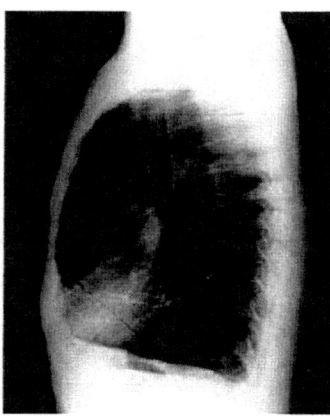

COPD

- COPD is a mixture of:
  - **Emphysema** (pink puffer)
    - Anatomic/Histologic diagnosis
  - **Chronic bronchitis** (blue bloater)
    - Epidemiologic diagnosis
      - Cough and sputum > 3 months for 2 years
  - **Asthma & COPD overlap syndrome** (ACOS)
- Most patients have characteristics of both with a predominance of one

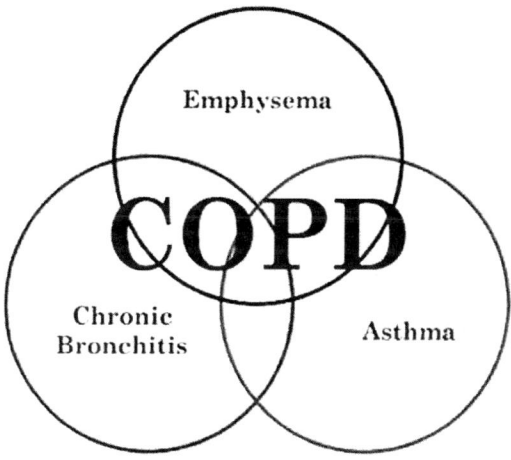

Treatment Categories and Options

- **Smoking cessation**
  - Varenicline titrating up to 2 mg daily for 12 weeks
  - Bupropion titrating up to 300 mg daily
  - Nicotine replacement
  - CBT
- **Bronchodilator therapy**
  - β_2-agonist
  - Anticholinergic
  - Methylxanthines
  - LABA & LAMA combinations
- **Corticosteroids**
  - Inhaled (controversial)
  - Systemic

- **Supplemental oxygen therapy**
  - OSA & the "overlap syndrome"
- **Drugs for reducing exacerbations**
  - Azithromycin
  - Roflumilast
- **Pulmonary rehabilitation**
- **Surgical therapy**
  - Lung volume reduction surgery (LVRS)
  - Lung transplant

Bronchodilator Treatment

1) **Anticholinergic agents**
   - Short-acting (GOLD stage I)
     - Ipratropium bromide
   - Long-acting
     - Tiotropium: **UPLIFT** trial, reduced exacerbations
2) **β_2-agonists**
   - Short-acting (GOLD stage I)
     - Albuterol, levalbuterol
   - Long-acting
     - Combination therapy reduced exacerbations
     - **SUN, TORCH**, and **SHINE**
3) **Methylxanthines**
   - Theophylline
     - 200 mg extended release PO daily

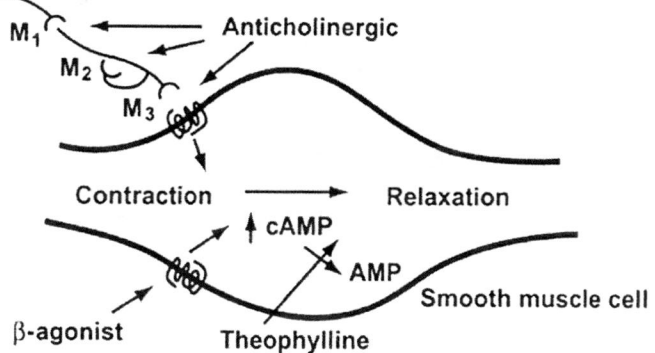

Oxygen Therapy for COPD

- Criteria for starting home oxygen (**mortality reduction**):
1) Resting P_aO_2 < 55 or
2) O_2 sat (S_aO_2) < 88% or
3) P_aO_2 < 59 mmHg (O_2 sat > 89%) with evidence of:
   - Cor pulmonale
   - Erythrocytosis
     - Hematocrit > 55%
- Decreases morbidity and mortality in severe **chronic** COPD
  - Keep these patients on supplemental oxygen 24 hours/day
    - Long-term continuous oxygen treatment in COPD: Nocturnal Oxygen Treatment Trial (NOTT)

Lung Volume Reduction Therapy

- **Lung volume reduction surgery**
  - The idea is that removing ruined areas of the lung:
    - Reduces dead space
    - Improves chest wall and diaphragm dynamics
  - There was no overall survival advantage in the LVRS group, <u>except</u> for mainly upper-lobe emphysema + poor exercise capacity

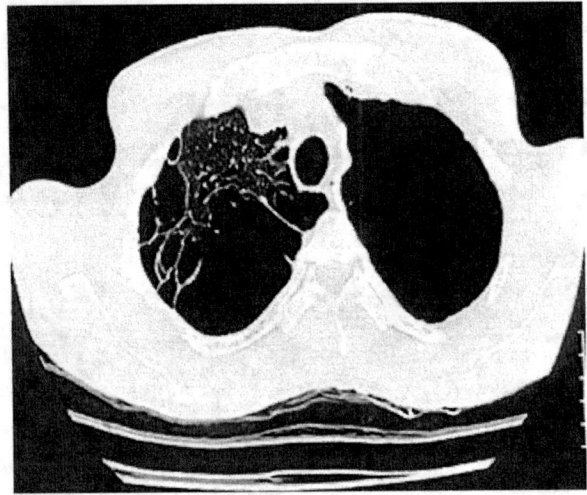

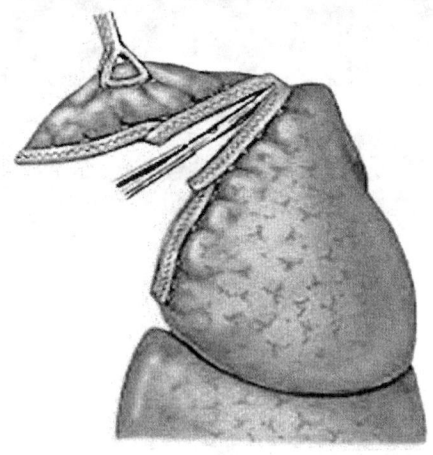

N Engl J Med. 2003;348(21):2059.

Lung Transplant

- Substantial improvement in exercise tolerance and quality of life
- Transplantation (over the past few years) **has convincingly** been shown to prolong survival from this disease
- Transplant recipients face
  - Infection secondary to immunosuppression
  - Toxic effects of immunosuppressant drugs
  - Acute and chronic rejection of lung allograft
- Can get **single** and double lung transplant

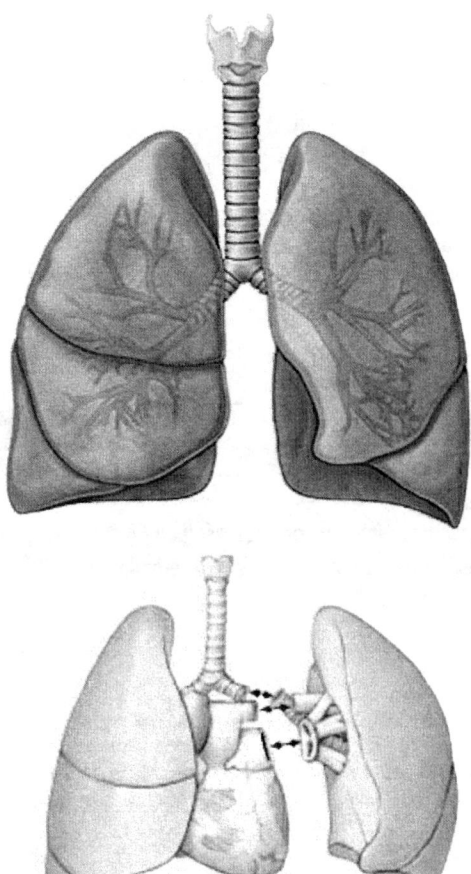

AR 14

59-year-old man who has a long-standing history of COPD with **chronic bronchitis** is evaluated in follow-up of his most recent exacerbation 6 weeks ago, which necessitated a visit to the ER. At that time, he was treated with a 7-day outpatient course of oral prednisone and azithromycin. His symptoms are now at baseline, but he still has a productive morning cough, which is "minimal."

The patient reports that he has dyspnea climbing stairs, but he is able to work as an accountant without difficulty. He smoked 2 packs of cigarettes daily for 20 years, before quitting at 50 years of age. He has had **2 COPD exacerbations** in the past year. His current therapeutic regimen is tiotropium, 18 mcg daily, and salmeterol/fluticasone propionate, 50/250 mcg twice daily.

On exam, temp 98.6° F (37.0° C), HR 78 bpm, RR 12 bpm and BP 130/80 mmHg.
Spirometry reveals FEV_1 45%, FVC 58%, and FEV_1/FVC 61%.
Oxygen saturation 93% at rest on RA.
Serum α_1-antitrypsin levels are normal.

AR 14 (cont.)

Which of the following should you recommend to reduce the frequency of this patient's exacerbations?

A. Add prednisone, 5 mg daily.
B. Add roflumilast, 500 mcg daily.
C. Change salmeterol/fluticasone to 50/500 mcg bid.
D. Discontinue salmeterol/fluticasone, and addition of roflumilast, 500 mcg daily.

Answer: _____

AMERICAN JOURNAL OF
Respiratory and Critical Care Medicine

Effect of Roflumilast and Inhaled Corticosteroid/Long-Acting β₂-Agonist on Chronic Obstructive Pulmonary Disease Exacerbations (RE²SPOND)
A Randomized Clinical Trial

American Journal of Respiratory and Critical Care Medicine Volume 194 Number 5 | September 1 2016

Conclusions: Roflumilast failed to statistically significantly reduce moderate and/or severe exacerbations in the overall population. Roflumilast improved lung function and reduced exacerbations in participants with frequent exacerbations and/or hospitalization history. The safety profile of roflumilast was consistent with that of previous studies.

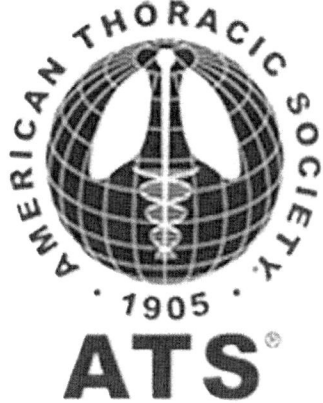

Bonus Question

Which tool is used by health care professionals to help predict COPD mortality (i.e., how long a patient will live after diagnosis)?

Answer

BODE Index Scoring

		Points		
Variable	0	1	2	3
FEV_1 (% predicted)	≥ 65	50-64	36-49	≤ 35
Walk distance in 6 min (m)	≥ 350	250-349	150-249	≤ 149
MMRC dyspnea scale	0-1	2	3	4
Body mass index	>21	≤ 21		

MMRC=Modified Medical Research Council.
Celli et al. *N Engl J Med*. 2004;350:1005-1012.

- Body mass index
- Obstruction of airflow
- Dyspnea
- Exercise capacity
Total of **10 points**

AR 15A

A 68-year-old man with a history of COPD (FEV_1 and P_aCO_2 measured under **stable conditions** of 550 mL and 58 mmHg respectively) is admitted with a 3-day history of increasing cough, purulent sputum, and dyspnea.
His only medications are an inhaled β₂-agonist and an inhaled anticholinergic agent; The patient weighs 65 kg; Temp 100.9° F (38.3° C), RR 28 bpm, irregular HR 120 bpm, and BP 100/65 mmHg.
He is using his accessory muscles of respiration and appears anxious; Heart sounds are diminished and breath sounds are decreased bilaterally.

CXR shows hyperinflation but no evidence of PNA, CHF, PNX, or rib fracture.
ABG drawn on 5 L/min of nasal oxygen shows a pH of 7.22, P_aCO_2 74 mmHg, and P_aO_2 92 mmHg.
ECG shows MAT.

AR 15A (cont.)

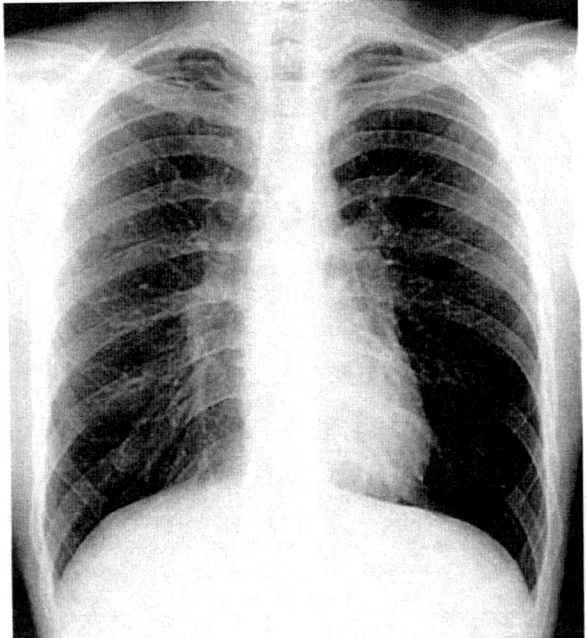

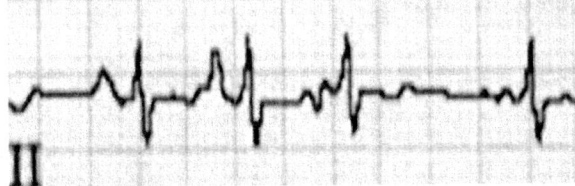

AR 15A (cont.)

All of the following would be expected to lower his P_aCO_2 except?

A. Reducing the FiO_2
B. Applying a BiPAP
C. Administering a benzodiazepine
D. Administering acetaminophen

Answer: _____

AR 15B

In the management of the previous patient, which of the following reduces mortality in <u>severe</u> acute exacerbations of COPD?

A. Oxygen
B. Smoking cessation
C. Corticosteroids
D. A & B
E. Other

Answer: _____

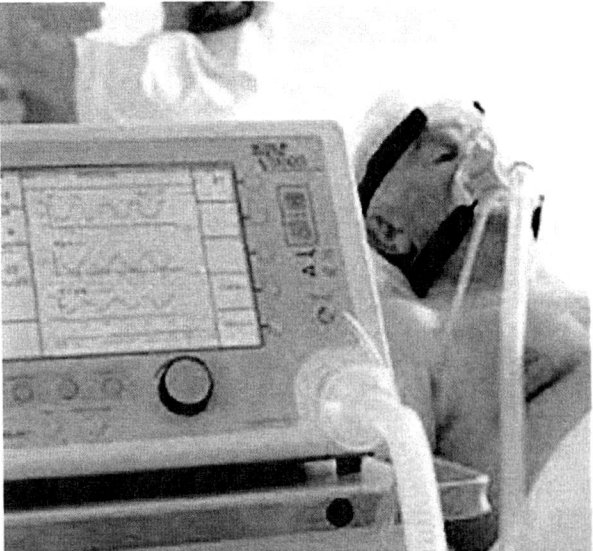

Annals of Int Med. 2003;138(11);861–870.

AR 16

A 62-year-old woman is evaluated in the ED for a 2-day history of increased dyspnea. She has advanced COPD with an FEV_1 of 35% of predicted.
She has a 75-pack-year smoking history and continues to smoke. Her current medications are tiotropium bromide and albuterol.
Exam: She is difficult to arouse; Temp 98.6° F (37.0° C), BP 145/90, HR 95, RR 25, and BMI 30
Lung exam discloses prolonged expiration and wheezing. Bilateral pitting leg edema is noted.
Oxygen saturation by pulse oximetry is 93%.

Which of the following is the most appropriate diagnostic test to perform next?

A. Arterial blood gas studies
B. Chest CT scan
C. Complete blood count
D. Echocardiography

Answer: _____

AR 16 (cont.)

With the presence of somnolence, there is a high chance that she has arterial hypoxemia and alveolar hypoventilation with carbon dioxide retention; Both are best evaluated by obtaining ABG

AR 17

A 63-year-old woman who has had COPD for 10 years is evaluated because of **easy bruising** that is making her increasingly **self-conscious**. Three years ago, the patient had 1 hospitalization related to an exacerbation. One year ago, she had an exacerbation that was treated with oral medications at **home**. She has had no exacerbations since. The patient **quit smoking** 3 years ago, and she does not have cough and sputum. She is **physically active** and able to do her own shopping and housework. Her current medications are fluticasone/salmeterol, 250/50 mcg twice daily, and tiotropium, 18 mcg daily. This regimen has been **unchanged** since her hospitalization 3 years ago.

On physical examination, temperature is 98.6° F (37.0° C). Pulse rate is 78 beats per minute, respirations are 14 breaths per minute, and blood pressure is 110/70 mmHg. FEV_1 is 1.4 L (45% of predicted), unchanged during the past 3 years. S_aO_2 is 92% on ambient air.

Which of the following is the best next step in this patient's management?
A. Make no changes in medications.
B. Taper and discontinue fluticasone/salmeterol.
C. Taper and discontinue fluticasone/salmeterol and add formoterol/budesonide.
D. Taper and discontinue fluticasone/salmeterol and add indacaterol.

Answer: _____

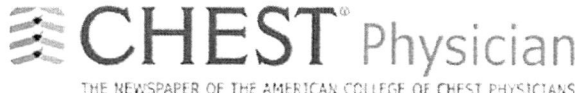

CHEST Physician

THE NEWSPAPER OF THE AMERICAN COLLEGE OF CHEST PHYSICIANS

LAMA/LABA may allow withdrawal of inhaled steroids

An option in severe but stable COPD.

BY SHARON WORCESTER
Frontline Medical News

AT CHEST 2014

AUSTIN, TEX. – Inhaled corticosteroids can be successfully withdrawn without increasing the risk of exacerbations in patients who have chronic obstructive pulmonary disease and are receiving dual bronchodilator therapy with a long-acting muscarinic antagonist and a long-acting beta₂-agonist, according to findings from the WISDOM study.

However, inhaled corticosteroid (ICS) withdrawal should be conducted with caution, as a small but statistically significantly greater decrease in lung function occurred in patients who withdrew completely, compared with those who did not during the 12-month, double-blind, parallel-group study, Dr. Helgo Magnussen reported at the annual meeting of the American College of Chest Physicians.

"In patients with severe but stable COPD who are receiving combination therapy with tiotropium, salmeterol and ICS, a stepwise withdrawal of ICS was noninferior to continuation of ICS with respect to the risk of moderate or severe

See **COPD** · *page 5*

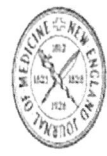

The NEW ENGLAND JOURNAL of MEDICINE

ORIGINAL ARTICLE

Withdrawal of Inhaled Glucocorticoids and Exacerbations of COPD

Helgo Magnussen, M.D., Bernd Disse, M.D., Ph.D., Roberto Rodriguez-Roisin, M.D., Anne Kirsten, M.D., Henrik Watz, M.D., Kay Tetzlaff, M.D., Lesley Towse, B.Sc., Helen Finnigan, M.Sc., Ronald Dahl, M.D., Marc Decramer, M.D., Ph.D., Pascal Chanez, M.D., Ph.D., Emiel F.M. Wouters, M.D., Ph.D., and Peter M.A. Calverley, M.D., for the WISDOM Investigators
N Engl J Med 2014; 371:1285-1294 October 2, 2014 DOI: 10.1056/NEJMoa1407154

Bronchiectasis

Bronchiectasis (Focal & Diffuse)
- Definition/Etiology
  - Persistent, pathologic dilatation of the bronchi due to breakdown of bronchial elastic and muscular elements
  - Suspect it if the patient has a long history of cough with a large amount of purulent, foul-smelling sputum ± blood
  - It is almost always caused by infection
    - Acute or recurrent pneumonia
    - Necrotizing, lung abscess
    - Occasionally by a chronic smoldering infection
    - Frequently see it in old TB areas of involvement

- Signs and Symptoms
  - Patients will have persistent cough
  - Purulent copious sputum production
    - "Multi-layering"
  - Wheezes and/or crackles
- Patient history
  - Significant history of recurrent pneumonias that commonly involve gram-negative bacteria
    - *Pseudomonas*

- Seen with:
  - Cystic fibrosis
    - Most common associated disease state
  - Hypogammaglobulinemia
    - Consider this entity with recurrent sinopulmonary infections and chronic cough with purulent sputum
      - Check IgA, IgM, and IgG (with subtypes)

  - ABPA (acute bronchopulmonary aspergillosis)
    - Associated with bronchiectasis of upper/central lung fields
    - Occurs in patients with asthma and CF
  - Immotile cilia syndromes
    - Kartagener
    - Ciliary dysmotility

- Diagnosis
  - Chest x-ray in advanced cases may show crowding of the bronchi (tram-tracking)
  - Can be confirmed by seeing the typical morphologic changes seen with a high-resolution CT (HRCT) with 1–2-mm cuts
  - During the workup
    - Check for low gamma globulin
    - Check for high sweat chloride

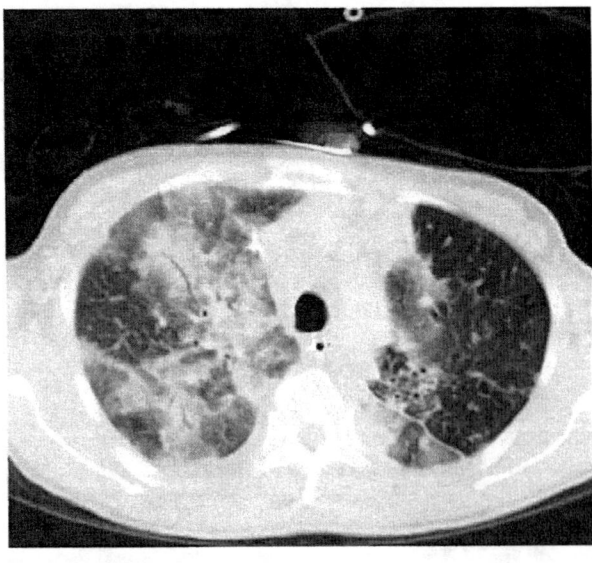

- Treatment
  - Patients with bronchiectasis do benefit from:
    - Bronchodilators
    - Physiotherapy
      - Flutter valve therapy
      - Pulmonary toilet
      - Percussion vest
      - Cough assist device

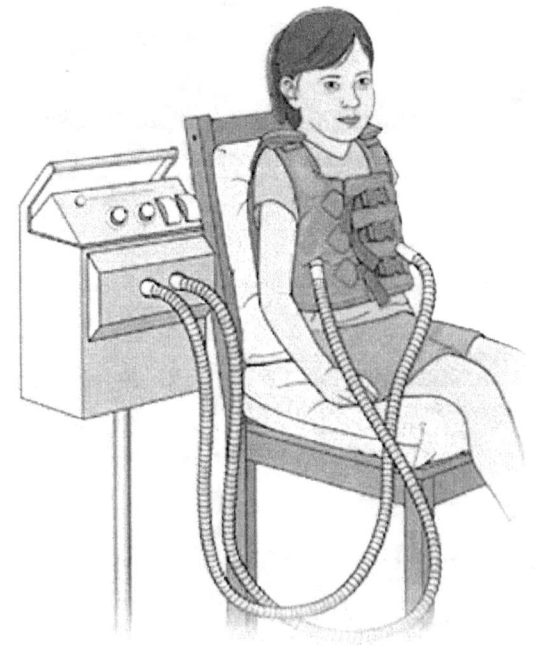

Bronchiectasis (cont.)

- Antibiotics should cover gram-negative rods
  - Double coverage for *Pseudomonas*
    - Aminoglycosides
    - Quinolones
    - Piperacillin-tazobactam
    - Cephalosporins
      » Ceftazidime (Fortaz) 3rd
      » Cefepime (Maxipime 4th, Ceftaroline [Teflaro]) 5th (covers MRSA)
    - Carbapenems
      » Doripenem

Question
Why is the disease named "cystic fibrosis"?

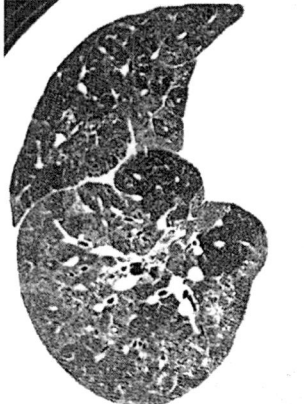
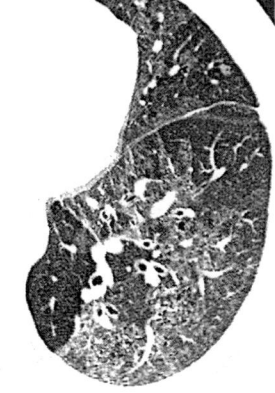

Answer

- It is a misnomer that the name "cystic fibrosis" refers to the characteristic scarring (fibrosis) and cyst formation within the **pancreas**, first recognized in the **1930s**
- Difficulty breathing is the most serious symptom and results from frequent lung infections

Cystic Fibrosis

- Autosomal recessive genetic disorder that affects most critically the:
  - Lungs
  - Pancreas
  - Liver
  - Intestine
- It is characterized by abnormal transport of chloride and sodium across an epithelium, leading to thick, **viscous secretions**

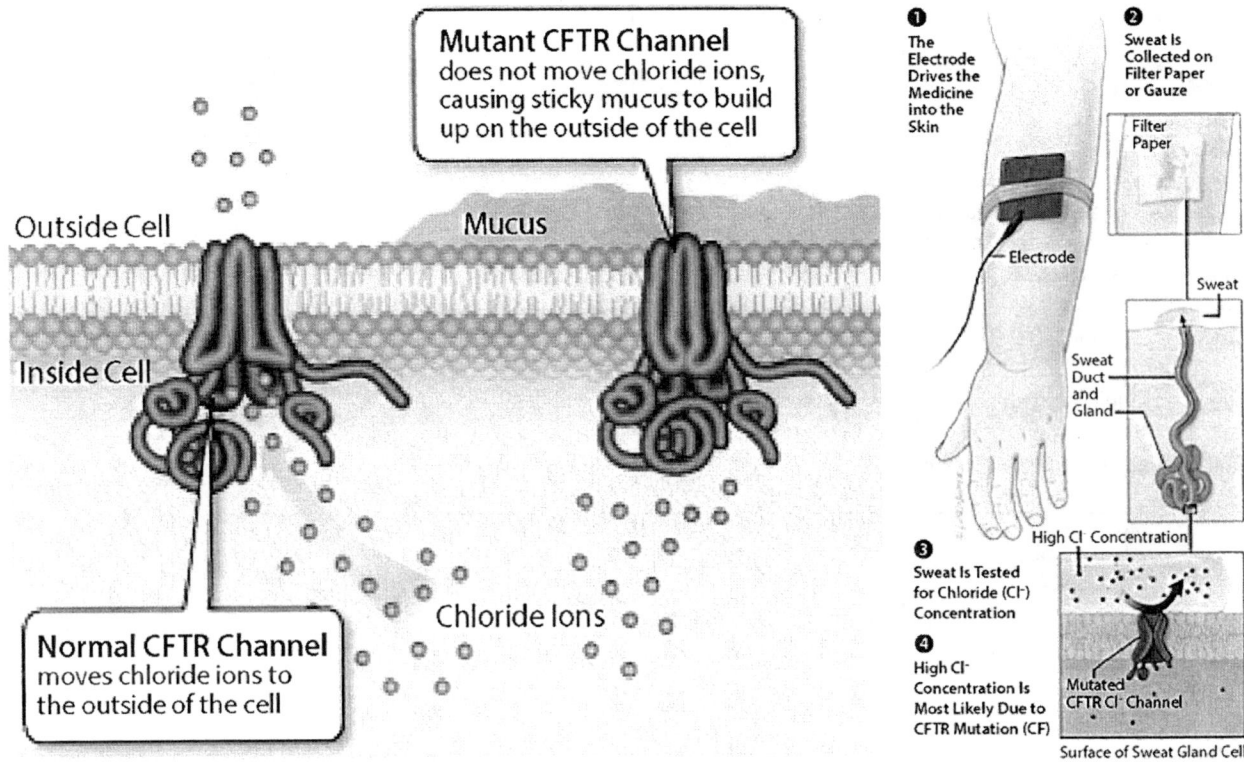

Mutant CFTR Channel does not move chloride ions, causing sticky mucus to build up on the outside of the cell

Outside Cell

Mucus

Inside Cell

Normal CFTR Channel moves chloride ions to the outside of the cell

Chloride Ions

❶ The Electrode Drives the Medicine into the Skin

Electrode

❷ Sweat Is Collected on Filter Paper or Gauze

Filter Paper

Sweat

Sweat Duct and Gland

High Cl⁻ Concentration

❸ Sweat Is Tested for Chloride (Cl⁻) Concentration

❹ High Cl⁻ Concentration Is Most Likely Due to CFTR Mutation (CF)

Mutated CFTR Cl⁻ Channel

Surface of Sweat Gland Cell

Cystic Fibrosis — Diagnosis

- **Requires 2 parts:**
  1) Clinical symptoms consistent with CF in at least 1 organ system
  2) Evidence of CFTR dysfunction:
     - Elevated sweat chloride
     - Presence of disease-causing mutations in CFTR
- For most individuals, a normal sweat chloride result is sufficient to rule out CF

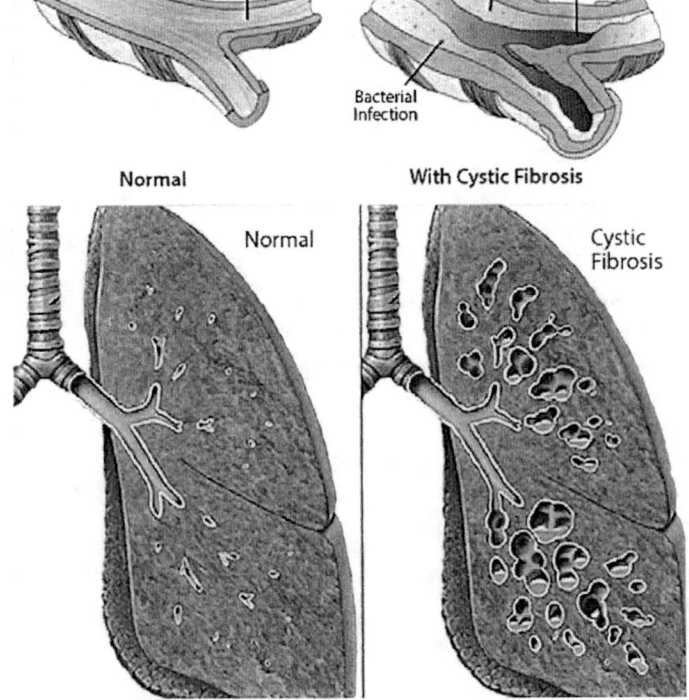

Airway Wall Thin Layer of Mucus

Thick Mucus Blocks Airway

Blood in Mucus

Bacterial Infection

Normal

With Cystic Fibrosis

Normal

Cystic Fibrosis

Question
Are there drugs that treat the underlying cause of cystic fibrosis?

Answer
Ivacaftor
- Kalydeco
- FDA approved January 2012
- Targets a very specific mutation of the *CFTR* gene
- STRIVE study improvement in FEV_1 and lung function

Lumacaftor-ivacaftor
- Orkambi
- FDA approved July 2015
- For patients with 2 copies of the *F508del* mutation
- Improves lung function and reduces hospitalization

Cystic Fibrosis — Bacterial Pathogens

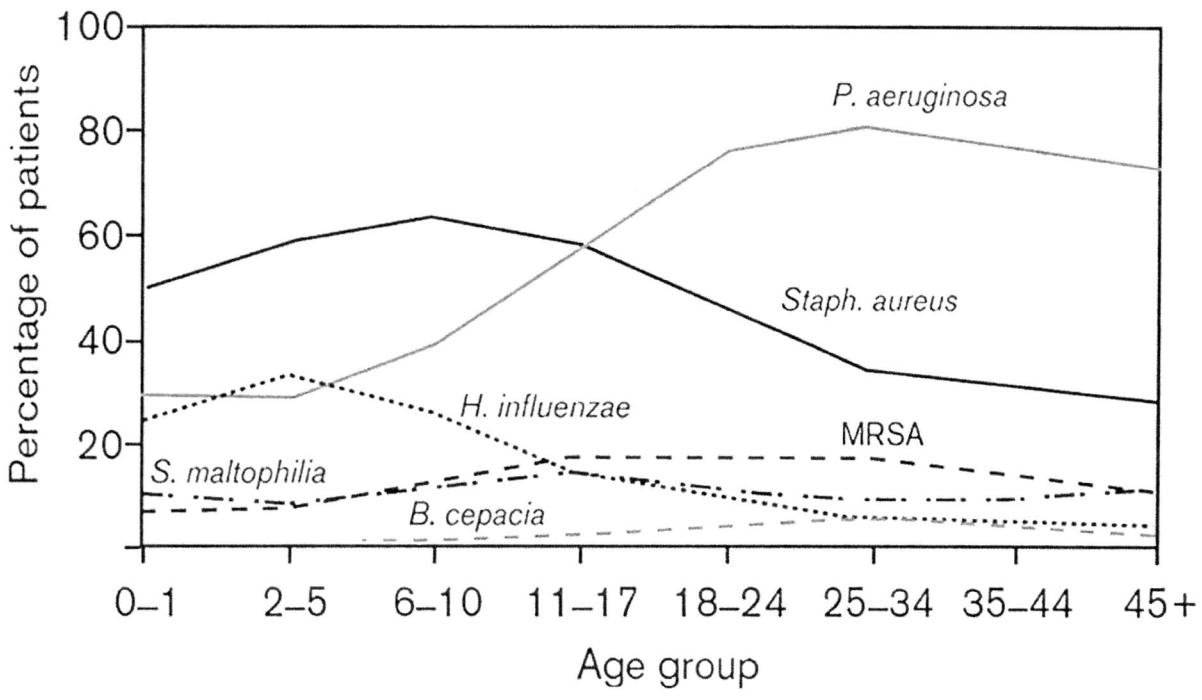

Question
Why does *Burkholderia cepacia* complex prevent CF patients from getting a lung transplant?

Answer
- Transplant recipients infected with ***Burkholderia cepacia*** have a worse survival rate after lung transplantation than those who are not infected with this organism
- The decreased survival is predominantly due to recurrent *B. cepacia* infection, with the majority of affected recipients succumbing within 3 months after transplant
- Almost universally fatal necrotizing pneumonic illness known as *"**Cepacia** syndrome"*

CF — Treatment
- **CFTR Modulators: 2 options**
  1) Ivacaftor (Kalydeco)
  2) Lumacaftor-ivacaftor (Orkambi)
- **Chronic antibiotics: 2 options**
  1) Chronic PO azithromycin mainly for patients with mucoid *Pseudomonas* and evidence of airway inflammation, such as chronic cough or any reduction in FEV_1
  2) For persistent *Pseudomonas* infection, recommend chronic treatment with inhaled tobramycin cycled between 28 days on and 28 days off treatment
     - Inhaled aztreonam lysine is a reasonable alternative, as is inhaled colistin

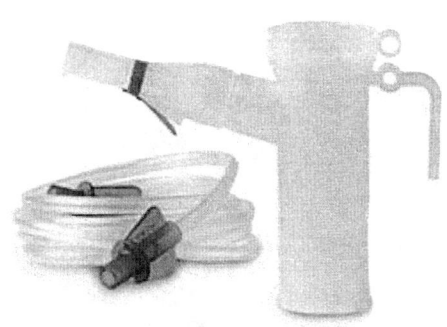

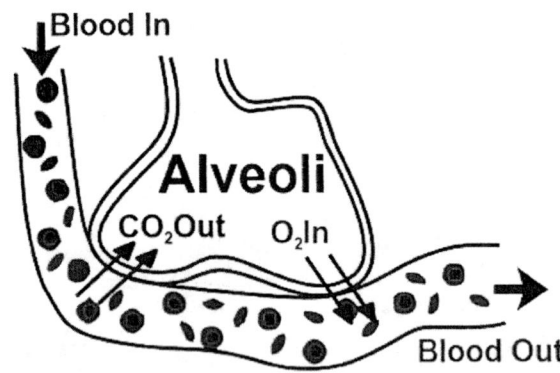

CF — Treatment (cont.)

- **Bronchodilators**
  - Short-acting inhaled beta-2-agonists prior to inhalation of hypertonic saline, antibiotics, or initiating chest physiotherapy
- **Agents to promote airway clearance**
  - DNase I (dornase alfa)
  - Hypertonic saline (hyper-sal)
- **Chest physiotherapy**
  - Acapella flutter valve
  - AeroriKA
  - Vest therapy
- **Antiinflammatory therapy**
  - For patients with CF but without asthma or ABPA, recommend against treating with inhaled corticosteroids
  - Recommend against chronic treatment with systemic glucocorticoids
- **Lung transplant**

Interstitial Lung Disease

Interstitial Lung Disease
- **Overview**
  - Diffuse parenchymal lung disease (DPLD)
  - Diverse (> 100) group of disorders that affect the **interstitium**, a potential space between the capillaries and the alveoli
  - Partly a **misnomer**, because there is often bronchial and alveolar involvement

Interstitial Lung Disease (cont.)
- **Common factors in their clinical presentation:**
  1) Dyspnea on exertion
  2) Diffuse disease on chest imaging
     - Reticulonodular disease on CXR
     - Ground-glass on CT scan
  3) Restrictive intrinsic PFTs
  4) Elevated A-a gradient
- **Diagnosis:**
  1) Bronchoscopy
     - BAL
     - TBB
     - EBUS
  2) Surgical biopsy
     - VATS
     - Thoracotomy

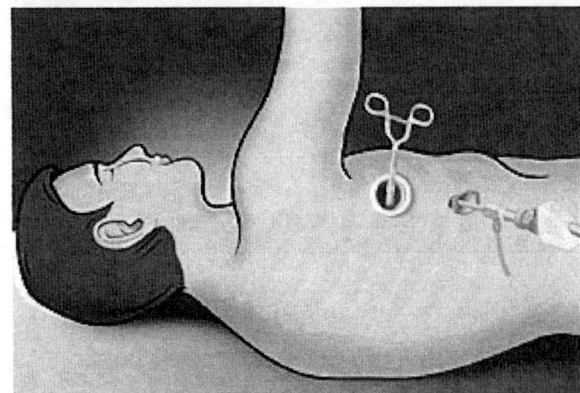

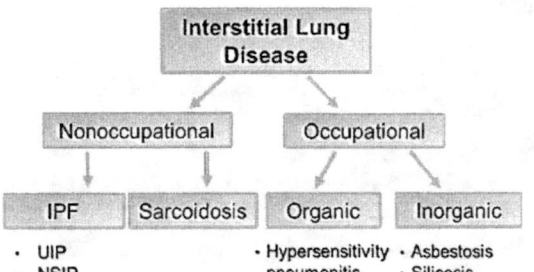

Sarcoidosis
- **Definition**
  - A systemic disease of unknown etiology
  - Characterized by the presence of noncaseating granulomas
- **Clinical manifestations**
  - Can involve almost any organ system
    - Ocular, skin, myocardial, rheumatologic, GI, and CNS
  - Pulmonary involvement is most common

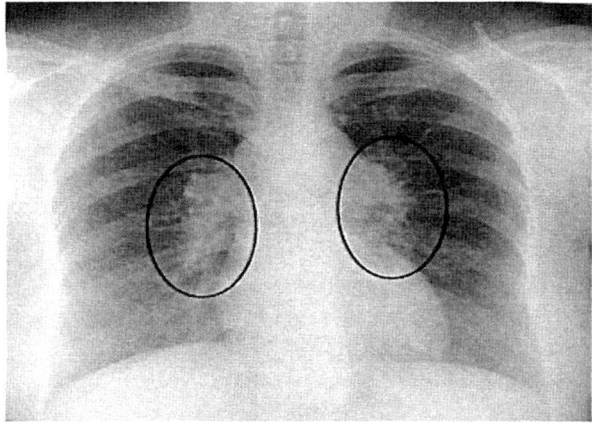

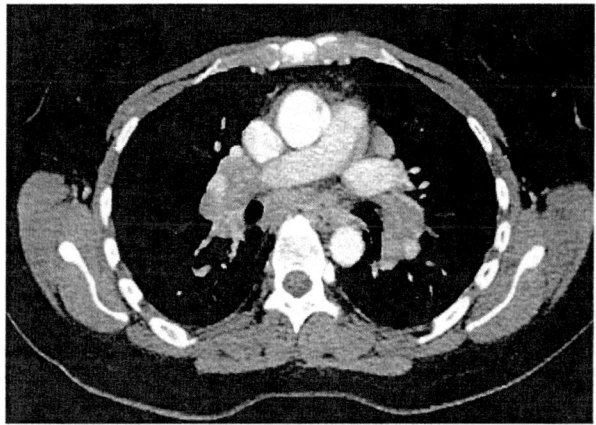

Two Distinct Syndromes
Löfgren Syndrome
- Acute
- Erythema nodosum
- Arthritis
- Hilar adenopathy

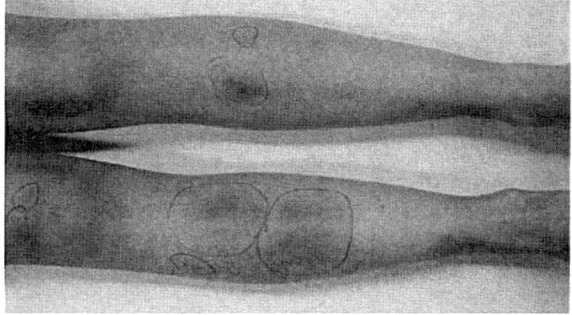

Heerfordt-Waldenström
- Subacute to chronic
- Fever
- Parotid enlargement
- Uveitis
- Facial palsy

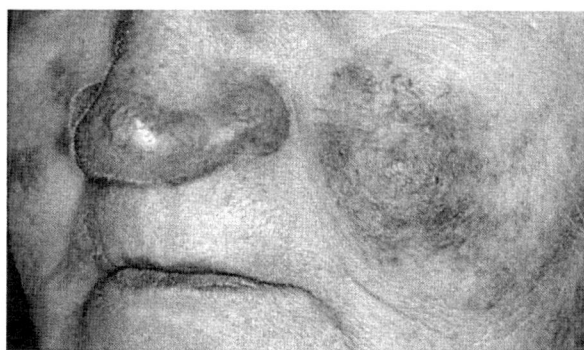

Sarcoid Diagnosis
- **Exclude the other granulomatous diseases**
  - Hypersensitivity pneumonitis
  - Berylliosis
  - Infectious diseases caused by mycobacteria and fungi
- **Bronchoscopy with TBB ± EBUS**
  - Noncaseating granulomas

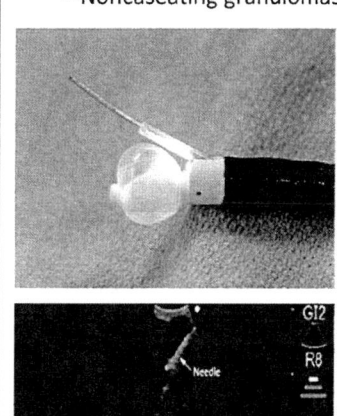
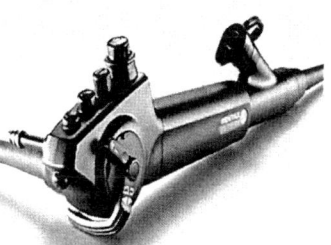
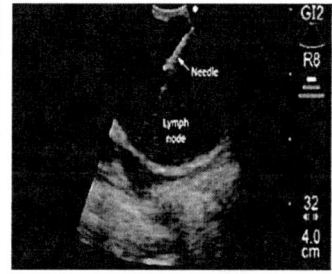
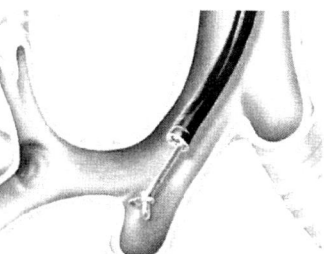
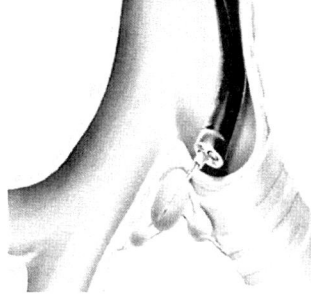
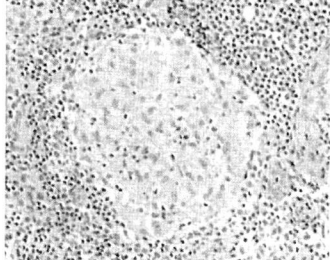

© 2017 MedStudy Internal Medicine Video Board Review – Pulmonary Medicine • Raj Dasgupta, MD

Sarcoid Treatment
- Treat severe disease with corticosteroids
- Corticosteroids:
  - Do not induce remission or alter the course of disease
  - Decrease symptoms
  - Improve PFTs
- **Indications** for systemic corticosteroids
  - Eyes
  - Heart
  - CNS
  - Pulmonary
  - Hypercalcemia
- Steroid-sparing agents
  - Hydroxychloroquine, infliximab, MTX, azathioprine, mycophenolate mofetil

Sarcoid Steroid-Sparing Agents
- The evidence in support of individual 2nd line agents is largely **observational**
- The agents that appear to have the greatest likelihood of benefit with an acceptable side-effect profile are:
  - Methotrexate
  - Azathioprine
  - Leflunomide
  - Antimalarial

Methotrexate
- Most commonly used steroid-sparing agent
- For lungs, skin, eyes, and CNS
- Oral or intramuscularly
- Begin PO **7.5 mg weekly**
- Dose is gradually increased by 2.5 mg q 2 weeks until a dose of **10–15 mg** per week
- Intramuscular MTX for refractory nausea

Azathioprine
- Start at **50 mg PO daily** to max of 200 PO daily
- Increase slowly by 25 mg every 2–3 weeks to reduce GI side effects
- Toxicity is largely related to its metabolites, which are broken down by the enzyme thiopurine-S-methyltransferase (**TPMT**)
- TPMT enzyme activity can be genotyped or measured

Leflunomide
- Start at **10 mg** and increase to 20 mg daily
- Nausea, diarrhea, abdominal pain, hepatotoxicity
- Common practice is to **combine** MTX and leflunomide

Antimalarials
- Chloroquine and hydroxychloroquine are antimalarial drugs with immunomodulating properties
- For **cutaneous** sarcoidosis, but several reports have described its use in pulmonary disease

- Glucose-6-phosphate dehydrogenase (**G6PD**) levels must be determined prior to initiating therapy
- Side effects retinopathy and blindness require exam at baseline and q 6–12 months

TNF Inhibitors
- Studies of the efficacy of TNF-α antagonist agents in the treatment of sarcoidosis have yielded **mixed results**
  - Infliximab (Remicade)
  - Adalimumab (Humira)
  - Etanercept (Enbrel)
  - Golimumab (Simponi)

Mycophenolate mofetil (MMF)
- Inhibitor of lymphocyte proliferation and activity has been used to treat a variety of ILDs associated with rheumatic disease
- Data regarding the use of MMF in sarcoidosis is **limited**
- Start at 500 mg PO bid up to 2 grams daily
- Nausea and diarrhea may be dose limiting

Corticotropin Injection (Acthar)
- **FDA approved** for pulmonary sarcoid and uveitis
- Work on **melanocortin** receptors
- 40–80 units sub-Q 2–3 times per week

AR 18

A **65-year-old** female is evaluated for a 10-month history of cough and dyspnea. She reports no other symptoms or medical problems and takes no medications. She is a **former smoker** with a 20-pack-year history. She has **no pets**.

On exam, BP 120/70 mmHg, HR 80 beats per minute, and RR 24 breaths per minute. Oxygen saturation is 87% on RA. There is **no JVD**. Cardiac examination is normal. Lung exam—bilateral **inspiratory crackles** at the lung bases. Digital **clubbing** is present.

PFT: Decreased TLC, decreased FEV_1, decreased FVC, normal FEV_1/FVC, and a decreased DLCO

CT scan is done.

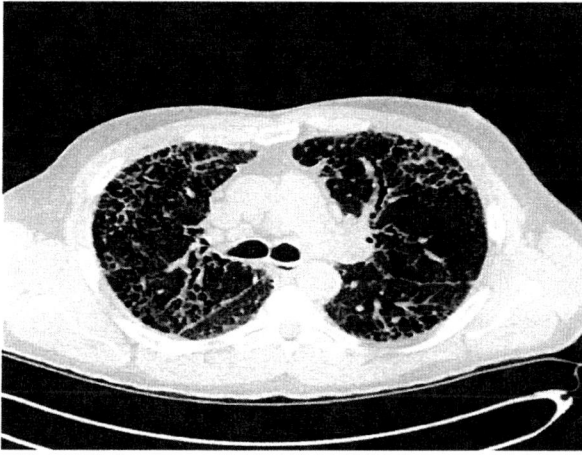

AR 18 (cont.)

Which of the following is the most likely diagnosis?

A. Emphysema

B. Heart failure

C. Hypersensitivity pneumonitis

D. Idiopathic pulmonary fibrosis

Answer: _____

AR 18 (cont.)

Idiopathic pulmonary fibrosis has the classic CT findings of basal and peripheral disease with evidence of honeycomb changes.

Idiopathic Pulmonary Fibrosis
- Etiology is unknown
- Diagnosis of exclusion
  - Occupation and exposures
  - Drugs
    - Bleomycin, amiodarone, MTX
  - Rheumatologic symptoms
- Physical exam
  - Velcro rales & clubbing

- Diagnostic workup includes:
  - CXR/CT Chest
  - PFTs
    - Intrinsic restrictive pattern
  - ABG
    - A-a gradient
  - Histologic tissue diagnosis
    - TBB & wedge resection

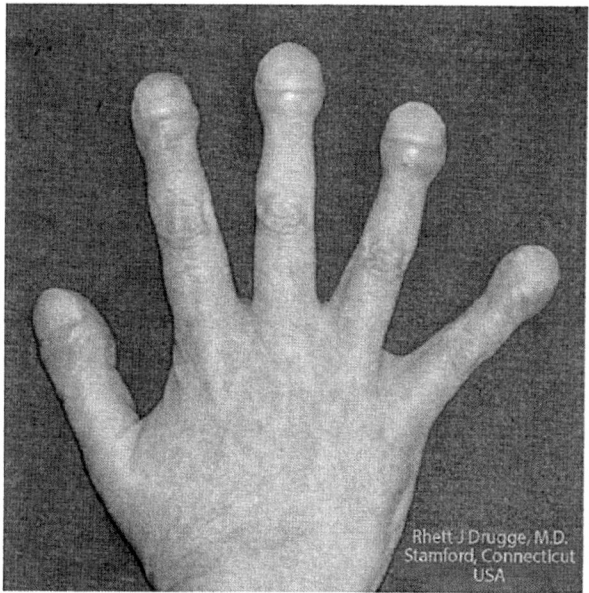

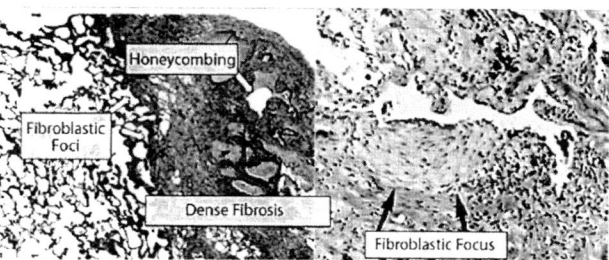

The histologic hallmark and chief diagnostic criterion is a heterogeneous appearance with alternating areas of normal lung, interstitial inflammation, fibroblast foci, and honeycomb change.

GERD and Chronic Microaspiration
- Up to **90%** of patients with IPF have GERD
- GERD is an important risk factor for the **progression** of IPF
- In a review, 67–76% of patients with IPF assessed with **ambulatory pH** probe had GERD
- Classic symptoms of GERD were **poor predictors** of increased esophageal acid exposure among patients with moderate-to-severe IPF

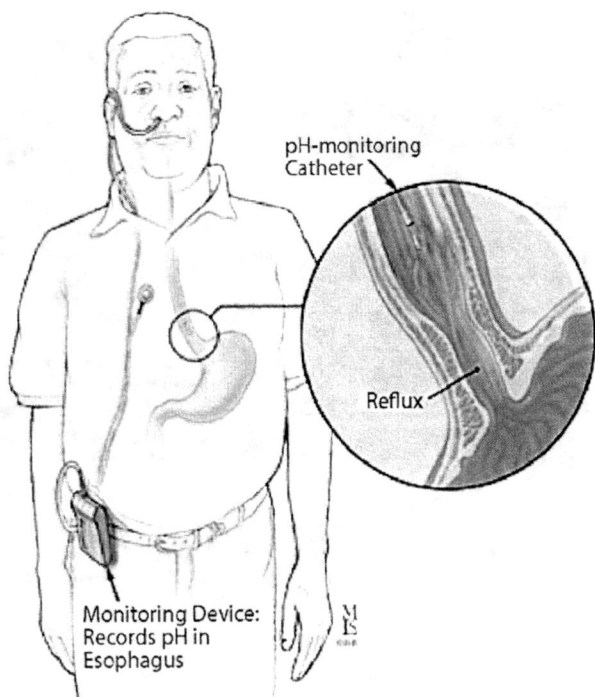

pH-monitoring Catheter

Reflux

Monitoring Device: Records pH in Esophagus

Am J Respir Crit Care Med. 1998;158:1804.
Eur Respir J. 2006;27:136.
Ann Thorac Surg. 2006;82:1570; author reply 1570.

AR 19

Which of the following is the most common side effect of nintedanib in the treatment of idiopathic pulmonary fibrosis?

A. Diarrhea
B. Headache
C. Hypertension
D. Liver enzyme elevation

Answer: _____

AR 19 (cont.)

Nintedanib
- Tyrosine kinase inhibitor
- Slows rate of disease progression in IPF
- 150 mg PO twice daily
- Side effects:
  - Diarrhea 62%
  - Nausea 24%
  - Vomiting 12%
  - Elevation in LFTs 14%

Pirfenidone
- Antifibrotic agent
- Slows rate of disease progression in IPF
- Start 267mg (1 capsule) PO tid
  - After 1st week increased to 534 mg PO tid
  - After 2nd week increased to 801 mg PO tid

- Side effects:
  - Rash 30%
  - Photosensitivity 9%
  - Nausea 36%
  - Diarrhea 26%
  - Abdominal discomfort 24%

IPF Treatment (Part 1)
- **Supportive care:**
  - Supplemental oxygen
  - Pulmonary rehabilitation
  - Vaccinations
  - Information regarding participation in randomized trials
- **For patients who desire active therapy rather than support care and are not interested in participating in a clinical trial:**
  1) Pirfenidone; The dose ranges up to 40 mg/kg per day in 3 divided doses
  2) Nintedanib
- **Do not use for chronic therapy:**
  1) Glucocorticoid monotherapy
  2) Combination therapy with azathioprine, prednisone, and *N*-acetylcysteine

IPF Treatment (Part 2)
- **Trial of sildenafil in patients with:**
  1) DLCO < 35%
  2) Echocardiographic evidence of right-ventricular dysfunction
  3) No contraindications to sildenafil
- **Early referral for lung transplantation evaluation**
- **In patients with an acute exacerbation of IPF, can consider:**
  - Broad-spectrum antibiotics
  - High-dose glucocorticoids in combination with a cytotoxic agent, such as azathioprine

AR 20

A **77-year-old** man is evaluated in the hospital for idiopathic **pulmonary fibrosis**. He was diagnosed 3 years ago and has gradually worsened despite therapy with prednisone, azathioprine, and *N*-acetylcysteine. All therapy has been discontinued over the past 6 months because of failure to respond and side effects. He has been **homebound** on high-flow oxygen and has been hospitalized 3 times in the past year. He just finished 7 days of levofloxacin. He has indicated that he **does not want** additional aggressive therapy.

On exam, patient is in severe respiratory distress. BP 144/80, HR 118, RR 28, and afebrile. Oxygen saturation is 88% with the patient breathing 100% oxygen by nonrebreather. Patient with neck retraction and accessory muscles use. Bilateral crackles are noted posteriorly.

AR 20 (cont.)
WBC is 5,000 with a normal differential count.
CXR and CT chest are shown (next).

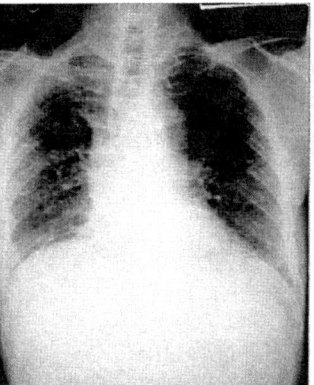
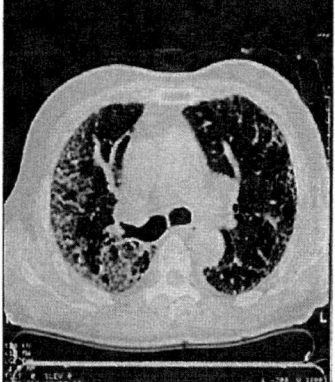

Which of the following is the most appropriate recommendation?
A. Intravenous methylprednisolone 120 mg IV q 6 hours
B. Mechanical ventilation with pressure control mode
C. BiPAP with initial settings of 10/5 cm H_2O
D. Palliative care consult

Answer: _____

AR 20 (cont.)
End-of-life care should be discussed with all patients with idiopathic pulmonary fibrosis, ideally in the outpatient setting with family present and when there is no urgency to intervene.

45-year-old male with increasing shortness of breath

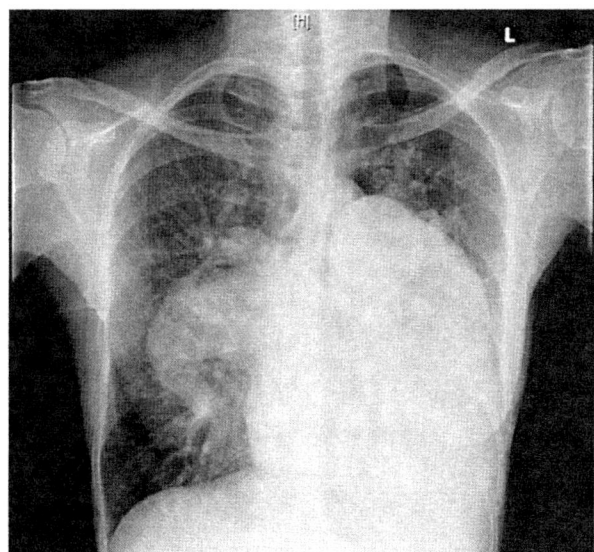

CT chest with contrast performed

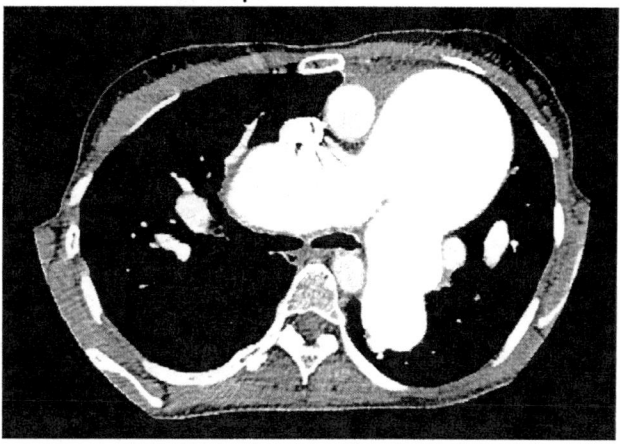

Pulmonary Hypertension (PH) — Introduction
- PH refers to elevated pulmonary arterial pressure
  - Can be due to a primary elevation of pressure in the pulmonary arterial system alone (pre-capillary PH)
  - Secondary to elevations of the pulmonary venous and pulmonary capillary pressures
- PH can be a progressive, fatal disease if untreated

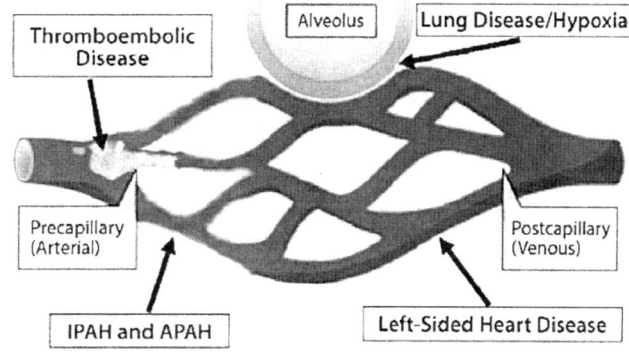

Pulmonary HTN — Definition
- PH is defined by a mean pulmonary arterial pressure (mPAP) ≥ 25 mmHg at rest usually confirmed by right heart catheterization
- Although PH can be measured on echocardiography, the gold standard for diagnosis is right heart catheterization

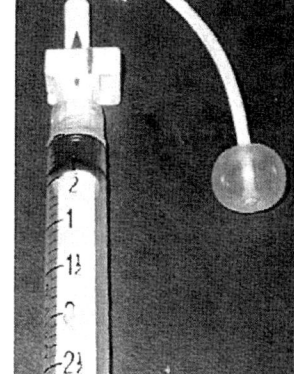

Pulmonary HTN — Classification
- **Group 1:** PAH
  - Drugs, connective tissue disease, HIV, portal HTN, congenital heart disease
- **Group 2:** PH due to left heart disease
- **Group 3:** PH due to chronic lung disease and/or hypoxemia
- **Group 4:** Chronic thromboembolic pulmonary hypertension (CTEPH)
- **Group 5:** PH due to unclear multifactorial mechanisms
  - Sickle cell, sarcoidosis

Pulmonary HTN — Screening
- Echocardiography for assessment of pulmonary artery systolic pressure (PASP)
- Modified Bernoulli equation:
  - $4 \times (TRV)^2 + RA$ pressure
- Estimated right atrial pressure (RAP) must be added to this obtained value

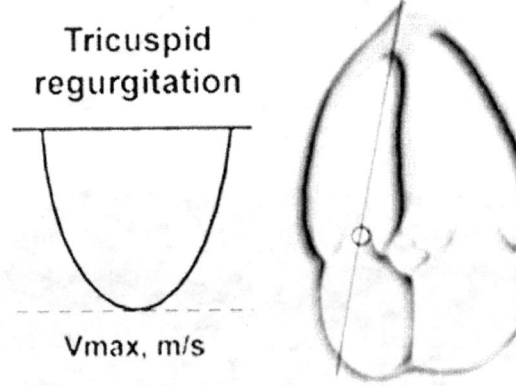

Tricuspid regurgitation

Vmax, m/s

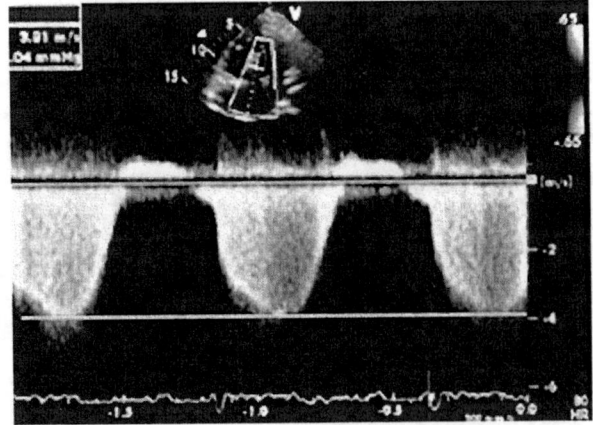

Pulmonary HTN — Diagnosis

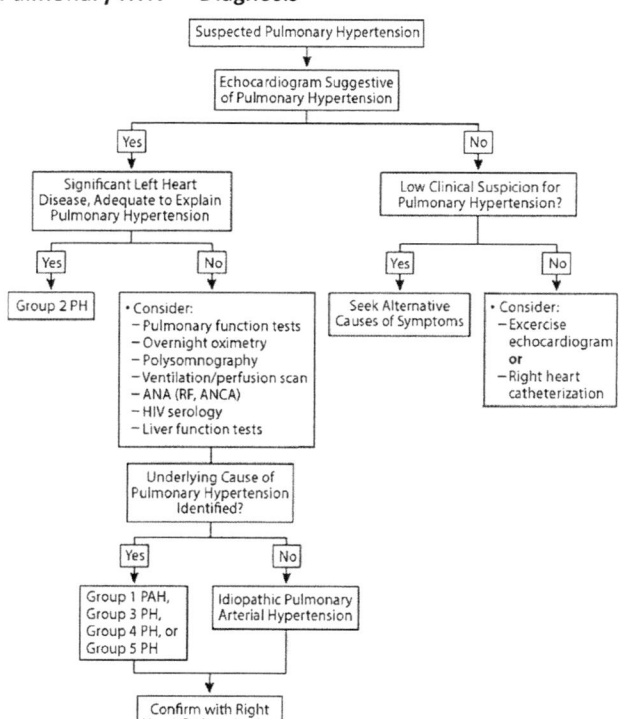

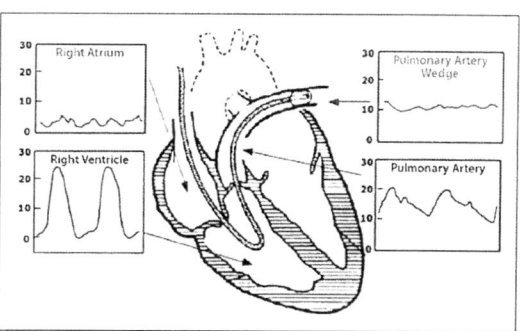

mPAP (↑), PVR (↑), PCWP (nl), CO (nl)

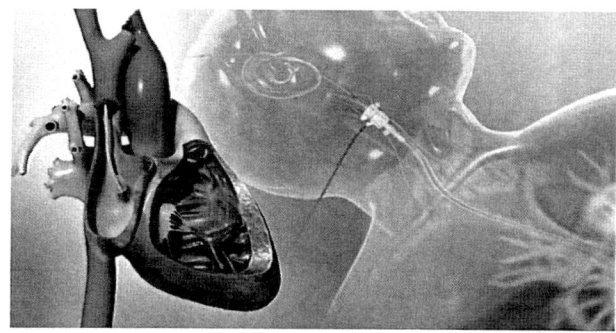

WHO (NYHA) Functional Class

Functional Class	Symptomatic profile
I	Patients with pulmonary hypertension but without resulting limitation of physical activity. Ordinary physical activity does not cause dyspnoea or fatigue, chest pain, or near syncope
II	Patients with pulmonary hypertension resulting in slight limitation of physical activity. They are comfortable at rest. Ordinary physical activity causes undue dyspnoea or fatigue, chest pain, or near syncope
III	Patients with pulmonary hypertension resulting in marked limitation of physical activity. They are comfortable at rest. Less than ordinary activity causes undue dyspnoea or fatigue, chest pain, or near syncope.
IV	Patients with pulmonary hypertension with inability to carry out any physical activity without symptoms. These patients manifest signs of right heart failure. Dyspnoea and/or fatigue may even be present at rest. Discomfort is increased by any physical activity

© 2017 MedStudy Internal Medicine Video Board Review – Pulmonary Medicine • Raj Dasgupta, MD

Pulmonary HTN — Treatment

Treatment of the underlying cause, and for some cases advanced PAH-specific therapy

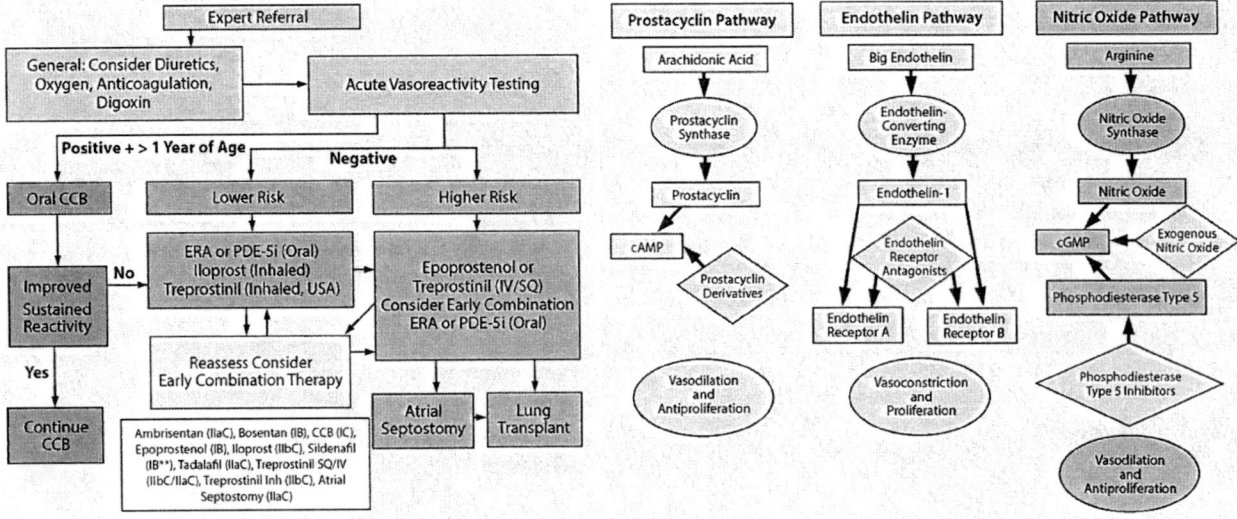

Pulmonary Embolism and DVT

Overview of Pulmonary Embolism & DVT

- Most pulmonary emboli are self-limited and resolve quickly
- PE is still the 3rd most common cardiovascular cause of death
- The incidence has **not** declined
  - Inadequate prophylaxis of hospitalized patients

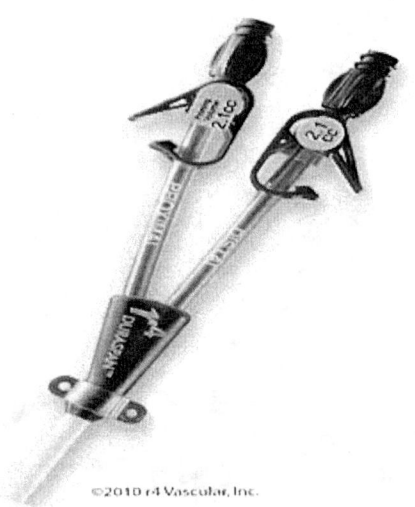

©2010 r4 Vascular, Inc.

Overview of Pulmonary Embolism & DVT (cont.)

- The majority of emboli are from the lower extremities
  - Virtually all from above the knee
- Newer data demonstrates the significance of **upper extremity** DVT being a more frequent cause of PE than previously expected
  - Internal jugular vein
  - Subclavian vein

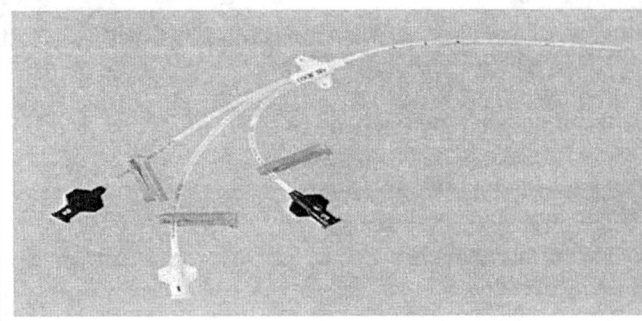

Risk Factors for PE and DVT (Part 1)

- Pregnancy
- Smoking
- Birth control
- Nephrotic syndrome
- Paroxysmal nocturnal hemoglobinuria
- Perioperative
- Virchow's triad:
  1) Alternations in blood flow
  2) Injury to the vascular endothelium
  3) Hypercoagulability
- Diabetes mellitus
- Age (> 60)
- Obesity
- Prolonged immobility
- CHF
- IBD
- Rheumatoid arthritis
- COPD

Risk Factors for PE and DVT (Part 2)
Occult cancer

- 8% of idiopathic DVT develop cancer in 2 years
- 17% of recurrent idiopathic DVT associated with malignancy
  - Especially lung and GI
- Routine screening and exam recommended
  - Not extensive cancer search

Coagulation

- *Factor 5 Leiden* gene mutation
  - **Not** deficiency
  - Most common inherited hypercoagulable disorder
  - Resistance to activated protein C
- Protein C and S deficiency
- Antithrombin III deficiency
- *G20210A* prothrombin mutation
- Elevated homocysteine levels
- Antiphospholipid antibodies
  - Lupus anticoagulant
  - Anticardiolipin
  - Beta 2 microglobulin

Overuse of the Hypercoagulable Workup
Controversy

- Not for 1st episode of unprovoked VTE
- If thrombophilia is detected in a patient with no history of VTE, anticoagulation is usually not necessary
- Conversely, patients with recurrent VTE should be anticoagulated even if their workup is negative

Indications

- Recurrent thromboembolic episodes
- Thromboembolism at a young age (< 40 years)
- Family history for thromboembolism
- Thrombosis in an unusual site

Specific Recommendations for a Hypercoagulable Workup

- Hepatic or portal vein thrombosis should be evaluated for:
  - *JAK2* mutations
  - Paroxysmal nocturnal hemoglobinuria (CD 55 & CD 59)
- Patients with VTE who have a history of warfarin-induced skin necrosis test for **protein C deficiency**
- For arterial thrombosis test for **antiphospholipid syndrome**
- Most of the hypercoagulable tests should be performed **2 weeks** following the discontinuation of anticoagulation

DVT Diagnosis

- **Venography**
  - Nonpractical gold standard
- **D-dimer**
  - Elevated D-dimer nonspecific in chronically ill and hospitalized
  - If pretest probability of DVT is low, DVT can be safely excluded in patients with a normal D-dimer
  - 2 main assays:
    1) Latex agglutination (no value)
    2) ELISA

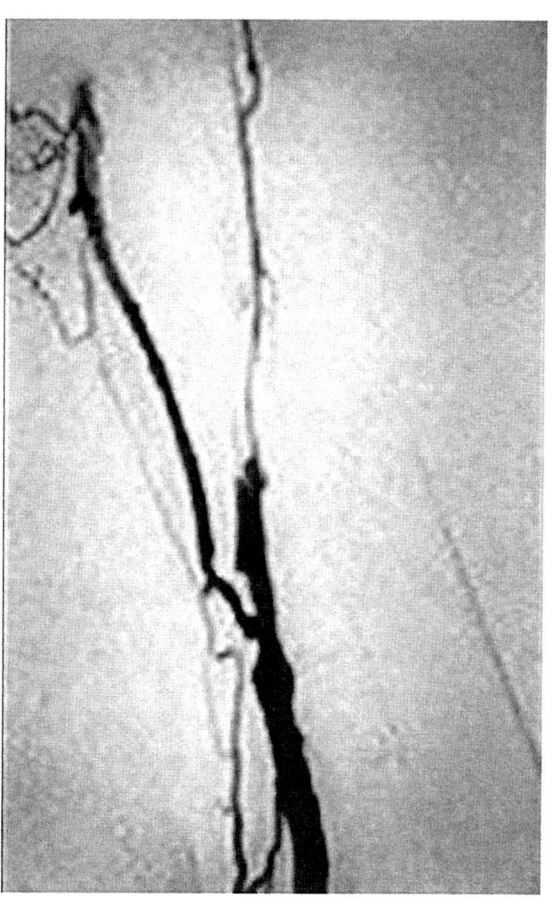

© 2017 MedStudy Internal Medicine Video Board Review – Pulmonary Medicine • Raj Dasgupta, MD

DVT Diagnosis (cont.)
- **Compression ultrasonography**
  - Has become the procedure of choice
- **MRI**
  - Advantage for renal, iliac, and pelvic veins

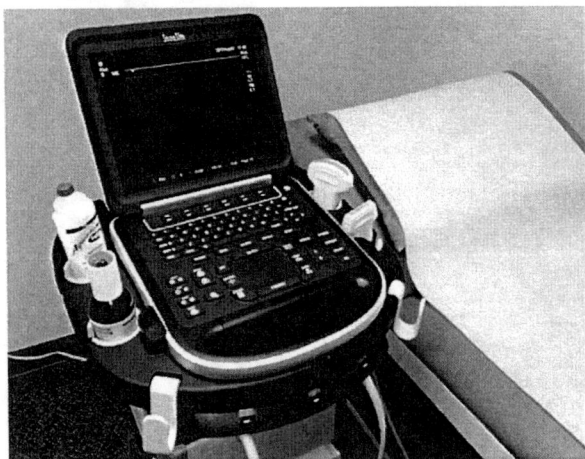

Clinical Question
Are DVTs more common in the left or right lower extremity?

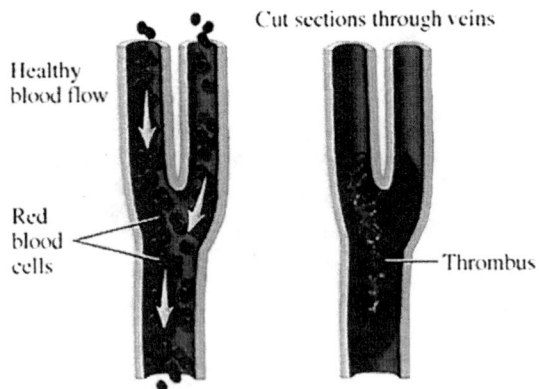

Answer
Left
- **May-Thurner syndrome**
  - In contrast to the right common iliac vein, which ascends almost vertically to the IVC, the left common iliac vein takes a more transverse course
    - Along this course, it underlies the right common iliac artery, which may compress it against the lumbar spine

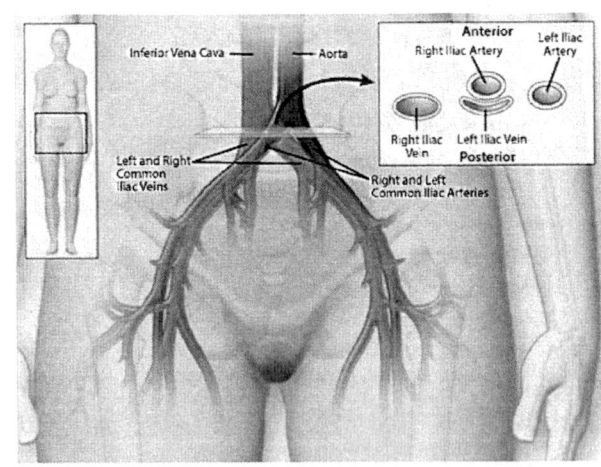

Pulmonary Embolism
- There are 10 techniques used in the evaluation of possible PE:
  1) ABG
  2) CXR
  3) ECG
  4) V/Q scan
  5) Venous studies
     - Venography
       - Invasive
       - Noninvasive
     - Ultrasonography
  6) D-dimer
  7) Pulmonary angiography
  8) CT angiogram
  9) MRI/MRA
  10) Echocardiography

- **ABG**
  - Indicate hypoxia
  - Necessitating further inquiry
  - A-a gradient

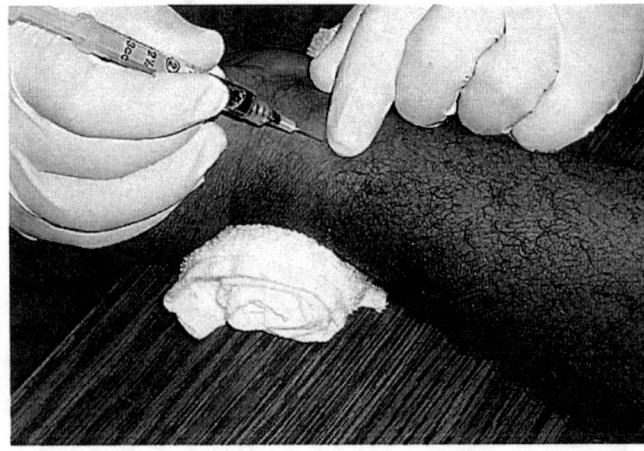

Pulmonary Embolism (cont.)

- Chest x-ray
  - Helps rule out other causes in the differential
  - "Hampton's hump"
    - Pleural based wedge shape defect from infarction just above the diaphragm
  - "Westermark's sign"
    - It is a lack of vascular markings in the area downstream of the embolus
  - "Fleischner lines"
    - Atelectasis
  - Pleural effusions
  - The most common CXR finding in PE
    - Normal (controversial)

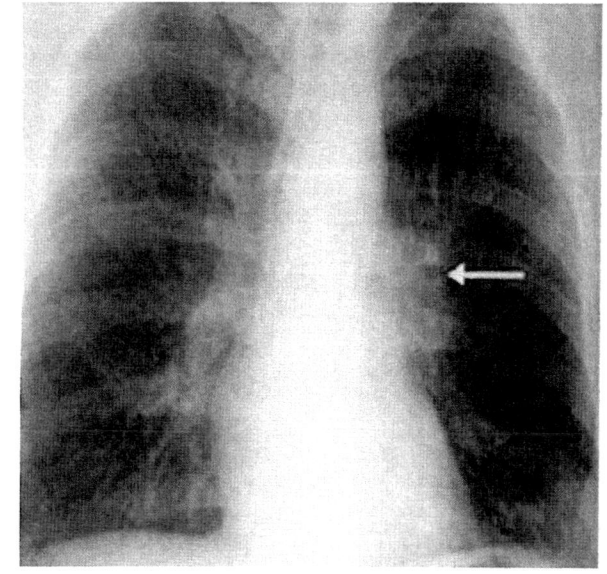

Hampton's Hump

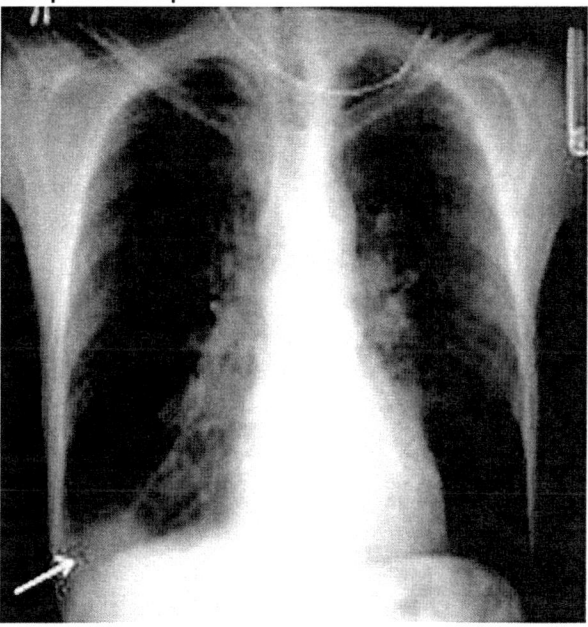

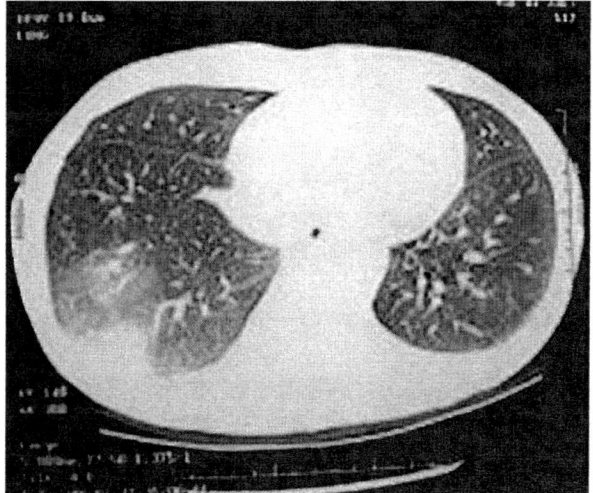

Westermark's Sign

© 2017 MedStudy Internal Medicine Video Board Review – Pulmonary Medicine • Raj Dasgupta, MD

Pulmonary Embolism (cont.)

- **ECG**
  - Right-axis deviation
  - S_1, Q_3, T_3
    - Deep S in lead I
    - Q wave in lead III
    - Inverted T wave in lead III
  - Sinus tachycardia is the most common ECG change

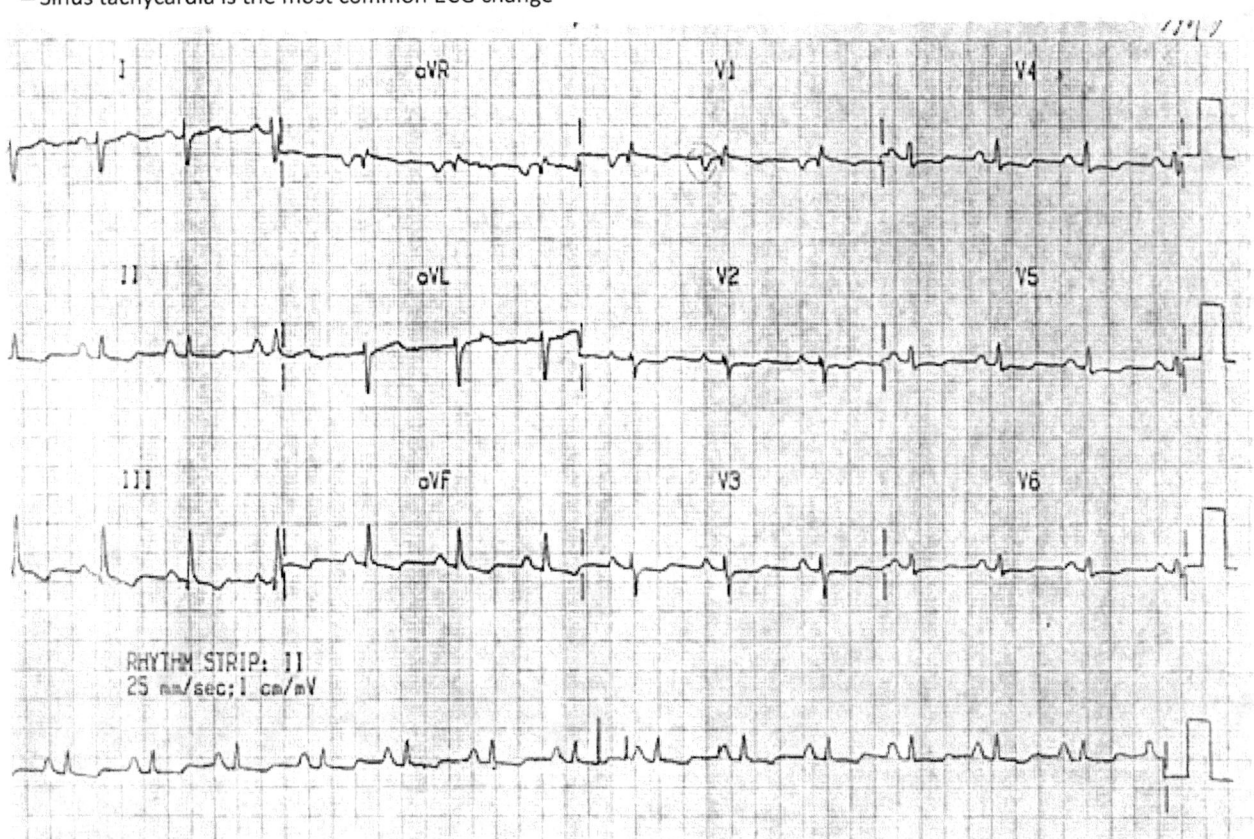

Pulmonary Embolism (cont.)

- **Ventilation/Perfusion lung scan**
  - 2 parts to the V/Q scan:
    1) Tagged albumin is injected into the pulmonary circulation
    2) Patient inhales a tagged gas that is distributed into the airways
  - Results
    - Normal
    - Low-probability
    - Moderate-probability
    - High-probability

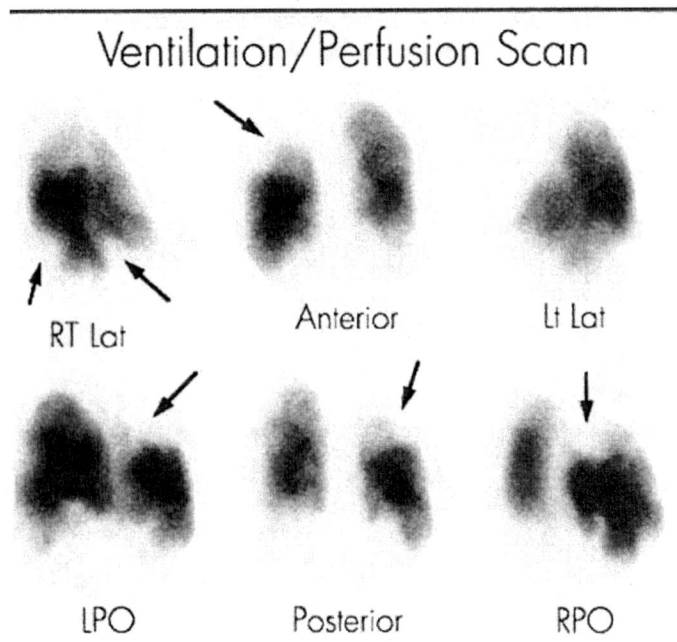

Pulmonary Embolism (cont.)
- **Venous studies**
  - PE and DVT are 2 manifestations of the same disease process
    - Venography
      - Invasive
      - Noninvasive
    - Ultrasonography

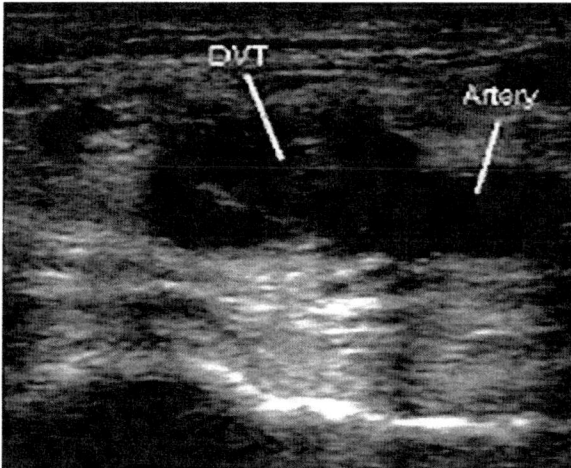

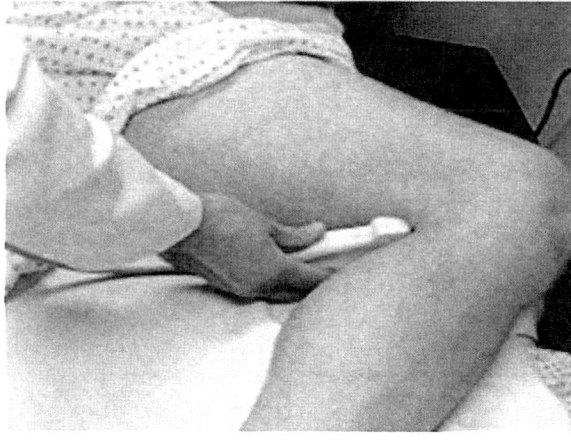

Pulmonary Embolism (cont.)
- **CT angiogram**
  - Limited to 4th order vessels
  - Requires contrast
  - Requires a 10- to 20-second breath hold
    - May lead to motion artifact
  - Is now often used in place of a V/Q scan

- **Question**
  - What study answered the question that a CT scan and **clinical suspicion** is the best combination to diagnose PE?

Pulmonary Embolism (cont.)
- **PIOPED II**
  - "The Prospective Investigation of Pulmonary Embolism Diagnosis"
    - Patients with suspected PE (n = 773)
    - All got
      - CT scan
      - Lower extremity ultrasound
      - V/Q
      - Angiogram when diagnosis not made by U/S or V/Q scan
    - CT sensitivity 83%, specificity 96%

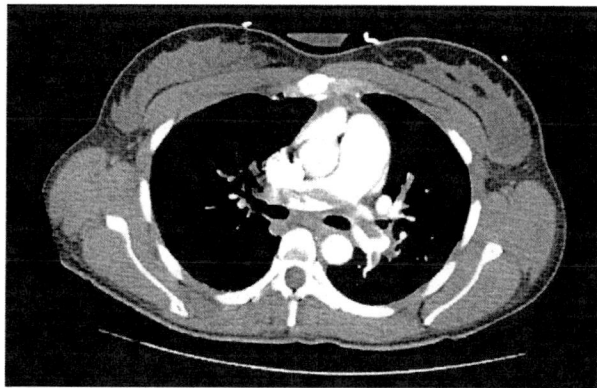

AR 21
Majority of patients with PE identified by CT have negative leg ultrasound
A. True
B. False

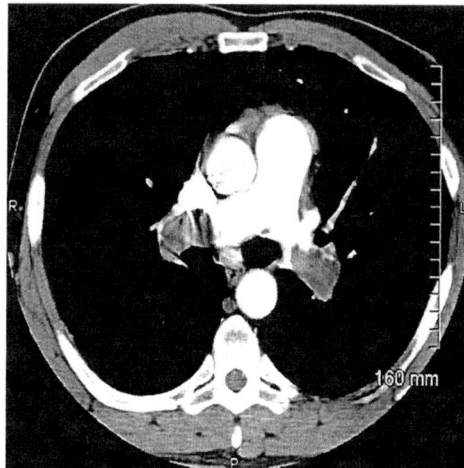

AR 21 (cont.)
Excluding the diagnosis of PE based on negative LE ultrasound makes no sense

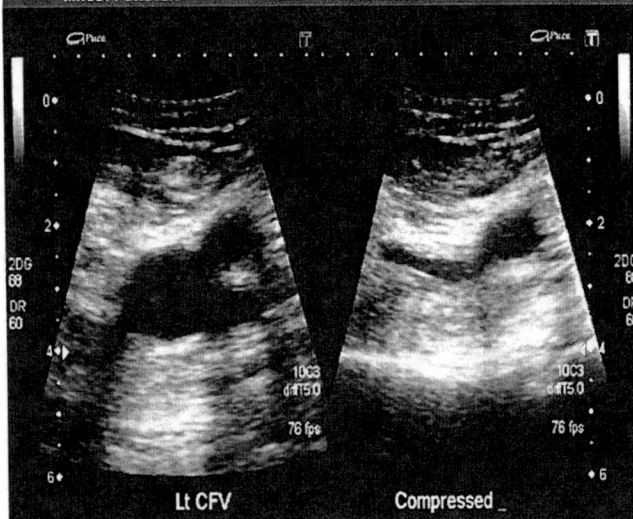

Pulmonary Embolism (cont.)
- **TTE/TEE**
  - Not indicated for the diagnosis of PE
  - Useful for determining right ventricular strain
  - Evaluate other etiologies for the patient's symptoms

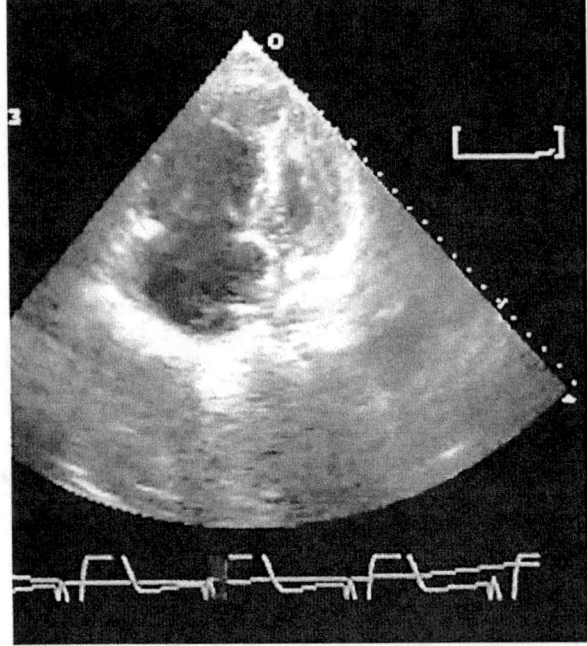

Pulmonary Embolism (cont.)
- **Pulmonary angiogram**
  - An invasive test
  - Consider for patients with:
    - High probability of PE but negative workup
    - Chronic thromboembolic pulmonary hypertension

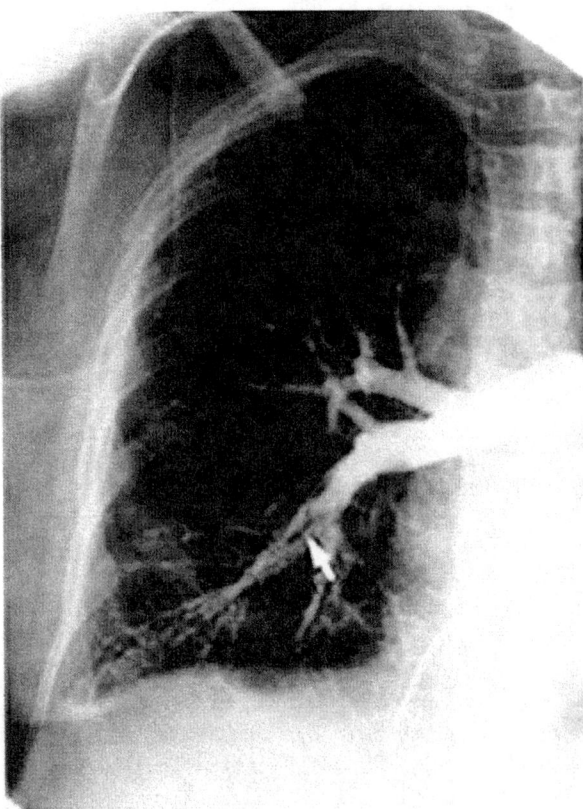

Clinical Question
Can you treat pulmonary embolism as an outpatient?

Answer: Yes
- **Pulmonary Embolism Severity Index (PESI)**
  - 11 variables
    1) Age
    2) Sex
    3) Cancer
    4) CHF
    5) Chronic lung disease
    6) HR > 110 beats/minute
    7) SBP < 100 mmHg
    8) RR > 30 breaths/minute
    9) Temp < 96.8° F (36.0° C)
    10) Altered mental status
    11) S_aO_2 < 90%

AR 22

26-year-old man is evaluated in the ED for a 24-hour history of swelling of the left leg and calf. Medical history is unremarkable, but he reports his uncle had a DVT. He takes no meds.
On exam, temp 98.0° F (36.7° C), BP 120/75 mmHg, HR 85 bpm, RR 14 breaths/min. Swelling of the left lower extremity is noted, and dorsiflexion of the foot elicits pain. Doppler ultrasonography confirms acute left lower extremity **DVT** of the **popliteal vein**.

Based on updated American College of Chest Physicians guidelines, which of the following is the most appropriate initial management?
A. Compression stockings
B. Rivaroxaban
C. Tissue plasminogen activator
D. Warfarin

Answer: _____

AR 22 (cont.)

According to recent guidelines from the American College of Chest Physicians, the use of a target-specific anticoagulant (apixaban, rivaroxaban) alone is recommended over warfarin in patients with proximal deep venous thrombosis

AR 23

28-year-old man is evaluated in the ED for a 24-hour history of swelling of the left lower extremity. Medical history is noncontributory, and he takes no meds.
On exam, temp 97.0° F (36.1° C), BP 120/75 mmHg, HR 80 bpm, and RR 14 bpm. Pulses are intact. He has a swollen left calf that is slightly tender to palpation. Labs show an activated partial thromboplastin time of 32 seconds, platelet count of 256,000 cells/mm³, and INR of 1.0. Doppler ultrasonography of the left leg shows an acute **DVT** in the left popliteal vein extending to the iliac vein.
The patient expresses significant concern about anticoagulant therapy. An uncle died of a **cerebral hemorrhage** while being treated for acute coronary syndrome.

According to several trials on treatment of venous thromboembolism, which of the following is the most appropriate treatment for this patient?
A. Apixaban
B. Aspirin
C. Clopidogrel
D. LMWH followed by warfarin

Answer: _____

AR 23 (cont.)

A meta-analysis of numerous studies shows that target-specific oral anticoagulants, such as apixaban, were associated with a lower odds ratio of fatal bleeding, case fatality due to bleeding, and a higher likelihood of survival following a major bleed compared with LMWH and warfarin

Introduction — Importance of Initial Anticoagulation
- Venous thromboembolism (**VTE**) is comprised of 2 entities, DVT and PE
- VTE has significant morbidity and **mortality** for both the inpatient and outpatient population
- The risk of recurrent thrombosis and embolization is highest in the **1st few days & weeks** following diagnosis
- Thus, initial anticoagulation during the 1st few days (**0–10 days**) is critical in the prevention of recurrence and VTE-related death

Barritt DW, Jordan SC. Anticoagulant drugs in the treatment of pulmonary embolism: A controlled trial. *Lancet.* 1960;1(7138):1309

Indications for Anticoagulation
- Patients with ultrasound-proven **proximal** DVT
  - Popliteal, femoral, or iliac vein
- Most cases of symptomatic **distal** DVT
  - Below the knee and in the calf veins
- Pulmonary embolism
- For each patient, the decision to anticoagulate must weigh the risk of morbidity and mortality without anticoagulation against the risk of **bleeding** on anticoagulation

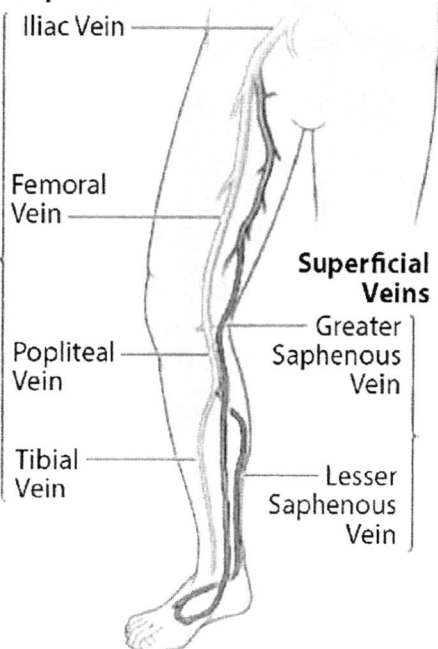

Deep Veins
Iliac Vein
Femoral Vein
Popliteal Vein
Tibial Vein
Superficial Veins
Greater Saphenous Vein
Lesser Saphenous Vein

Traditional Treatment of DVT / PE

- **UF heparin** (IV & sub Q) nomogram ± bolus
  - Adjusted by aPTT to 1.5–2 times control
  - HIT
- **LMWH** 1 mg/kg bid or 1.5 mg/kg daily
  - Renal adjustment
    - GFR < 30
- Warfarin
  - Begin on day 1
  - Overlap by 5 days and INR 2–3
    - Takes 5 days to suppress the activity of the intrinsic pathway
    - Factor **7** shortest half-life

Selection of Agent — Warfarin

- Warfarin **cannot** be administered as the only initial anticoagulant for the treatment of patients with VTE
- However, when chosen as the long-term anticoagulant, it must be coadministered with heparin so that **full anticoagulation** is assured
  - Studies have shown that patients on LMWH for VTE after **2 weeks** have almost total resolution showing the importance of immediate therapeutic anticoagulation

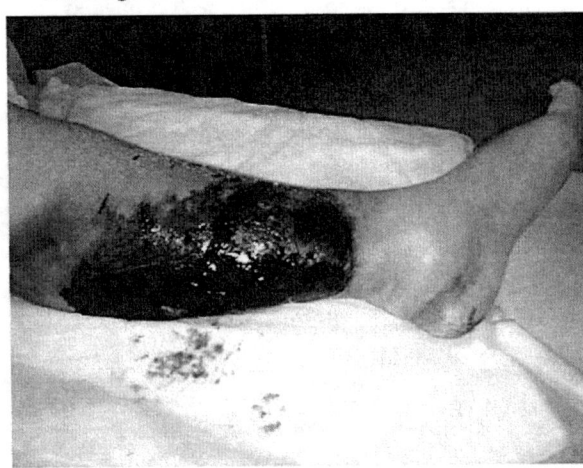

Options for initial anticoagulation include the following:

1) Unfractionated heparin (UFH)
2) LMWH
3) Fondaparinux
4) Oral Factor 10a inhibitors

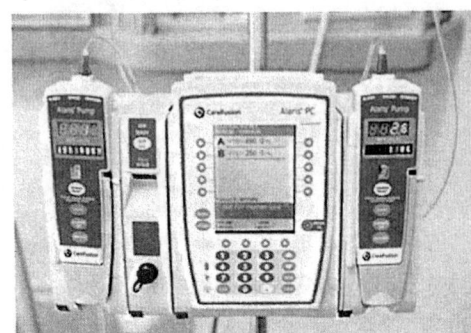

New Nomenclature

- Factor 10a and direct thrombin inhibitors have a variety of names including:
  - New/Novel oral anticoagulants
  - Non–vitamin K-antagonist oral anticoagulants
  - Direct oral anticoagulants (DOA)
  - Target-specific oral anticoagulants

Fibrin Formation

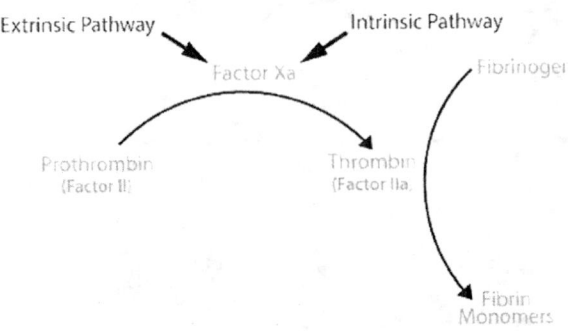

Bleeding Risk

- Tools are available for estimating the risk of bleeding in anticoagulated individuals (**HAS-BLED score**)
- However, none of these tools have been validated in patients anticoagulated for **VTE**
- Many clinicians use a **gestalt** estimate for assessing bleeding risk

HAS-BLED

Letter	Clinical Characteristic	Points
H	Hypertension	1
A	Abnormal Liver or Renal Function	1 or 2
S	Stroke	1
B	Bleeding	1
L	Labile INR	1
E	Elderly (age > 65)	1
D	Drugs or Alcohol	1 or 2
Maximum Score		9

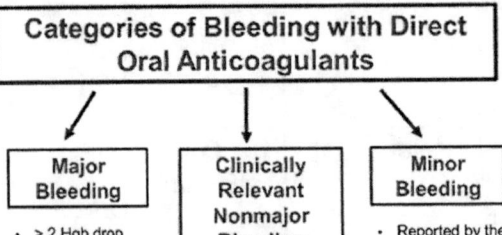

Bleeding Risk with Direct Oral Anticoagulant Therapy
Intracranial Hemorrhage
- All DOA have decreased risk compared to warfarin
- Studies are predominantly in atrial fibrillation patients

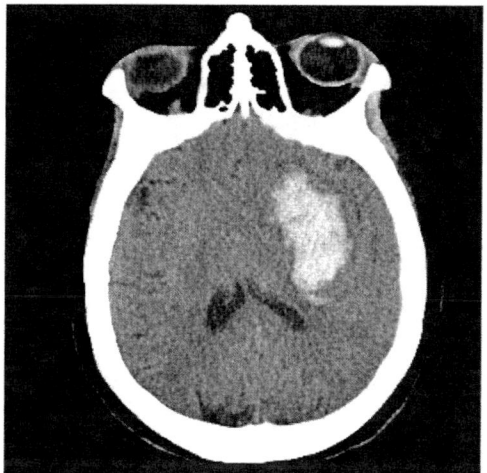

GI Bleeding
- All DOA have increased risk compared to warfarin except apixaban
- Apixaban had the same risk as warfarin
- Dabigatran as the highest risk of GI bleed

AR 24
A 54-year-old woman is evaluated in the emergency department after she consumed half a bottle of **dabigatran** 6 hours ago in a suicide attempt. Medical history is notable for **atrial fibrillation** and depression. Medications are dabigatran, paroxetine, and metoprolol. On exam, temp 98.0° F (36.7° C), BP **80/60 mmHg**, HR **125 bpm**, and RR 12 bpm. She has bleeding of the oral mucosa and gross blood per rectum. The remainder of the examination is normal.

Activated partial thromboplastin time	87 seconds
Hemoglobin	11.2 g/dL
Platelet count	185,000 cells/mm^3
Thrombin time	> 65 seconds

AR 24 (cont.)
In addition to intravenous normal saline, which of the following is the most appropriate treatment?
A. Andexanet alfa
B. Cryoprecipitate
C. Fresh frozen plasma
D. Idarucizumab
E. Prothrombin complex concentrate (Kcentra)

Answer: _____

AR 24 (cont.)
- Idarucizumab, a monoclonal antibody that rapidly absorbs dabigatran and causes a rapid reduction of available dabigatran in the body
- FDA approved as a reversal agent for patients with life-threatening bleeding from dabigatran

- Kcentra is the 1st FDA-approved 4-factor prothrombin complex concentrate (4F-PCC) for urgent warfarin reversal in adult patients with:
  1) Acute major bleeding
  2) Need for urgent surgery or other invasive procedure
- Kcentra replaces only those clotting factors needed for urgent warfarin reversal
- Infusion time with Kcentra is about 7x faster than with FPP and with less volume

Direct Oral Anticoagulants — Dosing
- **Rivaroxaban**
  - 15 mg bid (for the 1st three weeks) then 20 mg **daily**
  - Downside of once daily dosing is longer acting if bleeding occurs
- **Apixaban**
  - 10 mg bid (for 1st seven days) then 5 mg bid
  - Safest in renal failure, majority of drug is metabolized by the liver
- **Dabigatran**
  - 5–10 days of **parenteral anticoagulation**
  - 150 mg bid
  - Lowers pH in the stomach for adequate absorption therefore increased upper GI bleeding and dyspepsia
- **Edoxaban**
  - 5–10 days of **parenteral anticoagulation**
  - 60 mg **daily** (CrCl > 50) or 30 mg **daily** (CrCl 15–50)

General Population
- For most patients with VTE who are **hemodynamically stable**, suggest instead of IV UFH:
  - LMWH or fondaparinux
  - Oral Factor 10a inhibitors, rivaroxaban or apixaban
- Preference is based upon limited data that suggest that LMWH and fondaparinux are **superior** to UFH
- Data that also suggest that the direct oral anticoagulants have **similar** efficacy to LMWH/warfarin

- However, in practice, a decision between these agents is usually made based upon:
  - Clinician experience
  - Risk of bleeding
  - Patient comorbidities
  - Preferences
  - Cost
  - Convenience

Special Populations —Initial Anticoagulation
- **Renal failure:**
  - IV UFH is preferred anticoagulant in those with severe renal failure (CrCl < 30 mL/min)
- **Hemodynamic instability & extensive clot burden:**
  - IV UFH for extensive DVT or those with massive or submassive PE based upon an anticipated need for a procedural or surgical intervention
  - Direct oral anticoagulants and LMWH have not been adequately tested in this population

- **Anticipated need for discontinuation or reversal:**
  - IV UFH has a short half-life and a known reversibility agent (protamine sulfate)
- **Obesity or poor subcutaneous absorption:**
  - No preferred agent in patients who are obese or have massive edema; However, therapeutic anticoagulation can be assured with IV UFH
- **Malignancy:**
  - LMWH
- **Pregnancy:**
  - LMWH has a more favorable safety profile, especially when compared with warfarin

IVC filter for DVT / PE
- IVC filter
  - If anticoagulation contraindicated
  - If recurrence despite adequate anticoagulation
  - Bleeding requires discontinuation of anticoagulation
- There currently are **insufficient data** to compare the safety and efficacy of specific types of IVC filters (retrievable vs. permanent)

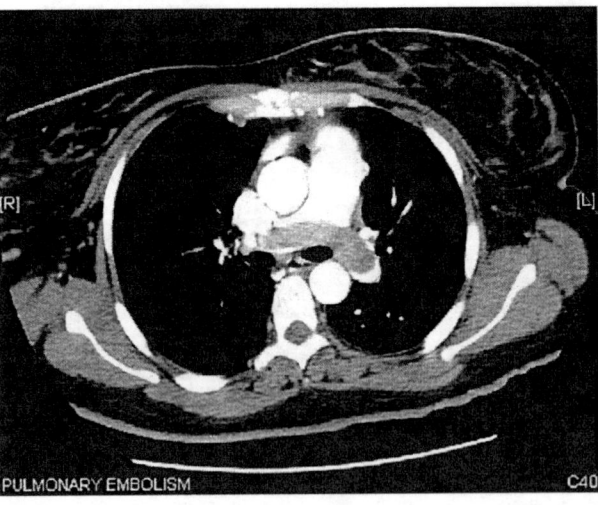

PULMONARY EMBOLISM

Thrombolytic Therapy for PE
- **Systemic** and **direct catheter**
  - 2 indications (FDA approved):
    1) Persistent hypotension
    2) Persistent severe hypoxemia despite maximization of oxygen therapy
  - tPA (FDA approved)
    - 100 mg as a continuous IV infusion administered over 2 hours
      - Can give a 40-mg bolus
  - Used to treat DVT (direct catheter)
    - Prevent postphlebitis syndrome

Thrombectomy for PE
- **Mechanical Thrombectomy**
  - Qualifies for thrombolytic therapy but has contraindications
  - Fails thrombolytic therapy
  - Associated with a high operative mortality rate

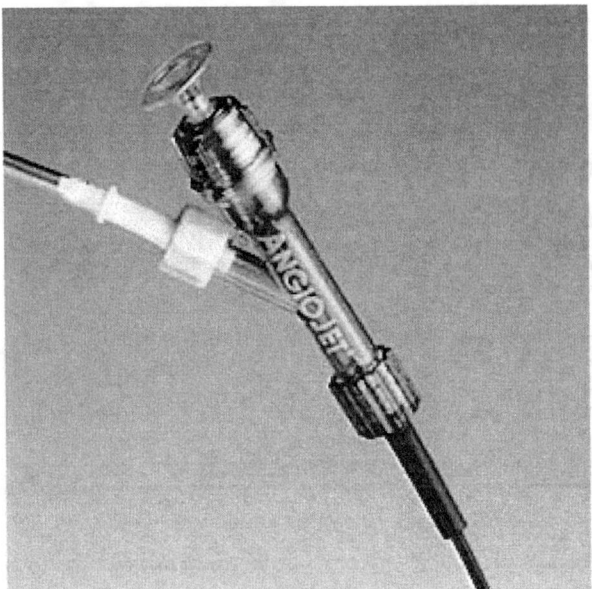

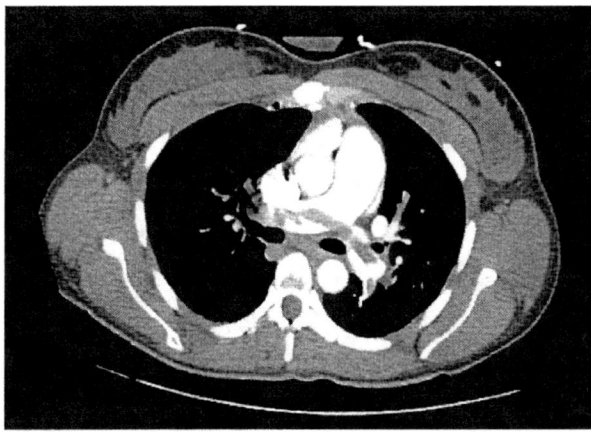

Systemic Thrombolysis of a Massive Pulmonary Embolism

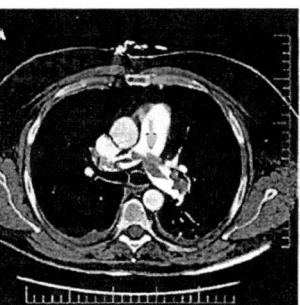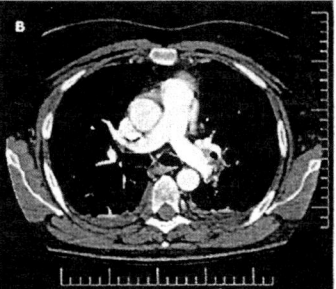

AR 25

Radiology calls you to say the CT scan reveals emboli in the right lower and middle segmental arteries. You begin LMWH and warfarin. The patient asks how long they need to take the warfarin. You tell the patient ...

A. 3 months
B. 6 months
C. 12 months
D. Indefinitely
E. Not enough information to determine this

Answer: _____

AR 26

A 44-year-old man is evaluated in follow-up for an episode of **unprovoked** left proximal leg DVT 3 months ago. Following initial anticoagulation with LMWH, he began treatment with warfarin. INR testing done every 3–4 weeks has shown a stable therapeutic INR. He has mild left leg discomfort after a long day of standing, but it does not limit his activity level. He tolerates warfarin well. Family history is unremarkable, and he takes no other medications.
On physical exam, vital signs are normal. He has mild edema of the left leg below the knee, with postthrombotic pigmentation. The remainder of the examination is unremarkable.

Which of the following is the most appropriate management?
A. Continue anticoagulation indefinitely.
B. Discontinue warfarin in another 3 months.
C. Discontinue warfarin now.
D. Discontinue warfarin and perform thrombophilia testing.

Answer: _____

AR 26 (cont.)

Long-term anticoagulation therapy is recommended for patients with unprovoked proximal leg deep venous thrombosis or pulmonary embolism who have low or moderate bleeding risk

Clinical Question
Does aspirin prevent the recurrence of venous thromboembolism?

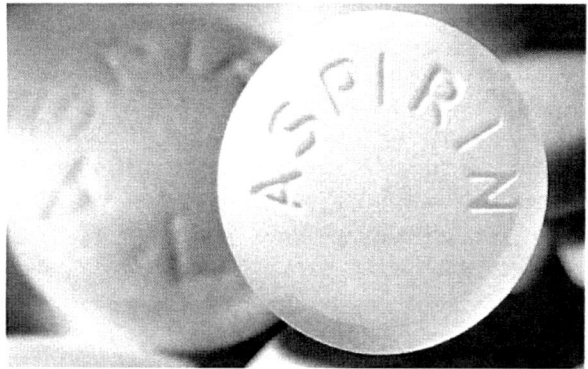

Answer
• **Yes**
• "Aspirin for Preventing the Recurrence of Venous Thromboembolism" *NEJM*, May 30, 2012.
  – The risk of recurrence of venous thromboembolism persists for many years after anticoagulant treatment is withdrawn
  – This risk is particularly high among patients with **unprovoked** venous thromboembolism, about **20% of whom have a recurrence within 2 years** after treatment with vitamin K antagonists has been discontinued
  – Extending treatment with these agents reduces the risk of recurrence but is associated with an increased risk of bleeding, as well as the inconvenience and expense of laboratory monitoring and dose adjustments

Prospectively planned combined analysis of the WARFASA and ASPIRE trials reported that aspirin as compared with placebo, significantly reduced the rate of VTE reoccurrence by 32% with no excess risk of bleeding

Clinical Question
Does D-dimer predict the recurrence of an unprovoked venous thromboembolism?

Answer
- Yes
  - Verhovsek M, et al. Systematic review: D-dimer to predict recurrent disease after stopping anticoagulant therapy for unprovoked venous thromboembolism. *Ann Intern Med.* 2008 Oct 7; 149(7):481–90, W94.

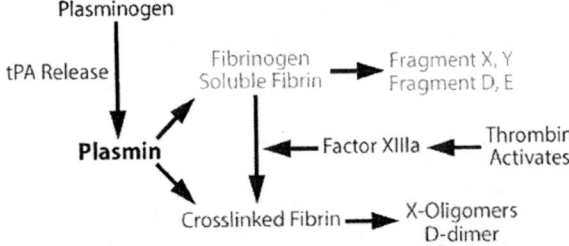

D-dimer is a **fibrin degradation product** (FDP), a small protein fragment present in the blood after a blood clot is degraded by fibrinolysis (the main enzyme is plasmin)

Clinical Question
Is gender a risk factor for recurrence of an unprovoked venous thromboembolism (VTE)?

Answer: Yes

Annals of Internal Medicine

ESTABLISHED IN 1927 BY THE AMERICAN COLLEGE OF PHYSICIANS

D-Dimer Testing to Select Patients With a First Unprovoked Venous Thromboembolism Who Can Stop Anticoagulant Therapy: A Cohort Study

Ann Intern Med. 2015;162(1):27-34. doi:10.7326/M14-1275

 The NEW ENGLAND JOURNAL of MEDICINE

ORIGINAL ARTICLE

The Risk of Recurrent Venous Thromboembolism in Men and Women

Paul A. Kyrle, M.D., Erich Minar, M.D., Christine Bialonczyk, M.D., Mirko Hirschl, M.D., Ansgar Weltermann, M.D., and Sabine Eichinger, M.D.
N Engl J Med 2004; 350:2558-2563 | June 17, 2004 | DOI: 10.1056/NEJMoa032959

- The risk for recurrence in patients with a first unprovoked VTE who have **negative D-dimer** results is not low enough to justify stopping anticoagulant therapy in **men** but may be low enough to justify stopping therapy in women
- The risk of recurrent venous thromboembolism is higher among men than women
- Why the women had a low risk of recurrent venous thrombosis is **unknown**

Common Clinical & Exam Questions

"What about IV Direct Thrombin Inhibitors for DVT and PE?"
- IV direct thrombin inhibitors include:
  - Bivalirudin (Angiomax)
  - Argatroban (Argatra)
- These agents have very short half-lives and specific clinical indications such as:
  - Percutaneous coronary intervention (**PCI**)
  - Heparin-induced thrombocytopenia (**HIT**)

"What labs should I check before starting the new oral anticoagulants?"
- DOA are generally administered at fixed doses without lab monitoring
- Lab testing prior to administration of these agents should include:
  - Prothrombin time (**PT**) and activated partial thromboplastin time (**aPTT**), to assess and document coagulation status before anticoagulation
  - Measurement of serum **creatinine**

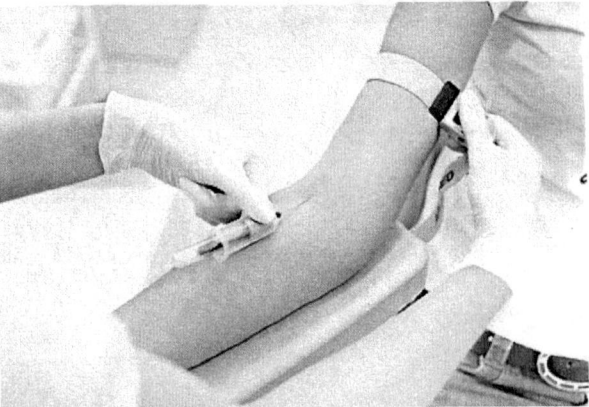

"How do I transition to the DOA?"
- **LMWH:**
  - Stop LMWH and wait till **next dose** to start DOA
- **Warfarin:**
  - Stop warfarin and wait till **INR < 2.0**, then start DOA

AR 27

When do most PE deaths occur after diagnosis?

A. 1 hour
B. 24 hours
C. 3 days
D. 1 week

Answer: _____

AR 27 (cont.)

- **1 hour**
  - Remember prophylaxis
    - Fondaparinux
    - Warfarin
    - Rivaroxaban
    - Dabigatran etexilate
    - Heparin
    - Apixaban
    - Enoxaparin

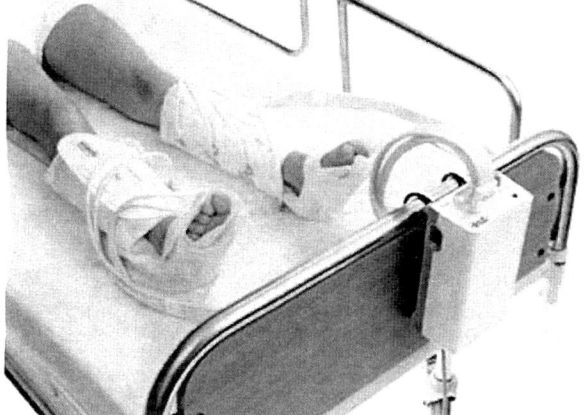

Pleural Effusions

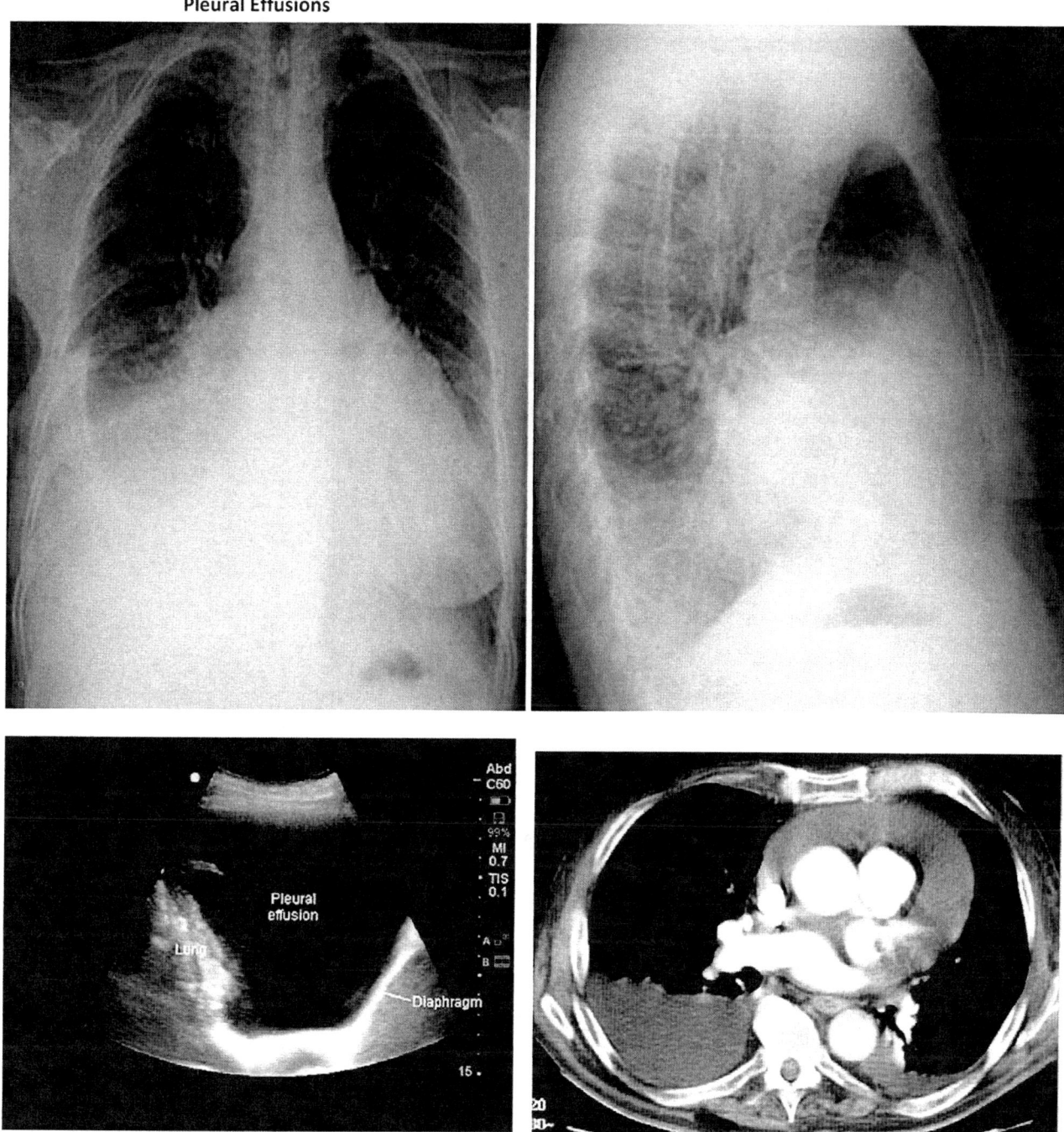

Light's Criteria

If Any **One** of the Following Criteria Is Met, the Fluid Is an **Exudate:**

Pleural Protein/Serum Protein > 0.5

Pleural LDH/Serum LDH > 0.6

Pleural LDH > 2/3 Upper Limit of Normal for Serum LDH

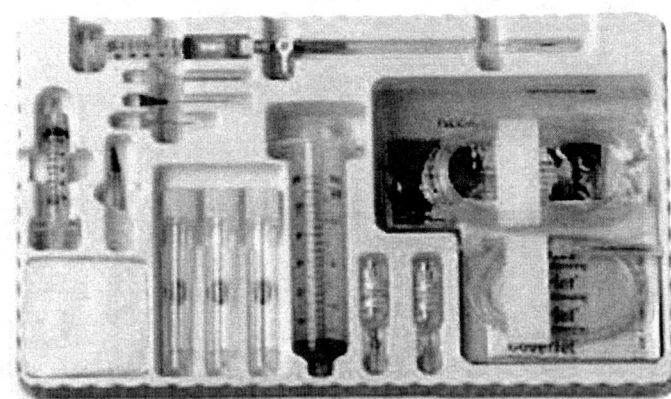

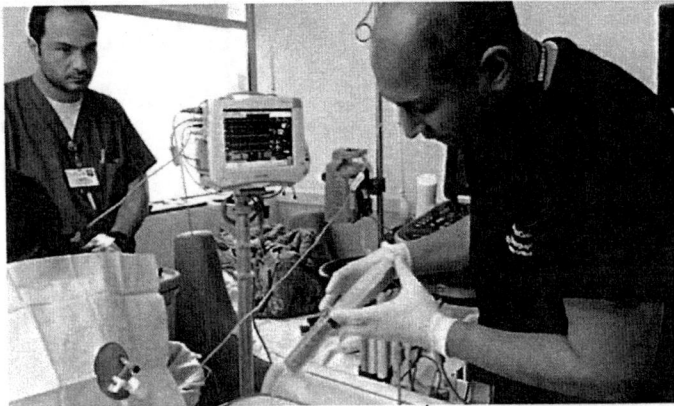

Pleural Effusions

Transudative Effusions
- CHF (LV failure)
  - Increased hydrostatic pressure
- Hypoalbuminemia (decreased oncotic pressure)
  - Cirrhosis
  - Nephrotic syndrome
- Atelectasis
- Pulmonary embolism

Exudative Effusions
- Pneumonia and malignancy
  - 80% of all exudates
- Pulmonary embolism
- Tuberculosis
- Chylothorax
- Dressler's syndrome
- Pancreatitis
- Rheumatologic disease

- **Indications for a chest tube:**
  1) Pus in pleural space
  2) Positive culture on pleural space fluid
  3) Complicated parapneumonic effusion

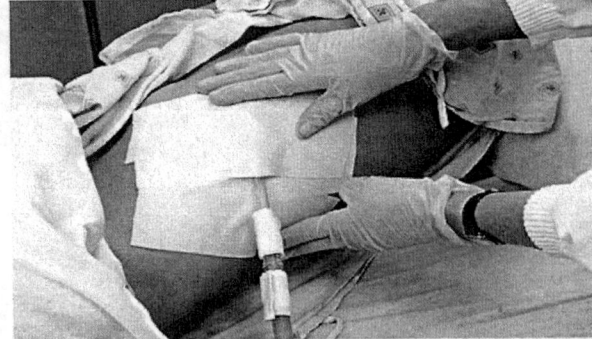

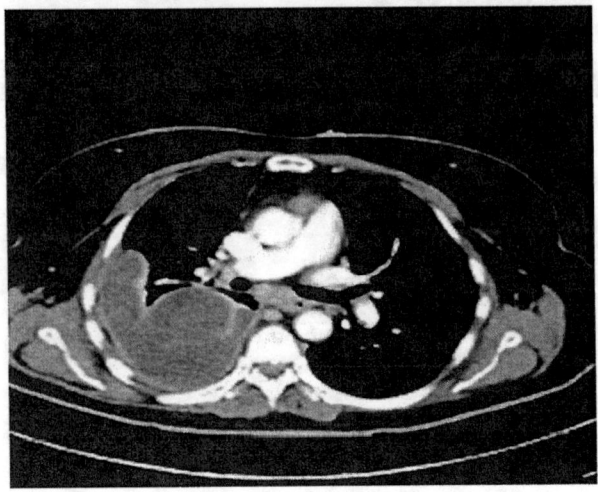

Pleural Effusions (cont.)
- **Mesothelial Cells**
  - Normally line the cavity
  - No mesothelial cells, think tuberculous effusion
- **Eosinophils**
  - Drug reaction, parasites
- **Lymphocytes**
  - TB (pleural biopsy)
  - Malignancy (cytology)
- **Neutrophils**
  - Pneumonia

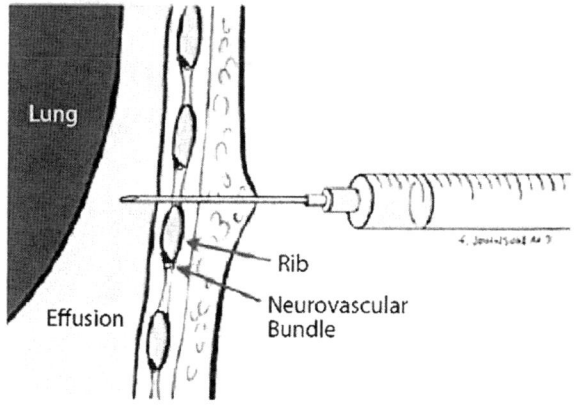

Lung

Effusion

Rib

Neurovascular Bundle

Pleural Effusions (cont.)
- **Glucose**
  - Low in RA and empyema
- **Amylase**
  - Pancreatitis (fistula)
  - Esophageal rupture
  - Tumor
- **pH**
  - pH > 7.0 suggests complicated effusion and **possible need for chest tube** or seen in RA
- **ANA**
  - Drug-induced SLE and native SLE
- **Triglycerides**
  - Chylous effusions
    - Associated with leakage of thoracic duct
    - Trauma, lymphoma, LAM

AR 28

A **62-year-old** male complains of a nonproductive **cough** and **weight loss** of 20 lbs over the last 3–4 months. He has also noted a hoarse voice for the last month. He has a 45- to 50-pack-year smoking history but quit recently. On exam, vitals are WNL; BMI is 19. Auscultation reveals decreased breath sounds with dullness to percussion on the right along with (+) egophony and decreased tactile fremitus prolonged expiration. The remainder of the exam is unremarkable.

- Chest CT shows a **pleural effusion** on the right and a **right upper lobe mass**
- Diagnostic thoracentesis is performed, and 100 mL of fluid is removed that reveals a lymphocytic exudate
- Cytology is negative for malignancy

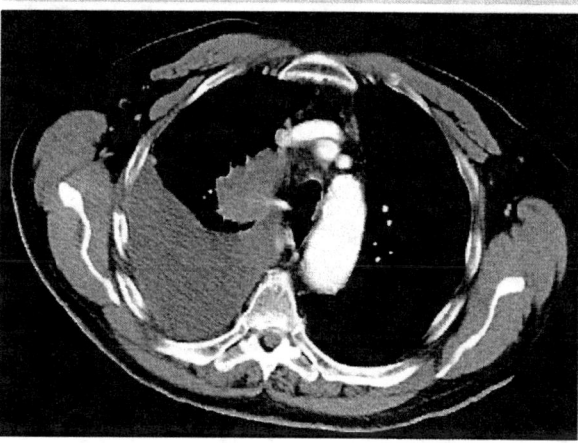

AR 28 (cont.)
Which of the following is the most appropriate next step in the evaluation of this patient?
A. Bronchoscopy ± EBUS.
B. Closed pleural biopsy.
C. PET scan.
D. Repeat thoracentesis and pleural fluid cytology.

Answer: _____

AR 28 (cont.)
- Imaging demonstrates a unilateral pleural effusion with an ipsilateral **lung mass** suspicious for bronchogenic carcinoma with pleural metastasis
- Initial evaluation is with thoracentesis, because positive cytology for non–small-cell carcinoma will effectively establish a diagnosis and simultaneously establish the malignancy as **Stage IV**
- The overall sensitivity of pleural fluid cytology averages 60%, with 65% of positive results obtained on the initial sampling; An additional **27%** are identified on the 2nd sampling, and **5%** on the 3rd

For Malignant Effusions
- Indwelling pleural catheter (PleurX catheter)
  - For symptomatic reaccumulating malignant pleural effusions
  - Can combine with chemical pleurodesis

For Malignant Effusions (cont.)

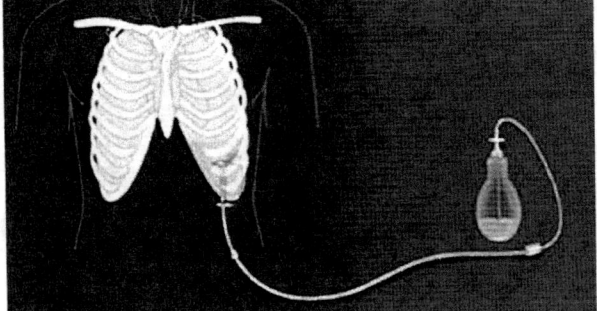

Bonus Case

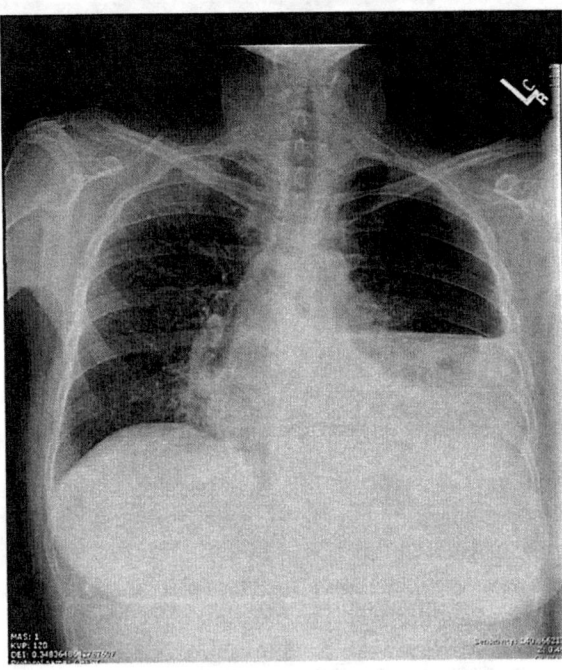

Chest Tube Placed at the Bedside

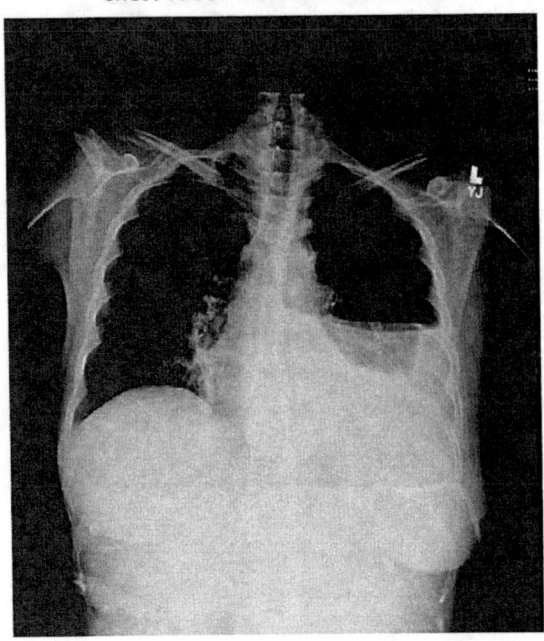

**No Improvement in the Patient's Shortness of Breath …
What is the Diagnosis?**

Chest Tube in the Spleen

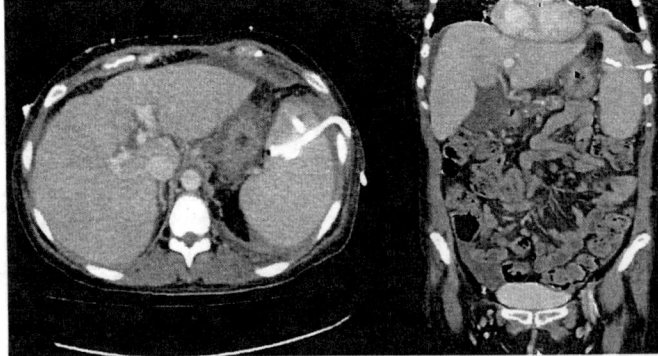

Pneumothorax — Chest X-Ray & CT Chest

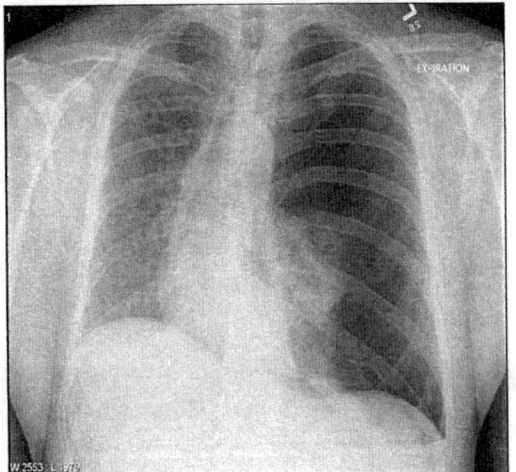

If patient is stable, prefer an upright expiratory film

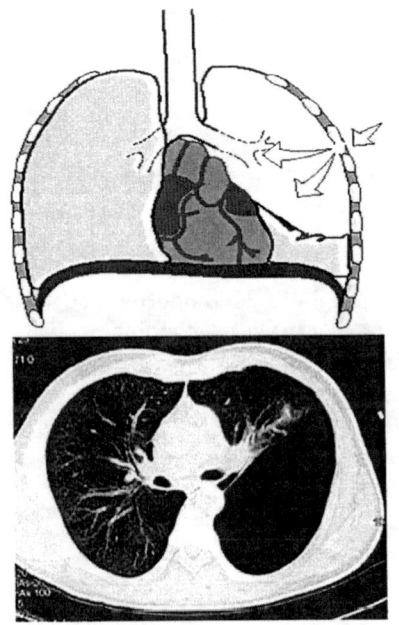

© 2017 MedStudy Internal Medicine Video Board Review – Pulmonary Medicine • Raj Dasgupta, MD

Pneumothorax — Ultrasound

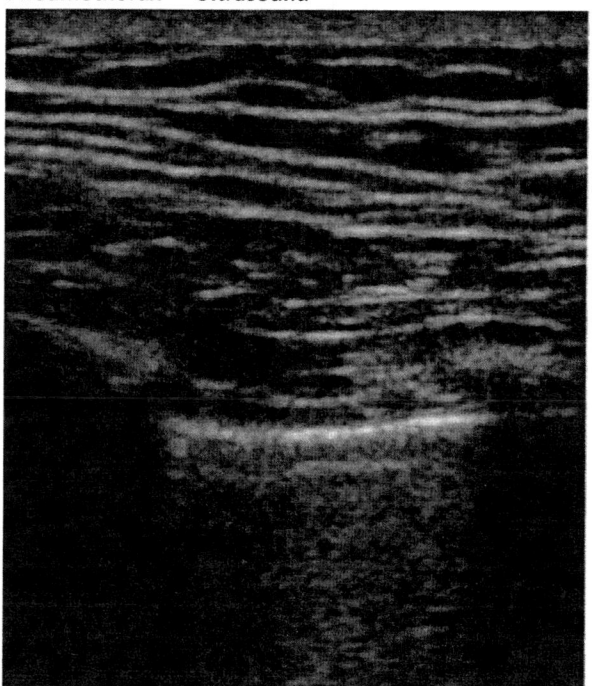

Pneumothorax — Types
- **Primary**
  - No history of lung disease or smoking
  - Tall slender body habitus
  - Pectus excavatum
- **Secondary**
  - COPD
  - Asthma
  - Cystic Fibrosis
  - Infections
- **Traumatic/Latrogenic**
  - MVA
  - Central line placement
- **Tension**
  - Positive pressure ventilation

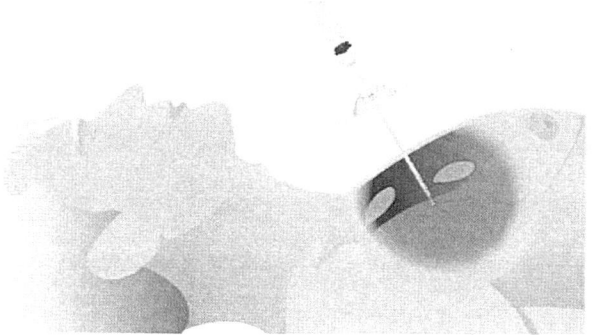

Pneumothorax — Treatment
- O_2 and observation if patient is stable and PNX is small
  - Distance between the lung and the chest wall is ≤ 2–3 cm on CXR
  - Nitrogen washout
- Pleural aspiration as initial therapy rather than chest tube insertion if patient is stable and PNX > 3 cm
  - Chest tube should be inserted if aspiration fails
  - Heimlich valve

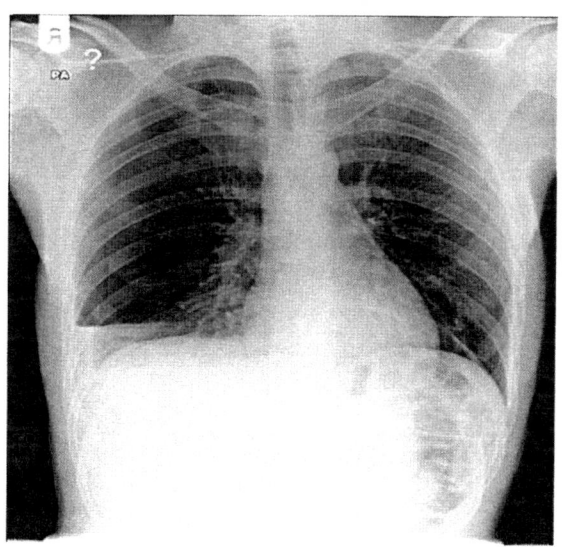

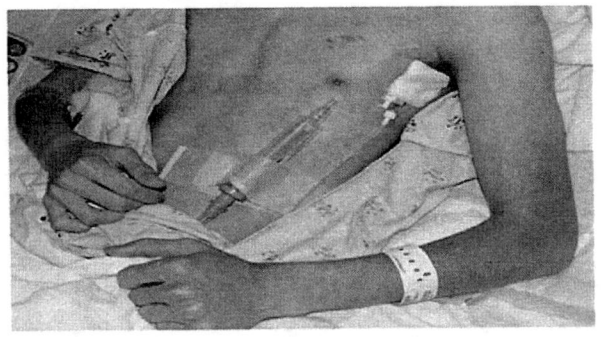

Pneumothorax — Treatment (cont.)
- Patients who are stable with a recurrent PNX should have a chest tube inserted
- Recurrent PNX should be evaluated for a preventive intervention
- Chemical pleurodesis should be performed through a chest tube if VATS is not readily available or patient declines

Talc Pleurodesis

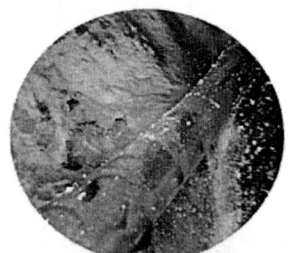

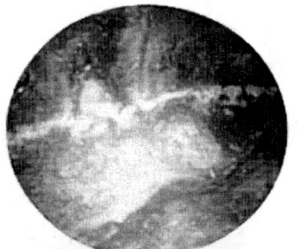

THORACOSCOPIC INSUFFLATION

SLURRY THROUGH CHEST TUBE

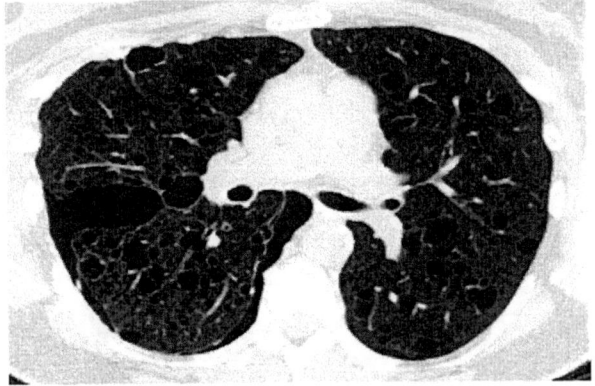

© 2017 *MedStudy Internal Medicine Video Board Review – Pulmonary Medicine* • Raj Dasgupta, MD

Pneumothorax — Pleural Aspiration

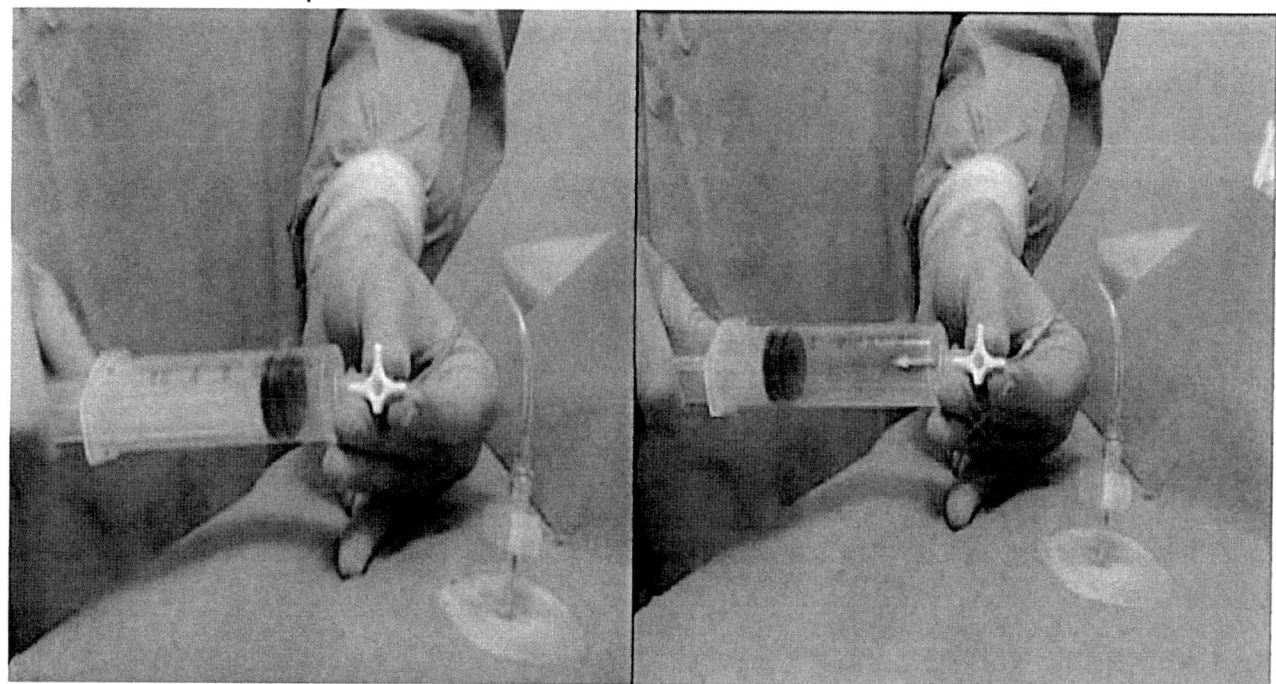

Pneumothorax — Pigtail Catheter

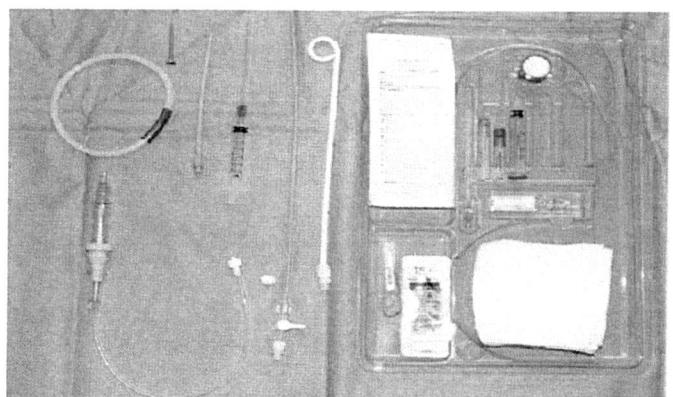
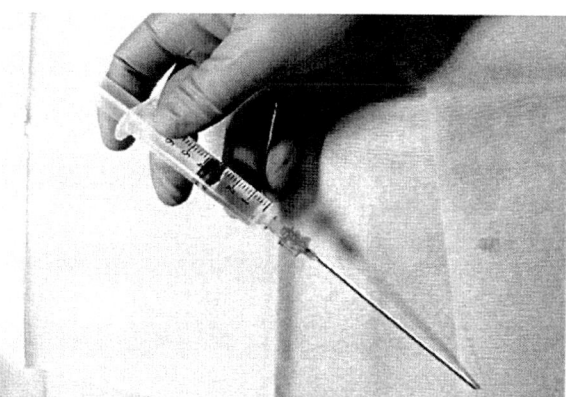
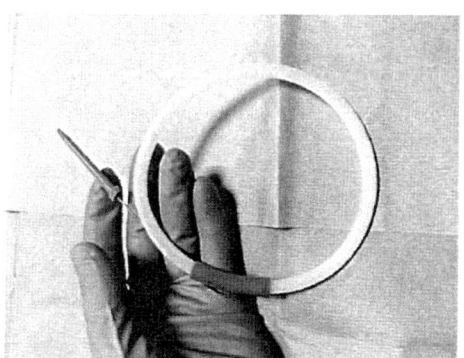
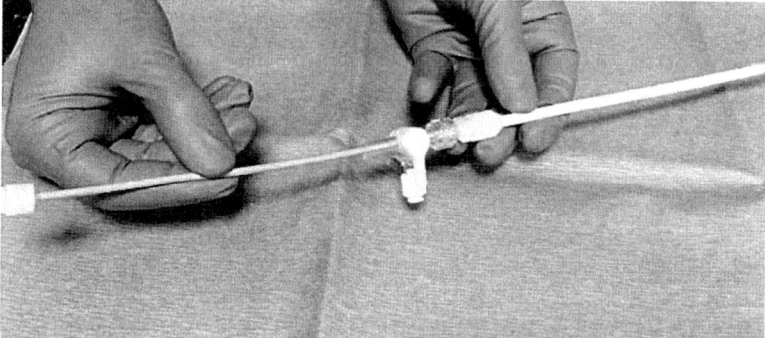

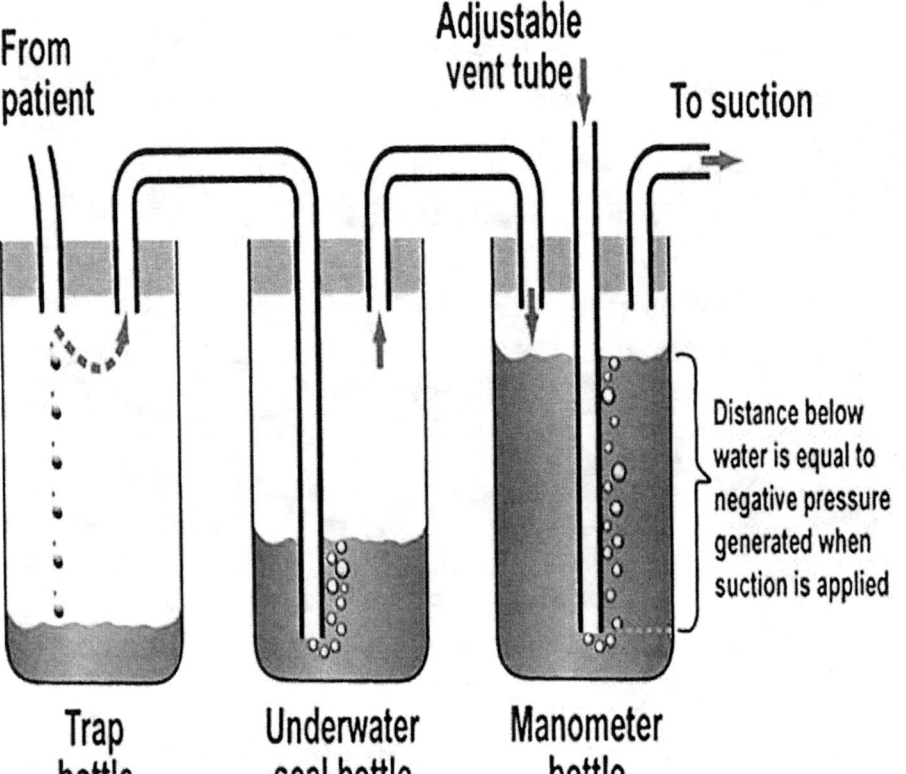

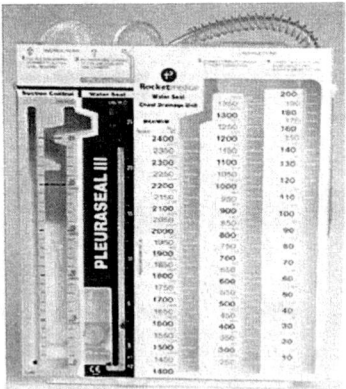

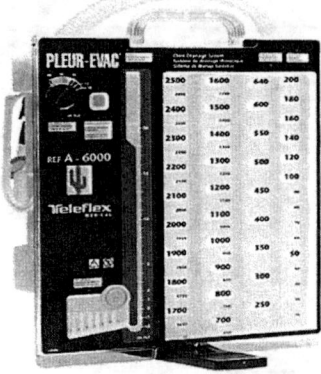

Chest Tube — Contraindications
- No absolute contraindications, particularly if the patient is in respiratory distress or has a tension pneumothorax
- Anticoagulation or bleeding diathesis is a relative contraindication

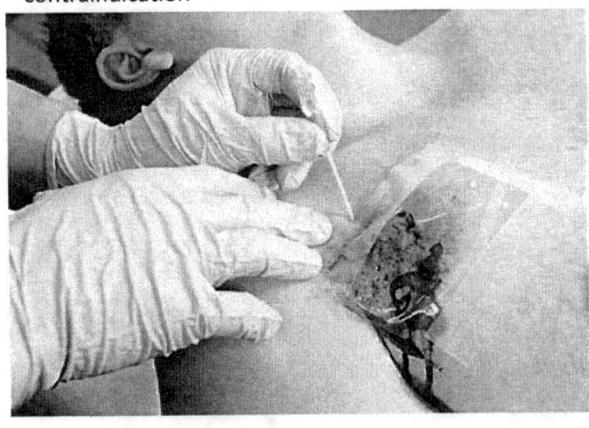

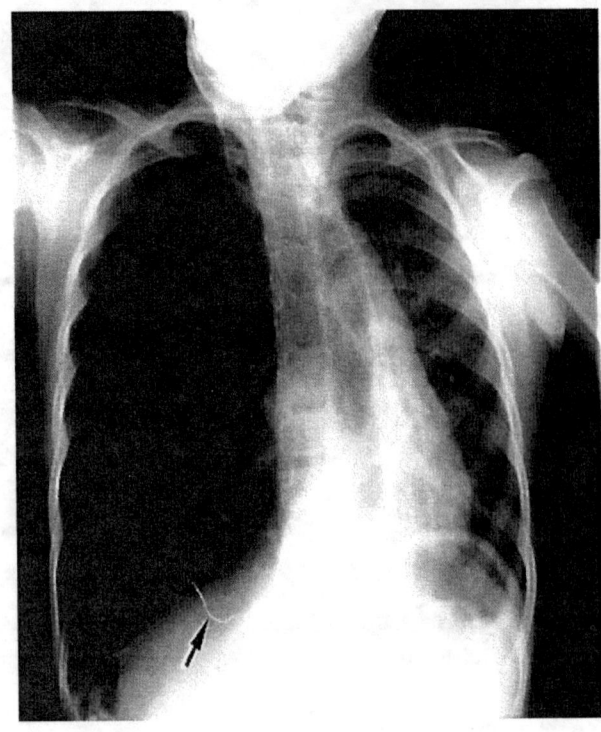

High-Yield Bacterial Pneumonias for IM Exams
- *Streptococcus pneumoniae*
  - Gram (+) lancet-shaped cocci or diplococci
  - Rust-colored sputum
  - Urinary antigen
- *Staphylococcus aureus*
  - Gram (+) cocci in clusters
  - CA-MRSA: Panton-Valentine leukocidin (PVL)
  - HA-MRSA

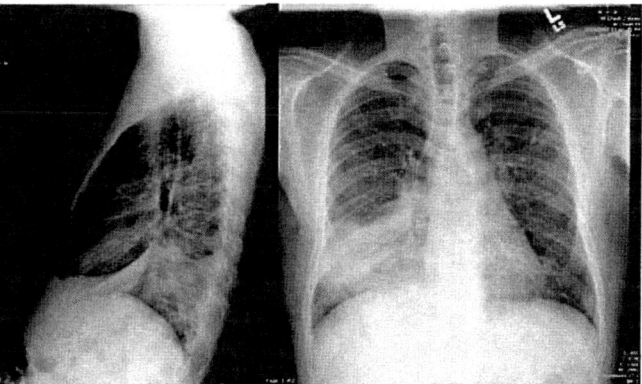

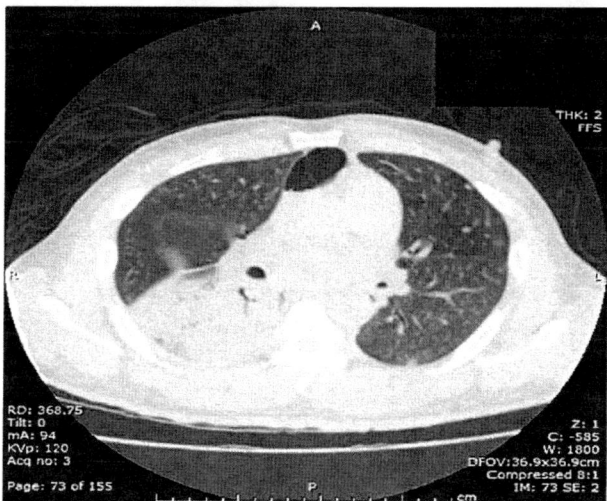

High-Yield Bacterial Pneumonias for IM Exams (cont.)
- *Coxiella burnetii*
  - Cattle, goats, and sheep are most commonly infected
  - **Q-fever**
    - The "Q" stands for "query" and was applied at a time when the causative agent was unknown
- *Chlamydophila psittaci*
  - **Intracellular bacteria**
  - **Psittacosis** also known as parrot fever
- *Francisella tularensis*
  - Intracellular gram (–) rod-shaped coccobacillus
  - Discovered in squirrels in Tulare County, California (Tularemia)

- *Pseudomonas aeruginosa*
  - Gram (–) rod
  - Nosocomial infection
  - Immunocompromised
- *Klebsiella pneumoniae*
  - Gram-negative rod encapsulated
  - Currant jelly sputum
  - Alcoholism
  - "Bulging fissure"

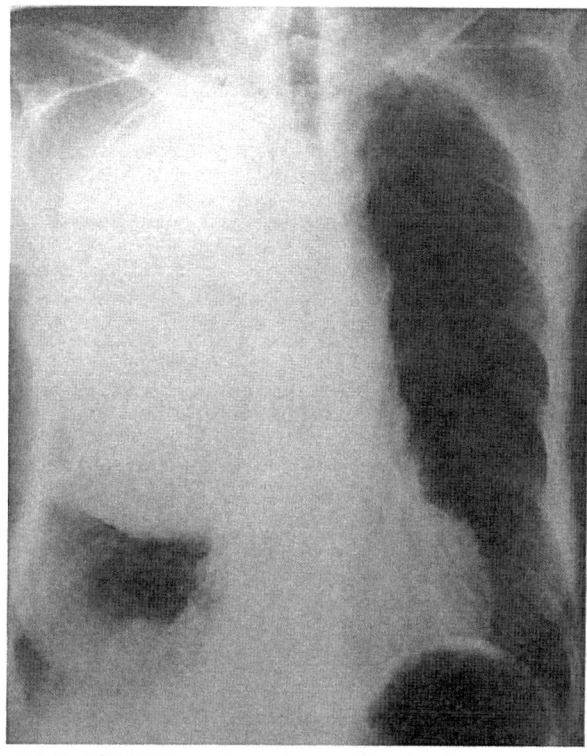

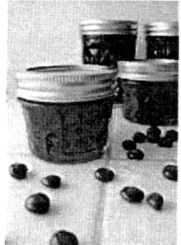
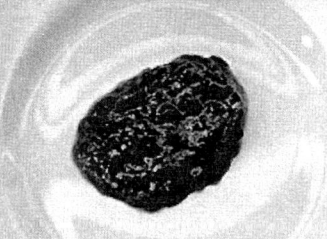

High-Yield Bacterial Pneumonias for IM Exams (cont.)
- *Mycoplasma pneumoniae*
  - Walking pneumonia
  - Extrapulmonary manifestations:
    - Cold agglutinin (IgM)
    - Arthritis
    - Erythema multiforme
- *Legionella pneumophila*
  - Gram (–) flagellated
  - Urinary antigen
  - Hyponatremia & relative bradycardia
  - Cruise ships

High-Yield Bacterial Pneumonias for IM Exams (cont.)
- *Nocardia asteroides*
  - Gram (+) rod
  - Weakly acid fast
  - Common disease sites
    - Lung (cavitation)
    - CNS
    - Skin
  - Trimethoprim/sulfamethoxazole
- *Actinomyces israelii*
  - Gram (+) rod
  - Forms characteristic sulfur granules in infected tissue but not *in vitro*
  - Cervicofacial abnormalities
  - Penicillin

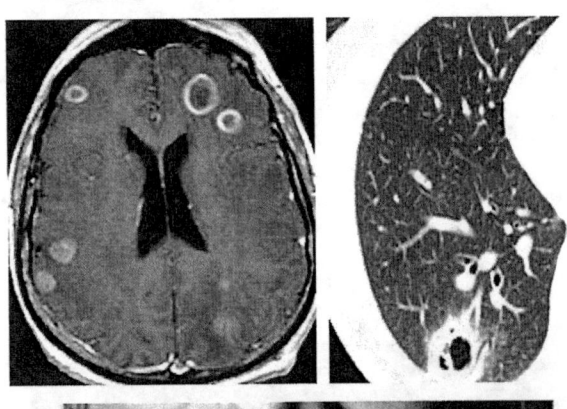

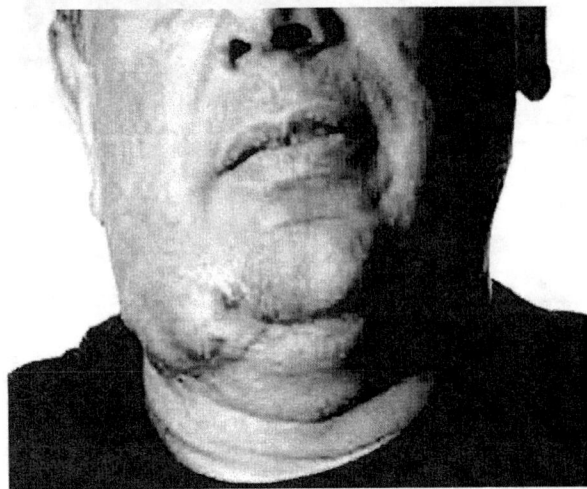

Lumpy Jaw Syndrome

Fungal Histology

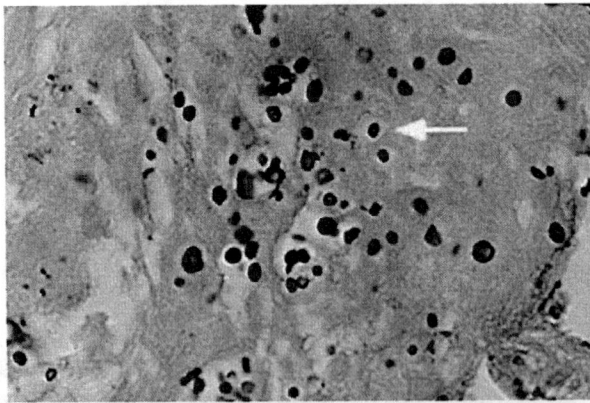

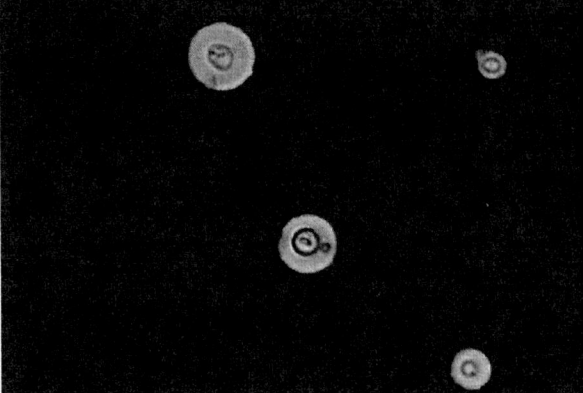

Fungal Histology (cont.)

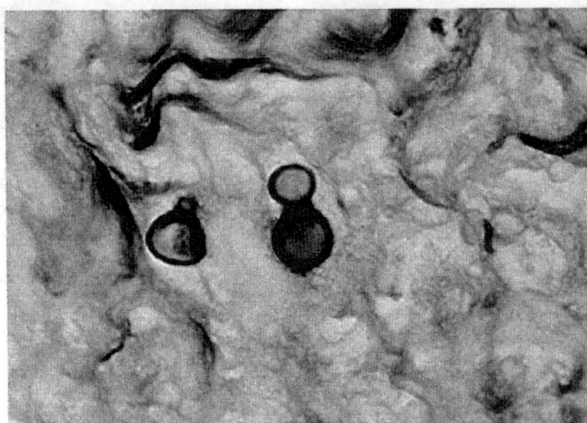

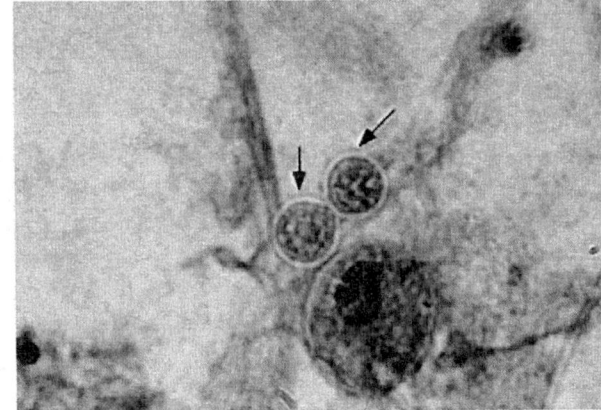

Fungal Histology (cont.)

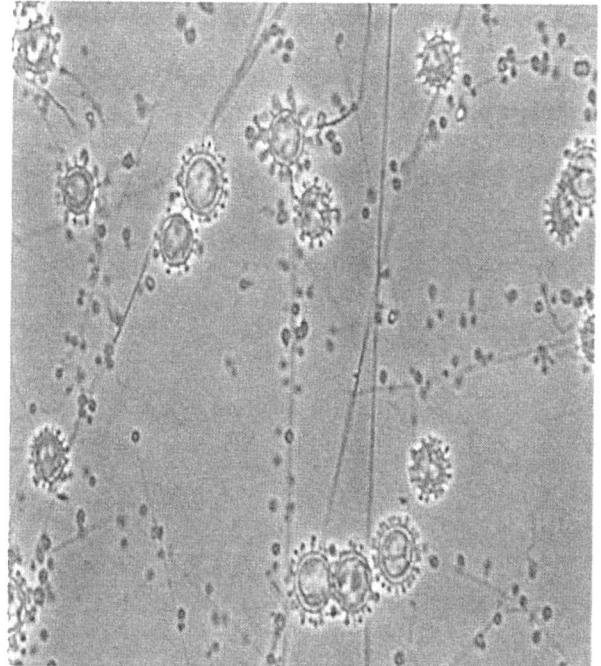

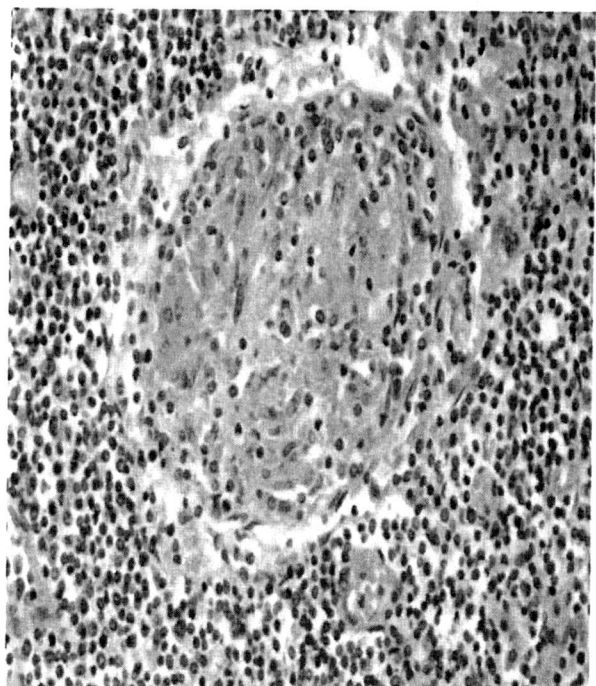

Fungal Histology (cont.)

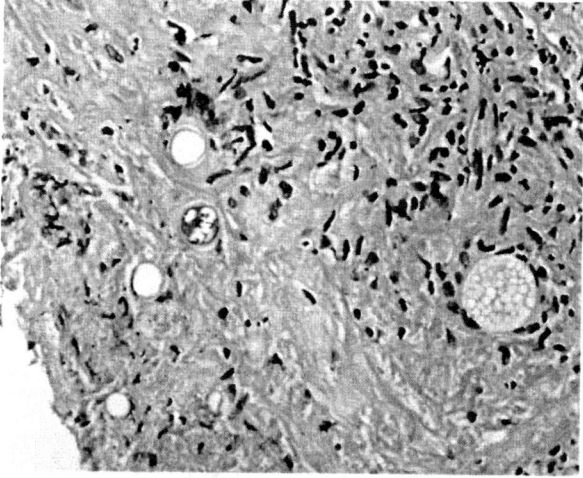

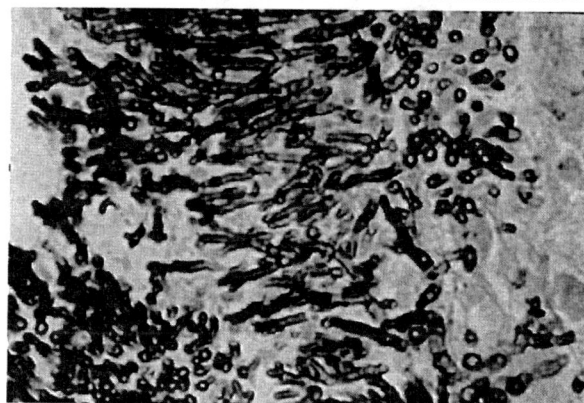

Common Fungi for IM Exams
- *Aspergillus* spp.
  - *A. fumigatus*
  - *A. flavus*
  - *A. niger*
- *Cryptococcus* spp.
  - *C. neoformans*
    - "Cannon ball" peripheral skin lesions
    - CSF antigen or India ink
  - Flucytosine
- *Blastomyces*
  - Arkansas & Wisconsin
- *Sporothrix*
  - *S. schenckii*
    - Gardeners

- *Mucor* spp. *& Rhizopus* spp.
  - *Zygomycosis*
    - In DM, sinusitis is more common
- *Histoplasma*
  - *H. capsulatum*
    - Mediastinal fibrosis
    - Splenomegaly
- *Coccidioides* spp.
  - *C. immitis*
    - "Valley fever"
    - Flu-like illness with arthralgias/erythema nodosum

What is Tuberculosis?

- Tuberculosis (TB) is a disease caused by a bacterium called *Mycobacterium tuberculosis* that is spread from person to person through the **air**
- TB usually affects the lungs (a.k.a. **primary or pulmonary TB**), but it can also affect other parts of the body, such as the brain, kidneys, or spine
- Not everyone infected with TB bacteria becomes sick; As a result, 2 TB-related conditions exist:
  1) Latent TB
  2) Active TB

What is Latent Tuberculosis?

- Persons with latent TB infection do not feel sick and **do not** have any symptoms
- They are infected with *M. tuberculosis*, but do not have active TB disease
- The only sign of TB infection is a positive reaction to the tuberculin skin test or TB blood test
- Persons with latent TB infection are **not infectious** and cannot spread TB infection to others

Screening for Latent TB Infection

- The Mantoux test
  - **Intradermal** injection of 0.1 mL of purified protein derivative (PPD) in the forearm
  - The injection site is evaluated in 48–72 hours after injection
  - The reading is based on the diameter of the induration/swollen area (**not the red area**)
  - Measure **perpendicularly** to the long axis of the forearm

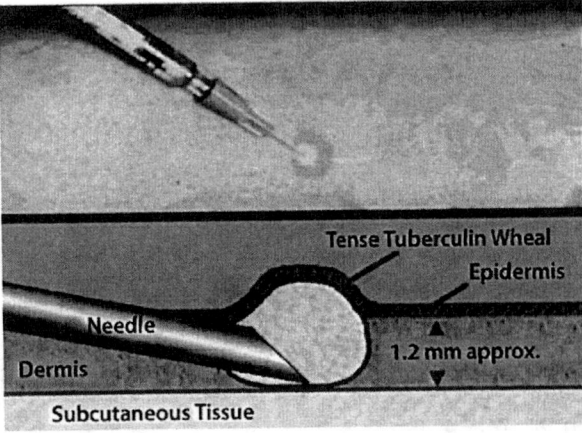

Screening for Latent TB Infection (cont.)

- Current recommendations from the **CDC** as to what constitutes a (+) reading
- Take into account the degree of **clinical suspicion** of LTBI
- Never PPD first in acutely symptomatic patients

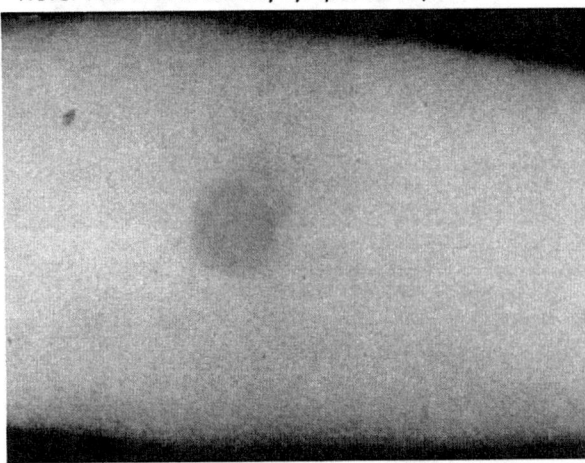

Screening for Latent TB Infection (cont.)

5 mm
- Is positive for those in the high-risk group
  - **HIV** or major cell-mediated dysfunction
  - Fibrotic changes on CXR consistent with prior TB
  - Close contact with a documented case
  - Patients with organ transplant and other immunosuppressed patients
    - Receiving the equivalent of > 15 mg/day of prednisone for ≥ 1 month

15 mm
- Is positive for the low-risk group
  - No known risk factors

10 mm
- Is positive for those in the moderate-risk group
  - Homeless persons
  - Recent immigrants
    - Within 5 years from high prevalence countries
  - IV drug abusers who are HIV negative
  - Prisoners
  - Health care workers
  - Nursing home patients and staff
  - **Diabetics**
  - Renal failure
  - Hematologic malignancy
  - Immunosuppressive therapy
    - < 15 mg/day prednisone

Summary
- Who should be tested in general?
  - Asymptomatic patients who are at risk
- What is a positive test?
  - > 5 mm
    - HIV, CXR (+), close contacts, severely immunocompromised
  - > 15 mm
    - No risk factors
  - > 10 mm
    - All the rest

Screening for Latent TB Infection (cont.)
- "New converter" and "booster effect"
  - Are terms to discuss patients who are monitored with yearly PPD
- Booster effect
  - Stimulating T cells with bad memory
  - Significant induration on the 2nd test but not the 1st
  - Effect can **persist for several months**, so it becomes difficult to diagnose a "new converter"
- 2-step TB skin test:
  - For patients with annual screening on the **1st screening**
  - Help diagnose "new converter" by getting a "**baseline**" with the 2nd step if the 1st is nonreactive
  - The risk of TB reactivation is highest in the 1st two years of a new converter

- What is treatment for a positive test?
  - 9 months of isoniazid (**4 options per CDC**)*
- Who should be treated?
  - Everyone (**controversial**)*
- What is the risk of developing TB with a positive test?
  - 10% lifetime risk (**5% in the 1st two years**)*
  - HIV (+) the risk is 10% per year
  - After INH treatment, the lifetime risk is 1–2%
- What is the effect of previous BCG vaccination on these recommendations?
  - Means nothing (**use gamma release assay**)*
- When is anergy testing the answer?
  - Never

Anergy Skin Testing
- Persons who do not mount a delayed-type hypersensitivity response are considered to be **anergic**, such as HIV
- The **1991** guidelines recommended the use of companion or "control" antigens in conjunction with PPD testing to provide additional information about a person's ability to mount a DTH response
- If the PPD is (−), and at least 1 antigen from the anergy panel is reactive, this individual's immune system is considered **healthy** enough to mount an immune response

Screening for Latent TB Infection (cont.)
- 2 IGRAs are approved by the U.S. Food and Drug Administration (FDA) and are available in the United States:
  1) QuantiFERON-TB Gold In-Tube (QFT-GIT) test
  2) T-SPOT.*TB* (T-SPOT) test

QuantiFERON-TB Gold
- Approved by the FDA in **2005** as a means of diagnosing tuberculosis
- The CDC considers the test to be an alternative to skin testing
- Incubating the patient's blood for 16–24 hours with synthetic peptides representing 2 TB-specific antigens
  - These antigens will stimulate interferon-gamma release from the patient's white blood cells, which is then measured by ELISA
  - Results are reported as positive, negative, or **indeterminate**

T-SPOT
- FDA approved in **2008**
- The T-SPOT is a unique, single-visit blood test for tuberculosis (TB) screening, also known as an interferon gamma release assay (IGRA)
- The T-SPOT is the only blood test for latent TB that has demonstrated both sensitivity and specificity exceeding **95%**

- Positive > 8 spots
- Negative < 4 spots
- Borderline 5, 6, or 7 spots

Advantages of QuantiFERON-TB Gold and T-SPOT
- The patient does not need to return for a reading
- Results are available within 24 hours
- There is no booster phenomenon
- There is no reader bias (as can affect skin test interpretation)
- The result is not affected by prior BCG vaccination
- Not affected by HIV (anergy)

Latent TB Treatment
- It is essential to rule out **active TB**
- Latent TB treatment to someone with active TB presents a serious risk of developing **drug-resistant** strains of TB
- There are 4 (CDC 2014) treatment regimens:
  1) 9 months of isoniazid is the gold standard (93% effective)
  2) 6 months of isoniazid based on cost effectiveness, patient compliance, and drug toxicity
  3) 4 months of rifampin for those who are unable to take INH or had exposure to INH-resistant TB
  4) 3-month (12-dose) regimen of weekly rifapentine and isoniazid

Latent TB Facts
- It isn't easy to catch TB; You need consistent exposure to the contagious person for a long time; For that reason, you're more likely to catch TB from a relative than a stranger
- It is assumed by most medical doctors that latent tuberculosis is the normal or regular strain of tuberculosis
- There are 3 other types of tuberculosis recognized in the world today:
  1) Multidrug-Resistant Tuberculosis (**MDR TB**)
     - Resistant to at least INH and rifampin
  2) Extensively Drug-Resistant Tuberculosis (**XDR TB**)
     - INH and rifampin, plus any fluoroquinolone and at least 1 of 3 injectable 2nd line drugs
  3) Totally Drug-Resistant Tuberculosis (**TDR TB**)

Case — History & Physical Exam
A 39-year-old **homeless** man comes to the clinic with a several-month history of a productive cough. He also reported nightly fevers to **103.1° F (39.5° C)** associated with chills. During the past 6 months, he has had a **20-lb weight loss.**
He is a nonsmoker, and his medical history is significant for a hospitalization 4 months ago. He was lost to follow-up after discharge.
He is thin and unkempt appearing, in no acute distress; He has bitemporal wasting, poor dentition, and multiple **1- to 2-cm mobile cervical lymph nodes.**
Temp 101.1° F (38.4° C), BP 105/60 mmHg, HR 88 bpm, and RR 20 bpm

Cardiac and pulmonary examinations are normal. Examination of his abdomen is benign, and extremities are normal.

Case —History & Physical Exam (cont.)
- **Differential Diagnosis**
  - Active TB
  - Lung abscess
  - Bronchiectasis
  - Lung cancer
  - Pneumonia

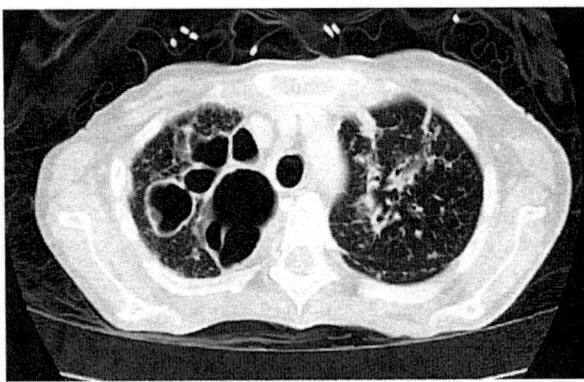

- **Initial Diagnostic Plan:**
  - Respiratory isolation
  - Sputum for culture and AFB
    - Induced
    - Bronch with BAL ± TBB
  - CXR/CT
- **Results:**
  - Cavitary lesion in the right upper lobe
  - Acid-fast bacilli on smear

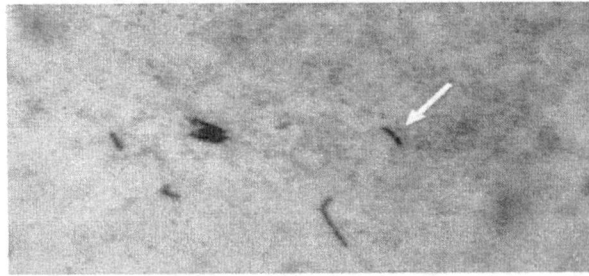

Case — Treatment
- **Suspect the diagnosis**
  - High-risk group
  - Worrisome chest x-ray
  - Consistent symptoms
- **Isolate early**
  - Airborne precautions
    - Negative pressure ventilation room
    - N95 respirator

- **Treatment Plan**
  1) Isoniazid (INH) with vitamin B_6
  2) Rifampin
  3) Pyrazinamide
  4) Ethambutol
- Used for the first 2 months; After that, isoniazid and rifampin are continued for 4 months, making it a 6-month total

Not All Acid-Fast Are TB
- *Mycobacterium* other than TB
- *M. avium complex* (MAC)
  - CT shows "tree-in-bud" pattern
  - Lady Windermere syndrome
- *M. kansasii*
- *M. scrofulaceum*
- *M. leprae*
  - Leprosy
- *M. marinum*
  - "Fish tank bacillus"
- *M. septicum*
- *M. abscessus*
- *M. xenopi*

Other acid-fast organisms
- *Nocardia*
- *Cryptosporidium*
- *Isospora belli*

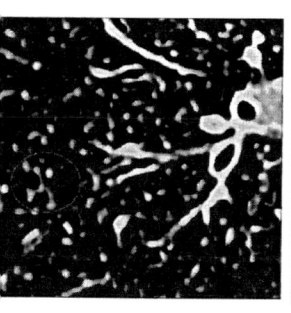
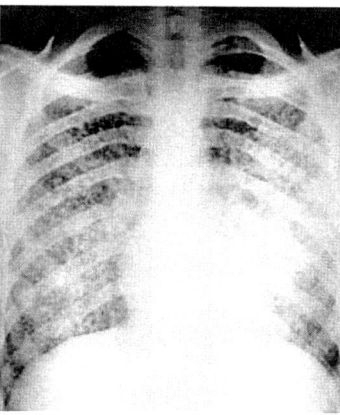

ATS / IDSA Criteria for Diagnosing NTM

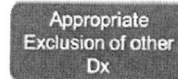

Pulmonary symptoms, nodular or cavitary opacities on chest radiograph, or a high-resolution computed tomography scan that shows multifocal bronchiectasis with multiple small nodules **+** Appropriate Exclusion of other Dx

Microbiologic

Positive culture results from at least **2** separate expectorated sputum samples **or** Positive culture results from at least **1** BAL **or** Typical biopsy + tissue culture **or** typical biopsy + positive sputum AFB culture

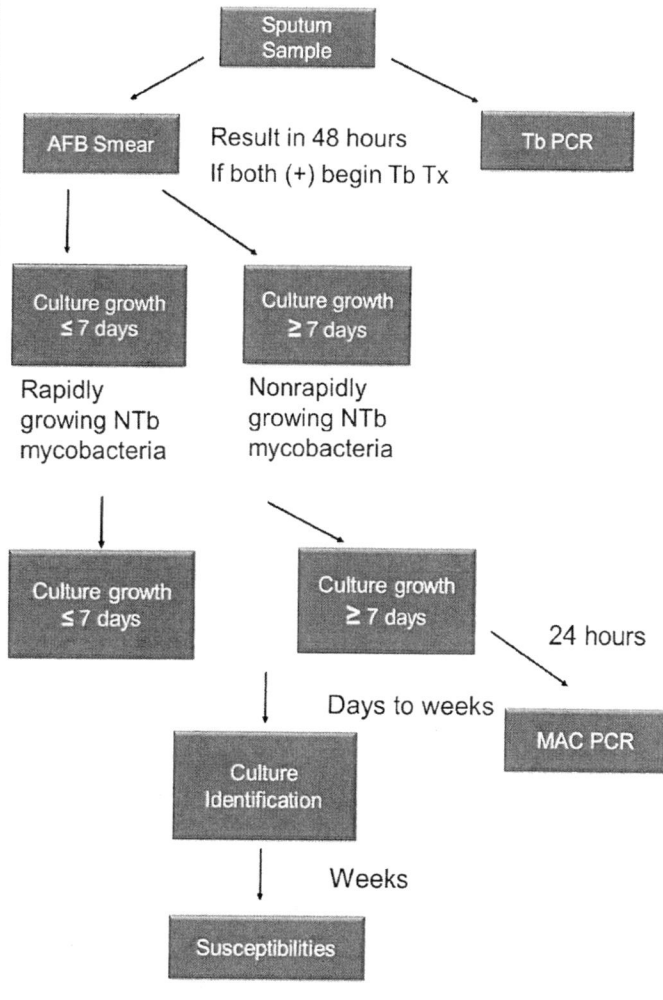

Sputum Sample → AFB Smear → Result in 48 hours / If both (+) begin Tb Tx → Tb PCR

AFB Smear →
- Culture growth ≤ 7 days — Rapidly growing NTb mycobacteria → Culture growth ≤ 7 days
- Culture growth ≥ 7 days — Nonrapidly growing NTb mycobacteria → Culture growth ≥ 7 days

Culture growth ≥ 7 days → 24 hours → MAC PCR

Days to weeks → Culture Identification → Weeks → Susceptibilities

Nontuberculous Mycobacteria (NTM)
Rapidly Growing
- *M. abscessus* (3rd most common in U.S.)
- *M. chelonae*
- *M. fortuitum*

Nonrapidly Growing
- **MAC** (most common in U.S.)
- *M. kansasii* (2nd most common in U.S.)
- *M. malmoense*
- *M. xenopi*
- *M. szulgai*
- *M. simiae*

Why is this important?
Rapidly Growing AFB Culture
- Resistant to antituberculous therapy
- Mortality up to 20% for severe infections

Nonrapidly Growing AFB Culture
- Resistant to conventional antibiotics
- Many regimens include rifampin or rifabutin

Active Tuberculosis
Epidemiology
- TB is still a leading cause of death in the world
- World Health Organization (WHO) estimates that about 1/3 of the world's population is infected
- The global incidence of active TB is increasing
  - Mainly due to TB associated with HIV infections

- **Sites of TB disease**
  - Lungs (**80–85%**)
  - Pleura
  - CNS
  - Lymphatic system
  - Genitourinary system
  - Bones and joints
  - Peritoneum

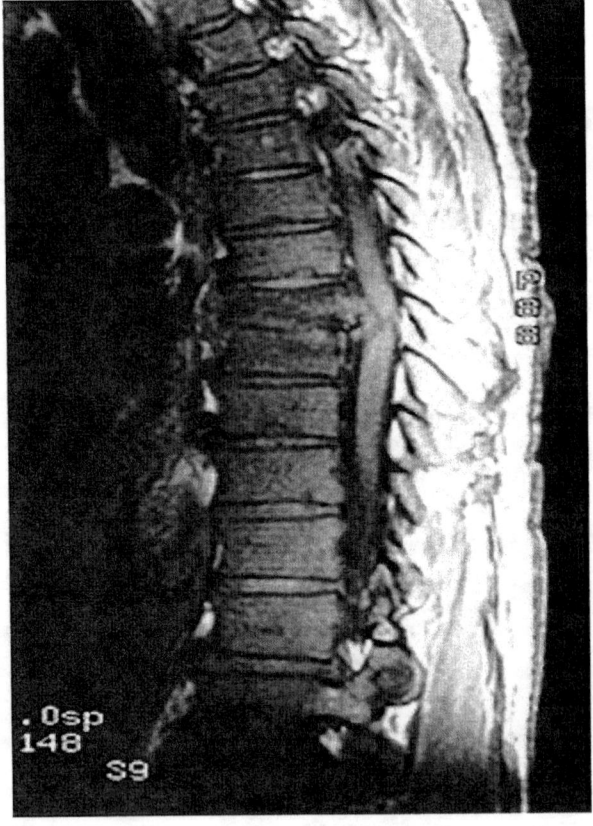

Active Tuberculosis (cont.)
- **Pulmonary complications of TB include:**
  - Hemoptysis
  - Pneumothorax
  - Bronchiectasis
  - Extensive pulmonary destruction
  - Malignancy
  - Chronic pulmonary aspergillosis

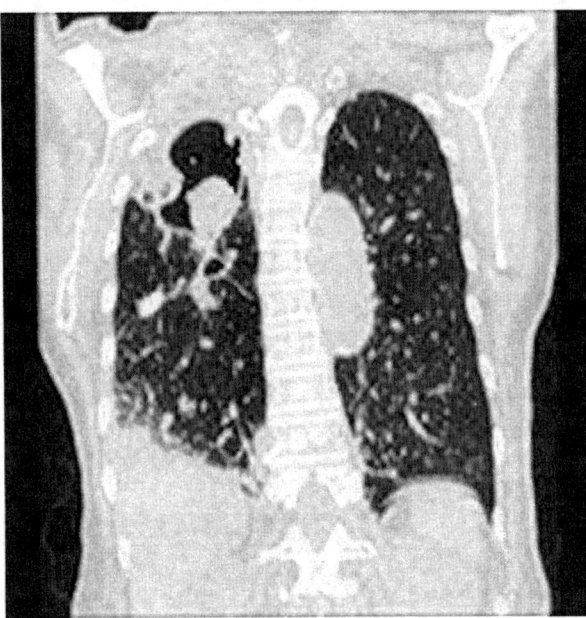

Historical Surgical Management

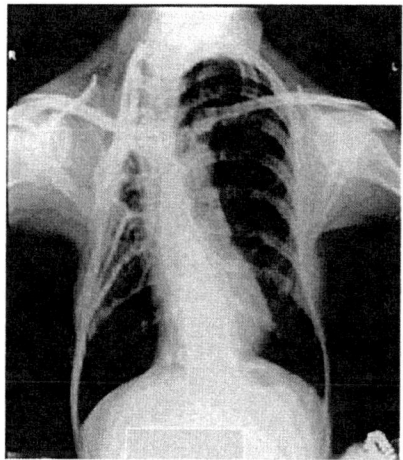

Phrenic Nerve Crush

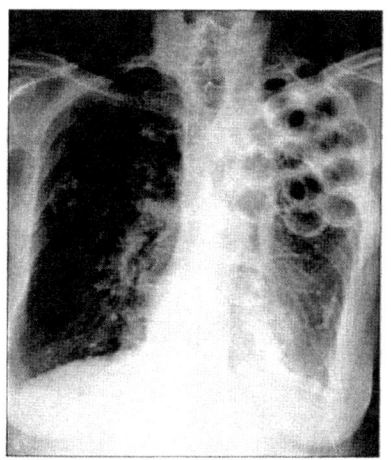

Plombage

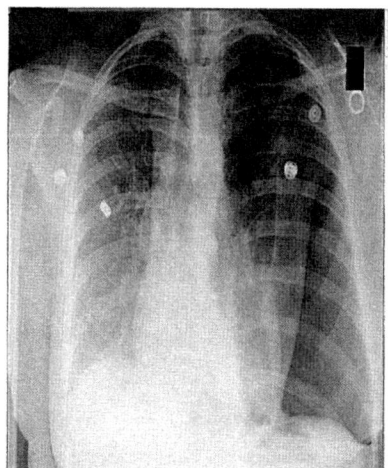

Pneumothorax

AR 29

A young male presents to the ED with symptoms consistent with community-acquired pneumonia, is started on antibiotics, and sent to the general medical floor. The patient significantly worsens over the next 24 hours.

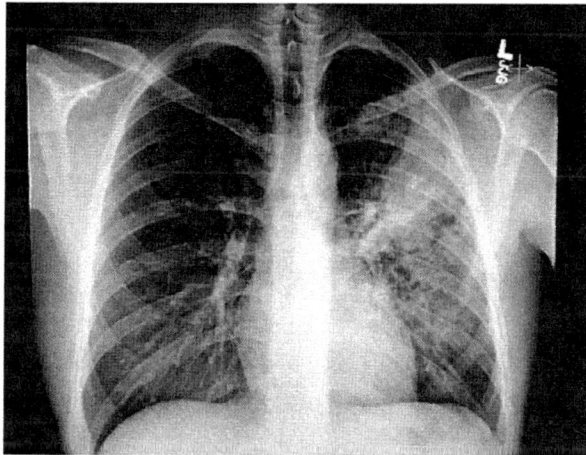

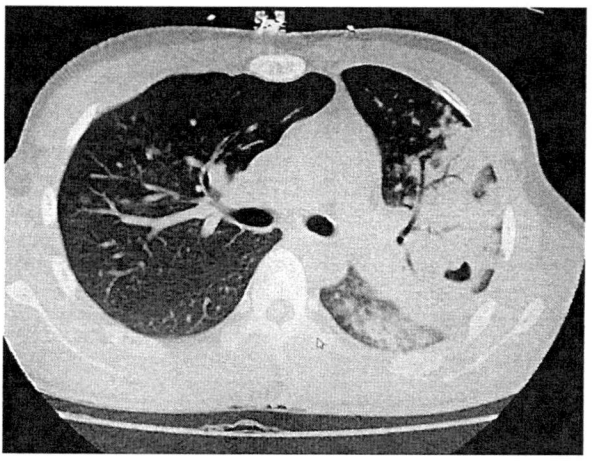

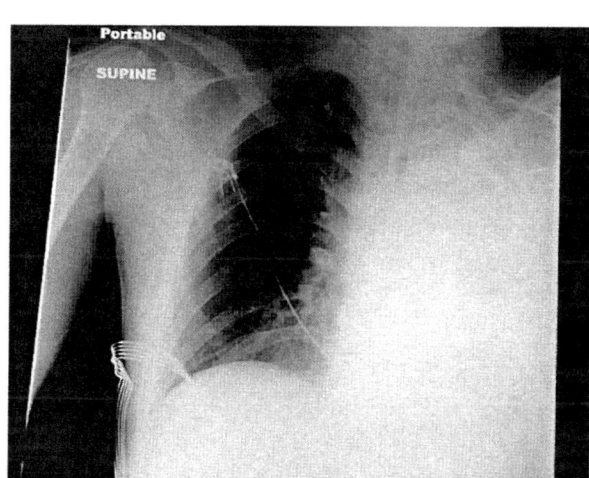

AR 29 (cont.)

During massive hemoptysis, a large single lumen ET tube should be placed in the mainstem bronchus of the ... ?

A. Bleeding lung
B. Nonbleeding lung

Answer: _____

AR 29 (cont.)

- To protect the patient from asphyxia by blood from the other lung
- To induce atelectasis of the bleeding lung

Critical Care Medicine

ARDS and Ventilator Management

Adult Respiratory Distress Syndrome (ARDS)
- **Classic Definition (American-European Consensus Conference's definition 1994)**
  1) Ratio of $P_aO_2/F_iO_2 < 200$
  2) Acute bilateral pulmonary infiltrates
  3) PCWP < 18 mmHg
     - Measured by Swan-Ganz catheter or no clinical evidence of left-heart failure

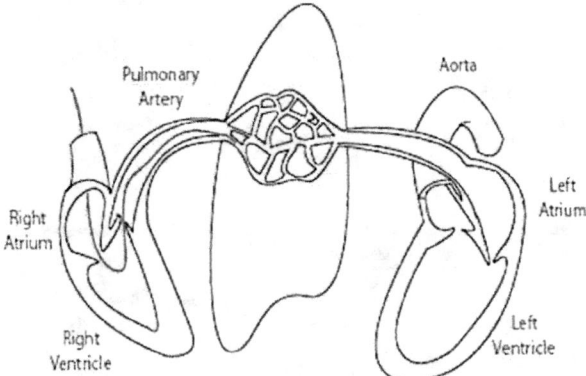

ARDS (cont.)
- **Direct causes**
  - Aspiration
  - Pneumonia
  - Inhalation injuries
- **Indirect causes**
  - Sepsis
  - Pancreatitis
  - TRALI
  - Trauma
- **Grouped together under the term ARDS due to similarities of:**
  - Clinical
  - Physiological
  - Pathological
  - Management

Berlin Definition of ARDS 2012
- The Berlin Definition of ARDS requires that **all of the following** criteria be present to diagnose ARDS:
  - Symptoms must have begun within 1 week of a known clinical insult
  - Bilateral opacities consistent with pulmonary edema must be present on CXR or CT
  - Respiratory failure must not be explained by cardiac failure or fluid overload

- The severity of the hypoxemia defines the severity of the ARDS:
  - **Mild ARDS**
    - P_aO_2/F_iO_2 is > 200 mmHg, but ≤ 300 mmHg, on ventilator settings that include PEEP ≥ 5
  - **Moderate ARDS**
    - P_aO_2/F_iO_2 is > 100 mmHg, but ≤ 200 mmHg, on ventilator settings that include PEEP ≥ 5
  - **Severe ARDS**
    - P_aO_2/F_iO_2 is ≤ 100 mmHg on ventilator settings that include PEEP ≥ 5

ARDS (cont.)
- **Overview**
  - ARDS is characterized by increased permeability if the alveolar-capillary membrane
    - Causing pulmonary edema
    - Leads to severe hypoxemia
    - Decreased pulmonary compliance
  - It is unknown what factors cause the leaky lungs
  - There is a 24- to 72-hour lag time between injury and ARDS
  - There is no prophylactic treatment for ARDS

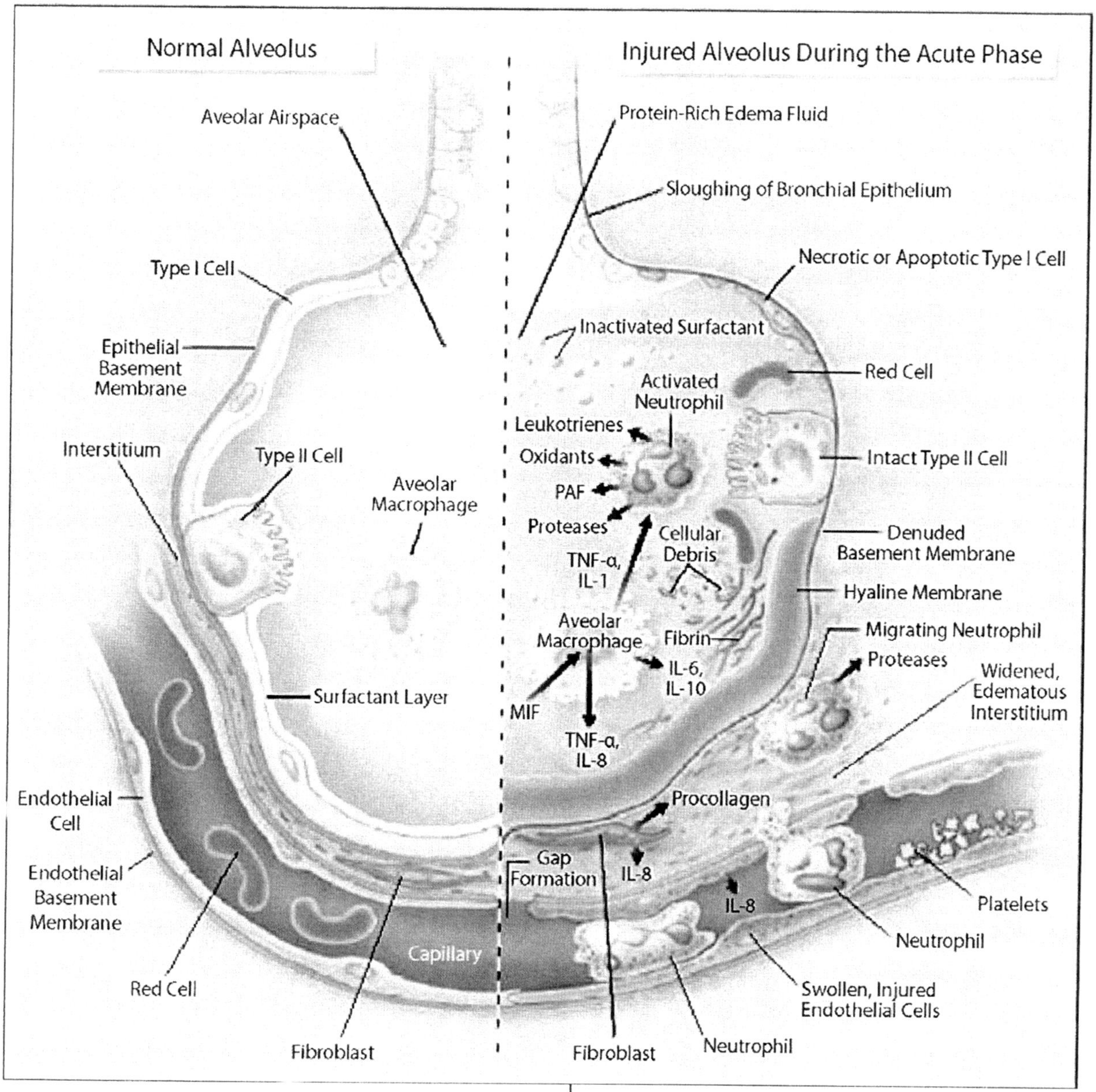

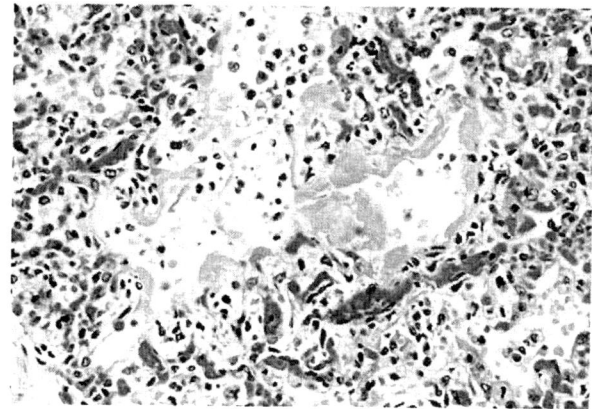

Normal Alveolus | Injured Alveolus During the Acute Phase

(Diagram labels, Normal Alveolus side)
- Aveolar Airspace
- Type I Cell
- Epithelial Basement Membrane
- Interstitium
- Type II Cell
- Aveolar Macrophage
- Surfactant Layer
- Endothelial Cell
- Endothelial Basement Membrane
- Red Cell
- Capillary
- Fibroblast

(Diagram labels, Injured Alveolus side)
- Protein-Rich Edema Fluid
- Sloughing of Bronchial Epithelium
- Necrotic or Apoptotic Type I Cell
- Inactivated Surfactant
- Red Cell
- Activated Neutrophil
- Leukotrienes
- Oxidants
- PAF
- Proteases
- Intact Type II Cell
- TNF-α, IL-1
- Cellular Debris
- Denuded Basement Membrane
- Hyaline Membrane
- Aveolar Macrophage
- Fibrin
- IL-6, IL-10
- Migrating Neutrophil
- Proteases
- MIF
- TNF-α, IL-8
- Widened, Edematous Interstitium
- Procollagen
- Gap Formation
- IL-8
- IL-8
- Platelets
- Neutrophil
- Swollen, Injured Endothelial Cells
- Fibroblast
- Neutrophil

ARDS (cont.)
- **Acute, diffuse, inflammatory lung injury that leads to:**
  - Increased pulmonary vascular permeability
  - Increased lung weight, and a loss of aerated tissue
- **Clinical hallmarks of ARDS are:**
  - Hypoxemia
  - Bilateral radiographic opacities
- **Pathological hallmark is "diffuse alveolar damage":**
  - Alveolar edema with or without focal hemorrhage
  - Acute inflammation of the alveolar walls
  - Hyaline membranes

Showing hyaline membranes, the key histologic feature of diffuse alveolar damage

ARDS Physiology
- Healthy lungs regulate the movement of fluid to maintain a small amount of interstitial fluid and dry alveoli
- This is interrupted by lung injury, causing excess fluid in both the **interstitium** and **alveoli**
- Consequences include impaired gas exchange, decreased compliance, and increased pulmonary arterial pressure

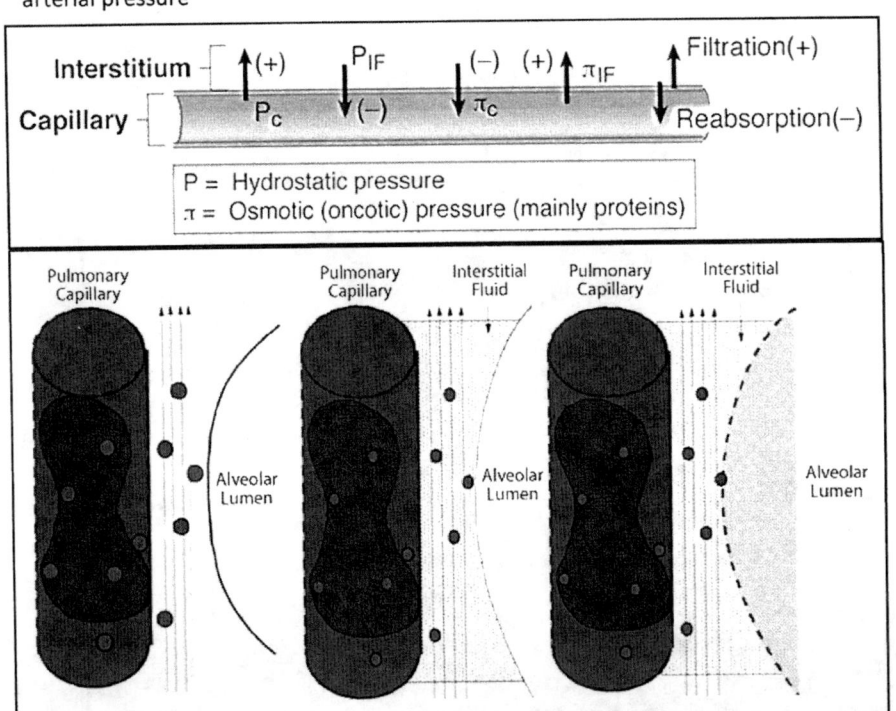

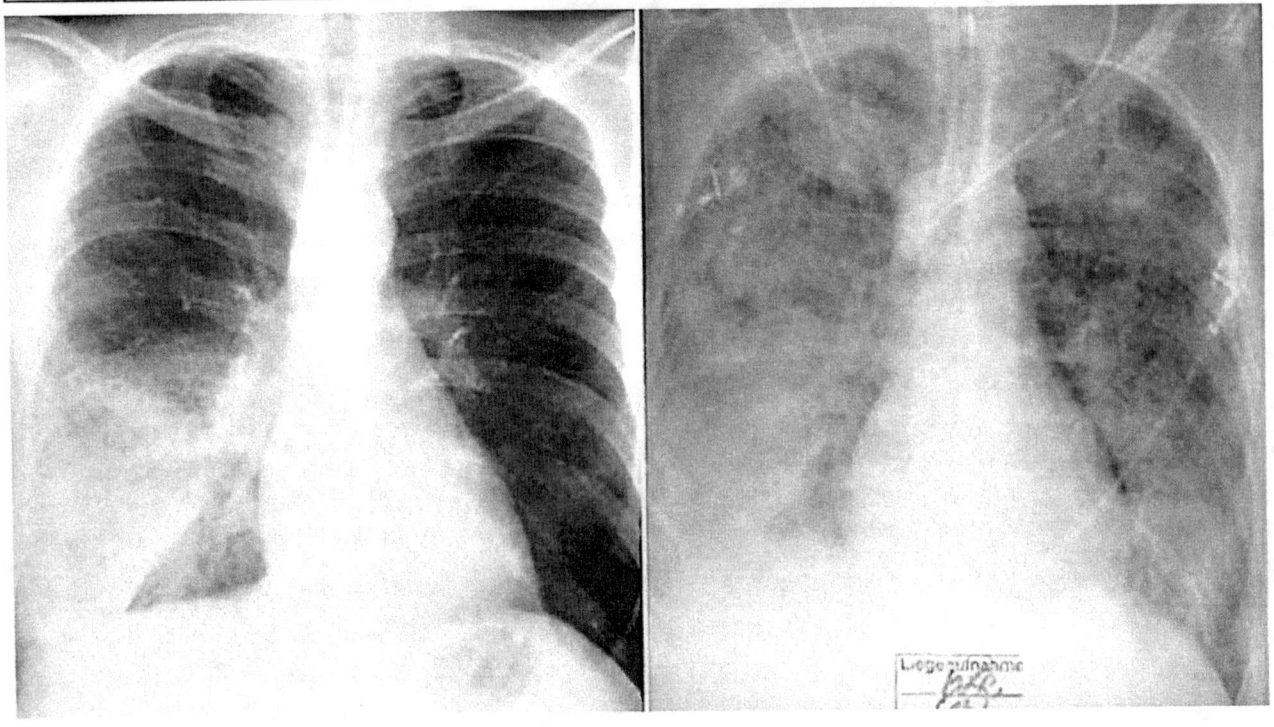

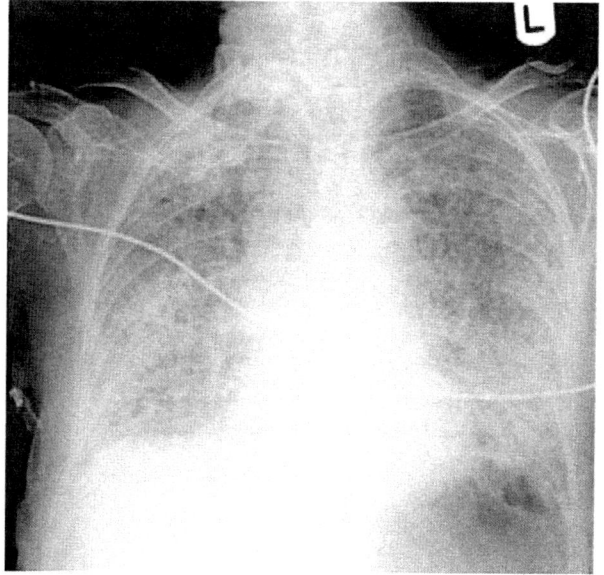

ARDS (cont.)
- **Treatment**
  - Treat the causative condition
    - If a patient has an abscess, push surgeons to remove it or IR to drain it
    - Give empiric antibiotics if **sepsis** is thought to be the cause
  - Optimize cardiopulmonary support
    - Maintain adequate cardiac output
    - Prevent worsening lactic acidosis
  - Nutrition
    - Should be enteral rather than parenteral
  - Medications
    - Glucocorticoids
      - Trials are ongoing

Efficacy and Safety of Corticosteroids for Persistent ARDS
- **Conclusions**
  - These results do not support the routine use of methylprednisolone for persistent ARDS despite the improvement in cardiopulmonary physiology
  - In addition, starting methylprednisolone therapy more than **2 weeks after** the onset of ARDS may increase the risk of death

The National Heart, Lung, and Blood Institute Acute Respiratory Distress Syndrome (ARDS) Clinical Trials Network. *New Engl J Med.* 2006; 354(16);1671–1684.

Methylprednisolone Infusion in Early Severe ARDS
- **Objective**
  - To determine the effects of low-dose prolonged methylprednisolone infusion on lung function in patients with **early** severe ARDS
  - Methylprednisolone infusion (1 mg/kg/d) vs. placebo
- **Conclusion**
  - Reduction in duration of mechanical ventilation and ICU length of stay

Meduri, et al. *Chest.* 2007; 131: 954–963.

ARDS Stages

1 Exudative Stage: Characterized by accumulation in the alveoli of excessive fluid, protein, and inflammatory cells that have entered the air spaces from the alveolar capillaries. The exudative phase unfolds over the first 2–4 days after onset of lung injury.

2 Fibroproliferative (or Proliferative) Stage: Connective tissue and other structural elements in the lungs proliferate in response to the initial injury. Under a microscope, lung tissue appears densely cellular. Also at this stage, there is a danger of pneumonia sepsis and rupture of the lungs causing leakage of air into surrounding areas.

3 Resolution and Recovery: During this stage, the lung reorganizes and recovers. Lung function may continue to improve for as long as 6–12 months and sometimes longer, depending on the precipitating condition and severity of the injury. It is important to remember that there may be (and often are) different levels of pulmonary recovery among individuals who suffer from ARDS.

Patients with ARDS tend to progress through 3 relatively discrete pathologic stages: the **exudative** stage, the **proliferative** stage, and the **fibrotic** stage.

ARDS Ventilator Management
- **ARDS is classic shunt physiology**
  - The only way to improve oxygenation is to recruit, or "pop open" some of the fluid-filled alveoli
  - To "pop open" alveolar unit use PEEP
- **Low tidal volumes**
  - 6 mL/kg is considered optimal
- **Permissive hypercapnia**
  - Low tidal volumes result in an elevated P_aCO_2
- **Positioning**
  - Lateral decubitus position is usually tried first

AR 30

A 63-year-old woman is admitted to the hospital for septic shock secondary to CAP. After antibiotics, fluids, and vasopressors, her condition stabilizes. However, she subsequently develops ARDS and is intubated. Her O_2 requirement increases until she is receiving 100% O_2. Vent settings are in the volume-controlled continuous mandatory ventilation mode with RR **22 breaths/min**, TV **330 mL** (6 mL/kg of ideal body weight), F_iO_2 **100%**, and PEEP **5**, peak pressure of 25 cm H_2O, and a plateau pressure of 22 cm H_2O.

On exam, temp 100.4° F, BP 115/60, HR 105/min, and RR 15.
The skin is cool. There is no JVD. Heart sounds are rapid and regular but otherwise unremarkable. Diffuse crackles are heard on pulmonary exam. There is no edema.
The remainder of the physical exam is noncontributory.
ABG show a pH **7.31**, P_aCO_2 **50 mmHg**, and P_aO_2 of **54 mmHg**.
CXR shows extensive patchy areas of opacification of the lung fields.

Which of the following is the most appropriate management?
A. Decrease the TV.
B. Implement a prone positioning maneuver.
C. Start inhaled NO.
D. Decrease the RR.
E. Increase the PEEP.

Answer: _____

 © 2017 MedStudy Internal Medicine Video Board Review – Pulmonary Medicine • Raj Dasgupta, MD

AR 30 (cont.)

In patients with severe acute respiratory distress syndrome, current recommendations are to use a positive end-expiratory pressure level that achieves adequate oxygenation with an F_iO_2 of < 0.6 and does not cause hypotension

AR 31

A patient with ARDS is on the ventilator with the settings of 12 mL/kg for the patient's tidal volume. This was switched appropriately to ARDSNet protocol of 6 mL/kg to improve survival.

What physiologic changes would you expect?

A. Increased compliance and oxygenation
B. Decreased compliance and oxygenation
C. No change in compliance and oxygenation
D. Decreased compliance and increased oxygenation
E. Increased compliance and decreased oxygenation

Answer: _____

Decreased Compliance

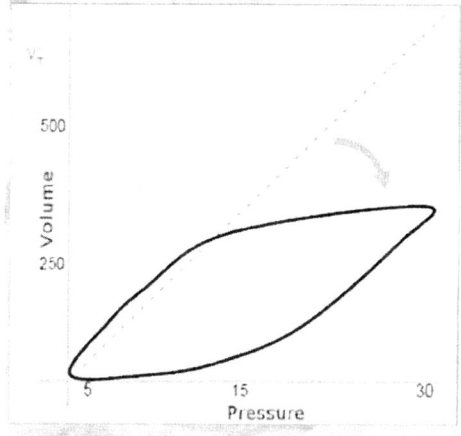

Example: ARDS, CHF, Atelectasis

Advance ARDS Management
- **ECMO** (extracorporeal membrane oxygenation)
  - VV or VA (for hemodynamic support)
- **High-frequency ventilation**
  - Combines a very high respiratory rate, very low tidal volumes (smaller than anatomical dead space) & high mean airway pressure (PEEP)
    - Brownian motion and pendelluft effect (different alveolar closing times)
    - Oxygenation (F_iO_2 and airway pressure), ventilation (frequency and piston amplitude "chest wiggle")
    - May increase in-hospital mortality
- **APRV** (airway pressure release ventilation)
- **Prone position**
- **Paralytics**: Careful of critical illness neuropathy/myopathy

Paralytics in ARDS

In patients with severe ARDS, early administration of a neuromuscular blocking agent improved the adjusted **90-day survival** and increased the time off the ventilator without increasing muscle weakness

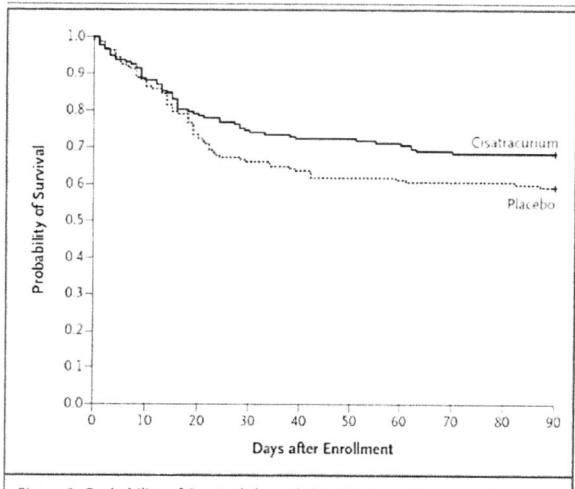

Figure 2. Probability of Survival through Day 90, According to Study Group.

Question
Does prone position ventilation decrease mortality in ARDS?

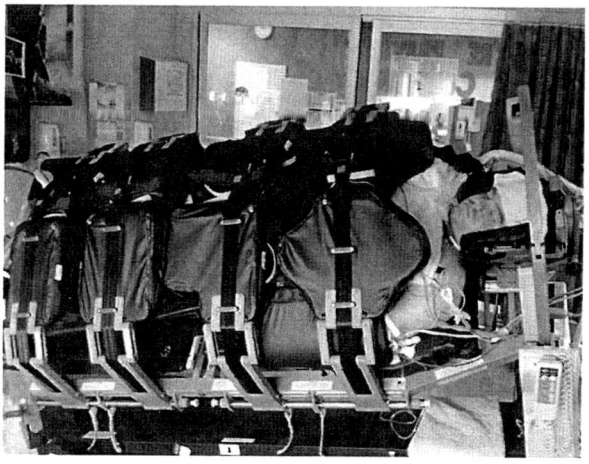

Answer
- **Yes**
  - "Prone Positioning in Severe Acute Respiratory Distress Syndrome" (*NEJM*, May 20, 2013)
    - Prospective, multicenter, randomized, controlled trial to explore
    - Showed that patients with ARDS and severe hypoxemia (as confirmed by a $P_aO_2:F_iO_2$ ratio of < 150 mmHg, with an F_iO_2 of ≥ 0.6 and a PEEP of ≥ 5 cm of water) can benefit from prone treatment when it is used early and in relatively long sessions

ARDS Ventilator Settings
- No 1 ventilator mode has **proven better** than another for ARDS
- Commonly recommend initial setting
  - Assist-control, volume-cycled
  - F_iO_2 = 100%
    - Lower to < 60% ASAP
  - Tidal volume = 6–8 mL/kg
  - Inspiratory flow = 60 L/min
  - PEEP = start at 5 cm H_2O
    - Usually goes up to 10–20 cm H_2O
    - Titrate to **plateau pressure** ≤ 30 cm H_2O

Peak and Plateau Pressures
- **If peak pressures are increasing:**
  - Check plateau pressures by allowing for an **inspiratory pause**
  - If peak pressures are high and plateau pressures are low, then you have an **obstruction**
  - If both peak pressures and plateau pressures are high, then you have a lung **compliance** issue

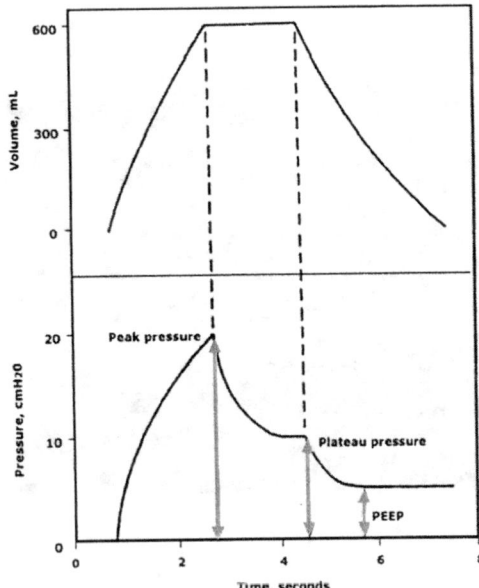

Peak and Plateau Pressures (cont.)

High Peak Pressures Low Plateau Pressures	High Peak Pressures High Plateau Pressures
Mucous Plug	ARDS
Bronchospasm	Pulmonary Edema
ET tube blockage	Pneumothorax
Biting	ET tube migration to a single bronchus
	Effusion

http://www.doctorrajd.com/#!videos/c15cu

What is "Early Goal-Directed Therapy" in the MICU?

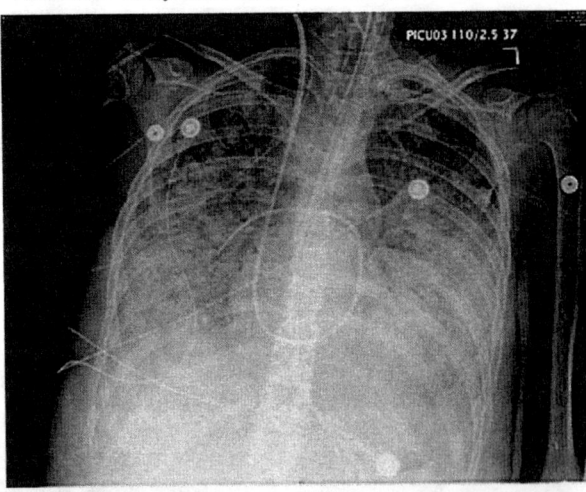

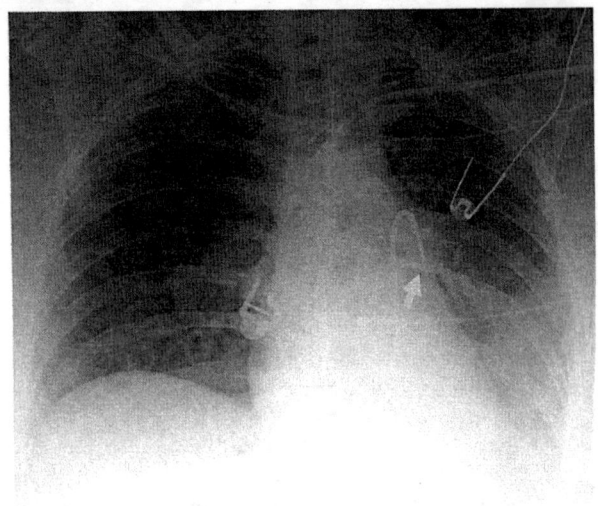

Back to the Basics

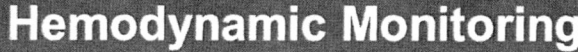
Hemodynamic Monitoring

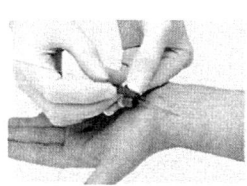

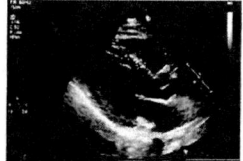

Invasive

Noninvasive

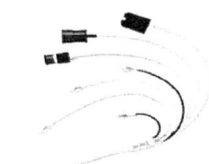

- Arterial line
- Central venous catheter
- Pulmonary artery catheter

- Transthoracic echocardiogram
- Jugular venous pressure (JVP)

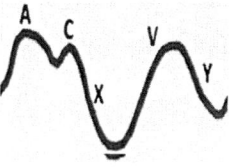

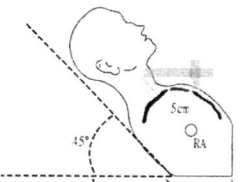

Back to the Basics (cont.)
- The goal of hemodynamic monitoring is to maintain adequate **tissue perfusion**:
  1) Oxygen delivery
  2) Oxygen consumption

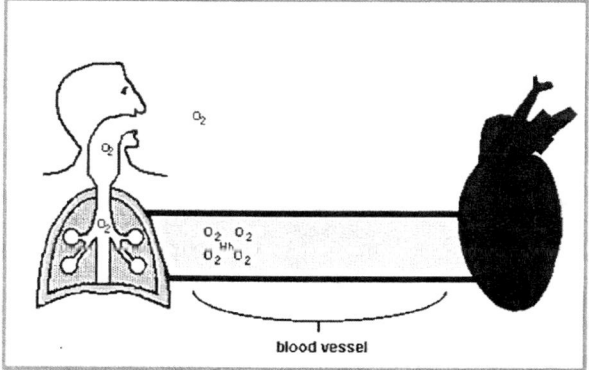

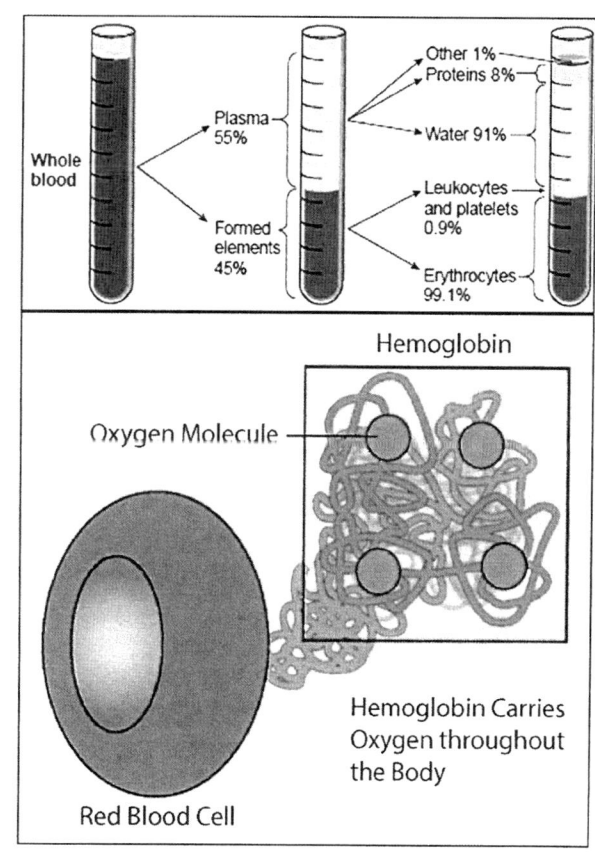

Back to the Basics (cont.)
- What is "**tissue perfusion**"?
  - The amount of blood volume that a tissue is receiving from the circulation
  - Blood carries oxygen
  - Inadequate perfusion leads to decreased oxygen delivery at the cellular level to the electron transport change that makes ATP
    - ATP is the basic unit of energy that cells use
  - Blood flow and tissue perfusion are not the same thing

Back to the Basics (cont.)
- What is impaired "**oxidative phosphorylation**"?
  - Pyruvate builds up, which starts to form lactic acid
  - Metabolic acidosis causes vasodilation
    - Secondary to a decreased response to stress hormones, such as epinephrine
  - Adenosine also builds up, which is a potent vasodilator

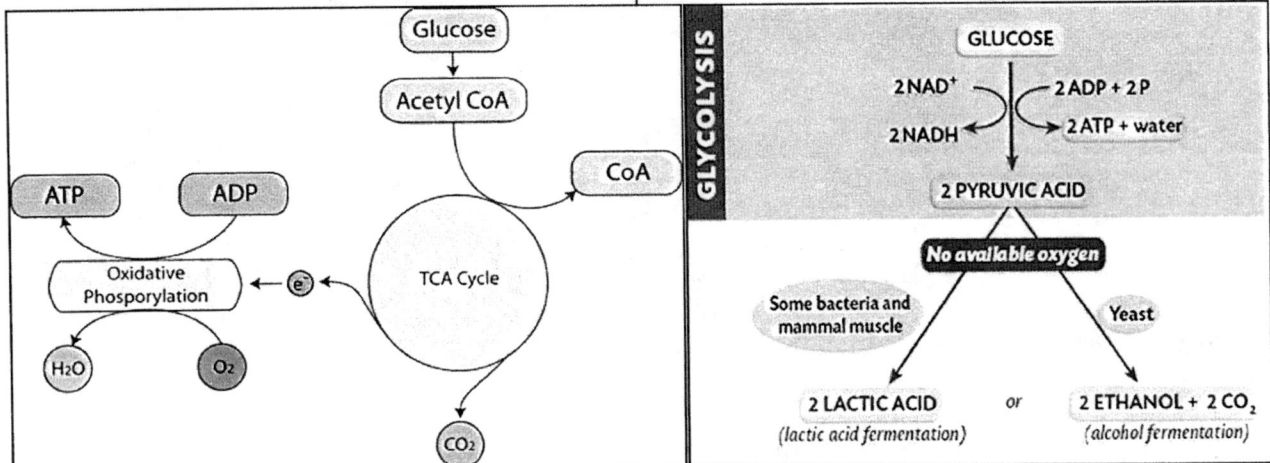

AR 32
Why are we interested in the mixed venous saturation (S_vO_2)?
A. Represents oxygen delivery
B. Represents oxygen consumption
C. Both A & B

Answer: _____

AR 32 (cont.)
S_vO_2 is a quick way of getting some idea about the adequacy of:
1) Oxygen delivery (DO_2)
2) Oxygen consumption (VO_2)

- Venous oxygen saturation reflects the balance between:
  - **Oxygen consumption (VO_2) = CO ($C_aO_2 - C_vO_2$)**
    - **"Fick Principle"**
      - C_aO_2 = (Hgb x 1.36 x S_aO_2) + (P_aO_2 x 0.0031)
      - C_vO_2 = (Hgb x 1.36 x S_vO_2) + (P_vO_2 x 0.0031)
- When tissues are poorly perfused, they will extract more O_2 from the blood, and the venous blood returning to the heart will be more deoxygenated
- Therefore, a low S_vO_2 can be used to diagnose hypoperfusion/shock

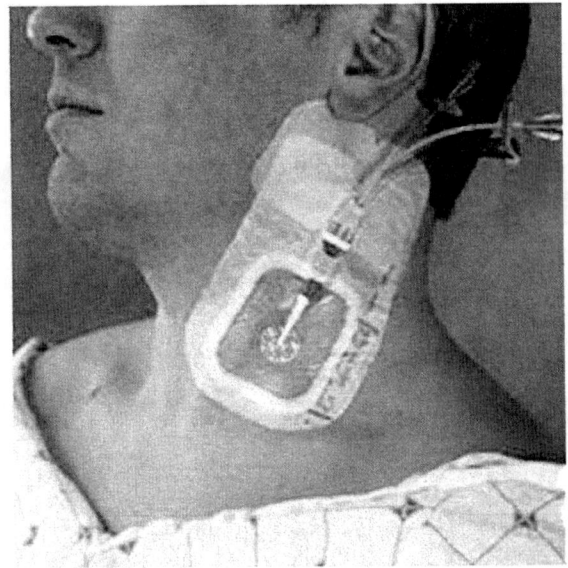

AR 33
Is a high mixed venous saturation (S_vO_2) always good?
A. Yes.
B. No.
C. It depends on the weather.

Answer: _____

AR 33 (cont.)
- Patients with septic shock are unable to properly extract and use oxygen, so venous blood returning to the heart will be very oxygen rich
- Normal S_vO_2 60–75%

AR 34

Which of the following approaches to treatment of sepsis has been demonstrated to <u>improve</u> outcomes?

A. Blood transfusion at hemoglobin levels of 7 g/dL compared with 9 g/dL
B. Early administration of appropriate antibiotics
C. Early goal-directed therapy
D. Protocol-based therapy
E. Target resuscitation to achieve a mean arterial blood pressure of 80–85 mmHg compared with 65–70 mmHg

Answer: _____

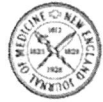

The NEW ENGLAND JOURNAL of MEDICINE

ORIGINAL ARTICLE

High versus Low Blood-Pressure Target in Patients with Septic Shock

CONCLUSIONS

Targeting a mean arterial pressure of 80 to 85 mm Hg, as compared with 65 to 70 mm Hg, in patients with septic shock undergoing resuscitation did not result in significant differences in mortality at either 28 or 90 days. (Funded by the French Ministry of Health; SEPSISPAM ClinicalTrials.gov number, NCT01149278.)

The NEW ENGLAND JOURNAL of MEDICINE

ORIGINAL ARTICLE

Lower versus Higher Hemoglobin Threshold for Transfusion in Septic Shock

In conclusion, patients with septic shock who underwent transfusion at a hemoglobin threshold of 7 g per deciliter, as compared with those who underwent transfusion at a hemoglobin threshold of 9 g per deciliter, received fewer transfusions and had similar mortality at 90 days, use of life support, and number of days alive and out of the hospital; the numbers of patients with ischemic events and severe adverse reactions to blood in the ICU were also similar in the two intervention groups

---

ORIGINAL ARTICLE

Goal-Directed Resuscitation for Patients with Early Septic Shock

The ARISE Investigators and the ANZICS Clinical Trials Group

CONCLUSIONS

In patients with septic shock who were identified early and received intravenous antibiotics and adequate fluid resuscitation, hemodynamic management according to a strict EGDT protocol did not lead to an improvement in outcome. (Funded by the United Kingdom National Institute for Health Research Health Technology Assessment Programme; ProMISe Current Controlled Trials number

The NEW ENGLAND JOURNAL of MEDICINE

ESTABLISHED IN 1812 · MAY 1, 2014 · VOL. 370 NO. 18

A Randomized Trial of Protocol-Based Care for Early Septic Shock

The ProCESS Investigators

CONCLUSIONS

In a multicenter trial conducted in the tertiary care setting, protocol-based resuscitation of patients in whom septic shock was diagnosed in the emergency department did not improve outcomes. (Funded by the National Institute of General Medical Sciences; ProCESS ClinicalTrials.gov number, NCT00510835.)

Practice Questions

AR 35

A 71-year-old male is admitted with hypotension, tachypnea, and tachycardia. His HR is 122 bpm, BP 83/48 mmHg, and RR 28 breaths/min.
A Swan-Ganz PA catheter is inserted:

- CO 9.3 L/min (normal 5–6)
- PCWP 8 mmHg (normal 8–12)
- SVR 550 dynes (normal 700–1,600)

What is the hemodynamic picture consistent with?

A. Hypovolemic shock
B. Distributive shock secondary to sepsis
C. Cardiogenic shock from left heart failure

Answer: _____

AR 36

What is the diagnosis of a patient with the following hemodynamic profile on Swan-Ganz monitoring?

- CO: 3.4 L/min (normal 5–6)
- PCWP: 6 mmHg (normal 8–12)
- SVR: 2,500 dynes (normal 700–1,600)

A. Distributive shock, secondary to anaphylaxis
B. Hypovolemic shock
C. Cardiogenic shock

Answer: _____

AR 37A

A 68-year-old male presents to the hospital with increasing shortness of breath, orthopnea, PND, and palpitations. He has a long history of recurrent CHF. Physical exam reveals bibasilar rales, and he is hypotensive with BP 70/40 mmHg.
- Swan-Ganz reveals the following:
  - Cardiac index 1.4 L/min/m² (normal 2.6–4.2)
  - PCWP 34 mmHg (normal 8–12)
  - SVR 2,400 dynes (normal 700–1,600)

What is the diagnosis?
A. Cardiogenic shock from left heart failure
B. Hypovolemic shock from blood loss
C. Distributive shock secondary to sepsis

Answer: _____

AR 37B

In the previous patient, what is the preferred drug of choice for this type of shock?
A. Norepinephrine
B. Dopamine
C. Dobutamine
D. Phenylephrine
E. Vasopressin

Answer: _____

AR 37C

In the same patient, what is the expected mixed venous O_2 saturation (S_vO_2)?
A. Low (< 60%)
B. Normal (60–75%)
C. High (> 75%)

Answer: _____

Sleep Medicine

Obstructive and Central Sleep Apnea

Sleep Apnea
- Obstructive **apnea** is defined as:
  - Cessation of airflow > 90% in the thermal sensor and 10 seconds duration; oxygen desaturation is <u>not</u> part of the definition
- Obstructive **hypopnea** has multiple definitions:
  - Medicare rule:
    - Cessation of airflow > 30%, 4% decrease in oxygenation and lasting 10 seconds
  - Alternative rule:
    - Cessation of airflow > 50%, 3% decrease in oxygenation or an arousal

- RERAs (**Respiratory Effort-Related Arousals**)
  - Last for 10 seconds; The event is not an apnea or hypopnea

Obstructive Sleep Apnea

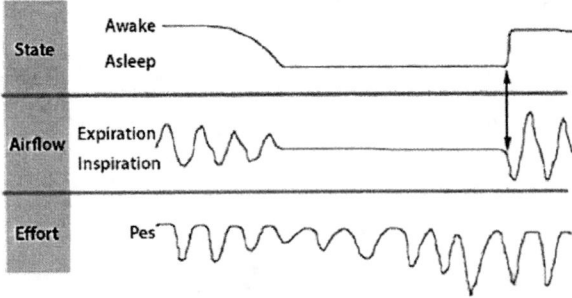

Continuing respiratory effort, as shown by esophageal pressure (Pes) at the time of cessation of airflow

Sleep Apnea (cont.)
- **Previously the best initial test**
  - Overnight pulse oximetry desaturation study
    - Good to evaluate **hypoxemia in patients using PAP**
- **Confirmation test**
  - Polysomnography (sleep study)
    - ECG, EEG, EMG, oximeter, tidal CO_2 recorder
    - Split study
    - Differentiates obstructive and central sleep apnea
      - Presence or absence of inspiratory effort during the apneic episodes
    - The frequency of hypoxic apneic episodes determines the severity of the disease
      - Normal < 5/hour
      - Mild 5–15/hour
      - Moderate 15–30/hour
      - Severe > 30/hour

- **Obstructive sleep apnea (OSA)**
  - Is sleep apnea occurring despite continuing ventilatory effort
  - Frequently associated with:
    - Abnormal airway
      - **Neck circumference**
        » Seems to be the most important determinant of OSA in both men and women
      - Tonsillar hypertrophy or lymphoma
      - Micrognathia
      - Acromegaly
      - Goiter
      - TMJ disease
    - Obesity
      - Not a necessary feature

Sleep Apnea (cont.)

- **Obesity-hypoventilation syndrome**
  - **Not all patients** with OHS have OSA
  - Pickwickian syndrome
    - These patients not only have extreme daytime sleepiness but also have hypoventilation (**high pCO_2**) while awake

Sleep Apnea Treatment

- **Lifestyle modifications**
  - Weight loss
  - Avoiding
    - Alcohol
    - Sedatives
    - Hypnotics
  - Not sleeping in the supine position

Mainstay Therapy

- **PAP ventilation**
  - **CPAP**
    - Continuous positive airway pressure
  - **BiPAP**
    - Bilevel positive airway pressure
  - **ASV**
    - Adaptive servo ventilation
  - **AVAPS**
    - Average volume assured pressure support

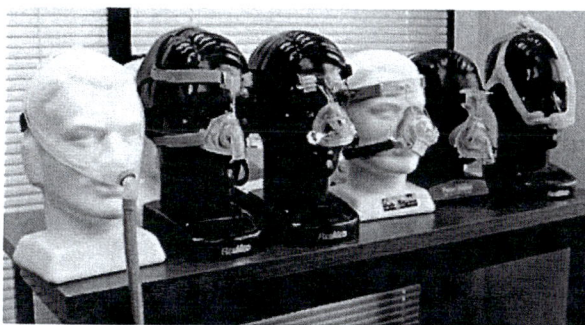

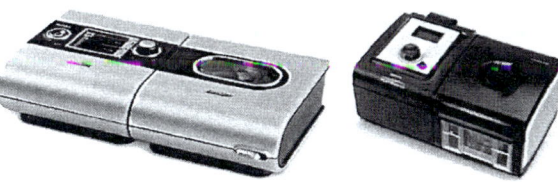

Unfortunately, Not Everyone Tolerates PAP Therapy

- Dental devices
- UPPP
- Tracheostomy
- Provent
- Inspire

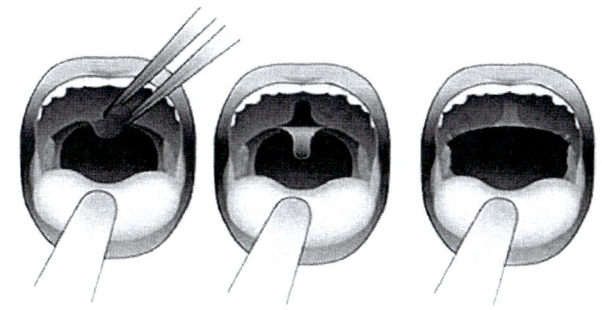

Uvulopalatopharyngoplasty

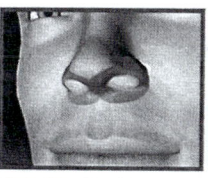 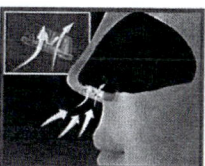 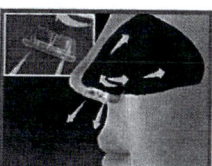

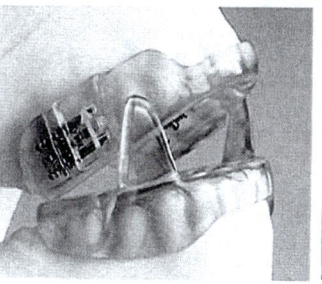 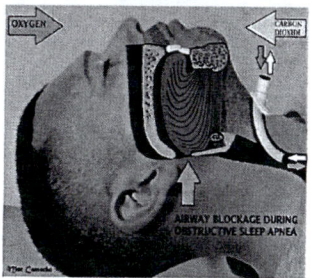

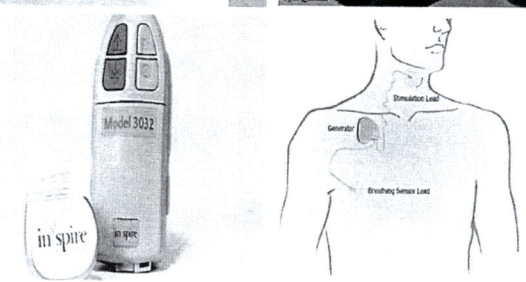

Central Sleep Apnea

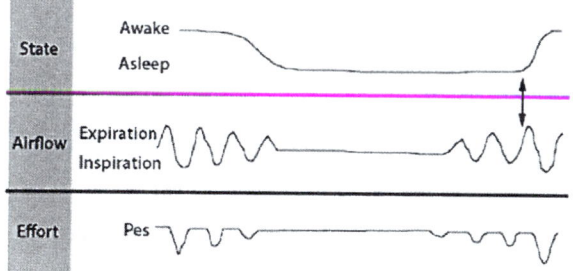

No respiratory effort, as shown by absence of changes in esophageal pressure (Pes), at the time of cessation of airflow

Central Sleep Apnea Classification — Hypercapnic
- High **sleep** and **waking** P_aCO_2
  Decreased ventilatory response to hypercapnia
- Causes:
  - Neuromuscular disorders
    - ALS, myasthenia gravis, Guillain-Barré, muscular dystrophy
  - Chronic use of long-acting opioids
    - Biot's respiration

Central Sleep Apnea Classification — Nonhypercapnic
- Normal or **low** waking P_aCO_2
  Increased ventilator response to hypercapnia
- Causes:
  - Primary or Idiopathic CSA
  - Sleep-onset CSA
  - Cheyne-Stokes respiration
  - High altitude periodic breathing
  - Complex sleep apnea

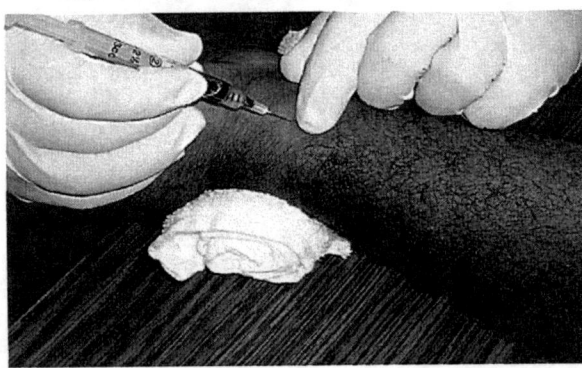

Central Sleep Apnea Treatment
- **Treatment**
  - Is not standardized
  - Try different therapies
    - Lifestyle modifications
      - Weight loss
      - Avoid alcohol
    - Supplemental oxygen
      - CPAP
      - BiPAP
      - ASV (controversial)
    - Medications
      - Acetazolamide (causes a metabolic acidosis)
      - Medroxyprogesterone (esp. for hypercapnia)

ORIGINAL ARTICLE

Adaptive Servo-Ventilation for Central Sleep Apnea in Systolic Heart Failure

Martin R. Cowie, M.D., Holger Woehrle, M.D., Karl Wegscheider, Ph.D., Christiane Angermann, M.D., Marie-Pia d'Ortho, M.D., Ph.D., Erland Erdmann, M.D., Patrick Levy, M.D., Ph.D., Anita K. Simonds, M.D., Virend K. Somers, M.D., Ph.D., Faiez Zannad, M.D., Ph.D. and Helmut Teschler, M.D.
N Engl J Med 2015; 373:1095-1105 | September 17, 2015 | DOI: 10.1056/NEJMoa1506459

Central Sleep Apnea (cont.)
- Congenital central alveolar hypoventilation syndrome (Ondine's curse)
  - Failure of autonomic control of breathing
  - Diminished responsiveness to O_2 and CO_2
  - Onset in infancy
  - Many cases involve mutations in **PHOX2B** gene

Pulmonary Nodules and Lung Cancer

Solitary Pulmonary Nodule
- Differential Diagnosis
  1) **Malignancy**
     - Bronchogenic carcinoma
     - Pulmonary metastases
  2) **Benign disease**
     - Granulomas
     - Benign tumors (hamartomas)
     - Resolving infarction
     - Rheumatoid and vasculitic nodules
     - AV malformations
     - Catamenial hemoptysis
     - Pulmonary sequestration
     - Rounded atelectasis
     - Rounded pneumonia

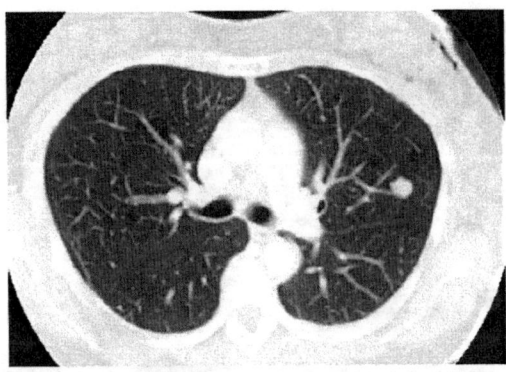

Granuloma

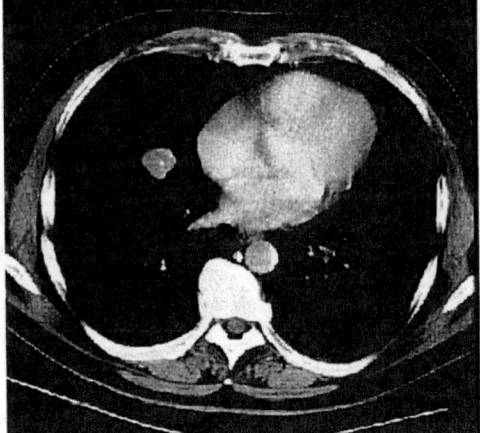

Target-like calcification in this right lower lobe granuloma

Pulmonary Hamartoma

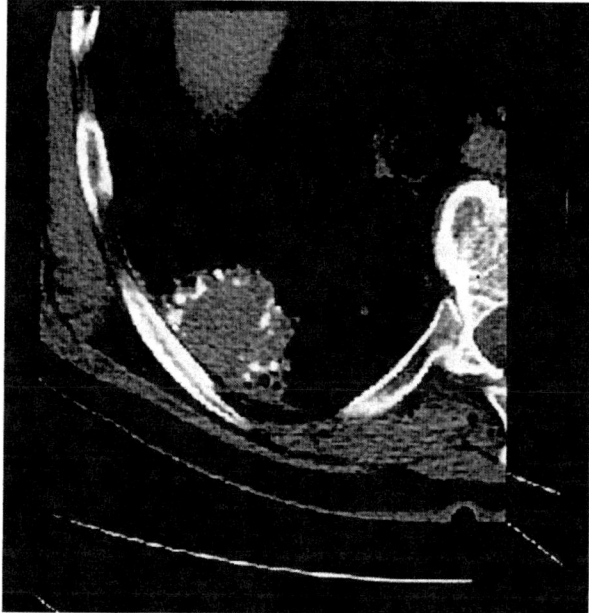

Characteristic popcorn configuration suggestive
of a hamartoma

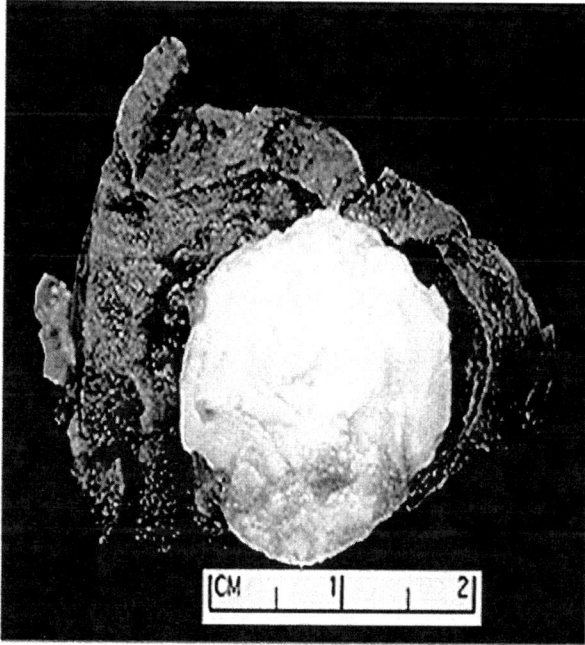

Well-circumscribed mass with a variegated yellow and
white appearance, which corresponds to fat and cartilage

Pulmonary AVM

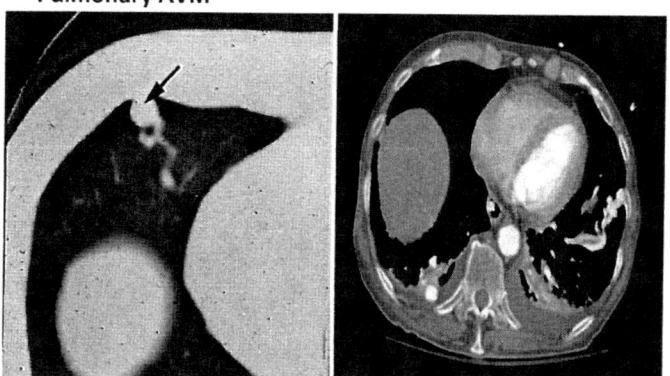

Hereditary Hemorrhagic Telangiectasia

Pulmonary Sequestration

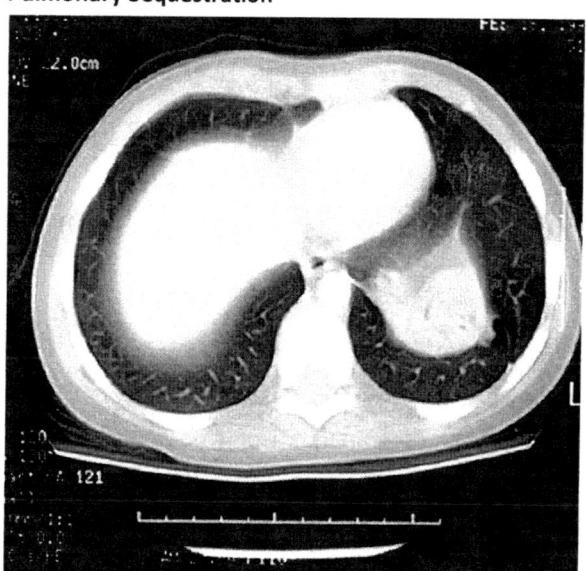

3.5 x 3 x 2.5-cm soft tissue mass located immediately
above the diaphragm on the left side of the chest; A large
artery from the descending aorta was identified

Rounded Atelectasis

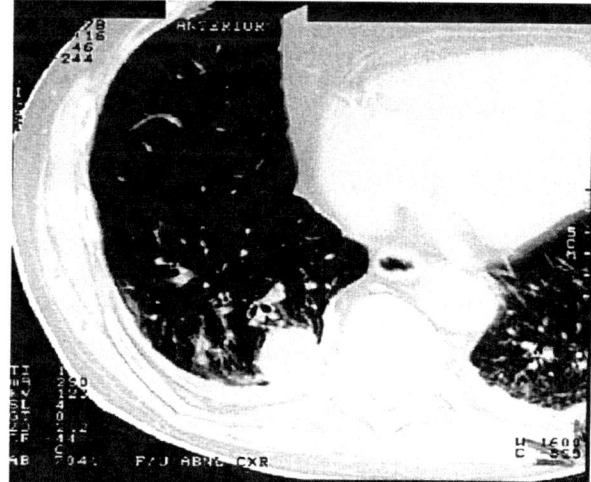

Seen in asbestosis and TB

Pulmonary Tuberculoma

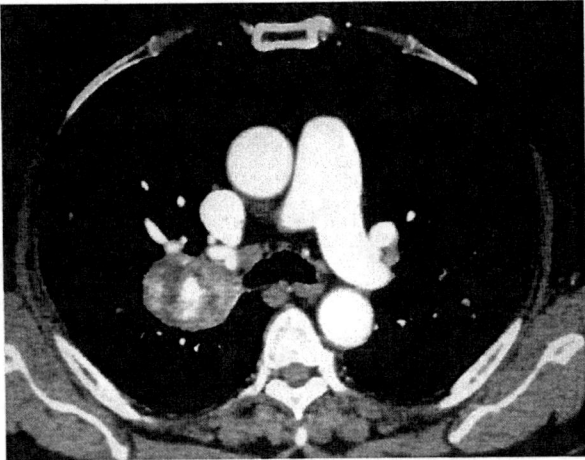

Pulmonary Nodule Evaluation
- **The 2 key elements are:**
  1) **History**
     - Smoking
     - Age > 30 years
     - Previous malignancy
  2) **Appearance of the nodule**
     - CT scan
     - Calcifications
- **Low risk**
  - Follow-up imaging
  - Fleischner Society recommendations
- **High risk**
  - Fine needle aspiration
  - Bronchoscopy/EBUS
  - Open-lung biopsy
- **Intermediate risk**
  - If nodules are > 1 cm diameter, 5-fluorodeoxyglucose + PET

Thoracic Positron Emission Tomography

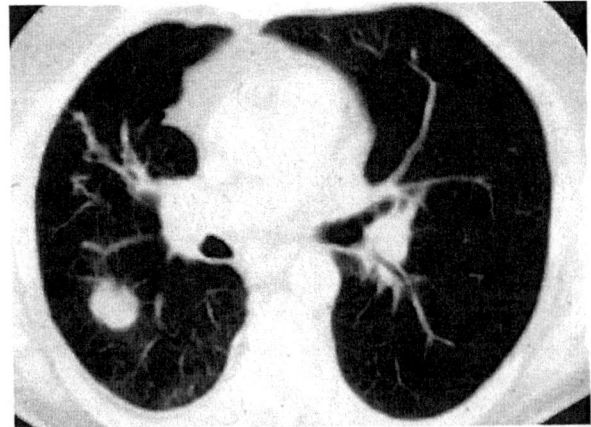

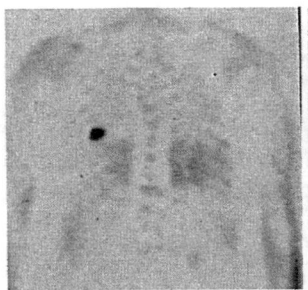 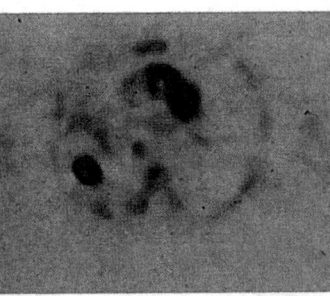

AR 38

In which of the following circumstances would a PET scan give the most useful clinical information in order to make a decision about proceeding to surgical resection?

A. A 45-year-old woman from Ohio, who has never smoked, who has a history of histoplasmosis, and is now found to have a 2.5-cm pulmonary nodule on chest CT; No prior radiographs are available

B. A 55-year-old man with a history of smoking who has a 2-cm left lower lobe nodule on chest CT with normal-sized mediastinal nodes

C. A 58-year-old woman with a 3.5-cm right lower lobe adenocarcinoma with new neurologic findings

D. A 46-year-old woman with a new 0.9-cm left lower lobe nodule with a history of adenocarcinoma *in situ* resected 1 year ago

E. A 52-year-old man with poorly controlled DM with HgbA1c of 10.2 and a 60-pack-year smoking history with an undiagnosed 3-cm right lower lobe nodule

Answer: _____

AR 39

A **57-year-old** man is evaluated after a **CXR** taken in a **preoperative assessment** for a knee replacement shows a **1-cm nodule** in the right lower lobe of the lung. The patient lives in Montana and has not traveled recently. He does not recall ever having been exposed to tuberculosis or having been tested for the disease. His most recent chest radiograph was 10 years ago. The result was normal, and the radiograph is no longer available. About 6 months ago, he had abdominal pain that was evaluated with an **abdominal CT scan**, and the pain has since resolved. The patient has a 20-pack-year history of cigarette smoking but quit 10 years ago. He is otherwise healthy.

On exam, VS are normal, lungs are clear, and there is no lymphadenopathy

© 2017 MedStudy Internal Medicine Video Board Review – Pulmonary Medicine • Raj Dasgupta, MD

Which of the following is the most appropriate next step in the management of this patient?
A. Fluorodeoxyglucose and positron emission tomography (FDG-PET) scan.
B. MRI of the chest.
C. Repeat CT scan in 3 months.
D. Review of lung images from CT scan of the abdomen.
E. Thin-section CT scan of the chest.

Answer: _____

AR 39 (cont.)
Evaluation of a pulmonary nodule should always begin by review of any previous images.

AR 40
A **52-year-old woman** is evaluated after a **screening** CT colonography detected a **3-mm nodule** in the right lower lobe of the lung. A tortuous colon prevented complete screening colonoscopy.
CT scan of the chest showed no additional nodules and was otherwise normal. The patient has **never smoked**. She works in the home and has not been exposed to potential carcinogens. She has not had a chest radiograph or other imaging procedure, except mammography.
Her medical history includes only hyperlipidemia, and her only medication is simvastatin. Her family history is unremarkable.
On exam, VS are normal. Examination of the skin is normal. There is no lymphadenopathy, and the lungs are clear.

Which of the following is the most appropriate next step in the management of this patient?
A. Chest radiograph in 3 months
B. CT scan of the chest in 3 months
C. CT scan of the chest in 6 months
D. CT scan of the chest in 12 months
E. No follow-up

Answer: _____

AR 40 (cont.)
Fleischner Society recommendations include no follow-up for low-risk patients with nodules 4 mm or smaller and follow-up CT at 12 months for patients with such nodules who are at risk for lung cancer. More frequent follow-ups are not recommended for nodules of this size.

Management of Nodules Smaller Than 8 mm Detected Incidentally at Nonscreening CT

Nodule Size (mm)*	Low-Risk Patient	High-Risk Patient
·≤ 4	No follow-up needed§	Follow-up CT at 12 mo; if unchanged, no further follow-up
·> 4–6	Follow-up CT at 12 mo; if unchanged, no further follow-up	Initial follow-up CT at 6–12 mo then at 18–24 mo if no change
·> 6–8	Initial follow-up CT at 6–12 mo then at 18–24 mo if no change	Initial follow-up CT at 3–6 mo then at 9–12 and 24 mo if no change
·> 8	Follow-up CT at around 3, 9, and 24 mo, dynamic contrast-enhanced CT, PET, and/or biopsy	Same as for low-risk patient

Nonsolid ("**ground-glass**") or partly solid nodules may require longer follow-up to exclude indolent adenocarcinoma.

Lung Cancer
- There are **4 major categories** of cancer:
  1) **Central lesions**
     - Squamous cell
     - Small cell
  2) **Peripheral lesions**
     - Adenocarcinoma
     - Large cell

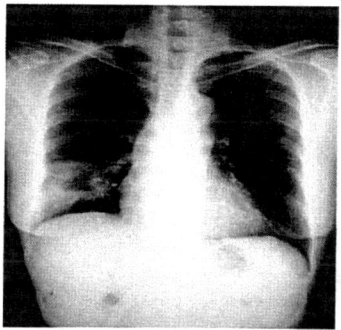
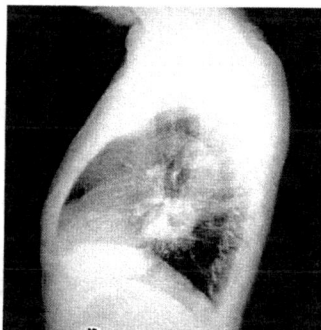
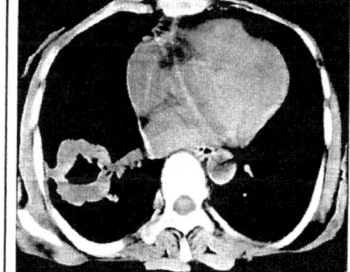
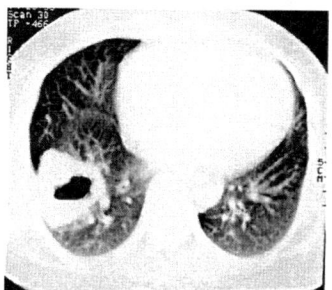

Lung Cancer (cont.)
- **Squamous cell**
  - Usually starts near a central bronchus
  - Associated with **cavitary lesions**
  - Usually metastasizes by direct extension into the hilar node and mediastinum
  - Associated with **hypercalcemia**
    - From secretion of a parathyroid hormone-like substance
  - Histologic
    - **Keratin** production by tumor cells
    - Intercellular desmosomes "intercellular bridges"

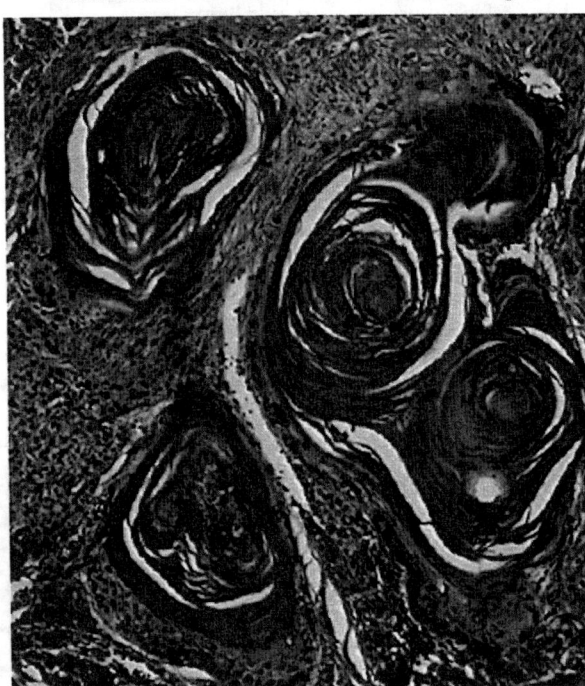

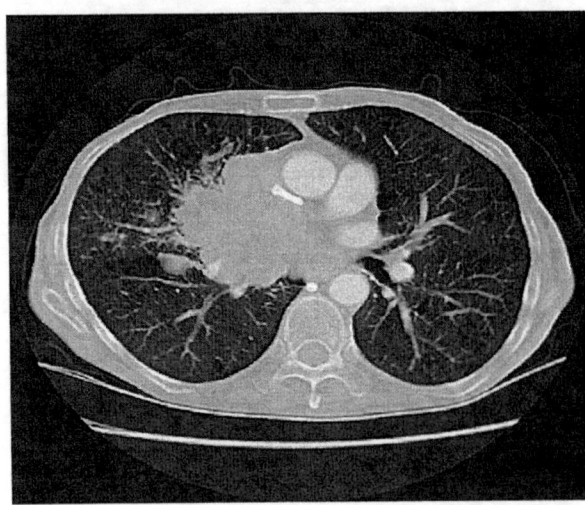

Lung Cancer (cont.)
- **Small cell**
  - Previously called "oat cell"
    - The "oat cell" contains dense neurosecretory granules
      - Vesicles containing neuroendocrine hormones
  - Extremely aggressive
    - 80% of patients have metastases at the time of diagnosis
  - Paraneoplastic syndromes
    - SIADH
    - Ectopic ACTH production
    - Lambert-Eaton syndrome
    - Most common cause SVC syndrome

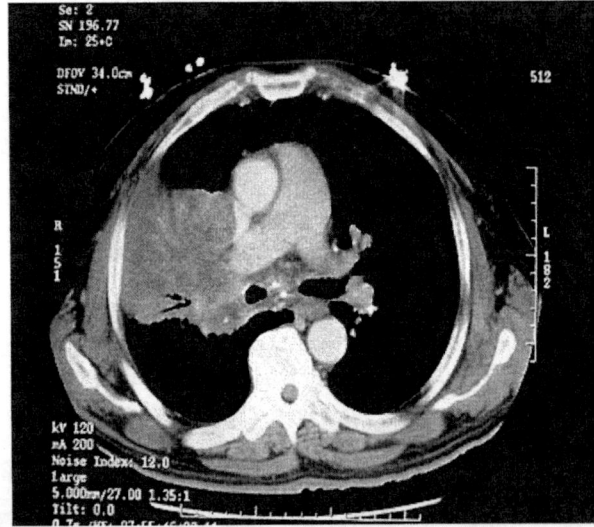

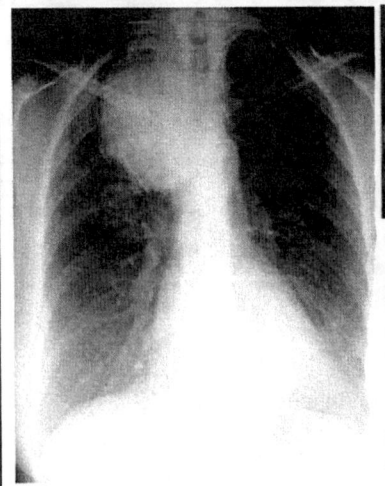

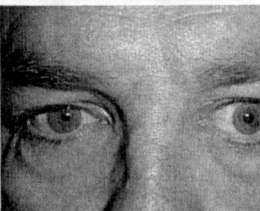

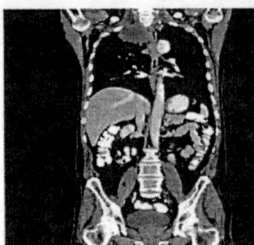

Lung Cancer (cont.)

- **Adenocarcinoma**
  - Pancoast tumor (superior sulcus tumor)
    - Named after the radiologist in 1924
    - Characteristic shoulder pain with weakness & numbness of the arm
    - Horner's syndrome
      - Ptosis, miosis, anhidrosis

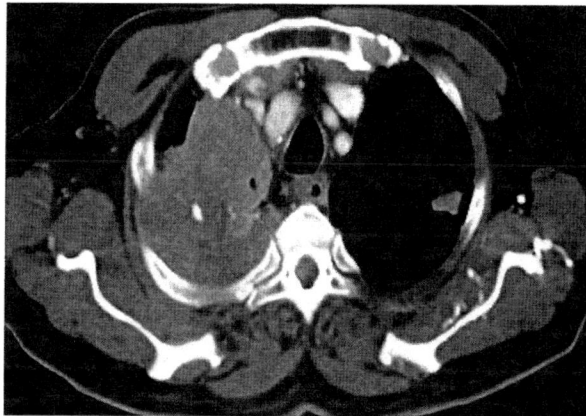

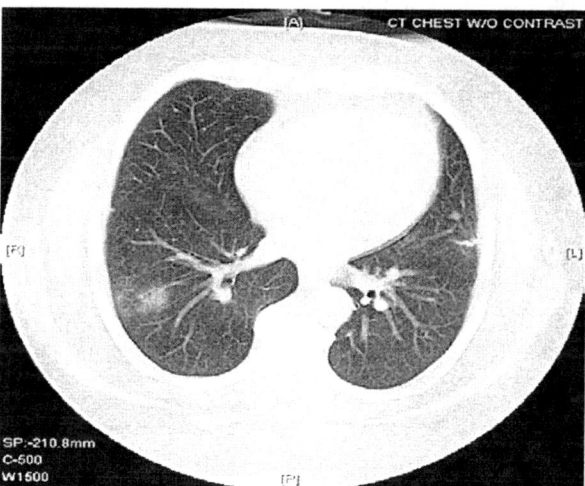

Lung Cancer (cont.)

- **Bronchoalveolar carcinoma (adenocarcinoma *in situ*)**
  - "The prostate cancer of the lung"
  - Least association with smoking
  - Up to 50% arises in the setting of preexisting lung disease
  - Usually PET negative
    - Low-glucose metabolism

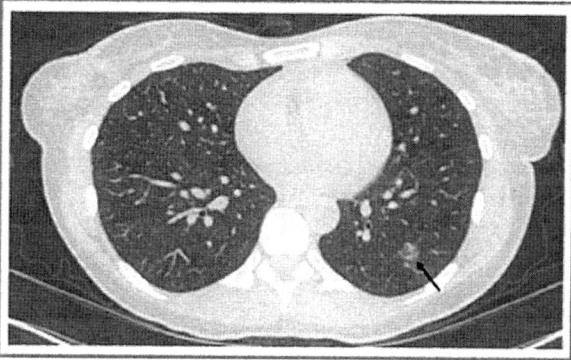

Lung Cancer Screening

- When should screening stop?
  1) Turns 81 years old **or**
  2) Has not smoked in 15 years **or**
  3) Develops a health problem that makes them unwilling or unable to have surgery if lung cancer is found
- The USPSTF recommends yearly lung cancer screening with low-dose CT scan for people who:
  1) Have a history of heavy smoking (≥ 30 pack years) **and**
  2) Smoke now or have quit within the past 15 years **and**
  3) Between 55 and 80 years old
- Radiation dose exposure is less than a 1/3 of a standard-dose diagnostic chest CT

Thank You

- Website: doctorrajd.com
- Facebook: Raj Dasgupta, MD
- Twitter: @DoctorRajD
- Instagram
- LinkedIn

Pulmonary Medicine
Audience Response Answers

Audience Response 1
Answer: A. Decreased atrial O_2 saturation (S_aO_2).

AR 2
Answer: B. Administer methylene blue.

AR 3
Answer: B. Neuromuscular disease.

AR 4
Answer: B. Mild lower airway obstruction
with reversibility.

AR 5
Answer: D. COPD.

AR 6
Answer: D. Fixed obstruction.

AR 7
Answer: A.

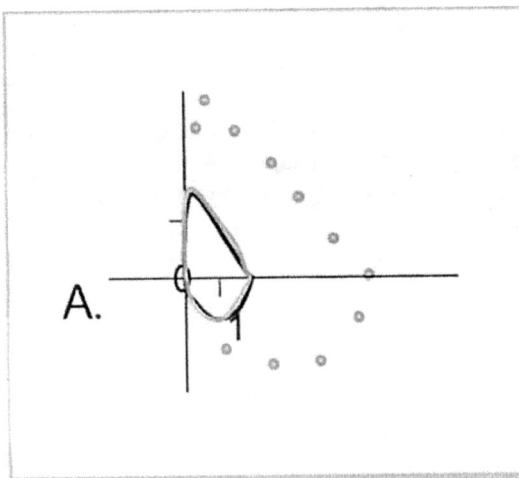

AR 8
Answer: D. Echocardiogram.

AR 9
Answer: C. Dendritic cell and macrophage.

AR 10
Answer: B. Eosinophil.

AR 11
Answer: D. Mepolizumab, omalizumab,
and bronchial thermoplasty; Yes/Yes/Yes.

AR 12
Answer: B. No.

AR 13
Answer: A. Yes.

AR 14
Answer: B. Add roflumilast, 500 mcg daily.

AR 15A
Answer: C. Administering a benzodiazepine.

AR 15B
Answer: E. Other.

AR 16
Answer: A. Arterial blood gas studies.

AR 17
Answer: D. Taper and discontinue
fluticasone/salmeterol and add indacaterol.

AR 18
Answer: D. Idiopathic pulmonary fibrosis.

AR 19
Answer: A. Diarrhea.

AR 20
Answer: D. Palliative care consult.

AR 21
Answer: A. True.

AR 22
Answer: B. Rivaroxaban.

AR 23
Answer: A. Apixaban.

AR 24
Answer: D. Idarucizumab.

AR 25
Answer: E. Not enough information to determine this.

AR 26
Answer: A. Continue anticoagulation indefinitely.

AR 27
Answer: A. 1 hour.

AR 28
Answer: D. Repeat thoracentesis and pleural
fluid cytology.

AR 29
Answer: B. Nonbleeding lung.

AR 30
Answer: E. Increase the PEEP.

AR 31
Answer: B. Decreased compliance and oxygenation.

AR 32
Answer: C. Both A and B.

AR 33
Answer: B. No.

AR 34
Answer: B. Early administration of appropriate antibiotics.

AR 35
Answer: B. Distributive shock secondary to sepsis.

AR 36
Answer: B. Hypovolemic shock.

AR 37A
Answer: A. Cardiogenic shock from left heart failure.

AR 37B
Answer: C. Dobutamine.

AR 37C
Answer: A. Low (< 60%).

AR 38
Answer: B. A 55-year-old man with a history of smoking who has a 2-cm left lower lobe nodule on chest CT with normal-sized mediastinal nodes.

AR 39
Answer: D. Review of lung images from CT scan of the abdomen.

AR 40
Answer: E. No follow-up.

MedStudy

Internal Medicine Video Board Review

Rheumatology

Presented by

Kathryn H. Dao, MD
Associate Director of Clinical Rheumatology
Baylor Research Institute
Dallas, Texas

Table of Contents

Rheumatology Abbreviations

AAU	Acute anterior uveitis
AC	Acromioclavicular
ADL	Activities of daily living
ANA	Antinuclear antibodies
ANCA	Antineutrophil cytoplasmic antibody
Anti-CCP	Anticyclic citrullinated peptide
Anti-dsDNA	Anti–double-stranded DNA antibody
Anti-Sm	Anti-Smith antibody
AS	Ankylosing spondylitis
AVN	Avascular necrosis
AZP	Azathioprine
AZT	Azidothymidine (a.k.a. zidovudine)
BCP	Basic calcium phosphate (crystal)
CCP	Cyclic citrullinated peptide
CKD	Chronic kidney disease
CMC	Carpometacarpal joint
CPK	Creatinine phosphokinase
CPPD	Calcium pyrophosphate deposition disease
CREST	Calcinosis, Raynaud phenomenon, esophageal dysmotility, sclerodactyly, telangiectasia
CRP	C-reactive protein
CTD	Connective tissue disease
CVA	Cardiovascular accident
CYA	Cyclosporine
CYP	Cyclophosphamide
DDD	Degenerative disc disease
DILS	Diffuse infiltrative lymphocytosis syndrome
DIP	Distal interphalangeal joint
DISH	Diffuse idiopathic skeletal hyperostosis
DJD	Degenerative joint disease
DLCO	Diffusing capacity of the lungs for carbon monoxide
DM	Dermatomyositis
DMARD	Disease-modifying antirheumatic drug
DVT	Deep venous thrombosis
EDS	Ehlers-Danlos syndrome
EGPA	Eosinophilic granulomatosis with polyangiitis
ELISA	Enzyme-linked immunosorbent assay
EntA	Enteropathic arthritis
EOA	Erosive osteoarthritis
FABER	Flexion, abduction, and external rotation
FM	Fibromyalgia
GC	Gonococcus
GCA	Giant cell arteritis
GH	Glenohumeral
GPA	Granulomatosis with polyangiitis
HBsAg+	Hepatitis B virus antigen
HBV	Hepatitis B virus
HCQ	Hydroxychloroquine
HTLV-1	Human T-cell lymphotropic virus Type 1
JAK	Janus kinase
La	La antibody (anti-SSB antibody)
LAC	Lupus anticoagulant
LDH	Lactate dehydrogenase
LEF	Leflunomide
LMWH	Low molecular weight heparin
MALToma	Mucus-associated lymphoid tissue lymphoma
MCP	Metacarpophalangeal joint
MCTD	Mixed connective tissue disease
MCV	Mean corpuscular volume
MD	Muscular dystrophy
MG	Myasthenia gravis
MMF	Mycophenolate mofetil
MPA	Microscopic polyangiitis
MTP	Metatarsophalangeal joint
MS	Multiple sclerosis
MSK	Musculoskeletal
MSU	Monosodium urate
MTX	Methotrexate
NCS	Nerve conduction study
OA	Osteoarthritis
PAN	Polyarteritis nodosa
PIP	Proximal interphalangeal joint
PM	Polymyositis
PMN	Polymorphonuclear leukocyte
PMR	Polymyalgia rheumatica
PNS	Peripheral nervous system
PPD	Purified protein derivative
PR3	Proteinase-3
PRPP	Phosphoribosyl pyrophosphate
Ps	Psoriasis
PsA	Psoriatic arthritis
PSS	Progressive systemic scleroderma
PTT	Partial thromboplastin time
PVNS	Pigmented villonodular synovitis
RA	Rheumatoid arthritis
ReA	Reactive arthritis
RF	Rheumatoid factor
RMSF	Rocky Mountain spotted fever
Ro	Ro antibody (anti-SSA antibody)
ROM	Range of motion
RPR	Rapid plasma reagin

SBE	Subacute bacterial endocarditis
SCLE	Subacute cutaneous lupus erythematosus
SGOT	Serum glutamic oxaloacetic transaminase (AST)
SkM	Skeletomuscular
SLE	Systemic lupus erythematosus
SNSA	Seronegative spondyloarthropathies
SSc	Systemic sclerosis
SSZ	Sulfasalazine
TIBC	Total iron-binding capacity
TNF	Tumor necrosis factor
TNFi	Tumor necrosis factor inhibitor

Rheumatology

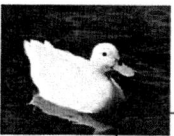
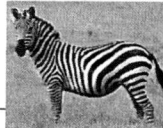

Common Dx Common S/Sx	Uncommon Dx Common S/Sx
Common Dx Uncommon S/Sx	Uncommon Dx Uncommon S/Sx

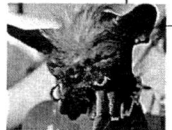
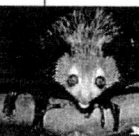

High-Yield Topics Covered Today:
- Classifying joint symptoms
- OA
- RA
- Spondyloarthritis
- Crystalline arthritis
- SLE, antiphospholipid syndrome, Sjögren's
- Systemic sclerosis
- Idiopathic inflammatory myopathies
- Fibromyalgia
- PMR & vasculitis
- Primary care orthopedics
- ... Other weird diseases

Rheumatologic Truths:
1) **No** single blood test can diagnose **any** rheumatologic disease
2) It is about **pattern recognition**!!!

Categorizing Arthropathies
- Inflammatory vs. noninflammatory
- Number of joints: Mono-, oligo-, or polyarthritis
- Acute vs. chronic
- Symmetric vs. asymmetric
- Specific joints/joint areas involved:
  - Axial (spine) vs. peripheral
  - Large vs. small joints
  - DIP vs. MCP
- Extraarticular features
  - Other organs involved
  - Systemic symptoms

Joint pain
- Arthralgia = joint pain
- Arthritis = joint inflammation

Cardinal signs of inflammation:
Erythema (rubor)
Swelling (tumor)
Heat (calor)
Pain (dolor)

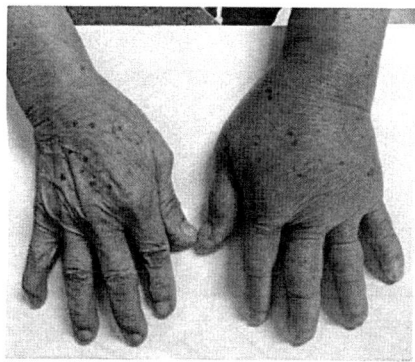

Source: Kathryn Dao, MD

Noninflammatory Arthropathies
- Osteoarthritis
- Trauma
- Neuropathy
- ± Metabolic disease

Inflammatory Arthritides
Noncrystalline arthritis:
- Rheumatoid arthritis
- Seronegative spondyloarthropathies (SNSA)
- Systemic lupus erythematosus (SLE)
- Mixed connective tissue disease (MCTD)
- Infectious arthritis

Crystalline arthritis:
- Gout
- Pseudogout
- Basic calcium phosphate

Classification of Synovial Effusions

Type of Fluid	Color	WBC/mm^3
Normal	Clear (colorless)	< 200 (< 25% PMN)
Noninflammatory	Clear Yellow	200–2,000 (< 25% PMN)
Inflammatory	Cloudy Yellow	2,000–100,000 (> 50% PMN)
Septic	Purulent	> 50,000 (> 75% PMN)

Joint Fluid Tests
Cell count with differential
Crystal analysis
Gram stain with culture and sensitivity

No protein, glucose, LDH
Most important are:

Crystals and culture

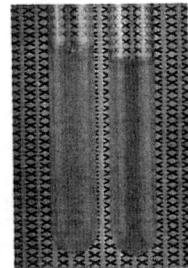

Definition
Osteoarthritis (degenerative joint disease)
- Affects an estimated 12% of the U.S. population between 25 and 75 years of age
- 80% of individuals > 75 years of age have radiographic evidence

Characterized by:
1) **Asymmetric** joint involvement
2) **Asymmetric** joint space narrowing
3) Joint hypertrophy
4) New bone formation (osteophyte)

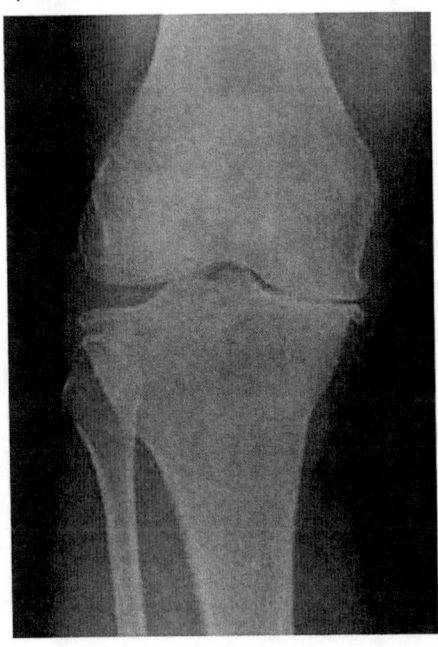

Typical OA History / Physical Exam
History
- Joint pain without inflammation, which is worse after use and relieved by rest
- Morning stiffness < 1 hour
- **No** constitutional symptoms (fever, malaise, fatigue)
Physical exam
- Not ill-appearing
- Bony joint enlargement
- Heberden and Bouchard nodes
- Joint tenderness with passive ROM
- ± Noninflammatory effusion

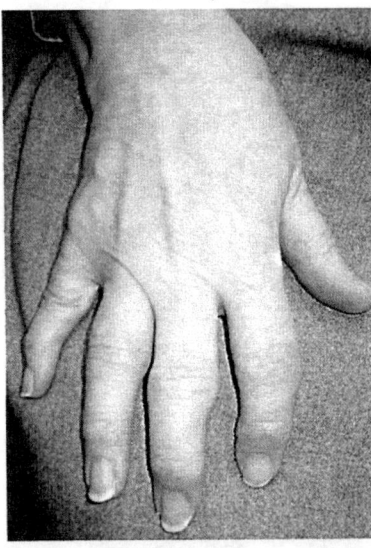

Osteoarthritis Etiology
1°: **No obvious underlying cause**
- Idiopathic
- Erosive osteoarthritis (EOA)

2°: **Resulting from prior joint disorders or systemic disease**
1) Joint trauma:
   - Congenital defect
   - Developmental defect — chondrodysplasias
   - Injury
   - Excessive loads
   - Charcot joint

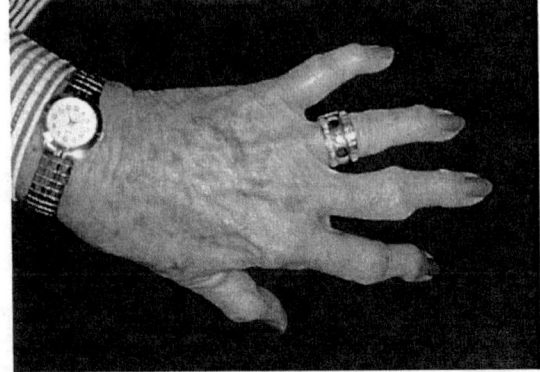

Source: Kathryn Dao, MD

Osteoarthritis Etiology (cont.)
  2) Prior inflammatory arthropathy:
     - Gout
     - CPPD
     - RA
  3) Metabolic disorders:
     - Hemochromatosis
     - Alkaptonuria
     - Wilson disease
     - Paget disease
     - Gaucher disease

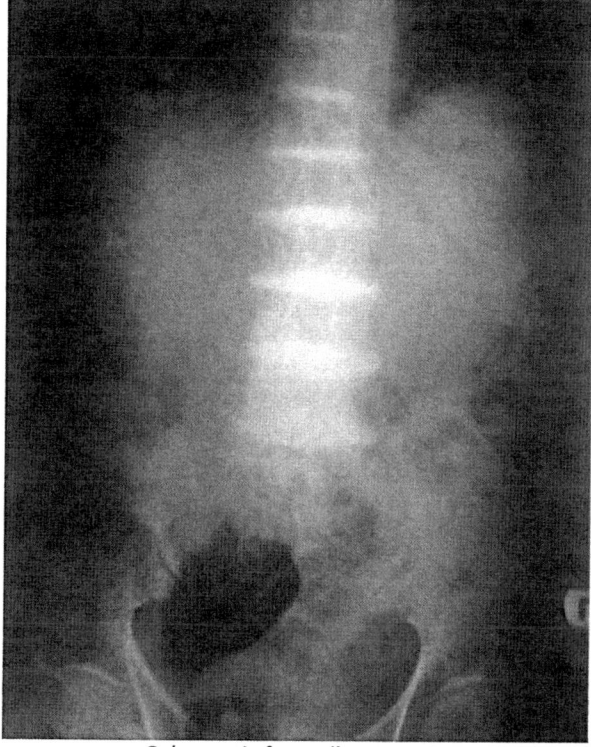

Ochronosis from alkaptonuria

Osteoarthritis Etiology (cont.)
  4) Endocrinopathies:
     - Diabetes mellitus
     - Acromegaly
     - Sex hormone abnormalities
     - Hyperadrenocorticism
  5) Collagen abnormalities:
     - Ehlers-Danlos syndrome (EDS)
  6) Miscellaneous:
     - Avascular necrosis
     - Hemophilia
     - Osteopetrosis

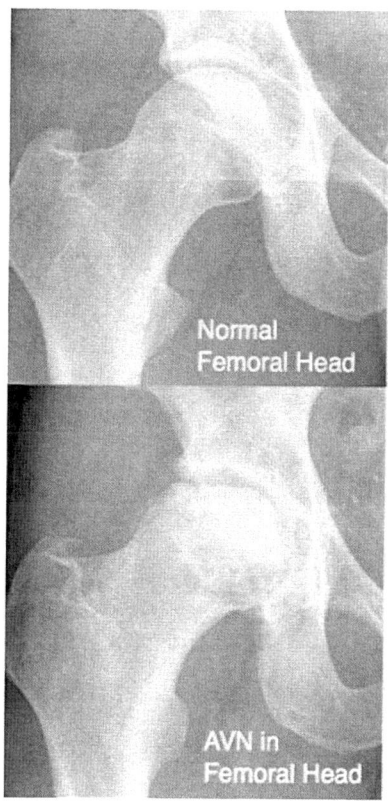

Typical OA Laboratories and Radiographic Changes
- <u>Labs</u>
  - ESR: Normal
  - Joint fluid: < 2,000 WBC
  - CBC: Normal
  - SMA-20: Normal
- <u>Radiographs</u>
  - Asymmetric/Nonconcentric joint space narrowing
  - Osteophytes
  - Bone enlargement

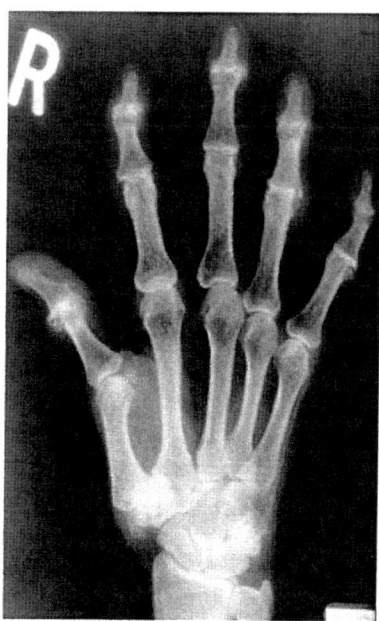

Knee Osteoarthritis

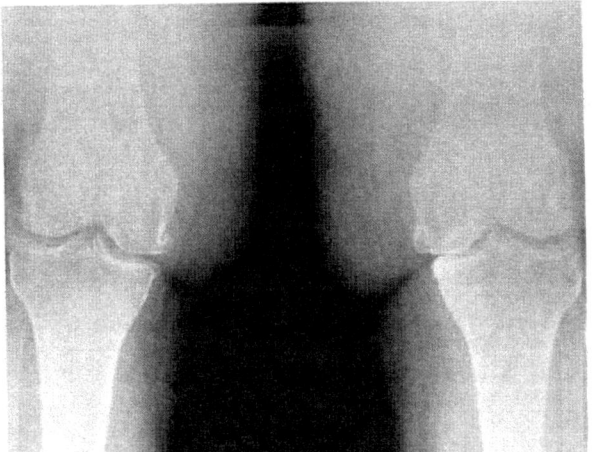

Audience Response 1

A 60-year-old Caucasian former professional football player with a h/o multiple knee injuries c/o left knee pain x 10 years reports 15–20 minutes morning stiffness.
He denies joint swelling, Raynaud phenomenon, sicca symptoms, fever, or chills.
The x-ray of his L knee is shown below.

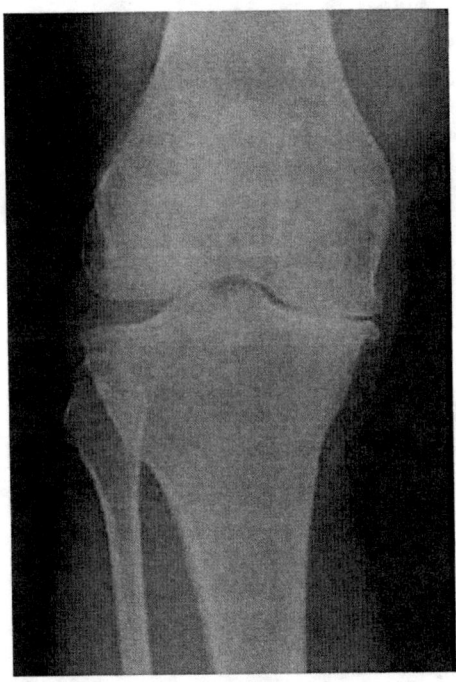

What is the diagnosis?

A. Fibromyalgia
B. RA
C. OA
D. Gout
E. Ankylosing spondylitis

Answer: _____

Contrast OA with RA

- **Rheumatoid arthritis:**
  - Affects 1–2% of the population worldwide
  - Male:female = 1:2.5
  - Peak age at onset: 25–55 years
- Rheumatoid arthritis is a systemic disease with:
  1) Autoantibody formation
  2) **Symmetric** joint inflammation

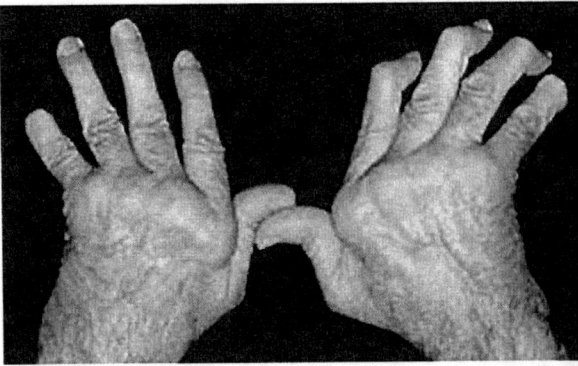

RA vs. OA

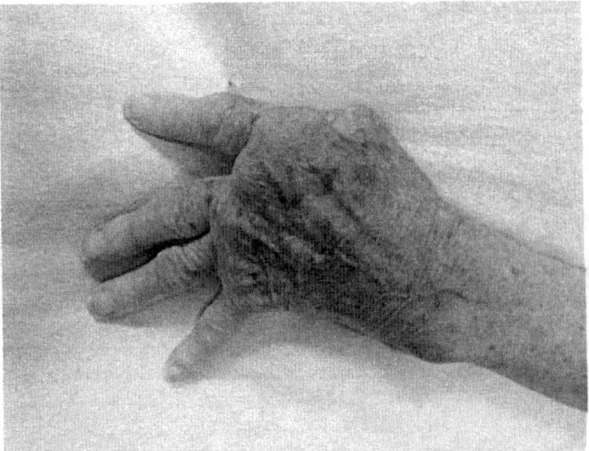

Source: James Heilman, MD

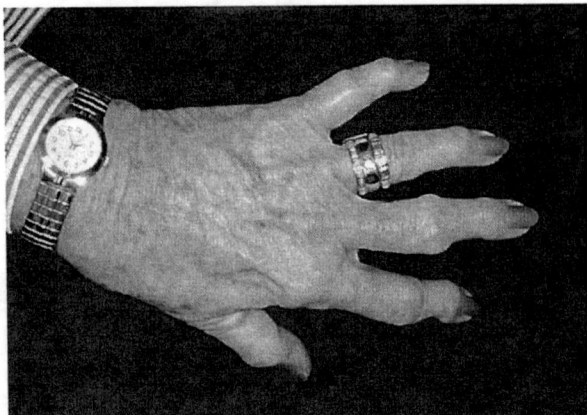

Source: Kathryn Dao, MD

© 2017 MedStudy Internal Medicine Video Board Review – Rheumatology • Kathryn H. Dao, MD

Renoir with RA

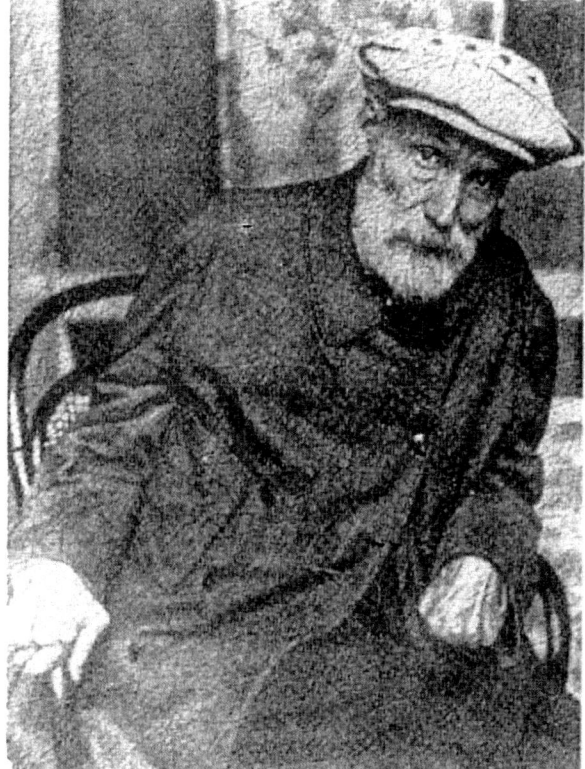

Pierre-Auguste Renoir
(February 25, 1841–December 3, 1919)

Typical RA History
- Symmetric joint swelling, warmth, redness
- Morning stiffness > 1 hour
- ± Constitutional symptoms (fever, weight loss, fatigue)

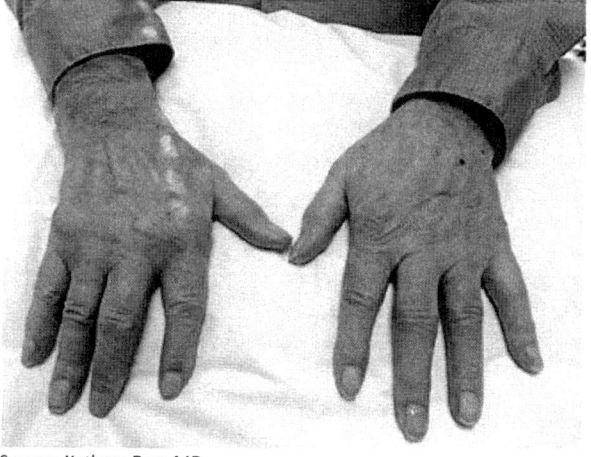

Source: Kathryn Dao, MD

Typical RA Physical Exam
- Ill-appearing
- Ulnar deviation
- Boutonnière and swan-neck deformity
- Limited joint range of motion

- Joint swelling, redness, warmth, and pain (arthritis)
- Extraarticular manifestations:

Rheumatoid nodule	Ocular	Pulmonary
Nervous system	Cardiac	Vasculitis

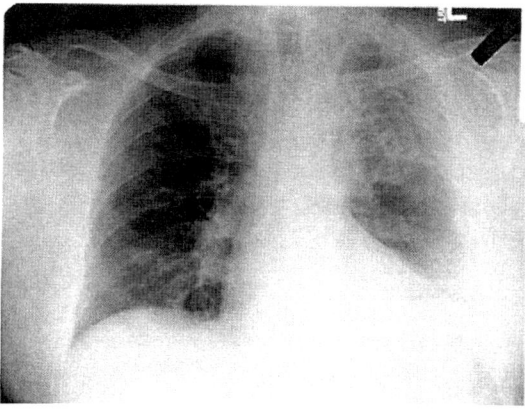

Complications of RA
- Lymphoma
- Scleritis (scleromalacia perforans)
- Atlantoaxial subluxation
- Interstitial lung disease
- Cardiovascular mortality
- Infections
- Death

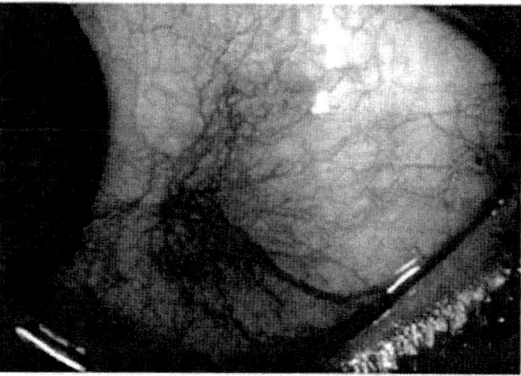

RA of the Hands

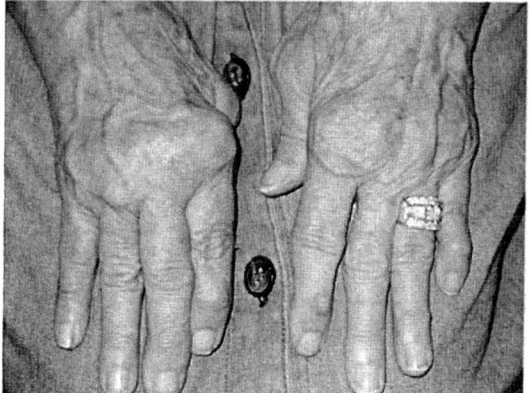

Source: Jack Cush, MD

Typical RA Laboratory Abnormalities
Inflammatory
- Normochromic normocytic anemia
- Elevated platelet count
- Elevated ESR
- Elevated C-reactive protein
- Elevated immunoglobulin concentration

- Joint fluid analysis — inflammatory
- Rheumatoid factor (RF) — antibodies directed against the Fc of IgG; Most common is IgM rheumatoid factor; 80% of patients are seropositive (RF+)
- CCP antibody — very specific for RA

Diseases with +RF

Autoimmune diseases
Cancers
Chronic bacterial infections
  Leprosy
  Lyme disease
  Subacute bacterial
    endocarditis
  Syphilis
  TB
	Viral infections
	  Cytomegalovirus
	  EBV
	  Hepatitis A, B, C
	  HIV
	  Influenza
	  Rubella
	Liver disease
	Mixed cryoglobulinemia
	Parasitic infection
	Pulmonary interstitial disease
	Sarcoidosis

Serologic Factors in RA — Anti-CCP & RF

	Sensitivity (%)	Specificity (%)
Anti-CCP*	40–60%	98%
RF	60–80%	84%
Anti-CCP + RF	33%	99.6%

No prognostic association with the ANA

* anticyclic citrullinated peptide

Bizzaro N, et al. *Clin Chem*. 2001;47:1089–1093.

Typical RA Radiographic Abnormalities
1) Periarticular osteopenia
2) Marginal erosions — where synovium attaches to bone
3) Target joints:
   - MCPs
   - PIPs
   - Wrists (carpal bones)
   - Cervical spine
   - MTPs
4) Soft tissue swelling

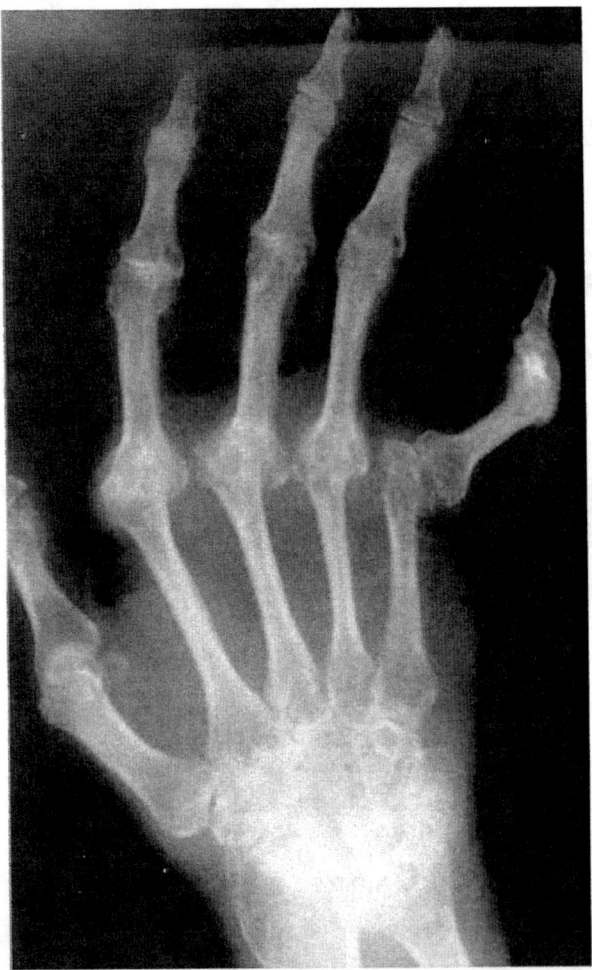

RA of the Knees

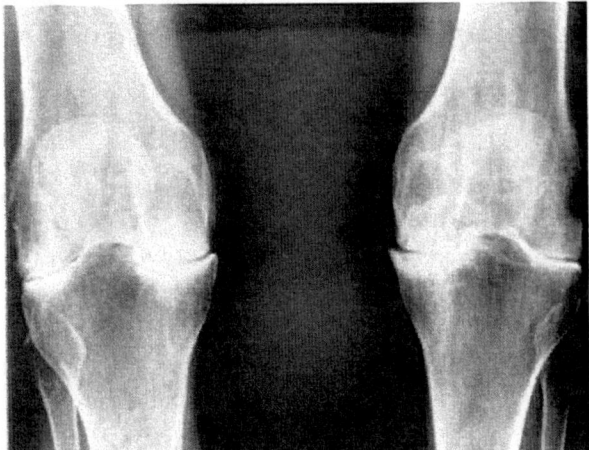

© 2017 MedStudy Internal Medicine Video Board Review – Rheumatology • Kathryn H. Dao, MD

AR 2

A 35-year-old female presents with a 3-month history of joint pain and swelling. She noted that it is hard to care for her new baby who is now 3 months old. She reported that stiffness is worse in the morning, lasting 1 hour. Other reviews of systems are negative.

Her hands are as shown:
Labs noted neg ANA, neg RF, +CCP, ESR 46.

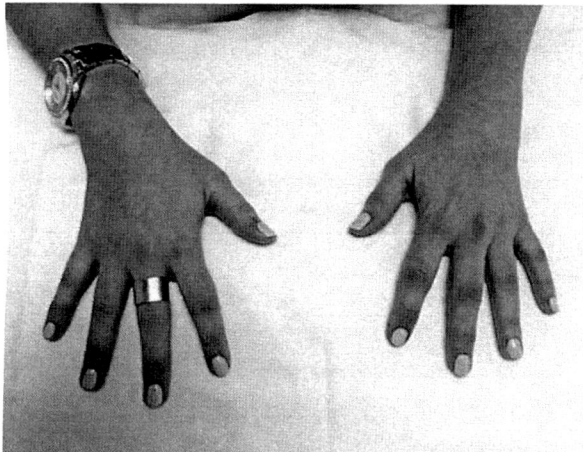

Source: Kathryn Dao, MD

She is at risk for which complication?

A. Gout
B. Ruptured Achilles tendon
C. Inflammatory bowel disease
D. Lymphoma
E. Systemic lupus erythematosus

Answer: _____

	OA	RA
Joint distribution	Asymmetric monoarticular, oligoarticular, polyarticular	Symmetric polyarticular
Synovitis	No, only bony enlargement	Yes
Inflammation	No	Yes
Target joint	DIP, PIP, CMC, Hips, Knees, Spine, Feet, Toes	PIP, MCP, Wrists, Elbows, C-spine, Knees, Hips, Ankles, Toes
Joints spared	MCP, Wrist, Ankles	DIP, CMC, T/L/S spine
AM Stiffness	< 45 minutes	> 1 hour
Labs	Noninflammatory	Inflammatory: Elevated Plt, anemia of chronic disease, ESR, +RF, +CCP
Bone changes	Bony enlargement with new bone formation (osteophytes)	Bone loss: Periarticular osteopenia, marginal erosions

Management Goal
OA: Relieve symptoms (pain); thus, maintain function
    and quality of life
RA: Suppress inflammation (synovitis) to minimize
    joint damage and preserve joint function

OA Management
Diet/Exercise
PT/OT
Analgesia
Surgery

Knee OA Treatment Guidelines

Table 4. Pharmacologic recommendations for the initial
management of knee OA*

We conditionally recommend that patients with knee OA
    should use one of the following:
Acetaminophen
Oral NSAIDs
Topical NSAIDs
Tramadol
Intraarticular corticosteroid injections
We conditionally recommend that patients with knee OA
    should not use the following:
Chondroitin sulfate
Glucosamine
Topical capsaicin
We have no recommendations regarding the use of
    intraarticular hyaluronates, duloxetine, and opioid
    analgesics

* No strong recommendations were made for the initial pharmacologic management of knee osteoarthritis (OA). For patients who
have an inadequate response to initial pharmacologic management,
please see the Results for alternative strategies. NSAIDs = nonsteroidal antiinflammatory drugs.

American College of Rheumatology 2012 Guidelines
    for Management of OA. *Arthritis & Rheumatism.*
    2012;64(4):465–474.

RA Management
Inflammation-suppression medications:
1) DMARDs: Disease-Modifying Anti-Rheumatic Drugs
2) Biologics
Analgesics — do not change the disease course:
    ASA, NSAIDs, acetaminophen, tramadol,
    codeine derivatives

• **DMARDs**
    – Gold (Au) and penicillamine — not used anymore
    – Cyclosporine (CYA)
    – **Methotrexate (MTX)**
    – **Sulfasalazine (SSZ)**
    – **Hydroxychloroquine (HCQ)**
    – Minocycline
    – **Leflunomide (LEF)**
    – Azathioprine (AZP)

    – Mycophenolate mofetil (MMF)
    – Cyclophosphamide (CYP)
    – **Tofacitinib (Xeljanz)**
        New: Intracellular signaling JAK inhibitor

Combination DMARD:
Triple therapy: HCQ + SSZ + MTX = efficacy TNFi
                    $ $$$

Biologics

TNF inhibitors	Etanercept (Enbrel)	Recombinant soluble TNF receptor
	Infliximab (Remicade)	Chimeric murine-human mAb
	Adalimumab (Humira)	Human mAb
	Certolizumab pegol (Cimzia)	Pegylated Fab' fragment from humanized mAb
	Golimumab (Simponi)	Human mAb
Non-TNF	Rituximab (Rituxan)	Chimeric Anti-CD20 mAb — targets B cells
	Abatacept (Orencia)	Recombinant CTLA4 Ig — targets T cells
	Tocilizumab (Actemra)	Anti-IL-6 receptor mAb
	Anakinra (Kineret)	Recombinant IL-1 receptor

Avoid live vaccines with biologics

Spondyloarthritis

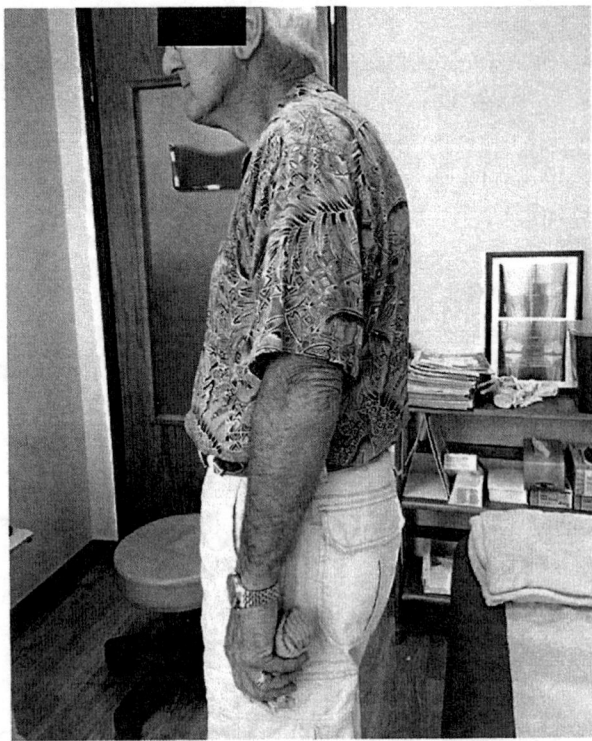

Source: Kathryn Dao, MD

© 2017 MedStudy Internal Medicine Video Board Review – Rheumatology • Kathryn H. Dao, MD

Spondyloarthritis

- **Seronegative spondyloarthritis (SNSA)** is a group of arthritides characterized by axial skeleton involvement (back pain), various degrees of peripheral joint arthritis, and inflammation and subsequent ossification of ligaments and tendons (enthesitis)
- Absence of RF or other specific antibodies (hence the term "**seronegative**")
- Associated with a variety of mucocutaneous, gastrointestinal, and ocular inflammatory disorders

Spondyloarthritides — The Spectrum

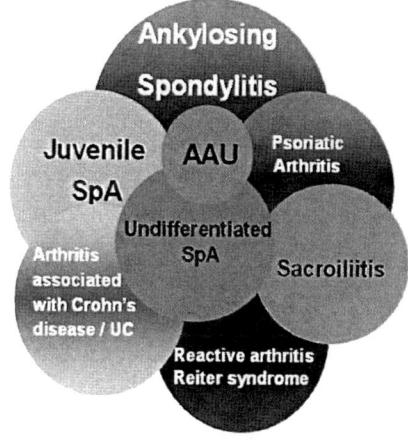

SNSAs — General Features

- Onset: Young adults
- Familial
- Inflammatory arthritis of spine or large (hips) and peripheral joints
- Peripheral arthritis, often asymmetric with "sausage" digits (dactylitis)
- Mucocutaneous manifestations:
  - Painless oral ulcers
  - Circinate balanitis
  - Keratoderma blennorrhagica
  - Psoriasis (Ps)
- Uveitis
- Enthesopathy (enthesitis)
- HLA-B27 is associated with spinal and eye disease

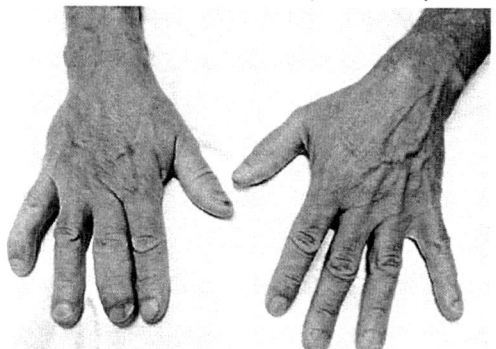

Source: Kathryn Dao, MD

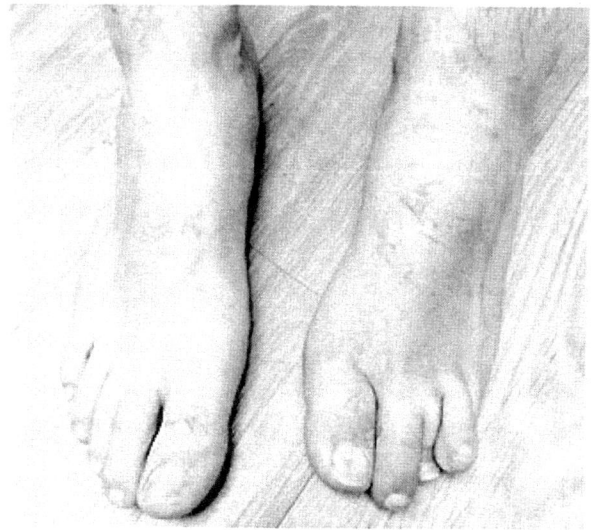

HLA-B27

- **HLA-B27** is positive in a large percentage of patients with SNSAs
- **However**, HLA-B27 is present in ~ 8–9% of the population, and back pain occurs in most people at some point in their lives
- Therefore, while HLA-B27 is associated with the SNSAs, it is **neither** specific nor diagnostic for the etiology of back pain nor for the diagnosis of spondyloarthropathy

Enthesitis

- Inflammation at the insertion of ligaments and tendons onto bone (entheses) = enthesitis
- Commonly occurs at Achilles insertion, within the plantar fascia, and at the epicondyles
- Manifests as tenderness of the posterior heel, plantar surface of the foot, spinous processes, epicondyles, and sausage digits
- The nail bed is an enthesis

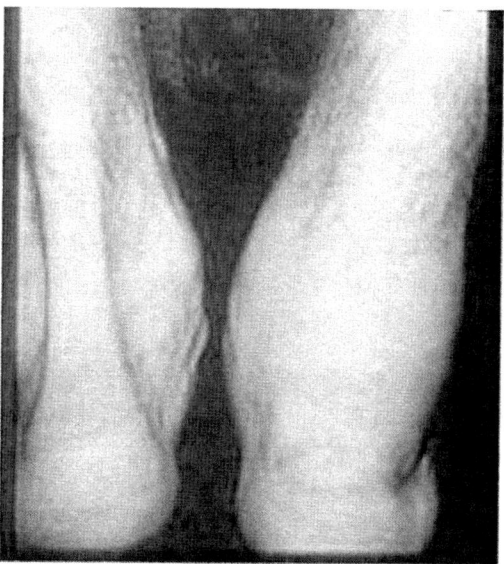

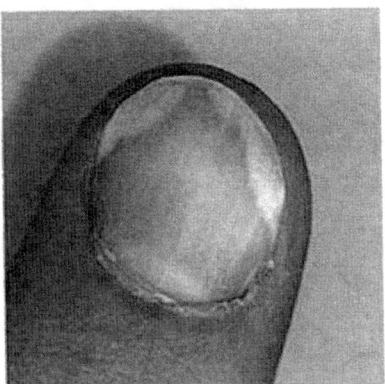

Ankylosing Spondylitis (AS) / Enteropathic Arthritis (EntA)

Both can have:

1) Symmetric spine radiographic changes
2) Symmetric SI joint radiographic changes
3) Bowel inflammation (colitis)
4) Minimal peripheral joint inflammation
5) Less enthesopathy

Psoriatic Arthritis (PsA) / Reactive Arthritis (ReA)

Both can have:

1) Asymmetric spine radiographic changes
2) Asymmetric SI joint radiographic changes
3) Prominent peripheral joint inflammation
4) Prominent enthesopathy and sausage digits
5) Rash which is psoriaform

Ankylosing Spondylitis (AS)
- Cardiac: Aortic insufficiency; conduction defects
- GI tract: Inflammatory bowel disease
- Lung: Apical fibrosis
- Musculoskeletal: Axial with symmetric SI joint changes with minimal peripheral joint arthritis
- Neurologic: Spine fracture dislocation, cauda equina syndrome
- Ophthalmologic: Acute anterior uveitis in 25% of patients

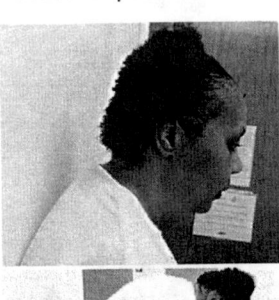

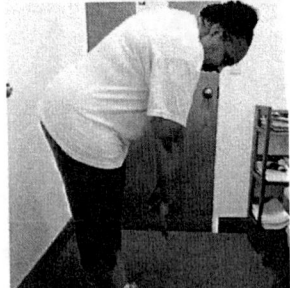

Source: Kathryn Dao, MD

Enteropathic Arthritis
Inflammatory bowel disease includes:
- Ulcerative colitis
- Crohn disease
- Whipple disease
- Intestinal bypass surgery
- Celiac disease

With arthritis:
- Oligoarticular
- Asymmetric, **and/or**
- Enthesitis — frequently looks like AS

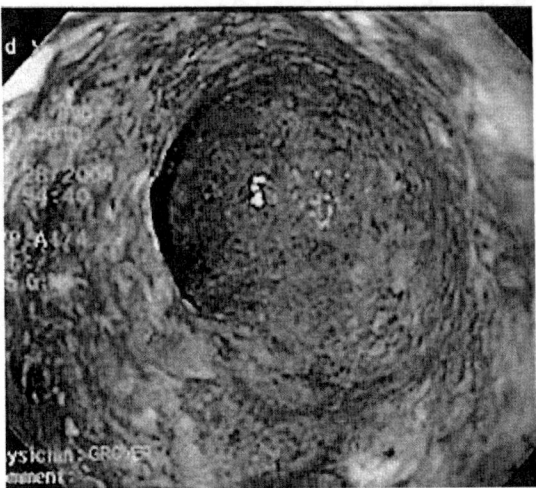

Reactive Arthritis (ReA)
Triad consisting of:

1) Arthritis (asymmetric, oligoarthritis)
2) Conjunctivitis
3) Urethritis (sterile)

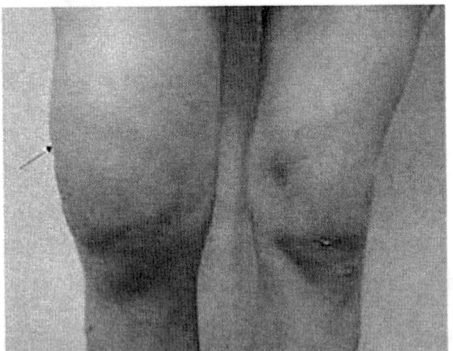

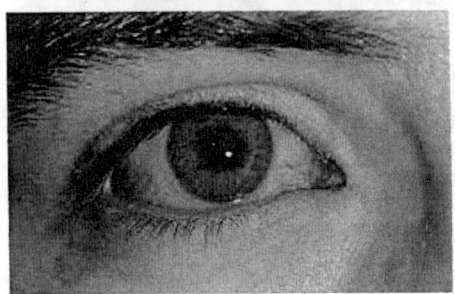

ReA (cont.)

Typically follows <u>GI or GU</u> infection with:
- *Campylobacter*
- *Shigella*
- *Salmonella*
- *Yersinia*
- *Chlamydia*

The arthritis represents an immune <u>reaction</u> to the infection and does <u>**not**</u> usually represent persistent infection.

ReA Mucocutaneous Manifestations
- Circinate balanitis
- Conjunctivitis
- Keratoderma blennorrhagica
- Painless oral ulcers

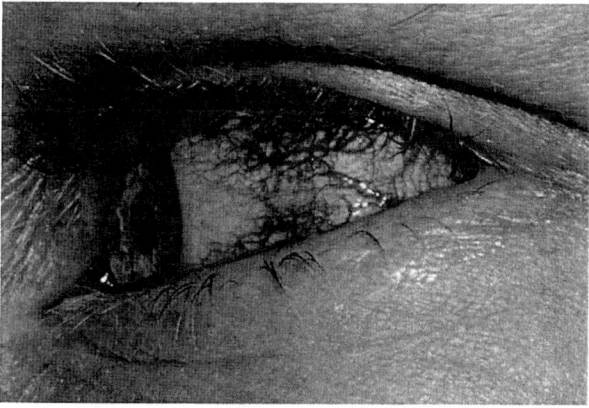

Source: CDC Library

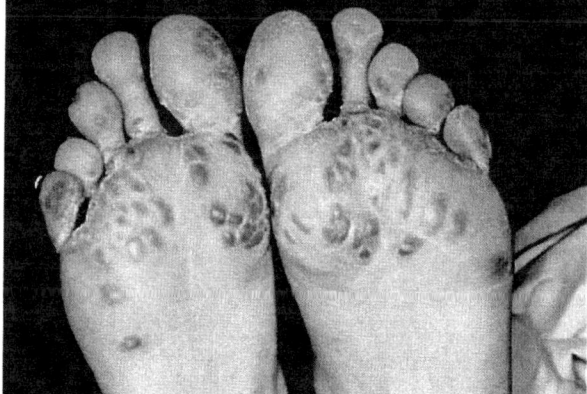

Source: CDC Library

Psoriatic Arthritis (PsA) — Characteristics
- Psoriasis or psoriatic nail changes (pitting or ridges) and
- Peripheral arthritis:
  - Axial
  - Oligoarticular/poly/symmetric/asymmetric
  - Pseudo-RA
  - Sausage digits

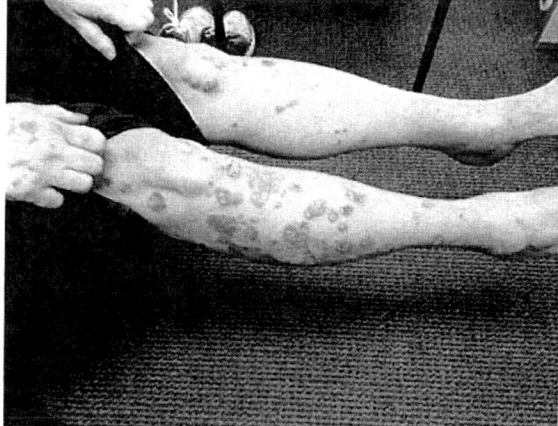

Source: John Cush, MD

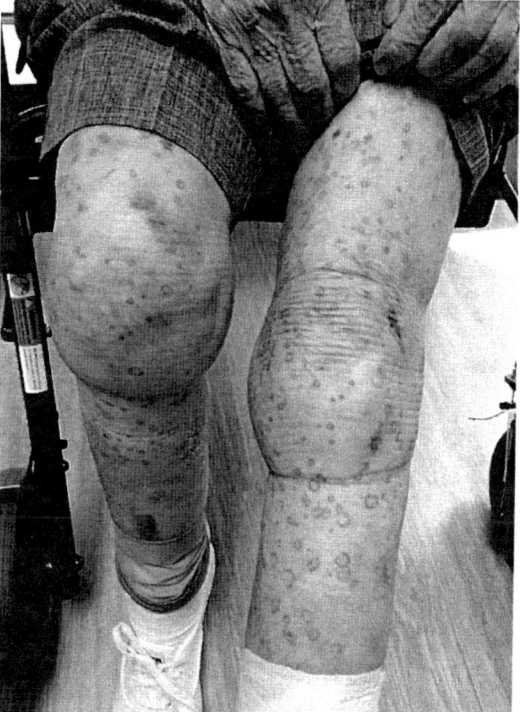

Source: Kathryn Dao, MD

Nail Changes in Psoriasis

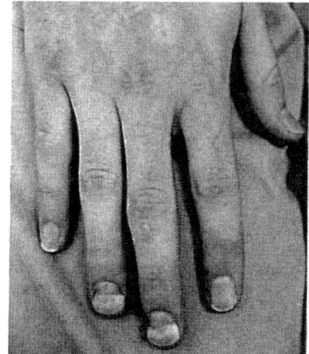 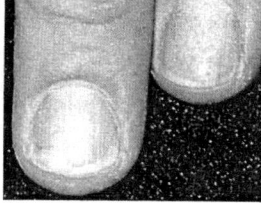

Source: Jack Cush, MD

Psoriasis
- Scalp — hairline
- Eyebrows/Eyelids
- Ears
- Extensor surfaces
- Umbilicus
- Gluteal folds

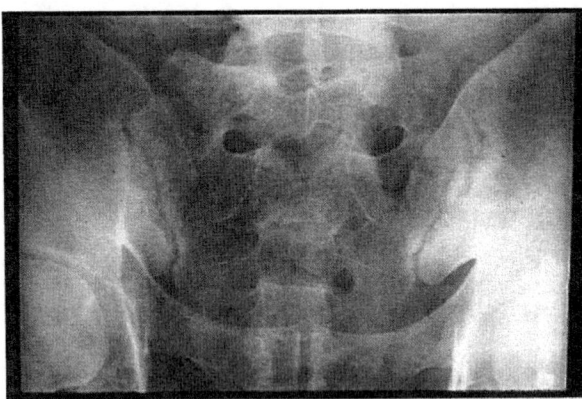

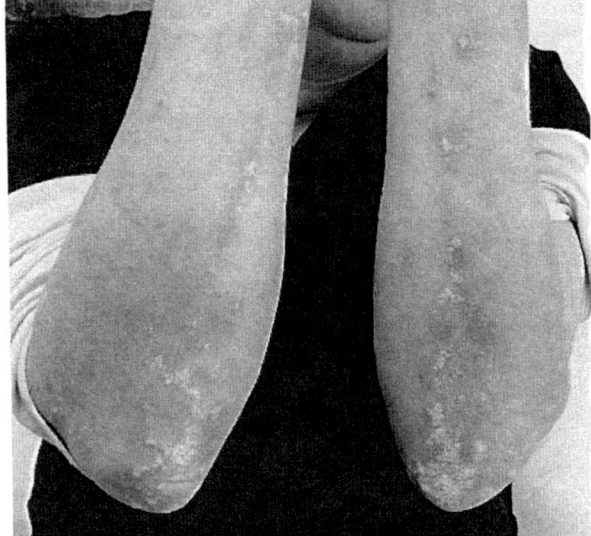

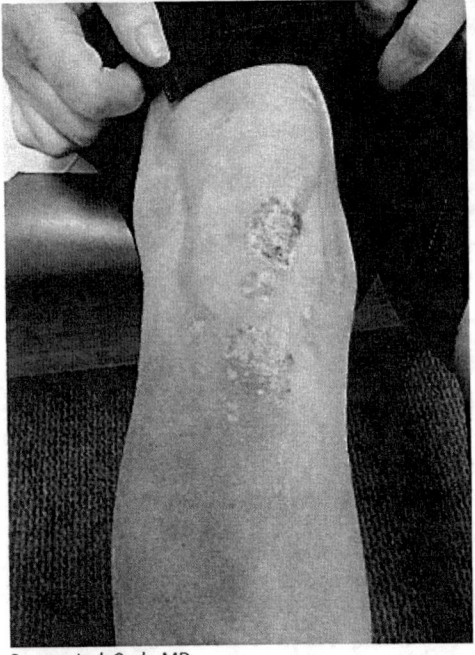

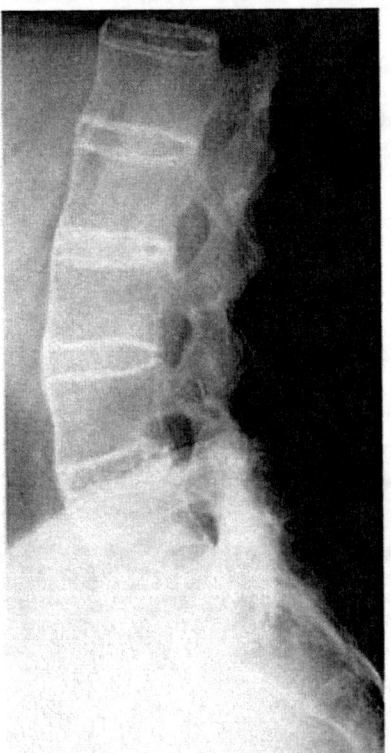

Source: Jack Cush, MD

SNSA Radiographic Findings
- Sacroiliitis
- Spinal fusion
- Bamboo spine
- Enthesitis

Recognize SNSAs by:
- Axial arthritis
- Mucocutaneous involvement
- Ocular involvement
- Peripheral arthritis:
  - Asymmetric
  - Non-nodular
  - DIP and/or "ray" involvement

Note: ESR and CRP may be normal even in the face of active inflammatory arthritis

Management of SNSAs
- Continued emphasis on postural training
- Similar to other immune-mediated inflammatory arthritides (RA):
  - For axial disease:
    - **NSAIDs**
    - **TNF inhibitors**
    - **IL12/23 inhibitor (ustekinumab)**
    - **IL-17 inhibitors (secukinumab)**
  - For peripheral disease:
    - **NSAIDs**
    - **Sulfasalazine**
    - **Methotrexate**
    - **Leflunomide**
    - **TNF inhibitors**
    - **IL12/23 inhibitor (ustekinumab)**
    - **IL-17 inhibitors (secukinumab)**

AR 3
A 45-year-old male presents with a 6-month history of R swollen foot and ankle. He has tried over-the-counter ibuprofen and naproxen as well as his wife's celecoxib over this period of time.

The antiinflammatories help some, but the pain and stiffness persist. His exam is as follows:

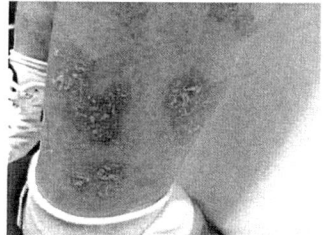 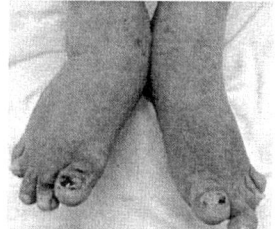

Source: Kathryn Dao, MD

What other issues might the patient have?
A. Iritis
B. Interstitial cystitis
C. *Clostridium difficile* colitis
D. Tinea pedis
E. Diffuse idiopathic skeletal hyperostosis

Answer: _____

Diffuse Idiopathic Skeletal Hyperostosis (DISH)
- Inappropriate ossification of the anterior longitudinal ligament
- Associated with morning stiffness, dorsolumbar pain, and reduced range of motion
- Most common: Thoracic spine; also see in lumbar and the cervical spine
- The ossification and the subsequent production of large osteophytes, may result in spinal stenosis and spinal stiffening, which increases the risk of fractures

DISH

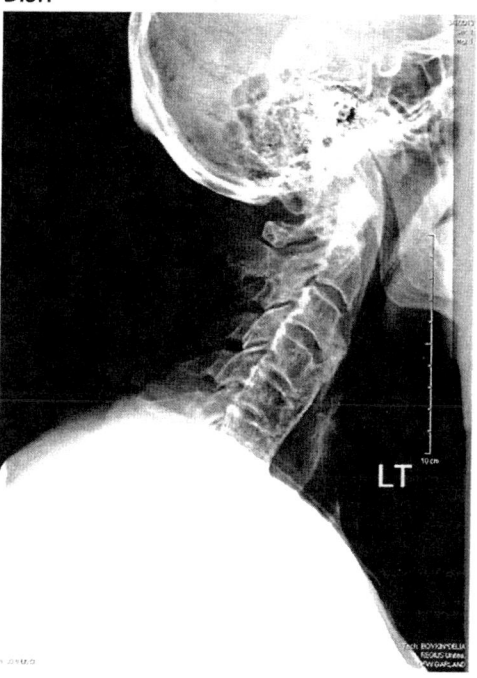

DISH (cont.)
Exostoses: Calcified enthesopathies

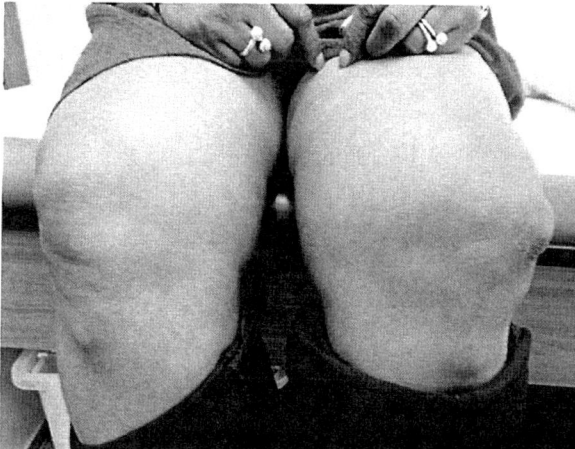

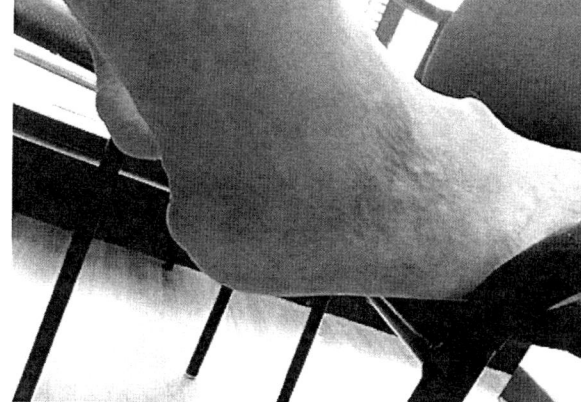

Source: Kathryn Dao, MD

Conditions Associated with DISH
- Non–insulin-dependent diabetes mellitus
- Obesity
- High waist circumference ratio
- Dyslipidemia
- Hypertension
- Hyperuricemia
- Hyperinsulinemia
- Elevated insulin-like growth factor-1
- Elevated growth hormone
- Use of retinoids
- Genetic predisposition

DISH (cont.)
1) The presence of flowing calcification or ossification along the anterolateral aspect of at least 4 contiguous vertebral levels
2) Relative preservation of intervertebral disk heights in the involved vertebral segments without the extensive changes of primary degenerative disc disease
3) The absence of apophyseal joint ankylosis or sacroiliac joint erosions, sclerosis, or widespread intraarticular bony ankylosis

DISH — X-Ray Findings

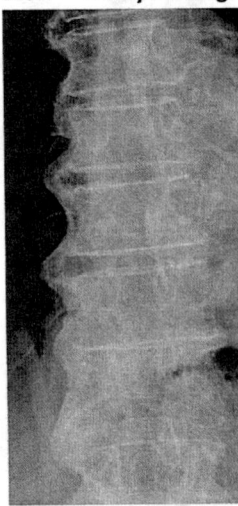 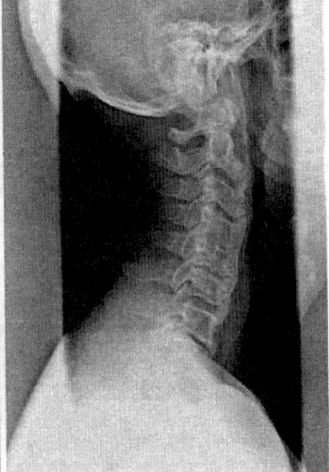

Therapeutic Targets in DISH
- Symptomatic relief of pain and stiffness (local heat, analgesia, NSAIDs)
- Prevent, retard, or arrest progression of heterotopic ossification:
  - Warfarin (Coumadin)
  - NSAIDs
  - Irradiation
- Treatment of associated metabolic disorder:
  - Hyperglycemia
  - Hyperinsulinemia
  - Hyperuricemia
  - Hypertension

- Prevent traumatic complications
- Prevent complications that might emerge during diagnostic or therapeutic procedures (i.e., endoscopy or intubation)

Crystalline Arthritis

Definition of Gout
- Acute arthritis resulting from monosodium urate (MSU) crystals in the joint
- Neutrophils phagocytose the crystals and degranulate
- The enzymes released cause the clinical manifestations of inflammation

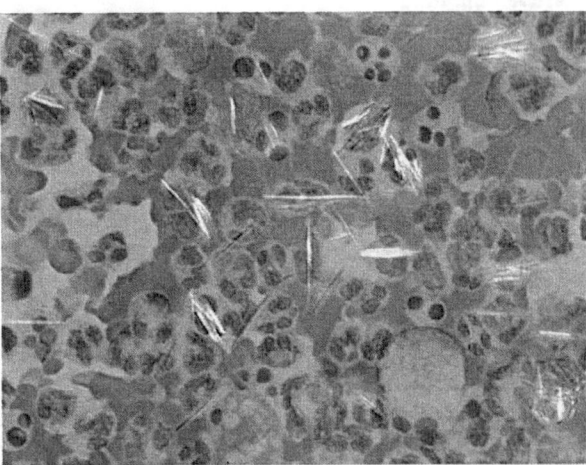

Some Famous People with Gout

Alexander Hamilton	Henry VIII	Nostradamus
Benjamin Franklin	Isaac Newton	Queen Anne
Charles V	John Calvin	Samuel Johnson
David Wells	John Hancock	Thomas Jefferson
George IV	John Milton	Wilkie Collins
George Mason	Karl Marx	William Pitt
Gottfried Liebniz	Kirk Reuter	???Sue, the T-Rex*
Henry Fielding	Mel Brooks	

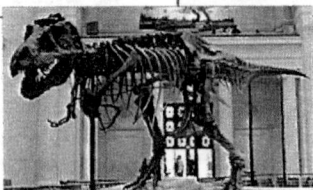

*Rothschild, BM, et al. "Tyrannosaurus Suffered from Gout." *Nature.* 387:357, 1997.

Patient History

A 56-year-old man with a h/o HTN, obesity, and regular alcohol intake presents to the ED on Sunday morning with a severely painful, red, swollen left great toe, which awakened him from a drunken sleep. The pain is so severe that he didn't even want the bed sheet touching it. He has had 5 similar episodes in the last year that resolved without treatment. He just completed 7 consecutive days of being too drunk to go to work. He takes a diuretic and 1 aspirin per day.

Patient Physical Examination

He is an obese male in obvious pain with a fever of 101.0° F (38.3° C).

On musculoskeletal examination, the right 1st MTP joint is purple-red and exquisitely tender.

The remainder of the physical examination is normal.

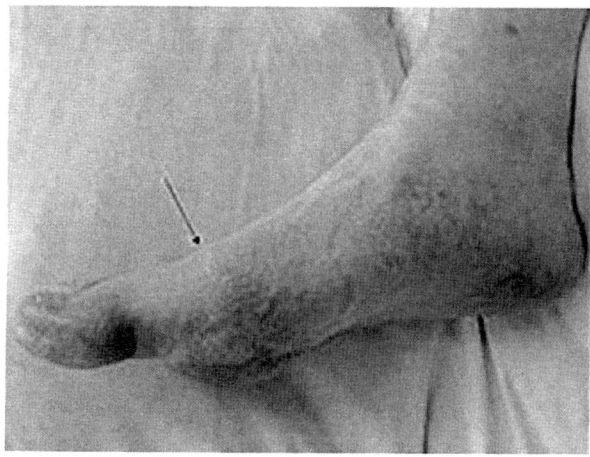

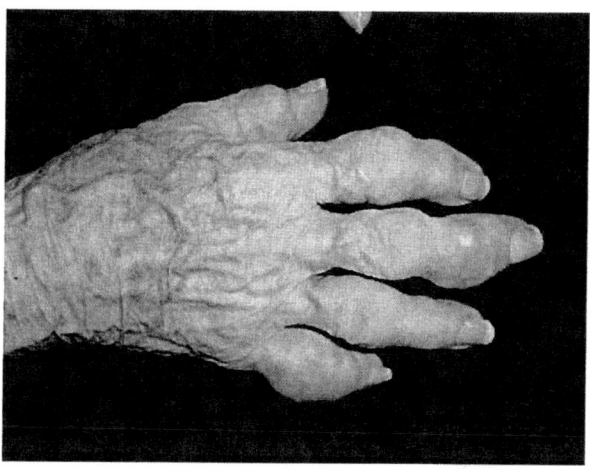

Common Symptoms of Gout

- Acute onset
- Severe inflammation (pain, swelling, warmth, and erythema)
- Monoarticular (initially) or pauciarticular
- Involvement of 1st MTP joint (Podagra) — occurs in 75% of patients
- Onset often at night
- Early attacks subside spontaneously in 3–10 days
- Attacks may be triggered by alcohol, trauma, drugs, surgical stress, or acute medical illness

Common Physical Examination Findings in Gout

1) Arthritis (joint inflammation):
   - Redness
   - Warmth
   - Tenderness
   - Swelling
2) Surrounding soft tissue inflammation
3) Tophi

Tophi

- Tophi are deposits of monosodium urate crystals
- Tophi occur in synovium, subchondral bone, olecranon bursa, along the extensor surface of forearms, overlying joints and tendons, and helix of the ear
- Cause the characteristic radiographic erosions
- Average onset is 10 years after first acute episode of arthritis but may occur earlier
- Often mistaken for rheumatoid nodules, which may be in similar locations
- Distinguished from rheumatoid nodules by aspirating and identifying MSU crystals under polarizing microscopy

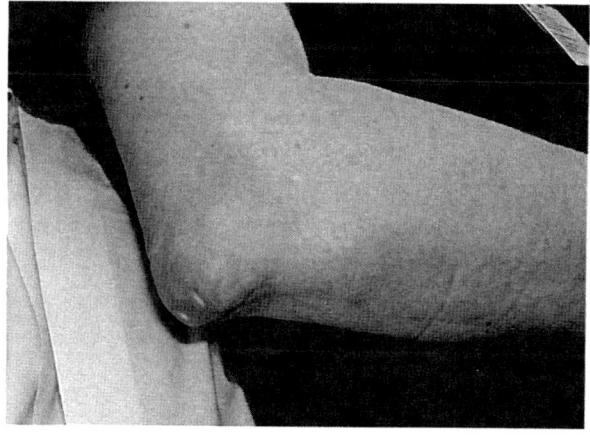

Differential Diagnosis
for
Acute-Onset Monoarticular Arthritis
Crystal-induced arthritis
Trauma
Septic arthritis

To Diagnose a Patient with Acute Monoarticular Arthritis
- <u>Joint aspiration</u> and inspecting synovial fluid or tophaceous material and demonstrating characteristic MSU crystals (intracellular, if joint fluid) is the only way to definitively diagnose gout; This will also allow Gram stain and culture to evaluate infectious arthritis
- <u>Foot radiographs</u> should be done to evaluate for possible fracture
- **Serum uric acid level is <u>not</u> helpful in making the diagnosis of gout**

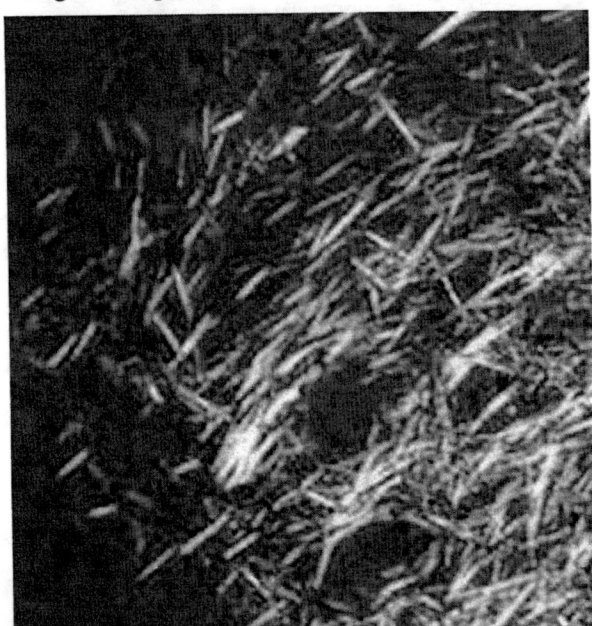

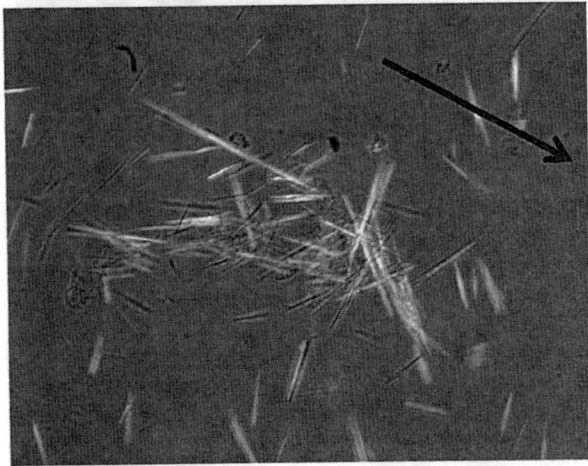

Pay attention to the direction of the red compensator. Gout is yellow — parallel.

Typical Laboratory Findings in Gout
- Inflammatory synovial fluid (**can be sterile pus**)
  - Cloudy
  - 20,000 to 100,000 WBC/mm
  - Predominately PMN

- Monosodium urate crystals in synovial fluid
  - Needle-shaped
  - Strong, negative birefringence with compensated polarized light

- Serum uric acid is elevated at some time in almost all patients; However, it is **not diagnostic**
- Urine uric acid > 750 to 1,000 mg/day suggests overproduction of uric acid (but clinically irrelevant)
- May have leukocytosis, high ESR, increased C-reactive protein during acute attack

Typical Radiographic Findings in Gout
- Soft tissue swelling during acute attack
- Soft tissue density **if** tophi are present
- Oval bone erosions with overhanging edge is classic abnormality

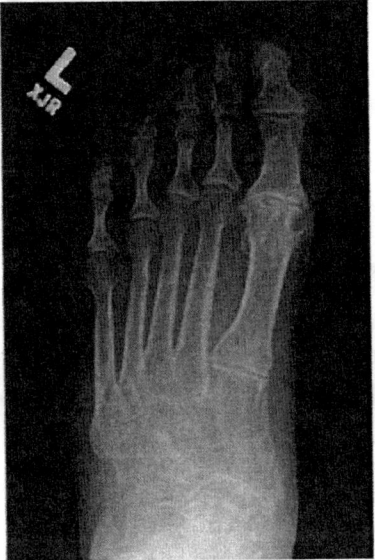

Hippocratic Aphorisms on Gout
- Eunuchs do not take the gout, nor become bald
- A woman does not take the gout, unless her menses be stopped
- A youth does not get gout before sexual intercourse
- In gouty affections, inflammation subsides within 40 days
- Gouty affections become active in spring and in autumn

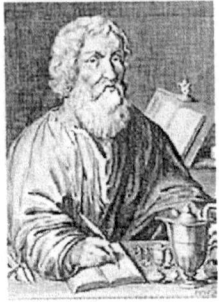

Hippocrates 5th century B.C.

Adapted from Nuki and Simkin. *Arthritis Research & Therapy.* 2006 8(Suppl 1):S1.

Why Does Gout Occur?
Too much urate in the body; Uric acid is a weak acid (pKa = 5.8)
<u>Overproduction</u> (metabolic) (10%)
  Primary
  Secondary
<u>Underexcretion</u> (renal handling of urate) (90%)
  Primary
  Secondary

Overproduction (10%)
<u>Primary</u>
1) Idiopathic
2) Specific enzyme defects (< 1% of primary gout)
   a) PRPP synthetase overactivity
   b) Partial deficiency of HGPRTase
   c) "Complete" deficiency of HGPRTase

Overproduction
<u>Secondary</u>
Increased cell turnover or destruction
(which increases nucleic acid release)
1) Lymphoproliferative or myeloproliferative disorders
2) Chemotherapy
3) Acute or chronic hemolysis
4) Psoriasis

Underexcretion (90%)
<u>Primary</u>
  Idiopathic
<u>Secondary</u>
1) Acute or chronic renal failure
2) Volume depletion
3) Altered renal tubular handling of uric acid
   due to drugs, volume status, or endogenous
   metabolic products:
   a) **Diuretic therapy**
   b) **Low-dose salicylate therapy**
   c) **Lactic acidosis**
   d) **Ketoacidosis**
   e) **Ethanol**

Dietary Influence

Risk factor	Relative risk
Meat[a]	1.41
Seafood[a]	1.51
Dairy[a]	0.56
Any alcoholic drink[b]	2.53
Beer[c]	1.49
Shot of spirits daily	1.15
Glass of wine daily	1.04
Fructose-containing soft drinks[d]	1.85
Coffee consumption[a]	0.41
Decaffeinated coffee consumption[a]	0.73
Tea, diet soft drinks, purine-rich vegetables	No increase in risk
Supplemental vitamin C[e]	0.55

[a] Highest *vs* lowest quintile
[b] Highest consumption, ≥50 g/day, *vs* no alcohol
[c] Per 12 oz daily serving, *vs* no alcohol
[d] Two or more servings daily, *vs* <1 per month
[e] Intake of 1000–1499 mg/d and 1500 mg/d or more

Bad: Alcohol, meat, seafood, high fructose corn syrup
Good: coffee, milk, vitamin C

ACR 2012 Gout Rx Recommendations
Counsel patients about lifestyle and diet
Treat the inflammation — ideally within 24 hours:
- <u>NSAIDs</u> are a treatment of choice for acute gout, preferably an NSAID with a short half-life, such as indomethacin or ibuprofen
- <u>Intraarticular corticosteroid injection</u> is effective for alleviating acute gouty arthritis in most cases; Injection into a small joint can be difficult and, rarely, the inflammation can recur when the steroid effect subsides; **Best if only 1 or 2 joints are affected**

Acute Treatment
- <u>Oral or intramuscular corticosteroids</u>
- <u>Oral low-dose colchicine</u> (<u>within 36 hours</u>):
  1.2 mg colchicine, followed by 0.6 mg in an hour; Note that high-dose colchicine is rarely used anymore due to the high frequency of adverse effects (diarrhea)
- <u>Intravenous colchicine should be avoided</u>
- **Avoid** increasing or starting a urate-lowering agent during an acute attack
Arthritis Care Res (Hoboken). 2012 Oct;64(10):1431–46.

Chronic Therapy
Start urate lowering therapy (ULT) when:
1) There have been 2 or more attacks/year
2) One attack and Stage 2 kidney disease or worse
3) Tophus/Tophi on exam or imaging
4) Past urolithiasis

Khanna D, et al. 2012 American College of Rheumatology guidelines for management of gout. Part 1: Systematic nonpharmacologic and pharmacologic therapeutic approaches to hyperuricemia. *Arthritis Care Res* (Hoboken). 2012 Oct;64(10):1431–46.
Khanna D, et al. 2012 American College of Rheumatology guidelines for management of gout. Part 2: Therapy and antiinflammatory prophylaxis of acute gouty arthritis. *Arthritis Care Res* (Hoboken). 2012 Oct;64(10):1447–61.

Chronic Therapy (cont.)
- Target uric acid < 6.0 mg/dL (< 5.0 mg/dL if tophi present or Sx still present)
- Use prophylaxis during ULT to prevent flares

Colchicine, NSAIDs, low-dose prednisone for prophylaxis
Prevent flares associated with changes in uric acid

Prophylactic Therapy During ULT
Duration of prophylaxis:
- 6 months after the last gout flare
- 3 months after reaching target urate level in patients without tophi
- 6 months after target urate level reached in patients with tophi

Choice of ULT

Xanthine Oxidase Inhibitors vs. Uricosurics
- **Uricosurics (probenecid, sulfinpyrazone, or high dose salicylate) may only be used in patients who are:**
  1) Underexcretors of uric acid, **and**
  2) Have normal renal function, **and**
  3) Have never had a kidney stone, **and**
  4) Do not have tophi
- However, their use requires patients drink > 1 gallon water/day
- The presence of tophi (such as in this patient) would indicate that the treatment of choice is a xanthine oxidase inhibitor (**allopurinol or febuxostat [Uloric]**)

Xanthine Oxidase Inhibitors
Allopurinol (cheap)
Febuxostat ($$$)
- Start allopurinol 100 mg/day (50 mg/day for Stage 4 renal disease)
- Titrate up to max dose of 800 mg (note that 300 mg dose is often insufficient and dose must be titrated up appropriately to reach the target)
- Check *HLA-B5801* allele in Han Chinese, Thai descent, or Koreans with CKD Stage 3 due to risk for severe allopurinol hypersensitivity
- Significant drug interactions w/ allopurinol: Theophylline, azathioprine, warfarin

Pegloticase (Krystexxa)
- Uricase
- Approved for patients with refractory chronic gout (failed oral urate-lowering agents/did not tolerate them)
- IV every 2 weeks
- Costly
- 26% of patients developed an infusion reaction and 6.5% of patients developed anaphylaxis
- Contraindicated in patients with G6PD deficiency

AR 4
A 70-year-old male with HTN, CAD, and renal insufficiency (creatinine 1.8) on lisinopril, ASA 81 mg/day, presents with acute pain and swelling of his L hand. He notes a history of pain and swelling in his R first toe that has occurred about twice a year for the last 5 years. His exam is as follows:

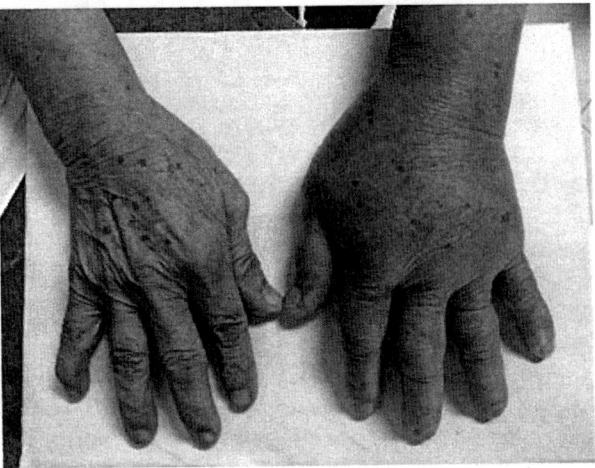

Source: Kathryn Dao, MD

What is the best way to manage this patient?
A. Start NSAIDs to treat the acute attack, then prescribe allopurinol for secondary prevention.
B. Start steroids to treat the acute attack, then start probenecid for secondary prevention.
C. Start colchicine to treat the acute attack, then counsel him on dietary changes only; he does not meet threshold for secondary prevention.
D. Start steroids to treat the acute attack, then prescribe allopurinol with a prophylactic agent for secondary prevention.
E. Start allopurinol immediately and titrate to uric acid < 6.0 mg/dL.

Answer: _____

Other Crystalline Diseases
CPPD (Pseudogout)
Hydroxyapatite

Clinical Pattern in CPPD Disease
- Pseudo-osteoarthritis — 50%
- Pseudogout — 25 %
- Lanthanic (asymptomatic) — 20%
- Pseudo-rheumatoid arthritis — 5%
- Pseudo-neurotropic joints — rare

Associated with aging

Pseudogout Clinical Features
Similar to gout
- Acute onset
- Initially monoarticular but becomes oligo- or polyarticular
- Self-limiting attacks last from 1 day to weeks
- **Knee** is most common joint
- May be precipitated by surgery, medical illness, or trauma
- CPPD crystals: Rhomboid, weak, positive birefringence

Pseudogout Radiographic Findings
- Chondrocalcinosis in 75%
- Calcification of cartilage
- Often associated with OA

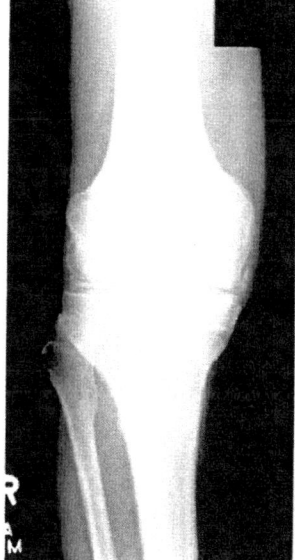
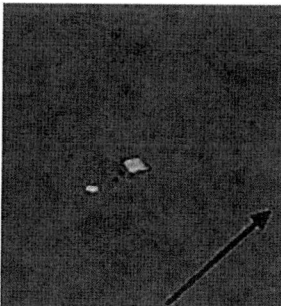

Pseudogout Therapy
Similar to acute gout therapy
- Arthrocentesis alone may be adequate
- Intraarticular corticosteroids
- Nonsteroidal antiinflammatory drugs (NSAIDs)
- Colchicine may be effective
- Maintenance therapy with NSAID and/or colchicine

CPPD — Associated with:
More commonly:
- Aging (primary — after 5th decade of life)
- Complication of primary OA/long-standing joint trauma
- Familial (3rd and 4th decades of life)
- Myxedematous hypothyroidism
- Hyperparathyroidism
- Hemochromatosis
- Dialysis-dependent renal failure

Less commonly:
- Familial hypocalciuric hypercalcemia
- Wilson disease
- Ochronosis

Hydroxyapatite
- Also known as basic calcium phosphate (BCP) crystal
- Associated with aging and:
  1) Acute synovitis rare
  2) Destructive arthropathy (Milwaukee shoulder — hemorrhagic shoulder effusion in elderly women)
  3) Calcific tendinitis/bursitis — more common
  4) Tumoral calcinosis/heterotrophic calcification
- 50% of patients with OA have BCP in the joint fluid
  (Is it pseudo-OA??)
- Only visualized by electron microscopy or alizarin red staining

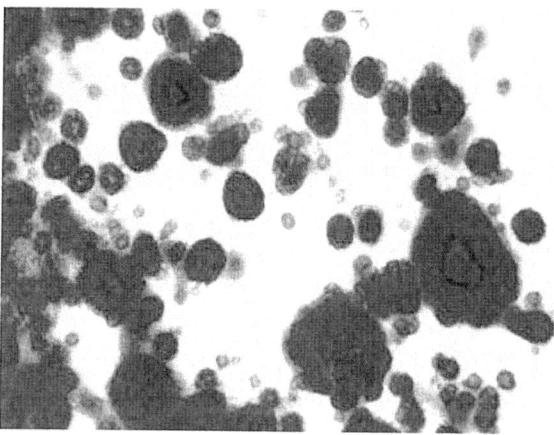

BCP Disease Associations
- Hyperparathyroidism
- Milk alkali syndrome
- Renal failure/Long-term dialysis
- Scleroderma
- Dermatomyositis
Treatment
Same as gout and CPPD

Infectious Arthritides

Disseminated Gonococcus (GC)
- Most common cause of monoarticular arthritis in sexually active adults < 35 years of age
- Migratory arthritis or tenosynovitis that settles in either a single joint or multiple joints
- Skin exam may show vesicular pustular skin lesions
- Joint fluid cultures are positive ≤ 25%; therefore, obtain vaginal, throat, or anal culture

Treatment:
Intravenous ceftriaxone
(and empirically treat *Chlamydia*)

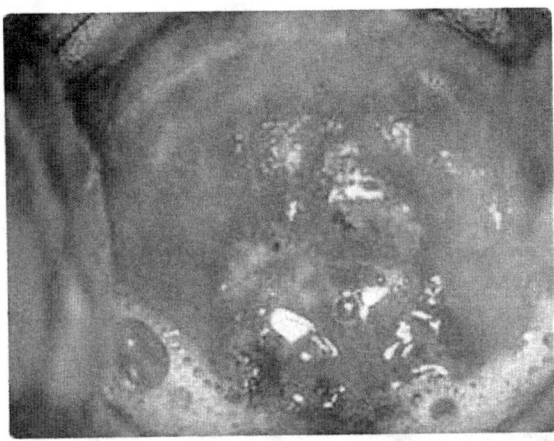

AR 5
A 25-year-old woman complains of severe right knee, wrist, and left ankle pain. She has several vesiculopustular skin lesions on her arms and legs. On physical examination, she has tenderness and swelling of the tendons of her right wrist without synovitis.

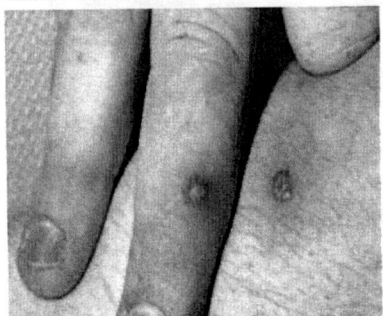

What will likely yield the correct diagnosis?
A. Arthrocentesis with culture
B. Pelvic exam with culture
C. PPD
D. Serum rheumatoid factor
E. Knee radiograph

Answer: _____

Septic Arthritis
- Monoarthritis is usually *Staphylococcus aureus*
  - WBC > 100,000
  - Patients with RA may have polyarticular septic joints
- **Sickle cell anemia:** *Salmonella* or Staph
- **IV drug use:** Sternoclavicular or sacroiliac MRSA or *Pseudomonas*
- **Lyme** arthritis usually requires appropriate exposure (endemic area), tick bite, and appropriate rash
  - +ELISA can be seen in SLE, RA, RMSF
  - +Western blot is used to confirm the Dx

Arbovirus Associated Arthritis
- Dengue fever (Latin America, Southeast Asia, and the Pacific Islands)
- Chikungunya virus* (Americas, Caribbean countries, SE Asia, Africa)
- Zika virus (South America, Puerto Rico, Mexico, Africa, Southeast Asia, and the Pacific Islands)

Incubation period: few days to a week
Fever, rash, joint pain, HA
Conservative management
*Joint pain mimics RA

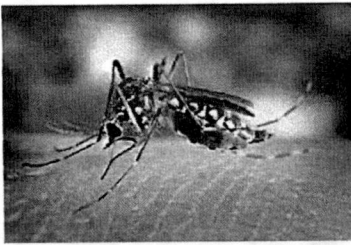

SLE, Antiphospholipid Syndrome, and Sjögren Syndrome

Systemic Lupus Erythematosus (SLE)
SLE is a chronic inflammatory disease characterized by loss of self-tolerance:
- **Overproduction** of pathogenic autoantibodies and immune complexes
- **Poor clearance** of pathogenic autoantibodies and immune complexes
- **Susceptibility to damage** by pathogenic autoantibodies and immune complexes

Any organ can potentially be affected.

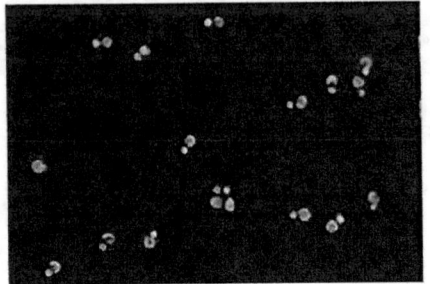

© 2017 MedStudy Internal Medicine Video Board Review – Rheumatology • Kathryn H. Dao, MD

SLE— 1997 Classification Criteria

Serositis	Blood dyscrasias	Malar rash
Oral ulcers	Renal disorder	Discoid rash
Arthritis	ANA	
Photosensitive rash	Immunologic disorder	
	Neurologic disorder	

Patient must have 4 of 11 criteria observed by physician.
- **SLICC 2012 Criteria:**
  - Acknowledges other skin manifestations of lupus
  - Antiphospholipid antibodies
  - Other neurologic manifestations of SLE

1997 ACR SLE Classification Criteria
- **Were patients being misclassified as having SLE while others were wrongly excluded?**
- Criticisms of the 1997 Criteria:
  - Not validated
  - Duplication of terms (e.g., malar rash and photosensitivity)
  - Omission of:
    - Other cutaneous manifestations of SLE
    - Other neurologic manifestations of SLE
    - New information on aPL Ab
    - Complements in the immunologic criteria

American College of Rheumatology. *Arthritis & Rheumatology.* 2012;64(8):2677–2686.

2012 SLICC Classification Criteria for SLE
Patients can be classified as having SLE if:

| Meet 4 out of 17 criteria, with at least 1 clinical and 1 immunologic criteria | **or** | Presence of biopsy-proven lupus nephritis and ANA or dsDNA |

Derivation	Validation
SLICC 2012: Sensitivity 94%; Specificity 92%	SLICC 2012: Sensitivity 97%; Specificity 84%
ACR 1997: Sensitivity 86%; Specificity 93%	ACR 1997: Sensitivity 83%; Specificity 96%

American College of Rheumatology. *Arthritis & Rheumatology.* 2012;64(8):2677–2686.

2012 SLICC Classification Criteria
New clinical criteria
ACLE:
- Malar rash
- Bullous lupus
- TEN variant
- Photosensitive lupus rash
- Maculopapular lupus rash
- SCLE

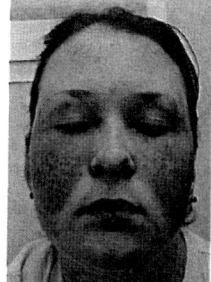
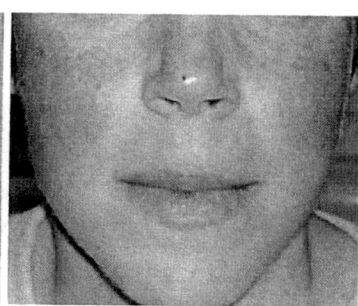

Source: Jack Cush, MD
American College of Rheumatology. *Arthritis & Rheumatology.* 2012;64(8):2677–2686.

2012 SLICC Classification Criteria (cont.)
Clinical criteria
CCLE:
- Localized/Generalized discoid
- Verrucous/Hypertrophic lupus
- Lupus panniculitis
- Mucosal lupus
- Lupus tumidus
- Chilblains lupus
- Discoid/Lichen planus overlap

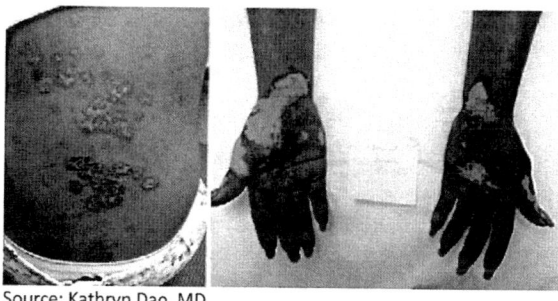

Source: Kathryn Dao, MD
American College of Rheumatology. *Arthritis & Rheumatology.* 2012;64(8):2677–2686.

2012 SLICC Classification Criteria (cont.)
Clinical criteria
Oral ulcers:
- Palate
- Buccal mucosa
- Tongue
- Nasal

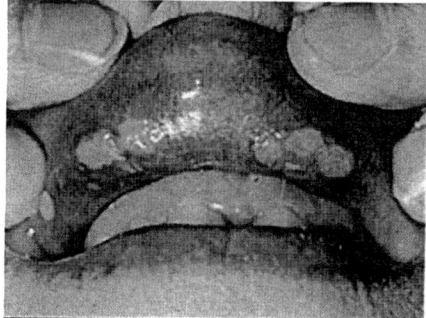

American College of Rheumatology. *Arthritis & Rheumatology.* 2012;64(8):2677–2686.

2012 SLICC Classification Criteria (cont.)
Clinical criteria
Nonscarring alopecia

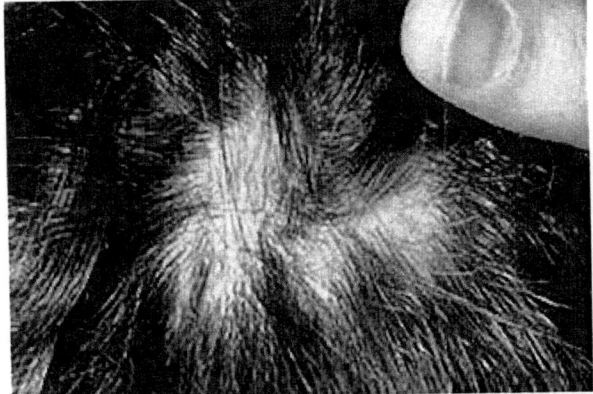

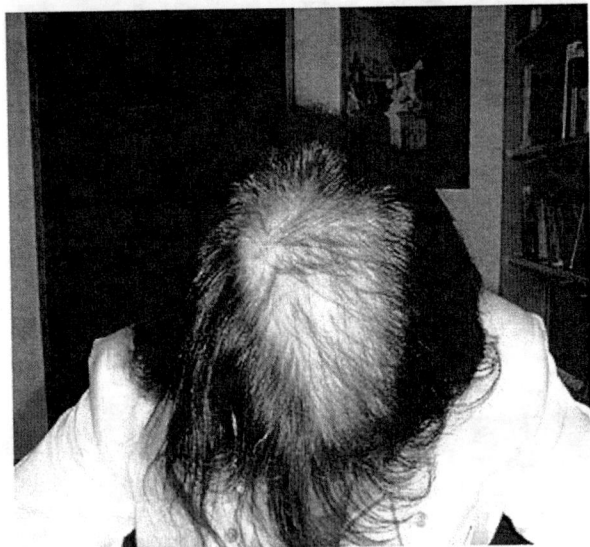

American College of Rheumatology. *Arthritis & Rheumatology.*
2012;64(8):2677–2686.

2012 SLICC Classification Criteria (cont.)
Clinical criteria
Serositis:
- Pleurisy > 1 day
- Pleural effusion
- Pleural rub
- Pericardial pain > 1 day
- Pericardial effusion
- Pericardial rub
- EKG evidence for pericarditis

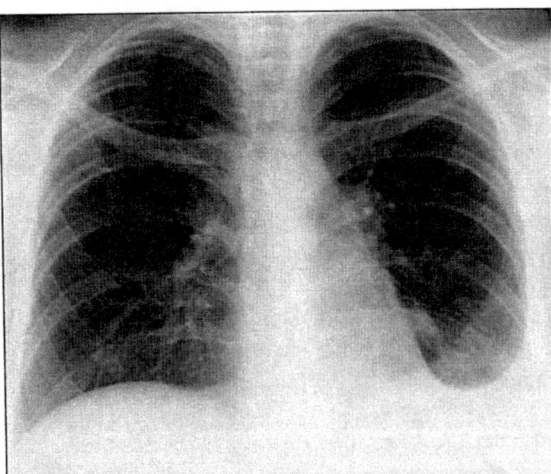

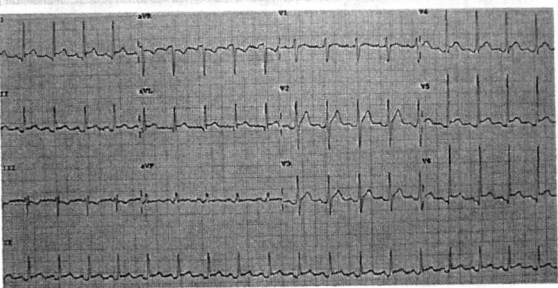

American College of Rheumatology. *Arthritis & Rheumatology.*
2012;64(8):2677–2686.

2012 SLICC Classification Criteria (cont.)
Clinical criteria
Synovitis:
- ≥ 2 joints with swelling/effusion
- ≥ 2 joints tender along the joint line with 30 minutes of a.m. stiffness

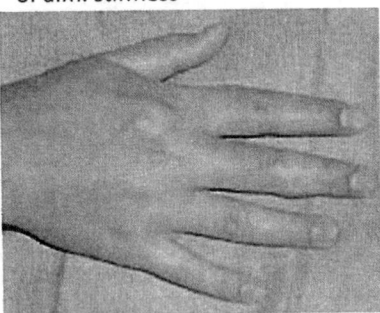

Jaccoud's deformity (can look like RA)

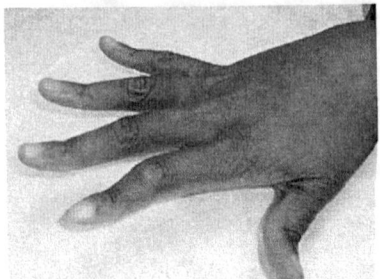

Source: Kathryn Dao, MD
American College of Rheumatology. *Arthritis & Rheumatology.*
2012;64(8):2677–2686.

2012 SLICC Classification Criteria (cont.)
Clinical criteria
Renal:
- Urine protein:Cr or 24-hour urine protein > 500 mg/24 hours
- Red cell casts
- Biopsy proven lupus

Lupus Nephritis
- Formerly WHO class
- Now ISN/RPS

American College of Rheumatology. *Arthritis & Rheumatology.* 2012;64(8):2677–2686.

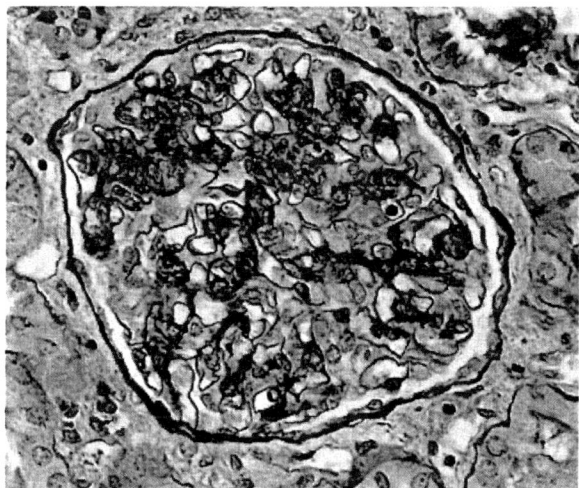

2012 ACR Lupus Nephritis Guidelines
ISN/RPS Classification of LN

Class I   Minimal mesangial LN — **Don't treat**
Class II   Mesangial proliferative LN — **Don't treat**
Class III Focal LN (< 50% glomeruli) — **Treat**
           A = active, C = chronic, A/C = active/chronic
Class IV   Diffuse LN (≥ 50% glomeruli) — **Treat**
           A = active, C = chronic, A/C = active/chronic
Class V   Membranous — **Treat**
Class VI   Advanced sclerosis LN (> 90% globally)

Hahn BH, et al. American College of Rheumatology guidelines for screening, treatment, and management of lupus nephritis. *Arthritis Care Res* (Hoboken). 2012 Jun;64(6):797–808.

2012 SLICC Classification Criteria (cont.)
Clinical criteria
Neurologic:
- Seizures
- Psychosis
- Mononeuritis monoplex
- Myelitis
- Neuropathy
- Acute confusional state

American College of Rheumatology. *Arthritis & Rheumatology.* 2012;64(8):2677–2686.

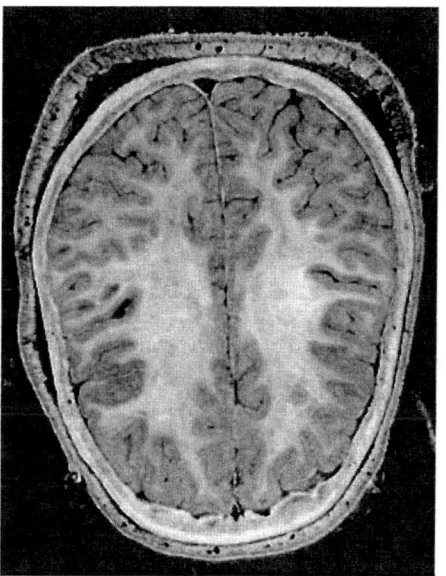

2012 SLICC Classification Criteria (cont.)
Each are separate clinical criteria*:
- Hemolytic anemia
- Leukopenia < 4,000/mm^3
- Lymphopenia < 1,000/mm^3
- Thrombocytopenia <100,000/mm^3

*Immune mediated

American College of Rheumatology. *Arthritis & Rheumatology.* 2012;64(8):2677–2686.

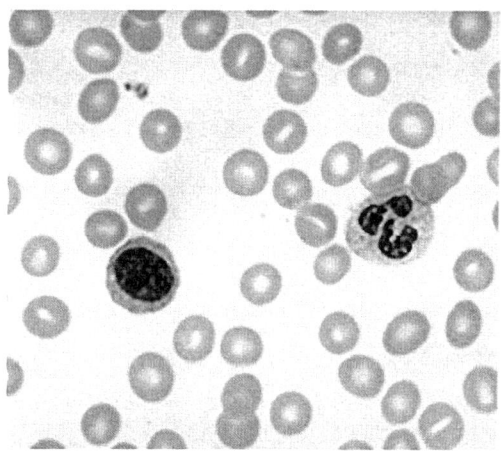

2012 SLICC Classification Criteria (cont.)
Immunologic criteria:
1) ANA+
2) Anti-dsDNA+
3) Anti-Sm+
4) Antiphospholipid Ab+ (LAC+, RPR false+, anticardiolipin IgG/M/A at mod to high titers, anti-B2gp1 IgG/M/A)
5) Low complement (CH50, C3, C4)
6) Direct Coombs+

American College of Rheumatology. *Arthritis & Rheumatology.* 2012;64(8):2677–2686.

2012 SLICC Classification Criteria (cont.)
Immunologic criteria:

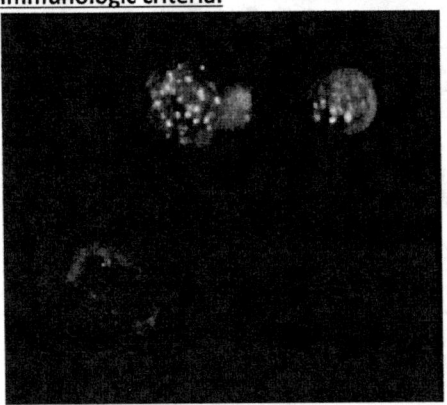

Antinuclear Antibody (ANA)
- Patterns typically do not matter
- Homogenous pattern — SLE
- Speckled — nonspecific
- Centromere — CREST

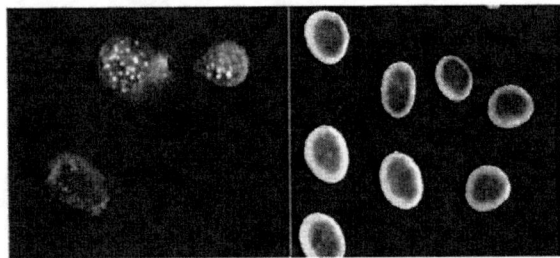

Frequency of Positive ANA (%)

	Hep 2 Cells
SLE	98
PSS	95
RA	50–75
Primary Sjögren's	75
Polymyositis	90
JRA	++
Chronic Active Hepatitis	++
Infectious Mono	+
Leprosy	+
Vasculitis	+
SBE	+

Antinuclear Antibody (ANA) (cont.)
- ANA is directed against nuclear components
- Significant titer is ≥ 1:80
- Found in 98% SLE patients but also:
  - RA
  - PSS
  - Polymyositis
  - Sjögren syndrome
  - MCTD
  - Procainamide/hydralazine/phenytoin (Dilantin)
  - Interstitial pulmonary fibrosis
  - Normal population

SLE therapy is based on the most severe manifestation.
Death is typically from:
- SLE disease (renal/brain)
- Infection
- CV mortality

SLE Therapy
- **Serositis**
  - NSAIDs
  - Corticosteroids
  - Immunosuppressive
- **Arthritis**
  - NSAIDs
  - Hydroxychloroquine
  - DMARDs
  - Corticosteroids
  - Immunosuppressive drugs
- **Blood dyscrasias**
  - Corticosteroids
  - Immunosuppressive drugs

- **Renal**
  - Corticosteroids
  - Immunosuppressive
- **Neurologic**
  - Symptomatic
  - Corticosteroids
  - Immunosuppressive
- **Rash**
  - Sunblock
  - Topical corticosteroids
  - Systemic steroids
  - Hydroxychloroquine, MTX
  - Immunosuppressive drugs

AR 6

22-year-old African American female nursing student with 1-year h/o arthralgias, alopecia, fatigue with sun exposure, +ANA, +dsDNA, WCB 3.1; U/A noted RBC casts and 3+ proteinuria

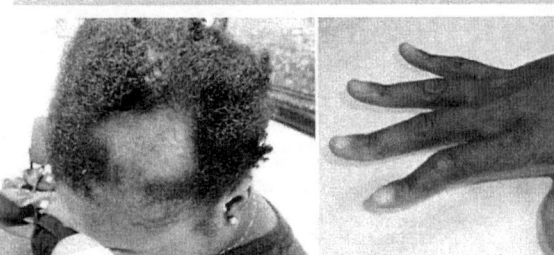

Source: Kathryn Dao, MD

AR 6 (cont.)
Which of the following increases her risk for morbidity/mortality?
A. +ANA
B. +dsDNA
C. Lupus nephritis
D. Inflammatory arthritis
E. Leukopenia

Answer: _____

Antiphospholipid Syndrome
Antiphospholipid ab = anticardiolipin ab = anti-beta-2 glycoprotein-1 ab
- Antibodies to phospholipid bind to and activate platelets resulting in aggregation and thrombosis
- Antiphospholipid antibodies are procoagulants despite the misnomer of also causing the "lupus anticoagulant" (falsely prolonged PTT)
- Can occur as a 1° illness or as part of SLE

Antiphospholipid Syndrome
- Arterial thrombosis
- Venous thrombosis
- Libman-Sacks endocarditis
- Livedo reticularis
- Recurrent fetal loss
- Thrombocytopenia

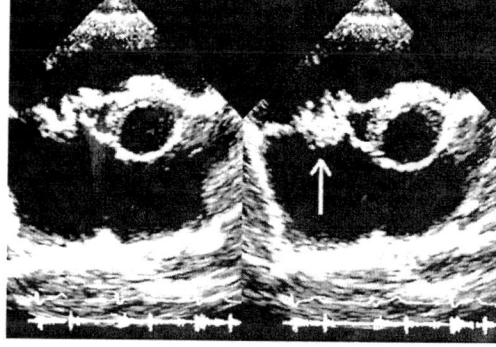

Therapy
- **Antiphospholipid antibody syndrome:** Usually lifelong
- **Pregnancy morbidity:** 81 mg/day ASA + DVT prevention dose LMWH
  1) ≥ 1 unexplained deaths of a normal ≥ 10-week fetus, or
  2) ≥ 1 births of a normal neonate before 34 weeks of gestation because of eclampsia, severe preeclampsia, or recognized features of placental insufficiency, or
  3) ≥ 3 consecutive spontaneous abortions before 10 weeks of gestation, with maternal anatomy/hormonal and paternal/maternal chromosomal causes excluded

- **First venous thrombosis:** INR of 2.0–3.0
- **Recurrent venous thrombosis:** INR > 3.0
- **Arterial thrombosis:** INR > 3.0
- **CVA:** 81 mg/day ASA
- **HCQ:** Lowers risk for thrombosis

Sjögren Syndrome
- **1° Sjögren's:** Dry mucous membranes (ocular, oral, vaginal dryness) due to exocrine gland inflammation and dysfunction
- **2° Sjögren's:** Sjögren's syndrome in the presence of another autoimmune rheumatologic disease (e.g., SLE, RA, SSc)

Incidence: 3.9/100,000 in Olmstead County, MN
50% are 1° Sjögren's (and 50% are 2° Sjögren's)
90% of the patients are women (mostly middle-age)

ACR/EULAR 2016 Classification Criteria for Primary Sjögren's Syndrome
- +SSA (Ro) (3 points)
- Focal lymphocytic sialadenitis focus score ≥ 1 foci/4 mm² (3 points)
- Abnormal ocular staining score ≥ 5 (1 point)
- Schirmer's test ≤ 5 mm/5 minutes (1 point)
- Unstimulated salivary flow ≤ 0.1 mL/minute (1 point)

Signs/Symptoms ≥ 4 meet criteria, sensitivity 96% (95% CI 92–98%), specificity 95% (95% CI 92–97%)
Ann Rheum Dis. 2017 Jan;76(1):9-16. doi: 10.1136/annrheumdis-2016-210571.

Differential Diagnosis for Sicca

Infiltrative processes
- Amyloidosis
- Fatty infiltration from alcohol, diabetes, pancreatitis
- Hemochromatosis
- Lipoproteinemia
- Lymphoma
- Sarcoidosis

Infectious processes
- Hepatitis B and C
- HIV (DILS)
- HTLV-1
- Syphilis
- Trachoma
- Tuberculosis

Neuropathic
- Cranial neuropathy
- Multiple sclerosis

Autoimmune disorders
- RA
- Sjögren syndrome
- SLE
- Systemic sclerosis

Others
- Aging
- Bulimia
- Fibromyalgia-like syndromes
- Graft vs. host disease
- Medications
- Radiation therapy

Sjögren Syndrome — Immunopathogenesis
- Decreased circulating T cells
- Increased circulating B cells

- Infiltration and destruction of glands by CD4+ T cells

- 75% patients have anti-SSA (anti-Ro) ab
- 40% patients have anti-SSB (anti-La) ab
- 66% patients have ANA
- 66% patients have rheumatoid factor

Sjögren Syndrome — Manifestations
Xeroses (dry mucous membranes):
- Dry eyes
- Dry mouth
- Dry vagina

Typical Sjögren's patient: A 55-year-old female complains of diffuse aches, fatigue, dry cough, paresthesias.
Exam: Injected conjunctiva, poor dentition, no salivary pooling, enlarged parotids, multiple FM tender points but no synovitis.
Labs show +ANA, +RF, +SSA or SSB, neg CCP, elevated LFTs.

Sjögren Syndrome — Systemic Manifestations
Musculoskeletal
Arthralgias, myalgias — FM is very common!
Cutaneous
Dry skin, hyperglobulinemic purpura, vasculitis
Pulmonary
Xerotrachea, pulmonary infiltrate
Gastrointestinal
Esophageal dysmotility, pancreatitis, hepatitis
Renal
Renal tubular acidosis, interstitial nephritis
Neurologic
Peripheral neuropathy, cranial neuropathy (especially 5th cranial nerve), CNS
Hematologic
Leukopenia, anemia, lymphoma

Sjögren Syndrome — Risk of Malignancy
- 1° Sjögren syndrome has between a 6x and 40x increased risk of developing non-Hodgkin's lymphoma (typically a B-cell lymphoma or MALToma)
- Heralded by the development of:
  - A monoclonal protein
  - New-onset leukopenia
  - New-onset anemia
  - Loss of previously present autoantibodies (ANA, Ro, La, RF)

Sjögren Syndrome — Treatment
Moisture replacement
- **Secretory stimulants** (secretagogues) stimulate muscarinic receptors in salivary glands and other organs, leading to enhanced secretion

(Caution should be used in patients with asthma, narrow-angle glaucoma, acute iritis, severe cardiovascular disease, biliary disease, nephrolithiasis, diarrhea, and ulcer disease.)
- **Pilocarpine** (Salagen) 5-mg tablets qid **and Cevimeline** (Evoxac) 30-mg capsules tid increase salivary flow rate

Prednisone/Immunosuppression does not improve mucous membrane gland secretion

Fox PC, et al. Prednisone and piroxicam for treatment of primary Sjögren's syndrome. *Clin Exp Rheumatol.* 11:149, 1993.

Systemic Sclerosis (SSc)

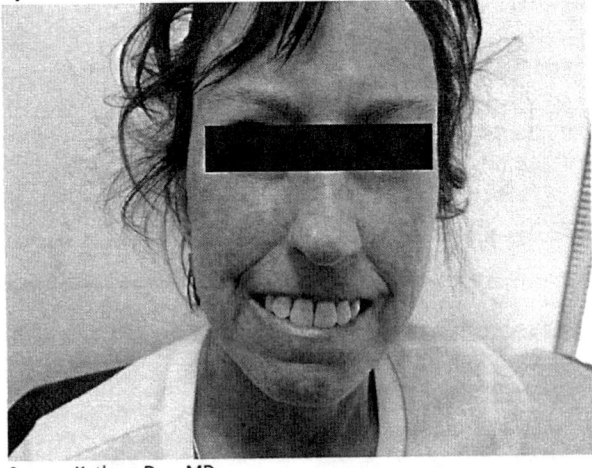

Source: Kathryn Dao, MD

Classification
Sclero = hard   **Derma** = skin
- Scleroderma (systemic sclerosis [PSS or SSc])
  - Limited scleroderma (formerly known as CREST)
  - Diffuse scleroderma (systemic sclerosis)
- Scleroderma-like illnesses — caused by:
  - Bleomycin
  - Eosinophilic fasciitis
  - Gadolinium in renal dysfunction (nephrogenic systemic fibrosis)
  - L-tryptophan (eosinophilic myalgia syndrome)
  - Tainted rapeseed (canola) oil
  - Vinyl chloride
- Localized scleroderma: Morphea and linear scleroderma

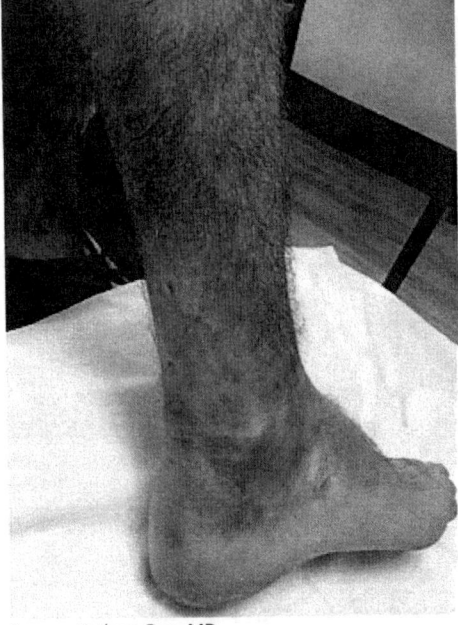

Source: Kathryn Dao, MD

Epidemiology
- Affects 19–75/100,000 population
- Peak occurrence 35–65 years of age
- Females:Males 7–12:1
- Choctaw Nation Native Americans 469/100,000

Pathology
- Inappropriate fibrosis of tissues and blood vessels
- Smooth muscle cells proliferate within the intima of small vessels (small arteries, arterioles, and capillaries), narrowing the lumen and causing tissue ischemia

Skin
Most common organ system involvement
- Earliest stage: Edema
- Fibrotic stage: Thick, hard skin develops
- **Limited PSS:** Affects hands, distal forearm, face
- **Diffuse PSS:** Entire extremity, trunk, face
- Hypo- and hyperpigmentation
- Subcutaneous calcinosis

Sclerodactyly

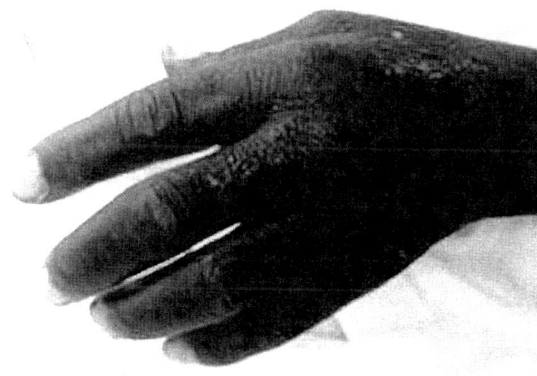

Source: Samina Hayat, MD

Telangiectasias

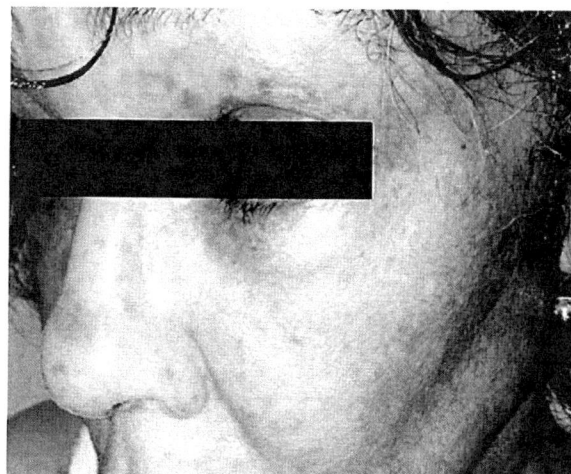

Source: Kathryn Dao, MD

Raynaud Phenomenon
- Caused by vasospasms/vasculopathy
- Tricolor change: White to blue to red
- Digital pitting scars and loss of digital pads
- Gangrene and autoamputation (acroosteolysis)
- Occurs in 90% of patients with scleroderma

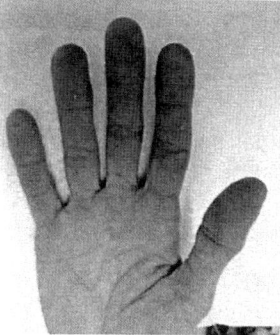
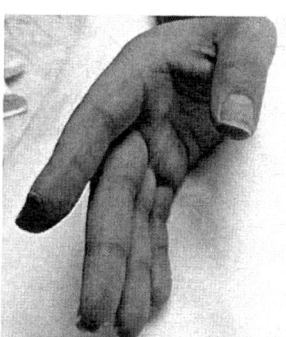

Source: Kathryn Dao, MD

Calcinosis and Acroosteolysis

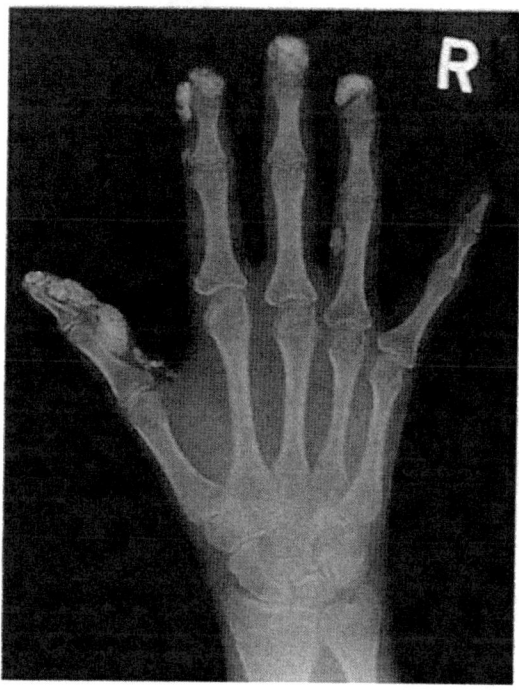

Gastrointestinal
2nd most common organ system involvement
- **Face**
  - Decreased oral aperture
  - Deep fissures around the mouth
  - Sicca
- **Esophagus**
  - Esophageal dysmotility (decreased peristalsis) causing dysphagia
  - GERD — 2° to decreased lower esophageal sphincter pressure
  - Esophagitis (with the potential for Barrett's)
  - Stricture formation

Gastrointestinal (cont.)

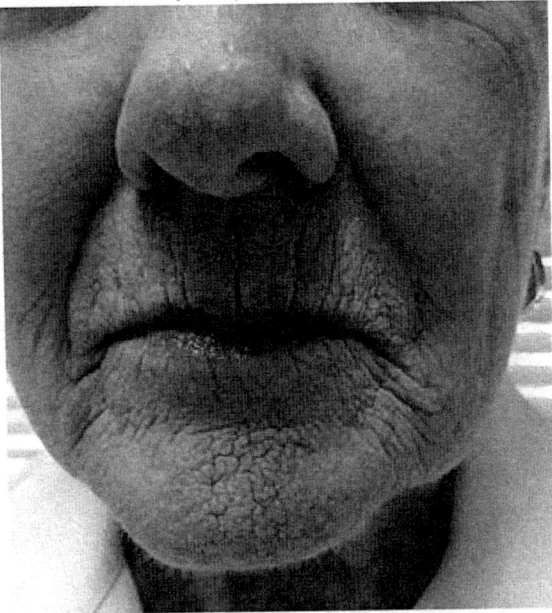

Source: Kathryn Dao, MD

Gastrointestinal (cont.)
- Chronic pseudoobstruction from decreased peristalsis
- GI bleeding from telangiectasias
- Malabsorption
- Diarrhea 2° to bacterial overgrowth
- **Large intestine**
  - Wide-mouth diverticular
  - Primary biliary cirrhosis

Pulmonary
- Serositis
- Alveolitis: Inflammation in alveoli
- Interstitial fibrosis: Presumably 2° to alveolitis
- Pulmonary Hypertension:
  - 30–35% in diffuse PSS
  - Up to 50% in limited PSS
  - Low DLCO
  - Low lung volumes on PFTs
  - Respiratory failure

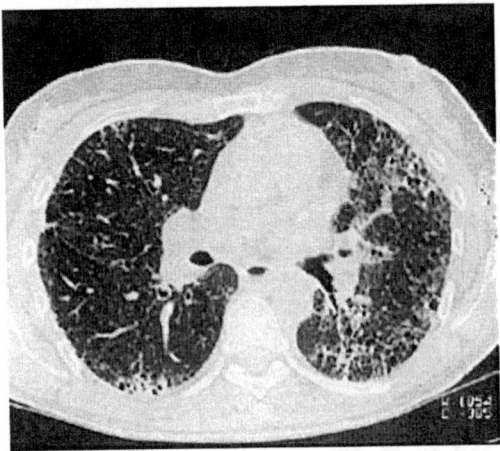

Renal
Kidneys are affected in patients with diffuse PSS.
Scleroderma Renal Crisis
- Only occurs in diffuse disease and appears to be related to steroid use
- 80% cases within first 5 years of diagnosis
- Characterized by:
  - Accelerated hypertension
  - Active urine sediment (nephritic)
  - Microangiopathic hemolysis
  - Rapidly progressive renal failure

Cardiac
- Primarily in diffuse PSS
- Pericarditis and effusion in 40% patients
- Band necrosis: Fibrosis of conducting pathways causing palpitations and dysrhythmias

Musculoskeletal
- Arthralgia
- Arthritis
- Atrophy and muscle weakness
- Acroosteolysis
- Tendon friction rubs and contractures

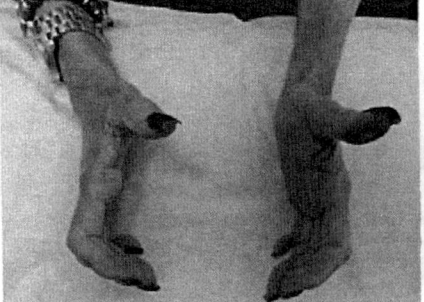

Source: Kathryn Dao, MD

Serology
- 95% of patients with PSS have an ANA
- Anti-Scl-70 (antitopoisomerase I) — antibody directed against a DNA processing enzyme
- Anti-Scl-70 ab is associated with diffuse PSS
- Anticentromere ab is associated with limited PSS
- Anti-Scl-70 is associated with a worse prognosis

Outcome
- Diffuse PSS has a 40–60% 10-year survival
- Limited PSS has a > 70% 10-year survival
  (if no pulm HTN)
- Cardiopulmonary disease is the leading cause of death
- Factors suggesting a poor prognosis include:
  - Diffuse skin involvement
  - Late age at disease onset
  - African Americans or Native Americans
  - Presence of tendon friction rubs
  - A diffusing capacity < 40% of predicted value
  - The presence of a large pericardial effusion
  - Renal failure or proteinuria or hematuria anemia
  - Elevated ESR
  - Abnormal ECG

2016 BSR / BHPR Treatment Guidelines for SSc
Raynaud phenomenon
- Local: Avoid cold exposure
- Systemic:
  - 1st line — CaChBlkr, ARB
  - 2nd line — SSRI, alpha blockers, statins, PDE type 5,
    IV prostanoid, digital sympathectomy (± botulinum)

Rheumatology (2016) 55 (10): 1906-1910.

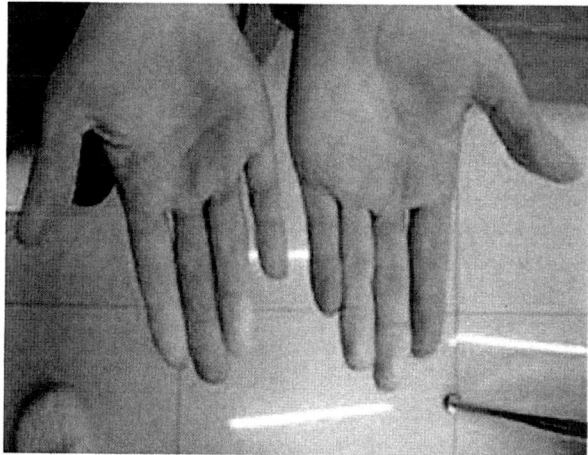

Treatment (cont.)
Renal
ACE inhibitors for HTN and management
of renal crisis
Gastrointestinal
- H_2 blockers
- Proton pump inhibitors
- Dilation of esophageal strictures
- Antibiotics for bacterial overgrowth
- Metoclopramide and erythromycin for dysmotility

Pulmonary
- Active lung inflammation (alveolitis)
  - **Steroids, cyclophosphamide, mycophenolate**
- Pulm HTN
  - **Endothelin-receptor antagonist**
    (bosentan [Tracleer]; ambrisentan [Letairis])
  - **Intravenous prostacyclin** (epoprostenol [Flolan])
  - **Phosphodiesterase-5 inhibitors** (sildenafil [Viagra, Revatio])
  - **Calcium channel blockers**
  - **O_2**
  - **Anticoagulation**

Rheumatology (2016) 55 (10): 1906-1910.

AR 7
33-year-old Caucasian female with systemic sclerosis diagnosed 6 months ago with skin tightness extending from shoulders down to her arms, thighs are also affected. She had been taking prednisone 30 mg/day. She presents with fatigue and headaches.
Her blood pressure measures 220/110 (normally her blood pressure runs 110/76).

What would you do next?
A. Stop her prednisone.
B. Give her a diuretic.
C. Measure blood pressure in her legs.
D. Admit her and give her IV enalapril.
E. Increase prednisone to 60 mg/day.

Answer: _____

Idiopathic Inflammatory Myopathies
PM/DM
- 0.5–8.4 cases/million
- African Americans:Caucasians = 2:1
- Women:men = 2:1
- Peak ages between:
  - 10 and 15 years in children
  - 45 and 60 years in adults

Cancer associated
Age > 50 years

Clinical Features of PM
- Begins insidiously (3–6 months)
- Manifests as **proximal** muscle weakness
  (shoulder, pelvic girdle/thigh, and neck)
- Dysphagia 2° to esophageal dysmotility
  (due to upper third of esophageal involvement)
- Raynaud phenomenon
- Pulmonary: Diaphragmatic weakness, interstitial pneumonitis, which causes fibrosis
- Cardiac: Supraventricular dysrhythmias, cardiomyopathy, CHF
- **Facial muscles, distal muscles, and sensation** are spared

Minimal pain, if any

Clinical Features of DM
Dermatomyositis has the same as PM plus:

- Rash
- Periorbital edema
- Heliotrope rash
- Gottron patches/papules
  - Scales and papules over joints and extensor surface of forearm and leg
- Shawl sign — erythema of shoulders and neck
- Calcinosis with long standing Dz

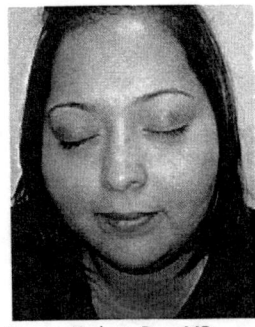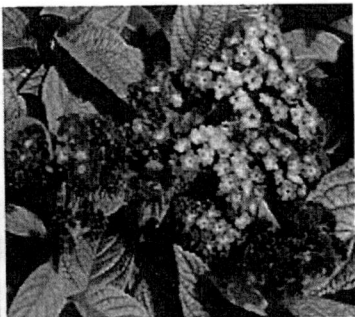

Source: Kathryn Dao, MD

Dermatomyositis

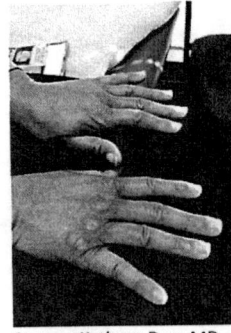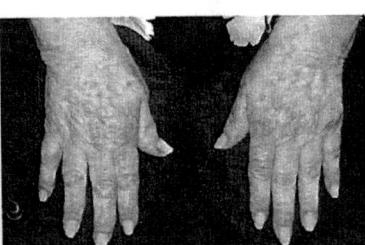

Gottron's papules

Source: Kathryn Dao, MD

Calcinosis

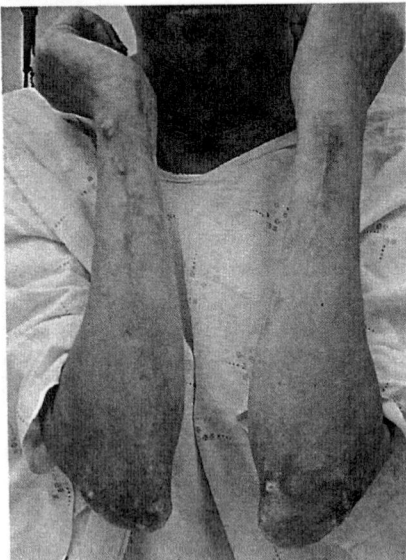

Source: John Cush, MD

Antisynthetase Antibody Syndrome
- Myosistis specific antisynthetase antibodies **and**
- Polymyositis/Dermatomyositis with:
  - Relatively acute onset
  - Interstitial lung disease
  - Fever
  - Arthritis
  - Raynaud phenomenon
  - "Mechanic's" hands (darkened or dirty-appearing cracking and fissuring of the lateral and palmar aspects of the fingers, as on an auto mechanic)

Evaluation
- **Elevated muscle enzymes:**
  - CPK, aldolase, SGOT, LDH
  - CPK usually in 1,000s
- **Unilateral EMG (in 85–90% patients) will show:**
  - Increased insertional activity fibrillations
  - Sharp positive waves
  - High-frequency discharges
  - Low-amplitude, short-duration polyphasic motor unit potentials
- **MRI shows muscle edema (inferring inflammation)**
- **Muscle biopsy**
  - Inflammation: Primarily lymphocytes and macrophages
  - Muscle fiber necrosis and regeneration

DDx — Myopathies
- Toxic/Drugs
  - EtOH, cocaine, steroids, hydroxychloroquine, penicillamine, colchicine, AZT, statins, clofibrate, tryptophan, paclitaxel, emetine
- Infectious
  - Coxsackie, HBV, HIV, Strep, Staph, *Clostridium*, *Toxoplasma*, *Trichinella*
- Inflammatory myopathies
- Congenital/Metabolic myopathies
- Neuropathic/Motor neuron disorders — MG, MD
- Endocrine/Metabolic — hypothyroidism
- Inclusion body myositis

Nonmyopathic Diagnoses
- Fibromyalgia/Fibrositis/Myofascial pain disorder
- Polymyalgia rheumatica
  - Caucasians, > 55 years of age, M = F
  - ESR > 100, normal strength, no synovitis
- CTD (SLE, RA, SSc)
- Vasculitis
- Adult Still's disease

Treatment for PM / DM
- Prednisone 1 mg/kg/day
- Methotrexate
- Azathioprine
- Mycophenolate mofetil
- IV IgG
- Plasmapheresis

Myositis Associated with Malignancy
- Controversial
- Reports range from 10% to 25%
- Men > age 50 years at greatest risk
- Common tumors: Breast, lung, ovary, stomach, uterus, colon
- 60% the myositis appears first, 30% neoplasm first, and 10% contemporaneously
- Avoid invasive, expensive searches for occult neoplasia

Other Rheumatology Topics

Fibromyalgia
- Noninflammatory disorder
- Diffuse pain
- Fatigue
- Nonrestorative sleep
- 2010 ACR diagnostic criteria WPI + SS score

Diagnosis of exclusion

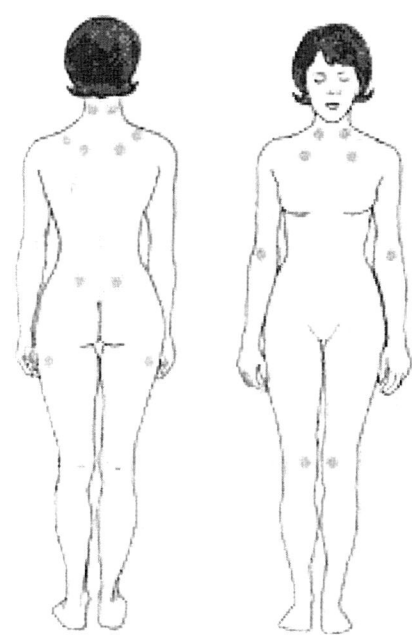

Fibromyalgia (cont.)
Treatment:
- Exercise
- Sleep restoration
- Stress reduction
- Antiepileptics
- Nonnarcotic analgesics (NSAIDs, acetaminophen, tramadol)
- Selective serotonin reuptake inhibitors (SSRIs)
- Serotonin-norepinephrine reuptake inhibitors (SNRIs)

FDA approved:
Pregabalin
Duloxetine
Milnacipran

Polymyalgia Rheumatica
- Women > men
- Extremely uncommon < 50 years of age
- Acute onset symmetric myalgias of neck, shoulders, lower back, hips, thighs, and occasionally trunk with an elevated ESR
- Patients may have trouble with ADL
- Weight loss, anorexia, depression, malaise are common
- Fevers would suggest GCA
- Men may have hand edema
- Traditionally, patients improve dramatically after a few days on 15–20 mg/day of prednisone
- **If they do not respond as expected, question the diagnosis**

Differential Diagnosis of Chronic Pain
- Anxiety/Stress/Depression
- Drug toxicity
- Folate/B_{12} deficiency
- Hepatitis B or C
- HIV
- Hypo- or hyperthyroidism
- Malignancy
- Multiple sclerosis
- Myasthenia gravis
- Obstructive sleep apnea
- Polymyalgia rheumatica (PMR)
- Syphilis
- Vasculitis
- Vitamin D deficiency

AR 8
A 36-year-old female is referred by her OB-GYN after experiencing 5 years of chronic, diffuse MSK pain. She states that her hands and fingers frequently swell, making it difficult to remove her rings. She has gained 30 pounds over the last year and is concerned about fatigue and poor, nonrefreshing sleep.

On physical exam:
She looks uncomfortable. Her vital signs are normal, and her exam is unremarkable except for diffuse tenderness on palpation of her upper and lower extremities.
Labs:
CBC, chemistry, CK, LDH, TSH, ESR are normal.

AR 8 (cont.)
Which of the following is the <u>most</u> appropriate next step?
A. Repeat the TSH.
B. Begin 10 mg of prednisone each a.m. to treat her PMR.
C. Order a full malignancy workup.
D. Order an ANA, RF, ANCA, CRP, dsDNA, CH50, C3, C4, SSA/SSB Ab, Sm/RNP Ab, and HLA-B27.
E. Recommend sleep hygiene, regular exercise, and stress management.

Answer: _____

Vasculitis

Definition
Vasculitis is a heterogeneous group of conditions characterized by inflammation and necrosis of blood vessel walls.

Arteries and veins of various sizes and in different locations may be involved, resulting in a great diversity of symptoms and findings.

Arteritis = **angiitis** = arterial inflammation
Venulitis = venule inflammation
Capillaritis = inflammation of the capillary

Small-vessel vasculitis
(eg, microscopic polyangiitis, Wegener's granulomatosis)

Medium-sized Vessel Vasculitis
(Polyarteritis nodosa, Kawasaki disease)

Large-vessel vasculitis
(Giant cell arteritis, Takayasu arteritis)

Capillary — Arteriole — Venule — Vein

Goodpasture's syndrome

Arteries — Henoch-Schönlein Purpura and Cryoglobulinemia

Aorta — Microscopic Polyangiitis, Wegener's granulomatosis, and Churg-Strauss syndrome

Typical presentation:
- Constitutional Sxs: Fever, malaise, night sweats
- Weight loss
- Claudication
- Pulselessness
- Necrosis
- Neuropathy

Vasculitis
- Large vessel vasculitis
  - Giant cell arteritis (temporal arteritis)
  - Takayasu arteritis
- Medium vessel vasculitis
  - Polyarteritis nodosa (PAN)

- Kawasaki (pediatric patients)
- Eosinophilic granulomatosis with polyangiitis (EGPA [Churg-Strauss])
- Small vessel vasculitis
  - Granulomatosis with polyangiitis (GPA)
  - Microscopic polyangiitis (MPA)

Large Vessel Vasculitis
- **Takayasu** arteritis (pulseless disease) and **Temporal** arteritis (cranial arteritis) are chronic vasculitis of aorta and large branches
- Histologically identical granulomatous inflammatory diseases (with multinucleated giant cells) of large/muscular arteries

Takayasu Arteritis (Pulseless Disease)
Epidemiology: Young Asian (esp. Japanese) females
Early Sxs (days–weeks):
- Constitutional symptoms
- Erythema

Weeks–months:
Narrowing occurs in carotid, cerebral, aortic, mesenteric, and subclavian arteries, resulting in vascular insufficiency

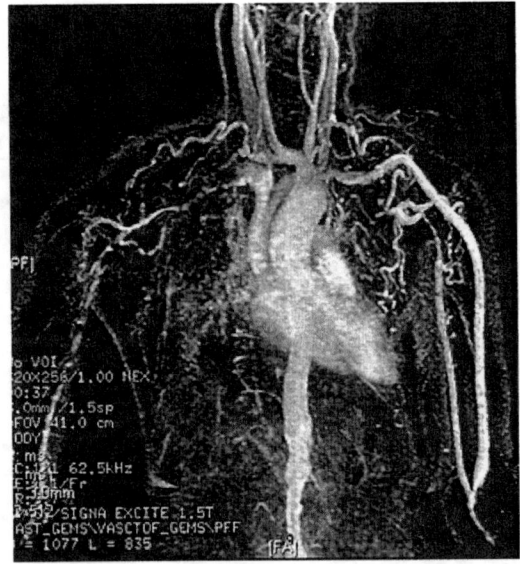

Takayasu Arteritis (cont.)
Vascular insufficiency (aortic arch syndrome):
- **Asymmetric BP: With differential > 10 mmHg**
- **Angina**
- **Aortic insufficiency** 2° aortic root dilatation
- **Bruits**
- **CNS ischemic symptoms:**
  - Headache
  - Dizziness
  - Amaurosis fugax
  - Diplopia
- **Hypertension 2° renal artery stenosis**

- **Labs:** Inflammatory
- **Diagnosis:** Angiogram or magnetic resonance angiography
- **Prognosis:** > 90% 5-year survival with treatment
- **Treatment:**
  - Steroids
  - Angioplasty (if not inflamed)
  - Bypass surgery

Temporal Arteritis
Rheumatologic emergency!!
Typical presentation: 75-year-old Caucasian female with headaches; achy shoulders/hips; scalp tenderness; difficulties chewing and swallowing; anorexia & weight loss over 2 months; fatigue; fever 99.0–100.0° F (37.2–37.8° C); tunnel vision on same side that scalp is tender

Exam: Prominent temporal artery, asymmetric temporal pulses with temporal wasting;
Labs show ESR > 100

Pathology Findings of Temporal Arteritis

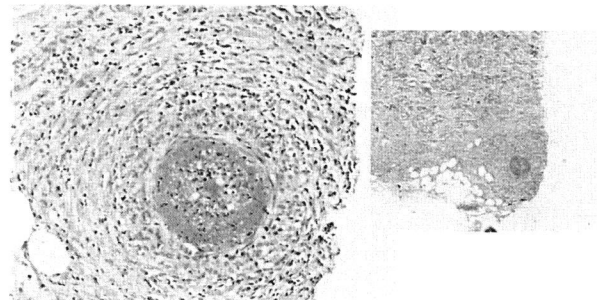

Source: Kathryn Dao, MD

Temporal Arteritis (cont.)
- > 50 years of age (mean age = 70 years)
- Female:male = 2:1
- Dry persistent cough
- North >> south
- 50% of patients have polymyalgia rheumatica (PMR)

- **Onset:** Gradual (weeks–months) **but** may be sudden onset with:
  - Flu-like symptoms
  - Fever to 104.0° F (40.0° C)
  - Weight loss

- **Symptoms 2° to vascular involvement:**
  - Headache
  - Scalp tenderness ± skin necrosis
  - Enlarged fibrotic tender temporal artery
  - Jaw/Tongue claudication
  - Visual symptoms/loss/diplopia
  - Sore throat/Cough
  - Aortic arch syndrome with asymmetric BP/bruits
  - Peripheral neuropathy

Distribution of the Carotid Artery

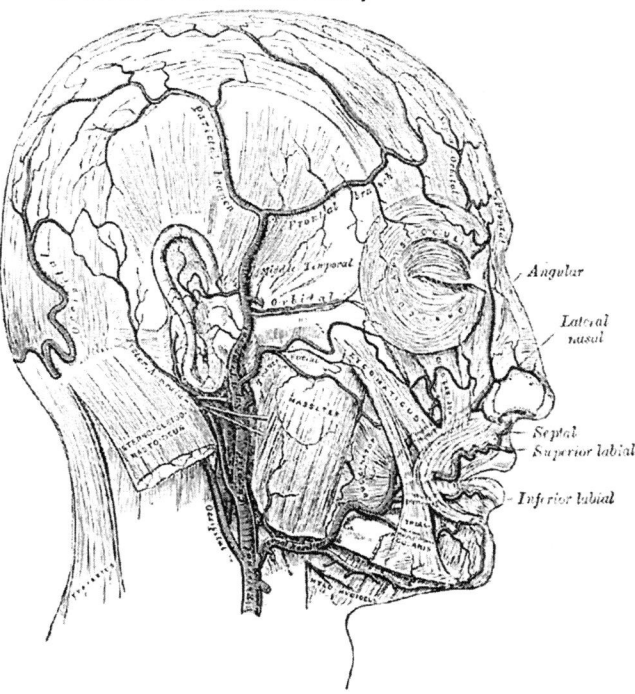

Temporal Arteritis (cont.)
- **Labs:** High platelets, low albumin, high ESR, ferritin, anemia chronic disease
- **Diagnosis:** Temporal artery biopsy — yield is higher in patients with jaw claudication; Bilateral temporal artery biopsy (additional 5% yield)*
- **Treatment:** High-dose steroids
- **Note: These patients are at risk for aortic aneurysms — screen 3–5 years after diagnosis**

Pless M, et al. Concordance of bilateral temporal artery biopsy in giant cell arteritis. *J Neuroophthalmol.* 2000 Sep;20(3):216–218.

Medium Vessel Vasculitis

Polyarteritis Nodosa (PAN)
- Necrotizing angiitis affecting small/medium-sized vessels characterized by granuloma and/or aneurysms at vessel bifurcations
- Most common age 40–60 years
- Male:female = 2:1
- 25% are caused by/related to hepatitis B virus antigenemia (HBsAg+)
- (Hepatitis C contributes to cryoglobulin vasculitis)

Onset: Abrupt or gradual with constitutional symptoms
- **GI tract:** Mesenteric vasculitis — **any GI symptoms** (70%)
- **Cardiac:** Coronary arteritis resulting in (50%) MI, CHF, Tachycardia
- **Skin:** Vasculitic/Vasculopathic rash: (50%) ischemic ulcers, livedo reticularis, palpable purpura

Polyarteritis Nodosa (PAN) (cont.)
- **PNS:** Multiple mononeuropathies
    (UE = LE) (50%)
    (mononeuritis multiplex)

- **Genitourinary:** Necrotizing glomerulonephropathy
- (50%) manifested as:
    - Proteinuria
    - Hematuria/RBC casts
    - HTN
    - Testicular pain/tender
- **Joints/Muscles:** Arthralgias/Myalgias (30%)

Cutaneous Vasculitis in PAN

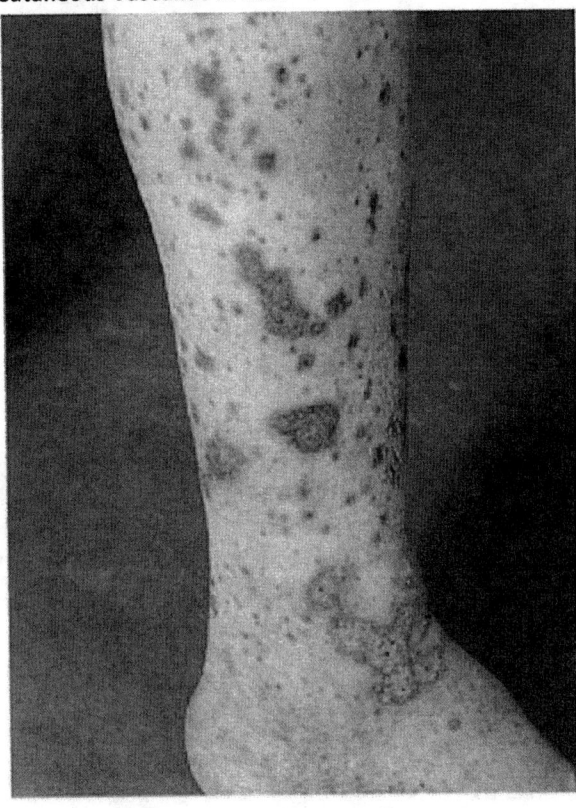

Polyarteritis Nodosa (PAN) (cont.)
Usually spares lungs

- **Labs:**
    - Hepatitis B surface Ag+ 25%
    - Hematuria/Proteinuria/RBC casts
    - Inflammatory

- **Diagnosis:**
    Obtain biopsy of any involved tissue or angiogram;
    ANCA typically not present (if p-ANCA present,
    think microscopic polyangiitis)

- **Treatment:**
    Steroids and cyclophosphamide
        or
    Steroids followed by plasmapheresis and antiviral
    agents (lamivudine) (if hepatitis B)
- **Prognosis:** 5-year survival when treated = 60%

AR 9
50-year-old Caucasian male with a 3-month h/o:
T = 100.3° F (38.0° C), 10-lb unintentional weight loss,
fatigue, achy joints and muscles, rash, indigestion,
and breathless with minimal activity
On PE:
Pt looks tired. BP = 155/93, HR = 92, T = 99° F (37.2° C);
Questionable numbness in hands with slightly decreased
grip strength o/w unremarkable exam
Laboratory results:
Hct = 31 (39–44)
ESR = 55 (< 20)
Plt = 450 (160–350)
U/A = 5–7 RBC/HPF

This patient has polyarteritis nodosa.
Which of the following helps in the diagnosis
of this patient?
A. Temporal artery biopsy
B. Mesenteric angiogram
C. ANCA
D. CRP
E. Electromyelogram/Nerve conduction studies
    (EMG/NCS)

Answer: _____

Eosinophilic Granulomatosis with Polyangiitis (Churg-Strauss)
Eosinophilic vasculitis
- Multiorgan disease involving small/medium-sized
  vessels in patients with allergies and/or asthma
- Most common in middle age
- Male > female

- **Presentation:**
    - **Initially:**
        1) Increased allergic manifestations (esp. asthma)
        2) Eosinophilia (> 10% WBC)
    - **Eventually:**
        - Vasculitis (typically
          develops
          as asthma/allergies
          improve)

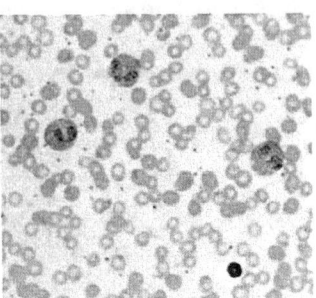

© 2017 MedStudy Internal Medicine Video Board Review – Rheumatology • Kathryn H. Dao, MD

Eosinophilic Granulomatosis with Polyangiitis (Churg-Strauss) (cont.)

- Manifestations:
  - **Sinopulmonary:**
    - Allergic rhinitis/Sinusitis
    - Chest discomfort
    - Shortness of breath
    - Asthma
  - **Skin, PNS, and GI** tract similar to PAN
  - **Renal and Cardiac** involvement less severe than PAN

- **Labs:**
  - Eosinophilia > 10% WBC
  - Inflammatory
- **Chest x-ray:**
  - Transient patchy or nodular infiltrates
- **Sinus x-ray:**
  - Opacification

- **Diagnosis:**
  - Obtain biopsy of any involved tissue
- **Prognosis:**
  - Better than PAN
- **Treatment:**
  - Steroids, DMARDs

Small Vessel Vasculitis

Granulomatosis with Polyangiitis (Wegener's)

- Necrotizing granulomatous vasculitis involving small arteries/arterioles/venules with classic triad of:
  1) Upper respiratory airway involvement **(sinus)**
  2) Lower respiratory airway involvement **(pulmonary)**
  3) Focal segmental glomerulonephritis **(renal)**

- Young to middle-aged adults
- Male = female

- Sinus/Nasal manifestations:
  Any sinus/nasal signs/Sxs including:
  - Saddle-nose deformity
- Pulmonary manifestations:
  Any chest signs/Sxs including:
  - Hemoptysis
  - Cough
  - Chest pain
  - Shortness of breath
  - Abnormal CXR
- Renal symptoms (2° to kidney inflammation)

Saddle Nose Deformity in GPA

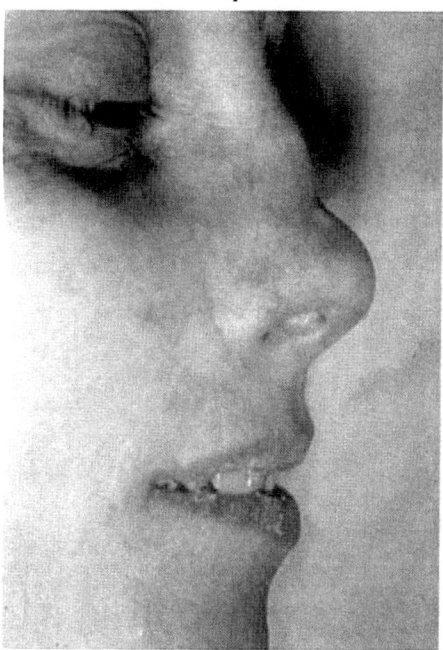

Source: Frederick Stucker, MD

Granulomatosis with Polyangiitis (cont.)

- **Other manifestations:**
  - Ocular — scleritis, episcleritis, keratitis, uveitis
  - PNS:
    - Cranial nerve deficits
    - Peripheral neuropathy
  - Skin:
    - Nodules
    - Palpable purpura
    - Vasculitic ulcers

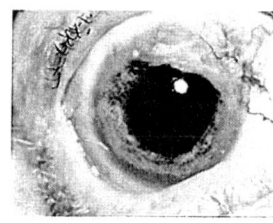

- **Labs:**
  - Inflammatory
  - Hematuria/Proteinuria/RBC casts
  - Antineutrophil cytoplasmic antibody (ANCA): 80% of patients have a c-ANCA with specificity against proteinase-3
- **Chest x-ray:**
  - Nodules and cavitary lesions
  - Diagnosis: Open lung biopsy or biopsy of other tissues
- **Treatment:**
  - Steroids
  - Cytoxan
  - Rituximab (FDA approved)
  - Methotrexate (in absence of life-threatening lung or kidney disease)

ANCA Immunofluorescence Patterns
1) **Perinuclear staining pattern (p-ANCA)**
   – > 70% of p-ANCA is directed against myeloperoxidase (MPO); Other p-ANCA antigens include cathepsin G, human leukocyte elastase, and lactoferrin
   – Associated with **MPA** and **Churg-Strauss**
2) **Cytoplasmic staining pattern (c-ANCA)**
   – > 90% of c-ANCA is directed against proteinase (PR3)
   – Associated with **granulomatosis with polyangiitis (Wegener's)**

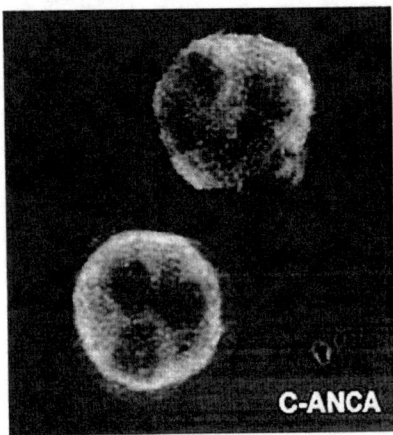

Summary
• **Polyarteritis nodosa (PAN):**
   – Middle-aged pt with weight loss, fever, fatigue, multiple organ involvement (PNS, GU, Skin, GI), spares the lungs, inflammatory labs, and HBsAg+
• **Eosinophilic granulomatosis with polyangiitis:**
   – Middle-aged pt with allergies/asthma, sinus Sxs, eosinophilia > 10% WBC, and systemic illness

• **Takayasu arteritis (pulseless disease):**
   – Young Asian (Japanese) women with asymmetric pulses, new HTN, bruits, vascular insufficiency symptoms
• **Temporal arteritis (cranial arteritis):**
   – > 50 years of age with weight loss, fever, fatigue, jaw claudication, vision change/loss, HA, asymmetric pulses, inflammatory labs with high ESR and PMR

• **Granulomatosis with polyangiitis:**
   – Young/middle-aged pt with pulmonary Sxs, sinus Sxs, abnormal urinalysis, inflammatory labs, and systemic illness; Strong association with c-ANCA and anti-proteinase-3 antibody

Red Flags of Vasculitis
1) Fever of unknown origin
2) Unexplained multisystem disease
3) Unexplained renal abnormality (especially with a nephritic urinalysis)
4) Unexplained cardiac/GI/CNS ischemia
5) Mononeuritis multiplex
6) Suspicious rash:
   a) Palpable purpura
   b) Maculopapular
   c) Nodules
   d) Ulcers
   e) Livedo reticularis

Office-Based Orthopedics

Back Pain
• <u>Origin of pain:</u>
   1) Vertebra
   2) Disc
   3) Facet joints
   4) Muscle
   5) Nerve root/Spinal cord
• <u>Terms:</u>
   1) Spondylosis: OA (DDD/DJD)
   2) Spondylolysis: Defect pars interarticularis/fractures leading to spondylolisthesis
   3) Spondylolisthesis: One vertebra slides over another

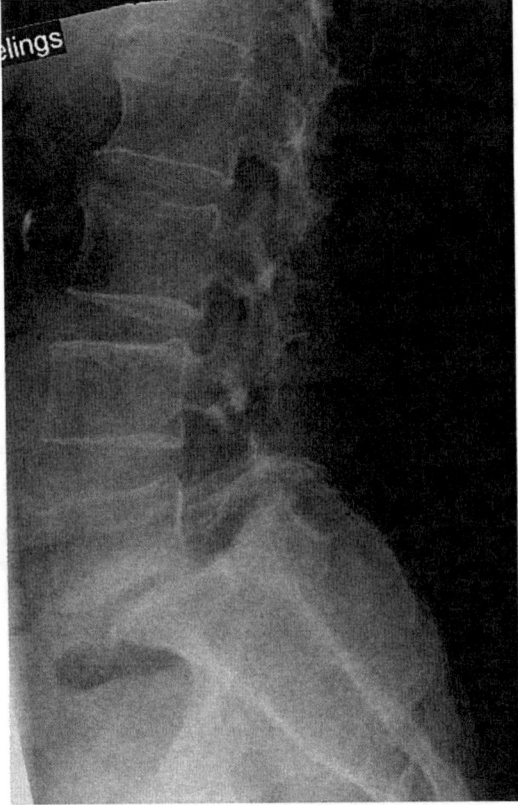

© 2017 MedStudy Internal Medicine Video Board Review – Rheumatology • Kathryn H. Dao, MD

Back Pain (cont.)
- **Red flags need urgent imaging (MRI):**
  - Known cancer diagnosis <u>or</u> suspicion for cancer is high
  - Recent infection/at risk for infection: Injection drug users, +TB exposure
  - Urinary retention/fecal incontinence
  - Saddle anesthesia
  - Progressive motor weakness

Refractory pain after 1 month conservative Rx → Get imaging

- **Common causes of back pain:**
  - Osteoarthritis
  - Muscle strain
  - Disc herniation
  - Spinal stenosis (neurogenic claudication)
  - Compression fracture
  - Infection (discitis, osteomyelitis)
  - Malignancy
  - Spondyloarthritis
  - DISH

Spinal Stenosis vs. Protruding Disc
- Prototypic **spinal stenosis** patient is:
  A little, old man hunched over a shopping cart to relieve his pseudoclaudication; Lower-extremity neuropathy or back pain, which radiates to the legs; It is relieved by back flexion (such as ascending stairs or sitting in a chair)
- A **protruding disc** is relieved by back extension (such as descending stairs) or worsened by ascending stairs
- LBP surgery is indicated only when the patient experiences lower-extremity sensory or motor abnormality

AR 10
A 72-year-old male complains of 40 years of back pain. Recently, his legs developed achiness and he felt as if they were filled with concrete after walking a block. These symptoms improve when he leans forward but return with activity.
On physical examination: He has normal pulses without bruits and a nonfocal neurologic examination.

What is the likely diagnosis?
A. Spinal stenosis
B. Protruding disc
C. Aortic aneurysm
D. Ankylosing spondylitis
E. Diffuse idiopathic skeletal hyperostosis

Answer: _____

Neck Pain
- Examination:
  - Muscle atrophy
  - Fasciculations
  - Hoffman's sign (flick the middle finger tips, noted thumb and 2nd finger flex)
  - Ankle clonus
  - Spurling's test (nerve root/radiculopathy)
  - Lhermitte's sign (dorsal column — MS)

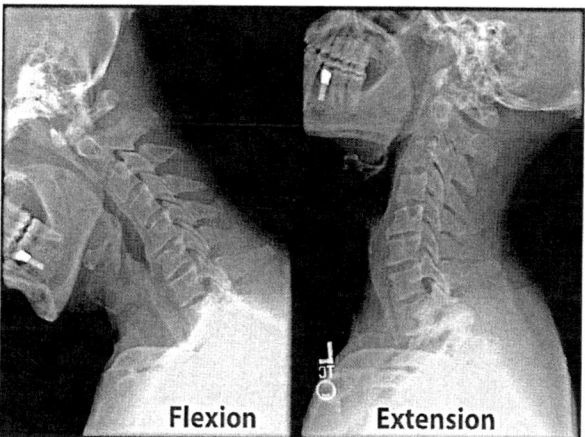

Flexion   Extension

Neck Pain (cont.)
Neck pain accounts for 15% of SkM problems in practice
- **Red flags:**
  - Trauma (fracture, dislocation)
  - History of RA (atlanto-axial subluxation)
  - Infectious symptoms (fever, night sweats, rash)
  - Systemic symptoms (anorexia, weight loss)
  - Neurologic symptoms (carotid dissection, cord compression, demyelinating disorders)
  - Intractable pain
  - Severe pain over the vertebral body

Dermatomes

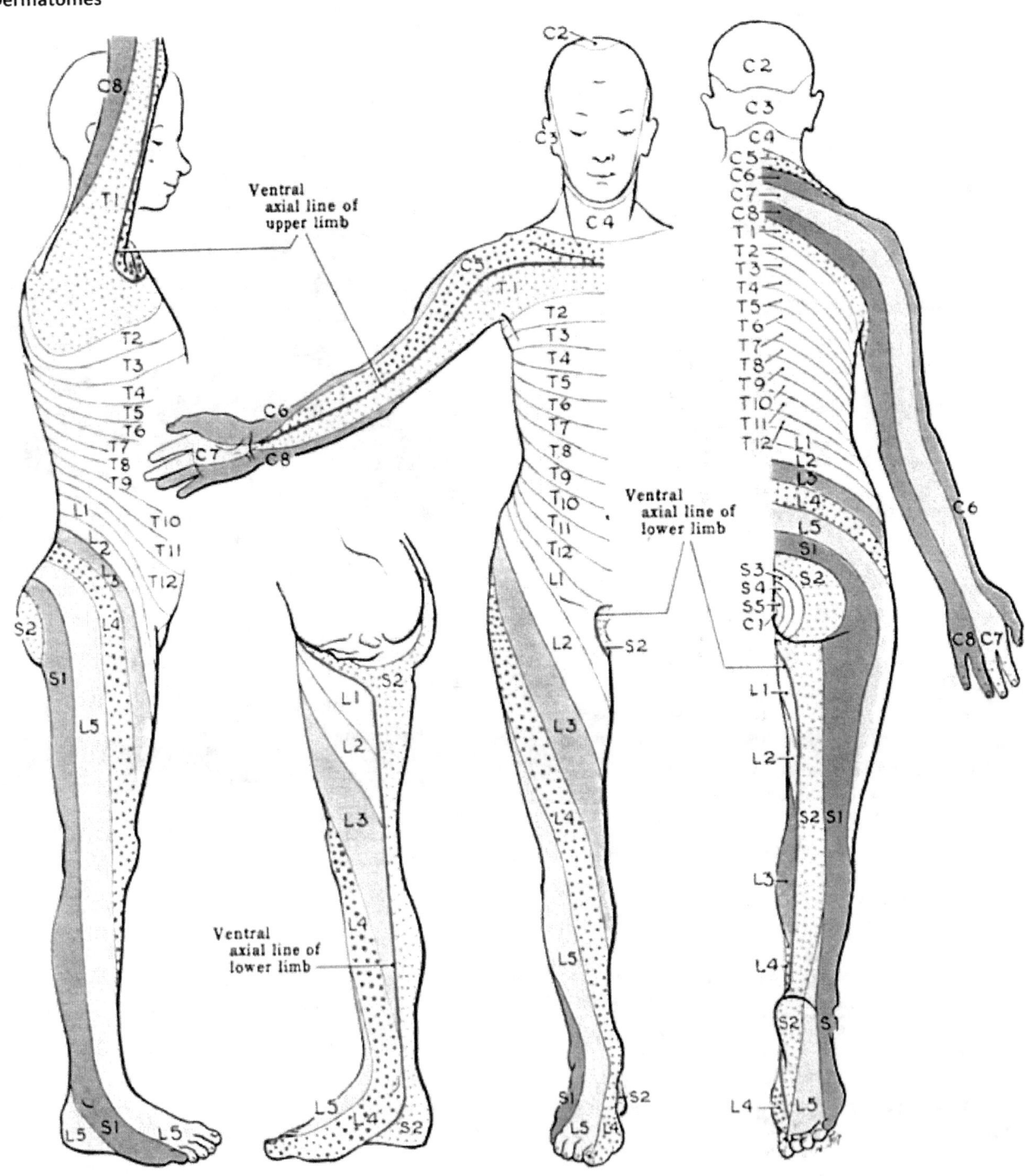

© 2017 MedStudy Internal Medicine Video Board Review – Rheumatology • Kathryn H. Dao, MD

Shoulder
- Rotator cuff injury
- Brachial plexopathy
- OA (GH joint, AC joint)
- Bursitis
- Crystalline arthritis
- Referred cervical pain
- Thoracic outlet syndrome

The Shoulder Joint

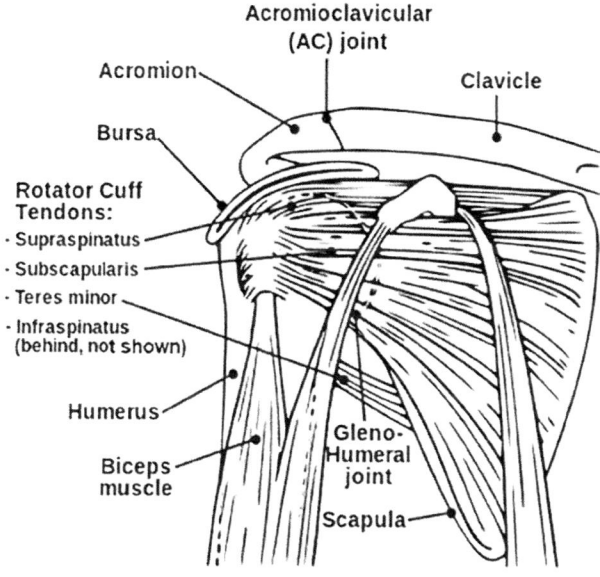

Thoracic Outlet Syndrome

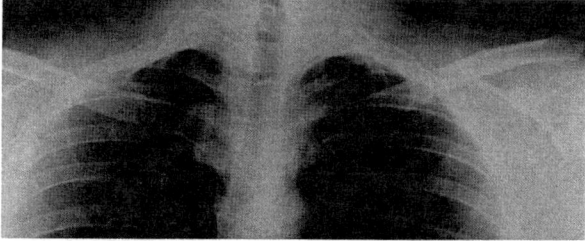

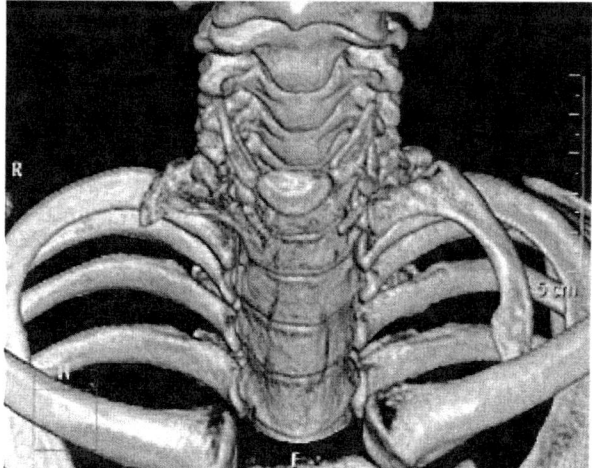

- Compression of the neurovascular structure (cervical rib, trauma, tumor, idiopathic)
- Arterial, venous, neurogenic (95%)
- Sx: Neck/Shoulder pain, paresthesias, weakness, Raynaud's
- Exam: Elevated arm test (3 minutes, open and close fist with raised arms), Roos test (90 degrees shoulder abduction, 90 degrees elbow flexion for 3 minutes), Adson test (radial pulse)
- Testing: EMG/NCS, CXR, ± MRI/CT
- Rx: PT, NSAIDs, surgery

Rotator Cuff — Impingement Syndrome
- Compression of the subacromial bursa or tendons between the acromion and humeral head
- Pain occurs when pt reaches overhead or pressure on the shoulder
- Diagnosis is clinical
- Exam: Neer test (stabilize scapula, passively forward flex GH joint)
- Hawkin's test (elbow flex, arm 90 degrees, internally rotate shoulder)
- Yocum test (pt touch other shoulder, lift flexed elbow)

The Shoulder Joint

Elbow Pain
- Olecranon bursitis
- Medial epicondylitis (golfer's elbow)
- Lateral epicondylitis (tennis elbow)
- Elbow OA
- Elbow synovitis (RA)

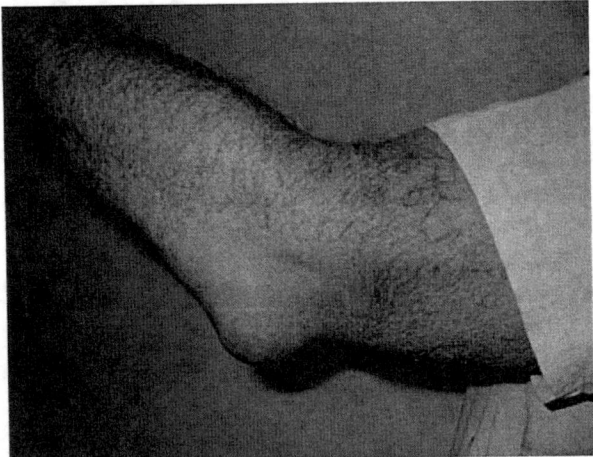

Hip Pain
- True hip pain is in the groin:
  - Hip OA
  - Avascular necrosis
- Supporting structures/DDx:
  - Trochanteric bursitis
  - Iliopsoas tendonitis
  - Piriformis syndrome
  - Iliotibial band syndrome (IT Band)
- Exam: FABER maneuver

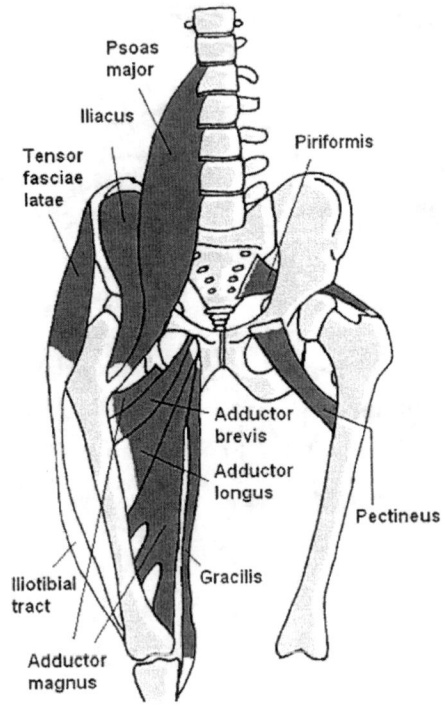

Knee Pain
- Knee OA
- Baker's cyst (popliteal cyst)
- Prepatellar bursitis
  (housemaid's knee/clergyman's knee)
- Pes anserine bursitis
- Avascular necrosis
- Pigmented villonodular synovitis
  (PVNS [recurrent hemarthrosis])

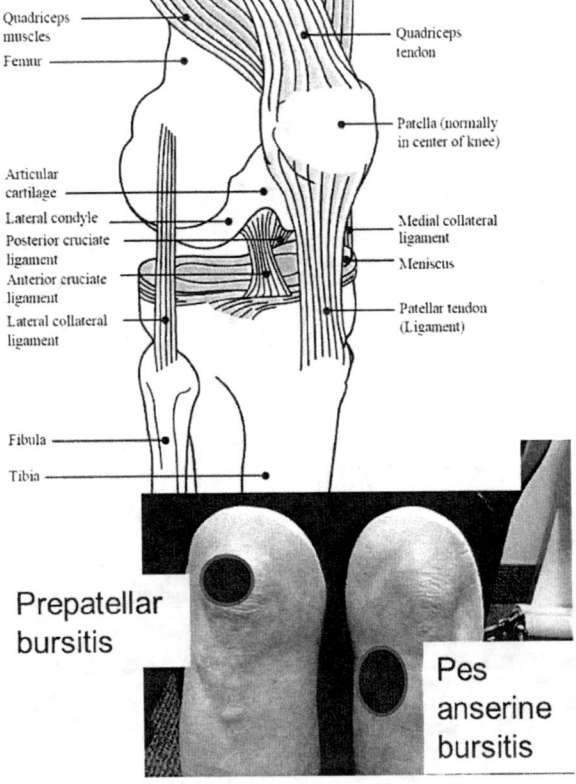

AR 11

57-year-old painter presents with pain in his right shoulder for about 6 months. He rested his arm and has not been able to work for the last month. Pain is worse at night. Exam notes slight atrophy of his R shoulder and also pain with internal rotation of the shoulder when the elbow is flexed and the arm is 90 degrees.

Which of the following is the likely cause of his pain?
A. Gout
B. Bicipital tendinitis
C. Shoulder impingement
D. Referred pain from his neck
E. Acromioclavicular joint osteoarthritis

Answer: _____

Compression Neuropathies
- **Etiologies**
  1) Repetitive trauma
  2) Pregnancy
  3) Hypothyroid
  4) Oral contraceptives
  5) Dialysis-related amyloid
  6) Synovitis (true inflammation)

Compression Neuropathies

	Carpal Tunnel	Cubital Tunnel	Radial Tunnel	Meralgia Paresthetica	Peroneal Nerve Palsy
Nerve involved	Median nerve	Ulnar nerve	Radial nerve	Lateral femoral cutaneous nerve	Peroneal nerve
Areas affected	Thumb, 2nd, 3rd, and part of 4th fingers	4th and 5th fingers, medial elbow	Finger extensors, anterior elbow (motor only)	Anterior thigh	Pain knee to dorsum of foot, loss of dorsiflexion of foot, toe extension and ankle eversion
Provocative maneuvers	Tinel's + @ volar wrist Phalen's at the wrist	Tinel's + @ medial epicondyle Elbow flexion	Weakness with extension of fingers (3rd and 4th — "Hook 'em horns")	Descending stairs, prolonged standing in erect posture Deep pressure medial to the anterior superior iliac spine	Tinel's fibular head (r/o L4/L5 radiculopathy)

Compression Neuropathies (cont.)

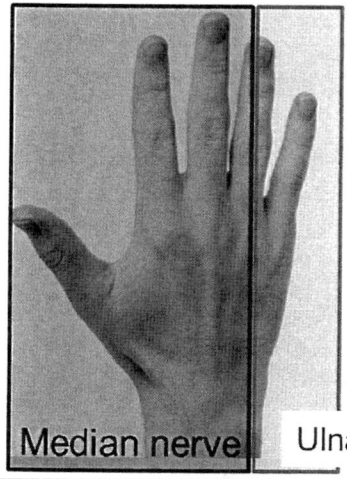

Median nerve / Ulnar nerve

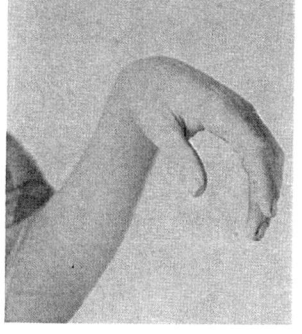

Radial nerve entrapment

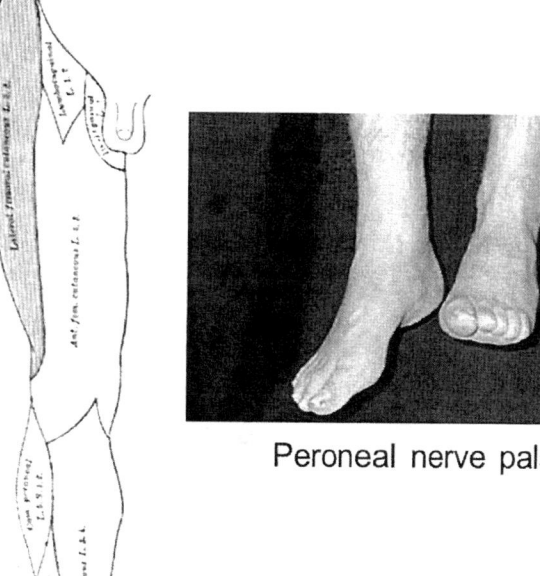

Peroneal nerve palsy

Lateral femoral cutaneous nerve (meralgia paresthetica)

Office-Based Miscellaneous
- **Dupuytren contractures:**
  - Fibrous thickening of flexor tendons of the fingers that cause palmar pain and limited extension of fingers
    1) Diabetes
    2) EtOH
- **AVN/Osteonecrosis:**
  - Hip pain (groin or buttock pain) with normal x-ray initially
    1) Steroids
    2) Alcoholism
    3) SLE
    4) HIV
    5) Pancreatitis hypercoagulability

- Genetic collagen disorders:
  - **Osteogenesis imperfecta** — blue sclera
  - **Pseudoxanthoma elasticum** — angioid streaks
  - **Marfan syndrome**
    - High-arched palate
    - Long limbs
    - Aortic root dilatation
    - Ectopia lentis
    - Pneumothorax
  - **Ehlers-Danlos — hypermobility**
    - **Classic**
      - Joint dislocation
      - Skin scarring
    - **Hypermobility** — hyperelasticity
    - **Vascular** — vascular rupture

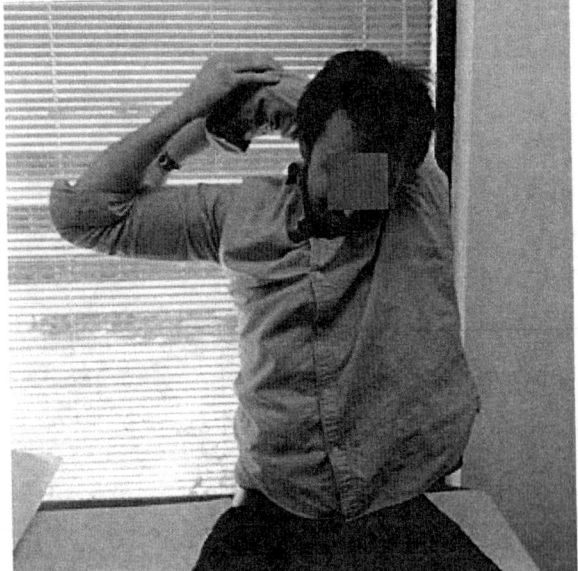

AR 12

23-year-old male comes for evaluation of his joint pains. He notes a sister recently diagnosed with Ehlers-Danlos syndrome and postural orthostatic tachycardia. He reports fatigue and pain in his shoulders, knees, neck and back. Exam: Height 6' 6" (78 cm), BP 98/66, noted a 2/6 diastolic murmur.
His exam is shown next.

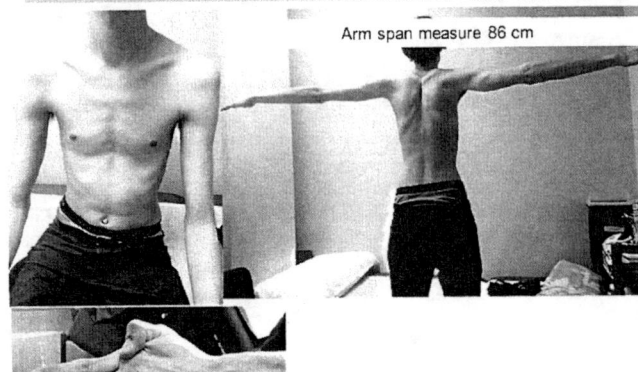

Source: Kathryn Dao, MD

Which of the following is the most appropriate next step?
A. Order physical therapy
B. Refer to a geneticist to rule out Ehlers-Danlos syndrome
C. Order an ECG
D. Order an echocardiogram
E. Prescribe an NSAID for his joint pain

Answer: _____

Pearls
- There is no lab that will make the diagnosis for you
- Recognize patterns of how diseases present
- Inflammatory arthritis = swelling, heat, pain, redness with prolonged morning stiffness, improves with activity
- The ANA is nonspecific, order it only if you have a high suspicion of an autoimmune disease (think lupus, Sjögren's)
- Rheumatoid arthritis = MCP + PIPs; Osteoarthritis DIP+ PIPs
- SLE mortality is from infection, the disease (renal/brain), cardiovascular disease

Pearls (cont.)

- Joint fluid with WBC > 2,000, think inflammatory
- **Pre**menopausal women **do not usually** suffer from gout; if they have gout, evaluate for underlying causes: Renal failure, high cell-turnover state, enzyme deficiency
- Quinolones have been associated with tendon ruptures
- Common things are common: fibromyalgia is more likely than normal CK polymyositis!
- Usually 1 autoimmune rheumatologic disease per patient
- Patients with temporal arteritis are at increased risk for aortic aneurysms

- Patients with PMR are at increased risk for strokes
- 90% of acute back pain without neurologic deficits improves within 2 months — no bed rest
- Patients with spinal stenosis like to lean on shopping carts
- Rotator cuff injuries are the most common cause of shoulder pain
- Baker/Popliteal cysts (knee) may mimic a DVT
- Morton neuroma causes burning paresthesias between the 3rd and 4th toes
- Review your dermatomes

Rheumatology
Audience Response Answers

Audience Response 1
Answer: C. OA.

AR 2
Answer: D. Lymphoma.

AR 3
Answer: A. Iritis.

AR 4
Answer: D. Start steroids to treat the acute attack,
then prescribe allopurinol with a prophylactic agent
for secondary prevention.

AR 5
Answer: B. Pelvic exam with culture.

AR 6
Answer: C. Lupus nephritis.

AR 7
Answer: D. Admit her and give her IV enalapril.

AR 8
Answer: E. Recommend sleep hygiene, regular exercise,
and stress management.

AR 9
Answer: B. Mesenteric angiogram.

AR 10
Answer: A. Spinal stenosis.

AR 11
Answer: C. Shoulder impingement.

AR 12
Answer: D. Order an echocardiogram.

MedStudy

Internal Medicine Video Board Review

Statistics

Presented by

Chris L. Knight, MD
Associate Professor of Medicine
University of Washington Medical Center
Seattle, Washington

Table of Contents

Statistics Abbreviations

CI	Confidence interval
FN	False negative
FOBT	Fecal occult blood testing
FP	False positive
LR	Likelihood ratio
NNT	Number needed to treat
NPV	Negative predictive value
PPV	Positive predictive value
TN	True negative
TP	True positive

Statistics
- Sensitivity
- Specificity
- Positive Predictive Value (PPV)
- Negative Predictive Value (NPV)
- Likelihood Ratio (LR)
- Absolute / Relative Risk
- Number Needed to Treat (NNT)
- p Value
- 95% Confidence Interval
- Study Designs

Statistics — Diagnostic Test
- Set up table!
- Disease goes on top, + to left of −
- Test goes down the side, + above −
- So, those with disease and have a positive test (true positives) go in upper left corner
- Those without disease and have a negative test (true negatives) go in lower right corner

Interpretation of Test Results

	Disease	No Disease
Test +		
Test −		

Interpretation of Test Results

	Disease	No Disease
Test +	True +	
Test −		True −

Interpretation of Test Results

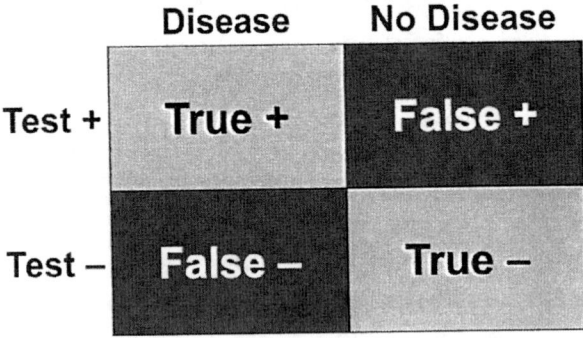

	Disease	No Disease
Test +	True +	False +
Test −	False −	True −

Math Overview
- Always true results over total results
- Sensitivity/Specificity: Use **columns**
- PPV/NPV: Use **rows**

$$\frac{\text{True}}{\text{Total}}$$

Sensitivity
- Proportion of diseased population with positive test results

- TP/(TP + FN)

$$\frac{\text{True +}}{\text{Total disease}}$$

- Use left column: (Top left) divided by (Total of column)!

Interpretation of Test Results

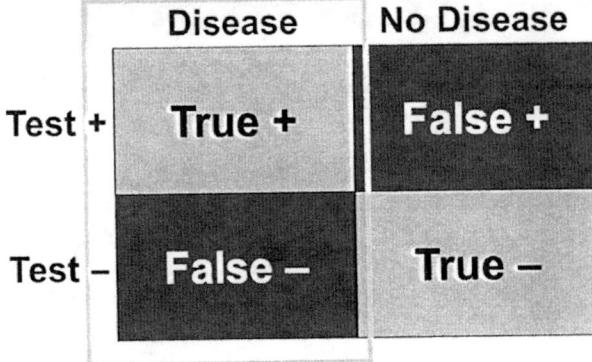

	Disease	No Disease
Test +	True +	False +
Test −	False −	True −

Specificity
- Proportion of healthy population with negative test results

- TN/(TN + FP)

$$\frac{\text{True −}}{\text{Total healthy}}$$

- Use right column: (Bottom right) divided by (Total of column)!

Interpretation of Test Results

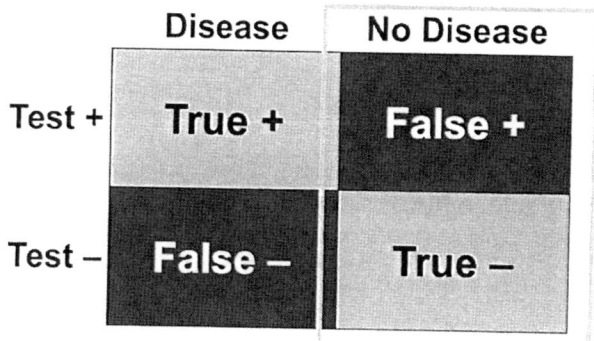

Rules of Thumb
- SpPin: A Positive result on a Specific test rules disease in
- SnNout: A Negative result on a Snsitive test rules disease out

Combining Tests
- A good testing strategy is to use a fast/cheap sensitive test followed by a slow/costly specific test
- HIV ELISA followed by WB
- D-dimer followed by CT-PA

Positive Predictive Value (PPV)
- Positive predictive value is the proportion of patients with positive tests who have the disease

$$\frac{True\ +}{Total\ +}$$

- PPV = TP/(TP + FP)

- Use top row: (Top left) divided by (total of row)

Interpretation of Test Results

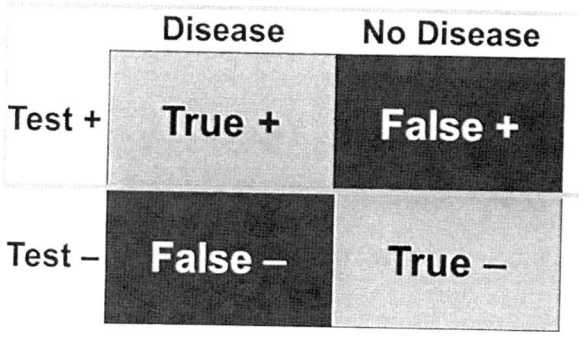

Negative Predictive Value (NPV)
- Negative predictive value is the proportion of patients with a negative test who are disease free

- NPV = TN/(FN + TN)

$$\frac{True\ -}{Total\ -}$$

- Use bottom row: (Bottom right) divided by (total of row)

Interpretation of Test Results

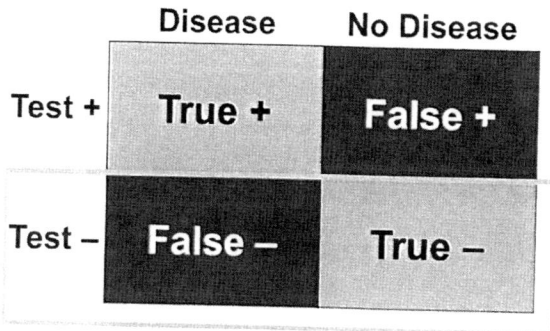

Influence of Disease Prevalence on PPV and NPV
- Prevalence of a disease within a screening population influences the performance of a screening test
- As prevalence of a disease falls, PPV drops and NPV rises
- The less common a disease, the more likely a positive test represents a false positive

Common — 20% Prevalence

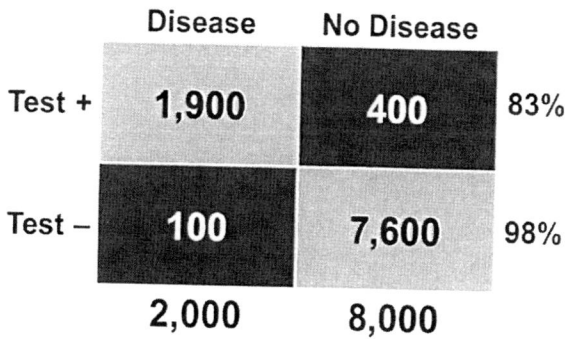

Rare — 0.2% Prevalence

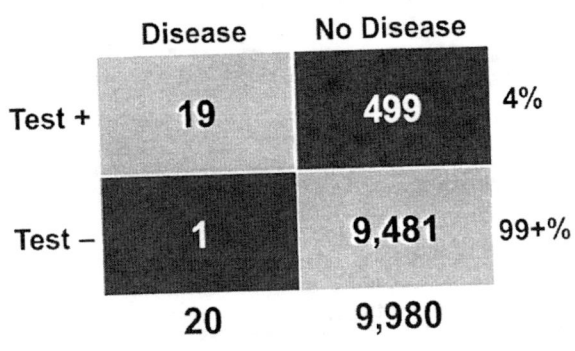

	Disease	No Disease	
Test +	19	499	4%
Test −	1	9,481	99+%
	20	9,980	

Likelihood Ratio (LR)
- Different way of looking at tests
- Combines sensitivity & specificity
- **Confusing:** Uses <u>odds</u> instead of <u>probability</u>

Odds — Coin Comes Up Heads

Flips	Probability	Odds
1	1/2	1:1
2	1/4	1:3
3	1/8	1:7
4	1/16	1:15
5	1/32	1:31

Odds — Coin <u>Doesn't</u> Come Up Heads

Flips	Probability	Odds
1	1/2	1:1
2	3/4	3:1
3	7/8	7:1
4	15/16	15:1
5	31/32	31:1

Positive Likelihood Ratio (LR+)
- Change in odds of disease being present with **positive** test result
- Post-test odds = pre-test odds x LR
- Higher LR+ = more powerful at ruling <u>in</u> disease

$$\frac{Sens}{1 - Spec}$$

Negative Likelihood Ratio (LR−)
- Change in odds of disease being present with **negative** test result
- Post-test odds = pre-test odds x LR
- Lower LR− = more powerful at ruling <u>out</u> disease

$$\frac{1 - Sens}{Spec}$$

LR for Those with No Calculator

LR	Δ Prob
10	+45%
5	+30%
2	+15%
1	0
0.5 (1/2)	−15%
0.2 (1/5)	−30%
0.1 (1/10)	−45%

Audience Response 1

In a study of 2,271 patients with a history of colon cancer, fecal occult blood testing (FOBT) is done to screen for recurrent colon cancer. 146 patients have positive FOBT, and 2,125 patients have negative FOBT. Colonoscopy is done on all the patients, finding 46 cancers. 12 patients with positive FOBT have colon cancer, and 34 with negative tests have colon cancer.

What is the sensitivity for FOBT?
A. 8.2%
B. 26.1%
C. 94%
D. 98.4%

Answer: _____

Interpretation of Test Results

	Cancer	No Cancer
FOBT+		
FOBT−		

© 2017 MedStudy Internal Medicine Video Board Review — Statistics Video Review • Chris L. Knight, MD

Interpretation of Test Results

	Cancer	No Cancer
FOBT+	12	Waste of time
FOBT−	34	

AR 2

A 67-year-old patient comes to the emergency department for cough and shortness of breath for the past 3 days. Past medical history is notable for prior MI and class II CHF.

VS: T 99.2° F, 116/78, P 92, R 26, SpO_2 88% RA
Chest: Crackles and scattered wheezes bilaterally
WBC 12.1, BNP 260

Procalcitonin blood test is positive.

Procalcitonin has a positive LR of 8.2 and a negative LR of 0.7.

Which statement best describes the diagnostic value of procalcitonin?
A. Good for ruling in disease, poor for ruling it out
B. Good for ruling out disease, poor for ruling it in
C. Good for both ruling disease in and out
D. Poor for both ruling disease in and out

Answer: _____

2 x 2 Table for Treatment

	Outcome	No Outcome
Tx		
Control		

Absolute / Relative Risk

- Risk in a study arm = number of events/total number of patients in that arm
- Absolute risk **difference** (reduction/increase) = Risk in control arm − risk in treatment arm
- Relative risk is a **ratio** = $\dfrac{\text{Risk in treatment arm}}{\text{Risk in control arm}}$

Number Needed to Treat (NNT)

- Number of people needed to treat to prevent 1 outcome
- NNT = 1/(absolute risk reduction)

Table for Treatment

	Dead	Not Dead	Total	
Tx	150	850	1,000	15%
Cntrl	200	800	1,000	20%
	RR = 15% / 20% = 0.75		ARR	5%

NNT = 1 / 0.05 = 20

AR 3

A study of colchicine for secondary prevention in CAD was recently completed. The treatment group had 250 patients, of whom 50 had an MI. The control group had 300 patients, of whom 90 had an MI.

What is the NNT for colchicine to prevent one MI?
A. 10
B. 25
C. 125
D. 1,000

Answer: _____

Table for Treatment

	MI	No MI	Total
Tx			
Cntrl			

Table for Treatment

	MI	No MI	Total	
Tx	50	Time	250	20%
Cntrl	90	Sink	300	30%
			ARR	10%

NNT = 1 / 0.10 = 10

---

p Value
- A p value is used to express a study's reliability
- A p value of 0.10 means the likelihood that the results are due to chance is 10%
- p values < 0.05 are generally considered statistically significant; The lower the p value, the better ($p < 0.001$ better than $p < 0.01$)

p Value — Coin Comes Up Heads

Flips	Probability	p
1	1/2	0.5
2	1/4	0.25
3	1/8	0.13
4	1/16	0.06
5	1/32	0.03

95% Confidence Interval
- Close cousin to p value
- 95% probability that the true result falls within the confidence interval
- Usually applied to the **difference** in outcomes between treatment and intervention group
- More patients in the study usually result in tighter confidence intervals and lower p values

---

Null Hypothesis
- The null hypothesis means no difference
- If talking about:
  - Treatment, test result, survival, or morbidity factor — look for "0"; If the confidence interval range includes 0, then it is **not** significant
  - Odds **Ratio**, Hazard Ratio, or Relative Risk — look for "1"; If the confidence interval range includes 1, then it is **not** significant

Forest Plots Made Simple
- Graphic of results from multiple studies
- Width of the bar represents confidence interval
- **Vertical line is the null hypothesis**
- If the bar touches the line, that study's result was not significant

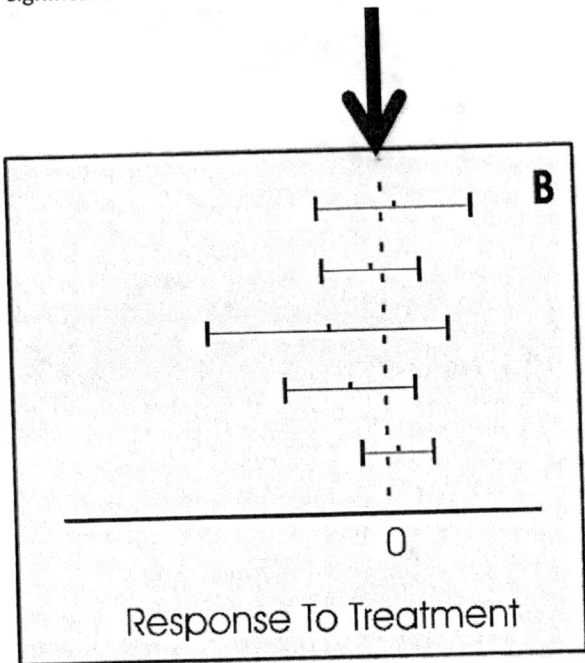

Response To Treatment

Meta-Analysis
- Mathematically combines multiple studies into a single result
- Look for a different shape (usually a diamond) at the bottom of the chart: That's the aggregate result
- **If the diamond touches the bar, the result is not significant**

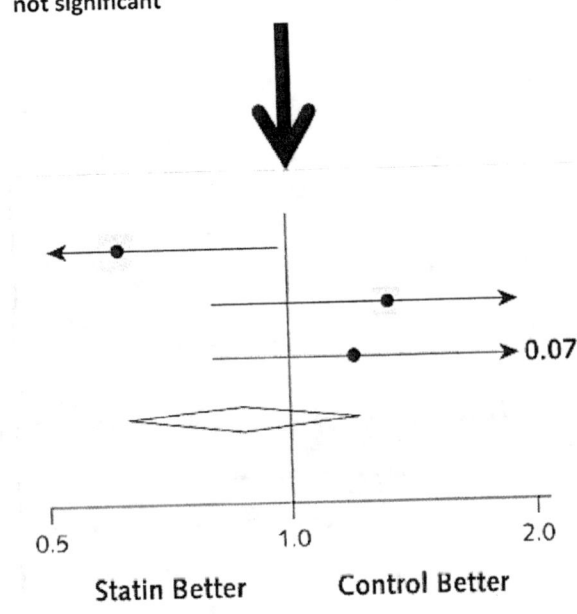

Statin Better   Control Better

AR 4

A meta-analysis is done to see if ordering diagnostic tests reduces patient anxiety. The forest plot of the odds ratio for reduced anxiety is shown.

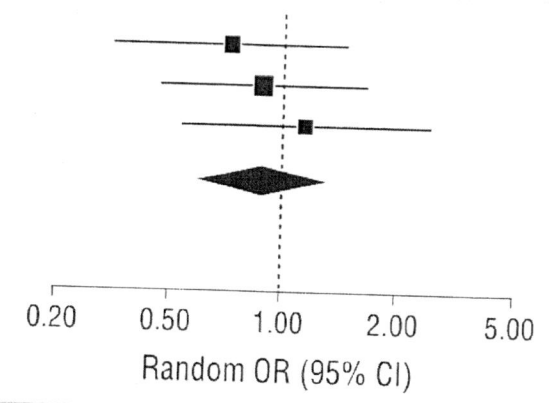

0.20   0.50   1.00   2.00   5.00

Random OR (95% CI)

What is a correct interpretation?
A. Ordering tests causes a statistically significant reduction in anxiety.
B. There is no significant difference in anxiety from ordering tests.
C. Ordering tests causes a statistically significant increase in anxiety.

Answer: _____

Study Designs
- Observational studies
  - Cross-sectional study
  - Cohort study
  - Case-control study
- Intervention studies
  - Randomized controlled trial

Cross-Sectional Study
- Weakest type of study
- Snapshot in time
- Difficult to draw conclusions about causation
- Example: Women have lower rates of MI than men; Maybe it has something to do with estrogen

Cohort Study
- Prospective or retrospective
- Identify **risk factors** first, then see who gets **disease**
- Unmeasured variables can confound results
- Good for potentially harmful exposures
- Example: Women who choose to take hormone replacement therapy have lower risk of MI than women who don't

Case-Control Study
- Always retrospective
- Identify **disease** first, then measure **risk factors**
- Good for initial studies of rare events
- Good for potentially harmful exposures
- Example: Women with endometrial cancer are 2.5x more likely to have taken unopposed estrogen in the past

Randomized Control Trials
- Always prospective
- Randomize into groups to either receive an intervention or not and blind the patient and the researcher to what was given; This reduces risk of confounding and bias
- Can't use for harmful exposures in humans
- Example: Women randomly assigned to take hormone replacement have **higher** risk of MI than those assigned to take placebo

Breaking It Down
- "Randomized" or "assigned" = intervention trial
- Was study a snapshot in time (cross-sectional), or did it look forward (prospective) or backward (retrospective)?
- What is the outcome/disease being studied?
- Did the authors find patients with risk factors first (cohort) or with outcome/disease first (case-control)?

AR 5

In a group of 99,187 patients with prior MI followed for 5 years, patients who took NSAIDs were found to have an increased risk of death compared to those who didn't; the hazard ratio is 1.59 (95% CI 1.49–1.69).

What type of study was this?
A. Cross-sectional study
B. Cohort study
C. Case-control study
D. Randomized controlled trial

Answer: _____

Statistics
Audience Response Answers

Audience Response 1
Answer: B. 26.1%.

AR 2
Answer: B. Good for ruling <u>out</u> disease,
poor for ruling it in.

AR 3
Answer: A. 10.

AR 4
Answer: B. There is no significant difference in anxiety
from ordering tests.

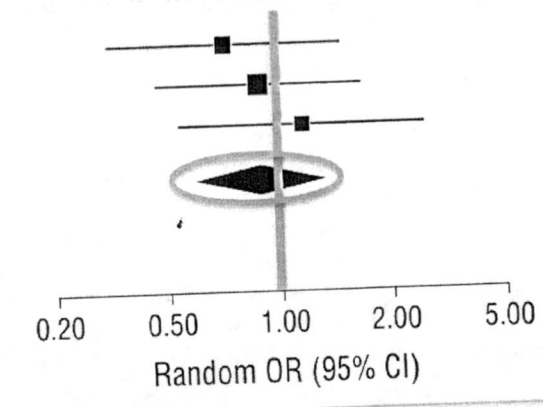

AR 5
Answer: B. Cohort study.